MAGNETIC RESONANCE IMAGING

Third Edition

MAGNETIC RESONANCE IMAGING

VOLUME I

DAVID D. STARK, MD, FACR
Professor and Chairman of Radiology,
University of Nebraska Medical Center,
Omaha, Nebraska

WILLIAM G. BRADLEY, JR., MD, PHD, FACR
Director, Magnetic Resonance Imaging and Radiology Research,
Long Beach Memorial Medical Center,
Long Beach, California;
Professor of Radiology,
University of California, Irvine,
Orange, California

with 6353 illustrations, including 272 in color

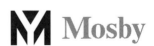 Mosby

St. Louis   London   Philadelphia   Sydney   Toronto

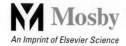
An Imprint of Elsevier Science

Please visit the Stark/Bradley home page at
www.Mosby.com/Stark-Bradley

Third Edition
Copyright © 1999 by Mosby, Inc.

Previous editions copyrighted 1992, 1988

Printed in China

Mosby, Inc.
11830 Westline Industrial Drive
St. Louis, Missouri 63146

Library of Congress Cataloging-in-Publication Data
Magnetic resonance imaging / [edited by] David D. Stark, William G.
  Bradley, Jr. — 3rd ed.
      p.   cm.
    Includes bibliographical references and index.
    ISBN 0-8151-8518-9
    1. Magnetic resonance imaging.   I. Stark, David D.   II. Bradley,
William G.
    [DNLM: 1. Magnetic Resonance Imaging.   WN 185M1959   1999]
  RC78.7.N83M333   1999
  616.07'548   dc21
  DNLM/DLC   98-36686

02 / 9 8 7 6 5 4 3

Contributors

DEREK C. ARMSTRONG, MB, BS, FRCP(C)
Associate Professor,
University of Toronto;
Staff, Division of Neuroradiology,
Hospital for Sick Children,
Toronto, Ontario, Canada

DENNIS J. ATKINSON, MD
Senior Scientist,
Siemens Medical Systems,
Iselin, New Jersey

SCOTT W. ATLAS, MD
Professor of Radiology,
Chief of Neuroradiology,
Stanford University Medical Center,
Stanford, California

ROBERT A.J. AVE'LALLEMANT, MD
Clinical Instructor—House Officer, Department of Urology,
Brown University School of Medicine,
Rhode Island Hospital,
Providence, Rhode Island

KIM B. BAKER, MD
Assistant Professor,
Allegheny University of the Health Sciences,
Hahnemann Hospital,
Philadelphia, Pennsylvania

RICHARD A. BAUM, MD
Assistant Professor of Radiology,
University of Pennsylvania;
Staff Interventional Radiologist,
Hospital of the University of Pennsylvania,
Philadelphia, Pennsylvania

CARLOS BAZAN III, MD
Clinical Associate Professor,
University of Texas Health Science Center at San Antonio,
San Antonio, Texas

JAVIER BELTRAN, MD
Professor of Clinical Radiology,
New York University School of Medicine;
Chairman, Department of Radiology,
Maimonides Medical Center,
Brooklyn, New York

LARISSA T. BILANIUK, MD
Professor of Radiology,
University of Pennsylvania School of Medicine;
Staff Neuroradiologist,
Children's Hospital of Philadelphia,
Philadelphia, Pennsylvania

DAVID A. BLUEMKE, MD, PhD
Assistant Professor,
Johns Hopkins University;
Clinical Director, Magnetic Resonance Imaging,
Johns Hopkins University School of Medicine,
Baltimore, Maryland

BRIAN C. BOWEN, MD, PhD
Associate Professor of Radiology,
University of Miami School of Medicine;
Attending Physician,
University of Miami Hospitals and Clinics,
Jackson Memorial Medical Center,
Miami, Florida

JERROLD L. BOXERMAN, MD, PhD
Instructor, Johns Hopkins University School of Medicine,
Johns Hopkins Hospital,
Baltimore, Maryland

OREST B. BOYKO, MD, PhD
Associate Professor of Radiology and Pathology,
Temple University School of Medicine;
Director of Neuroradiology,
Temple University Hospital,
Philadelphia, Pennsylvania

WILLIAM G. BRADLEY, JR., MD, PhD, FACR
Director, Magnetic Resonance Imaging
    and Radiology Research,
Long Beach Memorial Medical Center,
Long Beach, California;
Professor of Radiology,
University of California, Irvine,
Orange, California

MICHAEL N. BRANT-ZAWADZKI, MD
Clinical Professor of Diagnostic Radiology,
Stanford University,
Stanford, California;
Medical Director of Radiology,
Hoag Memorial Hospital,
Newport Beach, California

WILLIAM M. BROOKS, PhD
Research Associate Professor,
Center for Non-Invasive Diagnosis,
Department of Neurosciences,
University of New Mexico,
Albuquerque, New Mexico

JOACHIM BROSSMANN, MD
Privatdozent,
Christian-Albrechts-Universität,
Kiel, Germany

SHARON S. BURTON, MD
Associate Professor of Radiology,
University of Florida,
Gainesville, Florida

BRIAN BUSCONI, MD
Assistant Professor of Orthopaedics,
University of Massachusetts Medical Center,
Worcester, Massachusetts

KIM BUTTS, PhD
Assistant Professor,
Stanford University,
Stanford, California

GRAEME M. BYDDER, MB, ChB
Professor of Diagnostic Radiology,
MRC Clinical Sciences Centre,
Hammersmith Hospital,
London, United Kingdom

JEFFREY P. CARPENTER, MD
Associate Professor of Surgery,
University of Pennsylvania Medical Center,
Hospital of the University of Pennsylvania,
Philadelphia, Pennsylvania

MAURICIO CASTILLO, MD
Professor of Radiology,
Chief of Neuroradiology,
University of North Carolina School of Medicine,
Chapel Hill, North Carolina

DONALD W. CHAKERES, MD
Professor of Radiology,
Ohio State University College of Medicine and Public Health,
Columbus, Ohio

DAVID P. CHASON, MD
Associate Professor of Radiology,
University of Texas, Southwestern Medical Center at Dallas;
Chief of Neuroradiology,
Parkland Memorial Hospital,
Dallas, Texas

DAR-YEONG CHEN, PhD
MR Scientist,
Long Beach Memorial Medical Center,
Long Beach, California

DANIEL M. CHERNOFF, MD, PhD
Clinical Instructor,
University of California, San Francisco,
San Francisco, California

WILLIAM F. CONWAY, MD, PhD
Professor and Vice-Chairman of Radiology,
Director of Musculoskeletal Radiology,
Medical University of South Carolina,
Charleston, South Carolina

JOHN V. CRUES III, MD
Medical Director,
Radnet Management, Inc.,
Los Angeles, California

THOMAS M. CUMMINGS, MD
Associate Professor of Radiology,
Associate Vice Chairman of Radiology,
University of Massachusetts Medical Center,
Worcester, Massachusetts

JOEL K. CURÉ, MD
Associate Professor of Radiology,
Director of Magnetic Resonance Imaging,
Medical University of South Carolina,
Charleston, South Carolina

HUGH D. CURTIN, MD
Associate Professor of Radiology,
Harvard Medical School;
Chief of Radiology,
Massachusetts Eye and Ear Infirmary,
Boston, Massachusetts

LEO F. CZERVIONKE, MD
Associate Professor of Radiology,
Senior Consultant,
Mayo Clinic,
Jacksonville, Florida

ANGELA DAGIRMANJIAN, MD
Associate Staff, Neuroradiology,
Cleveland Clinic Foundation,
Cleveland, Ohio

MURRAY K. DALINKA, MD
Professor of Radiology,
University of Pennsylvania;
Chief, Musculoskeletal Radiology,
University of Pennsylvania Medical Center,
Philadelphia, Pennsylvania

DAVID L. DANIELS, MD
Professor of Radiology, Section of Neuroradiology,
Froedtert Memorial Lutheran Hospital,
Medical College of Wisconsin,
Milwaukee, Wisconsin

ELSE R. DANIELSEN, PhD
Senior Research Fellow, Magnetic Resonance
   Spectroscopy Unit,
Huntington Medical Research Institutes;
Boswell Fellow in Chemistry,
California Institute of Technology,
Pasadena, California;
Director of Clinical Magnetic Resonance Spectroscopy,
University Hospital Copenhagen,
Copenhagen, Denmark

ANGELO M. DEL BALSO, MD, DDS, FACR
Professor and Chairman, Department of Radiology,
State University of New York at Buffalo;
Director of Radiology,
Erie County Medical Center,
Buffalo, New York

ROSALIND B. DIETRICH, MB, ChB
Professor and Vice-Chair of Research,
Director of Magnetic Resonance Imaging,
University of California, Irvine,
Orange, California

ROBERT R. EDELMAN, MD
Magnetic Resonance Imaging Director,
Co-Chief of Radiology,
Beth Israel Deaconess Medical Center,
Boston, Massachusetts

ALLEN D. ELSTER, MD
Professor of Radiology,
Director of Magnetic Resonance Imaging,
Director of Teleradiology,
Wake Forest University School of Medicine;
Staff Radiologist,
North Carolina Baptist Hospital,
Winston-Salem, North Carolina

DIETER R. ENZMANN, MD
Professor and Chairman,
Department of Radiology,
Northwestern University Medical School,
Northwestern Memorial Hospital,
Chicago, Illinois

ROBERT E. EPSTEIN, MD
University of Medicine and Dentistry of New Jersey;
Director, Body Magnetic Resonance Imaging,
New Brunswick Affiliated Hospitals,
Lauric Imaging Center,
New Brunswick, New Jersey

SCOTT J.J. EVANS, MD
Assistant Professor of Radiology,
University of California, San Francisco;
Director, Computed Tomography,
San Francisco General Hospital,
San Francisco, California

JAMES L. FLECKENSTEIN, MD
Associate Professor of Radiology,
University of Texas Southwestern Medical Center,
Dallas, Texas

KAROLY FOLDES, MD
Research Fellow,
Harvard Medical School,
Brigham and Women's Hospital,
Boston, Massachusetts

JENS FRAHM, PhD
Professor,
Biomedizinische NMR Forschungs GmbH,
Goettingen, Germany

MOKHTAR H. GADO, MD
Professor of Radiology,
Washington University School of Medicine;
Attending Neuroradiologist,
Washington University Medical Center,
St. Louis, Missouri

ALISA D. GEAN, MD
Associate Professor of Radiology, Neurology,
    and Neurosurgery,
University of California, San Francisco;
Chief of Neuroradiology,
San Francisco General Hospital,
San Francisco, California

JOHN C. GORE, PhD
Professor of Diagnostic Radiology and Applied Physics,
Yale University,
New Haven, Connecticut

PENNY A. GOWLAND, PhD, MSc, BSc
Lecturer, Department of Physics,
Magnetic Resonance Centre,
University of Nottingham,
Nottingham, United Kingdom

ELLEN M. GRAVALLESE, MD
Assistant Professor,
Harvard Medical School;
Rheumatologist,
Brigham and Women's Hospital,
Boston, Massachusetts

DIETRICH H.W. GRÖNEMEYER, MD
Professor and Chairman,
Departments of Radiology and Microtherapy,
University Witten/Herdecke;
Director,
Institute of Microtherapy,
Bochum, Germany

WOLFGANG HÄENICKE, DIPL. MATH
Biomedizinische NMR Forschungs GmbH,
Goettingen, Germany

PETER F. HAHN, PhD
Associate Professor of Radiology,
Harvard Medical School;
Associate Radiologist,
Massachusetts General Hospital,
Boston, Massachusetts

JOSEPH V. HAJNAL, PhD
Professor, Imperial College School of Medicine,
Hammersmith Hospital Campus,
London, United Kingdom

CRAIG A. HAMILTON, PhD
Assistant Professor of Medical Engineering,
Wake Forest University School of Medicine,
Winston-Salem, North Carolina

L. JEAN FLOYD HARDIES, PhD
Assistant Professor,
University of Texas Health Science Center of San Antonio,
San Antonio, Texas

STEVEN E. HARMS, MD
Professor of Radiology,
University of Arkansas for Medical Sciences;
Director of Imaging Research,
Arkansas Cancer Research Center,
Little Rock, Arkansas

ANTON N. HASSO, MD, FACR
Professor and Chairman,
Department of Radiological Sciences,
University of California, Irvine,
Orange, California

VICTOR M. HAUGHTON, MD
Professor of Radiology and Biophysics,
Medical College of Wisconsin,
Milwaukee, Wisconsin

R. EDWARD HENDRICK, PhD
Professor and Chief,
Division of Radiological Sciences,
University of Colorado Health Sciences Center,
Denver, Colorado

R. MARK HENKELMAN, PhD
Professor, Departments of Medical Biophysics
   and Medical Imaging,
University of Toronto;
Vice President, Research,
Sunnybrook Health Science Centre,
Toronto, Ontario, Canada

SYLVIA H. HEYWANG-KÖBRUNNER, MD
Professor and Director, Diagnostic Radiology,
University Halle,
Halle, Germany

CHARLES B. HIGGINS, MD
Professor and Vice Chairman of Radiology,
University of California, San Francisco, School of Medicine;
University of California Stanford Health Care,
San Francisco, California

IBRAHIM A. HIRBAWI, MD
Resident, Department of Radiological Sciences,
University of California, Irvine,
Orange, California

BRIAN C. JACOBS, MD
Clinical Assistant Professor,
University of Washington School of Medicine;
Staff Radiologist,
Highline Community Hospital,
Seattle, Washington

MAUREEN C. JENSEN, MD
Staff Radiologist,
Hoag Memorial Hospital,
Newport Beach, California

J. RANDY JINKINS, MD, FACR
Director of Neuroradiology, Department of Radiology,
University of Texas Health Science Center,
San Antonio, Texas

BLAKE A. JOHNSON, MD
Director of CNS Imaging,
Center for Diagnostic Imaging,
St. Louis Park, Minnesota

EMANUEL KANAL, MD
Associate Professor,
University of Pittsburgh/UPMC Health System;
Director, Clinical and Educational Magnetic
   Resonance Imaging,
UPMC Health System,
Pittsburgh, Pennsylvania

EDWARD E. KASSEL, DDS, MD, FACR
Associate Professor, Department of Medical Imaging,
University of Toronto;
Senior Neuroradiologist,
Mount Sinai Hospital,
The Toronto Hospital,
Princess Margaret Hospital,
Toronto, Ontario, Canada

RICHARD P. KENNAN, PhD
Assistant Professor,
Department of Diagnostic Radiology,
Yale University School of Medicine,
New Haven, Connecticut

J. BRUCE KNEELAND, MD
Associate Professor of Radiology,
University of Pennsylvania;
Attending Radiologist,
Hospital of the University of Pennsylvania,
Philadelphia, Pennsylvania

LARRY A. KRAMER, MD
Associate Professor of Radiology,
University of Texas, Houston Medical School;
Co-Director of Magnetic Resonance Imaging,
Hermann Hospital,
Houston, Texas

MARK J. KRANSDORF, MD
Clinical Associate Professor of Radiology,
University of Virginia,
Charlottesville, Virginia;
Chief of Musculoskeletal Radiology,
Saint Mary's Hospital,
Richmond, Virginia

SURESH K. LAKHANPAL, MD
Neuroradiology Fellow,
University of Washington,
Seattle, Washington

CHARLES F. LANZIERI, MD
Professor of Radiology,
Case Western Reserve University;
Director of Neuroradiology,
University Hospitals of Cleveland,
Cleveland, Ohio

GERHARD LAUB, PhD
Siemens, Medical Engineering,
Erlangen, Germany

GHI JAI LEE, MD, PhD
Associate Professor,
Inje University;
Co-Director of Magnetic Resonance Imaging
and Staff Radiologist,
Seoul Paik Hospital,
Seoul, Korea

NADJA M. LESKO, MD
Instructor, Department of Radiology,
Wake Forest University School of Medicine,
Winston-Salem, North Carolina

JONATHAN S. LEWIN, MD
Vice Chairman for Research and Academics,
Associate Professor of Radiology,
Case Western Reserve University;
Director of Magnetic Resonance Imaging,
University Hospitals of Cleveland,
Cleveland, Ohio

JEFFREY D. LEWINE, PhD
Associate Professor of Radiology,
University of Utah;
Scientific Director,
Director, Magnetic Source Imaging Facility,
Center for Advanced Medical Technologies;
Director, Functional Brain Imaging Program,
Department of Radiology,
University of Utah Medical Center,
Salt Lake City, Utah

KERRY M. LINK, MD
Associate Professor of Radiology and Cardiology,
Co-Director of Magnetic Resonance Imaging,
Wake Forest University School of Medicine;
Winston-Salem, North Carolina

SCOTT A. LIPSON, MD
Attending Radiologist,
Long Beach Memorial Medical Center,
Long Beach, California

ANDREW W. LITT, MD
Assistant Professor of Radiology,
New York University School of Medicine;
Director of Neurologic Magnetic Resonance Imaging,
New York University Medical Center,
New York, New York

MARK J. LOWE, PhD
Assistant Professor,
Indiana University School of Medicine,
Indianapolis, Indiana

ROBERT B. LUFKIN, MD
Professor of Radiological Sciences,
Chief of Head and Neck Radiology,
University of California, Los Angeles, Medical Center,
Los Angeles, California

MASAYUKI MAEDA, MD
Assistant Professor, Department of Radiology,
Fukui Medical University,
Fukui, Japan

MAHMOOD F. MAFEE, MD
Professor of Radiology,
University of Illinois at Chicago;
Interim Head, Department of Radiology,
University of Illinois Hospital,
Chicago, Illinois

ELIZABETH P. MALTIN, MD
Staff Radiologist,
North Shore University Hospital at Plainview,
Plainview, New York

SALIM A. MANJI, MD, FRCP(C)
Radiologist,
University of Alberta,
Misericordia Hospital,
Edmonton, Alberta, Canada

KENNETH R. MARAVILLA, MD
Professor of Radiology and Neurological Surgery,
Director of Neuroradiology,
University of Washington,
Seattle, Washington

THOMAS J. MASARYK, MD
Professor of Radiology,
Ohio State University;
Head, Section of Neuroradiology,
Cleveland Clinic Foundation,
Cleveland, Ohio

VINCENT P. MATHEWS, MD
Associate Professor and Chief of Neuroradiology,
Indiana University School of Medicine,
Indianapolis, Indiana

GERALD B. MATSON, PhD
Adjunct Professor,
Department of Pharmaceutical Chemistry,
University of California, San Francisco;
Facilities Manager,
Magnetic Resonance Unit,
Department of Veterans Affairs Medical Center,
San Francisco, California

ROBERT F. MATTREY, MD
Professor of Radiology,
University of California, San Diego,
San Diego, California

NICHOLAS A. MATWIYOFF, PhD
Professor,
University of New Mexico,
Albuquerque, New Mexico

SHIRLEY M. MC CARTHY, MD, PhD
Professor of Radiology,
Vice-Chair of Academic Affairs,
Yale University School of Medicine,
New Haven, Connecticut

THOMAS R. MC CAULEY, MD
Associate Professor of Radiology,
Albany Medical College;
Attending Radiologist,
Albany Medical Center Hospital,
Albany, New York

VINCENT G. MC DERMOTT, MB, MRCPI, FRCR
Assistant Professor of Radiology,
Duke University;
Attending Radiologist,
Duke University Medical Center;
Durham Veterans Affairs Hospital,
Durham, North Carolina

MICHAEL S. MIDDLETON, PhD, MD
Assistant Clinical Professor of Radiology (Voluntary),
University of California, San Diego,
San Diego, California

DONALD G. MITCHELL, MD
Professor of Radiology,
Jefferson Medical College;
Director of Magnetic Resonance Imaging,
Thomas Jefferson University Hospital,
Philadelphia, Pennsylvania

BRYAN J. MOCK, PhD
Magnetic Resonance Applications Engineer,
GE Medical Systems,
Milwaukee, Wisconsin

MICHAEL T. MODIC, MD
Professor of Radiology,
Ohio State University;
Chairman, Division of Radiology,
Cleveland Clinic Foundation,
Cleveland, Ohio

SHEILA G. MOORE, MD
Clinical Assistant Professor of Radiology,
Stanford University;
Director of Pediatric and Orthopedic Radiology,
Cedars-Sinai Medical Center,
Los Angeles, California

MICHAEL E. MOSELEY, PhD
Associate Professor of Radiology,
Stanford University,
Stanford, California

SURESH K. MUKHERJI, MD
Assistant Professor of Radiology and Surgery,
Director, Head and Neck Radiology,
University of North Carolina School of Medicine;
Adjunct Assistant Professor of Diagnostic Sciences,
University of North Carolina School of Dentistry,
Chapel Hill, North Carolina

MARK D. MURPHEY, MD
Chief, Musculoskeletal Radiology,
Armed Forces Institute of Pathology,
Washington, District of Columbia;
Associate Professor,
Uniformed Services University of the Health Sciences,
Bethesda, Maryland;
Clinical Associate Professor of Radiology,
University of Maryland School of Medicine,
Baltimore, Maryland

ELIAS S. NAJEM, MD
Instructor and Fellow in Neuroradiology,
University of Texas Health Science Center at San Antonio,
San Antonio, Texas

KEVIN L. NELSON, MD
Chairman, Department of Radiology,
Clarkson Hospital,
Omaha, Nebraska

MARY C. OEHLER, MD
Assistant Professor of Radiology,
Ohio State University Hospitals,
Columbus, Ohio

WILLIAM W. ORRISON, JR., MD
Professor and Chairman,
Department of Radiology,
University of Utah,
Salt Lake City, Utah

ARTHUR M. PAPPAS, MD
Professor and Chairman,
Department of Orthopedics and Physical Rehabilitation,
University of Massachusetts Medical Center,
Worcester, Massachusetts

JOHN PERL II, MD
Staff, Neuroradiology,
Cleveland Clinic Foundation,
Cleveland, Ohio

ROBERT M. QUENCER, MD
Professor and Chairman,
University of Miami School of Medicine;
Chief of Radiology Services,
University of Miami/Jackson Memorial Medical Center,
Miami, Florida

SCOTT D. RAND, MD, PhD
Assistant Professor of Radiology,
Medical College of Wisconsin;
Co-Director of Magnetic Resonance Imaging,
Froedtert Memorial Lutheran Hospital,
Milwaukee, Wisconsin

DONALD L. RESNICK, MD
Professor of Radiology,
University of California, San Diego;
Chief, Musculoskeletal Imaging,
Veterans Affairs Medical Center,
San Diego, California

MATTHEW D. RIFKIN, MD
Professor and Chair of Radiology,
Professor of Surgery (Urology),
Albany Medical College;
Radiologist in Chief,
Albany Medical Center Hospital,
Albany, New York

PABLO R. ROS, MD
Visiting Professor of Radiology,
Director of Partners Radiology,
Harvard Medical School;
Vice Chair, Department of Radiology,
Brigham and Women's Hospital,
Boston, Massachusetts

ZEHAVA S. ROSENBERG, MD
Associate Professor of Clinical Radiology,
New York University School of Medicine;
Hospital for Joint Diseases,
New York, New York

BRIAN D. ROSS, MD, D PHIL (OXON),
　　FRCS (ENG), FRCP
Director, Clinical Magnetic Resonance Spectroscopy Unit,
Huntington Medical Research Institutes;
Professor of Clinical Medicine/Radiology,
University of Southern California;
Visiting Associate,
Chemistry and Chemical Engineering,
California Institute of Technology,
Pasadena, California

JEFFREY S. ROSS, MD
Head of Magnetic Resonance Research,
Staff Radiologist,
Cleveland Clinic Foundation,
Cleveland, Ohio

GERALD M. ROTH, MD
Assistant Adjunct Professor,
University of California, Irvine,
Orange, California

VAL M. RUNGE, MD
Professor of Diagnostic Radiology,
University of Kentucky,
Lexington, Kentucky

RICHARD K.N. RYU, MD
Chairman, Department of Orthopaedic Surgery,
Cottage Hospital,
Santa Barbara, California

DAVID J. SARTORIS, MD
Professor of Radiology,
University of California, San Diego;
Chief, Clinical Densitometry,
Thornton Hospital,
La Jolla, California

MITCHELL D. SCHNALL, MD, PhD
Associate Professor of Radiology,
University of Pennsylvania;
Section Chief, Magnetic Resonance Imaging,
Hospital of the University of Pennsylvania,
Philadelphia, Pennsylvania

CAROLINE PANGIE SCHWARTZ, MD
Assistant Professor of Radiology,
Albany Medical College;
Attending Radiologist,
Albany Medical Center Hospital,
Albany, New York

LESLIE M. SCOUTT, MD
Associate Professor,
Diagnostic Radiology,
Yale University School of Medicine,
Yale–New Haven Hospital,
New Haven, Connecticut

RAINER M.M. SEIBEL, MD
Professor of Radiology,
Chairman, Institute of Diagnostic
　　and Interventional Radiology,
Medical Computerscience,
University of Witten/Herdecke,
Mulheim, Germany

RICHARD C. SEMELKA, MD
Associate Professor and Director
　　of Magnetic Resonance Services,
University of North Carolina at Chapel Hill,
Chapel Hill, North Carolina

FRANK G. SHELLOCK, PhD
Clinical Professor of Radiology,
University of Southern California School of Medicine,
Los Angeles, California

EVAN S. SIEGELMAN, MD
Assistant Professor of Radiology,
University of Pennsylvania Medical Center,
Hospital of the University of Pennsylvania,
Philadelphia, Pennsylvania

ROBERT C. SIGAL, MD, PhD
Professor of Radiology,
Paris XI University;
Head of Diagnostic Radiology,
Institut Gustave Roussy,
Villejuif, France

JACK H. SIMON, MD, PhD
Professor of Radiology and Neurology,
Director of Neuroradiology and Magnetic Resonance Imaging,
University of Colorado Health Sciences Center,
Denver, Colorado

H. WAYNE SLONE, MD
Neuroradiologist,
Mount Carmel Health System,
Columbus, Ohio

PETER M. SOM, MD, FACR
Professor of Radiology and Otolaryngology,
Mount Sinai School of Medicine of the City University
   of New York;
Chief of Head and Neck Imaging Section,
Mount Sinai Hospital,
New York, New York

CHARLES E. SPRITZER, MD
Associate Professor of Radiology,
Duke University Medical Center,
Durham, North Carolina

DAVID D. STARK, MD, FACR
Professor and Chairman of Radiology,
University of Nebraska Medical Center,
Omaha, Nebraska

DAVID W. STOLLER, MD
Assistant Clinical Professor of Radiology,
University of California, San Francisco;
Director, California Advanced Imaging;
Director, Marin Radiology and National Orthopaedic
   Imaging Associates;
San Francisco, California

GORDON K. SZE, MD
Professor of Radiology,
Yale University School of Medicine;
Chief, Neuroradiology,
Yale-New Haven Hospital,
New Haven, Connecticut

JERZY SZUMOWSKI, PhD
Associate Professor,
Chief, Magnetic Resonance Imaging Physics,
Oregon Health Sciences University,
Portland, Oregon

ANNE A. TARDIVON, MD
Medical Doctor,
Institut Gustave Roussy,
Villejuif, France

LOUIS M. TERESI, MD
Associate Clinical Professor of Radiology,
University of California, Irvine,
Orange, California

JEAN A. TKACH, PhD
Adjunct Assistant Professor of Biomedical Engineering,
Case Western Reserve University;
Associate Professor of Radiology,
Ohio State University;
Head, Magnetic Resonance Imaging Research,
Cleveland Clinic Foundation,
Cleveland, Ohio

GLADYS M. TORRES, MD
Associate Professor of Radiology,
University of Florida,
Shands Hospital,
Gainesville, Florida

WILLIAM G. TOTTY, MD
Professor of Radiology and Orthopaedics,
Washington University School of Medicine;
Radiologist,
Barnes/Jewish Hospital,
St. Louis, Missouri

CHARLES L. TRUWIT, MD
Associate Professor of Radiology, Neurology, and Pediatrics,
University of Minnesota;
Director of Neuroradiology,
Fairview University Medical Center,
Minneapolis, Minnesota

PATRICK A. TURSKI, MD
Professor and Chairman,
University of Wisconsin Medical School;
Professor of Radiology,
University of Wisconsin Hospital and Clinics,
Madison, Wisconsin

JOHN L. ULMER, MD
Assistant Professor of Radiology,
Medical College of Wisconsin;
Director of Functional Magnetic Resonance Imaging,
Department of Radiology,
Froedtert Memorial Lutheran Hospital,
Milwaukee, Wisconsin

DANIEL VANEL, MD
Head, Department of Radiology,
Institut Gustave Roussy,
Villejuif, France

PETRA VIEHWEG, MD
Department of Diagnostic Radiology,
University Halle,
Halle, Germany

ELIZABETH VOGLER, MD
Resident in Radiology,
University of California, Irvine,
Orange, California

RICHARD J. WAITE, MD
Associate Professor of Radiology,
University of Massachusetts Medical School;
Director, Musculoskeletal Radiology,
University of Massachusetts Medical Center,
Worcester, Massachusetts

FELIX W. WEHRLI, PhD
Professor of Radiologic Science,
University of Pennsylvania Medical Center,
Philadelphia, Pennsylvania

MICHAEL W. WEINER, MD
Professor of Medicine, Radiology, and Psychiatry,
University of California, San Francisco;
Director, Magnetic Resonance Unit,
Department of Veterans Affairs Medical Center,
San Francisco, California

JEFFREY C. WEINREB, MD
Professor of Radiology,
New York University School of Medicine;
Director of Magnetic Resonance Imaging,
New York University Medical Center,
New York, New York

BARBARA N. WEISSMAN, MD
Professor of Radiology,
Harvard Medical School;
Vice-Chair of Radiology Ambulatory Services,
Head, Musculoskeletal Radiology,
Brigham and Women's Hospital,
Boston, Massachusetts

JANE L. WEISSMAN, MD
Associate Professor of Radiology and Otolaryngology,
University of Pittsburgh School of Medicine;
Director of Head and Neck Imaging,
University of Pittsburgh Medical Center,
Pittsburgh, Pennsylvania

ALAN L. WILLIAMS, MD
Professor and Chairman,
Department of Radiology,
St. Louis University;
Attending Neuroradiologist,
St. Louis University Health Sciences Center,
St. Louis, Missouri

ROBERT WILLIAMS, PhD
Associate Professor,
Department of Radiology,
University of Texas Health Science Center,
San Antonio, Texas

CARL S. WINALSKI, MD
Instructor in Radiology,
Harvard Medical School;
Director, Musculoskeletal Magnetic Resonance Imaging,
Department of Radiology,
Brigham and Women's Hospital,
Boston, Massachusetts

MICHAEL L. WOOD, PhD
Associate Professor,
University of Toronto,
Toronto, Ontario, Canada

BRIAN S. WORTHINGTON, BSc, LIMA, MBBS, DMRD, FRCR, FRS
Emeritus Professor of Diagnostic Radiology,
University of Nottingham,
Nottingham, United Kingdom

IAN R. YOUNG, PhD
Professor,
Imperial College School of Medicine,
Hammersmith Hospital,
London, United Kingdom

WILLIAM T.C. YUH, MD, MSEE
Professor of Radiology,
Director of Magnetic Resonance Imaging and Neuroradiology,
University of Iowa;
Iowa City, Iowa

MINGWANG ZHU, MD
Assistant Professor,
Chief of Magnetic Resonance Section,
Neuroimaging Center,
Beijing Neurosurgical Institute,
Beijing, People's Republic of China

ROBERT A. ZIMMERMAN, MD
Professor of Radiology,
University of Pennsylvania School of Medicine;
Chief, Neuroradiology and Magnetic Resonance Imaging,
Children's Hospital of Philadelphia,
Philadelphia, Pennsylvania

We dedicate this edition to the future of our profession and to our children:
Elizabeth and Emily (DDS), and David, Kristin, India, and Felicity,
and especially to Roz (WGB), who make it all worthwhile.

Foreword—*to the First Edition*

Magnetic resonance imaging (MRI) was introduced into clinical medicine in 1981, and in the short time since then it has assumed a role of unparalleled importance in diagnostic medicine. It is probably the most important imaging advance since the introduction of x-rays in 1895. MRI is unquestionably the imaging modality of choice for the central nervous system including the spinal cord, the musculoskeletal system including the spine and major joints, and the male and female pelvis.

Use of MRI in other parts of the body is also rapidly advancing. It is as good or better than other imaging modalities in the examination of the neck, heart, mediastinum, retroperitoneum, and liver. MRI is also rapidly gaining acceptance in the study of the spleen, and it shows promise in the evaluation of the pancreas.

These rapid successes and general acceptance of MRI result from its many physical imaging parameters: proton density, T1 and T2, proton bulk motion, chemical shift, diffusion coefficients, and magnetic susceptibility. Their multiplicity permits design of techniques that emphasize soft tissue contrast differences between normal and abnormal tissues.

This book is written by experts in their fields who treat their subjects knowledgeably and skillfully. The selection of the contributors shows the editors' familiarity with the research, engineering, and clinical skills worldwide. The orchestration of the whole by the two editors demonstrates their deep understanding of the subject.

It is particularly important to note that the editors have devoted a significant amount of space in the book to the physics and technical background of MRI, from spatial characteristics and physiologic basis of magnetic relaxation to special pulsing sequences and artifacts. The expert treatment of imaging of the body, an area that is rapidly catching up in importance with MRI of the central nervous system just as it did with CT, is another of the strengths of this book.

This spectacularly successful imaging modality is still immature and still has many accomplishments to deliver. For clinicians learning about or practicing MR imaging, this tightly woven and balanced book has the advantages of a treasure of references and the charm of being at the cutting edge of a dynamic diagnostic modality.

ALEXANDER R. MARGULIS
University of California, San Francisco, 1986

Foreword—*to the First Edition*

In the spring of 1972, 77 years after the discovery of x-rays by Konrad Roentgen in 1895, a startling announcement made by Godfrey Hounsfield and James Ambrose at the meeting of the British Institute of Radiology forever changed the manner in which cross-sectional imaging is carried out in diagnostic radiology. Tomography was well known since the early work of Vallebonna and others in the 1920s and early 1930s. The technique as then described was ingenious; it consisted in moving the x-ray tube and the x-ray film in opposite directions around an axis that was the only plane of the image in focus, everything above and below it being blurred. These analog images served us for many years, and apparatus was perfected to the point where we are able to obtain cross-sectional images with 1 mm resolution. Inherent to all radiography is an excellent spatial resolution but poor contrast resolution, which has not really been improved despite efforts carried out for over 90 years.

Computed tomography was significant because it changed the analog to digital images so that they could be manipulated at will and transmitted to several places simultaneously. In addition, there was more than 10-fold increase in contrast resolution in comparison to radiography. The marriage of the computer to the diagnostic imaging field was indeed a turning point. Only 1 year after the discovery of computer tomography (1973), Paul Lauterbur of New York published a paper indicating the possibility of localizing resonating nuclei in space. This opened a whole new vista. Scarcely 2 to 3 years later we learned that images were being produced and that some images, such as those of the wrist and hand published in *Nature* by Waldo Hinshaw and colleagues in 1977, were startling in the amount of detail observed. It soon became obvious that we were dealing with a method of cross-sectional imaging that was superior to x-ray computed tomography in depicting soft tissue contrast.

Like computed tomography, the first and principal applications of magnetic resonance have been in imaging of the central nervous system, brain, and spinal cord. The clarity of the images of the brain obtainable by magnetic resonance goes beyond our fondest expectations of only 4 years ago. It was several years, after extensive experience imaging the brain, before there was general acceptance of computed tomography to diagnose lesions in the rest of the body. I expect that the same will be true of magnetic resonance imaging. At present, approximately 85% to 90% of examinations involve the head and the spine, but in some institutions applications of magnetic resonance imaging diagnosis outside the brain and spine are increasing. This includes bone and joint diagnosis, pelvic pathology, and more recently the liver, mediastinum, and heart.

One area that will take some time to develop is that of magnetic resonance spectroscopy, where considerable research is required. The use of nuclei other than hydrogen, such as sodium, fluorine, and phosphorus, will continue to be investigated, and it is likely that they will be used for medical diagnosis in the future. I am happy to see this aspect of nuclear magnetic resonance included in this important volume.

The future of magnetic resonance in medical diagnosis and medical research is a bright one indeed, and this volume goes a long way toward accurately presenting the field as we know it in 1987.

JUAN M. TAVERAS
Massachusetts General Hospital, 1986

Preface—*to the Third Edition*

It has now been 25 years since the first magnetic resonance (MR) image was produced, yet magnetic resonance imaging (MRI) seems reluctant to mature from its tempestuous adolescence into predictable adulthood. Just about the time we think MRI has settled down and we begin to gather clinical experience worldwide, new software or hardware comes along, making previous techniques all but obsolete.

Consider the diagnosis of stroke. In the first edition of *Magnetic Resonance Imaging,* we showed conventional T2-weighted spin-echo images that were positive when the computed tomography (CT) scan was normal. In our second edition, we showed fluid-attenuated inversion recovery (FLAIR) images that were positive when the T2-weighted images were normal. In this third edition, we show echo-planar diffusion images that are positive when the T2-weighted and FLAIR images are normal. We imagine that in the future stroke treatment will be guided by findings on MR images.

Our goal in this third edition of *Magnetic Resonance Imaging* is to present mature techniques having indisputable clinical value alongside exciting but unproved developments. For example, our contributors teach the conventional MR appearance of brain tumors and also speculate on relationships between histopathological findings and MR spectroscopy. Liver and biliary system chapters include not only conventional and breath-hold sequences but MR cholangiopancreatography.

From the single neuroangiography chapter in the last edition, we have expanded to three chapters on angiography throughout the body and have added contrast-enhanced MR angiography, as well. Coverage of musculoskeletal MRI has risen from one chapter in the first edition and six in the second edition to a total 17 chapters in this third edition. Additional chapters on MRI of the breast (implants and cancer), functional imaging, magnetic source imaging, and interventional MRI have been added—all to keep you on the cutting edge! As always, we have updated the physics chapters to explain the basics of these new clinical developments.

You will notice a new look, with a "Key Points" listing at the beginning of each chapter for those wishing only an executive summary. Having suffered all manner of abuse over the last 10 years from the weight of our previous editions, we've slimmed each of the current three volumes to a more manageable size so we won't hear any more jokes about arm curls and toe raises.

We hope you like it!

WILLIAM G. BRADLEY, JR.
DAVID D. STARK
1998

Preface—*to the Second Edition*

Since the publication of the first edition of *Magnetic Resonance Imaging,* the field has virtually exploded. This has been reflected in the growth of this text. For example, one chapter on musculoskeletal MRI has been expanded to six. The coverage on MR angiography has grown from one tentative figure in the first edition to an entire chapter. New MR imaging techniques have been developed with improved speed, spatial resolution, signal-to-noise ratio, and image contrast. Tissue-specific MR contrast agents have been developed and are now being tested in humans. Magnetization transfer and other fundamentally new approaches to imaging and spectroscopy have been introduced. All are addressed here.

Magnetic resonance imaging is now used in virtually every part of the body, yet we seem to have barely scratched the surface of its potential. Clinical applications have expanded, and the sophistication of practitioners increases steadily. We have responded by increasing the number of technical chapters from 13 to 18. The fundamentals of MR physics are explained, beginning with the basic concepts needed to interpret clinical images. Advanced methods in high speed imaging, contrast media development, and spectroscopy are expertly summarized in the physics section.

As in the first edition of *Magnetic Resonance Imaging,* we have been fortunate to have contributions from so many of the leaders in technical development and clinical application. Elaine Steinborn, Peggy Fagen, and Anne S. Patterson of Mosby-Year Book share credit for the finished product, along with Kaye Finley, whose devotion and skill made this collaboration possible.

DAVID D. STARK

WILLIAM G. BRADLEY, JR.

1991

Preface—*to the First Edition*

This project was started during a period when clinical applications of magnetic resonance were under development in every organ system. Although instrumentation continues to improve, the fundamental principles of magnetic resonance are now familiar, and numerous variations are in routine clinical use. The major goal of this textbook is to provide practicing physicians a detailed guide to established clinical indications, insight into laboratory research methods, and a rational basis for evaluating new technology.

A complementary goal of this textbook is to provide physicists, chemists, and physiologists a guide to the clinical world of diagnostic imaging. Individual chapters focus upon the anatomy, pathophysiology, and clinical issues unique to each organ system. Trade-offs in diagnostic accuracy, patient acceptance, safety, and costs are analyzed with respect to existing diagnostic methods.

We have been blessed by contributions from 72 outstanding investigators who are technical experts and superb teachers. They not only document the state-of-the-art with specific case examples, data, and references; they also provide an indication of what is forthcoming.

Completion of this project on time can be attributed to the enthusiasm of our contributors and co-workers. The vision of our teachers and support of our colleagues have been invaluable. In particular, we are indebted to Joseph T. Ferrucci, Jr., MD, for this professional guidance. The quality of the text and images reflects the skills of Kaye Finley, Peggy Fagen, and George Stamathis.

DAVID D. STARK
WILLIAM G. BRADLEY, JR.
1986

Preface to the First Edition

Acknowledgments

A project of this magnitude involves much more than the efforts of the editors. We would like to thank several teams and individuals who were involved in the third edition of *Magnetic Resonance Imaging.*

First of all, the book most directly reflects the scientific knowledge and clinical experience of our chapter authors—a veritable Who's Who of MRI.

Organizing these scholarly contributions have been teams at Mosby, the University of Nebraska, and Long Beach Memorial Medical Center. Mosby fielded an editorial team in Philadelphia and a production, manufacturing, and design team in St. Louis. On the Philadelphia side, we'd like to thank Liz Corra, Editor for Radiology; Lauranne Billus and Mia Cariño, Developmental Editors; and Anne-Marie Hinds, Editorial Assistant. On the St. Louis side, we thank Carol Weis, Project Manager; Christine Carroll Schwepker, Project Specialist; David Graybill, Manufacturing Manager; and Jen Marmarinos, Designer.

At the University of Nebraska, we appreciate the efforts of Nancy Vahlkamp and Tina Clifton. And last but certainly not least, at Long Beach Memorial, we thank our most skillful veteran, Kaye Finley, who has been putting up with W.G.B. for the past 15 years.

D.D.S.
W.G.B.

Contents

VOLUME II

PART III   MUSCULOSKELETON

VOLUME III

PART IV   BRAIN

1 Principles of Magnetic Resonance Imaging

Michael L. Wood and Felix W. Wehrli

 KEY POINTS

- Very simply, MRI is an interaction between an external magnetic field, radiowaves, and hydrogen nuclei in the body (which are, themselves, little magnets).
- When placed in a magnetic field, the body temporarily becomes "magnetized"; that is, the hydrogen nuclei align with the magnetic field, creating "magnetization."
- At equilibrium, net magnetization is parallel to the z axis of the external magnetic field. This is called *longitudinal magnetization.*
- An RF pulse at the Larmor frequency tips longitudinal magnetization into the transverse plane, creating "transverse magnetization."
- Longitudinal magnetization recovers partially between RF pulses applied repeatedly at intervals of TR with time constant T1.
- Precession of transverse magnetization induces electrical signal in coil of wire, decaying at time constant T2.
- Imaging volume is restricted to a slice by specific frequencies in the RF pulse and magnetic field gradient.

Magnetic resonance (MR) is a phenomenon involving magnetic fields and radiofrequency (RF) electromagnetic waves. It was discovered in 1946 independently by Bloch and co-workers at Stanford and by Purcell at Harvard. Since then magnetic resonance imaging (MRI) has been a useful tool, especially for analytical chemistry and biochemistry, thanks to the discovery of the chemical shift.[1,2] MRI can produce images with excellent contrast between soft tissues and high spatial resolution in every direction. Similar to other imaging modalities, MRI uses electromagnetic radiation to probe inside the human body. Furthermore, the radiation has low energy and appears to be safe under normal operating conditions.

The idea to extend MR to studies on humans dates back to Jackson, who in 1967 produced what are believed to be the first MR signals from a live animal. The first two-dimensional (2D) proton MR image of a water sample was generated in 1972 by Lauterbur.[22] Before this, Gabillard had investigated one-dimensional (1D) distributions of the MR signal.[15] In 1974, Lauterbur produced the first image of a live animal.[23]

Subsequently, many groups began making contributions, and the technology blossomed.*

This chapter outlines the basic principles of MRI to provide background for the more specialized topics addressed subsequently. It begins with the phenomenon of MR to explain how the body can emit the radio waves that are measured to make an MR image. It then proceeds to strategies for localizing the source of these radio emissions. The description of the principles of MR is brief, and it assumes that the reader is already acquainted with the most elementary concepts of MR.[32]

NUCLEAR MAGNETISM
Properties of Atomic Nuclei

At the core of atoms and accommodating most of the elemental mass is the nucleus, consisting of neutrons and protons. Nuclei with an odd number of neutrons or protons possess spin-angular momentum, which was postulated by Pauli in 1924 to explain the fine structure of atomic spectra.[1,12] These nuclei have a magnetic moment, μ, characterizing the magnetic field surrounding the nucleus. The magnetic field attributed to a nucleus is analogous to that from a bar magnet (Figure 1-1).

Nuclei in a Magnetic Field

When exposed to a static magnetic field, the randomly oriented magnetic dipoles tend to align with the magnetic field. This phenomenon is explained by quantum mechanics, which assigns a quantum number, I, to the spin.[2,9] For the proton associated with a hydrogen nucleus, I = ½.

---

*References 6, 11, 17, 18, 25-28, 33, 38.

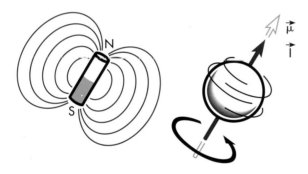

FIGURE 1-1   Nuclear magnetism. Nuclei with net spin *(I)* have a characteristic magnetic moment (μ) and an associated magnetic field, similar to a dipole, such as a bar magnet.

An external magnetic field, B_0, creates two states for this proton that are identified by the magnetic quantum numbers, $\mu = \pm \frac{1}{2}$. In general, μ can assume $2I + 1$ different states (Figure 1-2). The state $\mu = \frac{1}{2}$, in which the magnetic moment has a component parallel to the magnetic field, has lower energy than the antiparallel state.

Net Magnetization

The phases of an ensemble of magnetic moments are random, as shown in Figure 1-3. Therefore the individual magnetic moments make up the surface of a double cone, and their joint alignment creates the net magnetization, M. Many of the principles of MR can be understood from the behavior of the net magnetization.

The net magnetization is the vector sum of the individual magnetic moments, as follows:

(EQ. 1)

$$M = \Sigma p_i \mu_i$$

where μ_i is the magnetic moment of the *i*th state and p_i is its population, which follows Boltzman statistics. The two states for a nucleus, such as the proton, with spin ½, are almost equally probable because their energy difference is small. For protons in a magnetic field of 1.5 Tesla (T) (15,000 Gauss), the fractional excess population in the lower level is approximately 10^{-5}.

A dynamic balance, determined by magnetic field and temperature, exists between the two basic energy states. Nuclei are in thermal equilibrium when the number of transitions from the lower state to the upper state equals that in the opposite direction. The resulting magnetization is called the *equilibrium magnetization,* M_0.

Table 1-1 Magnetic Resonance Properties of Some Diagnostically Relevant Nuclei			
NUCLEUS	**RELEVANT ABUNDANCE (%)**	**RELATIVE SENSITIVITY***	**GYROMAGNETIC RATIO (MHz/T)**
^1H	99.98	1	42.58
^2H	0.015	9.65×0.00965	6.53
^{13}C	1.11	0.016	10.71
^{19}F	100	0.830	40.05
^{23}Na	100	0.093	11.26
^{31}P	100	6.6×0.066	17.23
^{39}K	93.1	5.08×0.000508	1.99

*At constant field for equal number of nuclei.

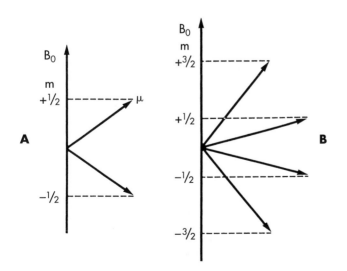

FIGURE 1-2   Quantization of nuclear spin in presence of magnetic field for spin quantum numbers, I of 1/2 **(A)** and 3/2 **(B).**

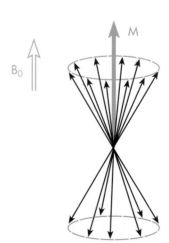

FIGURE 1-3   Development of net magnetization *(M)* by slight preference for magnetic moments to align parallel to magnetic field *(B₀)*. The transverse component of the net magnetization is zero because the phase of each magnetic moment is random.

Precession

The net magnetization experiences a torque from the magnetic field analogous to a spinning top in the earth's gravitational field. As a result, the magnetization precesses around the axis of the magnetic field at a special frequency called the *Larmor frequency,* f_L.

(EQ. 2)

$$f_L = (\gamma/2\pi)B_0$$

where $\gamma/2\pi$ is the gyromagnetic ratio characteristic of the nuclear isotope and B_0 represents the static magnetic field.

Gyromagnetic ratios, relative detection sensitivities, and isotopic abundances for a few relevant nuclei are listed in Table 1-1. The proton, which is the major isotope of hydrogen, is favored for MRI because of its abundance and sensitivity.

RESONANCE

Resonance is the induction of transitions between states of different energy ($\mu = \pm\frac{1}{2}$ for protons). The energy required to produce such transitions equals the difference in energy between the lower and upper states, which is $(\gamma/2\pi)hB_0$, where h is applied at the Larmor frequency, flipping magnetic moments from their $\mu = +\frac{1}{2}$ (lower energy) state to their $\mu = -\frac{1}{2}$ (higher energy) state (Figure 1-4). Such a process can deplete the longitudinal magnetization.

Radiofrequency Field

MR can be detected only if transverse magnetization (magnetization perpendicular to B_0) is created because this transverse magnetization

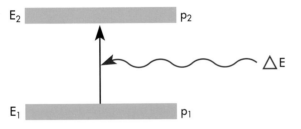

FIGURE 1-4   Transitions between energy states *(E_1 and E_2)* induced by radiation of energy *(ΔE)* exactly equal to the difference between the two states. At equilibrium, slightly more spins populate the lower energy state (i.e., p_1 greater than p_2).

is time dependent and thus, according to Faraday's law of induction, can induce a voltage in a receiver coil. The longitudinal magnetization in thermal equilibrium is static and therefore does not meet the criteria for magnetic induction. Transverse magnetization is created when an RF field of amplitude B_1, rotating synchronously with the precessing spins, is applied (Figure 1-5, *A*). When this RF field is directed perpendicular to the main field, the net magnetization rotates away from its equilibrium orientation. If the B_1 field rotates the net magnetization by 90 degrees, all of the longitudinal magnetization is converted to transverse magnetization, as in Figure 1-5, *B*.

Rotating Frame of Reference

In Figure 1-5, *B*, the motion of the net magnetization vector during the action of the B_1 field is shown in a coordinate system in which the x and y axes rotate in synchronism with the B_1 field. Such a rotating frame of reference greatly simplifies the description of the motion of the magnetization vector. In a static frame of reference, the tip of the magnetization vector spirals from the z axis onto the xy plane.

Free-Induction Decay

Once the RF pulse is removed, the magnetization precesses about the static magnetic field at the Larmor frequency. The precessing magnetization can be detected as a time-varying electrical voltage across the ends of a coil of wire oriented as shown in Figure 1-6. The magnetization also decays exponentially with time-constant T2. A simple model for this induced voltage is shown here:

(EQ. 3)

$$V = \kappa \, M_0 exp(i2\pi f_L t) \, exp(-t/T2)$$

where κ is a constant and $i = (-1)^{1/2}$.

The precessing transverse magnetization is represented by a complex number, which is composed of two numbers—the *real* part and the *imaginary* part. No special significance is attached to the terms real and imaginary. The induced voltage has the characteristics of a damped cosine and hence is also called *free-induction decay* (FID). In Figure 1-6 the imaginary component of the transverse magnetization has the same phase as the B_1 RF field and the real component is 90 degrees out of phase.

T1 Relaxation

RF stimulation causes nuclei to absorb energy, lifting them to the excited state. The nuclei can return to the ground state only by dissipating their excess energy to their surroundings, which is called the *lattice.*

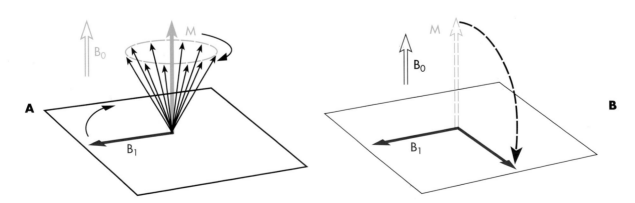

FIGURE 1-5   Tipping of longitudinal magnetization into transverse magnetization by a magnetic field, B_1, associated with an RF wave or pulse. **A,** For appreciable tipping to occur, the B_1 field must rotate synchronously with the precessing transverse magnetization. This condition is met by a circularly polarized RF pulse at the Larmor frequency. **B,** All of the longitudinal magnetization is tipped into the transverse plane by an RF pulse that is strong enough and applied long enough to tip the magnetization 90 degrees (90-degree RF pulse).

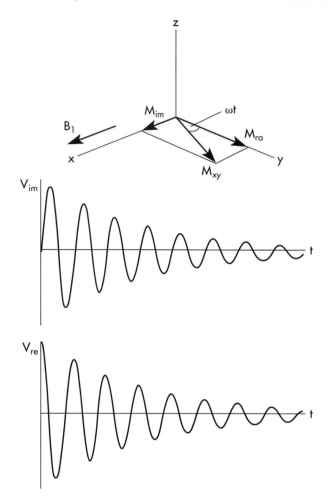

FIGURE 1-6 Transverse magnetization and MR signals. Transverse magnetization is depicted in a frame of reference rotating at the Larmor frequency. The transverse magnetization is regarded as a complex number, with real and imaginary components representing the components aligned along the y and x axes in the rotating frame of reference, respectively. The real component of the transverse magnetization is 90 degrees out of phase relative to the B_1 field, whereas the imaginary component is in phase with B_1.

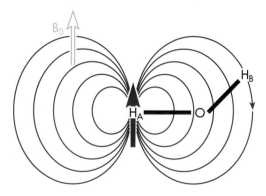

FIGURE 1-7 Perturbation of local magnetic field by magnetic field from neighboring protons. The nuclear magnetic moment creates a dipole field in a water molecule. Proton H_A perturbs the magnetic field near proton H_B. Molecular motion causes the time dependence necessary for these fields to induce relaxation.

The process, which is aptly named *spin-lattice relaxation,* describes the recovery of the longitudinal magnetization toward its equilibrium value. It depends on the lattice having a magnetic field that fluctuates at the Larmor frequency. Such a fluctuating magnetic field comes from rotation and translation of the nuclei in molecules of the lattice undergoing

Table 1-2 Relaxation Times for Different Brain Tissues at 1.4 T From 5-mm Slice at the Level of the Lateral Ventricles in Three Normal Volunteers

ORGAN	T1 (ms)	T2 (ms)
Putamen	747 ± 33	71 ± 4
Caudate nucleus	822 ± 16	76 ± 4
Thalamus	703 ± 34	75 ± 4
Cortical gray matter	871 ± 73	87 ± 2
Corpus callosum	509 ± 39	69 ± 8
Superficial white matter	515 ± 27	74 ± 5
Internal capsule	559 ± 18	67 ± 7
Cerebrospinal fluid (lateral ventricle)	1900 ± 353	250 ± 3

From reference 39.

Brownian motion (Figure 1-7). The average frequency of this Brownian motion depends on the size of the molecules in the lattice. Small molecules reorient more rapidly than larger molecules. The frequency of rotation in medium-size molecules, such as lipids, is closest to typical Larmor frequencies. Therefore the magnetization associated with lipids relaxes faster than that associated with pure water or much larger molecules, such as proteins. Moreover, T1 relaxation times depend on magnetic field strength because the latter affects the Larmor frequency. Table 1-2 lists approximate relaxation times at 1.4 T. Note that white matter in the corpus callosum has a shorter T1 than gray matter, presumably because of white matter's lower water content.

T2 Relaxation

The transverse magnetization decays because its component magnetic moments get out of phase as a result of their mutual interaction. Anything that changes the magnetic field strength also changes the precessional frequency and causes a loss of phase coherence (dephasing) and shrinking of the transverse magnetization. A process called *T2 relaxation* denotes the loss of phase coherence caused by interactions between neighboring magnetic moments. The T2 relaxation time, which differs for some tissues, characterizes the rate at which the transverse magnetization shrinks.

Unlike T1 relaxation, no energy is transferred from nuclei to the lattice in T2 relaxation. Nuclei in the excited and ground state may exchange energy with each other. However, in biological tissues the main contribution to T2 relaxation is from the relatively static magnetic field from neighboring protons. Large molecules, which tend to reorient more slowly than small molecules, promote T2 relaxation and have shorter T2 times. Free water has a longer T2 than water associated with macromolecules. The magnetic field strength influences T2 much less than T1, at least under the conditions encountered in MRI. Typically, T2 in biological tissue ranges from approximately 50 to 100 ms (Table 1-2).[39]

Repeated Tipping of Magnetization

Most MR techniques tip the magnetization repeatedly by using a train of RF excitation pulses. Repeated tipping is usually necessary to accumulate all of the desired data for an MR image. Moreover, because the longitudinal magnetization recovers only partially between closely spaced RF pulses and to an extent depending on T1, repeated tipping provides a mechanism to achieve contrast between tissues with different T1s.

Repetition Time

The time between repeated RF excitation pulses is called the *repetition time* (TR). The TR can be chosen from a certain minimum value, depending on the imaging technique and the MR system, to very long times. Under steady state conditions, the longitudinal magnetization recovers approximately to a fraction $(1 - e^{-TR/T1})$ of its equilibrium value between RF pulses. Longer values of TR allow more T1 relaxation to occur, and this property can be exploited to manipulate the contrast between tissues with different T1s or the signal-to-noise ratio in an image.

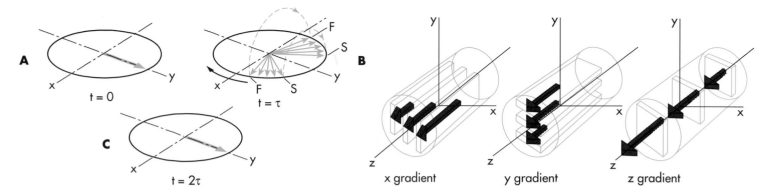

FIGURE 1-8   Refocusing of transverse magnetization into a spin echo. **A,** The spins composing the transverse magnetization are in phase immediately after a 90-degree RF pulse at time t = 0. **B,** At time t = τ, the partly dephased transverse magnetization is turned into mirror-image positions by a 180-degree RF pulse that tips the magnetization about the y axis in the rotating frame. **C,** The fastest precessing spins *(F)* catch up with those precessing more slowly *(S),* leading to refocusing at time t = 2τ.

FIGURE 1-9   Magnetic field gradients in the x, y, and z directions within a cylindrical magnet. The size and direction of each arrow represent the strength and direction of the magnetic field within a plane. The arrows would be identical if there were no magnetic field gradients. All of the arrows point along the bore of the magnet, signifying that the x, y, and z gradients produce magnetic fields with the same orientation as the static magnetic field from the magnet. The strength of the gradients is exaggerated.

Refocusing of Transverse Magnetization into Spin Echo

The transverse magnetization in an FID shrinks more rapidly than expected from T2 relaxation alone. The faster decay is characterized by a constant T2*, which is less than T2. Magnetic field inhomogeneities are the culprit. However, a 180-degree RF pulse applied at time τ after the 90-degree excitation pulse can reestablish phase coherence another time τ later in a spin echo, as shown in Figure 1-8. Spin-echo formation can be compared with a horse race. When the race starts (time τ = 0), all of the horses are lined up at the starting line. After some time, τ, the horses have run different distances, according to their speed. If the horses reverse direction and maintain their individual speeds, they will return to the starting line together at time t = 2τ.

Echo Time

The time from the center of the RF excitation pulse to the center of the echo is the echo time (TE). The amplitude of the transverse magnetization at the echo peak depends on TE and T2 of the tissue. In a spin echo this amplitude typically is proportional to $e^{-TE/T2}$. If TE equals T2, the transverse magnetization has decayed to 37% of its amplitude immediately after the RF pulse. As TE is prolonged, the transverse magnetization becomes weaker. Usually the operator of an MR unit can adjust TE from a certain minimum value to a much longer time. Adjusting TE influences the contrast between tissues that have different T2s. Strategies to create contrast between tissues or otherwise exploit the basic principles of MR outlined earlier are described in subsequent chapters.

IMAGING OF MAGNETIZATION
Spatial Characteristics of Magnetic Resonance Images

Almost every MR image arises from Fourier imaging, which is an efficient and versatile technique for identifying the location of MR signals emanating from various regions of the body.[21] It can create 2D and 3D MR images with various sizes and spatial characteristics. The images are calculated from digitized MR signals, which are usually echoes. The next section describes how spatial information is encoded into these MR signals and then decoded during the calculation of an MR image in a process called *image reconstruction.*

Most MR images are presented as 2D planes partitioned into a grid of picture elements (pixels). The intensity of a pixel represents the strength of the MR signals emanating from the corresponding region. Pixels are also referred to as *voxels* to acknowledge that an MR image represents a slice rather than a plane. The most common MR images consist of 256 columns and 256 rows of pixels or voxels, each repre-

sented by an integer number called *intensity.* Most often the intensity is proportional to the amplitude of the MR signals emitted from the region corresponding to the pixel. There is no standard scale for the intensity of pixels in MR images. Each pixel occupies two bytes (16 bits) in a computer file, allowing a more-than-adequate 2^{16} (65,536) possible intensity values.

Magnetic Field Gradients

Magnetic field gradients are activated briefly as pulses at carefully timed moments during MRI. A magnetic field gradient is a magnetic field that increases in strength along a particular direction. There are x, y, and z gradients, according to the direction along which the magnetic field changes strength (Figure 1-9). The strength of a gradient refers to the rate at which its magnetic field changes with distance. Regardless of the direction of a gradient, its magnetic field is always directed along the z axis in the geometry depicted in Figure 1-9.

SLICE SELECTION
Mechanism

Slice selection combines a magnetic field gradient and a specially shaped RF pulse to restrict MR signals to a slice instead of the entire region influenced by the transmitter coil. The gradient spreads out the Larmor frequency so that the frequencies contained in the RF pulse affect only a slice. Certain characteristics of the RF pulse and gradient affect the orientation, position, thickness, and actual shape of the slice.[7,20]

Slice Orientation

The orientation of a slice depends on which of the three magnetic field gradients is activated during the RF pulse. If a patient is positioned head first and supine in a magnet, such as in Figure 1-9, an RF pulse in the presence of the z gradient creates a transverse slice. The x and y gradients select slices in the sagittal and coronal orientations, respectively. Transverse, sagittal, or coronal slices can be created with similar ease and without any mechanical movements. Oblique slices are created by activating two or more gradients during an RF pulse. If turning on the x gradient selects a slice in the sagittal orientation and the y gradient is also turned on, the slice would be tilted toward the coronal plane through an angle, depending on the relative strength of the x and y gradients.[10]

Slice Position

Slices are located where the Larmor frequency matches the frequency of the RF pulse. The slice-selection gradient lowers the Larmor frequency on one side of the center of the magnet and raises it on the other side. Slice position is controlled by changing the frequency of the RF pulse because changing the amplitude of the slice-selection gradient would inadvertently alter the thickness of the slice. If the strength of the slice-selection gradient is 5 mT/m, the frequency of an RF pulse to position a slice 100 mm from the center needs to be 21 kHz (5 mT/m $\times$ 0.1 m $\times$ 42.58 MHz/T) higher than the Larmor frequency at the center.

Slice Thickness and Profile

RF pulses perturb magnetization within a band of Larmor frequencies matching the frequencies contained within the RF pulse, which is called its *bandwidth* (Figure 1-10). The bandwidth depends on the shape and duration of an RF pulse. Many shapes are possible for the RF pulses used for selective excitation in MRI.

The most widely cited RF pulse shape is the sinc function (Figure 1-11). Sinc-shaped RF pulses excite an approximately rectangular distribution of spins, which is the ideal slice shape (Figure 1-12).

Longer RF pulses, which have a lower bandwidth, produce thinner slices. Unfortunately, longer RF pulses prolong the minimum TE. An alternative is to use a pulse with fewer lobes, as in Figure 1-11, *C*. How-

ever, such a pulse fails to define slices as sharply as either of the other pulses.

The strength of the slice-selection gradient is altered to adjust the slice thickness. Suppose that a 5-mm slice is desired using a pulse sequence in which the RF pulse has 1-kHz bandwidth. The strength of the slice-selection gradient should be 1 kHz /(42.58 MHz/T $\times$ 5 mm), which is 4.7 mT/m.

Multiple Slices

The data for many slices can be acquired concurrently if TR is much longer than the time needed to acquire data from one slice. Usually, applying the RF pulses and gradient pulses and then measuring the resulting echo occupy only a small fraction of TR. The rest of TR is spent waiting for recovery of longitudinal magnetization in the particular slice. This inactive period can be used productively by acquiring data from adjacent slices (Figure 1-13). The maximum number of slices is limited by the time required to acquire data for each slice, power deposition, hardware, and software.

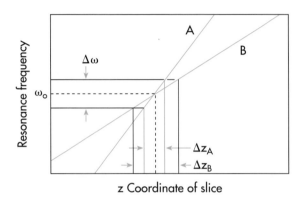

FIGURE 1-10   Effect of gradient amplitude and bandwidth on slice thickness. For an RF pulse with a given bandwidth $(\Delta\omega)$ the gradient strength determines slice thickness. Slice A, corresponding to the stronger gradient, is thinner than slice B.

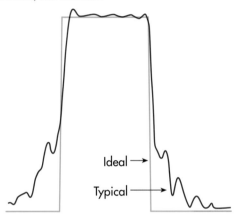

FIGURE 1-12   A slice profile, which is a side view of a slice, displaying the strength of MR signals through its thickness. An MR image collapses this side view into one number related to the area under the slice profile. The ideal slice profile starts abruptly at one edge, reaches a plateau immediately, stays constant from the front edge to the back edge of the slice, and then drops suddenly to zero. Typical slice profiles are neither sharp nor flat. This slice profile was measured from a uniform phantom under realistic conditions. Regions beyond the presumed edge of a slice contribute to MR signals, which would interfere with adjacent slices.

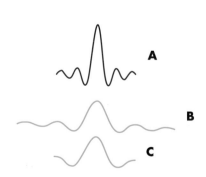

FIGURE 1-11   *A,* Common shape for envelope of slice-selective RF pulses in MRI (sinc function). The slice thickness depends on the bandwidth, which is the range of frequency components contained within the RF pulse. *B,* RF pulse with the same shape but bandwidth reduced by half because length is doubled. *C,* RF pulse with the same bandwidth as *B* but fewer lobes so that it has the same duration as *A.* Slices from *B* and *C* would be half as thick as slices from *A.*

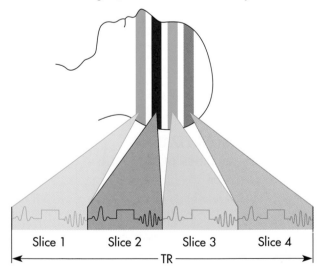

FIGURE 1-13   Interleaved acquisition of multiple slices during dead time within TR. After the RF pulses and magnetic field gradient pulses have generated an echo and the echo has been sampled, a similar procedure is repeated three more times to generate data from three other slices before new data for the first slice are acquired. Data acquisition typically includes several hundred TR intervals such as the one shown here. More slices can be acquired if the TR is longer.

SPATIAL ENCODING THROUGH κ SPACE
Sinusoidal Patterns from κ-Space Points

Images can be decomposed into thousands of sine and cosine waves of different frequency and orientation. An array of numbers called κ *space* holds the weighting factor for each of these waves (Figure 1-14).[24,29-31,37] The coordinates of κ space are called *spatial frequencies,* and their units are cycles per unit length. Each spatial frequency represents a sine or cosine wave across the entire image. The spatial frequencies κ_x and κ_y correspond to a 2D image with coordinates x and y. Note that spatial frequency is completely different from Larmor frequency.

κ Space presents information about the intensity of various edges in an image rather than the spatial relationship of anatomical structures. The spatial domain is the usual representation for MR images. Images are transformed from κ space to the spatial domain by an inverse Fourier transformation, which is described later. In MRI, κ space is interesting because the MR signals that are acquired are actually samples of κ space.

Each data sample in κ space affects an entire MR image. Figure 1-14 shows the contribution of six particular data samples to MR images. An MR image acquires a pattern of lines if the data sample is displaced in either direction from the center of κ space. The distance of the data sample from the center of κ space determines the frequency of the repeated lines.

Influence of κ-Space Regions on Spatial Properties

The center of κ space encodes coarse features in an image. Regions farther from center encode finer detail (Figure 1-15). Low and high spatial frequencies represent an object's overall shape and fine details, respectively. The transition from coarse structures to fine detail occurs gradually from the center of κ space to its edges. An MR image produced from only low spatial frequencies is blurry. If κ space contains higher spatial frequencies, the associated image has higher spatial resolution (Figure 1-16). The image in Figure 1-16, *A* and *C,* omits most of the negative κ_y, which makes the image noisier but not more blurred. The data for negative κ_y are redundant, so they contribute somewhat like averaging. Methods such as half-Fourier imaging produce images successfully from data essentially composed of κ_y of one polarity.[13] This is significant because, as shown later, it takes less time to acquire κ-space data that include a smaller range of κ_y.

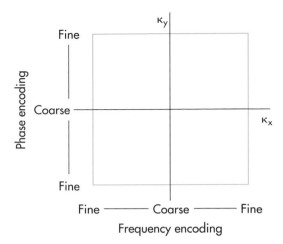

FIGURE 1-15 Influence of κ-space regions on spatial properties. Each κ-space sample affects an entire MR image. The samples in each row of κ space resolve the frequency-encoding direction of an MR image. The data in the columns are responsible for spatial information along the phase-encoding direction. Small values of κ_x and κ_y, which are called *low spatial frequencies,* are in the center of κ space. Low spatial frequencies encode coarse features in an MR image. Conversely the edges of κ space contain the high spatial frequencies, which add fine detail to images. The transition from coarse to fine detail occurs gradually from the center to the edges of κ space.

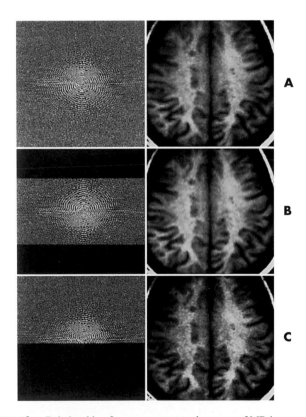

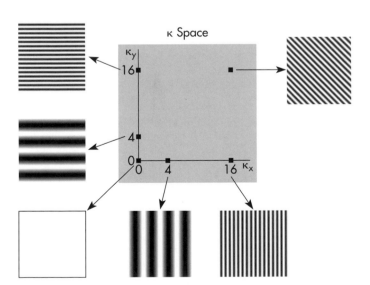

FIGURE 1-14 Definition of κ space, which holds the weighting factor for each of the sine waves into which any picture can be decomposed. These sine waves have a different frequency and orientation. A single point in κ space corresponds to a sinusoidal pattern of a specific frequency and orientation in an MR image. Six simulated images are shown, each arising from κ-space data containing a single nonzero spatial frequency at the coordinates shown. For simplicity, only one of four κ-space quadrants is shown here. Figure 1-15 shows all four quadrants, including negative values of κ_y and κ_x.

FIGURE 1-16 Relationship of κ-space extent to sharpness of MR images. **A,** Reference κ space and image. This κ space contains nonzero samples in 256 rows, corresponding to κ_y from −127 to 128. **B,** κ Space with nonzero samples for κ_y between −63 and 64. The corresponding image has only half as much spatial resolution along the vertical direction (anteroposterior) but is less noisy because the pixels are twice as large. **C,** κ Space with nonzero samples for κ_y from −127 to 8 and image formed by half-Fourier imaging. The image has similar spatial resolution as **A,** but it is noisier. Compared with **A,** κ spaces **B** and **C** would take half as long to acquire.

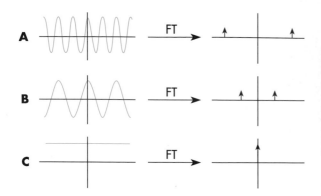

FIGURE 1-17   Fourier transformation of sine waves. The Fourier transformation is a mathematical tool that decomposes an object into cosine waves and sine waves. The three curves on the left are cosine waves of different frequency and the same amplitude. The Fourier transformation of each curve is shown on the right; the axes are amplitude and frequency. These graphs consist of spikes because each curve on the left is simply a cosine wave. There are two spikes because cosine waves are identical for positive and negative frequencies. The spikes are half as far apart in **B** because the frequency of the curve on the left is half as large as the frequency of the curve in **A.** The two spikes converge in **C** to a single spike at zero frequency.

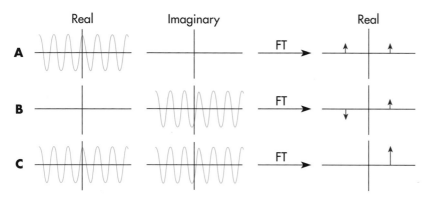

FIGURE 1-18   Fourier transformation of complex sinusoids, which resolves ambiguity between positive and negative frequencies. The Fourier transformation operates on complex numbers, which consist of real and imaginary parts, and generally returns complex numbers. However, the result is purely real for the special cases shown here. The Fourier transformation of curves **A** and **B** consists of two spikes centered on positive and negative frequencies. Both curves are added in **C,** and the Fourier transformation is also equal to the sum of the pattern of spikes from **A** and **B** separately.

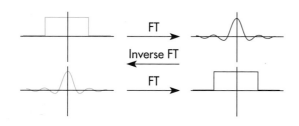

FIGURE 1-19   Fourier transformation and its inverse. The Fourier transformation of a rectangular pulse is a sinc function. Conversely the Fourier transformation of a sinc function is a rectangular pulse. The inverse Fourier transformation converts the curves on the right back to the curves on the left. The inverse Fourier transformation of each curve is similar to the Fourier transformation.

Fourier Transformation

Fourier transformations decompose signals or curves into a distribution of cosine waves and sine waves of different frequency.[3] The Fourier transformation evaluates the match between a curve and sinusoidal waves of a particular frequency. The Fourier transformation of a cosine wave is simply a pair of spikes (Figure 1-17). A spike along the frequency axis is equivalent to a cosine wave plotted against time. The height of the spike is proportional to the amplitude of the cosine wave. There are two spikes in the Fourier transformation of cosine or sine waves because of their symmetry for positive and negative frequencies.

The Fourier transformation used in MRI expects the data to be complex numbers. Figure 1-18 shows that the Fourier transformation of a complex exponential (for which the real and imaginary parts are cosine and sine waves, respectively) resolves the ambiguity between positive and negative frequencies. The Fourier transformation of a wave of complex numbers is also complex. However, if the data possess Her-

mitian symmetry (real part even and imaginary part odd), the Fourier-transformed result is purely real (Figure 1-18).

A curve that continues for a long time has a compact Fourier transformation. For example, the Fourier transformation of the square pulse in Figure 1-19 is a sinc function. The sinc function has lobes that extend forever, although they become smaller farther away from the center.

Inverse Fourier Transformation. Fourier transformation has an inverse, aptly called *inverse Fourier transformation.* Properties of inverse Fourier transformation are similar to those of Fourier transformation (Figure 1-19). Differences between Fourier transformation and its inverse are subtle, and either one could be used to reconstruct MR images from κ space.

Discrete Fourier Transformation. An inverse discrete Fourier transformation (DFT), rather than a continuous Fourier transformation, is used to reconstruct MR images because κ space consists of discrete samples. The DFT and its inverse are defined as a mathematical series, with the number of terms equal to the number of data samples. The terms in the series are summed to calculate one pixel of an MR image. The fast Fourier transformation (FFT) is an efficient algorithm for computing a DFT. An inverse DFT can be evaluated at more frequencies than the number of data samples by appending zeroes to the data in a procedure called *zero filling.* The additional pixels that result after inverse DFT are between the pixels that would have resulted without zero filling. Thus zero filling causes interpolation.

Two-Dimensional Fourier Transformation. An inverse 2D DFT reconstructs a 2D MR image from a 2D κ space. An inverse 2D DFT is implemented as many separate inverse DFTs, applied in turn to the collection of samples across each κ-space row and then to the collection of samples down each column. If the κ space has 256 columns and 256 rows, a 2D inverse DFT consists of 512 separate inverse DFTs. A 3D inverse Fourier transformation, which is used to reconstruct 3D MR images, is a straightforward extension of the 2D transformation.

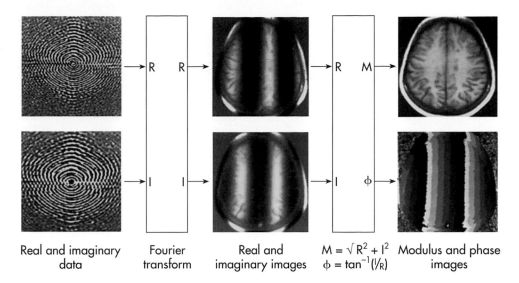

Real and imaginary data — Fourier transform — Real and imaginary images — $M = \sqrt{R^2 + I^2}$ $\phi = \tan^{-1}(I/R)$ — Modulus and phase images

FIGURE 1-20   Reconstruction of 2D κ space into 2D MR image. A 2D inverse Fourier transformation of κ space (displayed using gray scale) of complex numbers generates an MR image of complex numbers (real and imaginary parts shown). The symbols *R, I, M,* and Π represent real, imaginary, modulus, and phase, respectively. The image intensity is distributed between the real and imaginary images. The amplitude and phase are extracted from the real and imaginary images and presented in modulus and phase images, respectively.

Image Reconstruction

κ Space contains complex numbers, which have real and imaginary parts. Both parts are passed to an inverse 2D DFT, as pictured in Figure 1-20, and the output is a matrix of complex numbers split into real and imaginary images. Usually, neither the real nor imaginary images are displayed because the image intensity is distributed indiscriminately between them. Instead the real and imaginary images are combined into a modulus (or magnitude) image. The modulus is appropriate for most MR images because pixels represent the magnitude of MR signals from that location.

Phase Correction

After a 2D inverse DFT, the image intensity is distributed between the real and imaginary images in a way that reflects the pulse sequence more than the patient. Such is the case for the vertical stripes in Figure 1-21. The phase image indicates how the intensity is distributed between the real and imaginary images. If all of the intensity in the imaginary image could be moved into the real image, the real image could be displayed alone without the annoying vertical stripes, which occur when the phase jumps between 360 and 0 degrees. This is accomplished by phase correction.

FILLING OF κ SPACE
Phase-Sensitive Detection

Phase-sensitive detection removes the Larmor frequency at the center of the field of view (FOV) from MR signals. The resulting lower-frequency signals can be measured more slowly, which is less demanding of equipment and allows for less noise. After phase-sensitive detection, the MR signals are directed to a low-pass filter with a cut-off frequency tailored to the reject frequencies higher than those in the MR signals.

After phase-sensitive detection, positive and negative frequencies correspond to MR signals from different sides of the FOV. The cosine wave from the phase-sensitive detector is identical for MR signals on either side of the center. The ambiguity is resolved by using two detectors, as shown in Figure 1-22. The outputs from both detectors have the same frequency but are always 90 degrees out of phase. Separately, neither output can distinguish between positive and negative frequencies. The outputs from the two detectors are combined as complex numbers, which allows for the separation of positive and negative frequencies (Figure 1-18). Outputs from the two detectors are channeled to either

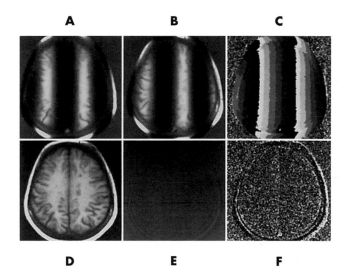

FIGURE 1-21   Phase correction to move image intensity from the imaginary part into the real part of a complex image. **A, B,** and **C,** Real, imaginary, and phase images before correction. The vertical stripes are a pattern of cosine or sine waves. The stripes in **A** and **B** are equally wide but 90 degrees out of phase. **D, E,** and **F,** Real, imaginary, and phase images after phase correction. The imaginary and phase images are essentially blank.

the real or imaginary part of κ space. Phase-sensitive detection is also known as *quadrature detection* because of the manner in which the two outputs are combined.

Sampling

MR signals are digitized in a process called *sampling*. The value of each sample is proportional to the voltage of the MR signal. There are many possible sampling patterns, but as a rule MR signals are sampled at equally spaced intervals of time. Continuous MR signals can be represented accurately by their samples if the interval between each sample is small enough. The time between consecutive samples is called the *sampling interval* (Figure 1-23). Sampling intervals in MRI can be as short as 5 μs or longer than 100 μs. The number of samples from each MR signal ranges from 128 to 1024. The total time necessary to collect these samples is called the *sampling time*. Sampling times can

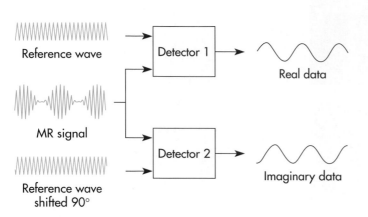

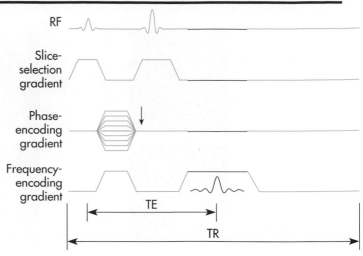

FIGURE 1-22 Phase-sensitive detection converts MR signals from radio frequencies to audio frequencies. A phase-sensitive detector (PSD) combines an MR signal with a reference wave from the frequency synthesizer. The reference wave is a sinusoidal wave of the same frequency as the Larmor frequency at the center of the FOV. The signal emerging from the PSD has a frequency equal to the difference between the frequencies of the MR signal and the reference wave. The second PSD uses a copy of the reference wave shifted in phase by 90 degrees. This shifted reference wave makes the output of the second PSD a sine wave instead of a cosine wave. The outputs from both detectors have the same frequency but are always 90 degrees out of phase.

FIGURE 1-24 Pulse timing diagram for spin-echo pulse sequence in conventional Fourier imaging. The horizontal axis tracks the passage of time from the RF pulse to the end of TR, after which the sequence is repeated. The vertical axis indicates the strength and polarity of each pulse. The second RF pulse is a 180-degree RF pulse, which inverts the phase of the transverse magnetization. The diagram is divided into the following three sections: (1) preparation of transverse magnetization, (2) sampling of echo, and (3) recovery for next repetition. The ladderlike appearance of the phase-encoding gradient pulse signifies that this pulse assumes different amplitudes upon subsequent repetitions.

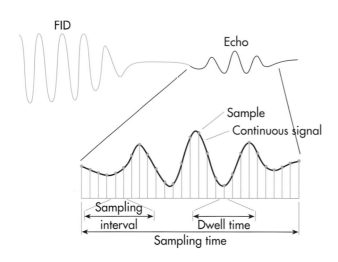

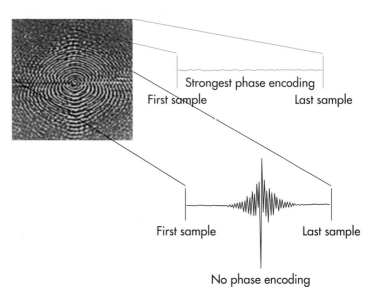

FIGURE 1-23 Sampling of an echo to fill part of κ space. An echo produces a continuous electric voltage across the ends of a receiver coil. The time necessary to acquire one sample is called the *dwell time,* which is much shorter than the sampling interval. The sampling time is the necessary time to acquire all of the samples.

FIGURE 1-25 κ Space regarded as a stack of echoes with different phase encoding. Each row stores the samples from one echo. There is a new row for every echo. The first row contains the echo following the strongest phase-encoding gradient. This echo tends to be the weakest because of the defacing caused by the phase-encoding gradient. The strongest echo is the center of κ space. There is no phase-encoding gradient for this echo. The echoes in the bottom half of κ space correspond to progressively stronger phase-encoding gradient pulses of opposite polarity to the gradient pulses applied for the top half.

be as short as 1 ms or as long as 50 ms, depending on the sampling interval and the number of samples.

Conventional Fourier Imaging

Fourier imaging resolves spatial information by three distinct procedures, called *selective excitation, phase encoding,* and *frequency encoding* (Figure 1-24).[5,19,21,34,35] As explained earlier, the slice-selection gradient spreads out the Larmor frequency over a broad range so that the frequencies contained in the RF pulse affect only a slice. The phase-

encoding gradient is pulsed briefly after the RF excitation pulse has been turned off, making the Larmor frequency depend on spatial position along the phase-encoding direction. Afterward, magnetization components everywhere in the slice regain the same Larmor frequency, but the phase depends on their position along the phase-encoding direction. Spatial information in the phase-encoding direction can be resolved if many separate MR signals are collected. The amplitude of the phase-encoding gradient for each signal is decreased systematically. Each of these signals is measured as an echo while the frequency-encoding gradient is active, which creates a distribution of Larmor fre-

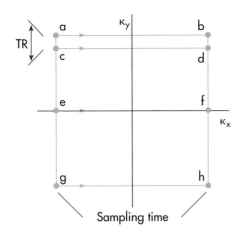

FIGURE 1-26   Filling of κ space in Fourier MRI. Each sample from an echo has a different value of κ_x. The peak of the echo occurs at $\kappa_x = 0$. If there are 256 samples and the echo forms midway through sampling, $\kappa_x = -127$ for the first sample and $\kappa_x = 128$ for the last sample. Each row in κ space is associated with a phase-encoding gradient pulse of different amplitude. Normally the top row of κ space is the first to be filled. Sample a is the first sample in the echo after the strongest phase-encoding gradient. The last sample from this echo is stored at position b. The time between a and b is the sampling time, which is typically about 10 ms. The second row of κ space is filled with samples from the next echo, for which the phase-encoding gradient is slightly weaker. The time between samples a and c is the repetition time, TR. The samples from e to f, acquired without a phase-encoding gradient having been applied, fill the row corresponding to $\kappa_y = 0$. Sample h marks the end of data acquisition.

quencies along the frequency-encoding direction. The first pulse of the frequency-encoding gradient is necessary for an echo to form during the middle of the second pulse.[30]

Data Acquisition Time.   The pulse sequence illustrated in Figure 1-24 must be repeated hundreds of times to fill the κ space for a 2D MR image, depending on the number of pixels and redundant data for averaging or canceling various artifacts. Moreover, the sequence is usually executed initially for several seconds to allow the longitudinal magnetization to reach a steady state. The time for data acquisition is simply the product of TR and the number of pulse-sequence repetitions.

κ-Space Trajectories.   In conventional Fourier imaging, each row of κ space holds an echo after a different phase-encoding gradient pulse (Figure 1-25). Filling the rows of κ space takes much longer than filling the columns (Figure 1-26). However, certain MR techniques skip rows, jump back and forth across rows or columns, or even produce data samples that do not fall exactly on the rectangular κ-space grid.[16] The sequence of spatial frequencies generated during data acquisition is known as the κ-*space trajectory*. κ-Space trajectories are informative because they show when each spatial frequency is measured. That knowledge, coupled with an understanding of how each sample or region of κ space affects MR images, helps optimize imaging conditions and correct artifacts.

FREQUENCY ENCODING
Mechanism

Frequency encoding resolves spatial information along one direction of an MR image by keeping a magnetic field gradient on while each MR signal is being measured. The magnetic field gradient is called the *frequency-encoding gradient, read-out gradient,* or *measurement gradient.* Similarly the direction of space that is encoded is called the *frequency-encoding direction.*

The frequency-encoding gradient spreads the Larmor frequency over a range wide enough to distinguish 128 or 246 different locations along one direction. (The actual number of locations is the number of pixels in an MR image.) The Larmor frequency at the center of the FOV remains unchanged by the frequency-encoding gradient. However, the

gradient increases the Larmor frequency on one side of the center and decreases it on the opposite side. If the x axis is the frequency-encoding direction, the frequency-encoding gradient makes the Larmor frequency linearly proportional to the x coordinate. As a result the frequency-encoding gradient affects the frequency of MR signals from tissues at different locations along the frequency-encoding direction. These signals are not detected separately. Instead they form a composite MR signal known as an *echo* (Figure 1-23).

Data from a Point

Instead of studying a composite MR signal from a human subject, it is informative to consider MR signals from points or at least very small regions. The frequency and phase of these MR signals are the important characteristics for identifying their location. That these signals also decay with time is of secondary importance here. Therefore MR signals from a point in space are modeled as cosine and sine waves, as shown in Figure 1-27.

Inverse Fourier transformation identifies the frequency of each MR signal. Given that the frequency of an MR signal is proportional to the strength of the frequency-encoding gradient, and that the resulting magnetic field varies linearly across the FOV, the frequency identifies the position along the frequency-encoding direction.

Signals from the edge of the FOV (regions a and e) have the highest frequency that can be sampled accurately. These signals complete one cycle between every two data samples. The Nyquist sampling theorem specifies that at least two samples be acquired within each cycle.[3] Inverse Fourier transformation indicates that the frequency of these MR signals is the highest that can be measured by positioning a spike at either end in Figure 1-27. These extreme locations are the edges of the FOV. Lower-frequency MR signals are emitted by tissues closer to the center of the FOV. Signals from regions b and d, which are midway between the center and an edge, complete one cycle after four samples are acquired. By definition, lower-frequency signals take longer to complete each cycle, so more samples are acquired during each cycle.

Together the real and imaginary parts of data allow structures on either side of the center to be distinguished. The real part of the data from positions b and d is identical. So too is the real part of data from regions a and e. However, the imaginary part is 180 degrees out of phase. Inverse Fourier transforming these data produces one spike on the correct side of the FOV. Inverse Fourier transforming only the real part or only the imaginary part produces spikes on both sides (Figure 1-18).

PHASE ENCODING
Mechanism

Spatial information along one direction is encoded into the phase of MR signals by phase encoding. The so-called phase-encoding direction is perpendicular to the frequency-encoding direction. Phase is encoded into MR signals by pulsing a magnetic field gradient briefly (1 ms to 5 ms) before each echo is sampled, as illustrated in Figure 1-24. While the phase-encoding gradient is on, the Larmor frequency becomes linearly proportional to the position along the phase-encoding direction. This is no different from the effect of the frequency-encoding gradient. The key is the phase shift that has accumulated by the time the phase-encoding gradient pulse is turned off.

Phase Shifts

Phase shifts caused by the phase-encoding gradient depend on the location of the magnetization and the amplitude and duration of the phase-encoding gradient pulse. A phase-encoding gradient pulse of 0.1 mT/m amplitude and 2 ms duration shifts the phase of the transverse magnetization located 20 mm from the center of the FOV by 61 degrees (360 degrees × 42.58 MHz/T × 0.1 mT/m × 2 ms × 20 mm). The phase shift would be double 40 mm from the center of the FOV and −61 degrees for a structure 20 mm on the other side of the center.

The phase-encoding gradient is pulsed to a different amplitude before each MR signal so that the different rows of κ space can be filled. Stronger phase-encoding gradient pulses cause phase shifts. Doubling the amplitude doubles the phase shifts everywhere. The amount by which the phase changes as the phase-encoding gradient steps through

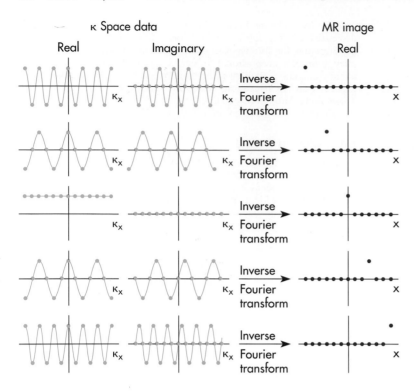

FIGURE 1-27   Sampled κ-space data originating from points at five different locations along the frequency-encoding direction. Locations a and e are at either edge of the FOV, c is in the center, and b and d are midway between an edge and the center. The continuous curves represent MR signals after phase-sensitive detection, and the dots are 13 consecutive samples. The frequency of each signal is unique to the location. An inverse FT of these complex κ-space samples creates 13 pixels along the frequency-encoding direction of an MR image, which is purely real in this case. Only the frequency and phase of the signals are modeled here and not their decay or relative amplitude.

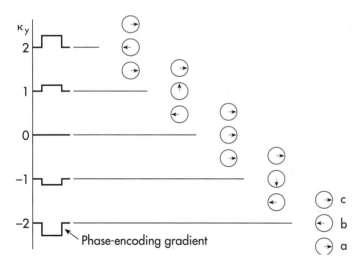

FIGURE 1-28   Characteristic phase advance for each location along the phase-encoding direction. Regions a, b, and c are at the edge of the field of view, midway between the edge and center, and the center, respectively. The position along the frequency-encoding direction is irrelevant. This diagram compares the phase of the transverse magnetization after three consecutive phase-encoding gradient pulses have been applied. Only the dependence on the location in the phase-encoding direction is modeled. The phase of the transverse magnetization is indicated by the angle between each arrow and the horizontal axis.

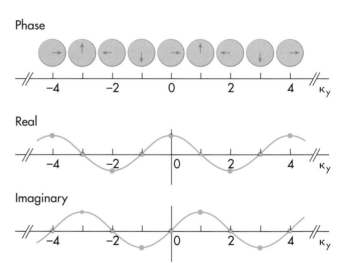

FIGURE 1-29   Transverse magnetization at the location midway between the edge and center along the phase-encoding direction (region b in Figure 1-28) after various phase-encoding gradient pulses. Each phase-encoding gradient pulse corresponds to a distinct value of κ_y, from a total of 256. The phase of the transverse magnetization from this region advances 90 degrees for each successive value of κ_y. The group of samples in the real and imaginary data form a cosine wave and sine wave, respectively. These data samples would be located in the same column of κ space. The data samples from each column of κ space are processed to decode spatial information in the phase-encoding direction.

its range of amplitudes is the key to identifying the location of structures along the phase-encoding direction.

The magnitude and sign of the phase shifts caused by the phase-encoding gradient pulses are identified by comparing a series of MR signals that have experienced a systematic progression of phase shifts (Figure 1-28). Regardless of the strength of the phase encoding, direction has zero phase. A 90-degree phase shift between subsequent phase-encoding gradient pulses characterizes locations halfway between the center and the edge of the FOV. Similarly the phase advances by 180 degrees at the edge of the FOV. The magnetization from tissues on the other side of the FOV experiences phase shifts of similar magnitude

but opposite polarity. For example, the FOV is 240 mm if the phase-encoding gradient pulses are 2 ms long and incremented by 0.05 mT/m (180 degrees /360 degrees × 42.58 MHz/T × 0.05 mT/m × 2 ms).

Data from a Point

The data samples that are compared to determine the phase shifts caused by successive phase-encoding gradient pulses are stored in the same column of κ space, so each sample has a different value of y. Usually each row of κ space has already been inverse Fourier transformed, in which case the data samples in any particular column have the same

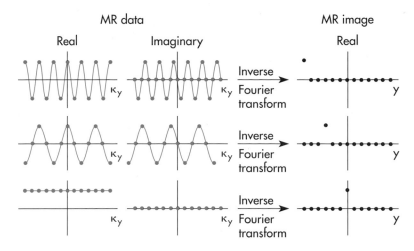

FIGURE 1-30   Sampled κ-space data from three different locations along the phase-encoding direction. Locations a, b, and c are at one edge of the FOV, midway between the edge and center, and the center, respectively. Each curve contains samples from one column of κ space, and each sample originates from separate MR signals following a phase-encoding gradient pulse of different amplitude. The samples are joined by a curve to demonstrate that the group of data samples resemble the data in Figure 1-26. The real and imaginary components of the κ-space data are cosine and sine waves of the variable, κ_y. The frequency of the curve connecting the data samples is identified by an inverse Fourier transformation, and this frequency is proportional to the y coordinate.

x coordinate. Otherwise the data samples in a column correspond to the same portion of different echoes. It is crucial that the only difference between data samples in each column be the phase shift imparted by the phase-encoding gradient pulse.

The frequency of a curve connecting the data samples in any particular κ-space column reveals the rate at which the phase changes with κ_y. Each sample along this curve originates from a different MR signal after a phase-encoding gradient pulse of different amplitude. The frequency components of this curve are identified by an inverse Fourier transformation, just as MR signals are resolved into frequency components. If the frequency is double, it means that each phase-encoding gradient pulse shifts the phase twice as much. Such a larger phase shift occurs twice as far from the center of the FOV along the phase-encoding direction. This is analogous to the frequency-encoding gradient doubling the frequency of an MR signal (after phase-sensitive detection) twice as far from the center.

The collection of data from a column of κ space follows a simple cosine curve or a sine curve if all of the structures are at one location along the phase-encoding direction. Although this is a hypothetical scenario, it is useful for demonstrating the mechanism of phase encoding (Figure 1-29). Each data sample is the cosine or sine of the phase angle. When $\kappa_y = 2$, the real part of the data attains its most extreme negative value because the phase is 180 degrees and the cosine (180 degrees) equals −1. The phase advances 90 degrees between each data sample in Figure 1-29.

Figure 1-30 shows the κ-space data samples from three regions. Their inverse Fourier transformation indicates the location from which the MR signals were emitted. The procedure is similar to reconstructing the frequency-encoding direction, demonstrated in Figure 1-27. Thus the frequency of the curve connecting the data samples for different κ_y identifies the location along the phase-encoding direction of the structure that emitted the MR signal. The inverse Fourier transformation determines that region c is at the edge of the FOV because the curve has the highest frequency that can be measured without aliasing. Namely the curve starts a new cycle at every second sample. Similarly the inverse Fourier transformation recognizes that the data samples from region a remain constant, so it assigns the location to the center of the FOV. Incidentally, real and imaginary data are necessary to resolve the ambiguity between data from both sides of the FOV.

System of Equations

Further insight into phase encoding is possible by regarding the κ space data as a system of algebraic equations. The number of frequencies that

an inverse Fourier transformation can identify depends on the number of different values of κ_y. The 13 values of κ_y in Figure 1-30 yield 13 pixels. If there are only three data samples (S_1, S_2, and S_3, corresponding to $\kappa_y = 0$, 1, and 2), there will be only three pixels in the phase-encoding direction, identified as a, b, and c. For simplicity, assume that pixels a, b, and c cover one side of the center of the FOV at coordinates FOV/2, FOV/4, and 0, respectively. Any column of the κ space contains three data samples representing κ_y equal to 0, 1, and 2.

Each κ-space data sample is a weighted sum of the MR signals from the three locations. The weight depends on the phase shift imparted by the phase-encoding gradient. Each data sample is a complex number, but its real part alone suffices to identify the location of the MR signals, assuming that all three pixels are on the same side of the FOV. Image reconstruction determines the intensity of pixels a, b, and c (denoted I_a, I_b, and I_c, respectively) by an inverse Fourier transformation, which is analogous to solving the following set of three equations for three unknowns:

(EQ. 4)

$$S_1 = I_a + I_b + I_c$$
$$S_2 = I_a \cos(180°) + I_b \cos(90°) + I_c \cos(0)$$
$$S_3 = I_a \cos(360°) + I_b \cos(180°) + I_c \cos(0)$$

The phase angles were obtained from Figure 1-28. As a specific example, if S_1, S_2, and S_3 are 6, −2, and 2, respectively, the solution to Equation 4 is $I_a = 3$, $I_b = 2$, and $I_c = 1$, which can be verified through substitution.

THREE-DIMENSIONAL IMAGING

Three-dimensional Fourier imaging produces MR images of an entire volume by a straightforward extension of 2D Fourier imaging (Figure 1-31).[8,36] If 128 slices are desired, the first phase-encoding gradient steps through 128 different amplitudes while the second phase-encoding gradient is pulsed to the same amplitude. Afterward the second phase-encoding gradient is assigned a new amplitude, and the pulse sequence is repeated another 128 times, covering the full range of the first phase-encoding gradient. The second phase-encoding gradient needs 256 steps to resolve 256 pixels in one direction of each slice. In this case the total number of phase-encoding gradient steps is 128 × 256, which is 32,768. Repeating a pulse sequence so many times to acquire the data for a 3D MR image is prohibitive unless TR is very short.[14]

The slices in a 3D MR image are resolved by inverse Fourier transforming a collection of κ-space data samples from MR signals corre-

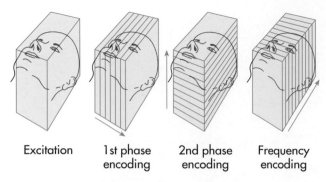

Excitation   1st phase   2nd phase   Frequency
              encoding   encoding   encoding

FIGURE 1-31   Procedures for creating a 3D MR image. An RF pulse excites the magnetization within a slab covering the middle of the head. Two directions are phase encoded separately. The first phase-encoding procedure partitions the slab into slices, which are in the sagittal orientation here. Each slice is resolved by a second phase-encoding procedure and frequency encoding, similar to 2D Fourier imaging.

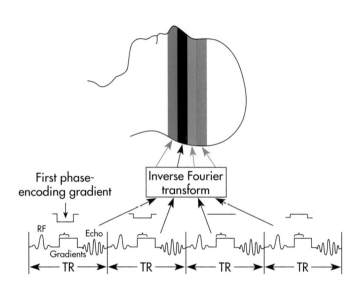

FIGURE 1-32   Encoding of slices in 3D Fourier imaging by an inverse Fourier transformation. The data samples that are inverse Fourier transformed belong to separate echoes. There is one data sample for each step of the first phase-encoding gradient. Each data sample corresponds to the same value of the second phase-encoding gradient and the same temporal position in each echo (i.e., same κ_x and κ_y).

sponding to every step of the first phase-encoding gradient. Figure 1-32 illustrates this procedure for four slices. The procedure is identical to phase encoding for a 2D MR image. Four MR signals arise from four repetitions of the pulse sequence, in which the first phase-encoding gradient has a different amplitude but all other pulses are the same. One data sample from each signal is collected, and then the four data samples are subjected to a 4-point inverse DFT. The process is repeated for every data sample in each group of four MR signals. The inverse Fourier transformation separates the four signals into four slices.

The most compelling attribute of 3D MRI is that it can cover extensive regions of anatomy with high resolution in all three directions. Each κ-space data sample for a 3D MR image contributes to every voxel, unlike 2D imaging, in which slices are excited separately. The fact that all of the data samples in 3D MRI are related helps increase the SNR, but it also makes 3D images vulnerable to artifacts.[4]

REFERENCES

1. Abragam A: The principles of nuclear magnetism, London, 1961, Oxford University Press.
2. Allen PS: Some fundamental principles of nuclear magnetic resonance. In Medical Physics Monograph No. 21: The physics of MRI: 1992 AAPM Summer School Proceedings, American Institute of Physics, 21:15, 1993.
3. Bracewell RN: The Fourier transform and its applications, ed 2, New York, 1978, McGraw-Hill.
4. Carlson J, Crooks L, Ortendahl D, et al: Signal-to-noise ratio and section thickness in two-dimensional versus three-dimensional Fourier transform MR imaging, Radiology 166:266, 1988.
5. Cho ZH, Kim HS, Song HB, et al: Fourier transform nuclear magnetic resonance tomographic imaging, Proc IEEE 70(10):1152, 1982.
6. Crooks L: Selective irradiation line scan technique for NMR imaging, IEEE Trans Nucl Sci NS-27, 1239, 1980.
7. Crooks LE, Hoenninger J, Arakawa M, et al: High-resolution magnetic resonance imaging: technical concepts and their implementation, Radiology 150:163, 1984.
8. den Boef JH, van Uijen CMJ, and Holzscherer CD: Multiple-slice NMR imaging by three-dimensional Fourier zeugmatography, Phys Med Biol 29:857, 1984.
9. Dixon RL, and Ekstrand KE: The physics of proton NMR, Med Phys 9(6):807, 1982.
10. Edelman RR, Stark DD, Saini S, et al: Oblique planes of section in MR imaging, Radiology 159:807, 1986.
11. Edelstein WA, Hutchison JMS, Johnson G, et al: Spin warp NMR imaging and applications to human whole body imaging, Phys Med Biol 25:751, 1980.
12. Farrar TC, and Becker ED: Pulse and Fourier transform nuclear magnetic resonance, New York, 1971, Academic Press.
13. Feinberg DA, Hale JD, Watts JC, et al: Halving MR imaging time by conjugation: demonstration at 3.5 kG, Radiology 161:527, 1986.
14. Frahm J, Hasse A, and Matthaei D: Rapid three-dimensional MR imaging using the FLASH technique, J Magn Reson 67:258, 1986.
15. Gabillard R: A steady state transient technique in nuclear resonance, Phys Rev 85:6794, 1952.
16. Henning J, Naureth A, and Friedburg H: RARE imaging: a fast method for clinical MR, Magn Reson Med 3:823, 1986.
17. Hinshaw WS: Image formation by nuclear magnetic resonance: the sensitive point method, J Appl Phys 47(8):3709, 1976.
18. Hinshaw WS, Bottomley PA, Holland GN, et al: Radiographic thin-section imaging of the human wrist by nuclear magnetic resonance imaging, Nature 270:722, 1977.
19. Hinshaw WS, and Lent AH: An introduction to NMR imaging: from the Bloch equation to the imaging equation, Proc IEEE 71(3):338, 1983.
20. Kucharczyk W, et al: Effect of multislice interference on image contrast in T2-weighted and T1-weighted MR images, Am J Neuroradiol 9:443, 1988.
21. Kumar A, Welti D, and Ernst RR: NMR Fourier zeugmatography, J Magn Reson 18:69, 1975
22. Lauterbur PC: Image formation by induced local interactions: examples employing nuclear magnetic resonance, Nature 242:190, 1973.
23. Lauterbur PC: Image formation by induced local interactions: examples employing nuclear magnetic resonance, Pure Appl Chem 40:149, 1974.
24. Ljunggren S: A simple graphical representation of Fourier-based imaging methods, J Magn Reson 54:338, 1983.
25. Macovski A: Volumetric NMR imaging with time-varying gradients, Magn Res Med 2:29, 1985.
26. Mansfield P: Proton spin imaging by nuclear magnetic resonance, Contemp Phys 17:553, 1976.
27. Mansfield P, and Pykett IL: Biological and medical imaging by NMR, J Magn Reson 29:355, 1978.
28. Maudsley A: Multiple-line-scanning spin-density imaging, J Magn Reson 41:112, 1980.
29. Mezrich R: A perspective on κ space, Radiology 195:297, 1995.
30. Pelc NH, and Glover GH: A stroll through κ space. In Medical Physics Monograph No. 21: The physics of MRI: 1992 AAPM Summer School Proceedings, American Institute of Physics 21:771, 1993.
31. Peters TM: An introduction to κ-space. In Medical Physics Monograph No. 21: The physics of MRI: 1992 AAPM Summer School Proceedings, American Institute of Physics 21:754, 1993.
32. Pykett IL, Newhouse JH, Buonanno FS, et al: Physical principles of nuclear magnetic resonance imaging, Radiology 143:157, 1982.
33. Pykett IL, and Mansfield P: A line scan image study of a tumorous rat leg by NMR, Phys Med Biol 23:961, 1978.
34. Riederer SJ: Spatial encoding and image reconstruction. In Medical Physics Monograph No. 21: The physics of MRI: 1992 AAPM Summer School Proceedings, American Institute of Physics 21:135, 1993.
35. Song HB, Cho ZH, and Hilal SK: Direct Fourier transform NMR tomography with modified Kuman-Welti-Ernst (MKWE) method, IEEE Trans Nuc Sci NS 29:493, 1982.
36. Sutherland RJ, and Hutchinson JMS: Three-dimensional NMR imaging using selective excitation, J Phys E Sci Instrum 11:79, 1979.
37. Twieg DB: The κ-trajectory formulation of the NMR imaging process with applications in analysis and synthesis of imaging methods, Med Phys 10(5):610, 1983.
38. Wehrli FW: The origins and future of nuclear magnetic resonance imaging, Physics Today, p 34, June 1992.
39. Wehrli FW, MacFall JR, and Prost JH: Impact of the choice of the operating parameters on MR images. In Partain CL, Price RR, and Patton JA, eds: Magnetic resonance imaging, Philadelphia, 1988, WB Saunders.

2 Instrumentation

Nicholas A. Matwiyoff and William M. Brooks

The Magnet
Origin of Magnetic Fields
Superconducting Magnets
Quenches
Resistive Magnets
Permanent Magnets
Magnetic Field Homogeneity
Passive shimming and shielding
Active shimming
Field Homogeneity and Quality of Images and Spectra
Summary of Conventional Magnet Characteristics
Open-Configuration Superconducting Magnets
The Gradient System
Functions and General Characteristics
Gradient Coils and Gradient Fields
Eddy Currents
Special Requirements for Fast Imaging and Spectroscopy
The Radiofrequency System
Functions and Characteristics
Noise, Signal-to-Noise Ratio, Magnetic Field Strength, and Radiofrequency Coils
Coil Geometry
Coil Quality
Transmitters and Receivers
Transmitter Frequency Bandwidth
Complete Transmitter System
Quadrature excitation
Receiver System
Detection in quadrature
Digital sampling rate
Bandwidth
Fast Imaging and Spectroscopy Revisited
Computer and Accessories

The objectives of this chapter are to describe magnetic resonance (MR) instrumentation and the interactions among its components in the context of the physics of the construction of MR images. The key steps taken in the generation of spin-echo proton magnetic resonance imaging (^{1}H MRI) are sketched in Figure 1-15. Common to the wide variety of MR instruments used to produce proton images of humans are the following basic components:

1. A magnet that has a bore size or gap large enough to accept the human torso, produces a stable homogeneous magnetic field (B_0) over the imaging volume of interest, and induces a weak magnetization (M) in the tissue as a result of alignment of fat and water proton magnetic dipoles with the field

The authors appreciate the permission of Dr. J. Bruce Kneeland to use material from the first edition of this book, especially Figures 2-7; 2-11; 2-14, *A* and *C*; 2-15; and 2-16. They are grateful to C. Gasparovic for a careful reading of the text and critical comments on it.

 KEY POINTS

- The key components of an MR system are the magnet, the gradient, the radiofrequency subsystem, and the computer.
- The magnet can be superconducting, resistive, or permanent. Superconducting magnets tend to have high fields in Tesla and therefore higher signal-to-noise. Resistive and permanent magnets tend to have a more open architecture, allowing interventional MRI applications and reduced claustrophobia.
- The gradients are resistive electromagnets consisting of metallic coils driven by power amplifiers. Gradient performance is measured in amplitude (in milliTesla per meter [mT/m] and rise time [in microseconds]), larger values of the former (>20 mT/m) and smaller values of the latter (<400 ms) being required for high-performance applications (e.g. EPI and first pass Gd-enhanced MRA).
- The RF subsystem consists of a transmitter, a receiver, and coils, which can be simple surface coils, double-saddle (Helmholtz) coils, quadrature-receive/quadrature excitation coils, or phased-array coils.
- The computer is required for data manipulation and to coordinate the RF and gradient subsystems.

2. A gradient coil that creates pulsed magnetic field gradients, which are required for selecting the imaging slice or slices and for frequency encoding and phase encoding of the magnetization within the slice
3. A radiofrequency (rf) transmitter/receiver (transceiver) for generating the RF (B_1) pulses, which rotate M away from alignment with B_0, and for detecting the MR signal produced by the precession of M
4. A computing system for managing the magnet, transceiver, and gradient coil components; for processing and storing the MR signal; and for constructing, storing, and displaying the image

MR instrumentation for diagnostic imaging is complex and expensive because of the following:
1. Intrinsic weakness (low intensity) of the MR signal
2. Time dependence of the MR signal (many tissue signals decay completely in less than 300 ms)
3. Signal characterization by amplitude, frequency, and phase[19,35,45,47,64]

THE MAGNET
Origin of Magnetic Fields

The heart of all MR systems is the magnet. There are three types of magnets in common use for MRI—permanent magnets, resistive electromagnets, and superconducting electromagnets. The most important criterion for a magnet is unchanging field strength with respect to both time and position; that is, it should be of consistent amplitude and be homogeneous. Magnetic fields are created in the space surrounding moving electrical charges (electrical currents). The intensity, strength, and homogeneity of the magnetic field generated depend on the current density and the path it traverses. These two properties of magnetic fields are of central importance in MRI. The shape and inhomogeneity of the magnetic field surrounding a long linear wire conducting an electrical current are illustrated in Figure 2-1, *A*. One method to produce a homogeneous magnetic field having the same number of magnetic field lines per unit area (constant flux density) at all points in space in an electromagnet is illustrated in Figure 2-1, *B* to *D*. The other basic type of magnet, the permanent magnet, does not require the supply of an external electrical current because it is constructed of ferromagnetic ma-

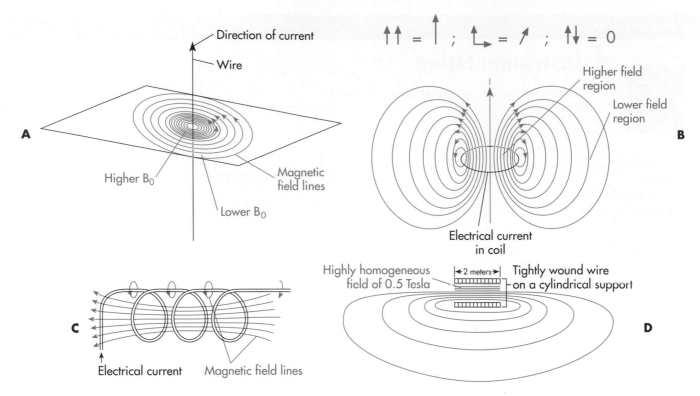

FIGURE 2-1 Magnetic field lines (fluxes) of wires carrying electrical current. **A,** A long straight wire has more magnetic field lines (flux) per unit area (higher field strength) near the wire. Overall the B_0 field is highly inhomogeneous. **B,** A circular wire (coil) conducting an electrical current. The flux density or magnetic field strength is stronger and more homogeneous inside the coil than outside it. This results from a reinforcement of the flux lines from opposite segments of the wire within the coil and a reduction of flux lines exterior to it. The magnetic field has the vector properties of amplitude and direction. The result of the interaction of two vectors ($\uparrow$) of equal amplitude but three different orientations is also illustrated in **C.** A loosely wound coil (solenoid) illustrating the evolution of a more homogeneous magnetic field caused by reinforcement of flux lines within the coil. **D,** An ideal tightly wound solenoid exhibiting a highly homogeneous magnetic field in the interior of the coil and a highly inhomogeneous field (a fringe field) exterior to the coil. Electrical current goes out of the paper at the top and into the paper at the bottom.

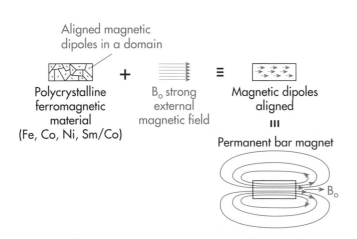

FIGURE 2-2 Creation of a permanent magnet from a ferromagnetic material. Before imposition of the external field the magnetization of the domains is random and there is little net magnetization of the bar, although each domain is magnetized as a result of alignment of electron magnetic dipoles within the domain. A ferromagnetic material "saturates" in that the induced magnetization levels off as B_0 increases.

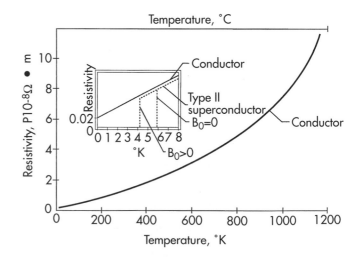

FIGURE 2-3 The temperature dependence of the resistivity of a hypothetical conductor and a hypothetical type II superconductor is plotted. The resistivity is directly related to resistance (high resistivity = high resistance). The temperature dependence of the resistivity of a typical conductor is a smooth function of temperature and does not become zero even at absolute zero (0° K). This is not the case for a type II semiconductor: Its resistivity drops precipitously to zero at a relatively high temperature. Strong magnetic fields, such as those generated by passing current through the conductor, can quench the superconductivity of some materials, but in type II superconductors it merely shifts the superconducting transition to a lower temperature, as shown in the insert.

terials that contain microcrystalline structures (domains) in which there is a permanent net flow of electrons in closed loops. These ferromagnetic materials (e.g., iron, cobalt, nickel, rare earth elements, or certain of their alloys) in certain crystalline forms thus contain magnetic domains that can be aligned by an external magnetic field. When the external field is removed, the domains remain aligned and a permanent magnet results; the magnet's field strength depends on the saturation field for the particular ferromagnetic materials (Figure 2-2). A single bar magnet has an extremely inhomogeneous B_0 field, but as illustrated in a later section the flux lines can be concentrated homogeneously.

The strength of the magnetic field is measured in Gauss (G) or Tesla (T) units (10,000 G = 1 T). Diagnostic MR systems usually employ magnets with operating field strengths ranging from 0.02 to 1.5 T. As reference points, the average magnetic field strength at the surface of the earth is approximately 0.5 G, or 0.00005 T (the field strength is different at the poles and the equator), and the field strength 1 cm from a wire carrying 1 amp of electrical current is 0.2 G, or 0.00002 T.

Superconducting Magnets

Fortunately some metals (e.g., Hg) and alloys (e.g., niobium/titanium, Nb/Ti; niobium/tin, Nb_3Sn; and vanadium/gallium, V_3Ga) lose their electrical resistance at very low temperatures and become superconductors. The electrical resistance of conductors is caused by the random motion of conducting electrons, which are "scattered" by core cations of the lattice. The scattering decreases as the temperature is lowered, leading to a decrease in electrical resistance (Figure 2-3). As shown in Figure 2-3, superconductors differ from normal conductors in the sharp loss of electrical resistivity at a critical temperature. This difference is due to the occupation by electrons of conducting bands in which the electrons are not scattered at all by core cations. There is no power loss in a superconductor, and once it has been energized the current continues in a loop as long as the superconducting wire is maintained below the critical transition temperature.

The superconductor most widely used in the construction of clinical magnets is Nb/Ti. This alloy becomes superconducting at 10° Kelvin (K) in the absence of an external magnetic field. Consequently, superconducting magnets are operated at temperatures provided by a bath of liquid helium (4° K). A schematic diagram of such a magnet is shown in Figure 2-4. After it has been cooled, the magnet is energized by connecting a section of superconducting wire across the end wires of the coil, heating this short section (switch) of the superconductor into the resistive state so that a voltage can be established and delivering current through an external power supply. After the current has stabilized to the desired value, the heater is removed, the switch is allowed to cool and

become superconducting, the power supply is turned off, and the current continues to circulate through the coil and the now superconducting (persistent) switch. The current and the field will be constant, subject only to a minor drift (0.001 G/hr) caused by minuscule resistance losses in imperfect wire joints (Figure 2-4, legend). However, because of heat leaks into the system, the cryogens steadily boil off and must be replenished on a regular basis. A compressor mounted to the magnet will reliquefy the cryogens, which often means that fills are required only after about 6 months.

Quenches. When the current in the magnet is lost through a resistive pathway in the conductor and the magnetic field is discharged by dissipation of the energy, a quench occurs. Such a pathway can be created by minor motions of the wire in the coil, resulting in sufficient frictional heating to drive the temperature of a small volume of the coil above the superconducting transition temperature. This effect is exacerbated by the very low heat capacities of materials at 4° K. Once the small volume is driven above the superconducting temperature, electrical resistance heating can rapidly drive larger and larger volumes of the coil above the transition temperature, resulting in a quick discharge of the coil energy. The heat created is rapidly transferred to the cryogens and causes a rapid discharge of helium gas (accompanied by a loud report). Quenches also can be caused by the heat released in flux jumping, which arises from currents induced in one part of the coil by magnetic fields generated in another part of the coil; the induced currents oppose the main current flow and cause resistive heating. Frictional and flux jump heating most often occur during the energization of a superconducting magnet, which sometimes will quench below the desired field as a result. This is particularly true of magnets in which the wires are not completely bonded by the epoxy; the magnetic forces on the conductor in an evolving field are very large. On reenergization (perhaps several times) the magnet is usually found to "train" to the desired field as a result of the windings having achieved a stable configuration. The copper matrix in which the Nb/Ti filaments are embedded (Figure 2-4, legend) makes the wire more workable and reduces flux jumping and the temperature rise in the superconducting filaments. Copper has a high thermal and electrical conductivity. Quenches, although dramatic, are uncommon because of the sophisticated engineering of modern magnets. Moreover, modern magnets are designed with protection to absorb the enormous energy dissipated during a quench so that the magnet itself is rarely damaged and may be recooled and energized.

All high-field MR systems are of the superconducting coil type. Low-field systems (less than 0.3 T) can be based on either resistive coils or permanent magnets. Magnets based on relatively low-weight–resistive coils can be built with a horizontal bore having B_0 parallel to the

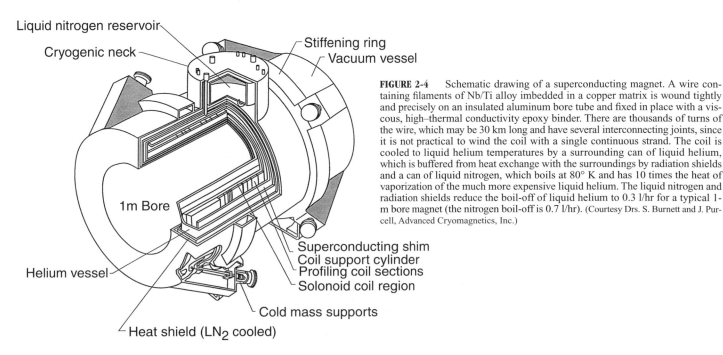

Liquid nitrogen reservoir
Cryogenic neck
Stiffening ring
Vacuum vessel
1m Bore
Helium vessel
Superconducting shim
Coil support cylinder
Profiling coil sections
Solonoid coil region
Cold mass supports
Heat shield (LN_2 cooled)

FIGURE 2-4 Schematic drawing of a superconducting magnet. A wire containing filaments of Nb/Ti alloy imbedded in a copper matrix is wound tightly and precisely on an insulated aluminum bore tube and fixed in place with a viscous, high–thermal conductivity epoxy binder. There are thousands of turns of the wire, which may be 30 km long and have several interconnecting joints, since it is not practical to wind the coil with a single continuous strand. The coil is cooled to liquid helium temperatures by a surrounding can of liquid helium, which is buffered from heat exchange with the surroundings by radiation shields and a can of liquid nitrogen, which boils at 80° K and has 10 times the heat of vaporization of the much more expensive liquid helium. The liquid nitrogen and radiation shields reduce the boil-off of liquid helium to 0.3 l/hr for a typical 1-m bore magnet (the nitrogen boil-off is 0.7 l/hr). (Courtesy Drs. S. Burnett and J. Purcell, Advanced Cryomagnetics, Inc.)

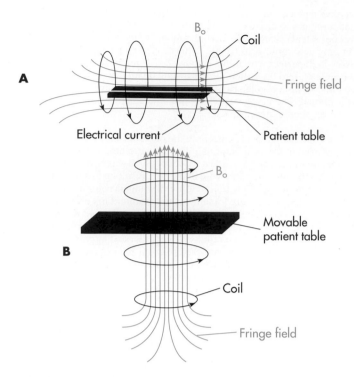

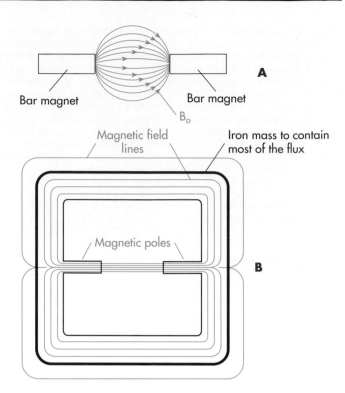

FIGURE 2-5   Two different configurations possible for a lightweight magnet based on four resistive coils. **A,** A tubular, horizontal bore in which the homogeneous portion of the field is parallel to the long axis of a prone patient. **B,** An "open" configuration in which the homogeneous portion of the field is perpendicular to the long axis.

FIGURE 2-6   Schematic diagrams of two idealized permanent magnets for MR systems. **A,** Two "bar" magnets with an air-return path for the magnetic flux lines. The divergence of the flux lines in air weakens the field and renders it inhomogeneous. **B,** A mass of iron "conducts" the flux lines and thereby increases the field strength and homogeneity between the poles between which the patient support table is inserted.

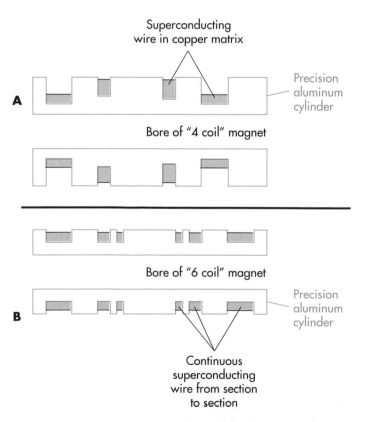

FIGURE 2-7   Schematics of solenoids containing coil segments of different radii, numbers of turns, or both. The segments are connected with a continuous wire. **A,** A so-called four-coil solenoid. **B,** A six-coil solenoid.

long axis of a prone patient or with a vertical bore perpendicular to the long axis of the patient. These two configurations are illustrated in Figure 2-5. Horizontal tubular bore magnets make patients feel isolated in a deep tunnel and limit access for monitoring and life-support systems. The open configuration (Figure 2-5, *B*) does not have these disadvantages and allows the use of efficient solenoidal RF coils to generate a B_1 perpendicular to B_0.

Resistive Magnets

A resistive magnet is an electromagnet in which the magnetic field is generated by the passage of electrical current through a wire, which is a good electrical conductor but nonetheless possesses a finite electrical resistance (Figure 2-3). One design for a 1-m, bore-resistive magnet having a 0.15 T field strength in the central bore requires 1500 turns of wire, through which 200 amps of electrical current is passed. Because all wires at normal temperature resist the passage of electrical current, high power (50,000 watts for the 0.15 T magnet described) is required to generate sufficient electrical current for the magnetic field desired. The supply of current must be steady, and a highly stable 50 kW power supply must be used because a highly homogeneous field is needed. The power to energize such a resistive magnet is dissipated as heat in the coil. This heat is removed by running cooled water through tubes passing over the ends of the coil. The power and cooling requirements are easily met for resistive magnets having a field strength of 0.15 T or less. However, the power rises as the square of the current, which in turn is proportional to the field strength. To generate a 1.5 T field in such a resistive magnet would require enormous power, presenting formidable cooling and power-supply problems.[24]

Permanent Magnets

The saturation field strength of ferromagnetic materials, the closed-loop nature of magnetic field lines, and the divergence of these lines in air relative to a conductor all limit the field strength of permanent magnets and substantially increase their mass relative to resistive coil magnets. The evolution of a permanent magnet with a homogeneity suitable for MRI is illustrated in Figure 2-6. The mass of iron required for flux confinement to generate a suitably homogeneous 0.2 T static magnetic field with a gap capable of accepting a human torso is nearly 23 tons, an enormous weight. Rare earth alloys produce a more intense magnetic field per unit weight than iron, and a permanent large-bore 9000-lb neodymium alloy magnet is capable of producing a static field of 0.2 T.[26] An advantage of these low-field permanent magnet systems is that they can be constructed in a variety of easy-patient-access configurations, and their openness circumvents the claustrophobic experiences common to solenoidal magnets.

Magnetic Field Homogeneity

The magnetic field at the interior of the ideal solenoid shown in Figure 2-1 is highly homogeneous. As Figure 2-1 suggests, a simple solenoid, even though tightly wound, would have to be extremely long compared with its diameter to generate such a homogeneous field because of the strong divergence of the field lines at the ends of the coil. To compensate for this divergence and generate a reasonably homogeneous field in a bore of acceptable length (2 m), the coil segments are wound with a smaller radius or with more turns at the end of the solenoid than in the middle. Cross sections through such multisegment solenoids are illustrated in Figure 2-7. To achieve the high homogeneity required for proton ^{1}H MRI, the magnetic field must be adjusted periodically at the site of diagnostic operations by a process called *shimming*. This process is necessary because of the difficulty of winding a "perfect" coil, slight variations of current densities within the wire, and the presence of metal in the environment, which concentrates flux lines compared with air.

Passive Shimming and Shielding. First-order corrections of field inhomogeneities caused by, for example, spot defects in wiring or metal structures in the environment of the magnet can be accomplished by placing small pieces of iron on the magnet (when it is deenergized) or symmetrically balancing (and removing) the field distortion of a fixed metal object in the environment with another of similar shape. This is called *passive shimming*. Indeed many modern superconducting magnets are designed to be shimmed in this way at installation. For a grossly metal-contaminated operating environment, an extreme form of passive shimming is used, whereby the magnet is surrounded symmetrically by large quantities of iron alloys (tens of thousands of kilograms), which concentrate the magnetic flux lines, thereby reducing the fringe fields by a factor of 5 to 10. This containment minimizes the effect of external metal on the homogeneity of the main field. The iron alloys can be fabricated into a modular open dome with an axis parallel to the B_0 field, into plates to enclose the magnet room, or into tubes surrounding the magnet.[4]

Active Shimming. The field homogeneity is further improved by passing current through appropriate gradient coils, which generate small magnetic field gradients superimposed on the main B_0 field. These gradients add to or subtract from the field at desired points along its axis or transverse to it, smoothing out field nonuniformities. These shim coils,[3,61] which are illustrated in Figure 2-8, fit within the main magnet coil on separate fiberglass cylindrical forms. They can be resistive windings located within the room-temperature bore of the magnet or superconducting windings located within the helium vessel. In either case the necessity to add shim coils to the system reduces the effective room-temperature bore size of the magnet.

Field homogeneity can be adjusted manually or by means of an interactive computer ("auto shim") program that analyzes an image produced by a uniform standard and calculates the correct current for each correction coil.[74] Modern imaging systems allow the field to be automatically shimmed on each patient at the beginning of each protocol. For MR spectroscopy, homogeneity requirements are especially stringent, and the field is shimmed on the localized region of anatomy to be examined by adjusting the current in the primary shim coils until the shape of the water-proton resonance in the tissue to be imaged is optimized (i.e., its line width is minimized).[71,76] Figure 2-9 shows the water-proton line shapes obtained from $10 \times 2 \times 2$–cm voxels in the brain of the same patient in a highly homogeneous and an inhomogeneous magnetic field at 1.5 T.

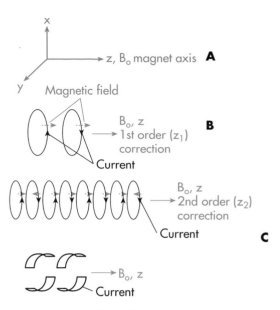

FIGURE 2-8   The shapes of shim coils for adjusting the homogeneity of the B_0 field in the axial and transverse directions. The coils are of varying orders of complexity and influence on the B_0 field. Higher-order coils are of more complex field shape and smaller influence on the static B_0 field. Only first- and second-order axial shims and a first-order transverse shim are shown. Ordinarily, shim coils to fourth order are employed. **A,** Coordinate system. **B,** Axial shims. **C,** Transverse shim.

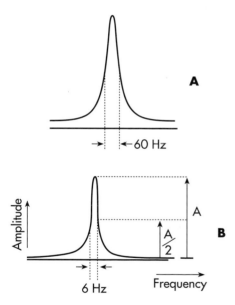

FIGURE 2-9   Line shapes of the water-proton resonance of the brain of a patient obtained at 1.5 T. **A,** Inhomogeneous magnetic field. The water-proton resonance is spread over a wide range of frequencies (v). The width of the line ?$v_{1/2}$ at half the maximum signal intensity (A/2) is 60 Hz. The frequency spread of the resonance is related to the time constant of the free-induction decay (FID) by Fourier transformation. A large spread in the frequencies is characterized by a small time constant for the FID, namely, $\pi \Delta v_{1/2} = 1/T2^*$ where T2* (5.3 ms = $1/\pi$ 60) is the time constant for the FID because of field inhomogeneities (T2$_{inh}$) and spin-spin relaxation (T2) ($1/T2^* = 1/T2_{inh} + 1/T2$). **B,** Magnetic field in **A** shimmed to homogeneity by minimizing the water proton line width and optimizing its shape. Width is 6 Hz, which corresponds to T2 of 53 ms, close to the intrinsic spin-spin relaxation time. T2$_{inh}$ is long, $1/T2_{inh}$ is small, and T2 $\approx$ T2*.

Field Homogeneity and Quality of Images and Spectra

The homogeneity of a magnet is often specified as the maximum deviation of the field in parts per million (ppm) over a spherical volume of a given diameter (dsv) and can be measured by plotting the field at a number of points through the volume of interest to find the maximum and minimum values. For the same field strength, a magnet with a homogeneity of 1 ppm over a 30-cm dsv is more homogeneous than one with a 10-ppm field deviation over a 30-cm dsv. In MRI the size and location of the imaging voxels are defined by field gradients specified in G/cm or Hz/cm, and the minimum homogeneity requirements are most unambiguously expressed in the same units (Hz/cm).

These minimum homogeneity requirements in Hz/cm are established by the size of the voxel and the strength of the gradients. For a gradient strength of 1 G/cm (10 mT/m) or 4257 Hz/cm ($\cong$ 1 G/cm $\times$ 42.57 MHz/T $\cong$ 1 G/cm $\times$ 4257 Hz/G) and 1 $\times$ 0.1–mm voxels, the field homogeneity over the voxel must be better than 425.7 Hz (4257 Hz/cm $\times$ 0.1 cm). Otherwise, voxels will be misregistered and the images will be blurred. At 1.5 T (63.86 MHz) this corresponds to a homogeneity of the magnetic field of 6.7 ppm, but at 0.35 T (14.90 MHz) this corresponds to a uniformity of only 28.6 ppm. Thus for a given gradient strength and voxel size, the minimum homogeneity requirements, expressed as a fraction of the field strength (ppm), become more stringent at higher field strengths. Of course in high-field imaging, higher gradient strengths, which can translate to more hertz per voxel, can compensate for large field inhomogeneities, but there is a practical upper limit to gradient strengths (1 to 2 G/cm) because of large power requirements and the necessity for short gradient rise and settling times. In this context it should be noted that high-field superconducting magnets can readily achieve homogeneities of 1 ppm or better.

Apart from the necessity of avoiding voxel misregistration, the desirability of high field homogeneities has assumed added importance in the gradient-echo imaging protocols.[33] For example, although the inhomogeneity of the field in Figure 2-9, *A* (60 Hz, or 1 ppm), might be acceptable for resolving anatomy in spin-echo imaging, it would lead to poor image quality in gradient-recalled echo imaging. This results from the fact that magnetization in the transverse plane dephased by field inhomogeneities is refocused in the spin-echo technique but is not refocused in gradient-echo imaging. In the example given in Figure 2-9 for the inhomogeneous field, the spin-echo image intensities would be weighted by the factor $e^{-TE/53}$ (or 0.83 for TE = 10 ms), but gradient-echo images would be weighted by the factor $e^{-TE/5.3}$ (or 0.15 for TE = 10 ms). Thus the signal-to-noise ratio (SNR), as well as contrast and resolution, would be much less in the latter. For this reason, gradient-recalled echo imaging techniques require a highly homogeneous static magnetic field.[72] Even with optimum shimming, however, there will be some unavoidable distortions in the image as a result of the different magnetic susceptibilities of structures within the body (e.g., water, lipids, bone, and cavities containing air). Local field inhomogeneities (10 ppm) arise from these differences and as discussed earlier have a greater impact on gradient-echo images than on spin-echo images. In proton spectroscopy a highly homogeneous magnetic field (0.1 ppm) is also required because the chemical-shift separation between adjacent proton resonances frequently is small (e.g., less than 10 to 20 Hz [at 1.5 T]). To distinguish one resonance from another requires that the line widths be less than the chemical-shift separation.

Summary of Conventional Magnet Characteristics

A summary of the major characteristics of the three types of magnets used in MR images is contained in Table 2-1. The question of the optimum field strength for MRI vis-à-vis cost, image contrast and resolution, and image chemical-shift and motion artifacts has been the subject of great controversy. Even though each case of magnet and system selection should be considered on its own merits in the context of long-range imaging objectives, recent developments have added fuel to this controversy. In general, increased field strength provides increased SNR. Although there is still debate about the exact functional dependence of SNR on the field strength in the clinical setting, there is consensus that it approximates a linear increase with B_0 for fields at least up to 1.5 T. This fact is of particular importance as more fast-scan protocols are being developed. Moreover, as faster scans are available, one of the major drawbacks to high-field imaging—movement artifact—is reduced because scan times are reduced.

Another issue that is becoming more important is clinical MR spectroscopy, which is showing increasing utility as a clinical tool and has recently been approved in the United States for routine clinical use. Proton spectroscopy can be accomplished as a short (10-min) add-on

Table 2-1	Magnet Characteristics	
MAGNET	**POSITIVES**	**NEGATIVES**
Permanent magnet	No electrical energy for operation Low capital cost Low operational cost High patient acceptance Low fringe field	Limited field strength Spectroscopy not possible Low SNR Field sensitive to temperature fluctuations
Resistive coil	Low capital cost Reliable No refrigerants Field can be readily and inexpensively turned on and off Variable geometry Easy seating and installation	Limited field strength High electrical power consumption Spectroscopy not possible Low SNR
Superconducting coil	High fields (0.35 to 4 T) readily attainable High field homogeneity, 0.1 ppm attainable High SNR Spectroscopy possible Fast scanning supported by high homogeneity and high SNR	High capital cost Large fringe fields Expensive refrigerants must be replaced regularly Elaborate seating and high site preparation costs Quenches possible Patient claustrophobia Field cannot be readily turned on and off

SNR, Signal-to-noise ratio; *T,* Tesla.

examination to a routine diagnostic imaging protocol.[23,30,54,62,71] For a variety of technical reasons, such as SNR and resolution, this type of add-on examination is optimally carried out at 1.5 T or higher. Most interventional MRI is performed in vertical V field permanent or resistive magnets (Figure 2-5, *B*).

Open-Configuration Superconducting Magnets

There is increasing interest in image-guided, interventional therapeutic procedures that employ MRI to locate surgical tools and determine the effects of interventions in real time (see Chapter 15). These procedures require extremely fast imaging sequences and open-configuration magnets. Split-coil, high-field, superconducting magnets that allow relatively free horizontal and vertical access to the patient (two 55-cm diameter-access coils, sharing interconnected cryostats and separated by a free access of 56 cm) can be used for interventional studies.[63] The coaxial split coils produce a 1.5 T field at each of their isocenters and a 0.5 T field at the center of the patient, a field that is sufficiently high to allow fast, nearly real-time imaging. As can be appreciated from Figure 2-1, *C,* a split-coil magnet (coil gap of 55 cm) cannot produce a magnetic field as homogeneous at the patient as a single-coil magnet can because of the diverging field lines at the coil extremities. Nonetheless, the recently described split-coil system[63] has an acceptable homogeneity over the patient volume: 12.3 ppm/30 cm dsv; 1.6 ppm/20 cm dsv; and less than 0.9 ppm/10 cm dsv. It is probable that the split-coil configuration can be used to produce magnetic fields as high as 0.9 T at the patient center, with the associated capability to produce interventional images at less than 1-sec intervals.

THE GRADIENT SYSTEM
Functions and General Characteristics

The gradient system consists of three sets of coils that can be switched on and off frequently to allow slice selection, phase encoding, and frequency encoding. In typical spin-echo imaging with high-field imaging systems, the slice-selection gradient is on for 3 ms, the phase-shift gradient for 4 ms, and the read gradient for 8 ms. These gradients must rise to full power quickly (<1 ms). In addition, the phase-selection and

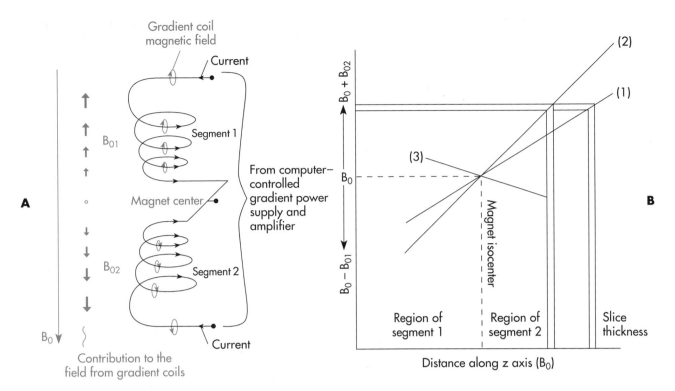

FIGURE 2-10   A general method for creating a gradient in the B_0 field along the z axis. **A,** A pulse of current from a computer-controlled power supply is passed through the gradient coils. For the direction of the current shown, the coil windings at the top of the diagram generate a field that is opposed to the main B_0 field and subtracts from it, whereas those at the bottom of the diagram generate a field that is parallel to B_0 and adds to it. The opposed fields in the two segments of the symmetrically wound coil ensure that the gradient-coil field at the magnet isocenter is zero. The field gradient so created is plotted in line (1) in **B.** If the current in the coils is doubled, the field gradient becomes steeper, as shown in line (2) in **B.** If the current in the coils is reversed, the direction of the field gradient is reversed, as shown in line (3) in **B. B,** Plots of the field gradients created by the system described in **A.** The magnet isocenter is the point at which none of the gradients makes a contribution to the static field and the magnetic field is just B_0. In the region of the field corresponding to segment 2 of **A,** the gradients make a positive contribution to the static field for lines (1) and (2) and the static field is $B_0 + B_{02}$, where B_{02} is a linear function of distance from the isocenter. For segment 1 of **A,** the gradients make a negative contribution to the static field for lines (1) and (2) and the static field is $B_0 - B_{01}$, where B_{01} is again a linear function of distance from the isocenter. Line (3) corresponds to a gradient that could be created if the current in the coils of **A** were switched relative to the current direction used to create the gradients corresponding to lines (1) and (2).

slice-selection gradients must be switched off and lose power quickly before the read gradient is turned on, and in some protocols the polarities of one or more gradients are rapidly switched. These operations put severe demands on the coils and gradient power supplies and amplifiers. The heating of the gradient coils is substantial during repetitive rapid gradient switching. Magnetic forces on the gradient coils during switching are also an important consideration.

Gradient Coils and Gradient Fields

For solenoidal magnets there are three gradient coils that fit coaxially within the room-temperature bore.[8,10,45] These coils create the gradients along the z, x, and y axes. The general method for this is illustrated in Figure 2-10 for the Z or B_0 gradient. As shown in Figure 2-11, the coils for creating gradients perpendicular to B_0 are more complicated than Z gradient coils. The steepness of the magnetic field gradient (change in magnetic field per unit distance, $\Delta B_0/\Delta Z = G/cm$) affects the slice thickness sampled and the minimum field of view (FOV) that can be employed. The slice thickness effects, which arise from the use of an RF pulse with a finite bandwidth, are illustrated in Figure 2-10, *B.* As shown in the figure, an RF pulse with a frequency width that corresponds to a specific range of values of the static field strength ($B_0 + B_{02}$) will correspond to a thicker slice if a weak gradient (line 1) is employed compared with a strong gradient (line 2). (Note that because we selected the same RF center frequency, we necessarily are comparing slices from different locations, but because the gradients are linear, the argument holds for slices from the same location along the z axis.) FOV effects are considered later in this chapter.

Other parameters that characterize the quality of the gradient subsystem are the gradient linearities and their rise and fall times. The linearity of the gradients refers to the maintenance of a constant slope of the plot of B versus distance over the FOV; that is, a straight line is obtained, as shown in Figure 2-10, *B.* If the gradient falls off nonlinearly on either side of the magnet isocenter, then the intensity in the image will not code linearly with the distance in the phase-encoding and frequency-encoding directions, and the image will be distorted. One such distortion, for example, is compression of the anatomy near the edge of the FOV. Particularly with large FOVs, perfect linearity of the gradients is impossible. However, with the most widely used method of image reconstruction, two-dimensional Fourier transformation (2D FT), the slightly nonlinear gradients encountered in most systems usually have no adverse effects on resolution in the images. In extreme cases these distortions can be corrected using experimentally measured nonlinearities or theoretical values calculated from the geometry of gradient coils.[31,52,73] Specialized gradient coils are under development for a variety of unique clinical applications.[13,21,40,43,51]

Eddy Currents

Eddy currents are a manifestation of Faraday's law of induction, which among other things states that any time-varying magnetic field will induce a current in a conductor that opposes the effect of the time-varying field. In this case the time-varying field is caused by switching the gradients on and off. This field induces an opposite time-varying electric current in the surrounding metal structure of the magnet and cryostat. The induced fields can be quite complex and specific to the mag-

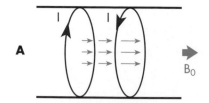

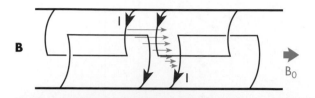

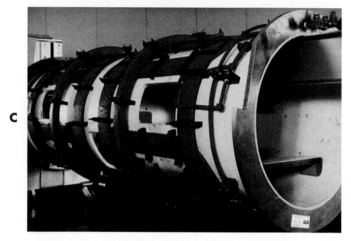

FIGURE 2-11 Typical gradient-coil configurations used to produce gradients parallel **(A)** and perpendicular **(B)** to the static field B_0. The configurations shown are a Maxwell pair **(A)** and Golay coils **(B)**. The arrows represent the fields produced by the gradient coils that are superimposed on the larger B_0 static field. The differences in field strength (i.e., the gradient), as indicated by the differences in the length of the arrows, are considerably exaggerated over those found in real systems (i.e., B_0 is typically 10,000 G, and the field gradient is approximately 1 G/cm). Gradient coils for a superconducting magnet **(C)**. These fit within a 1-m cryostat bore, reducing the diameter available for RF coils and patients.

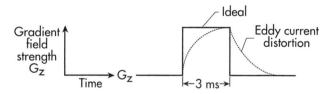

FIGURE 2-12 Time profile of an ideal rectangular gradient pulse and one distorted by eddy currents (and magnetic fields) induced in surrounding conductors.

net system and imaging protocol. Typically they have time constants ranging from a few milliseconds to several hundred milliseconds. Eddy currents with long time-constant components severely degrade the homogeneity of the field, whereas those with short time-constant components act more to distort the gradient time profile (Figure 2-12). Unless they are compensated, these effects can degrade image quality severely and preclude spectroscopic studies.

One method for compensating for eddy currents, called *preemphasis,* involves overdriving the gradient coil by as much as 30% for a short time just as the pulse is turned on to square up its leading edge (Figure 2-12) and then reversing the polarity of the pulse for a short time at its trailing edge. This method is implemented by reshaping the waveform that drives the coils by applying that waveform to a set of parallel high-

pass filters of varying time constants and gains before amplification. The parameters of the filter are then adjusted to obtain the appropriate gradient profile. This method of compensation is not completely effective because of the complex paths traversed by the eddy currents, which have diverse time constants.

A more satisfactory method for dealing with eddy currents is to eliminate them by using gradient coils that are shielded in such a way that the gradient fields are restricted to the interior of the magnet bore.[42,60,69] One method for accomplishing this is to construct a wire mesh screen around the gradient coil and pass the appropriate amount of current through it in a direction such that the magnetic field associated with the current in the wire mesh cancels that generated by the gradient coils. The price paid for the reduction in the eddy current fields by two orders of magnitude is an attenuation of the gradient field within the coil by approximately 40% compared with its unscreened value. These actively shielded gradients are widely used, especially since the demonstration of the clinical utility of rapid-scan imaging based on gradient echos and the increasing acceptance of gradient-localized proton spectroscopy in research protocols.

Special Requirements for Fast Imaging and Spectroscopy

For a variety of reasons there is a great demand for faster and faster imaging protocols. These reasons include the need for higher patient throughput in a time of financial constraint and the need for reducing motion artifacts in unstable patients. Moreover, the development of functional MRI (see Chapter 72) has argued for more rapid imaging capabilities. For a number of years, spin-echo imaging has been the mainstay of clinical diagnostic imaging. More recently, gradient-echo imaging and so-called fast imaging, where κ space is traversed more efficiently than in conventional spin-echo imaging (see Chapter 1), have led to more rapid image acquisition protocols[6,36,50] and allowed the reduction of the single-slice scan time to approximately 1 sec. Nonetheless, these sequences use standard gradient coils and do not place undue demands on the data processing and archiving hardware. For example, a conventional imaging system would be equipped with gradient coils capable of a maximum amplitude of 10 mT/m, a minimum rise time of 0.6 ms (slew rate of 0.01/0.0006 or ~17 T/m/s), and a duty cycle of 8% (percentage of time the gradients are on during a hypothetical repetition time) for conventional spin-echo imaging, whereas a fast imaging system would be equipped with gradient coils capable of a maximum amplitude of 15 mT/m, a minimum rise time of 0.3 ms (slew rate of 50 T/m/s), and a duty cycle of 25% for fast spin-echo imaging.

However, in echo-planar imaging (EPI) (discussed at length in Chapter 6)[18,41,66,67] and echo-planar spectroscopic imaging[56] the requirements for gradient strengths, rise times, and duty cycles are markedly increased because all of κ space can be traversed in a single excitation by using a rapidly oscillating readout gradient to create a train of phase-encoded gradient echoes. In single-shot, or "snapshot," EPI with a resolution of 128 $\times$ 128, there are 128 oscillations of the readout gradient to create the gradient-echo train in a period as short as 50 to 100 ms, which minimizes the effects of spin-spin relaxation. This method requires each phase-encoding "projection" to be acquired in less than 0.8 ms. This is accomplished using gradient coils capable of a maximum amplitude of 20 mT/m, a minimum rise time of 0.1 ms (slew rate of 200 T/m/s), and a duty cycle of 50% to 60%. This remarkable technical achievement was enabled by the marriage of resonant (rapidly switching) gradient technology to power supplies that are capable of catching a resonant mode at maximum amplitude and holding it there for a short period of time. In the particular case of rapid head imaging the required large gradient amplitudes and rapid gradient rise times can be accomplished with small local head coils[21,67] powered by conventional gradient amplifiers because the power required to drive the coil varies as the fifth power of its radius. EPI places stringent requirements on the RF system as well, and these are discussed in the next section.

THE RADIOFREQUENCY SYSTEM
Functions and Characteristics

The primary functions of the RF system are to generate and collect the MR signals. The processes that are involved are summarized in Figures 2-13 and 2-14. The MR signal is generated by the magnetization M un-

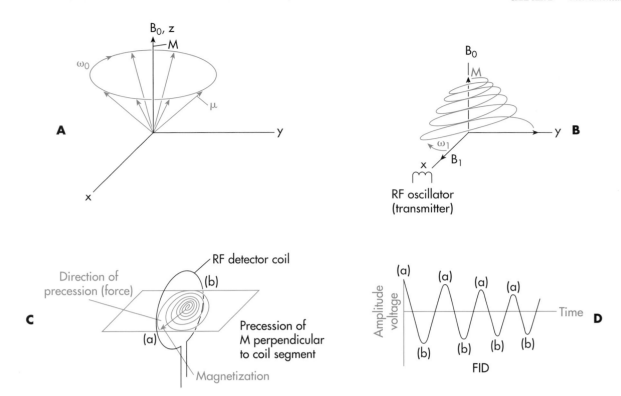

FIGURE 2-13   Generation and collection of the proton MR signal. **A,** When a tissue sample is placed in a strong static magnetic field B_0, some of the proton magnetic dipoles μ are forced to become aligned with it. This is analogous to aligning the magnetic dipole needle of a compass with the earth's field. Unlike the compass needle, the nuclear dipoles also precess about the B_0 field in random phase at a frequency ω_0, called the *Larmor frequency*. The precession or rotation arises from the quantum properties of small particles like the proton. Because of the forced alignment of the proton magnetic dipoles, the tissue acquires a slight magnetization M, which consists of the sum of the static (z) components of the individual magnetic moments μ. This magnetization is often referred to as *longitudinal magnetization*. **B,** If an oscillating or rotating magnetic field B1 is turned on a right angle to B_0 for a short time and it is rotating at the Larmor frequency ($\omega_1 = \omega_0$), then it maintains a constant phase with each of the precessing dipoles and exerts a torque on them that tilts them away from alignment with B_0 toward the xy (transverse) plane. The net tissue magnetization follows a complex spiral course during the time the B_1 field has been turned on for a period of time sufficient to rotate the net sample magnetization by 90 degrees (or $\pi/2$ radians). When the RF oscillator has been turned off, M continues to precess about B_0. **C,** During free precession of M in the transverse plane, it induces an alternating current in a sensitive RF receiver coil (the electrons in the coil are pushed in one direction when M passes [a] and in the opposite direction when M passes [b]). The resulting MR signal is depicted in **D. D,** The MR signal is the time-dependent AC voltage induced in the RF coil by the free precession of M. Magnetization starts along (a) (maximum + voltage), rotates to (b) (maximum − voltage), completes the cycle at (a), and then repeats the pattern.

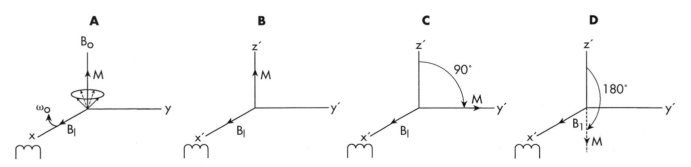

FIGURE 2-14   The rotating frame of reference simplifies the description of the response of M to B_1. **A,** Initial view of a stationary observer looking down the coordinate system; B_1 and μs are rotating about B_0 at the Larmor frequency. **B,** Initial view of an observer rotating with the B_1 field. Nothing is rotating, everything is stationary in a relative sense, and the B_0 field has disappeared! Now B_1 is the only field acting on M, and it will begin to precess about B_1 at a frequency $v_1 = \gamma B_1$, where $\gamma = 42.57$ MHz/T. The rotation or precession of M about B_1 is slower than the precession of μ about B_0 because B_1 is much less than B_0. A typical B_1 would be 0.004 mT (1 mT = 0.001 T). **C,** Initial view of an observer rotating with the B_1 field (0.004 mT) 1.47 ms after turning the B_1 field on. M will have rotated about B_1 by one-fourth cycle, or 90 degrees, in the 1.47 ms that B_1 was turned on (one-fourth cycle = $42.57 \times 10^{+6}$ cycles/sec T $\times$ 0.004 T $\times 10^{-3} \times 1.47 \times 10^{-3}$ sec). This is a so-called 90-degree or $\pi/2$ pulse. (There are 2π radians in 360 degrees, or one cycle.) **D,** Initial view of an observer rotating with the B_1 field (0.004 mT) 2.94 ms after turning the B_1 field on a 180-degree pulse.

dergoing free precession in the transverse plane after it has been rotated out of alignment from B_0 by a pulsed B_1 field of the correct frequency and amplitude. This precessing magnetization induces a voltage (MR signal) in a coil made of a suitable conductor. The RF system is an integrated, computer-controlled, transceiver unit, and its design, construction, and operation are driven by the weakness of the MR signal. Whereas the transmitter output is hundreds of volts, the voltage input to the receiver from the magnetization in an individual voxel is approximately one tenth of a microvolt (0.1 μV). Related considerations for the RF system are the relative orientations of the static B_0 field, the transmitter B_1 field, and the precessing magnetization M (Figures 2-13 and 2-14). These latter considerations limit the geometry of the transmitter and receiver coils: The B_1 transmitting coil must generate a rotating magnetic field that is perpendicular to B_0, and the receiver must be oriented such that it is perpendicular to the precessing M.

Noise, Signal-to-Noise Ratio, Magnetic Field Strength, and Radiofrequency Coils

Many sources of noise that affect MR system performance can be minimized by proper system design and construction. However, there is a noise floor provided by the inherent noise of the receiver coil and the patient that cannot be designed away. The inherent noise in the receiver is a random voltage arising from the thermal motion of the electrons in the conductor. This motion is related to the inherent resistance of the coil, which increases with its size (the length of the conductor). The origin of the noise in the patient is the high electrolyte content of cells and body fluids. For example, blood serum contains approximately 200 mmol of salt per liter. This high concentration of ions results in a relatively high conductivity for tissues, and as a consequence eddy currents are induced in the tissue by the application of an RF pulse.

These eddy currents dissipate power and contribute to the resistance of the coil through the resulting "back" electromotive force (EMF) in-

duced in the tissue. At low precessional frequencies (low B_0) the coil and the tissue resistance are comparable, but at high precessional frequencies (high B_0) the tissue resistance is higher than the coil resistance. This resistance is a result of the linear increase of the induced EMF with frequency, whereas the coil noise increases only slightly with increasing frequency. As a consequence, even though the signal strength increases with the square of the frequency, the SNR increases only linearly with precessional frequency.

These considerations provide the logic for the use of local coils as receivers. A coil that receives signal from the entire volume that is excited also receives noise from that volume and distributes it over each pixel in the image. Because the surface coil or each component coil in a phased array receives only noise from a small region of interest (ROI), the signal received is not degraded by noise in the large volume excited by, for example, a body coil. The body coil or another volume coil is used as a transmitter in the first place because the uniformity of its B_1 field ensures uniformity of excitation.

Coil Geometry

For a solenoidal magnet the transmit and receive coils are commonly saddle shaped (Figure 2-15, *A*) and have the volume of greatest B_1 field homogeneity along the linear portion of the coil, the ends being highly inhomogeneous.[29,45] An alternate design, called a *birdcage coil*[25] (Figure 2-15, *B*), has improved B_1 homogeneity and higher sensitivity and has found increasing use.[20,34] A number of other coil designs are available, notably the slotted resonator.[38] For a permanent magnet or a resistive one with the B_0 field perpendicular to the long axis of the patient (Figure 2-5, *B*), a solenoidal coil (Figure 2-15, *C*) is used because of its excellent B_1 homogeneity.

The coil shown in Figure 2-15, *A*, has a radius large enough to accept a human torso and is called a *body coil*. Because the noise detected by an RF coil increases with coil size and the signal decreases as the

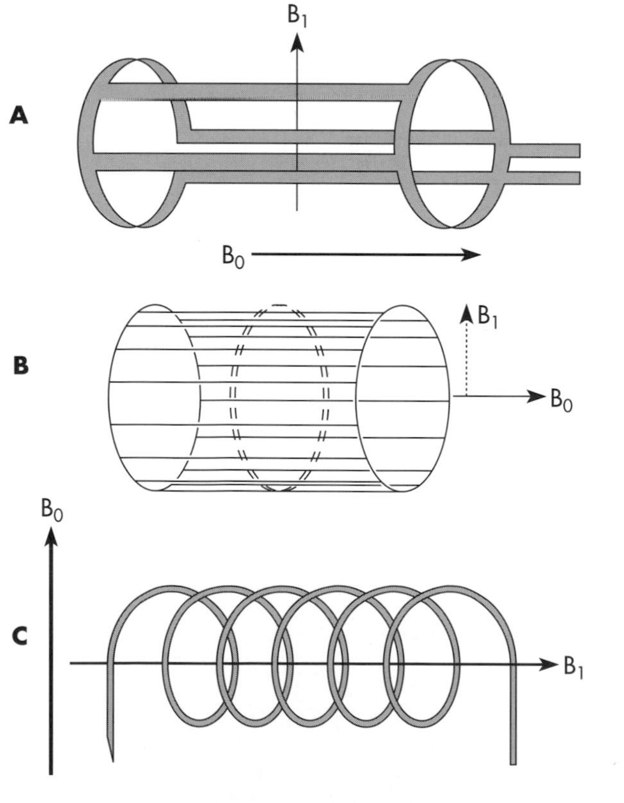

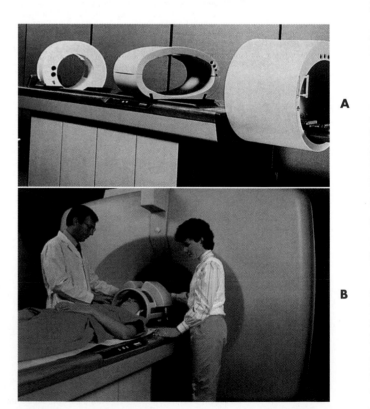

FIGURE 2-15 Volume coils for use in a solenoidal magnet. **A,** A saddle-shaped coil that would fit snugly all along the inside bore of a solenoid that already contains tightly fitting gradient and shim coils. **B,** A "birdcage" based on a closed-loop transmission line design. **C,** Typical design for a solenoid coil in which the relative directions of the magnetic component of the RF field (B_1) transmitted by the coil and static field (B_0) are shown. When used in permanent-magnet installations, the long axis of the subject is oriented along B_1.

FIGURE 2-16 Small-volume coils. **A,** Saddle-shaped RF coils (within plastic enclosure) for the head, a small body, and a large body. **B,** Positioning for a head examination in a saddle-shaped coil.

distance of the coil from the anatomy increases, numerous specialty smaller diameter (local) coils have been developed for studying the head and the extremities. These coils fit snugly over the body part imaged (Figure 2-16) and have high B_1 homogeneities for RF transmission and signal reception. An alternate form of a local coil is the surface coil[1] (Figure 2-17), which has a large B_1 inhomogeneity and is usually used only as a receiver (Figure 2-17, *B*). Nonetheless, they are used for a variety of special purposes in both imaging and spectroscopy and find general use as receivers for imaging, especially in the spine, where they are more closely coupled to the anatomy than a body coil and thus markedly improve the SNR and decrease motion artifacts.

Arrays of surface coils can be used to extend the effective FOV of the receiver coil while maintaining the improved SNR characteristics of the limited FOV of a single coil in the array.[32, 59,75] This development is extremely important because the exact region of interest in diagnostic imaging usually is not known beforehand. To ensure proper coverage of the ROI with a single surface coil requires either that the coil be large (thus reducing the SNR advantage) or that a smaller coil be repositioned after the ROI has been defined in a localizer image, a process that can be time consuming and uncomfortable for the patient. The array can be constructed such that the coils can be activated remotely as single receivers and cover a limited FOV in one or more specific ROIs. Alternatively, as in the so-called phased-array set of noninteracting coils, which have separate receiver channels,[60] MR signals can be collected from all coils in the array simultaneously, and the data can be combined from all channels to construct an image of the complete FOV, with SNR equivalent to that for a single coil in the array. In the latter arrangement the time saved in covering the complete FOV with a high SNR is purchased at the relatively high cost of the additional separate receiver channels.[55] As discussed in the following sections, fast-imaging protocols require operation of the receiver at larger bandwidths than in conventional imaging, with a consequent reduction in the SNR. One of the few ways this SNR can be recovered is with the use of phased-array coils, and a wide variety has become available.[2,15,48,70]

Coil Quality

The circuit diagram for a typical single-tuned RF coil is shown in Figure 2-18. For a well-tuned resonant circuit (coil) the inductance (L) of the coil is a measure of the stored magnetic energy and the capacitance

(C) of the stored electrical energy. When this stored energy is transferred to the sample as a $\mu/2$ pulse, some of it is dissipated through the resistance (r) of the coil. A good RF coil stores or receives a large amount of magnetic energy compared with resistance losses in the coil. Coils are characterized by a quality factor (Q), defined as:

(EQ. 1)

$$Q = \frac{\text{Maximum energy stored}}{\text{Average energy dissipated per radian}}$$

In general, coils with higher Qs deliver energy to the tissue magnetization more efficiently as a transmitter and result in higher signal strengths when the coil is used as a receiver. One expression for Q in terms of the coil parameters is the following:

(EQ. 2)

$$Q = \frac{1}{r\omega C}$$

where ω is the frequency in radians per second and is equal to $\frac{1}{\sqrt{LC}}$ (Figure 2-18, legend). This equation sets important design and operational limits, some obvious and others not so obvious, on the coils because the parameters ω, C, L, and r are interdependent.

Consistent with the discussion in the previous section, a high-Q coil must have a low r. Similarly the Q factor of a coil that is "loaded" with a patient is lower than that of an unloaded coil because the patient increases the resistance of the coil. Indeed, at high precessional frequencies ($B_0 \geq 0.5$ T) the Q factor of a loaded, high-quality coil is dominated by the resistance of the patient, who can have a discernible effect on the image SNR if there are especially high electrolyte contents in the imaging volume.

It is not so obvious in Equation 2 that a large, high-Q coil is more difficult to construct for operation at higher precessional frequencies. A high-frequency coil requires a low value of L and the stray C. The inductance of a wire-wound coil increases with the square of the number of turns constituting the coil. Although the L of a wire-wound coil can be reduced to the appropriate value at high ω by simply reducing the number of turns in the coil, this would result in a reduction of the homogeneity of the B_1 field to an unacceptably low value. Thus at high frequencies (>10 to 15 MHz), wide-sheet conductors, which have a lower surface-current density and inductance, are used to construct resonators.

Transmitters and Receivers

The RF coils described can be used to transmit only, receive only, or act as transceivers by first transmitting the B_1 field and, after a suitable delay, receiving the free-induction decay (FID) from the magnetization excited by B_1. Where appropriate the coil should be designed and constructed as a transceiver because in general, if a coil is optimized for the homogeneous transmission of B_1 to the tissue, then it is optimized for

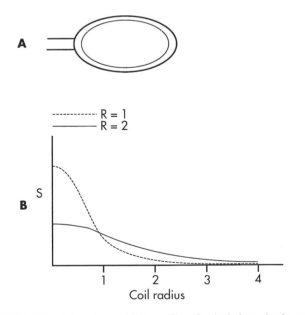

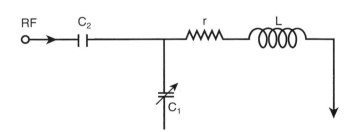

FIGURE 2-17   Schematic sensitivity profiles of a single-loop circular surface coil. **A,** Geometry of the surface coil. **B,** The sensitivity of the surface coil for both tissue MR signal and noise falls with distance from the coil, but a whole-volume coil has a uniform region of sensitivity. Axial signal intensity *(S)* versus tissue depth measured in coil radii. Sensitivity profile along line orthogonal to center of a receive-only single-loop circular surface coil shows calculated effects of doubling the coil radius (R = 2). For deep structures the larger coil yields slightly better SNR, although the measured difference in SNR between the two coils is smaller than this calculation would indicate.

FIGURE 2-18   An RF coil is equivalent to an electrical circuit having an inductance *(L)*, a capacitance *(C)*, a resistance *(r)*, and a voltage oscillating at the frequency ω. The peak current in the circuit (and in the coil magnetic field) will occur when $\omega = \frac{1}{\sqrt{LC}}$ (if R << L, a condition easily met). This is accomplished by adjusting C to achieve the resonance condition for the circuit (and the coil). Note that for MRI, ω of the coil is the precessional frequency of the nuclear spin moments. C_1 denotes an external capacitor that can tune the circuit to resonance.

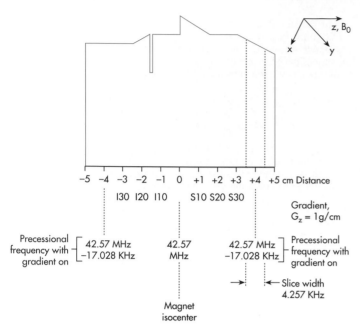

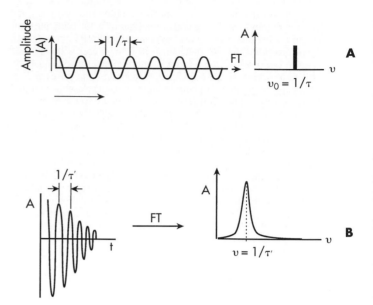

FIGURE 2-19 Selection of the imaging slice. The center of the field of view is delivered to the magnet isocenter, the point at which the gradient contribution to the net static field strength is zero even when the gradients are turned on. For a 1 T B_0 the proton precessional frequency is 42.57 MHz at the magnet isocenter. When a gradient is turned on, protons in imaging planes above the magnet isocenter acquire a higher precessional frequency, whereas those below the magnet's isocenter acquire a lower precessional frequency. For a Gz gradient of 1 G/cm (4257 Hz/cm, or 4.257 kHz/cm), protons in an imaging slice 4 cm (40 mm) above the isocenter (slice S40) will acquire a precessional frequency of 42.57 MHz plus the gradient contribution of 4 cm × 4.257 kHz/cm and can be excited to precession by an RF oscillator of frequency 42.57 MHz + 17.028 kHz, with a frequency width of 4.257 kHz corresponding to the 1-cm thickness of the desired slice. Similarly, protons in an imaging slice 4 cm below the magnet isocenter (I40) will acquire a lower precessional frequency (42.57 MHz to 17.028 kHz), and the protons in this slice can be excited to precession by an RF B_1 tuned to the appropriately lower frequency.

FIGURE 2-20 RF envelopes in the time and frequency domains are related by a mathematical operation called a *Fourier transformation* (FT). **A,** At the left is the cosine wave that the amplitude *(A)* of the B_1 magnetization traces out as a function of time if a single frequency transmitter is turned on. The frequency of the wave v (in cycles per second, Hz) is $1/\tau$ where τ (in seconds) is the time required to complete one cycle of the wave. The frequency of the wave in radians per second is $\omega = 2\pi v$. In the frequency domain the amplitude of the wave is characterized by a single sharp peak at the well-defined frequency v_0. The time and frequency domains are equivalent and are interconvertible by the mathematical operation, FT. **B,** The time response (A versus t) of the real part of the MR signal when the B_1 field of the appropriate frequency is applied then removed. This is the FID produced by the freely precessing spins, which have been flipped into the transverse plane by B_1. The response of the spins is measured with respect to a reference frequency in the rotating frame (Figure 2-14), and in the FT a single line of frequency v' is obtained where the frequency is the difference between the sample frequency and that of the reference. The FID is a damped oscillation and the line has a finite frequency width because the signal in the time domain can be sampled only for a short time.

collecting the signal homogeneously. In the operation of a transceiver, a pulse of high-voltage AC power is applied across the ends of the coil, during which time the receiver circuitry is protected by a large resistance (crossed diodes). After the pulse generator has been turned off, the coil requires time to deenergize and return to equilibrium. After this time has elapsed, the "resistor" is bypassed and the coil is now able to accept the signal from M, which is precessing in the transverse plane.

Generally, head imaging is accomplished with a transceiver head coil, and body imaging is often done with the body coil operating as a transceiver. However, as discussed earlier, the SNR can be improved for spine imaging by using a surface coil receiver for imaging the spine. In that case the body coil, which has a very homogeneous B_1 field distribution, serves as the transmitter, with the inhomogeneous B_1 reception characteristics of the surface-coil receiver causing only minor distortions and shadings of the image in the limited FOV. If a local coil is used as a receiver, it must be decoupled from the high-pulsed power from the transmitter to prevent damage to the receiver, to avoid saturating the receiver electronics so that it cannot accept signal in a timely fashion, and to prevent distortion of the transmitted B_1 field. A variety of flexible surface-coil receivers that conform to body contours, such as the shoulder, neck, and jaw, has been used.* Indeed, two noninteracting local coils can be used to receive signal from separate regions without loss of image quality.[32] The special coils discussed in the clinical chapters illustrate the full range of coil types available.

In selecting a local receiver coil to image a structure, the maximum region of B_1 homogeneity and sensitivity should be matched to the structure as closely as possible. For a round loop the most sensitive and

homogeneous B_1 region is in a slice parallel to the loop, extending nearly one diameter from the loop face (Figure 2-17, *B*). Close inspection of the shape of the sensitivity profiles in Figure 2-17, *B,* suggests that larger is not always better. For example, a 5-cm loop is better than a 10-cm loop for imaging the temporomandibular joint, a small structure 2 to 3 cm below the surface. On the other hand, to image the entire knee, the clinician may choose a volume coil that surrounds the entire knee. However, to image only a single meniscus, a small loop placed over the side of interest may be a better choice.

Transmitter Frequency Bandwidth

The frequency bandwidth is an important operational parameter of both the transmitter and receiver sections of the RF system. The transmitter bandwidth required is defined by the field gradient for slice selection, as illustrated in Figure 2-19. The transmitter excites the imaging slice by delivering a B_1 pulse of the proper center frequency, defined by the combination of the B_0 field and the gradient contribution to the field at the slice desired. Because the field gradient is finite, there is a finite range of frequencies across the selected slice. In the example of Figure 2-19 this frequency bandwidth is 4257 Hz (4.257 kHz), corresponding to the gradient of 1 G/cm (4257 Hz/cm) and the 1-cm slice thickness. For a gradient strength of 0.5 G/cm, a 1-cm slice would have a frequency bandwidth of 2148.5 Hz and a 0.5-cm slice would have a frequency bandwidth of 1574.2 Hz for the same gradient strength.

To excite magnetization uniformly across the slice, the transmitter must deliver a pulse having the proper center frequency and the appropriate bandwidth and shape. This delivery is accomplished by a process known as *pulse shaping,* the first step of which is switching the transmitter on and off rather than operating it continuously. An understand-

*References 7, 11, 12, 17, 37, 46, 58.

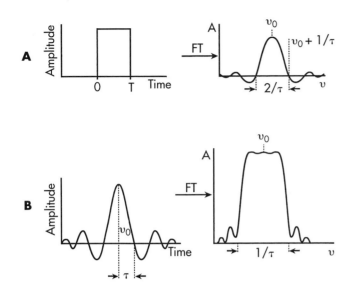

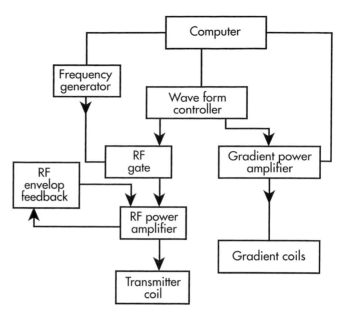

FIGURE 2-21 Shaping RF-transmitter pulses to cover a specific frequency range. **A,** If an RF transmitter at the single frequency v_0 is turned on at time t = 0 and then turned off after a few milliseconds time t = τ, then FT analysis of the amplitude as a function of frequency reveals that the output is not a single frequency v_0 but the spread of frequencies shown. The amplitude of the B_1 field as a function of time is shown as it would appear in the rotating frame (Figure 2-14), that is, as a constant. If the rotating-frame description were not used, as in the left of Figure 2-20, *A,* the operation would correspond to transmitting only a limited number of cycles of the oscillating RF wave. **B,** If the time-dependent amplitude waveform shown (A versus t) is imposed on the RF of frequency v_0 shown in **A,** then the FT analysis of B_1 in the frequency domain is an output such that the magnetization flipped into the transverse plane has the shape shown: It rises and falls relatively sharply with v and is centered about the frequency v_0 with a bandwidth of $1/\tau$ Hz.

FIGURE 2-22 Simplified flow chart of the transmitter section of an MR system. The reference frequency at very low power is provided by an extremely precise and stable frequency synthesizer or a fixed-frequency RF oscillator. The frequency generator generates the central RF frequency and provides for small shifts in this central frequency to move from selected slice to new selected slice. The digital pulse shape is provided from the computer to the waveform controller, which passes this waveform through precisely timed RF gates to the RF power amplifier. Driven by the waveform generator, the amplifier generates the appropriately shaped frequency-selective RF pulse of prescribed flip angle to the transmitter coil. It is critical that the energy from the power amplifier be transmitted efficiently into the RF coil. This requires that the antenna (the two circuits) be appropriately matched.

ing of pulse shaping is facilitated by considering the equivalence of the time and frequency domain representations of RF waves. Time and frequency domain descriptions of the amplitude of the B_1 transmitter field are illustrated in Figure 2-20, *A.* If the output of the transmitter is to be received as a wave with a single well-defined frequency, then the output must be measured (sampled) over many cycles of the RF wave in the time domain: It must be turned on for a long time. If the transmitter is merely switched on and off with constant amplitude, the frequency domain response will be as is shown in Figure 2-21, *A,* that is, a curved major excitation profile flanked by smaller oscillations of inverse phase. This "sinc" profile does not excite the spins within the slice uniformly, and the out-of-phase components from outside the slice actually cancel the slice signal. (Mathematically, sinc x = (sin x)/x.) However, the effects of this Fourier transformation are commutative; that is, the frequency domain response to a sinc excitation pulse is a square profile, as shown in Figure 2-21, *B.* In practice a perfectly square profile requires an infinitely long sinc pulse, which is impractical for an imaging sequence. Fortunately, more sophisticated pulse shapes have been developed and are commonly used to achieve optimum slice excitation characteristics. Once the pulse shape has been optimized, only the appropriate frequency and duration need to be determined.

Complete Transmitter System

A simplified flow chart for one type of transmitter is sketched in Figure 2-22. The transmitter must (1) generate a temporally stable basic frequency for the RF, (2) develop the appropriate waveform to drive the amplifier so that it delivers an RF pulse of the desired shape and flip angle to the coil, and (3) time the delivery of the pulses through an on/off

RF gate. These requirements are readily fulfilled by a variety of analog and digital methods.*

A critical factor in the quality of an MR system is the linearity of the transmitter. That is, the output of the power amplifier should be directly proportional to the input power. The importance of linearity is a result of the variety of pulse sequences that are combinations of pulses with different flip angles, such as the 90-degree—τ—180-degree spin-echo sequence. In a linear system a 180-degree pulse requires doubling the amplitude (quadrupling the power) of a 90-degree pulse. Because many amplifiers are nonlinear over this power range, a 180-degree pulse might require 5 times rather than 4 times the power for a 90-degree pulse. Consequently the amplifier "settings" for the spin-echo sequence need to be determined empirically by calibrating the individual 90- and 180-degree pulses. Similarly the linearity of the transmitter amplifier is important in gradient-recalled echo imaging, where the complete imaging protocol might require the use of a wide range of flip angles. In gradient-echo imaging the contrast can be a highly sensitive function of the flip angle for a particular TR/TE combination.

Fortunately, power amplifiers can be empirically adjusted to linearity through a process known as *envelope feedback* of the shape of the RF from the amplifier. The incoming RF is monitored and compared with a sample of the RF output envelope, and the incoming RF is adjusted to compensate for any differences between the two waveforms.

Quadrature Excitation. Figure 2-23, *A,* illustrates the linearly oscillating B_1 field generated by passing a pulse of alternating current through an RF coil having one resonant mode. As shown in Figure 2-23,

---

*References 28, 39, 44, 45, 64, 65, 68.

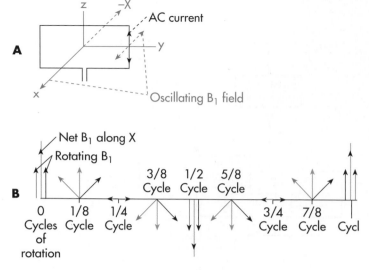

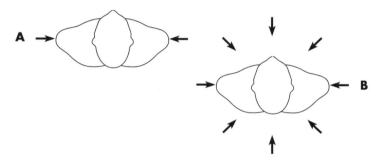

FIGURE 2-23 The oscillating B_1 field. **A,** An alternating current passed through a coil generates an oscillating B_1 magnetic field. The current flows in the xy plane, and the perpendicular B_1 field is generated along the x axis. **B,** A linear oscillating B_1 is caused by two B_1 fields rotating in opposite directions.

FIGURE 2-24 Diagrammatic representations of linearly **(A)** and circularly **(B)** polarized RF waves. The arrows represent the magnetic components (B_1) of the radio waves.

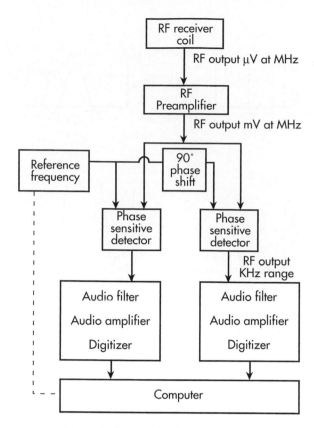

FIGURE 2-25 Schematic diagram of an RF receiver system. The low level (μV) output of the receiver is amplified in a broad-band, very low-noise preamplifier (extra noise at this stage is disastrous). The amplified RF signal is then mixed with the reference frequency v_T provided by a computer clock or frequency synthesizer generating the signals $v_T - v_i$, which are the different audio signals detected by a quadrature detector. The audio signals are passed by an audio filter into a high-power audio amplifier and then digitized and stored in the computer.

B, this linearly oscillating field is equivalent to two B_1 fields rotating at the same frequency but in opposite directions. The B_1 field rotating at the Larmor frequency in the same direction as the precessing magnetic moments tilts the magnetization away from alignment with B_0 into the transverse plane. The B_1 field rotating in the opposite direction cannot maintain a constant phase with the precessing moments and has no effect on the magnetization. In effect the RF power put into the latter mode of opposite rotation is lost. Double coils are also constructed in which there are two resonant coil components that are geometrically and electrically orthogonal but have identical resonant frequencies.[14,22] If these coil components are excited with AC pulses of identical amplitude but phases that differ by 90 degrees, then the counter-rotating B_1 component is not activated and a "standing wave" of constant amplitude B_1 is set up in the coil as a whole (Figure 2-24). This type of coil is called a *quadrature coil,* and it increases the SNR by a factor of $\sqrt{2}$ and offers an additional advantage as a transmitter. It requires only one half the power to generate the circularly polarized B_1 field compared with the linearly polarized one, thereby reducing power deposition in tissue.

Receiver System

A schematic of an RF receiver system is shown in Figure 2-25. A central feature of MR receivers is that the final signal output is in the low-frequency audio range (kHz), whereas the transmitter output and the initial RF receiver coil signal collection are in the much higher RF range (MHz). The processing of an audio signal is desirable because it allows flexible filtering of system noise and digitizing of the audio signal at high rates relative to the signal frequency. With an RF signal in the MHz range, noise filtering is more difficult, and rapid digitization of the signal compared with its frequency is not practical. Audio MR sig-

nal detection is possible because, although the proton spins must be excited with a transmitter that operates at the Larmor frequency with a bandwidth sufficient to include the precessional frequencies of all the protons in the slice selected, the receiver or detector system need monitor only the amplitudes and phases of the proton frequencies within the bandwidth defined by the readout field gradient (after slice selection, all magnetization in the transverse plane is precessing at the Larmor frequency). For example, with respect to the receiver, for a frequency-encoding gradient of 0.5 G/cm over a 15-cm FOV, this requires that only the frequencies 0 to 32 kHz (0.5 G/cm $\times$ 15 cm $\times$ 4257 Hz/G = 31,027 Hz [~32 kHz]) be monitored, not the higher-frequency range (e.g., 42,570,000 to 42,602,000 [for a 1 T field at which the proton precessional frequency is 42.57 MHz]). This is accomplished in an MR system by mixing, in the phase-sensitive detector, the output signal with a reference frequency, which in the simplest illustrative case is v_o, the B_1 transmitter frequency. The output of the phase-sensitive detector is a wave of the form cos $[2 \pi (v_i - v_o) t + \Phi]$, where $v_i - v_o$ is the MR signal expressed as a difference between the RF of the signal and the reference, and π is the phase angle between the signal and reference. The difference signals $v_i - v_o$ in the audio range are then amplified, digitized, and stored in the computer.

Detection in Quadrature. As shown in Figure 2-25, two phase-sensitive detectors (PSDs) differing in phase by 90 degrees (a quadrature arrangement) are often used in MR systems. The advantages of quadrature detection include an improvement of the SNR by the factor $\sqrt{2}$ relative to detection with a single PSD channel. An appreciation of the origin of this improvement requires a more detailed consideration of the time dependence of the transverse magnetization M, as illustrated in Figure 2-26. Because of the operation of the frequency-encoding gra-

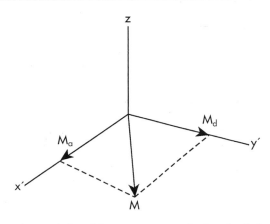

FIGURE 2-26 Depiction of the transverse magnetization of a pixel away from the magnet isocenter during collection of a spin echo while a frequency-encoding gradient is turned on. The coordinate system is the rotating frame (Figure 2-14), in which x and y are rotating at the Larmor frequency ν_0. For a pixel at the isocenter where $2\pi\nu_0 = \gamma B_0$ (there is no gradient field) the magnetization would be exactly along y and would be detected as a steady magnetization by a detector along x. The magnetization (M) depicted in the figure experiences B_0 and the gradient field, and correspondingly it will be precessing faster than ν_0 in the rotating frame. It will alternately get in and out of phase with y and x, and it is actually this in- and out-of-phase pattern that causes the oscillatory pattern of the detected signals (Figures 2-13, *D*, and 2-20). The magnetization in the plane has x and y components, either of which can be detected. The component along x is called the *absorption component* (Ma), or the "real" (u) mode, and the component along y is called the *dispersive component* (Md), or the "imaginary" (v) mode. The real and imaginary designation owes to the fact that the magnetization M can be expressed as a complex number u + i v.

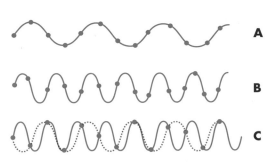

FIGURE 2-27 Sampling rate and the fidelity of digitizing the frequency components of an FID. The components **A** (frequency = 300 Hz), **B** (frequency = 476 Hz), and **C** (frequency = 600 Hz) are sampled by an ADC at a rate of 1000 Hz. Component A is sampled 3 to 4 times per cycle, and component **B** is sampled 2 to 3 times per cycle. The frequency of each component will be faithfully represented by the sampling process. However, component **C** has a frequency "ghost" (alias) that can be fit equally well to the sampling points. This aliased component (400 Hz) will appear in the image at a frequency equal to the sampling rate (1000)—the true frequency (600). In this case a frequency width of 600 Hz could be sampled without aliasing if a sampling or digitization rate of 1200 Hz or greater is used. Even when the sampling rate is appropriate, a sharp cut-off, high-frequency filter is used to improve image quality by eliminating aliasing or fold-back of high-frequency noise.

dient and the effect of magnetic field inhomogeneities, the magnetization of all pixels off isocenter is spread out in the transverse plane, with components 90 degrees out of phase along x and y, either of which can be detected with a single PSD. In quadrature detection, both components are collected using two PSDs 90 degrees out of phase—one channel collecting a wave of the form cos [2 p ($\nu_i - \nu_o$) t + Φ] and the second a wave of the form sin [2 p ($\nu_i - \nu_o$) t + Φ]. These signals are separately amplified, digitized, and manipulated in the computer to create the image. Because the signal from each channel is correlated but the noise is not (the noise in each channel is random), the SNR will be increased by a factor of $\sqrt{2}$ compared with a single PSD.

There is a related effect of quadrature detection that is worthy of note. Because the cosine term cannot distinguish positive and negative values of $\nu_i - \nu_o$ [cos x = cos(−x)], a single PSD cannot distinguish a ν_i that is higher in frequency than ν_o from one that is lower. Because quadrature detection operates with both the cosine and sine terms, positive and negative frequencies can be distinguished, thereby allowing a smaller detector bandwidth because the reference frequency can be centered in the band of detected signals. The advantages of smaller bandwidths are discussed later.

Digital Sampling Rate. The majority of the components of an MR system are analog devices that generate or are triggered by continuous signals. However, the computer that monitors and directs the system[5,16,27,53] operates in a digital manner through multiple electronic logic gates, which are either open (the message cannot get through) or closed (the message gets through to the next logic gate or triggers an output signal). Therefore a translation between the analog and digital signals is required. These translations are provided by rapid, accurate, analog-to-digital converters (ADCs) and digital-to-analog converters (DACs), which are characterized by their speed (data-conversion rates) and resolution (number of bits). The speed at which these devices operate is especially important in MRI because the audio-MR signal must be sampled at a rate that is twice the frequency of the highest-frequency MR signal present. This is the Nyquist frequency, and the requirement follows from information theory. If the data are sampled at less than the Nyquist frequency, aliasing or fold-back occurs in the image. This finding is illustrated in Figure 2-27. A rate of data conversion of approximately 1 ms/bit, or a total of 16 ms for a 16-bit converter, represents a data-sampling rate of 60,000 events/sec, or 60 kHz, and a maximum effective audio-frequency range for the MR signals of 30 kHz

before aliasing occurs. For a readout gradient of 0.5 G/cm and a 20-cm FOV the audio range of MR signals that must be sampled is 42.57 kHz (0.5 G/cm × 20 cm × 42.57 MHz/T [4257 Hz/G]). In this frequency range aliasing can be a problem unless the conversion rate of the ADC is less than 1 ms (and the sampling rate is greater than 60 kHz). (MR systems can have ADCs and DACs with sampling rates as high as 250 kHz.) Alternatively the FOV or the field gradient could be changed to bring the range of frequencies sampled below 42.57 kHz. Because the MRI parameters are highly interdependent, changes in the FOV, sampling rate, and gradient strength cannot be considered in isolation, a subject for the next section.

Bandwidth. The manner in which frequency encoding is accomplished in most MR systems requires that the following relationship be satisfied:

(EQ. 3)

$$\text{(Readout field gradient, Hz/cm)} \times \text{(FOV, cm)}$$
$$\leq \text{(Receiver bandwidth, Hz)}$$

The receiver bandwidth is equivalent to the digital sampling rate, which is determined by the ratio of the number of points sampled to the amount of time the receiver is on. For example, if 256 complex points in the frequency-encoding direction are sampled by the receiver in 8 ms, then the sampling rate or receiver bandwidth is 32,000/sec, or 32 kHz (with quadrature detection, the receiver bandwidth is ± 16 kHz). With this fixed receiver bandwidth, the FOV is fixed by the field gradient used. For a 12-cm FOV the readout gradient that must be used is

(EQ. 4)

$$32,000 \text{ Hz}/12 \text{ cm} = 2667 \text{ Hz/cm or } 0.6 \text{ G/cm}$$
$$(2667 \text{ Hz/cm} \div 4257 \text{ Hz/G})$$

To increase the FOV to 24 cm with the same receiver bandwidth, the readout gradient strength must be reduced by a factor of 2 to 0.3 G/cm. If this reduction is not done, frequencies (61.3 kHz = 0.6 G/cm × 4257 Hz/G × 24 cm) will be generated outside the receiver bandwidth, and severe aliasing will result. Similarly a decrease in the FOV to 6 cm, keeping the receiver bandwidth constant, requires an increase in the readout gradient strength (to 1.2 G/cm). In some MR systems it is possible to alter the bandwidth for special purposes.[49] In the aforementioned example a readout gradient strength of 1.2 G/cm might not be achievable, but a match of the receiver bandwidth and the distribution of frequencies in the 6-cm FOV could be accomplished by keeping the gradient strength at 0.6 G/cm and reducing the receiver bandwidth to 16 kHz (0.6 G/cm × 6 cm × 4257 Hz/G). The bandwidth would be decreased by increasing the sampling time from 8 to 16 ms.

A decrease in the bandwidth reduces the noise received (random noise varies as the square root of the bandwidth). Although this is a salutary effect, the increased sampling time required to narrow the bandwidth has important consequences in spin-echo imaging. The minimum possible echo time for a spin-echo sequence is the sum of the sampling time and one and a half times the duration of the RF pulse (i.e., the sum of the time required for execution of the pulse and the time required for rephasing by short gradient reversal). For an 8-ms sampling time and an RF pulse width of approximately 2 ms, the minimum TE is 11 ms. An increase of the sampling time to 16 ms would increase the minimum TE to 19 ms. For a tissue sample with a T2 relaxation time of 60 ms this increase would result in a diminution of signal for the longer TE of 12% relative to the shorter TE. In this particular example the trade-off would be a good one, all other things being equal, but for a tissue sample with a shorter T2 the longer sampling time might be unacceptable.

Fast Imaging and Spectroscopy Revisited

Some applications of EPI and echo-planar spectroscopic imaging require MR systems to perform at their operational limits,[18,56] and it is instructive to consider one of these at greater length. Single-shot EPI has become a popular technique in functional imaging of the brain because images can be obtained so rapidly (in less than 100 ms) that the nearly instantaneous hemodynamic response in the brain to sensory and cognitive stimuli can be measured. In this technique a single excitation is followed by successive blips of a weak phase-encoding gradient and rapid switches in polarity of a strong readout gradient to create gradient echoes that contain all the phase and frequency information necessary to create the image (all of κ space is covered in one excitation). During the 50- to 100-ms encoding and sampling period, the signal decays as a result of spin-spin relaxation processes in the tissue, inhomogeneities in the static magnetic field, and magnetic susceptibility gradients in the sample. The results are phase and frequency shifts unrelated to the imposed phase- and frequency-encoding gradients and signal decays as κ space is traversed (T2 and T2* range from 20 to 100 ms). This decay results in image blurring and distortion in the phase-encode direction.

The blurring can be described by a point-spread function, the width of which (2/πT2 [or T2*]) is a measure of how far each point or edge in the image is spread out in space. To minimize the blurring, the point-spread function is made less than the pixel width by keeping the total gradient readout time less than the inverse of the point-spread function. For a tissue T2 of 70 ms this means that the readout time must be less than 110 ms ≈ πT2/2, and if there are 128 phase-encoding steps (128 lobes in the readout gradient), the time between each lobe must be 110/128 ms, or 860 μs. In this time period the gradient must rise to its maximum and fall from it. These numbers put into perspective the importance of high gradient slew rates and high gradient amplitudes for EPI discussed previously; the resolution is a function of the gradient strength, which in turn depends on the area of the lobe of the gradient versus time plot. Imaging a large area in a short time requires a large amplitude achieved quickly. This assessment also underscores the importance of highly homogeneous static magnetic fields for EPI. If the inhomogeneity of the static field in this ideal example actually amounted to 6 Hz over a pixel, then T2* would be about 30 ms (1/T2* = 1/0.1 + 6 π) and the point-spread function would require a readout time of less than ≈46 ms, with the requirement that the slew rates and maximum gradient amplitudes be raised accordingly to preserve the resolution.

Another extremely important reason for highly homogeneous fields in EPI is the sensitivity of the technique to off-resonance effects, which can cause geometric artifacts and ghosting in EP images. These effects, which arise from chemical shifts present in water and lipid protons and induced in tissue protons by inhomogeneous magnetic fields, cause miscentering of gradient echoes and spatially varying phase shifts. They can be reduced by increasing the homogeneity of the field and by de-

creasing the echo spacing in the readout gradient, which again requires high slew rates and maximum gradient amplitudes. When the off-resonance effects arise from the intrinsic chemical shifts of water and lipid protons, they can be avoided by presaturating the lipid proton resonances.

The large gradient amplitudes required for high-resolution EPI place large requirements on the RF system as well. For example, a maximum gradient amplitude of approximately 20 mT/m over a 12-cm FOV would require a digital sampling rate of approximately 100 kHz, nearly at the limit of the capability (125 kHz) of digitizers available today. The larger bandwidth also causes a significant drop in the SNR because noise increases as the square root of the bandwidth. The noise in a 125-kHz bandwidth EPI receiver is nearly twofold higher than in a 32-kHz receiver that might be used in conventional spin-echo imaging. This finding, combined with the signal decay during data acquisition in EPI, puts severe limitations on the technique. Fortunately, the use of phased-array surface coils can boost the SNR significantly in many applications.

COMPUTER AND ACCESSORIES

The computer and accessories constitute the command and control center of the MR system, performing myriad functions in data collection, manipulation, storage, retrieval, and multiformat presentation and selecting the VOI, shaping and timing the RF pulses, turning the gradients on and off, instructing the receiver to collect data, and providing data for the diagnosis of the state of the MR system components. A simplified block diagram of a computer-controlled MR system is drawn in Figure 2-28. In addition to the host computer, a fast-array processor for high-speed computations and magnetic disks for data storage are essential. A well-equipped system might consist of a host computer having at least 32 megabytes (MB) (1 byte = 8 bits) of core memory in 32-bit words, disk drives with gigabyte (GB) capacity, a floating-

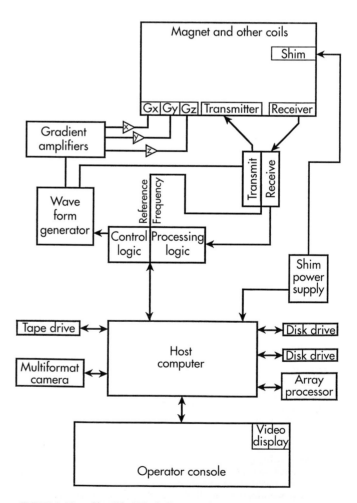

FIGURE 2-28 Simplified block diagram of a representative MR system.

point–array processor, a real-time data acquisition subsystem micro-processor with 1 MB of memory, and a status and calibration 1-MB subsystem. Other possible configurations are used. The need for this computational power and speed should be considered in the context of the storage and computational demand on the computer systems. Of particular importance is the fact that an MR system operates both in real time and in "pseudo–real-time," in the sense that raw image data are being acquired at the same time that other raw data are being processed into digital images that are stored for later film processing. To acquire a single image with 512 × 512, or 262,144, pixels with 1024 discrete gray levels, approximately 0.5 MB of storage in core memory is required, assuming that each pixel is encoded by 2 bytes. If 10 to 20 patients are studied each day, the requirement for off-line storage in disks (one for raw data, another for processed images) is appreciable; the daily data-storage requirements are in the range of 50 to 200 MB of information. Also the central processing unit must have access to more than the 0.5 MB of core memory necessary to store a "current" image data set; it must also have sufficient memory available for operating software and the codes for the RF and gradient-pulse programmer.

Processing the raw data for construction of a 256 × 256 pixel image by fast Fourier transformation (FFT) requires about 2 million floating-point operations in real time. This requires more speed than a mini-computer is capable of but is within the capabilities of an appropriate parallel-array processor (18,000,000 operations/sec). Unlike the host computer, which to maximize versatility requires that calculations be performed serially (one after the other), the array processor is designed for speed and simplicity so that multiple simple arithmetic operations in FFT can be performed simultaneously. Even so the task in pseudo–real time is not without complications. The computer system must give top priority to the acquisition of real-time data (this means execution of RF and gradient pulse sequences and the timely transfer of incoming data from buffer to core).

For long-term data storage the processed images are transferred from the disk to either magnetooptical disk (MOD) or digital magnetic tape (DAT), each of which has a typical capacity of about 1 GB per disk or cassette. The number of images that can be stored in the processed-image file disk is approximately 2000 (for a matrix size of 256 × 256). Approximately 12,000 compressed 256 × 256 images fit on an MOD or DAT (about one fourth as many 512 × 512 images will fit).

REFERENCES

1. Ackerman JJH, Grove TH, Wong GG, et al: Mapping of metabolites in whole animals by ^{31}P NMR using surface coils, Nature 283:167, 1980.
2. Alley MT, Grist TM, and Swan JS: Development of a phased-array coil for the lower extremities, Magn Reson Med 34:260, 1995.
3. Anderson WA: Electrical current shims for correcting magnetic fields, Rev Sci Instr 32:241, 1961.
4. Andrew ER, and Szczesniak E: Magnetic shielding of magnetic resonance systems, Magn Reson Med 10:373, 1989.
5. Arenson RL, Chakraborty DP, Seshadri SB, et al: The digital imaging workstation, Radiology 176:303, 1990.
6. Atlas SW, Kackney DB, and Listerud J: Fast spin echo imaging of the brain and spine, Magn Reson Q 9:61, 1993.
7. Axel L: Surface coil magnetic resonance imaging, J Comput Assist Tomogr 8:381, 1984.
8. Bangert V, and Mansfield P: Magnetic field coils for NMR imaging, Journal of Physics E 15:235, 1982.
9. Bittoun J, Saint-James H, Querleux BG, et al: *In vivo* high resolution MR imaging of the skin in a whole body system at 1.5T, Radiology 176:457, 1990.
10. Bottomley PA: A versatile magnetic field gradient control system for NMR imaging, Journal of Physics E 14:1081, 1981.
11. Bydder GM, Curati WL, and Gadian DG: Use of closely coupled receiver coils in MR imaging: practical aspects, J Comput Assist Tomogr 9:987, 1985.
12. Carlson JW, Gyori M, and Kaufman L: A technique for MR imaging of the knee under large flexing angles, Magn Reson Med 8:407, 1990.
13. Carlson JW, and Roos MS: Shielded gradient coils on hyperbolic surfaces of revolution, Magn Res Med 34:762, 1995.
14. Chen CN, Hoult DI, and Sank VJ: Quadrature detection coils: a further $\sqrt{2}$ improvement in sensitivity, J Magn Reson 54:324, 1983.
15. Constantinides CD, Westgate CR, O'Dell WG, et al: A phased array coil for human cardiac imaging, Magn Reson Med 34:92, 1995.
16. Cooper JW: The computer in Fourier-transform NMR. In Levy GC, ed: Topics in ^{13}C NMR spectroscopy, vol 2, New York, 1976, Wiley Interscience.
17. Doornbos J, Grimbergen HAA, Booijen PE, et al: Applications of anatomically shaped surface coils in MRI at 0.5T, Magn Reson Med 3:270, 1986.
18. Farzaneh F, Riederer S, and Pelc NJ: Analysis of T2 limitations and off-resonance effects on spatial resolution and artifacts in echo-planar imaging, Magn Reson Med 14:123, 1990.
19. Gadian D: Nuclear magnetic resonance and its application to living systems, Oxford, 1982, Clarendon Press.
20. Gasson J, Summers IR, Fry ME, et al: Modified birdcage coils for targeted imaging, Magn Reson Imaging 13:1003, 1995.
21. Gideon P, Danielsen ER, Schneider M, et al: Short echo time spectroscopy of the brain in healthy volunteers using an insert gradient head coil, Magn Reson Imaging 13:105, 1995.
22. Glover GH, Hayes CE, Pelc N, et al: Comparison of linear and circular polarization for magnetic resonance imaging, J Magn Reson 64:255, 1985.
23. Griffey RH, and Flamig DP: Vapor for solvent suppressed short echo, volume localized proton spectroscopy, J Magn Reson Imaging 88:161, 1990.
24. Hanley P: Magnets for medical applications of NMR, Br Med Bull 40:125, 1984.
25. Hayes CE, Edelstein WA, Schenck JF, et al: An efficient highly homogeneous radiofrequency coil for whole body NMR imaging at 1.5T, J Magn Reson Imaging 63:622, 1985.
26. Holsinger RF, Lown RR, Remillard PA, et al: Novel light weight permanent ring magnet MR imaging system: design, installation, and clinical experience. In Book of abstracts, Society for Magnetic Resonance in Medicine, Fifth Annual Meeting, Montreal, Aug 19-22, 1986.
27. Horowitz P, and Hill W: Digital electronics, and Digital meets analog. In The art of electronics, Cambridge, 1980, Cambridge University Press.
28. Hoult DI: The solution of the Bloch equations in the presence of a varying B1 field: an approach to selective pulse analysis, J Magn Reson Imaging 35:69, 1979.
29. Hoult DI: Radiofrequency coil technology in NMR scanning. In Witcofski R, Karstaedt N, and Partain CL, eds: NMR imaging, Winston Salem, NC, 1982, Bowman Gray School of Medicine.
30. Howe FA, Maxwell RJ, Saunders DE, et al: Proton spectroscopy *in vivo,* Magn Reson Q 9:31, 1994.
31. Hutchison JMS, Sutherland RJ, and Mallard JR: NMR imaging: image recovery under magnetic fields with large non-uniformities, Journal of Physics E 11:217, 1978.
32. Hyde JS, Jesmanowicz A, Froncisz W, et al: Parallel image acquisition from non-interacting local coils, Magn Reson Med 70:512, 1986.
33. Jezzard P, and Balaban RS: Correction for geometric distortion in echo planar images from B$_0$ field variations, Magn Res Med 34:65, 1995.
34. Jin J, Shen G, and Perkins T: On the field inhomogeneity of a birdcage coil, Magn Reson Med 32:418, 1994.
35. Keller PJ: Basic principles of magnetic resonance imaging, Pub. No. 7798, Milwaukee, 1988, General Electric Medical Systems.
36. Keller PJ, Heiserman JE, Fram EK, et al: A Nyquist modulated echo-to-view mapping scheme for fast spin-echo imaging, Magn Reson Med 33:838, 1995.
37. Kneeland JB, Jesmanowicz A, Froncisz W, et al: High resolution MR imaging using loop gap resonators: work in progress, Radiology 158:247, 1986.
38. Leroy-Willig A, Darasse L, Taquin J, et al: The slotted cylinder: an efficient probe for NMR imaging, Magn Reson Med 2:20, 1985.
39. Locher PR: Computer simulation of selective excitation in NMR imaging, Philos Trans R Soc Lond B Biol Sci 289:537, 1980.
40. Maier CF, Chu KC, Chronik BA, et al: A novel transverse gradient coil design for high resolution MR imaging, Magn Reson Med 34:604, 1995.
41. Mansfield P: Multi-planar image formation using NMR spin echoes, J Phys Chem 10:55, 1977.
42. Mansfield P, and Chapman B: Active magnetic screening of gradient coils in NMR imaging, J Magn Reson 66:573, 1986.
43. Mansfield P, Chapman BLW, Bowtell R, et al: Active acoustic screening: reduction of noise in gradient coils by Lorentz force balancing, Magn Reson Med 33:276, 1995.
44. Mansfield P, Maudsley AA, Morris PG: Selective pulses in NMR imaging: a reply to criticism, J Magn Reson Imaging 33:261, 1979.
45. Mansfield P, and Morris PG: NMR imaging in medicine and biology, New York, 1982, Academic Press.
46. Marshall EA, Listinsky JJ, Ceckler TL, et al: Magnetic resonance imaging using a ribbonator: hand and wrist, Magn Reson Med 9:369, 1989.
47. Matwiyoff N: Magnetic resonance workbook, New York, 1990, Raven Press.
48. Monroe JW, Schmalbrock P, and Spigos DG: Phased array coils for upper extremity MRA, Magn Reson Med 33:224, 1995.
49. Mugler JP, and Brookman JR: Implementation of mixed bandwidth MRI pulse sequences using a single analog low pass filter, Magn Reson Imaging 7:487, 1989.
50. Nishimura DG, Irarrazabal P, and Meyer CH: A velocity κ-space analysis of flow effects in echo planar and spiral imaging, Magn Reson Med 33:549, 1995.
51. O'Dell WG, Schoeniger JS, Blackband SJ, et al: A modified quadruple gradient set for use in high resolution MRI tagging, Magn Reson Med 32:246, 1994.
52. O'Donnell M, and Edelstein WA: NMR imaging in the presence of magnetic field inhomogeneity and gradient field non-linearities, Med Phys 12:20, 1985.
53. Pickens DR, and Erickson JJ: Computers in computed tomography and magnetic resonance imaging, Radiographics 5:32, 1985.
54. Podo F, Bovee WMM, DeCertaines J, et al: Quality assessment in *in vivo* NMR spectroscopy. I. Introduction, objectives, and activities, Magn Reson Imaging 13:117, 1995.
55. Porter JR, Wright SM, Famili A: A four-channel domain multiplexer: a cost-effective alternative to multiple receivers, Magn Reson Med 32:499, 1994.
56. Posse S, Tedeschi G, Risinger R, et al: High speed H1 spectroscopic imaging in human brain by echo planar spatial-spectral encoding, Magn Reson Med 33:34, 1995.
57. Reeder SB, and McVeigh ER: The effect of high performance gradients on fast gradient echo imaging, Magn Reson Med 32:612, 1994.
58. Requardt H, Offermann J, and Erhard P: Switched array coils, Magn Reson Med 13:385, 1990.
59. Roemer PB, Edelstein WA, Hayes CE, et al: The NMR phased array, Magn Reson Med 16:192, 1990.
60. Roemer PB, Edelstein WA, and Hicks JS: Self shielded gradient coils. In Book of abstracts, Society for Magnetic Resonance in Medicine, Fifth Annual Meeting, Montreal, Aug 19-22, 1986.
61. Romeo F, and Hoult DI: Magnetic field profiling: analysis and correcting coil design, Magn Reson Med 1:44, 1984.

62. Ross B, and Michaelis T: Clinical applications of magnetic resonance spectroscopy, Magn Reson Q 10:191, 1995.

63. Schenck JF, Jolesz FA, Roemer PB, et al: Superconducting open-configuration MR imaging system for image guided therapy, Radiology 195:805, 1995.

64. Shaw D: Fourier transform NMR spectroscopy, New York, 1984, Elsevier.

65. Skinnar M, Bolinger L, and Leigh JS: The synthesis of soft pulses with a specified frequency response, Magn Reson Med 12:88, 1990.

66. Slavin GS, Butts K, Rydberg JN, et al: Dual-echo interleaved echo-planar imaging of the brain, Magn Reson Med 33:264, 1995.

67. Song AW, Wong EC, and Hyde JS: Echo volume imaging, Magn Reson Med 32:668, 1994.

68. Sutherland RJ, and Hutchison JMS: Three dimensional NMR imaging using selective excitation, Journal of Physics E 11:79, 1978.

69. Van Zijl PCM, Moonen CTW, Alger JR, et al: High field localized proton spectroscopy in small volumes: greatly improved localization and shimming using shielded strong gradients, Magn Reson Med 10:256, 1989.

70. Wald LL, Carvajal L, Moyher SE, et al: Phased array detectors and an automated intensity correction algorithm for high resolution MR imaging of the brain, Magn Reson Med 34:433, 1995.

71. Webb PG, Sailasuta N, Kohler SJ, et al: Automated single-voxel proton MRS: technical development and multisite verification, Magn Reson Med 31:365, 1994.

72. Wehrli FW: Fast scan magnetic resonance: principles and applications, Magn Reson Q 6:165, 1990.

73. Weis J, and Budinsky L: Simulation of the influence of magnetic field inhomogeneity and distortion correction in MR imaging, Magn Reson Imaging 8:483, 1990.

74. Wen H, and Jaffer FA: An *in vivo* automated shimming method taking into account current constraints, Magn Reson Med 34:898, 1995.

75. Wright SM, Magin RL, and Kelton JR: Arrays of mutually coupled receiver coils: theory and application, Magn Reson Med 17:252, 1991.

76. Yongbi NM, Payne GS, and Leach MO: A gradient scheme suitable for localized shimming and in vivo $^1H/^{31}P$ STEAM and ISIS NMR spectroscopy, Magn Reson Med 32:768, 1994.

3 Physical and Physiological Basis of Magnetic Relaxation

John C. Gore and Richard P. Kennan

Relaxation Theory in Solutions
Relaxation in Multicompartment Systems and the Effects of
  Exchange
Relaxation in Solutions of Macromolecules and Tissues
Magnetization Transfer
Summary

 KEY POINTS

- Most of the contrast in MR images comes from variations in relaxation times T1 and T2.
- T1 is the longitudinal, or spin-lattice, relaxation time. It is longer in pure water than in proteinaceous solutions or tissues or when paramagnetic species capable of dipole-dipole interactions are present. T1 is a first-order exponential time constant that reflects the molecular tumbling rate of protons and the strength of local magnetic fields they experience.
- T2 is the transverse, or spin-spin, relaxation time. It is also longer in pure water than in proteinaceous solutions or tissues or when paramagnetic species capable of dipole-dipole interactions are present. T2 is also shorter when protons exchange between different chemical environments or diffuse between regions of different susceptibility. T2 is also a first-order exponential time constant so that 63% of the initial transverse magnetization or signal is lost during one T2 period.

The contrast that is apparent in magnetic resonance (MR) images of soft tissues usually arises from the heterogeneous distribution of tissue-proton densities and relaxation times. The sensitivity of magnetic resonance imaging (MRI) to pathological changes and variations in tissue composition, which underlies its clinical usefulness, most often relies on detecting small changes in tissue-water relaxation rates, albeit indirectly via pulse sequences that also depend on other tissue and technical parameters. Thus it is of immense practical importance to understand the mechanisms responsible for proton relaxation in heterogeneous media, such as tissues, and to be able to explain the changes that occur in tissue relaxation in disease. A complete understanding of tissue relaxation may then permit a proper interpretation of clinical MR images and also may provide guidance on the development of improved imaging techniques for more specific characterization of tissues. Theoretical descriptions provide an understanding of the physical processes that account for water-proton relaxation in tissues. Many detailed aspects of relaxation in complex biological media are not well understood in a quantitative sense, meaning there are no adequate models that can be used to account precisely for the observed relaxation in practical cases. Furthermore, because tissues are heterogeneous, have complex structures, and vary widely in their detailed composition and because different pathological processes involve different types of change in tissue composition and character, often it is not possible to explain observations of changes in relaxation in terms of specific underlying causes. However, we do possess a reasonably complete understanding of the various processes and factors that contribute to relaxation in

aqueous biological media. These factors are described later in some detail. Changes in relaxation that occur, for example, in disease then correspond to structural or chemical modifications that in turn modulate one or more of these contributing processes.

In this chapter the fundamental concepts of relaxation are reviewed first, and the atomic view of relaxation of protons in liquids, such as water, is described. Human tissues are 70% to 90% water, so most MR signals are derived from water, and understanding relaxation in pure water is a necessary first step in understanding relaxation in more complex situations. We then consider what changes to relaxation arise as a result of adding simple macromolecules and other solutes and show that these are insufficient to explain all the relaxation phenomena observed in tissues. However, studying what happens to proteins and biopolymers when they become organized into larger-scale and less-mobile structures provides additional insights into the causes of relaxation in tissues.

RELAXATION THEORY IN SOLUTIONS

Relaxation connotes the recovery back toward equilibrium of nuclear dipoles that have been disturbed by radiofrequency (RF) excitations. First, reconsider some underlying basic concepts of nuclear magnetization and MR. Each hydrogen nucleus (proton) possesses spin, which in turn gives rise to a magnetic dipole moment, so it can be considered like a small bar magnet with separate poles. When a large number of such magnetic nuclei are placed in an external magnetic field, they tend to align themselves in the direction of the field. Quantum theory constrains the nuclear magnetic energy states so that only certain energy levels are permitted, analogous to the behavior of electrons orbiting the nucleus in shells. For protons in a magnetic field this results in only two orientations of the nuclear magnet relative to the field direction being allowed, which naively can be described as parallel and antiparallel to the magnetic field. These two states correspond to two allowed energy levels (see Figure 1-4). Because the aligned position corresponds to a lower energy level, a slightly larger number of protons populate this energy level, and they produce a net magnetization in the direction of the field.

The populations of the two energy levels in equilibrium depend on the energy difference between them (ΔE), which is proportional to the static applied field strength (B_0). In practice, ΔE is very small. For example, for protons in a magnetic field of 1 Tesla (T), ΔE is only 1.76×10^{-7} eV, which is an insignificant energy difference on the chemical or molecular scale. Because the energy difference is so small, the preference for taking one alignment rather than the other is also very weak so that the difference in numbers of spins pointing up rather than down is very small (about one in a million).

NMR experiments involve inducing transitions between the two energy levels by absorption or emission of quanta with energy ΔE, which is analogous to the transitions of electrons between orbits in an atom. In the presence of a static field and an additional alternating field of frequency ω_0, where ω_0 satisfies the relation

(EQ. 1)

$$\Delta E = \hbar \omega_0$$

and $\hbar$ is Planck's constant, the spin system absorbs energy so that the population of the upper energy level increases while that of the lower level decreases. Because only radiation of a precisely defined frequency (the Larmor frequency) is effective, the process is called a *resonant process*. For hydrogen nuclei in a field of 1.5 Tesla (T) the Larmor frequency is 63.9 MHz, which is an RF field. If the energy absorbed is sufficient to equalize the populations of the two levels, saturation has occurred and no further absorption will take place. A completely or partially saturated system will return to equilibrium because of two simultaneous processes. First, the absorbed energy will be redistributed within the spin system by processes in which every transition of a nucleus from a higher to a lower level is accompanied by a transition of a nucleus from the lower to the higher state, called *spin-spin relaxation.* Second, there will be a gradual loss of energy to the other nuclei and electrons in the material collectively called the *lattice,* resulting from transitions of nuclei from the upper to the lower state. This second process is called *spin-lattice relaxation.* The time constants characterizing these two processes are T2 and T1, respectively, the spin-spin (or transverse) and spin-lattice (or longitudinal) relaxation times.

Although we have introduced relaxation as the recovery from saturation, it more generally describes the return to equilibrium after any disturbance of the spins, such as occurs in MRI pulse sequences. Spin-lattice relaxation is also the process that limits the time it takes for the equilibrium magnetization to become established when the sample is first subjected to the magnetic field. The time constants T1 and T2 yield valuable information about the local interactions experienced by nuclei.

T1 describes the rate at which a nonequilibrium spin distribution exponentially approaches equilibrium after absorption of RF energy. However, because the energy change involved is so small, an excited nuclear spin does not spontaneously lose its energy (or rather, it would do so at an exceptionally slow rate) but relies almost entirely on interaction with the surrounding material. Spin-lattice relaxation, where the lattice is the environment surrounding the nucleus and includes the remainder of the host molecule and other solute and solvent molecules, occurs because of interactions of the excited nuclear-spin dipole with the random fluctuating magnetic fields that exist on an atomic scale inside tissues. These fields originate from neighboring nuclei and are modulated by the motion of other surrounding dipoles in the lattice, which have components fluctuating with the same frequency as the resonance frequency (ω_0). Spin-lattice relaxation is a type of stimulated recovery in which the spins that have been excited to the upper energy level by the transmitted RF pulse are encouraged to return to the lower level by the action of an alternating magnetic field of appropriate frequency. This stimulated recovery is very efficient when there is a local fluctuating field that can provide a magnetic perturbation at the Larmor frequency, so there is a quantum of energy available exactly equal to the difference in levels of the nuclear-spin states. A suitable source of stimulating interaction can be discovered by close inspection of the atomic environment of the protons in tissue. For example, each proton in a water molecule has a neighboring proton that is also a magnetic dipole, which generates a magnetic field at the proton of about 5 Gauss (0.5 milliTesla [mT]) (Figure 3-1). This field, however, is constantly changing in amplitude and direction as the water molecule rotates rapidly and moves about in the liquid. It also changes as a result of intermolecular collision, translation, or chemical dissociation and exchange.

The magnetic field experienced by any nucleus therefore fluctuates with a frequency spectrum that is dependent on the molecular tumbling because of the random thermal motion of the host and surrounding molecules (Figure 3-2). The mean strength of the local field is determined by the strength of the magnetic dipoles in the medium and how closely they approach the hydrogen nuclei. Only the component of the frequency spectrum that is equal to the resonant frequency ω_0 (or, for reasons beyond our discussion, $2\omega_0$) is effective in stimulating an energy exchange to induce transitions between nuclear-spin states and lead to thermal equilibrium, that is, T1 relaxation. In liquids such as water the characteristic frequencies of thermal motion are approximately 10^{11} Hz or higher, much greater than nuclear magnetic resonance (NMR) frequencies of 10^7 to 10^8 Hz. Consequently the component of the frequency spectrum from molecular motion that can induce T1 relaxation is small, and the process is relatively slow. As the molecular motion becomes slower, either because of lower temperature or increased molecular size, the intensity of the fluctuations of the magnetic field at the resonance frequency increases, reaches a maximum, and then decreases again as the energy of the motion becomes increasingly concentrated in frequencies lower than the NMR range. Thus T1 passes through a minimum value as the molecular motion becomes slower (Figure 3-3).

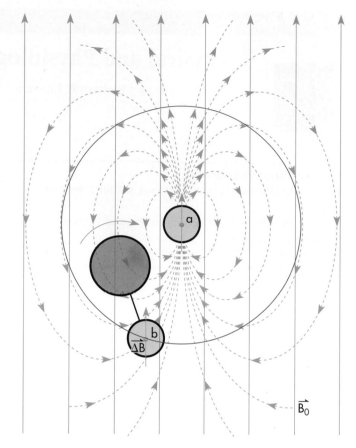

FIGURE 3-1 Schematic diagram of dipolar coupling between two hydrogen nuclei within a water molecule. Each proton generates a field pattern similar to that from a thin bar magnet that falls off as the inverse third power of the distance. The magnetic field around hydrogen nucleus *(a)* therefore varies in space, and the effect on the neighboring nucleus *(b)* in the same molecule changes with time as the molecule moves or rotates, for example, if *b* moves around the circular path shown, which occurs in about 10^{-12} seconds. The dashed lines represent the additional field *(ΔB)* as a result of *a.*

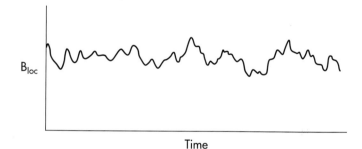

FIGURE 3-2 The local magnetic field experienced at any proton varies as the molecule rotates or as other nuclei that generate magnetic fields move past. In water the field is dominated by the neighboring proton within the same water molecule, but in solutions of proteins the field also may be due to the effects of protons at the surface of the macromolecule. The rate of change of the field is described by the correlation time, τ_c.

The effect of the molecular motion is usually expressed by a correlation time, characteristic of the time of rotation of a molecule or of the time of its translation into a neighboring position. Relaxation rates in simple liquids are affected, for example, by viscosity, temperature, and the presence of dissolved ions and molecules, which alter the correlation times of molecular motion, as discussed later. In addition, relaxation will be faster if the amplitudes of the local dipolar fields increase, which is the case when water molecules pass close to paramagnetic

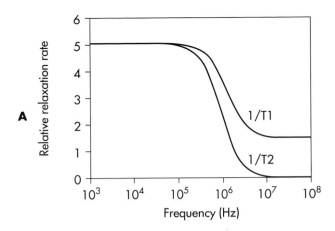

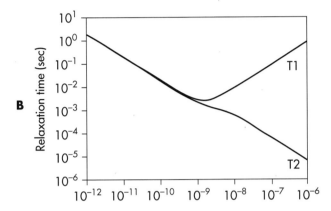

FIGURE 3-3   Schematic dependence of relaxation rates on frequency (**A**) and relaxation times on correlation time (**B**), as predicted by the theory of Bloembergen, Purcell, and Pound.[3] The correlation time, c, in water is inversely related to the temperature.

ions, such as gadolinium, an effect that is exploited in the design of MRI contrast agents.

Whereas T1 is sensitive to RF components of the local field, T2 is also sensitive to low-frequency components. When an ensemble of nuclei is excited with RF, a transverse component of magnetization, orthogonal to the applied field direction, may develop, and this component rotates with the Larmor frequency and induces the MR signal in a receiver coil. T2 reflects the time it takes for the ensemble to become disorganized and for the transverse component to decay. Because any growth of magnetization back toward equilibrium must correspond to a loss of transverse magnetization, all contributions to T1 relaxation affect T2 at least as much. In addition, components of the local dipolar fields that oscillate slowly, at low frequency, may be directed along the main field (B_0) direction and thus can modulate the precessional frequency of a neighboring nucleus. Such frequency perturbations within an ensemble of nuclei result in rapid dephasing of the transverse magnetization and accelerated spin-spin relaxation. Because the low-frequency content of the local dipolar field increases monotonically as molecular motion progressively slows, although T1 passes through a minimum value, T2 continues to decrease and then levels off so that T1 and T2 then take on quite different values.

In the picture developed in the previous paragraph, relaxation results from the action of fluctuating local magnetic fields experienced by protons, which stimulate the return to equilibrium of an excited population of spins. In pure water the dominant source of such effects is the dipole-dipole interaction between neighboring protons, mainly between hydrogen nuclei in the same water molecule. The tumbling of each water molecule then causes the weak magnetic field produced by each proton to fluctuate randomly, and at the site of a neighboring proton these random alterations in the net field produce relaxation. The time scale

characteristic of the dipolar interaction reflects molecular motion and clearly is expected to influence the efficacy of relaxation. Qualitatively, when there is a concentration of kinetic motion in the appropriate frequency range, relaxation will be efficient. We can envisage other types of motion that will be too rapid or too slow to be effective. The key important descriptor is the correlation time (τ_c), which measures the time over which the local fluctuating field appears continuous and deterministic. It represents the time it takes on average for the field to change significantly.

In simple liquids, such as water, the molecular motion is rapid and on average is isotropic. The motions are so fast that relaxation is not very efficient. The dipolar fields fluctuate too rapidly to be very efficient, and the motion averages out any net effects of the local fields (so-called motional averaging). In pure water, T1 is measured to be approximately 3 to 4 sec, and T2 is about equal. A simple demonstration that water relaxation is dominated by intramolecular magnetic dipole-dipole interactions between the two protons on the same water molecule is given by dilution of H_2O with heavy water (D_2O) so that most protons find themselves in hybrid HDO molecules. The dipolar coupling between H and D is much weaker than between H and H, and consequently the relaxation rate for the residual protons is much lower than in water.[1]

This qualitative description of relaxation can be given a more formal mathematical basis. For water the relaxation rates may be written as follows:

(EQ. 2)

$$\frac{1}{T1} = \frac{3}{2}\gamma^4\hbar^2 I(I+1)\{J(\omega) + J(2\omega)\}$$

$$\frac{1}{T2} = \frac{3}{4}\gamma^4\hbar^2 I(I+1)\left\{\frac{1}{2}J(0) + 5J(\omega) + \frac{1}{2}J(2\omega)\right\}$$

ω = The Larmor frequency for protons
γ = The proton gyromagnetic ratio
I = Angular momentum quantum number
$\hbar$ = Planck's constant
$J(\omega)$ = The strength of the local field fluctuating at frequency ω, the so-called spectral density

Spectral densities represent the frequency distribution of components of the local fields experienced by nuclei, obtained by Fourier analysis of the random changes in molecular orientation and position that cause the local field to fluctuate. For intramolecular relaxation in water these changes arise from random walks of water molecules undergoing self-diffusion in the liquid and are characterized by a single correlation time (τ_c). The corresponding spectral densities then can be calculated, and we obtain

(EQ. 3)

$$\frac{1}{T1} = \frac{2}{5}\gamma^4\hbar^2\frac{(I)(I+1)}{r^6}\left[\frac{\tau_c}{1+\omega^2\tau_c^2} + \frac{\tau_c}{1+4\omega^2\tau_c^2}\right]$$

$$\frac{1}{T2} = \frac{1}{5}\gamma^4\frac{\hbar^2 I(I+1)}{r^6}\left[3\tau_c + \frac{5\tau_c}{1+\omega^2\tau_c^2} + \frac{2\tau_c}{1+4\omega^2\tau_c^2}\right]$$

where r is the distance between nuclei. It can be seen that when $\omega^2\tau_c^2$ <<1, T1 = T2. In water, intramolecular effects do not completely describe the relaxation. For example, translational motions also may modulate dipolar interactions between nuclei in different molecules. In these circumstances other spectral densities have to be included. In pure water, such intermolecular interactions (rather than intramolecular effects) account for approximately 30% of the total relaxation rate.

Provided that the relevant physical quantities (such as magnetic moments and interatomic distances) are known, the measured relaxation rate for protons in solutions can be used to infer the correlation time for reorientation of a water molecule. This time effectively indicates the viscosity on a molecular scale and is longer in fluids in which tumbling is slowed by interatomic forces. The behavior of relaxation rates is shown in Figure 3-3 as a function of correlation time and NMR frequency. T1 is always greater than or equal to T2. There is a strong dependence of T1 on temperature because, as the temperature is increased, the kinetic and vibrational energy of molecules increases so that the local dipolar fields fluctuate more rapidly, making them less effective at inducing relaxation. The correlation time and T1 are reduced until $\tau_c = \dfrac{0.616}{\omega_c}$ and T1 is a minimum; that is, spin-lattice relaxation is fastest when the molecular rotational frequencies are near the NMR frequency, a type of resonance behavior. Below this temperature the motions are too slow compared with the NMR frequency to be effective at promoting T1 relaxation, though T2 continues to decrease via the low-frequency component of the dipolar field, J(0) in Equation 2. For example, in solid ice the correlation time $\tau_c \approx 10^{-5}$ so that $\omega\tau_c \gg 1$ and T1 is very long (many seconds), whereas T2 is very short (a few microseconds). From this we may infer that the observation of a T1 significantly longer than T2 (which is the case for most tissues) likely indicates the presence of a long correlation time for some motions. Furthermore, the frequency (field) dependences of T1 and T2 at constant temperature reflect the intensity of the local field at different frequencies and thus are a direct visualization of the spectral density. The frequency at which T1 increases rapidly depends on the correlation times of water in the sample. Special instrumentation has been developed and used by various workers, most notably Koenig and colleagues,[18] to measure the variation of T1 with field, the so-called T1 dispersion, efficiently to probe relaxation in various systems.

The theory just discussed was first developed by Bloembergen, Purcell, and Pound[3] and describes the behavior of relaxation rates in simple homogeneous liquids well, as functions of temperature and NMR frequency. However, solutions of macromolecules and biological tissues are chemically heterogeneous, and thus water in such media may experience a wide variety of different environments and chemical species with which to interact. Even in simple protein solutions there may be different ranges and distributions of correlation time, coupling strengths, and molecular dynamics that affect the local dipolar fields experienced by water protons. An even greater variety of different scales and types of constituents occur within cells and whole tissues. Tissues contain diverse, freely tumbling solute ions and molecules, such as small proteins and lipids, as well as relatively immobilized or even rigid macromolecular assemblies, such as membranes and mitochondria. Tissues are also spatially inhomogeneous, containing many different types of cells or structures, and there may be multiple compartments that are not connected or in which water transport is restricted. Nonetheless, although tissues are markedly heterogeneous at the cellular level, NMR relaxation still reflects the average character of local dipolar fields experienced by water protons.

RELAXATION IN MULTICOMPARTMENT SYSTEMS AND THE EFFECTS OF EXCHANGE

If at any time only a small proportion of water protons are in close juxtaposition to efficient relaxation sites, then the average water-proton relaxation will depend on how effectively and at what rate these effects are spread through the rest of the water population. There has been considerable debate about the precise nature of water in different environments in tissue and the degree to which these pools differ and exchange. However, as shown later, it is clear that in tissue some water molecules can be found in strongly absorbing, or binding, sites on relatively immobile macromolecular constituents; in a so-called bulk aqueous phase, which is separated by more than one water diameter from these constituents; or in "interfacial" regions between the macromolecular constituents and the bulk aqueous phase. The motions and relaxation interactions experienced by the water and ions while they are in these various environments are different. However, water molecules may migrate (or exchange) among these environments by diffusion, and such exchange processes have profound effects on the observable NMR relaxation phenomena. In 50 ms, water molecules diffuse distances of approximately 20 μm, so they sample many different environments on the cellular level during relaxation. The following discussion of exchange effects is based on the classification of processes originally described by Woessner[21] and illustrates how such exchange processes may affect the relaxation observed.

The simplest illustration of exchange effects is the case of two different environments when the residence time of a molecule in either is greater than the correlation time in each environment. These environments are labeled a and b, with their respective population fractions, P; average residence times, τ; and relaxation times, T. The environment

with the shorter relaxation time is arbitrarily labeled b. This basic example was considered by Zimmerman and Brittin.[25] The decay of transverse and longitudinal nuclear magnetism toward the equilibrium values is given by

(EQ. 4)

$$M(t) = P_a'\exp(-t/T_a')+P_b'\exp(-t/T')_b$$

where

$$1/T_a' = C_1 - C_2$$
$$1/T_b' = C_1 + C_2$$
$$P_b' = \left(\frac{1}{2}\right)-\left(\frac{1}{4}\right)\left[(P_b-P_a)\left(\frac{1}{T_a}-\frac{1}{T_b}\right)+\frac{1}{\tau_a}+\frac{1}{\tau_b}\right]/C_2$$
$$P_a' = 1 - P_b'$$

in which

$$C_1 = \left(\frac{1}{2}\right)\left[\frac{1}{T_a}+\frac{1}{T_b}+\frac{1}{\tau_a}+\frac{1}{\tau_b}\right]$$
$$C_1 = \left(\frac{1}{2}\right)\left[\left(\frac{1}{T_b}-\frac{1}{T_a}+\frac{1}{\tau_b}-\frac{1}{\tau_a}\right)^2+4/(\tau_a\tau_b)\right]^{\frac{1}{2}}$$

These equations describe both T1 and T2 when the NMR frequencies of a and b are equal. When the NMR frequencies are unequal, only T1 obeys these equations. In the general case, without further restrictions, Equation 4 is biexponential, reflecting the different relaxation time values in the two different environments. The degree to which this departure from exponential recovery is apparent depends on the precise conditions, some special cases of which are now considered.

There are several special cases relating to the relative values of the inherent relaxation times in each compartment and the average residence times of the molecules in the environments. In the case of very slow exchange in which

(EQ. 5)

$$\left[\frac{1}{\tau_a}+\frac{1}{\tau_b}\right] \ll \left[\frac{1}{T_b}-\frac{1}{T_a}\right]$$

the P_a' and P_b' values are very close to P_a and P_b, but the apparent relaxation times are slightly decreased.

(EQ. 6)

$$\frac{1}{T_a'} = \frac{1}{T_a}+\frac{1}{\tau_a}$$
$$\frac{1}{T_b'} = \frac{1}{T_b}+\frac{1}{\tau_b}$$

The two components may be distinguished in multiecho (T2) or multiple inversion-time (T1) experiments by appropriate analysis of the recovery curves. Such multicomponent behavior is most frequently observed for T2, especially when exchange is limited by low membrane permeability or if the physical dimensions of the compartments are larger than the distance over which molecules can diffuse in the time of the decay.

In the contrasting case of very rapid exchange obeying the condition

(EQ. 7)

$$\left[\frac{1}{\tau_a}+\frac{1}{\tau_b}\right] \gg \left[\frac{1}{T_b}-\frac{1}{T_a}\right]$$

the observable relaxation is single exponential with the weighted average relaxation rate

(EQ. 8)

$$\left(\frac{1}{T}\right)_{av} = P_a/T_a + P_b/T_b$$

which is independent of the precise value of the exchange rate. Thus if even a small fraction of water-occupying sites have relaxation much greater than the rest (e.g., water in which tumbling is slowed so that correlation times are lengthened to be much greater than in pure water), the average relaxation rate may still be dominated by this small pool. For example, if 1% of water relaxes with a rate of 100 sec^{-1} and the remainder acts like near-pure water with T1 = 1 sec, then the average T1 of the whole is reduced to 500 ms. This is an example of the third special case, which arises when $T_b \ll T_a$ and $P_a \approx 1$ (which also means $\tau_b \ll \tau_a$). The observed relaxation is then approximately single exponential with

(EQ. 9)

$$\frac{1}{T'_a} = \frac{1}{T_a} + P_b/(P_a T_b + P_b \tau_a)$$

A fourth special case is when the exchange rates are intermediate between the relaxation rates (i.e., $T_b \ll \tau_b, \tau_a \ll T_a$). In this case the observed relaxation is biexponential, with $P'_a = P_a$, $P'_b = P_b$ and

(EQ. 10)

$$T'_a = \tau_a$$
$$T'_b = T_b$$

These special cases show that even in simple two-component systems the observable relaxation phenomena can have many different dependencies on population fractions and exchange rates. Furthermore they show that relaxation may not be simple exponential when exchange is slow or intermediate.

It is common to assume that very rapid exchange occurs between bulk water and bound and interfacial water in biological systems. If 1 g of the dry-weight biological material directly decreases the relaxation times of C g of water, we obtain

(EQ. 11)

$$\left(\frac{1}{T}\right)_{av} = \frac{1}{T_a} + C(g/h)\left(\frac{1}{T_b} - \frac{1}{T_a}\right)$$

in which g is the number of grams of dry-weight biological material and h is the total weight of water in the sample. Small variations in the ratio of g/h (i.e., in the ratio of dry matter to water) may then markedly affect the relaxation rate, since $\frac{1}{T_b} - \frac{1}{T_a}$ is large. This is believed to be the origin for many increases in T1 or T2 in various pathologies, such as edematous changes after insults to tissue, or in rapidly dividing cells that have higher water fractions. Changes in tissue water content in general affect relaxation.

The effect of exchange on the observable transverse relaxation is different from Equation 4 when the NMR frequencies in the various environments are unequal. This fact is important when considering what additional processes shorten T2 compared with T1 because several surface groups (e.g., amides) on proteins may exchange protons with water and have different NMR chemical shifts. This frequency difference causes a further increase in the transverse relaxation rate. Under the condition of rapid exchange between two environments such that

(EQ. 12)

$$\left(\frac{1}{\tau_a} + \frac{1}{\tau_b}\right) \gg |\omega_a - \omega_b|, \left(\frac{1}{T_b} - \frac{1}{T_a}\right)$$

a single NMR frequency

$$\omega_{av} = P_a\omega_a + P_b\omega_b$$

is observed, representing the weighted average of the two components.[20,21]

$$\frac{1}{T2} = P_a/T2_a + P_b/T2_b + P_aP_b\tau_a\tau_b(\tau_a + \tau_b)^{-1}(\omega_a - \omega_b)^2$$

The assumed rapid exchange results in a weighted average NMR frequency and a transverse relaxation rate contribution that depends on the square of the difference in NMR frequencies. Chemical exchange contributes significantly to relaxation effects of tissue constituents, and when important it can account for some of the shortening of T2 that occurs at higher field strengths.[23]

RELAXATION IN SOLUTIONS OF MACROMOLECULES AND TISSUES

In general the relaxation times of hydrogen (and other nuclei) are significantly shortened in biological systems compared with pure water. In addition, the T2 values are several times smaller than T1. Such observations indicate that the average environments that the water molecules experience over time are significantly altered compared with pure water and dilute solutions. These changes may be partially explained by considering what happens when macromolecules, such as proteins or polysaccharides, are dissolved in solution. Usually the relaxation rates of the water increase linearly in direct proportion to the amount of solute present. The rate increase per gram is the relaxivity of the substance, and this depends strongly on the molecular weight of the solute and the nature of the chemical groups that characterize the surface exposed to the solvent. For example, Table 3-1 contains data on measured relaxation rate increases for pure proteins of different molecular weights, measured at 20 MHz. These data are plotted in Figure 3-4.

Larger proteins on average shorten relaxation times to a greater degree. Large polysaccharides, such as glycogen, also shorten relaxation times, so variations in the cellular concentrations of such molecules will likely affect relaxation rates.[11] Such effects have a straightforward interpretation, at least in principle. For example, water molecules in biological media are often in the vicinity of cellular constituents that contain hydroxyl and amine groups, which can strongly bind water mole-

Table 3-1   Relationship of Molecular Weight to Longitudinal Relaxivity for Selected Pure Proteins*

MOLECULAR WEIGHT (Daltons)	RELAXIVITY (sec^{-1}M^{-1}) AT 20 MHz
1,400	0.017
14,000	0.043
30,000	0.025
37,100	0.056
64,500	0.106
68,500	0.033
102,000	0.046
153,000	0.036
178,000	0.098

From reference 24.
*For comparison, liver relaxivity equals 0.19.

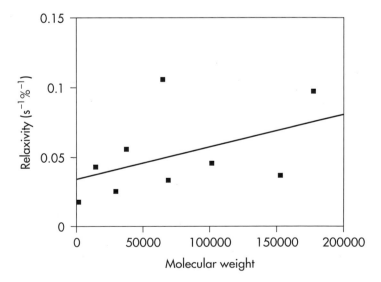

FIGURE 3-4   The dependence of protein relaxivity on molecular weight for a selection of proteins of molecular weight 1000 to 200,000 Daltons as measured at 20 MHz. In general there is an increase in the efficacy of proteins at shortened relaxation times as the individual molecules become larger and tumble more slowly.

cules. Water molecules bound to such hydrophilic groups have altered hydrogen bonding characteristics compared with bulk water and reduced hydrogen bonding overall because the accessibility to other water molecules is reduced. This is consistent with the well-documented observation that part of the water in biological cells does not freeze at 0° C. (Hydrogen bonding raises the freezing temperature of water compared with that of non–hydrogen-bonded water.) While associated with the macromolecule in this fashion, water protons may experience intermolecular dipolar relaxation interactions with the protons and nitrogen nuclei at the surface, as first shown by Edzes and Samulski[4] and as described later. They also may exchange protons with labile groups at the surface. In addition, the strongly binding sites on the relatively immobile macromolecules may increase the correlation times for the hydrogen atoms in the water of hydration. The dipolar field they experience there may be modulated by the rate at which the host macromolecule tumbles, which depends on its size, and perhaps by local motions of molecular segments. In a well-mixed system the influence of such sites may then be propagated through the sample via exchange mechanisms described later. Several workers have proposed detailed models to distinguish water molecules in different, well-defined environments within tissue, but there is little compelling evidence that such models are realistic or of general application to most situations. However, the aforementioned processes can explain much of the observed decrease of relaxation times in solutions of proteins or other macromolecules.

The precise natures of surface groups and the structures to which they are attached are clearly each expected to affect water relaxation in tissue, but precisely how the slower motions and relaxation properties of the macromolecules are communicated to the water is complex and still somewhat controversial. Two processes that can be important, collectively termed *magnetization transfer processes,* are considered later. However, although large proteins have significant relaxivities, quantitative comparisons of the rate increases per gram of dry material of pure proteins (Table 3-1) with the relaxation rates found for whole tissues reveals some major discrepancies. For example, for a tissue such as heart muscle, which is approximately 9% protein, with a spin-lattice relaxation rate at 20 MHz of approximately 2 sec^{-1}, the relaxivity of the solid component must on average equal approximately 0.2 $sec^{-1}\%^{-1}$, much beyond the typical relaxivities found for individual constituent proteins.[9,24] Earlier conjectures that relaxation in tissues can be derived from "an appropriately weighted superposition of the relaxation rates of homogeneous solutions of the cellular constituents"[17] are clearly inaccurate. Superimposing the relaxation rates of individual constituents underestimates the relaxation by at least a factor of 2 and more often an order of magnitude, particularly for T2. Consequently, although understanding the precise nature of relaxation in pure protein solutions is important, there are additional mechanisms and factors that must be invoked to explain relaxation in tissues. The most obvious difference lies in the manner in which macromolecules form larger assemblies and become immobilized in biological media compared with simple solutions. This supramolecular organization is essential to produce the range of relaxation behaviors seen in tissues but still relies on some form of exchange or mixing mechanism to affect most of the water.

MAGNETIZATION TRANSFER

We have suggested that relaxation in tissues is affected by interactions that occur between water protons and protons at or near the surface of macromolecules. Longitudinal proton magnetization can be exchanged between water and neighboring nuclei (whether interfacial water that is hydrogen bonded to the surface or protons within other chemical groups that are part of the macromolecule) by direct through-space dipolar couplings and so-called chemical exchange of protons. Such effects can be easily demonstrated in simple systems. For example, Figure 3-5 shows the effect of selectively inverting the water magnetization in a solution of polyethylene glycol. The water spin population is inverted, and this magnetization change is communicated via dipolar coupling to the nonexchangeable, nonpolar methylene protons in the polymer.[10] The magnetization of the CH_2 resonance in the high-resolution NMR spectrum then shows a transient increase and recovery as the spins reestablish equilibrium–a transient nuclear Overhauser enhancement effect. There is ample clear evidence that such through-space dipolar cross-relaxation can occur between water and other protons at

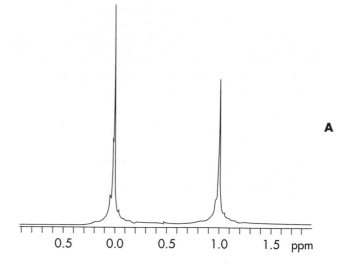

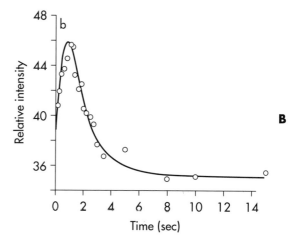

FIGURE 3-5   Magnetization transfer in polyethylene glycol (PEG). **A,** High-resolution NMR spectrum of solution of 8000 Daltons molecular weight PEG at 200 MHz. The two peaks correspond to water (H_2O) and methylene (CH_2) protons. **B,** Time course of the amplitude of the methylene resonance line after selective inversion of the water. The transient increase from equilibrium value indicates transfer of magnetization from the water pool via dipolar coupling. (From reference 10.)

the surface of macromolecules. In addition, chemical dissociation of protons can occur at rates that are pH dependent, providing possible interchanges between water and surface sites (hydroxyls, amides, and so forth) as intact water molecules move constantly in and out of the hydration layers of macromolecular surfaces and exchange protons. Collectively these processes have been termed *corporeal exchange*[20] to distinguish them from cross-relaxation.

A good deal of evidence supports the notion that cross-relaxation and chemical exchange are important in tissues. For example, substitution of most of the water and labile protons with deuterons (e.g., by soaking tissue samples in D_2O) reduces the relaxation rate of the remaining water protons but only by approximately 20%[24] even at high degrees of deuteration. This result may be interpreted as evidence that water relaxation does not depend much on the so-called hydrodynamic effects produced within the sample (i.e., alterations in the tumbling of the water molecules in the bulk phase that influence water proton–proton interactions from simple viscosity effects) that should be dramatically reduced by substitution of H with D (in contrast to the case for pure solutions described earlier). Instead it demonstrates that the dominant mechanism for relaxation of protons is unaffected by such replacement, implying that dipolar coupling to nonexchanging protons within the solute plays a major role.

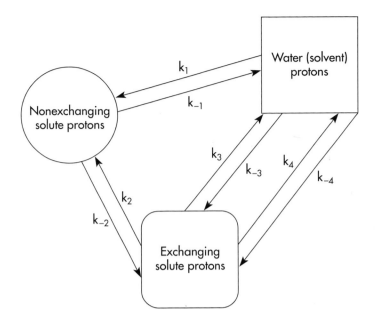

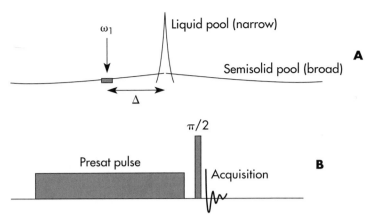

FIGURE 3-6   **A,** Schematic representation of the high-resolution proton spectrum of a sample containing water (narrow resonance) and a semisolid component (broad background). **B,** In magnetization-transfer experiments, a conventional $\pi/2$ RF pulse is preceded by a saturating pulse transmitted with amplitude ω_1 at an offset frequency Δ.

This figure summarizes magnetization transfer pathways in a three-compartment system composed of water and exchanging, as well as nonexchanging, macromolecular (solute) protons.

Different rate constants are included to differentiate chemical exchange (k_4) from dipolar interactions (k_1, k_2, k_3) between protons. In dilute solutions of proteins the dipolar cross-relaxation rate for water is negligible, and between exchangeable and nonexchangeable protons it is very slow.[15] The nonexchanging pool gives a separable, faster-relaxing component of magnetization if T1 is measured. In addition, the average T1 for the water and exchanging proton pools will show a T1-field dispersion when the NMR frequency is the reciprocal of the rotational correlation time of the protein.[18] When the lifetime of exchanging protons is short or when the rotational motion of the macromolecule is rapid, the dipolar fields that might contribute to cross-relaxation fluctuate rapidly, and cross-relaxation is negligible. However, more significant contributions to relaxation arise when proteins are immobilized or constrained in a more rigid matrix, and the protons in the matrix become more solidlike (or icelike) and may undergo spin exchange with neighbors. This exchange can propagate a form of spin diffusion deep into the structure until efficient relaxation sites are encountered. Such effects are believed to be very important in tissues, and special techniques have been devised to quantify such mechanisms. The supramacromolecular organization within tissue is a key feature that explains why the relaxation rate per gram of solid content for tissue is much greater than for isolated proteins.[9] Tissue relaxation partially reflects the larger-scale organization of macromolecules into more complex structures, and when this occurs, cross-relaxation and magnetization transfer become important contributions to the overall behavior. Some of the evidence and methods used to study these processes are described later.

We have seen that relaxation in tissues is strongly influenced by the presence of solidlike protons that occur in organized structures, such as proteins and lipids. These protons are normally invisible in MRI experiments because of their inherently short transverse relaxation times. However, indirect effects of the solidlike pool may be detected and visualized in MRI. This type of image contrast is broadly characterized as magnetization-transfer contrast (MTC). There are a variety of ways to measure or demonstrate magnetization-transfer effects. One such approach is to selectively excite the longitudinal magnetization in the water-proton pool and monitor its transfer into the other pools, as shown earlier for polyethylene glycol. In practice this transfer may occur via chemical exchange or dipolar cross-relaxation into nonexchanging protons, and it is often difficult to identify which of these processes dominates in biological samples. Magnetization transfer was first demonstrated in the 1970s by Edzes and Samulski[4] using an inversion recovery experiment to investigate relaxation mechanisms in hydrated collagen. The experiment involved changing the length of the inversion

pulse in a T1 measurement such that the pulse varied from a short nonselective pulse (which inverted all protons in the sample) to a long selective pulse (which inverted only free water protons while leaving those of the solid pool unaffected). As the inversion pulse becomes less selective, the solid and liquid pools are placed in different energy states, and the resultant biphasic decay can then be used to calculate the magnetization exchange between these two different pools. An initial rapid decay component yielded a direct measure of magnetization exchange in collagen with a rate of about 40 sec^{-1}. After this transient period the water and protein pools were equilibrated and the observed relaxation decay is simply that of the free water pool.

Another useful way of measuring transfer rates can be used when, as in tissues, the transverse relaxation time of the exchanging component is much less than that of the water protons. Goldman and Shen[8] used three nonselective 90-degree pulses, $90_{+x} - t - 90_{-x} - T - 90_{+x}$. By setting the interval t between the first and second pulses to be several times the transverse relaxation time of the solidlike component but still much less than the water relaxation time (i.e., approximately 100 μs), all transverse magnetization in the nonexchanging proton pool is lost. The second pulse realigns only the water and exchangeable protons with the field, and then magnetization transfer occurs between the pools in the interval T. The third pulse produces a signal that depends on T and the rate of magnetization transfer, and by fitting the recovery curve as a function of the mixing time T, Gochberg et al[7] have been able to directly measure cross-relaxation rates in tissues and tissue models.

More recent magnetization transfer pulse sequences have exploited the idea of partially saturating the semisolid pool with respect to the liquid pool through the use of preparation pulses.[22] This is illustrated schematically in Figure 3-6, *A*, where the separate but overlapping NMR line shapes of the macromolecular and water protons are shown. If a long, low-amplitude RF pulse is applied many kilohertz off-resonance to water, as shown in Figure 3-6, *B*, we can take advantage of the fact that the macromolecular spins have a much shorter T2 (approximately 10 μs) and a much broader resonance line width (10 s of kHz) than the water. The preparation pulse will therefore preferentially saturate the solidlike protons while barely affecting the water protons. Magnetization exchange between the two pools then transfers saturation into the water pool so that a subsequent measurement returns a reduced signal intensity from the water. This technique lends itself to imaging quite readily, and a variety of related methods have been used to produce MTC. Partial saturation of the water can occur from the off-resonance irradiation, but by using a series of prepulses the rate of magnetization transfer can be measured. Indeed a quantitative model to interpret magnetization transfer behavior that is relevant to imaging studies has been developed[13] and may be usefully considered to illustrate the concepts introduced earlier.

The sample is treated as consisting of two pools—a liquid pool of free water (denoted as pool a) and a solidlike pool (denoted as pool b) (Figure 3-7). This model makes no distinction between protons actually on the macromolecule or associated water, which may have solidlike characteristics. The equilibrium magnetization densities of the two pools are denoted M_{0a} and M_{0b}, respectively. The two pools are coupled by a constant (R), which defines the rate of magnetization exchange between the two pools. The intrinsic longitudinal relaxation rates for each pool are denoted by R_a and R_b, and the transverse relaxation times for each pool are $T2_a$ and $T2_b$. The first-order rate constant for magnetization transfer (k_{MTC}) is given by the product RM_{0b},[13] and corresponds to the rate at which magnetization is transferred from pool a to pool b. Under steady state equilibrium conditions, the Bloch equations can be solved in terms of the system parameters (R, M_{0a}, M_{0b}, $T2_a$, $T2_b$, R_a, and R_b) and the pulse-sequence parameters (offset frequency, Δ, and presaturation amplitude, $\omega_1 = \gamma B_1$). The measured magnetization of the free water pool a is then given by

(EQ. 13)

$$M_{za} = \frac{R_b RM_{0b} + R_{rfb}R_a + R_bR_a + RR_a}{(R_a + R_{rfa} + RM_{0b})(R_b + R_{rfb} + R) - RRM_{0b}}$$

where

(EQ. 14)

$$R_{rfa} = \frac{\omega_1^2 T2_a}{1 + (2\pi\Delta T2_a)^2}$$

is a rate that accounts for the direct saturation of the liquid pool, and its transverse magnetization is assumed to decay exponentially. The direct saturation of the solidlike pool can be modeled in different ways that represent the altered characteristics of these less-mobile protons. For example, the resonance line shape may be chosen to be either a lorentzian (Equation 15A) or a gaussian (Equation 15B) line shape:

(EQ. 15A)

$$R_{rfb} = \frac{\omega_1^2 T2_b}{1 = (2\pi\Delta T2_b)^2}$$

(EQ. 15B)

$$R_{rfb} = \omega_1^2 \sqrt{\frac{\pi}{2}} T2_b \exp\left(-\frac{(\pi\Delta T2_b)^2}{2}\right)$$

The choice of solid-pool line shape depends on the degree of mobility of the macromolecular pool: A lorentzian is more appropriate to describe liquidlike environments, and a gaussian line shape is more suitable for a rigid lattice. Recent experiments have shown that for certain tissues a more complex line shape is required to adequately describe experimental data.[14] Experimentally the characteristic rates and pool sizes for a given system can be obtained through a steady state saturation transfer technique by measuring the water magnetization (M_{za}) as a function of both the presaturation power level (ω_1) and offset frequency (Δ). Fitting the data to the form given by Equations 13 through 15 allows the determination of the other magnetization transfer parameters.

This procedure has been used to characterize a variety of systems ranging from agar gels to various tissue types.[6,13,14] For the case when the solid pool is completely saturated ($M_{zb} = 0$), the first-order rate constant can be evaluated using an expression that is often quoted in the literature, that is,

(EQ. 16)

$$k_{MTC} = RM_{0b} \cong \left(1 - \frac{M_{za}}{M_{za}(0)}\right)\frac{1}{T1_{sat}}$$

where M_{za} is the measured magnetization in the presence of the saturating pulse, $M_{za}(0)$ is the magnetization without a saturation pulse, and $T1_{sat}$ is the measured longitudinal relaxation when the solid pool is saturated. Equation 16 often has been used to define the rate of magnetization transfer in vivo, but the condition of complete saturation of the semisolid pool is rarely if ever attained in magnetization-transfer imaging sequences, and more time-consuming experiments are needed to accurately represent the system.

Using a quantum-mechanical–based analysis, it has been shown that at the high fields used in clinical MRI the contribution of dipolar cross-relaxation to the first-order rate constant for magnetization transfer (k_{MTC}) is simply proportional to the probability of a so-called zero-order quantum transition induced by magnetic dipolar interactions. The zero-order transitions correspond to mutual spin flips of two adjacent nuclei, which thereby transfer energy between the coupled pools without a loss of energy to the surroundings. Such zero-order transitions also account for transverse relaxation (see earlier discussion) but do not directly contribute to longitudinal relaxation. This correlation between dipolar coupled T2 and MT effects can be observed in practical MRI at high field because in many cases magnetization-transfer image contrast follows T2 contrast very closely.

Because supramolecular organization is key for magnetization effects and adequately explaining relaxation times in tissue, it is instructive to consider some of the factors that may be important for its regulation. For this purpose, model biopolymers, in which some of the factors can be varied in controlled fashion, have been studied in detail. For example, Figure 3-8 shows the effects of cross-linking on magnetization transfer between water and the globular protein, bovine serum albumin (BSA), which forms cross-links when it is denatured chemically or after heating. Figure 3-8 shows the water signal intensity as a

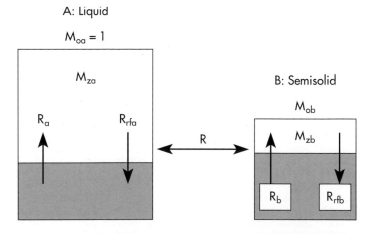

FIGURE 3-7 Schematic diagram of the two-pool model used to interpret magnetization-transfer measurements. M_{0a}, Total number of liquid spins; M_{0b}, total number of semisolid spins; R, MTC transfer rate (RM_{0b}, rate of transfer from A to B; RM_{0a}, rate of transfer from B to A); R_a, longitudinal relaxation rate of pool A; R_b, longitudinal relaxation rate of pool B; R_{rf}, rate of loss of longitudinal magnetization because of direct saturation from the off-resonance irradiation.

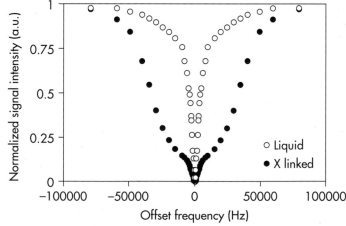

FIGURE 3-8 Z spectrum of BSA. The water signal amplitude is measured as a function of the frequency offset from resonance of the preirradiation pulse for a 20% BSA solution and for a heat-denatured cross-linked BSA gel.

function of presaturation pulse offset frequency for dissolved liquid BSA and a sample that has been heated to form a gel. The data representing the dependence of longitudinal magnetization on offset frequency are referred to as a *Z spectrum*.[12] In this case it is apparent that as the BSA becomes immobilized through cross-linking, the Z spectrum broadens.

To more clearly illustrate the role of solute mobility, other model polymer systems in which the degree of structure can be carefully controlled also have been studied. An example of such a polymer system is polyacrylamide gel (PAG) composed of acrylamide (AC) and N,N′-methylene-bis-acrylamide (BIS). PAGs are used extensively for gel electrophoresis in biochemistry for macromolecular separations. The structures of the monomer AC, cross-linking agent BIS, and PAG are illustrated in Figure 3-9. The cross-linking agent forms bridges between acrylamide chains in the polymer, thereby making the system more rigid. Figure 3-10, *A* and *B*, shows results of relaxation and magnetization transfer measurements as a function of cross-linker density.[16] In Figure 3-10, *B*, mixtures of the monomers demonstrate only a weak relaxation rate dependence on the amount of cross-linking agent, whereas the polymers demonstrate a much stronger dependence. The transverse relaxation rate shows a biphasic dependence, increasing rapidly above 40% cross-linking, at which point (Figure 3-10) magnetization-transfer effects between the water pool and the polymer also are measurable. The change in the gel behavior is consistent with a structural change as cross-linking density is increased. At greater than 30% cross-linking density, small beadlike structures begin to form as the hydrophobic BIS molecules cross-link tightly with each other and with the residual AC.[16] Such structures are more rigid than the structures formed at low cross-linking density, which can be considered a flexible network of chain structures. Once this structural change occurs in PAG, the increased rigidity allows efficient spin diffusion. The change in magnetization transfer with BIS corresponds to a linear increase in the density of these structures.

The presence of specific groups on the surface of macromolecules is another important determinant of relaxation and magnetization transfer. It appears, for example, that for lipid systems a primary conduit is via the hydroxyl groups. In lipid bilayer samples where hydroxyl groups on the lipid head were replaced by relatively inert chlorine, magnetization transfer was much reduced.[5] Further work has shown that hydroxyl groups in cholesterol are largely responsible for magnetization transfer in white matter,[19] and loss of these specific species may account for the altered relaxation of white matter in demyelinating diseases. The amide group is clearly an important determinant in the relaxation of polyacrylamide. Substituting amides with other groups, such as carboxyls, or changing the pH so that chemical exchange is slowed alters the rate

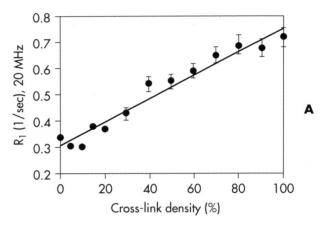

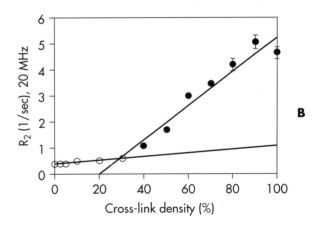

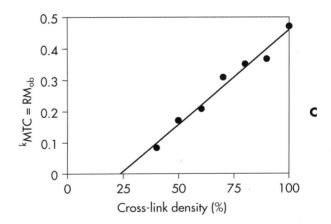

FIGURE 3-9   Structures of AC **(A)**, BIS **(B)**, and two possible forms of cross-linked PAG **(C** and **D)**. The amide protons are indicated in bold.

FIGURE 3-10   Results of measurements of relaxation rates and magnetization transfer on PAG for different cross-linking densities. **A,** Longitudinal relaxation rate. **B,** Transverse relaxation rate. **C,** Rate of magnetization transfer, $RM_{0b} = k_{MTC}$.

and importance of magnetization transfer.[7] Work is currently in progress to further quantitate what specific sites on macromolecules are responsible for magnetization transfer to understand the molecular biology of relaxation processes.

SUMMARY

We have emphasized only the general features of proton relaxation in complex media and have introduced most of the types of processes that are believed to be involved in water relaxation in biological tissues. This chapter is not a comprehensive survey of all phenomena; notably, we have not included effects from anisotropic ordering of structures that can occur and have small effects on the transverse relaxation of some tissues[2] or many specific examples of precise explanations of changes that occur in pathology because these are not of general application. Tissue is a highly complex and heterogeneous collection of water environments, and it is probably naive to expect to be able to interpret gross changes in the bulk relaxation times of tissue water in anything other than gross pathological changes, such as increases in water content or loss of cellular integrity. The signals from water that are depicted in MR images reflect a myriad of interactions at the atomic level. Water molecules sample a wide variety of tissue subcompartments, and what we measure is the net, time-averaged effect of these multiple interactions. Relaxation times are not found nor expected to be sensitive to individual biological processes that might dramatically alter the specificity of MRI. However, it remains to be seen whether more detailed understanding of the factors that affect relaxation can add to the utility of MR measurements in clinical practice.

REFERENCES

1. Abragam A: The principles of nuclear magnetism, London, 1969, Oxford University Press.
2. Berendsen HJC: Nuclear magnetic resonance study of collagen hydration, J Chem Phys 36:3297, 1962.
3. Bloembergen N, Purcell EM, and Pound RV: Relaxation effects in nuclear magnetic resonance absorption, Phys Rev 73:679, 1948.
4. Edzes HT, and Samulski ET: Cross relaxation and spin diffusion in the proton NMR of hydrated collagen, Nature 265:521, 1977.
5. Fralix TA, Ceckler TL, Wolff SD, et al: Lipid bilayers and water proton magnetization transfer: effect of cholesterol, Magn Reson Med 18:214, 1991
6. Gochberg DF, Kennan RP, and Gore JC: Quantitative studies of magnetization transfer by selective excitation and T1 recovery, Magn Reson Med 38:224, 1997.
7. Gochberg DF, Kennan RP, Maryanski MJ, et al: The role of specific side groups and pH in magnetization transfer in polymers, J Magn Reson 131:191, 1998.
8. Goldman M, and Shen L: Spin-spin relaxation in LaF_3, Phys Rev 144:321, 1966.
9. Gore JC, Brown MS, Mizumoto CT, et al: Influence of glycogen on water proton relaxation times, Magn Reson Med 3:463, 1986.
10. Gore JC, Brown MS, and Armitage IM: An analysis of magnetic cross-relaxation between water and methylene protons in a model system, Magn Reson Med 9:333, 1989.
11. Gore JC, and Brown MS: The pathophysiological significance of relaxation. In Partain CL, Price RR, Patton JA, et al, eds: Magnetic resonance imaging, vol 2, Philadelphia, 1988, WB Saunders.
12. Grad J, and Bryant RG: Nuclear magnetic cross-relaxation spectroscopy, J Magn Reson 90:1, 1990.
13. Henkelman RM, Huang X, Xiang Q, et al: Quantitative interpretation of magnetization transfer, Magn Reson Med 29:759, 1993.
14. Henkelman RM, and Morrison C: A model for magnetization transfer in tissues, Magn Reson Med 33:475, 1995.
15. Hills BP: The proton exchange cross-relaxation model of water relaxation in biopolymer systems, Mol Phys 76:489, 1992.
16. Kennan RP, Richardson KA, Zhong J, et al: The effects of cross-link density and chemical exchange on magnetization transfer in polyacrylamide gels, J Magn Reson 110(B):267, 1996.
17. Koenig SH, and Brown RD: Relaxometry of tissue. In Gupta RK, ed: NMR spectroscopy of cells and organisms, vol 2, Boca Raton, 1987, CRC Press.
18. Koenig SH, and Brown RD: Field-cycling relaxometry of protein solutions and tissue: implications for MRI, Prog Nucl Magn Reson Spectr 22:487, 1990.
19. Koenig SH, Brown RD, Spiller M, et al: Relaxometry of brain: why white matter appears bright in MRI, Magn Reson Med 14:482, 1990.
20. Winkler H, and Michel D: Exchange processes in NMR, Adv Colloid Interface Sci 23:149, 1985.
21. Woessner D: Relaxation theory with applications to biological systems. In Pettegrew JW, ed: NMR: principles and applications to biomedical research, New York, 1989, Springer-Verlag.
22. Wolff SD, and Balaban RS: Magnetization transfer contrast (MTC) and tissue water proton relaxation in vivo, Magn Reson Med 10:135, 1989.
23. Zhong J, Gore JC, and Armitage IM: Relative contributions of chemical exchange and other relaxation mechanisms in protein solutions and tissues, Magn Reson Med 11:295, 1989.
24. Zhong J, Gore JC, and Armitage IM: Quantitative studies of hydrodynamic effects and cross-relaxation in protein solutions and tissues with proton and deuteron longitudinal relaxation times, Magn Reson Med, 13:192, 1990.
25. Zimmerman JR, and Brittin WE: Nuclear magnetic resonance studies in multiple phase systems: lifetimes of a water molecule in an absorbing phase in silica gel, Phys Chem 6:1328, 1957.

4 Image Contrast and Noise

R. Edward Hendrick

 KEY POINTS

- All MRI pulse sequences include a combination of hydrogen spin density, T1, and T2 (or T2*) contrast. The particular weighting of these inherent sources of tissue contrast is determined by RF pulse intensity "tip angles," pulse sequences, and interpulse timing parameters.
- SE image T1-weighting is determined by the TR and T2-weighting by the TE; hydrogen spin-density weighting is always present.
- Inversion recovery image T1-weighting is determined by TI, while TR has a minor effect and TE controls T2-weighted contrast.
- Gradient-echo image contrast is determined primarily by the tip angle (θ). Short TR values permit rapid planar (2D FT) imaging and volume (3D FT) imaging.
- Statistical noise is usually more apparent at low magnetic field strengths; it can be minimized by increasing the number of acquisitions per phase-encoding step, by decreasing the bandwidth, and by decreasing the sensitive volume of the receiver coil.
- Systematic noise is usually more apparent at high magnetic field strengths; it can be decreased by minimizing patient motion, by eliminating signal-producing tissues lying outside the field of view in the acquired plane, and by increasing the number of averages per phase-encoding step.
- Detection of pathology is improved by maximizing signal and contrast relative to noise.

The author thanks Dr. Ulrich Raff for providing the computer-generated color contour plots and synthetic images used in this chapter and is grateful to Drs. Anne Osborn, Lawrence Jacobs, and Jack Simon for providing the clinical examples and Ms. Paula Nichols for providing the artwork.

OVERVIEW

Adequate contrast among normal tissues is necessary for good anatomical definition, and adequate contrast between normal and diseased tissues is essential for sensitivity to disease. The basis of inherent tissue contrast in computed tomography (CT) is electron density, which varies by as much as 100% between soft tissues and bone but by only a small percentage among soft tissues. The primary sources of inherent tissue contrast in magnetic resonance imaging (MRI) are threefold—hydrogen spin densities (N[H]), longitudinal recovery times (T1), and transverse relaxation times (T2). Although hydrogen densities within soft tissues typically vary by only a few percent, the hydrogen contributing to the measured MR signal (referred to as the *hydrogen spin density*) tends to vary by a greater amount, up to 30% among soft tissues. T1 and T2 relaxation times often vary even more widely, sometimes varying among soft tissues by more than 100%. For example, the T1 and T2 values of cerebrospinal fluid (CSF) are several times the T1 and T2 values, respectively, of white matter and gray matter (Table 4-1).

What stands between inherent tissue contrast and resultant image contrast on a given MR system are a number of user-selectable imaging parameters, such as the choice of imaging pulse sequence and timing parameters within a selected pulse sequence (Figure 4-1). The effect of varying user-selectable imaging parameters is shown in Figure 4-2, which depicts brain images of a 39-year-old woman with multiple sclerosis (MS). Depending on the choice of interpulse delay times, MS lesions appear slightly darker than, isointense with, or brighter than normal brain tissues.

On both CT and MRI, image noise is the primary deterrent to the discrimination of tissues and the detection of low-contrast lesions. The ratio of signal difference (or contrast) to noise, the contrast-to-noise ratio (CNR), is an accepted figure of merit indicating how well a given pulse sequence and choice of imaging parameters will perform in revealing disease.[7,16]

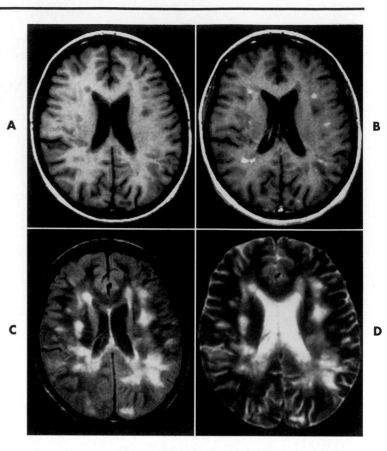

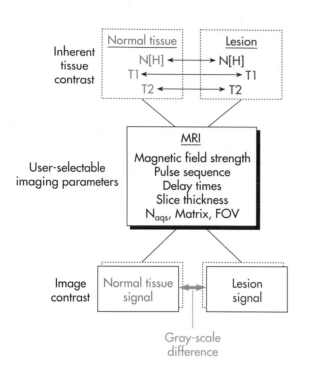

FIGURE 4-1   User-selectable (extrinsic) imaging parameters determine translation of inherent tissue contrast (determined by N[H], T1, and T2 values of tissues) into image contrast.

FIGURE 4-2   SE images of a 39-year-old woman with clinically proven MS. Only a single slice within the full brain study is shown. **A,** SE 600/20 image, precontrast. Several MS plaques show up as darker regions within white matter. **B,** SE 600/20 postgadolinium study shows contrast enhancement of some, potentially new growth, MS regions. **C,** SE 2000/30 image shows many extensive areas of MS involvement and clearly differentiates MS from brain and CSF. **D,** SE 2000/90 image. Increased CSF signal intensity matches that of MS plaques, complicating lesion definition. (Courtesy J. Simon and L. Jacobs.)

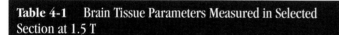

Table 4-1   Brain Tissue Parameters Measured in Selected Section at 1.5 T

TISSUE	T1 (ms)	T2 (ms)	N[H]
White matter	510	67	0.61
Gray matter	760	77	0.69
Edema	900	126	0.86
Cerebrospinal fluid	2650	280	1.00
Upper cystic fluid (extracellular methemoglobin)	1080	215	1.12
Lower cystic fluid (intracellular deoxyhemoglobin)	720	43	1.02
Methemoglobin	460	106	0.96

(EQ. 4-1)

$$C_{N[H]} = \frac{N[H_B] - N[H_A]}{N[H_B] + N[H_A]}$$

(EQ. 4-2)

$$C_{T1} = \frac{T1_B - T1_A}{T1_B + T1_A}$$

(EQ. 4-3)

$$C_{T2} = \frac{T2_B - T2_A}{T2_B + T2_A}$$

MRI, however, is constantly pushing toward faster scan times, thinner slices, higher in-plane spatial resolution, and more specialized techniques, such as three-dimensional (3D) gradient-echo, fast spin-echo (FSE), and echo-planar imaging (EPI) to facilitate the detection of smaller lesions. All of these imaging demands tend to reduce both the signal-to-noise ratio (SNR) and CNR, placing a premium on maximizing SNR and CNR.

Inherent Tissue Contrast

Tissue contrast derives primarily from inherent N[H], T1, and T2 differences. Other sources of tissue contrast, such as flow, magnetic susceptibility inhomogeneities, and chemical shift, are discussed more extensively in other chapters.

Inherent N[H], T1, and T2 contrast between two tissues (A and B) can be defined in terms of the characteristics of the two tissues as follows:

Expressed in this manner, inherent N[H], T1, and T2 contrasts are dimensionless quantities, with each source of tissue contrast on an equal footing regardless of the different physical dimensions of different tissue parameters.

Inherent tissue properties remain essentially unchanged regardless of the imaging method. Although defined only for MRI, T1, T2, and N[H] will not change simply because a different pulse sequence or a different set of timing parameters is chosen.

Most tissue T1 values increase with increasing magnetic field strength.[1,2] This is analogous to the situation in plain radiography or CT, where linear attenuation coefficients (also inherent tissue properties) change with the effective energy of the x-ray beam. The T1 values of different tissues also increase at different rates as the applied magnetic field is increased,[1,2] so inherent T1 contrast (C_{T1}) may be different at different magnetic field strengths. This is analogous to the change in subject contrast with a change in effective x-ray energy in radiography or CT.

Available data on most tissues indicate that inherent T2 values and therefore inherent T2 contrast remain approximately constant with changing magnetic field strength.[1,2]

The dependence of N[H] on magnetic field strength depends on its definition. If N[H] is strictly defined to be the amount of hydrogen per unit volume, then N[H] is independent of magnetic field strength. More often, however, N[H] is defined to be proportional to the tissue magnetization in a given voxel, which increases with magnetic field strength as a result of a greater imbalance of hydrogen nuclei pointing along the externally applied magnetic field. Defined in this way, the N[H] value of each tissue increases proportionately with increasing magnetic field strength, whereas the inherent N[H] contrast, defined by Equation 4-1, remains constant with increasing magnetic field strength.

Image Contrast

Image contrast may be defined analogously to inherent tissue contrast in terms of the signals from the two tissues (A and B):

(EQ. 4-4)

$$C_{image} = \frac{|S_B - S_A|}{|S_B + S_A|}$$

where S_A and S_B are the signal strengths from the two tissues between which contrast is being measured. In MRI as in CT, however, negative signals are sometimes possible, and in some cases, especially when $S_A + S_B$ is small, this definition of contrast does not accurately reflect the level of tissue differentiation observed in the image. A more acceptable definition of contrast in MR images is analogous to that used in CT[31]:

(EQ. 4-5)

$$C_{image} = \frac{|S_B - S_A|}{S_{ref}}$$

where S_{ref} is some reference signal that remains constant, independent of the choice of tissues, pulse sequences, or interpulse delay times. In CT, S_A and S_B represent CT numbers in Hounsfield units (HU), and S_{ref} is generally taken to be 1000 HU. In MRI, S_A and S_B are signal strengths in arbitrary units that vary from sequence to sequence and from scanner to scanner. No standard has been established for S_{ref} in MRI. In both CT and MRI, image contrast defined in this way is directly proportional to the signal difference between tissues. Consequently the terms *contrast* and *signal difference* are used interchangeably.[16]

Extrinsic (user-selectable) imaging parameters, such as the choice of pulse sequences, interpulse delay times, and number of acquisitions per phase-encoding step (N_{aqs}, or N_{ex}), can dramatically affect the signal from each tissue and the image contrast between tissues. It is important to understand the effect of user-selectable imaging parameters on the translation of inherent tissue contrast into image contrast.

Image Noise

Image noise is the primary obstacle to the detection of low-contrast lesions. There are two main categories of image noise: (1) statistical (or random) noise, and (2) systematic (nonrandom or structured) noise. Figure 4-3 illustrates both types of noise in MR images. Statistical noise is the pixel-to-pixel variation in signal intensities, apparent even for uniform tissues, caused by random signal fluctuations measured during signal sampling. At magnetic field strengths used for imaging, most statistical image noise is the result of eddy currents set up in the patient, producing spurious background signals that add to or subtract from true signals caused by precessing tissue magnetization.[22] The results are random fluctuations in pixel intensities spread across the entire reconstructed image (Figure 4-3, *A* and *B*). Statistical noise is reduced relative to signal by increasing the voxel volume (slice thickness or in-plane pixel size), by increasing the number of acquisitions per phase-encoding step, by decreasing the sensitive volume of the receiver coil, or by decreasing the bandwidth, thereby narrowing the range of frequencies over which noise can be recorded.

Except for extremely low SNR situations, systematic noise is usually more perverse and more confusing to image interpretation. Systematic noise consists of nonrandom signal variations that arise from a number of possible sources, including patient motion, such as respiration, vascular, and CSF pulsations; receiver-coil or gradient-coil motion; aliasing; and data truncation (Gibbs) artifacts. Although sometimes useful to the experienced radiologist, such systematic noise

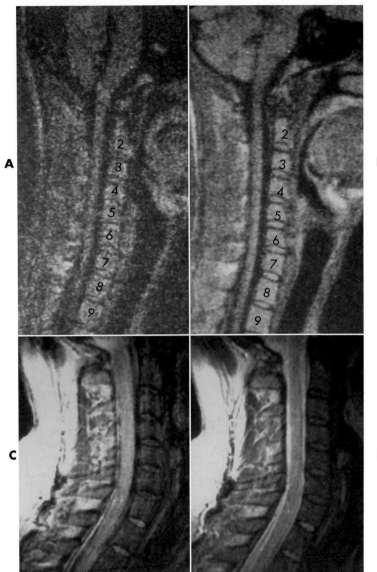

FIGURE 4-3 Cervical spine images illustrating statistical and systematic noise. **A,** Suboptimal cervical spine image collected in 1985 on a low-field (0.15 T) scanner using a body receiver coil rather than a specialized cervical spine receiver coil. Pulse sequence is an SE 500/30, 5-mm slice thickness, 256 × 256 matrix. Image shows a high level of statistical noise. **B,** Identically acquired cervical spine image, but with a 10-mm slice thickness. The SNR is improved by a factor of approximately 2. **C,** High-field (1.5 T) acquisition using an SE 2000/80, 256 × 256, without any motion suppression or gating. **D,** Identically acquired image to **C,** but with cardiac gating and first-order (constant velocity) flow compensation, reducing the level of systematic noise.

reveals itself as spurious signals in the image that do not reflect but tend to mask true inherent tissue properties. Figure 4-3, *C* and *D,* shows cervical spine images illustrating systematic noise resulting from CSF and spinal cord pulsations.

Both statistical and systematic noise tend to mask the detection of low-contrast lesions. In most imaging situations the CNR governs the ability to detect low-contrast lesions.[7] This chapter concludes with a discussion of CNRs to provide an understanding of the effect of user-selectable imaging parameters on CNRs and low-contrast lesion detection. The chapter begins with a simple discussion of the mechanisms affecting signal and contrast in MR images.

Contrast Model

A brain example is used to illustrate the concept of tissue contrast. The example consists of a brain section of a 41-year-old woman with a history of breast cancer who had imaging performed because of flulike symptoms. Figure 4-4, *A*, is a labeled schematic drawing of the brain section; Figure 4-4, *B* to *D*, displays three original images acquired in the same section of brain using different SE timing parameters on a 1.5-Tesla (T) scanner. Table 4-1 lists tissue parameters extracted numerically from these three primary images for white matter, gray matter, edema, CSF, and the two cystic fluids: the upper fluid identified as extracellular methemoglobin and the lower cystic fluid identified as intracellular deoxyhemoglobin in packed, intact cells. No metastatic breast cancer is visible in the selected section.

T1 and T2 relaxation times are listed in units of milliseconds; spin densities are listed in dimensionless units, scaled so that CSF has a spin density of 1.0. The tissues listed (other than the blood products) are typical of most cellular tissues in that tissues with higher T1 values also have higher T2 values and often have higher hydrogen spin densities. Intracellular deoxyhemoglobin differs from this rule by having a smaller T2/T1 ratio than the other brain tissues, whereas methemoglobin differs by having a larger T2/T1 ratio. These variations in T2/T1 can be explained by the relaxation effects of iron in deoxyhemoglobin and methemoglobin on hydrogen.[10,11]

The brain model is typical in that lesions or edematous regions within normal tissues usually have longer T1 and T2 relaxation times than the normal tissues themselves. (Note that in Table 4-1 edema has higher T1 and T2 values than normal white matter.) Only a few types of lesions, such as lipomas, melanomas, and fibrous lesions, deviate from this general rule of having higher T1 and T2 values than surrounding normal tissues.

Although data on hydrogen spin densities are limited, hydrogen spin densities are usually directly correlated with relaxation times (i.e., tissues with longer T1 and T2 values also tend to have higher spin-density values). This correlated behavior between hydrogen spin densities, T1 values, and T2 values has been demonstrated for brain white matter lesions[9] and appears to be generally true for most other lesions. In some types of lesions, such as metastatic liver cancer, however, although the T1 and T2 values for the lesion are almost always higher than those of the normal liver; N[H] values for lesions are variable from patient to pa-

tient and not consistently correlated with T1 and T2 values (Stark DD: personal communication, 1987).

There are a number of interesting tissues in the brain section of Figure 4-4. The appearances of the cystic fluids in the images that appear throughout the chapter illustrate the effect of pulse sequences and timing parameters on blood products. However, as a more basic illustration of contrast between tissues, two representative tissues—edema and white matter—are examined. The model of edema versus white matter is representative of contrast between other pathological and normal tissues, such as MS lesions versus white matter, most tumors versus normal brain tissues, and liver cancer versus normal liver. Inherent T1, T2, and spin-density contrast between edema and white matter in this example can be calculated by substituting the appropriate tissue parameters from Table 4-1 into Equations 4-1 to 4-3, with white matter as tissue A and edema as tissue B:

(EQ. 4-6)
$$C_{T1} = \frac{T1_B - T1_A}{T1_B + T1_A} = \frac{900 - 510 \text{ ms}}{900 + 510 \text{ ms}} = 0.277$$

(EQ. 4-7)
$$C_{T2} = \frac{T2_B - T2_A}{T2_B + T2_A} = \frac{126 - 67 \text{ ms}}{126 + 67 \text{ ms}} = 0.306$$

(EQ. 4-8)
$$C_{N[H]} = \frac{N(H_B) - N(H_A)}{N(H_B) + N(H_A)} = \frac{0.86 - 0.61}{0.86 + 0.61} = 0.170$$

Based on these measured tissue parameter values, inherent T1 and inherent T2 edema–white matter contrast values are comparable with one another and are 63% to 80% greater than the inherent N[H] edema–white matter contrast. If individual pulse sequences existed that could produce pure T1, pure T2, and pure spin-density images (e.g., signals that are directly proportional to the T1, T2, and spin-density values alone, respectively, without any contribution from other tissue parameters), then the pure T1 and the pure T2 images would present nearly twice as much contrast between edema and white matter as the

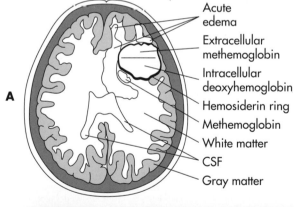

A

Acute edema
Extracellular methemoglobin
Intracellular deoxyhemoglobin
Hemosiderin ring
Methemoglobin
White matter
CSF
Gray matter

FIGURE 4-4 Brain images of a 41-year-old woman with a history of breast cancer and complaint of flulike symptoms. Only a single section of a full brain study is shown. **A,** Schematic of brain tissues in the selected section. **B,** SE 600/20 image. **C,** SE 2700/20 image. **D,** SE 2700/80 image. (Courtesy Dr. Anne Osborn.)

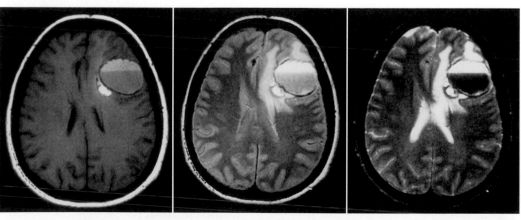

B **C** **D**

pure N[H] image. Although these pure T1, T2, and N[H] images cannot be acquired directly, they can be numerically calculated from the three primary images. Figure 4-5 shows synthetic pure T1, T2, and N[H] images of the brain section corresponding to the acquired images in Figure 4-4. Figure 4-5, *A,* displays the pure T1 image, with long T1 tissues displayed brightest. This is the opposite of the appearance of the T1-weighted short-TR/short-TE SE image in Figure 4-4, *B,* in which the shortest T1 tissues have the strongest signals. Figure 4-5, *B,* is a pure T1 image but with contrast reversed so that tissues with the shortest T1 values are displayed brightest. Note the similarity between soft tissues of the brain in Figure 4-5, *B,* and in the T1-weighted image of Figure 4-4, *B.* Figure 4-5, *C* and *D,* shows the pure N[H] and pure T2 images of the model brain section with signal intensities in direct proportion to N[H] and T2 values, making the appearance of these pure images similar to the appearance of N[H]-weighted and T2-weighted images (Figure 4-4, *C* and *D*).

Directly acquired MR images have contrast based on some combination of T1, T2, and N[H] parameters. For most choices of pulse sequences and interpulse delay times, some of these sources of inherent tissue contrast work against one another (interfere destructively), reducing the level of contrast in the resultant image. The best solution is to choose user-selectable parameters so that one or two sources of tissue contrast dominate and add constructively, minimizing the negative effect of other inherent sources of contrast. This is most easily discussed in the context of specific MR pulse sequences.

SPIN-ECHO IMAGING

The SE pulse sequence devised by Hahn for nuclear magnetic resonance (NMR) spectroscopy in 1950[15] is the most commonly used pulse sequence in clinical MRI. The SE sequence, as applied in two-dimensional Fourier transform (2D FT) reconstruction imaging, is shown in Figure 4-6. The pattern of the basic pulse sequence is the same from one repetition to the next, except for changes in the strength of the phase-encoding gradient.[6] Figure 4-6 shows the timing pattern of radiofrequency (RF) pulses, the magnetic gradient used to select a particular planar section (the slice-select gradient), the gradients used to resolve the signals from all voxels within the selected section (the phase-encoding and frequency-encoding gradients), and the measurement of RF signal from the patient on each sequence repetition.

The behavior of the magnetization in a voxel of tissue during the SE sequence is sketched in Figure 4-7. Before each 90-degree RF pulse, a certain amount of tissue magnetization points along the direction of the

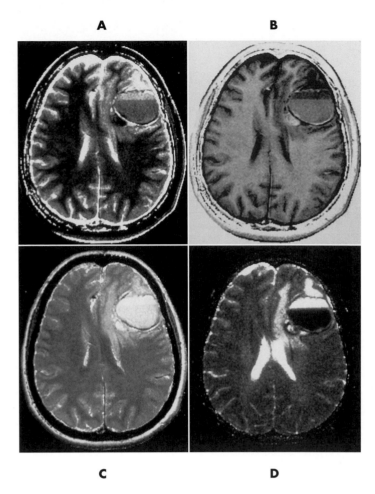

A **B**

C **D**

FIGURE 4-5 Synthetically derived pure tissue parameter images corresponding to same patient and section described in Figure 4-4. **A,** Pure T1 image with intensity directly proportional to tissue T1 values. **B,** Pure T1 image with intensity inversely proportional to tissue T1 values. **C,** Pure N[H] image. **D,** Pure T2 image. In **C** and **D,** intensities are directly proportional to tissue N[H] and T2 values.

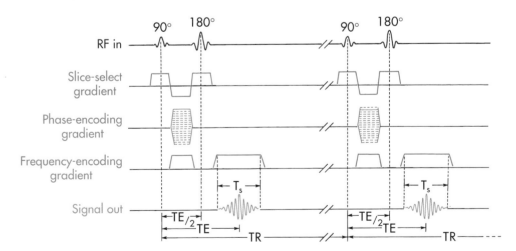

FIGURE 4-6 Multislice SE pulse sequence. Horizontal direction represents time line, with time progressing from left to right. Top line of pulse sequence shows the timing of RF pulses sent into the patient. In the SE sequence the two pulses are a 90-degree pulse followed by a 180-degree pulse. Second line indicates the timing of the slice-select gradient. The slice-select gradient is turned on only when slice-selection RF pulses are sent into the patient. Third line shows the timing of the phase-encoding gradient, which is turned on sometime between signal excitation (90-degree pulse) and signal measurement. Horizontal hatchmarks indicate that the phase-encoding gradient is turned on to a different strength for each repetition of the basic sequence (only two repetitions are shown). Fourth line shows the timing of the frequency-encoding (or readout) gradient, which is turned on during signal measurement. Bottom line is the signal from the patient, which is measured by receiver coils during the total sampling time (T_s), while the readout gradient is turned on.

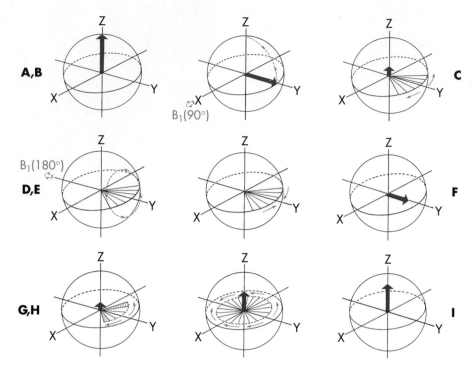

FIGURE 4-7   SE pulse sequence: Behavior of the magnetization in a voxel (see text).

static magnetic field B_0 (the +z direction in Figure 4-7, *A*). The magnetization projecting along the z direction is called the *longitudinal magnetization;* the magnetization projecting perpendicular to B_0 (i.e., projecting in the x-y plane) is called the *transverse magnetization.* The longitudinal magnetization cannot be measured directly. The 90-degree pulse in each repetition of the SE sequence tips all available longitudinal magnetization into the transverse plane, where it can be measured (Figure 4-7, *B*). Transverse magnetization is measurable because of the precession of magnetization tipped away from the longitudinal direction. A properly placed and sufficiently sensitive receiver coil can measure the strength of the precessing transverse magnetization by detecting the changing magnetic field it produces. After being tipped into the transverse plane, the transverse magnetization precesses (not shown) and decreases in total strength because of the dephasing of magnetic dipoles within the voxel (Figure 4-7, *C*). This dephasing occurs because different dipoles are located in slightly different local magnetic field environments, even within the same voxel. A short time (TE/2) after the 90-degree pulse, a 180-degree pulse is applied to reorient each component of the transverse magnetization (Figure 4-7, *D*). This reorientation makes the transverse magnetic dipoles that were precessing slightly faster "reorient" to the direction of slower transverse magnetic dipoles, and the slower dipoles are reoriented to the direction that faster components used to have. Although the directions of magnetic dipoles have changed, the local magnetic inhomogeneities have not changed; thus the dipoles that previously precessed faster still precess faster. Therefore, aside from the dephasing resulting from true irreversible T2 effects, there is a rephasing: The faster magnetic dipoles continue to precess faster and catch up, and the slower dipoles continue to precess slower and fall back (Figure 4-7, *E*). In a single instant a maximum number of dipoles are rephased as they precess, forming an echo at time TE/2 after the 180-degree pulse (Figure 4-7, *F*) or at time TE after the 90-degree pulse. The signal is measured for a time period (T_S) before, during, and after peak echo formation. As time progresses, the transverse magnetization continues to rapidly dephase to zero (Figure 4-7, *G* and *H*), and the longitudinal magnetization slowly regrows, reflecting the fact that T2 is much shorter than T1 (Figure 4-7, *G* to *I*). The remaining time un-

til the next repetition of the pulse sequence is required to permit sufficient recovery of the longitudinal magnetization (Figure 4-7, *I*), taking a total time of TR from one 90-degree pulse to the next.

The expression for the signal in SE imaging from a voxel with tissue parameters T1, T2, and N[H], assuming a rectangular slice profile, is as follows:

(EQ. 4-9)

$$S_{se}(TE,TR) = \underbrace{N[H]}_{\substack{\text{Spin-density} \\ \text{factor}}} \underbrace{[1 - 2e^{-(TR-TE/2)/T2} + e^{-TR/T1}]}_{\text{T1 factor}} \underbrace{e^{-TE/T2}}_{\text{T2 factor}}$$

By varying the two user-selectable delay times, the echo delay time (TE), and the sequence repetition time (TR), the SE sequence can be used to highlight T1, T2, or spin-density effects.

As indicated by Equation 4-9, the full SE signal expression can be thought of as the product of three factors—a spin-density factor, a T1 factor, and a T2 factor. The spin-density factor is proportional to the effective number of hydrogen nuclei per unit volume, contributing a fixed factor (independent of TE and TR) to the signal from each voxel. Because TR is the dominant user-selectable parameter appearing with T1 in the T1 factor, TR controls the amount of T1-weighting of the SE pulse sequence. Because TE is the only user-selectable parameter appearing with T2 in the T2 factor, TE controls the amount of T2-weighting of the SE signal from each voxel.

T1 Relaxation and the Effect of Varying Repetition Time

The contributions of the spin-density, T1, and T2 factors to the SE signals from edema and white matter as a function of TE and TR are illustrated in Figure 4-8. Figure 4-8, *A*, plots the T1-induced recovery of longitudinal magnetization (the T1 factors in Equation 4-9) for edema and white matter as a function of TR. The shorter T1 of white matter produces a faster recovery of the longitudinal magnetization at a given

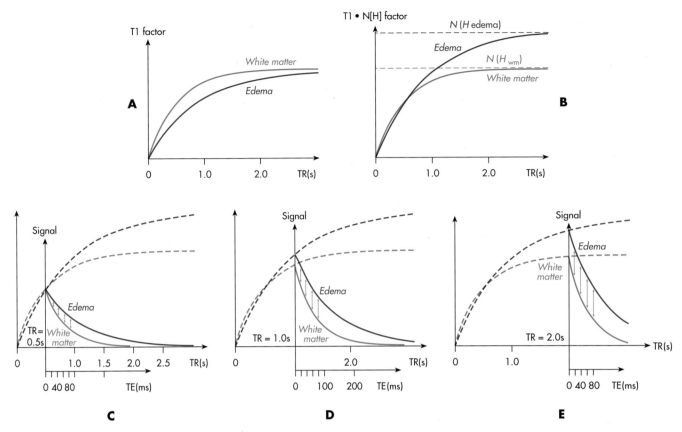

FIGURE 4-8   Factors contributing to measured signal strength from white matter *(blue)* and edema *(red)* in SE imaging. **A,** T1 factors versus TR. **B,** T1 factors multiplied by N[H] factors versus TR. The dotted lines represent different spin-density factors for white matter and edema. **C,** T1, N[H], and T2 factors combined. Dotted curves represent the product of T1 and N[H] factors. Solid T2 decay curves are plotted, assuming TR of 500 ms. Vertical green arrows indicate edema–white matter signal difference at TE values of 20, 40, 60, and 80 ms. **D,** T1, N[H], and T2 factors combined, with TR of 1000 ms. Vertical green arrows indicate edema–white matter signal difference at TE values of 20, 40, 60, and 80 ms. **E,** Same as D but with TR of 2000 ms. In **C** to **E**, scale of the TE axis has been expanded by a factor of 5 relative to the TR axis.

TR value. This produces a potentially stronger signal from white matter on successive repetitions of the pulse sequence and therefore a brighter signal from the white matter in the reconstructed image. The signal difference between white matter and edema is illustrated by the vertical separation of the two curves. Figure 4-8, *A,* indicates that to maximize the effect of inherent T1 contrast between white matter and edema in the image (the T1 factor difference), an intermediate TR value should be chosen. Thus intermediate- to short-TR values (comparable to or less than the T1 values of tissues of interest) are chosen in T1-weighted SE imaging. Figure 4-8, *A,* also shows that to minimize inherent T1 contrast in the image, a long-TR value should be chosen so that T1 factors from both tissues are equal. Thus long-TR values are chosen in T2-weighted SE imaging. Figure 4-8, *A,* however, illustrates only the T1 factor contributions to the SE signal. The contributions of spin-density and T2 factors also must be considered.

Spin-Density Effects

If the spin densities of white matter and edema were equal, the products of T1 and N[H] factors would match the curves shown in Figure 4-8, *A,* approaching the same values for long TR. Because the measured spin density of normal white matter is only about 70% of the measured spin density of edema (Table 4-1), the inclusion of spin-density effects decreases the signal from white matter relative to the signal from edema at all TR values. Consequently, when both spin-density and T1 factors are taken into account, the white matter and edema curves approach different maxima (see the two dotted horizontal lines in Figure 4-8, *B*). The higher spin density (along with the higher T1 value) of edema reduces the contrast between white matter and edema for shorter-TR values (TR ≤ 600 ms) and reverses the contrast between white matter and

edema for longer-TR values (TR > 600 ms, where edema becomes brighter than white matter). In this example, as in all SE imaging with directly correlated spin-density and T1 values (i.e., where tissues having higher T1 values also have higher spin-density values), inherent spin-density contrast and inherent T1 contrast interfere destructively, reducing the resultant image contrast for short-TR values.

T2 Relaxation and the Effect of Varying Echo Time

Full consideration of image contrast is incomplete because T2 factors have not been included. Note in Equation 4-9 that the T2 factor $e^{-TE/T2}$ multiplies spin-density and T1 factors and is controlled by the user-selectable parameter TE. This T2 factor has a value of 1 at a TE of 0 and decreases exponentially toward zero as TE increases. For shorter-T2 values the T2 factor decreases to zero more rapidly. Because white matter has a shorter T2 value than does edema (Table 4-1), the T2 factor decreases more rapidly for white matter than for edema. T2 factors are combined with N[H] and T1 factors for white matter and edema in Figure 4-8, *C* to *E*. Figure 4-8, *C,* is a plot of signals from white matter and edema as a function of TE for a user-selected TR value of 500 ms. Arrows indicate the signal differences at TE values of 20, 40, 60, and 80 ms. Figure 4-8, *D,* is a plot of signals from white matter and edema for a TR of 1000 ms, with arrows again indicating the signal differences at four different TE values. Figure 4-8, *E,* is a similar plot for a TR value of 2000 ms. In each plot the time scale on the TE axis has been expanded by a factor of 5 relative to the TR axis.

The collective effects of spin-density, T1, and T2 values on signals from each tissue are illustrated in Figure 4-8, *C* to *E*. Solid curves indicate the signal from each tissue for a fixed TR value and any TE set-

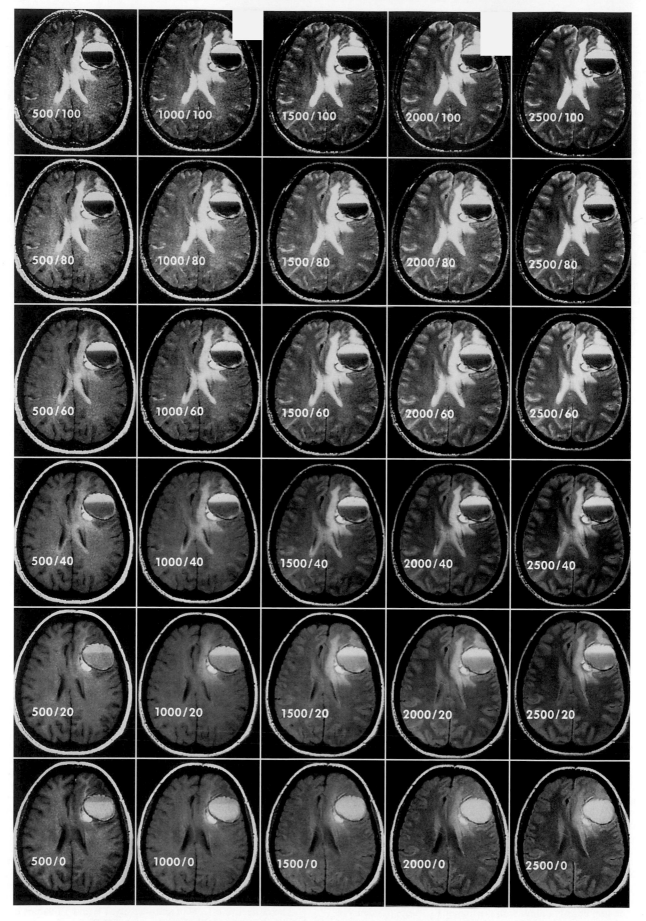

FIGURE 4-9 Synthetic SE images of the brain model section at a matrix of TR and TE settings (TR/TE), including the timing parameters corresponding to the vertical arrows in Figure 4-8, *C* to *E*.

ting. After including T1, T2, and spin-density factors, the vertical separations between (solid) curves are an accurate representation of signal differences or tissue contrast between edema and white matter.

These figures indicate the difficulty in obtaining heavily T1-weighted sequences with the SE sequence in tissues with correlated T1, T2, and N[H] values. The effect of a shorter-T1 value, which makes the T1 factor greater (and therefore works to make the signal stronger) for a short-TR setting, is canceled by a lower N[H] value, which reduces the signal from that tissue, and by a shorter-T2 value, which also reduces the signal from that tissue, with a more pronounced reduction as TE is increased. The practical constraint of a nonzero TE value (typically, TE ≥ 10 ms in SE imaging) is that correlated T2 values and correlated N[H] values interfere destructively with inherent T1 contrast to reduce the T1-induced contrast between two tissues. This reduction of inherent T1 contrast between tissues resulting from spin-density and T2 effects is typical of T1-weighted sequences in general because diseased tissues or lesions typically have greater T1, T2, and spin-density values than surrounding normal tissues.

The same difficulty does not exist for T2-weighted scanning (Figure 4-8, *E*). At a TR value of 2000 ms, the greater spin density of lesion over that of normal brain tends to enhance the T2-induced contrast between the two tissues. The curves suggest that a substantial part of the contrast between edema and normal brain at long-TR values is the result of inherent spin-density contrast, with inherent T2 contrast adding coherently to inherent spin-density contrast as TE is increased. Whereas inherent T1 contrast works opposite to both spin-density and T2 contrast, the use of a long-TR value minimizes the adverse effect of inherent T1 contrast on image contrast.

Examples: Clinical Images

Numerically derived SE images at a variety of TE and TR settings for the model brain section of Figures 4-4 and 4-5 are shown in Figure 4-9. Figures 4-8 and 4-9 show good agreement between the edema–white matter contrast predicted by the SE-sequence equation at specific TR/TE combinations and the contrast present in the SE images acquired or simulated at those TR/TE settings. The signal graphs in Figure 4-8 assume that the same number of acquisitions per phase-encoding step (N_{aqs} or N_{ex}) have been acquired, regardless of the TR/TE choices. Although the images shown in Figure 4-9 have been calculated with this constraint, this often is not the case clinically. Because TR, N_{aqs}, and the number of phase-encoding steps (N_{pe}) all have the effect of increasing the total scan time (T_{total}):

(EQ. 4-10)

$$T_{total} = (TR) (N_{aqs}) (N_{pe})$$

it is often more efficient to use higher N_{aqs} (2 or 4) for short-TR values and reduce N_{aqs} (to 1 or 2) for long-TR values. Signal and contrast are increased in direct proportion to the number of acquisitions per phase-encoding step:

(EQ. 4-11)

$$S(N_{aqs}) = S(1) - N_{aqs}$$

and

(EQ. 4-12)

$$C_{image} (N_{aqs}) = C_{image}(1) - N_{aqs}$$

where $S(1)$ and $C_{image}(1)$ are the signal and contrast resulting from a single planar acquisition at each phase-encoding step. Most MR scanners scale the measured signal so that the improvement suggested by Equations 4-11 and 4-12 is not apparent in region-of-interest (ROI) measurements. In these cases the improvement in signal or contrast with N_{aqs} is apparent only if signals or signal differences are referred to the level of noise in the image.

Although Figure 4-8 gives an indication of the signal difference between white matter and edema in SE imaging at several clinically relevant TR/TE settings, it may be difficult to visualize edema–white matter contrast over the full range of TE and TR values. Brain edema signal difference or contrast over the full range of TR/TE settings is more easily presented in the form of contour or 3D plots. The contours represent lines of equal contrast plotted versus TR and TE (Figure 4-10). Figure 4-10 is plotted under the assumption of a fixed number of acquisitions per phase-encoding step. Therefore imaging time increases in direct proportion to TR, so as the plot moves farther out along the TR axis, total imaging time increases.

The contrast between white matter and edema is maximized in two distinct regions of Figure 4-10—a short-TR/short-TE region where white matter is brighter than edema and a long-TR/long-TE region where edema is brighter than white matter. Often these two regions are referred to as the *T1-* and *T2-weighted regions,* respectively, but because of possible confusion about the underlying sources of contrast, use of this terminology is not being encouraged in the literature. For instance, in the brain example a large part of the edema–white matter contrast at long-TR/long-TE settings is derived from spin-density differences rather than just T2 differences between tissues; thus it is misleading to refer to the long-TR/long-TE region simply as being "T2-weighted."

A contour plot of the signal difference between white matter and edema under the assumption of fixed total imaging time is shown in Figure 4-11. The constraint of fixed total imaging time means that as TR is increased, N_{aqs} is decreased proportionally, while N_{pe} is kept constant, so the total time required to collect the image remains the same (Equation 4-10). Long-TR/long-TE settings continue to provide far greater edema–white matter contrast under the constraint of fixed total imaging time (Figure 4-11). (Figures 4-8 to 4-11 also indicate that long-

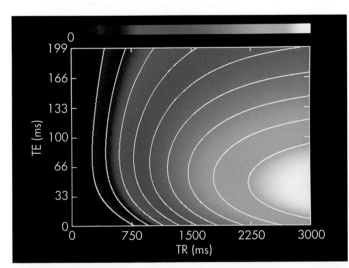

FIGURE 4-10 Edema–white matter contrast (or signal difference) in SE imaging displayed on a contour plot as a function of TR and TE, a fixed number of acquisitions per phase-encoding step (N_{aqs}). Pseudocolor contrast scale ranges from black (zero contrast) to white (maximum contrast).

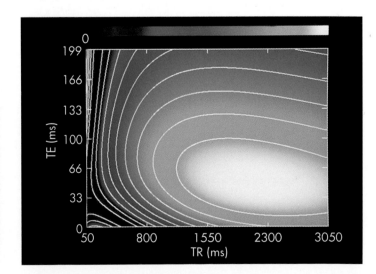

FIGURE 4-11 Edema–white matter contrast in SE imaging. Assumes a fixed total imaging time (T_{total}). Under this more realistic condition, maximum contrast is achieved at a finite TR value.

TR/long-TE settings are more forgiving in that there are wide ranges of TR and TE settings in the long-TR/long-TE region that preserve a large amount of edema–white matter contrast.) Conversely it is more difficult to distinguish edema from white matter with a short-TR/short-TE setting because it requires an accurate prescription of the best short-TR/short-TE delay times.)

Table 4-2 summarizes the TR and TE settings used to weight the SE image toward a particular source of inherent tissue contrast. If T1 is sought as the major source of image contrast between two or more tissues, it is essential to use short-TE settings (to minimize T2 relaxation effects and T2 differentiation of tissues) and TR settings comparable to the T1 values of the two tissues (to preserve some degree of T1 differentiation). If T2 is sought as the major source of image contrast, it is desirable to use longer-TE values (to permit some T2 decay) and long-TR values (to minimize the T1 differentiation between tissues). If N[H] is sought as the major source of image contrast, it is essential to use short-TE values (to minimize T2 differentiation) and long-TR values (to minimize T1 differentiation); what remains are spin-density differences as the major source of image contrast.

Carr-Purcell-Meiboom-Gill Sequence

The Carr-Purcell-Meiboom-Gill (CPMG) sequence is a modification of Hahn's SE sequence, proposed by Carr and Purcell[5] and refined by Meiboom and Gill,[24] to collect multiple SEs. In imaging applications, each echo signal is stored separately to reconstruct images at each of several different TE values. Any number of echoes may be collected by applying additional consecutive rephasing 180-degree pulses after the initial 90-degree pulse. Figure 4-12 illustrates a CPMG sequence with two echoes. The signal expressions for CPMG sequences with two, three, and four equally spaced echoes are listed as follows:

(EQ. 4-13)

$$S_{CPMG-2echoes} = N[H]e^{-nTE/T2} [1 - 2e^{-(TR-3TE/2)/T1} + 2e^{-(TR-TE/2)/T1} - e^{-TR/T1}]$$

(EQ. 4-14)

$$S_{CPMG-3echoes} = N[H]e^{-nTE/T2} [1 - 2e^{-(TR-5TE/2)/T1} + 2e^{-(TR-3TE/2)/T1} - 2e^{-(TR-TE/2)/T1} + e^{-TR/T1}]$$

(EQ. 4-15)

$$S_{CPMG-4echoes} = N[H]e^{-nTE/T2} [1 - 2e^{-(TR-7TE/2)/T1} + 2e^{-(TR-5TE/2)/T1} - 2e^{-(TR-3TE/2)/T1} + 2e^{-(TR-TE/2)/T1} - e^{-TR/T1}]$$

where n denotes the echo number and TE the time between the initial 90-degree pulse and the first echo (and the time between successive echoes).

Minor modifications in the T1 factor occur if different numbers of echoes are collected, owing to the effect of additional 180-degree rephasing pulses on the longitudinal magnetization. In the limit n_{max} TE << T1, where n_{max} is the largest number of echoes collected, the T1 factor may be assumed to be identical to the T1 factor in single-echo SE imaging, both signal expressions reducing to:

(EQ. 4-16)

$$S_{se} (TE,TR) = N[H] [1 - e^{-TR/T1}] e^{-TE/T2}$$

where TE is the effective delay time between the 90-degree pulse and signal collection, regardless of the echo collected. Thus the contrast between tissues in CPMG sequences with a given TR and TE value is nearly identical to the contrast in single-echo SE imaging with the same TR/TE setting.

Although multiecho SE sequences are common in clinical MRI, their use typically is restricted to the collection of a few echoes at long-TR values. The first echo, acquired at short TE, is interpreted as a spin density–weighted or "balanced" image. Second or later echoes are acquired at significantly longer TEs to provide a T2-weighted image. Even the first echo in a CPMG or multiecho sequence will contain some T2 weighting, and all echoes will contain spin-density weighting (Figure 4-8, C to E).

In clinical applications, accumulation of a large number of CPMG echoes for each slice in a multislice protocol has proved cumbersome because of the large number of images that require reconstruction and archiving, while providing little additional diagnostic information beyond that achieved with one long-TR/short-TE image and one long-TR/long-TE image. More often, asymmetrical echoes, one at a short TE (10 to 20 ms) and one at a long TE (60 to 100 ms), are preferable to a larger number of evenly spaced echoes (e.g., TE = 30, 60, 90, 120

Table 4-2	Effect of TE and TR on Image Contrast in Spin-Echo Imaging	
CONTRAST SOURCE	**TE SETTING**	**TR SETTING**
T1	As short as possible, limited by bandwidth and noise (≤15 ms)	Comparable to T1s of the two tissues (better toward the shorter T1)
T2	Comparable to T2s of the two tissues (better toward the longer T2)	Long compared with the T1s of the two tissues (≥2000 ms)
N[H]	As short as possible (≤15 ms)	Long compared with the T1s of the two tissues (≥2000 ms)

TE, Echo time; *TR*, repetition time; *N[H]*, hydrogen spin density.

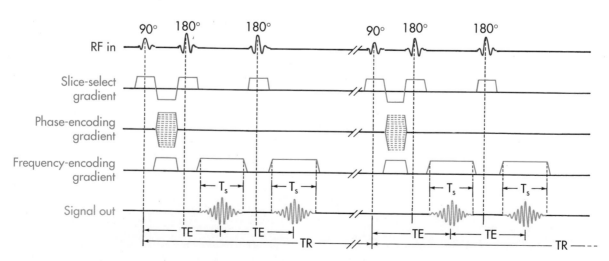

FIGURE 4-12   Carr-Purcell-Meiboom-Gill (CPMG) pulse sequence with two echoes per excitation. Second or later echoes are acquired at significantly longer TEs to provide a T2-weighted image.

ms) using the CPMG concept. For asymmetrical SE images the 180-degree pulses are unevenly spaced. For example, asymmetrical echoes at 20 and 80 ms would require placing the two 180-degree pulses in Figure 4-12 at 10 and 50 ms after the 90-degree pulse. The signal expression is still well approximated for each echo by Equation 4-16.

INVERSION RECOVERY IMAGING

The inversion recovery (IR) sequence commonly used in MRI consists of an inverting 180-pulse, a 90-degree pulse, and a rephasing 180-

degree pulse. The timing pattern of these pulses, the gradients used for section selection and voxel resolution within the selected section, and signal measurement are shown in Figure 4-13.

The behavior of the magnetization within a selected voxel during the IR sequence is shown in Figure 4-14. Before the start of each sequence repetition, the magnetization projects along the +z axis and is therefore only longitudinal magnetization, with no transverse component (Figure 4-14, *A*). The initial 180-degree RF pulse tips the positive longitudinal magnetization into negative longitudinal magnetization (along the −z direction; Figure 4-14, *B*). Over a time interval (TI) be-

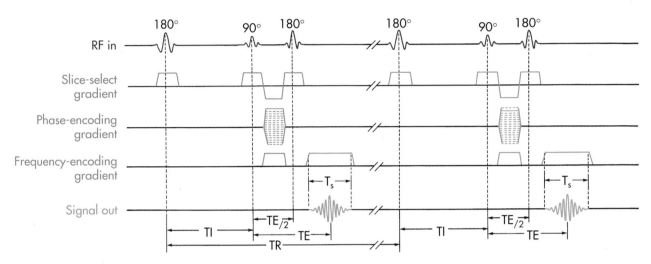

FIGURE 4-13   Inversion recovery (IR) pulse sequences.

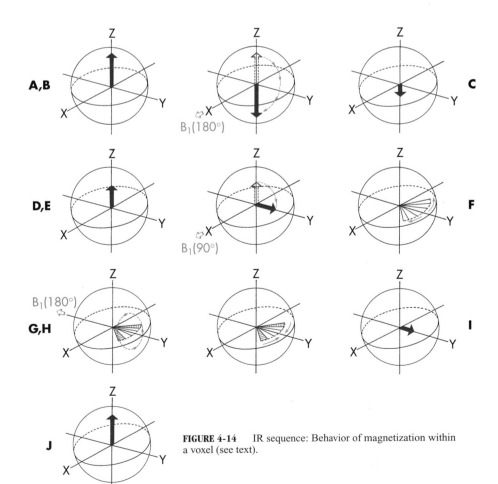

FIGURE 4-14   IR sequence: Behavior of magnetization within a voxel (see text).

tween the initial 180-degree pulse and the 90-degree pulse, the longitudinal magnetization shrinks along the $-z$ direction and then regrows along the $+z$ direction as a result of TI recovery. If a short TI is used, the longitudinal magnetization may still be negative at the time of the 90-degree pulse (Figure 4-14, *C*); if a longer TI is used, the longitudinal magnetization will be positive (Figure 4-14, *D*). The purpose of the 90-degree pulse is the same in IR as in SE: to take the longitudinal magnetization, which is unmeasurable, and tip it into the transverse plane, where it can be measured (Figure 4-14, *E*). The transverse magnetization then dephases (Figure 4-14, *F*) because of irreversible T2 relaxation and other, reversible causes for transverse dephasing, such as magnetic field inhomogeneities and applied magnetic gradients. Like the SE sequence, the IR sequence makes use of a rephasing 180-degree pulse (Figure 4-14, *G*) to reverse the orientation of transverse magnetic components and rephase the reversible components (Figure 4-14, *H*), forming an SE for signal collection (Figure 4-14, *I*). IR imaging sequences that collect signal by forming an echo are sometimes referred to as *inversion recovery spin-echo (IRSE) sequences.* Signal measurement is performed just before, during, and just after the peak echo signal. After signal measurement, a long interval of inactivity occurs (at least for that particular slice) to permit a reasonable amount of T1-induced recovery of the longitudinal magnetization before the sequence is repeated (Figure 4-14, *J*).

The expression for the signal from a voxel having tissue parameters N[H], T1, and T2, assuming a rectangular slice profile, in IR imaging is:

(EQ. 4-17)

$$S_{IR}(TI, TE, TR) = \underbrace{N[H]}_{\substack{\text{Spin-density} \\ \text{factor}}} \underbrace{[1 - 2e^{-TI/T1} + 2e^{-(TR-TE/2)/T1} - e^{-TR/T1}]}_{\text{T1 factor}} \underbrace{e^{-TE/T2}}_{\text{T2 factor}}$$

The following three interpulse delay times in principle can be controlled by the user: TI (the time between the initial 180-degree pulse and 90-degree pulse), TE (the echo-rephasing time between the 90-degree pulse and the echo peak), and TR (the full-sequence repetition time, including the time after signal measurement allowed for recovery of the longitudinal magnetization). The IR signal expression in Equation 4-17 can be factored into spin-density, T1, and T2 factors similarly to the SE signal expression. The spin-density and T2 factors in the two sequences are identical. There is a difference between T1 factors in SE and IR sequences.

T1 Relaxation and the Effect of Repetition Time and Inversion Time

The IR T1 factor is a function of both TR and TI, and both user-selectable delay times can influence the amount of T1-induced contrast in the image. If a real reconstruction of IR data is used, the IR T1 factor is negative for shorter-TI values and positive for longer-TI values. A potential advantage of real-reconstructed IR over T1-weighted SE imaging is that the range of the TI factor is doubled, potentially ranging from -1 to $+1$ in IR, rather than from 0 to 1 in SE imaging. This greater dynamic range in TI factors has the potential of providing greater T1-weighted contrast between tissues. The range of the T1 factor is -1 to $+1$ only if TR is chosen to be infinitely long (or much, much greater than TI). For finite TR values the T1 factor has a reduced range from $-(1 - e^{-TR/TI})$ to $+(1 - e^{-TR/TI})$.

The T1 factor for the edema–white matter model in the case of real-reconstructed IR images is shown graphically in Figure 4-15, *A*. The left side of Figure 4-15, *A*, plots the factor $(1 - e^{-TR/TI})$, the effect of TR on the T1 factor. This curve represents the amount of recovered longitudinal magnetization between successive 90-degree pulses, which depends only on the selected TR value and the T1 of the tissue. As in SE imaging the tissue with shorter T1 (in our example, white matter) has a greater recovery of longitudinal magnetization at each TR setting. (A TR value of 2000 ms gives the amount of recovery shown at the vertical line in the middle of the graph.) The inverting 180-degree pulse then takes the recovered longitudinal magnetization and tips it along the $-z$ direction (pointing opposite to the main magnetic field B_0), from which T1 recovery begins again (see the right side of Figure 4-15, *A*). The tissue with more recovered longitudinal magnetization before the invert-

ing 180-degree pulse has a larger negative longitudinal magnetization after the 180-degree pulse. The selected TI value then controls the amount of T1 recovery that occurs after inversion: A short TI (<350 ms) yields a negative longitudinal magnetization for both tissues; a longer TI (>550 ms) yields a positive longitudinal magnetization for both tissues. The vertical separation of the two curves indicates the T1 factor difference that contributes to image contrast at any selected TI value (assuming TR = 2000 ms). Selection of a particular TI value sets the amount of recovered longitudinal magnetization that is tipped by the 90-degree pulse into the transverse plane for signal measurement. A crossover of the signal curves (a point of no T1 contrast) occurs at a TI value of about 50 ms, since the white matter is initially more negative just after the 180-degree pulse but also recovers more quickly after the 180-degree pulse because of its shorter-T1 value.

Spin-Density Effects

Figure 4-15, *A*, plots only the T1 factors in Equation 4-17. The inclusion of spin-density factors multiplying the T1 factors for each tissue results in the curves shown in Figure 4-15, *B*. As can be seen by comparing Figure 4-15, *A* and *B*, correlated T1 and N[H] values increase the available T1-induced image contrast between tissues for negative signals (TI values <350 ms) and decrease image contrast for positive signals (TI values >550 ms). This indicates that correlated N[H] and T1 values add constructively to image contrast for short TI IR (STIR) imaging, while interfering destructively to decrease image contrast for conventional, longer-TI IR.

Real Reconstruction Versus Magnitude Reconstruction

Real reconstruction of IR images is illustrated in Figure 4-15, *A* and *B*. Real reconstruction preserves sign information in the acquired IR data and image reconstruction. Because phase-shift artifacts can occur in real-reconstructed IR images, most clinical IR images are magnitude (modulus) reconstructed (i.e., sign or phase information is ignored in the reconstruction process and only the magnitude of the recorded signals is used in image reconstruction). The effect of magnitude reconstruction is that negative signals are recorded as positive signals of the same strength. Hence the negative signals on the right side of Figure 4-15, *A* and *B*, are replaced by the positive signals on the right side of Figure 4-15, *C* and *D*, respectively. Instead of crossing the zero signal axis, in modulus-reconstructed images each tissue has an inflection point (or null point) where the signal from that tissue is zero, occurring at $TI_{null} = (T1) \cdot \ln[2/(1 + e^{-TR/T1})]$, found by solving for the TI value that makes the T1 factor zero. For TR set to several times the T1 of the tissue, the null point is $TI_{null} \approx T1\ln(2)$ or ≈ 0.7 T1, so the longer the T1 of the tissue, the longer the null point for that tissue.

The use of modulus reconstruction in IR automatically compresses the range of the T1 factor to be between 0 and 1, just as for SE imaging. Thus modulus reconstruction eliminates a major potential advantage of conventional IR imaging: the greater range of available T1 image contrast. Magnitude reconstruction also has the potential disadvantage of reducing or eliminating contrast between tissues having different T1 values for certain choices of TI, as described later.

The nulling of signal from a particular tissue in magnitude-reconstructed IR may be used to specific advantage, such as the nulling of signal from fat and the elimination of motion-induced ghosting of fat elsewhere in the image. The short-TI values used in STIR imaging are selected specifically for this purpose (see later discussion).

T2 Relaxation and the Effect of Varying Echo Time

T2 relaxation effects can be illustrated by adding the T2 decay curves as a function of TE for specific TI and TR values (Figure 4-15, *E* to *H*). As demonstrated by the graphs, two distinct situations exist. For the longer-TI values used in conventional IR imaging, correlated inherent T1 and T2 contrast interfere destructively (Figure 4-15, *E*). The shorter-T1 value of white matter tends to make white matter brighter than edema (through the T1 factor), whereas the shorter T2 of white matter tends to reduce the brightness difference (through the T2 factor). This destructive interference may be minimized by operating with short-TE values. Short-TE values also ensure maximum signal strength from both tissues.

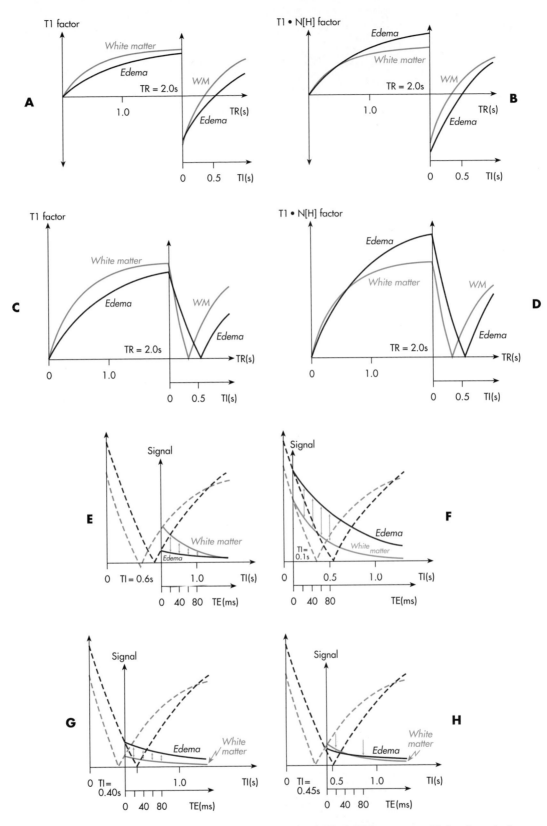

FIGURE 4-15   T1, T2, and N[H] factors for IR signal (Equation 4-17). **A,** TI factors versus T1 for edema *(red)* and white matter *(blue),* assuming sign information is preserved in image reconstruction (real reconstruction); TR of 2000 ms. **B,** T1 factors multiplied by N[H] factors for edema and white matter, assuming real reconstruction of the image. **C,** T1 factors alone for edema and white matter, assuming the image is reconstructed without maintaining sign information (magnitude reconstruction). **D,** T1 factors multiplied by N[H] factors for edema and white matter, assuming magnitude reconstruction. **E,** T1, N[H], and T2 factors for edema and white matter in magnitude-reconstructed IR. T1 factors multiplied by N[H] factors are shown by dashed curves. T2 factors multiplied by the T1 and N[H] factors are shown by solid curves; TR of 2000 ms, TI of 600 ms. **F,** Same as **E** but TI of 100 ms. **G,** Same as **E** but TI = 400 ms. **H,** Same as **E** but TE = 450 ms. In **E** to **H,** TE scale is expanded by a factor of 5 relative to TR and T1 scale.

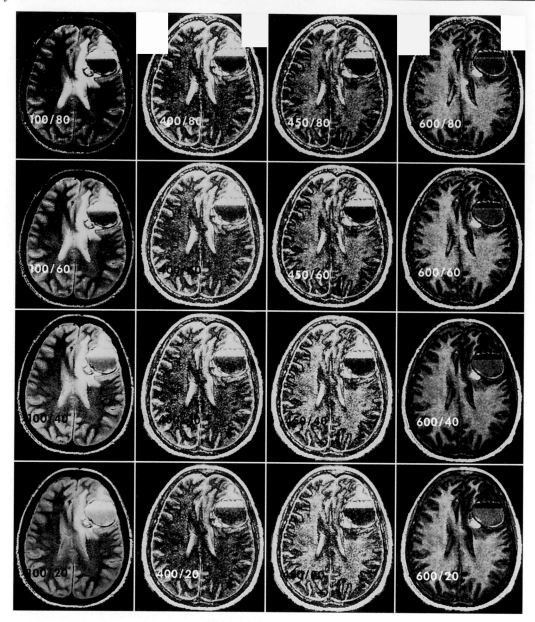

FIGURE 4-16   Synthetic magnitude-reconstructed IR images of the brain model section at a matrix of TI and TE values (TI/TE); TR of 2000 ms for all images.

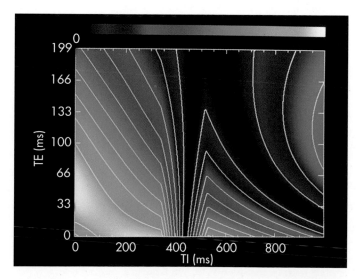

FIGURE 4-17   Edema–white matter contrast (or signal difference) in IR imaging as a function of TI and TE displayed on contour plot; TR of 2000 ms.

Short Inversion Time Inversion Recovery

For shorter-T1 values (below the null point of white matter), inherent T1 contrast adds constructively to inherent T2 contrast, producing increased image contrast (Figure 4-15, *F*). With TI short, the shorter T1 of white matter works in concert with the shorter T2 of white matter, both contributing to make edema brighter than white matter. A comparison of Figure 4-15, *C* and *D*, illustrates that the higher spin density of edema also contributes significantly and, in a manner constructive with the contributions of T1 and T2, makes edema brighter than white matter for short-TI values.

The suppression of signal from fat, a primary source of motion-induced ghosting, can be achieved by choosing TI ≈ 0.7 TI$_{fat}$ in magnitude-reconstructed IR. Because fat has a TI value shorter than that of other tissues of interest, it also has a shorter null point than other tissues. The result is that a selection of TI that nulls the signal from fat also produces constructive T1, T2, and spin-density contributions to image contrast.[4,33] Alternatively, selection of TI of 0.7 T1$_x$ for other tissues will similarly null their signal intensity. This technique is commonly performed to null the intensity of CSF, where T1$_x$ ≈ 2000 ms, in conjunction with increasing TE to 30 ms or more to add T2 weighting.

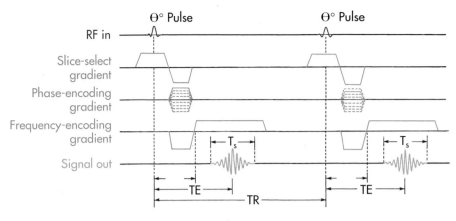

FIGURE 4-18   Generic gradient-echo pulse sequence, without rephasing (or "rewinding") of phase-encoding gradients after signal measurement.

Contrast Loss in Magnitude-Reconstructed Inversion Recovery

If TI is set between the null points of the tissues of interest, image contrast is reduced between the tissues using magnitude-reconstructed IR.[17] This is illustrated in Figure 4-15, *G* and *H*, which plots edema–white matter contrast with TI settings of 400 and 450 ms, respectively, between the null points of white matter and edema. At a TI value of 400 ms, edema is predicted to be slightly brighter than white matter, whereas at a TI value of 450 ms, almost no contrast exists between the two tissues because of the contrast lost due to magnitude reconstruction.

Examples: Clinical Images

Numerically generated IR images are shown in Figure 4-16 for the same patient and section as the SE images presented in Figure 4-9. These images have been calculated assuming magnitude reconstruction because it is the more commonly used IR image reconstruction method. For all images in Figure 4-16, TR has been fixed at 2000 ms, whereas TI and TE have been varied to correspond to the settings illustrated in Figure 4-15, *E* to *H*. For TI above the null points of white matter and edema (TI = 550 ms), edema and white matter present contrast similar to that in short-TR/short-TE SE imaging. However, other tissues in the image, especially long-T1 tissues such as CSF, present signal uncharacteristic of T1-weighted SE images. For TI below the null point of both tissues (e.g., TI = 100 ms, the STIR imaging domain), a more T2-weighted appearance occurs, although image contrast in this short-TI (STIR) domain is related to the additive effects of correlated T1, T2, and N[H]-inherent contrast. Also, in the images in Figure 4-16, this choice of TI has not completely nulled the signal from subcutaneous fat. Finally, the noisier appearance of images generated with a TI setting between the null points of white matter and edema (TI = 400 or 450 ms) reflects the lower signals from both tissues and a general loss of contrast between the two tissues relative to image noise.

A more complete illustration of the dependence of contrast in magnitude-reconstructed IR on TI and TE (at fixed TR) is illustrated by the contour plot in Figure 4-17. The dark vertical band marks the region of contrast lost because of the use of magnitude-reconstructed IR.[17] The lobe of increased contrast to the right (longer-TI values) is the conventional IR T1-weighted contrast region where white matter is brighter than edema. The lobe of increased contrast to the left (shorter-TI values) is the STIR region, where T1, T2, and N[H] contrast add constructively to make edema brighter than white matter.

GRADIENT-ECHO IMAGING

Gradient-echo imaging techniques provide methods of accumulating images in much shorter total times than conventional pulse sequences. Gradient-echo pulse sequences for MRI were introduced by Haase et al in 1985.[13,14] The basic idea of gradient-echo pulse sequences is to replace the 180-degree rephasing pulses used to form an echo in SE sequences with gradient reversals, in particular reversal of the frequency-encoding or "readout" gradient, as diagrammed in Figure 4-18. The initial negative lobe of the frequency-encoding gradient dephases transverse magnetization; reversal to the positive lobe rephases reversible components of the transverse magnetization to form an echo at time TE when the area under the positive lobe of the frequency-encoding gradient equals the area under the negative lobe. All other gradient manipulations are the same in gradient-echo imaging as in SE imaging. As in SE imaging, the basic gradient-echo pulse sequence must be repeated a large number of times (e.g., 128, 192, or 256, depending on the desired spatial resolution in the phase-encoding direction), each repetition with a different degree of phase encoding so that a sufficient number of phase-encoding "views" is collected to form an image.

The behavior of magnetization in a gradient-echo pulse sequence is illustrated in Figure 4-19. With replacement of 180-degree pulses by gradient reversals, it becomes efficient to use smaller tip-angle excitations (<90 degrees) rather than 90-degree pulses as the initial pulse in each sequence. The use of tip angles less than 90 degrees leaves a component of the longitudinal magnetization unperturbed, still pointing along the +z direction, while tipping a component of magnetization into the transverse plane (Figure 4-19, *B*). In conventional SE or IR pulse sequences, most of the pulse sequence repetition time (TR) is used to allow sufficient recovery of the longitudinal magnetization. In gradient-echo imaging the use of reduced tip angles, leaving a substantial portion of the longitudinal magnetization unperturbed, obviates the need for long TR values to provide sufficient T1-induced recovery. As shown in Equation 4-10, the shortening of TR values from seconds (in conventional SE or IR sequences) to tens of milliseconds (in gradient-echo sequences) greatly reduces scan times, from minutes for conventional imaging to seconds for planar gradient-echo imaging.

The formation of a signal echo by gradient reversal has one distinction from the formation of an SE by a 180-degree pulse. In SE imaging the 180-degree pulse reverses the direction of all transverse magnetization, making the relaxation that occurs between the initial 90-degree RF pulse and signal echo immune to fixed magnetic field inhomogeneities. These magnetic field inhomogeneities may be static magnetic field nonuniformities, any unreversed gradients applied during the time interval TE, or magnetic-susceptibility inhomogeneities. As a result, the transverse relaxation measured in SE sequences is related entirely to "true" T2 relaxation effects, the irreversible dephasing of transverse magnetization resulting from nuclear, molecular, and macromolecular magnetic interactions with hydrogen dipoles.

In gradient-echo imaging, formation of an echo by gradient reversal does not eliminate the dephasing effects of magnetic field inhomogeneities. Therefore the signal decay between the initial (θ-degree pulse and gradient echo depends on "true" T2 relaxation plus relaxation caused by magnetic field inhomogeneities and is governed by a different relaxation time, T2*, which is shorter than T2:

(EQ. 4-18)

$$1/T2^* = 1/T2 + \gamma\pi\Delta B_0$$

where y is the gyromagnetic ratio and ΔB_0 is the magnetic field inhomogeneity across a voxel. In extremely homogeneous magnets using

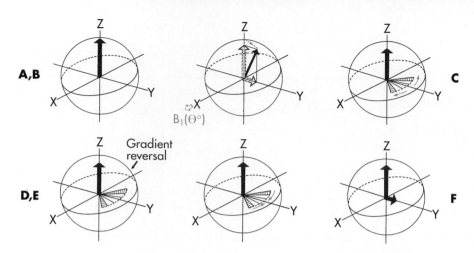

FIGURE 4-19 Gradient-echo pulse sequence: Behavior of magnetization within a voxel. **A,** Initially, magnetization is along +z direction. **B,** θ-Degree pulse tips some fraction of longitudinal magnetization in the transverse plane. If θ is less than 90 degrees, some magnetization will remain in the longitudinal direction. **C,** Transverse component of magnetization dephases during initial period TE/2. **D,** At time TE/2 after the θ-degree pulse, some transverse dephasing is reversed by switching the frequency-encoding gradient from negative to positive. **E,** During the second TE/2 period, transverse magnetization rephases. **F,** At time TE after the θ-degree pulse, a rephasing or echo of transverse magnetization occurs. Signal is measured just before, during, and just after formation of the gradient echo.

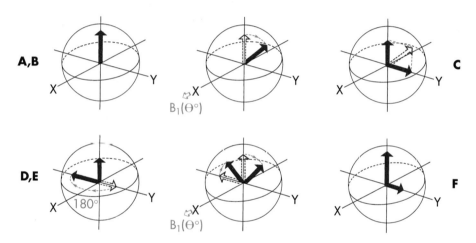

FIGURE 4-20 Steady state gradient-echo pulse sequences: Behavior of the magnetization. **A,** Before the first θ-degree pulse. **B,** θ-Degree pulse tips longitudinal magnetization by θ degrees. **C,** This rotates a component of the tipped magnetization into the transverse plane and leaves a component of the tipped magnetization along the longitudinal direction. **D,** With correct choice of gradient strength, during time period TR, the transverse component of magnetization can precess through a 180-degree phase shift. **E,** Next, the θ-degree pulse tips a component of the 180-degree phase-shifted transverse magnetization back along the +z axis so that it adds to the component of longitudinal magnetization that is unperturbed by the θ-degree pulse **(F).** Condition of steady state equilibrium is that with each θ-degree pulse, longitudinal magnetization feeds into transverse magnetization while transverse magnetization feeds into longitudinal magnetization.

properly designed pulse sequences and in tissue regions without magnetic susceptibility inhomogeneities, T2* values are approximately equal to T2 values. In voxels with magnetic inhomogeneities, including susceptibility inhomogeneities, T2* will be much shorter than T2.

Alternative Methods of Gradient-Echo Imaging

The signal resulting from gradient-echo imaging depends on three independent user-selectable parameters—the sequence repetition time (TR), the echo delay time (TE), and the tip angle (θ). At sufficiently short TR values (TR <100 ms), the measured signal from gradient-echo sequences also depends on the user's choice of treating transverse magnetization after signal measurement. Transverse magnetization can be rephased or destroyed after signal measurement. The following discussion describes the two separate cases.

Rephasing of Transverse Magnetization

The case of rephased transverse magnetization can be depicted by the gradient-echo sequence shown in Figure 4-18 if, after signal measurement, a rephasing (or rewinder) phase-encoding gradient is applied opposite the originally applied phase-encoding gradient (not shown).[32] This reforms a maximum amount of transverse magnetization before repetition of the pulse sequence. With a proper choice of gradient strength and TR values, the reformed transverse magnetization can be used to partially replenish the longitudinal magnetization during the next θ-degree pulse (Figure 4-20). This concept is behind gradient-echo sequences with steady state equilibrium (with vendor acronyms of GRASS, FISP, and FAST): The rephased transverse magnetization is typically permitted to go through a 180-degree phase shift during the TR, so when the next θ-degree pulse occurs (tipping some portion of longitudinal magnetization into the transverse plane where it can form

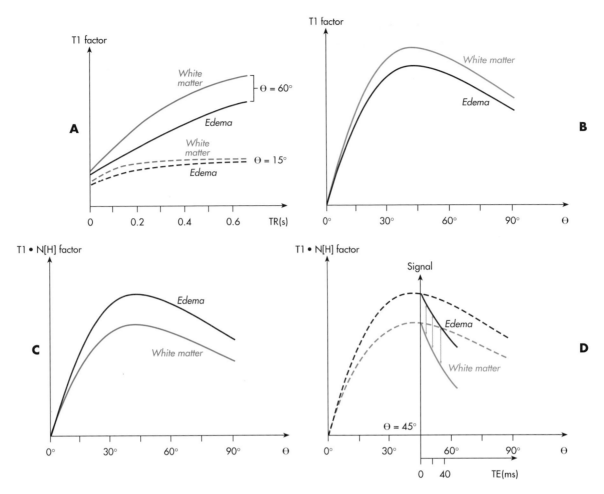

FIGURE 4-21   "T1," N[H], and T2* factors contributing to signal in steady state gradient-echo imaging. **A,** "T1" factors for edema *(red)* and white matter *(blue)* as a function of TR for θ of 15 degrees and 60 degrees. **B,** "T1" factors for edema and white matter as a function of θ for TR of 50 ms. **C,** "T1" factors multiplied by N[H] factors as a function of θ for TR of 50 ms. "T1" and N[H] factors multiplied by T2* factors as a function of TE *(solid lines).* Solid lines are plotted assuming TR of 50 ms, θ of 45 degrees. Vertical distance between solid lines *(green arrows for TE = 10, 20, and 33 ms)* is the edema–white matter contrast at those delay time. In **D,** T2* is assumed to be equal to T2 for edema and white matter.

a signal), some portion of the transverse magnetization is tipped into the +z direction, where it adds to the unperturbed longitudinal magnetization.[26,32,34] The amount of transverse magnetization fed back into longitudinal magnetization, and therefore the degree of steady state equilibrium, increases as the tip angle is increased up to 90 degrees.

Assuming gradient-echo imaging with steady state equilibrium and a 180-degree phase shift of rephased transverse magnetization during the time interval TR and assuming rectangular slice profiles at all tip angles, the signal expression is:

(EQ. 4-19)

$$S_{GE_{ss}}(\theta, TE, TR) = N[H]e^{-TE/T2*} \cdot$$

$$\cdot \frac{[1 - e^{-TR/T1}]\sin\theta}{[1 - e^{-TR/T1}e^{-TR/T2} - (e^{-TR/T1} - e^{-TR/T2})\cos\theta]}$$

The gradient-echo signal from each voxel is a function of four intrinsic tissue parameters in the voxel—N[H], T1, T2, and T2*—and a function of three user-selectable parameters—TR, TE, and θ. The first two terms in the signal expression are similar to the spin-density and T2 factors in SE imaging, with the replacement of T2 (in the T2 factor for SE) by T2* (for gradient echo) because T2* governs the decay of transverse magnetization in gradient-echo imaging. The remaining factors in the gradient-echo signal expression have a complicated dependence on intrinsic tissue parameters T1 and T2 and on user-selectable parameters TR and θ. This set of factors will be referred to as the "T1 factor." Quotation marks are added to indicate that there is a dependence on T2, as well as T1, within the "T1 factor."

To illustrate the effect on contrast of each of the factors in Equation 4-19, we return to the edema–white matter brain model. Figure 4-21, *A,* plots "T1 factors" for edema and white matter as a function of TR for two different tip angles (15 and 60 degrees). There is a minor change in contrast between edema and white matter as a function of TR and a much greater effect of θ on signal and contrast from the "T1 factor." Figure 4-21, *B,* plots the same "T1 factor" as a function of tip angle (θ) for a fixed TR of 50 ms. From the "T1 factor" alone, white matter would produce a higher signal than edema at all tip angles, with the greatest "T1 factor" difference between the two tissues at a tip angle of 37 degrees. Figure 4-21, *C,* illustrates the effect of including the N[H] factor with the "T1 factor": The higher spin density of edema reverses the T1-induced contrast between edema and white matter, making edema brighter at all tip angles, with the greatest edema–white matter signal difference at a tip angle of 43 degrees. This finding indicates that in gradient-echo imaging, just as in SE imaging, correlated N[H] and T1 values interfere destructively in their contribution to image contrast. The inclusion of the T2* factor with "T1" and N[H] factors is illustrated in Figure 4-21, *D,* which shows that T2* decay reduces signal from both tissues, but T2* contrast adds constructively to N[H] contrast, with both T2* and N[H] making edema brighter than white matter. Steady state, gradient-echo edema–white matter contrast as a function of θ and TE, with TR fixed at 50 ms, is more completely illustrated by the contour plot in Figure 4-22.

The general rules gleaned from this steady state gradient-echo example are as follows:

1. The signals from tissues increase only weakly with increasing TR for small tip angles, within the steady state regime. Even for

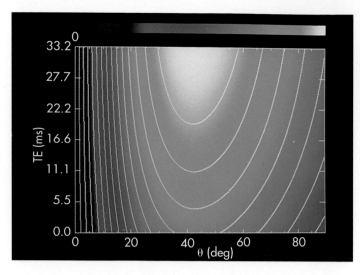

FIGURE 4-22 Contour plot of steady state edema–white matter contrast as a function of TE and θ; TR of 50 ms.

larger tip angles the increase in signal from a single tissue or in contrast between two tissues with increasing TR is so slow that when SNRs or CNRs per unit time are taken into account, SNRs and CNRs decrease or remain approximately constant with increasing TR. Therefore the shortest achievable TR values are most effective.

2. In steady state gradient-echo imaging, correlated N[H] and T1 values interfere destructively, yielding reduced image contrast. Whether T1 effects or N[H] effects dominate depends on the relative inherent contrast between each. Inherent spin-density contrast, however, has a more pronounced effect on image contrast, as exemplified by our brain model, where inherent T1 contrast exceeds inherent N[H] contrast by 63% (Equations 4-6 and 4-8), but N[H] contrast dominated image contrast at all tip angles (Figure 4-21, B and C).

3. As the tip angle θ is increased to 90 degrees, the amount of steady state equilibrium is increased, and the signal from each tissue in steady state gradient-echo sequences assumes an increased dependence on the T2/T1 ratio of tissue relaxation times. Because most tissues, including many lesions, maintain a relatively narrow range of T2/T1 ratios (as do our model tissues of white matter and edema, T2/T1 = 0.13 and 0.14, respectively), short TE, steady state gradient-echo sequences may be limited to relying on relative N[H] as the primary source of image contrast. As TE is increased (up to a practical limit of 2[TR]/3 for symmetrical sampling about the echo peak), the T2* weighting of the sequence is increased. These effects are demonstrated by the simulated gradient-echo steady state images of the brain model appearing in Figure 4-23 for a number of different TE and θ values at a fixed TR value of 50 ms.

Only for very short TR values (TR < T2*) is steady state equilibrium possible. For TR >> T2*, sufficient time exists after signal measurement for the transverse magnetization to completely disappear as a result of T2* relaxation. In that case steady state equilibrium is lost and the signal expression of Equation 4-19 reduces to the signal expression that appears in Equation 4-20 for the case of no transverse magnetization at the time TR.

Finally, a brief word of caution about considering Equation 4-19 completely accurate. Equation 4-19 assumes that all magnetization in a voxel has gone through a 180-degree phase shift during the time interval TR (Figure 4-20). This will be true for some but not all magnetization within a voxel during a steady state, gradient-echo pulse sequence. In general there will be a range of phase shifts that occur during the time interval TR. Therefore Equation 4-19 is only a rough approximation of the signal expression in steady state, gradient-echo imaging.[30,32]

Destroying Transverse Magnetization

Two alternatives exist to produce gradient-echo sequences without the effect of residual transverse magnetization. One is to make TR sufficiently long to ensure that transverse magnetization is completely dephased before the start of the next pulse sequence, as previously mentioned. The other alternative is to keep TR short and intentionally dephase the transverse magnetization after signal measurement. A number of methods to intentionally destroy transverse magnetization have been used, including spoiler gradients applied in a stepped or random manner and RF excitation pulses stepped in phase to avoid phase coherence.[8] Pulse sequences with vendor acronyms, such as FLASH and spoiled GRASS, intentionally destroy transverse magnetization.

The resulting signal expression for gradient-echo imaging with long TR values or with spoiled transverse magnetization, assuming rectangular slice profiles at all tip angles, is:

(EQ. 4-20)

$$S_{GE_{Spoiled}} (\theta, TE, TR) = N[H] e^{-TE/T2^*} \cdot \frac{[1 - e^{-TR/T1}]\sin\theta}{[1 - e^{-TR/T1}\cos\theta]}$$

The signal from each pixel is a function of three intrinsic tissue parameters—N[H], T1, and T2*—and a function of the three user-selectable parameters—θ, TE, and TR. Again, signal strength separates into N[H], T1, and T2* factors, and in this case the T1 factor really is a T1 factor, with dependence on only the inherent tissue parameter T1 and the user-selectable parameters TR and θ.

The contribution of each factor in spoiled gradient-echo imaging is shown in Figure 4-24. Although not shown in Figure 4-24, the dependence of the "T1 factor" on TR in spoiled gradient-echo imaging is quite similar to that in steady state gradient-echo imaging (Figure 4-21, A), with the modification that all signals start at zero for TR of 0 in spoiled gradient-echo imaging. The T1 factor as a function of θ in spoiled gradient-echo imaging for a fixed TR value of 50 ms is shown in Figure 4-24, A. Comparison of Figures 4-21, B, and 4-24, A, illustrates the sizable effect of T2 on the "T1 factor" in steady state gradient-echo imaging. The T2 effect that occurs in steady state equilibrium causes the signal from each tissue to peak at a higher tip angle. In spoiled gradient-echo imaging, signals peak at smaller tip angles. The product of T1 and N[H] factors for white matter and edema is shown in Figure 4-24, B. Note the crossover at a tip angle of 28 degrees. Below the crossover, edema dominates because of its higher spin density (with a peak difference at a 10-degree tip angle), whereas above the crossover white matter dominates because of its shorter-T1 value (with a peak difference at 56 degrees).

Figure 4-24, C and D, shows the T2* factor contributions on top of the T1 and N[H] factors. For smaller tip angles (Figure 4-24, C), T2* effects add constructively to the dominant N[H] effects to make edema brighter than white matter. For tip angles above the crossover (Figure 4-24, D), T2* effects interfere destructively with the dominant T1 effects, tending to reduce image contrast, with a crossover in edema–white matter signal (a total loss of contrast) at θ of 45 degrees, TE of 18 ms.

Figure 4-25 is a contour plot of edema–white matter contrast in spoiled gradient-echo imaging as a function of TE and θ for TR fixed at 50 ms, showing the crossover of edema and white matter signals (dark band) more generally. In the region to the left of the dark band (smaller tip angles) edema is brighter than white matter, whereas to the right of the dark band (larger tip angles), for sufficiently short-TE values, white matter is brighter than edema.

Some general rules can be stated for the contrast in spoiled gradient-echo imaging. At short TR, short TE, and small tip angles, N[H] makes the dominant contribution to image contrast. Increasing TR for small tip angles does not increase image contrast significantly. Increasing TR for larger tip angles shows some increase in image contrast, but the CNR per unit time (contrast divided by TR) remains approximately constant. Increasing the tip angle θ increases the amount of T1 weighting of the image. Increasing TE increases the T2* weighting of the image. For fixed TR and symmetrical signal sampling, however, TE cannot be increased beyond approximately 2(TR)/3 (Figure 4-18). For realistic gradient rise times and RF excitation times, the longest possible TE is slightly less than 2(TR)/3.

As in SE imaging, in tissues where N[H], T1, and T2 are correlated, inherent N[H] and T2* contrast tend to add constructively to image contrast, whereas inherent T1 contrast interferes destructively with inherent N[H] and T2 contrast. These general rules are illustrated by the simulated, spoiled gradient-echo images of the brain model in Figure 4-26 at a matrix of TE and θ values for a fixed TR of 50 ms.

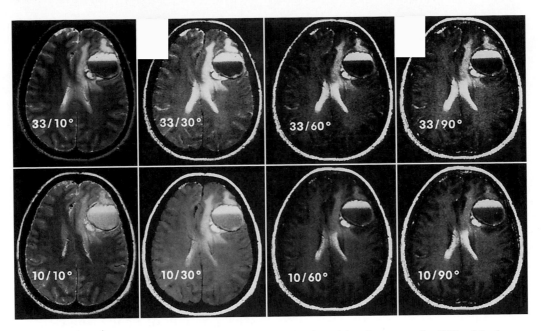

FIGURE 4-23   Synthetic steady state gradient-echo images of brain model section at a matrix of TE and θ values (TE/θ); TR of 50 ms for all images. These images have been reconstructed assuming T2* is equal to T2 for all tissues.

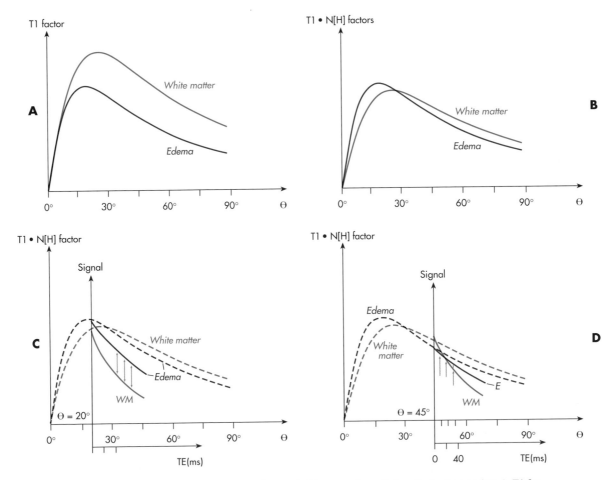

FIGURE 4-24   T1, N[H], and T2* factors for edema and white matter in spoiled gradient-echo imaging. **A,** T1 factors as a function of θ for TR of 50 ms. **B,** T1 factors multiplied by N[H] factors as a function of θ for TR of 50 ms. **C,** T1 and N[H] factors as a function of θ *(dotted lines)* multiplied by T2 factors as a function of TE *(solid lines).* Solid lines are plotted assuming TR of 50 ms, θ of 20 degrees. Vertical distance between solid lines (green arrows for TE = 10, 20, and 33 ms) is edema–white matter contrast at those delay times. **D,** Same as **C** but θ of 45 degrees. In **C** and **D,** T2* is equal to T2 for both tissues.

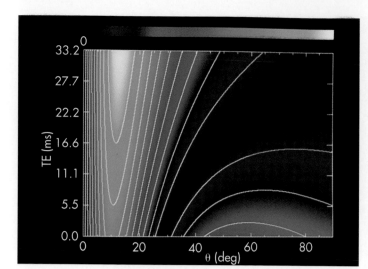

FIGURE 4-25   Spoiled gradient-echo edema–white matter contrast displayed as a function of TE and θ; TR of 50 ms.

Although the simulated gradient-echo images of Figures 4-23 and 4-26 can approximate the image contrast resulting from N[H], T1, and T2 effects, they cannot fully simulate the effects of T2* (which are to some extent scanner dependent), flow, magnetic susceptibility, and chemical shift in gradient-echo imaging. Systematic evaluation of steady state and spoiled gradient-echo imaging at a variety of θ, TE, and TR settings should be performed on a scanner to assess its clinical viability.

Previous studies indicate that gradient-echo imaging offers a moderate advantage in SNR and CNR per unit time over conventional SE imaging.[3,20,29,30] Contrast and CNRs in planar gradient-echo imaging are reduced from that in conventional planar SE imaging, however, because total scan times are much shorter. Because of lower image CNRs and increased artifacts, gradient-echo imaging has not replaced SE imaging for most 2D FT clinical imaging applications. These fast-scanning sequences are of more value because of their ability to capture flow-induced contrast for MR angiography (see Chapter 19), separate CSF from bone and white-gray matter in spine imaging (see Chapter 85), permit more rapid imaging of MR contrast agents (see Chapter 12), and shorten the time required for 3D (volume) image acquisition (see Chapter 6).

NOISE AND ITS EFFECT ON LOW-CONTRAST LESION DETECTION

So far this chapter has described the effect of pulse sequence selection, interpulse delay time selection, and the number of planar acquisitions per phase-encoding step on the signal from a single tissue and the signal difference (or contrast) between tissues. However, because image noise masks low-contrast lesions, it is important to understand how image noise is affected by the imaging technique. After a discussion of the factors affecting image noise, contrast and noise are discussed together, and the effect of imaging techniques on CNRs is considered.

Both statistical noise and systematic noise contribute to the total noise in an MR image. In general, for a given ROI, the two sources of noise add in quadrature:

(EQ. 4-21)

$$\sigma_{total} = \sqrt{(\sigma^2_{statistical} + \sigma^2_{systematic})}$$

where σ is the standard deviation of signal intensity in a prescribed ROI. It is difficult to give general rules for the relative importance of statistical noise versus systematic noise. Statistical noise is present in every MR image; systematic noise occurs in imaging situations in which motion (such as conventional body imaging); truncation, or Gibbs, artifacts (too few matrix elements are selected in a given direction); or aliasing (such as imaging with signal-generating tissue in the

selected plane but outside the prescribed field of view) is a problem. The use of motion-suppression techniques, adequate matrix size, and anti-aliasing techniques can be effective in reducing systematic noise but will not suppress statistical noise.

As in CT, it is reasonable to normalize the noise in an MR image by some reference signal, just as signal difference was normalized by a reference signal to form the image contrast expression in Equation 4-5:

(EQ. 4-22)

$$Noise = \sigma_0/S_{ref}$$

Combining the ratios of Equations 4-5 and 4-22 to form the CNR eliminates the reference signal:

(EQ. 4-23)

$$CNR = \frac{|S_A - S_B|}{\sigma_0}$$

Thus using the definition of contrast given by Equation 4-5 and that of normalized noise given by Equation 4-22, the CNR is identical to the signal difference-to-noise ratio, which frequently is used to assess the ability of MRI to detect low-contrast lesions.[7,16]

Measurement of Image Noise

The 2D FT image reconstruction methods used in planar MRI and the three-dimensional Fourier transform (3D FT) reconstruction methods used in volume MRI have the property of propagating statistical noise from the measured signals uniformly across the reconstructed image. Consequently, random variations in any of the signals used in the reconstruction of a particular plane or volume will show up as random statistical image noise spread evenly throughout the image plane or volume. Hence a simple way to measure statistical image noise is to measure the standard deviation of signal in a background ROI, outside the signal-producing tissue. This measurement is best made in the air-filled region outside the patient in the frequency-encoding direction because background regions in the frequency-encoding direction are less likely to be contaminated with motion-induced or aliasing-induced systematic noise, therefore giving a more accurate estimate of statistical noise alone.

In 2D FT and 3D FT imaging, systematic noise is typically propagated in the phase-encoding direction (or directions) (one direction in 2D FT imaging, two directions in 3D FT imaging). Although the degree of systematic noise (such as motion-induced ghosting) may vary as a function of distance from the source of the noise (the high signal-producing moving tissues), it is possible to estimate the degree of systematic noise by measuring the standard deviation of signal in background regions of interest in the phase-encoding direction from the patient. These ROI measurements estimate total image noise; systematic noise can be estimated by separately measuring and subtracting the contribution of statistical noise according to Equation 4-24.

(EQ. 4-24)

$$\sigma_{systematic} = \sqrt{(\sigma^2_{total} - \sigma^2_{statistical})}$$

Effect of Pulse Sequence and Delay-Time Selection

The statistical noise in an image does not depend on the choice of pulse sequences or interpulse delay times. The primary source of statistical noise (the receiver electronics at very low magnetic field strengths and eddy currents in the patient at mid and high magnetic field strengths) is independent of the pulse sequence and delay times selected by the user. ROI measurements indicate the independence of statistical noise within images acquired with different pulse sequences and delay times.

Systematic noise resulting from both respiratory and cardiac motion has been studied for dependence on interpulse delay times in SE imaging.[28] Results indicate that changing TR alone has no effect on the level of motion-induced systematic noise. Decreasing TR while increasing N_{aqs} (to keep the total imaging time fixed) significantly decreases the level of motion-induced noise. Decreasing TE also decreases the amount of motion-induced systematic noise. Pulse

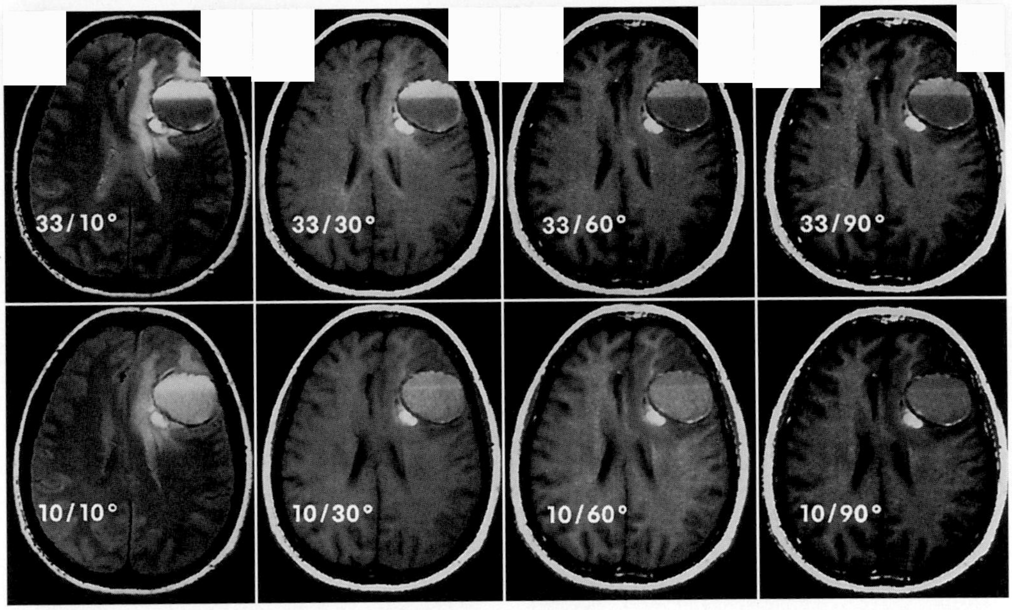

FIGURE 4-26 Synthetic spoiled gradient-echo images of the brain model section, a matrix of TE and θ values (TE/θ) TR of 50 ms for all images and T2* is equal to T2 for all tissues.

sequences (such as STIR) that suppress unwanted signals from moving tissues (such as fat)[4,33] and more general motion-suppression techniques, such as gradient-moment nulling,[25] can be very effective in reducing systematic noise and improving the detection of low-contrast lesions or other subtle anatomical differences.

Effect of Signal Averaging

There is a clearly demonstrated effect of signal averaging on both statistical and systematic noise. Equation 4-11 indicates that the signal from a tissue increases in direct proportion to the number of planar acquisitions per phase-encoding step (N_{aqs}) because signals add coherently. Statistical noise, on the other hand, accumulates incoherently, producing an increase in noise in proportion to the square root of N_{aqs}:

(EQ. 4-25)

$$\sigma_{statistical} \; \alpha \sqrt{N_{aqs}}$$

(The symbol α means "is directly proportional to.") This means that the overall SNR from a single tissue will increase as the square root of N_{aqs}:

(EQ. 4-26)

$$SNR \; \alpha \; \sqrt{N_{aqs}}$$

Investigations into the dependence of motion-induced systematic noise on N_{aqs} indicate that systematic noise also increases in proportion to the square root of N_{aqs}. Other more detailed studies of motion artifacts indicate that the displacement and intensity of motion artifacts depend on the correlation between N_{aqs}, TR, and the periodicity of the moving structure (see Chapter 6).

In most clinical imaging situations, total image noise is approximately independent of interpulse delay times for fixed N_{aqs} but is not independent of N_{aqs}. Therefore an easy way to increase signal or contrast in proportion to noise is to increase N_{aqs}. The SNRs and CNRs increase with N_{aqs} as follows:

(EQ. 4-27)

$$SNR(N_{aqs}) = SNR(1) \cdot \sqrt{N_{aqs}}$$

and

(EQ. 4-28)

$$CNR(N_{aqs}) = CNR(1) \cdot \sqrt{N_{aqs}}$$

where SNR(1) and CNR(1) are the SNR and CNR measured with N_{aqs} equal to 1. Increasing N_{aqs} is particularly effective in situations in which TR can be shortened so that the total imaging time is not too long.[27]

Effect of Sampling Time or Bandwidth

During each repetition of the pulse sequence, the time-varying signal emitted by a selected plane or volume of tissue is measured (or sampled) a large number of times, N_{samp} (e.g., 256 or 512), with a sampling interval between measurements, δt, that is on the order of microseconds. The total sampling time over which the signal is measured (T_s) is the product of the number of samples and the sampling interval:

(EQ. 4-29)

$$T_s = N_{samp} \cdot \delta t$$

Total sampling time is inversely proportional to bandwidth, the range of radiofrequencies over which the signal is measured. A roughly equal amount of noise exists at each frequency. As the bandwidth is widened (the total sampling time is decreased), more noise is included in the measured signal because of the wider range of frequencies recorded. The noise level in the time-varying signal (and the statistical noise level in the image reconstructed from time-varying signals) varies in proportion to the square root of the bandwidth or in inverse proportion to the square root of the sampling time.

(EQ. 4-30)

$$\sigma_{statistical} \; \alpha \sqrt{(Bandwidth)} \; \alpha \; 1/\sqrt{T_s}$$

If statistical noise is the dominant source of image noise, then bandwidth or sampling time will have a major effect on the noise level in the resultant image.

In most imaging situations, sampling time is unaffected by the choice of TR. However, in many pulse sequences, sampling time and TE are interrelated. As shown in the schematics of pulse sequences (Figures 4-6, 4-13, and 4-18, for example), for symmetrical sampling about the echo peak, TE must exceed the sampling time by some minimum time constant, T_c.

(EQ. 4-31)

$$TE \geq T_s + T_c$$

For example, in SE imaging, $T_c/2$ is the minimum time required to complete the second half of the 180-degree rephasing pulse, switch off

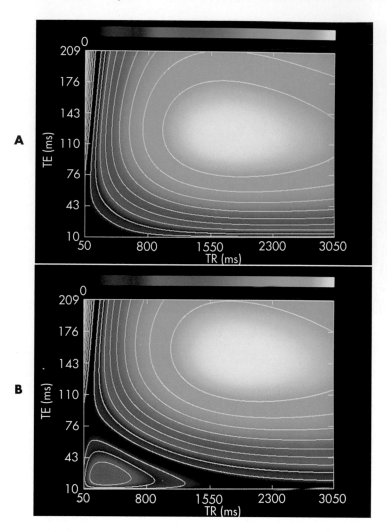

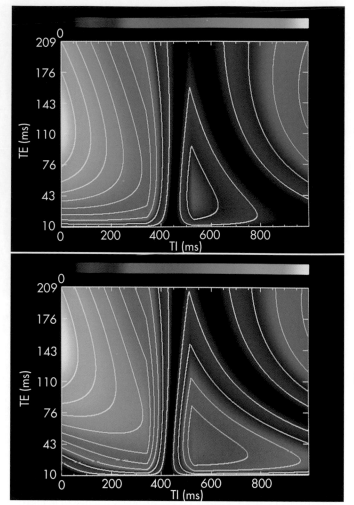

FIGURE 4-27   SE imaging with fixed total imaging time: Edema–white matter CNR is plotted as a function of TR and TE. **A,** Measured, unequal hydrogen spin densities of edema and white matter (Table 4-1). **B,** Equal spin densities for edema and white matter.

FIGURE 4-28   IR imaging with fixed total imaging time: Edema–white matter CNR is plotted as a function of TI and TE with TR of 2000 ms. **A,** Measured, unequal hydrogen spin densities of edema and white matter (Table 4-1). **B,** Equal spin densities for edema and white matter.

slice-select gradients, and switch on read gradients before beginning signal measurement. Minimum T_c values range from 1 to 10 ms on most commercial scanners.

A strategy now used by most MR-scanner manufacturers is to match the sampling time (and bandwidth) to the TE value, so $T_s = TE - T_c$, with T_c a fixed minimum value, up to some maximum sampling time value. Then sampling time may be increased linearly as TE is increased. This means using a short sampling time (wider bandwidth) in short-TR/short-TE imaging (where there is usually adequate signal to overcome the extra noise) and longer sampling times (narrower bandwidths) with long-TR/long-TE images (where there is less signal, and therefore reduced image noise is desirable). Sampling times cannot be increased indefinitely without penalty. Loss of spatial resolution can occur when sampling times exceed the T2 values of the imaged tissues.[12,21] This limit for sampling times, however, is rarely reached using conventional MR pulse sequences.

Effect of Voxel Volume

Voxel volume is determined by the user-selected image matrix, field of view, and slice thickness. If N_x is the number of pixels in the frequency-encoding direction (usually $N_x = 256$), N_y is the number of pixels in the phase-encoding direction (usually $N_y = N_{pe}$, the number of distinct phase-encoding steps), L_x is the length of the field of view in the x direction, L_y is the length of the field of view in the y direction, and δ_z is the slice thickness, then the voxel volume is

(EQ. 4-32)

$$V = \left(\frac{L_x}{N_x}\right)\left(\frac{L_y}{N_y}\right)(\delta_z)$$

The voxel volume can be increased by increasing the field of view (in the x or y direction), by using a coarser image matrix (fewer pixels in x or y), or by increasing the slice thickness. Because for a uniform tissue the amount of hydrogen per voxel is linearly proportional to the voxel volume, the signal per voxel is also linearly proportional to the voxel volume.[23] Noise, however, originates from eddy currents in the patient over the entire sensitive volume of the receiver coil and is independent of the voxel volume. Therefore, assuming uniform tissues in each voxel, SNR and CNR are linearly proportional to voxel volume.

SIGNAL-TO-NOISE AND CONTRAST-TO-NOISE RATIOS

Now the factors affecting signal, contrast, and noise can be combined into individual expressions for SNRs and CNRs in MRI.

Defining Signal-to-Noise and Contrast-to-Noise Ratios

The SNR and CNR are:

(EQ. 4-33)

$$SNR \propto \frac{S(1)}{\sigma_0}\sqrt{(T_{tot}/TR)}\sqrt{(TE - T_c)} \cdot V$$

(EQ. 4-34)

$$CNR \propto \frac{|S_A(1) - S_B(1)|}{\sigma_0}\sqrt{(T_{tot}/TR)}\sqrt{(TE - T_c)} \cdot V$$

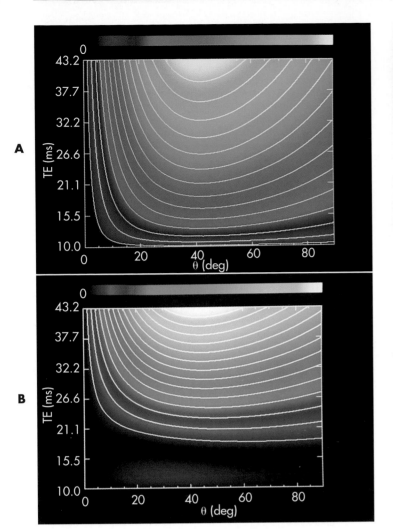

FIGURE 4-29 Steady state gradient-echo imaging: Edema–white matter CNR is plotted as a function of TE and θ with TR of 50 ms. **A,** Measured, unequal hydrogen spin densities of edema and white matter (Table 4-1). **B,** Equal spin densities for edema and white matter.

where $S(1)$, $S_A(1)$, and $S_B(1)$ are signals from a single acquisition per phase-encoding step from a prescribed pulse sequence (as given by Equation 4-9 for SE imaging, Equation 4-17 for IR imaging, or Equations 4-19 and 4-20 for gradient-echo imaging), and V is the voxel volume in Equation 4-32. Each signal term contains an implicit dependence on spin density, T1, and T2 values; interpulse delay times, and possibly tip angles, as given previously in the chapter. The denominator is the noise level per unit time from a single repetition of the pulse sequence. The term $\sqrt{(T_{tot}\, / \, TR)}$ is proportional to the square root of the number of acquisitions per phase-encoding step (excluding the spatial factor N_{pe}), and the term $\sqrt{(TE - T_c)}$ is the sampling time (or bandwidth) factor, assuming that sampling time is adjusted with TE according to the relation:

(EQ. 4-35)

$$T_s = TE - T_c$$

where T_c is fixed. The echo-delay time TE must exceed T_c to permit sampling of the signal.

The SNR and CNR expressions of Equations 4-33 and 4-34 can be used to determine the pulse sequences, interpulse delay times, and, if relevant, tip angles that maximize the SNR from a single tissue or maximize the CNR between a pair of tissues. Maximization of the SNR from a single tissue might be relevant when a small lesion or other signal-producing tissue is located on a background producing little or no signal, such as an acoustic neuroma on a background of CSF and bone.[18] More often, a lesion or tissue of interest is surrounded by background tissues producing some comparable signal; in such cases it is the CNR between the lesion and background tissues that should be maximized.[7,16,19]

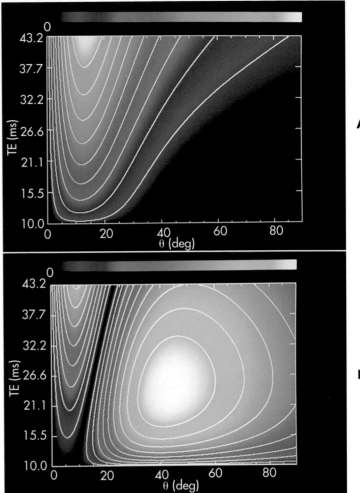

FIGURE 4-30 Spoiled gradient-echo imaging: Edema–white matter CNR is plotted as a function of TE and θ; TR of 50 ms. **A,** Measured, unequal hydrogen spin densities of edema and white matter (Table 4-1). **B,** Equal spin densities for edema and white matter.

Maximizing Contrast-to-Noise Ratios in Clinical Imaging

To illustrate the maximization of the CNR between two tissues, the edema–white matter model previously discussed is considered. Equation 4-34 can be used to maximize the CNR between white matter and lesion using various pulse sequences under the assumption of a fixed total imaging time, a fixed number of phase-encoding steps (e.g., N_{pe} = 256), and a fixed T_c value. As described earlier, in the case of a fixed total imaging time, when a shorter TR value is chosen, a greater number of planar acquisitions per phase-encoding step (N_{aqs}) are acquired and averaged.

Edema–white matter CNRs from SE, IR, and gradient-echo sequences are shown in Figures 4-27 to 4-30. All CNR plots are done under the conditions of a fixed total imaging time with sampling time (or bandwidth) adjusted with TE according to Equation 4-35 and a T_c of 10 ms.

In the SE plot (Figure 4-27, *A*) a broad maximum CNR per unit time (center of the white region) occurs at TR/TE of 1770/120 ms. In this entire long-TR/long-TE region, edema will be brighter than white matter because of the constructive contributions of inherent N[H] and T2 contrast to image contrast. The broad maximum of CNR per unit time in TR and TE makes long-TR/long-TE SE imaging forgiving to the user's choice of delay times. For TR/TE selections within the first white band surrounding the maximum (roughly, TR ranging from 1000 to 3000 ms and TE ranging from 75 to 160 ms), at least 90% of the maximum CNR per unit time will be achieved.

Although not visible in Figure 4-27, *A*, a short-TR/short-TE CNR maximum occurs at TR/TE of 110/15 ms but with a CNR per unit time of only 3% of that at the long-TR/long-TE maximum. At this short-TR/short-TE maximum, edema appears darker than white matter (see the inverse pure T1 image in Figure 4-5, *B*). However, the cancellation of inherent T1 contrast by both inherent N[H] and T2 contrast makes the detection of edema by short-TR/short-TE pulse sequences impractical.

To evaluate the effect of the measured, unequal hydrogen spin densities on CNR and on the optimal selection of TR/TE values in SE imaging, the CNR plot of Figure 4-27, *A,* is recalculated for the hypothetical case of equal spin densities for edema and white matter. This CNR contour plot, again assuming a fixed total imaging time, is shown in Figure 4-27, *B*. With spin densities of the two tissues artificially set equal, there are two distinct maxima—a short-TR/short-TE maximum with a peak in TR/TE at 300/24 ms and a long-TR/long-TE maximum with a peak at 1915/150 ms. With equal spin densities, the CNR at the short-TR/short-TE maximum is about 40% of that at the long-TR/long-TE maximum.

By comparing Figure 4-27, *A* and *B,* it can be seen qualitatively that the measured, unequal spin densities have a pronounced effect, suppressing the CNR at the short-TR/short-TE peak. (The correlated, unequal spin densities have a CNR at short-TR/short-TE that is a factor of 8 smaller than the CNR for equal spin densities.) The effect of spin densities on CNR at the long-TR/long-TE settings is opposite in direction and less dramatic. (The measured, unequal spin densities produce CNR at the long-TR/long-TE peak that is 24% higher than that for the case of equal spin densities.) This is one more demonstration that spin densities correlated with T1 and T2 interfere destructively with T1-induced contrast but add constructively to T2-induced contrast.

Magnitude-reconstructed IR CNR as a function of two of the independent interpulse delay times (TE and TI) is illustrated in Figure 4-28. The third user-selectable delay time (TR) is fixed at a value of 2000 ms, fixing the total imaging time as well. Figure 4-28, *A,* plots CNR for the measured, unequal spin densities. Figure 4-28, *B,* plots CNR for a hypothetical case of equal spin densities. In either case there are three TI/TE regions of distinct contrast. The short-TI/long-TE maximum is the STIR region, where T1, T2, and N[H] effects add constructively to produce the greatest image contrast, with edema brighter than white matter. This STIR maximum in CNR occurs at TI values as short as possible and at long-TE values (TE = 115 ms for the measured, unequal spin densities; TE = 140 ms for equal spin densities).

The second maximum is the conventional T1-weighted IR maximum, where edema is darker than white matter, occurring at intermediate TI and shorter-TE values. For equal or unequal spin densities the maximum edema–white matter CNR occurs at TI/TE of 520/43. This conventional IR maximum is approximately 30% of the STIR maximum in the case of measured, unequal spin densities and is approximately 50% of the STIR maximum in the hypothetical case of equal spin densities. The dark band between the STIR and conventional IR regions reflects the loss of edema-white matter contrast caused by the use of magnitude reconstruction in IR imaging.[17] The dark band to the right of the conventional IR maximum is the crossover that occurs for longer-TE values, resulting from the destructive interference between correlated T1 and T2 values in conventional IR imaging. The region of increased CNR in the upper right-hand corner of both figures is a T2-weighted contrast region occurring at long TI and long TE. Long-TI/long-TE delay times are seldom used in IR imaging because of the cancellation of contrast by T1 and T2, the loss of signal at long TE, and the reduction in the number of slices that can be obtained with long-TI and long-TE settings.

CNRs in steady state gradient-echo imaging are shown by the contour plots of Figure 4-29, *A,* for measured, unequal spin densities and by Figure 4-29, *B,* for the hypothetical case of equal spin densities. Both contour plots are similar in shape, showing broad maxima at longer-TE values and intermediate tip angles. The peak CNR in the measured, unequal spin-density case occurs at the longest attainable TE, θ = 42 degrees, and in the equal spin-density case at the longest attainable TE, θ = 44 degrees. At the peak the CNR is approximately a factor of 3 greater in the case of measured, unequal spin densities than in the case of equal spin densities, indicating that the contrast is largely derived from spin-density differences, with T2* and T2 as weaker sources of edema–white matter contrast.

CNR in the case of spoiled gradient-echo imaging is illustrated by the contour plot of Figure 4-30, *A,* for unequal spin densities and by Figure 4-30, *B,* for equal spin densities. In measured, unequal spin den-

sities there is a much narrower edema–white matter CNR maximum as a result of correlated N[H] and T2* differences (occurring at the longest attainable TE, θ = 13 degrees), again with edema brighter than white matter. There is also a very weak T1-induced maximum (edema darker than white matter) for short-TE values ($\approx$15 ms) and larger tip angles (50 to 90 degrees), but this maximum is not visible in Figure 4-30, *A,* because it has at most approximately 5% of the CNR of the N[H] − T2*-induced maximum.

Artificially setting spin densities of edema and white matter equal in the spoiled gradient-echo case markedly alters the contrast between tissues. Setting spin densities equal pushes the N[H] T2*-induced CNR peak to smaller tip angles ($\approx$10 degrees), again peaking for the longest attainable TE values, and creates a broad T1-induced CNR region where edema is darker than white matter, peaking for intermediate TE values (20 to 30 ms) and intermediate tip angles (40 to 50 degrees) (Figure 4-30, *B*). For this hypothetical case of equal spin densities in spoiled gradient-echo imaging, the edema–white matter CNR at the T1-induced peak is approximately double the CNR at the N[H] T2*-induced peak.

SUMMARY

The following criteria should be used in choosing pulse sequences and interpulse delay times for MRI of disease:

1. It is important to choose pulse sequences and delay times that come as close as possible to maximizing CNR per unit time between the tissues of interest.
2. It is important that the choices be forgiving, with broad maxima that will still produce adequate CNR even if delay times are not chosen precisely to maximize CNR for a given pair of tissues. Often, delay times will be adjusted for reasons other than the optimization of CNR, such as the need to obtain a sufficient number of slices to cover the anatomy of interest without doubling the total imaging time. In most cases the imaging task will be to distinguish a number of tissues within the same image, not just to maximize the CNR between two tissues. For example, in imaging MS (Figure 4-2) the goal is to maximize contrast between MS and white matter, while also maximizing the contrast between MS and CSF. Choosing delay times that fall within a broad maximum has a far greater chance of achieving a reasonable amount of contrast among several tissues.
3. It is important to recognize that tissue N[H] can vary widely, having just as much effect on resultant image contrast as tissue T1 and T2 values. If disease states are known to have consistent trends toward elevated spin densities (such as MS[9]), knowledge of elevated spin densities can be used to advantage in the choice of pulse sequences and timing parameters (such as the collection of long-TR/short-TE SE sequences to ensure the distinction of MS from brain and CSF in Figure 4-2, *C*). In disease states in which spin densities are unknown or are widely variable, the best approach still is to collect a variety of pulse sequences, including those weighted to emphasize T1-, T2-, and N[H]-induced contrast. This approach ensures the greatest likelihood that disease will be detected, regardless of the particular correlation among tissue parameters.

REFERENCES

1. Bottomley PA, Foster TH, Argersinger RE, et al: A review of normal tissue hydrogen NMR relaxation times and relaxation mechanisms from 1-100 MHz: dependence on tissue type, NMR frequency, temperature, excision and age, Med Physics 11:425, 1984.
2. Bottomley PA, Hardy CJ, Argersinger RE, et al: A review of H nuclear magnetic resonance relaxation in pathology: are T1 and T2 diagnostic? Med Physics 14:1, 1987.
3. Buxton RB, Edelman RR, Rosen BR, et al: Contrast in rapid MR imaging: T1- and T2-weighted imaging, J Comput Assist Tomogr 11:7, 1987.
4. Bydder GM, and Young IR: MRI clinical use of the inversion recovery sequence, J Comput Assist Tomogr 8:588, 1985.
5. Carr HY, and Purcell EM: Effects of diffusion on free precession in nuclear magnetic resonance experiment, Phys Rev 94:630, 1954.
6. Edelstein WA, Hutchison JMS, Johnson G, et al: Spin warp imaging and applications to human whole-body imaging, Phys Med Biol 25:756, 1980.
7. Edelstein WA, Bottomley PA, Hart HR, et al: Signal, noise, and contrast in nuclear magnetic resonance (NMR) imaging, J Comput Assist Tomogr 7:391, 1983.
8. Frahm J, Merboldt KD, and Hanicke W: Transverse coherence in rapid FLASH NMR imaging, J Magn Reson 27:307, 1987.
9. Geis R, Hendrick RE, Lee S, et al: White matter lesions: the role of spin density effects in MR imaging, Radiology 170:863, 1989.

10. Gomori JM, and Grossman RI: Mechanisms responsible for the MR appearance and evolution of intracranial hemorrhage, Radiographics 8:427, 1988.

11. Grossman RI, Gomori JM, Goldberg HI, et al: MR imaging of hemorrhagic conditions of the head and neck, Radiographics 8:441, 1988.

12. Haacke EM: Effects of finite sampling in spin-echo or field-echo magnetic resonance imaging, Magn Reson Med 4:407, 1987.

13. Haase A, Frahm J, Matthaei D, et al: Rapid images and NMR movies. In Proceedings of the 4th Annual Meeting of the Society of Magnetic Resonance in Medicine, 1985.

14. Haase A, Frahm J, Matthaei D, et al: FLASH imaging: rapid NMR imaging using low flip angle pulses, J Magn Reson 67:217, 1986.

15. Hahn EL: Spin echoes, Phys Rev 80:580, 1950.

16. Hendrick RE, Nelson TR, and Hendee WR: Optimizing tissue contrast in magnetic resonance imaging, Magn Reson Imaging 2:193, 1984.

17. Hendrick RE, Nelson TR, and Hendee WR: Phase detection and contrast loss in magnetic resonance imaging, Magn Reson Imaging 2:279, 1984.

18. Hendrick RE, Newman FD, and Hendee WR: MR imaging technology: maximizing the signal-to-noise ratio from a single tissue, Radiology 156:749, 1985.

19. Hendrick RE: Sampling time effects on signal-to-noise and contrast-to-noise ratios in spin-echo MRI, Magn Reson Imaging 5:31, 1987.

20. Hendrick RE, Kneeland JB, and Stark DD: Maximizing signal-to-noise and contrast-to-noise ratios in FLASH imaging, Magn Reson Imaging 5:117, 1987.

21. Hoult D: Field, contrast, and sensitivity in imaging. In James TL, and Margulis AR, eds: Biomedical magnetic resonance, San Francisco, 1984, Radiology Research and Education Foundation.

22. Hyde JS, and Kneeland JB: High-resolution methods using local coils. In Wehrli FW, Shaw D, and Kneeland JB, eds: Biomedical magnetic resonance imaging: principles, methodology, and applications, New York, 1988, VCH Publishers.

23. Kanal EM, and Wehrli FW: Signal to noise ratio, resolution, and contrast. In Wehrli FW, Shaw D, and Kneeland JB, eds: Biomedical magnetic resonance imaging: principles, methodology, and applications, New York, 1988, VCH Publishers.

24. Meiboom S, and Gill D: Modified spin-echo method for measuring nuclear relaxation times, Rev Sci Instr 29:688, 1958.

25. Pattany PM, Philips JJ, Chiu LC, et al: Motion artifact suppression technique (MAST) for MR imaging, J Comput Assist Tomogr 11:369, 1987.

26. Patz S: Steady state free precession: an overview of basic concepts and applications, Adv Mag Reson Imaging 1:73, 1989.

27. Stark DD, Wittenberg J, Edelman RR, et al: Detection of hepatic metastases: analysis of pulse sequence performance in MR imaging, Radiology 159:365, 1986.

28. Stark DD, Hendrick RE, Hahn PF, et al: Motion artifact reduction by fast spin echo imaging, Radiology 164:183, 1987.

29. Tkach JA, and Haacke EM: A comparison of fast spin echo and gradient field echo sequences, Magn Reson Imaging 6:373, 1988.

30. van der Muelen P, Groen JP, Tinus AMC, et al: Fast field echo imaging: an overview and contrast calculations, Magn Reson Imaging 6:355, 1988.

31. Wehrli F, McFall JR, Glover GH, et al: The dependence of nuclear magnetic resonance (NMR) image contrast on intrinsic and pulse sequence timing parameters, Magn Reson Imaging 2:3, 1984.

32. Wehrli FW: Fast MR imaging. In Kressel HY, Modic MT, and Murphy WA, eds: Syllabus, special course: MR 1990, Oak Brook, Ill, 1990, RSNA Publications.

33. Young IR, Burl M, and Bydder GM: Comparative efficiency of different pulse sequences in MR imaging, J Comput Assist Tomogr 10:271, 1985.

34. Zur Y, Stokar S, and Bendel P: Analysis of fast imaging sequences with steady state transverse magnetization refocusing, Magn Reson Med 6:175, 1988.

ADDITIONAL READINGS

Books

Bradley WG: Fundamentals of magnetic resonance image interpretation. In Bradley WG, Adey WR, and Hasso AN, eds: Magnetic resonance imaging of the brain, head, and neck: a text atlas, Rockville, Md, 1984, Aspen.

Bradley WG, Crooks LE, and Newton TH: Physical principles of NRM. In Newton TH, and Potts DG, eds: Advanced imaging techniques, vol 2, San Francisco, 1983, Clavadel Press.

Hendrick RE, Russ Pd, and Simon JH: MRI: principles and artifacts, New York, 1993, Raven Press.

Mansfield P, and Morris PG: NMR imaging in biomedicine, New York, 1982, Academic Press.

Rose A: Vision: human and electronic, New York, 1973, Plenum Press. (See especially Chapter 1.)

Runge VM: Enhanced magnetic resonance imaging, St Louis, 1989, Mosby.

Smith H-J, and Ranallo F: A non-mathematical approach to basic MRI, Madison, Wis, 1989, Medical Physics.

Wehrli FW, MacFall J, and Newton TH: Parameters determining the appearance of NMR images. In Newton TH, and Potts DG, eds: Advanced imaging techniques, vol 2, San Francisco, 1983, Clavadel Press.

Wehrli FW, Shaw D, and Kneeland JB: Biomedical magnetic resonance imaging: principles, methodology, and applications, New York, 1988, VCH Publishers.

Young SW: Magnetic resonance imaging: basic principles, ed 2, New York, 1988, Raven Press.

Articles

Bradley WG: Effect of relaxation times on magnetic resonance image interpretation, Non-invasive Med Imaging 1:193, 1984.

Bradley WG, and Waluch V: Blood flow: magnetic resonance imaging, Radiology 154:443, 1985.

Brant-Zawadzki M: MR imaging of the brain, Radiology 166:1, 1988.

Hendrick RE, Kanal E, and Osborn AG: Basic MR physics. In Kressel HY, Modic MT, and Murphy WA, ed: Syllabus, special course: MR 1990, Oak Brook, Ill, 1990, RSNA Publications.

Mitchell MR, Tarr RW, Conturo CL, et al: Spin echo technique selection: basic principles for choosing MRI pulse sequence timing intervals, Radiographics 6:245, 1986.

Pavlicek W: MR instrumentation and image formation, Radiographics 7:809, 1987.

Perman WH, Hilal SK, Simon HE, et al: Contrast manipulation in NMR imaging, Magn Reson Imaging 2:23, 1984.

5 Use of the Inversion Recovery Pulse Sequence

Graeme M. Bydder, Joseph V. Hajnal, and Ian R. Young

Basic Form of the Inversion Recovery Sequence
Short TI Inversion Recovery Sequence
Medium TI Inversion Recovery Sequence
Long TI Inversion Recovery Sequence
Flow Effects, Angiography, and Perfusion
Other Variants of the Inversion Recovery Sequence
Summary

 KEY POINTS

- Inversion recovery accomplishes selective nulling of a specific tissue based on its T1 relaxation time and the chosen inversion time TI.
- Short TI: High-contrast, fat-nulled T1- and T2-weighted sequences for imaging of the head and neck, abdomen, pelvis, and musculoskeletal systems (e.g., fast STIR or turbo STIR).
- Medium TI: Highly T1-weighted sequence with high sensitivity to contrast enhancement (e.g., MP-RAGE).
- Long TI: CSF-nulled sequence with high sensitivity to acute subarachnoid hemorrhage and parenchymal disease, especially disease at the brain–CSF interface, such as multiple sclerosis, cortical infarcts, infection, and tumors (e.g., fast FLAIR or turbo FLAIR).

The inversion recovery (IR) pulse sequence (180 degrees–90 degrees–data collection) has been used to provide heavily T1-weighted images since the earliest days of clinical magnetic resonance imaging (MRI). The initial 180-degree pulse inverts the stored magnetization so that it becomes antiparallel to the main magnetic field. During the inversion time (TI) after the initial pulse and before the subsequent 90-degree pulse, the magnetization recovers back toward its equilibrium value as a function of T1. The IR sequences first used for clinical studies produced high contrast between normal and pathological tissues based on differences in T1. The sequence was used in the first studies that showed the advantage of MRI over ultrasound[92] and x-ray computed tomography (CT)[116] and was the single most effective imaging technique available from 1980 until 1982.

In 1982 the heavily T2-weighted spin-echo (SE) sequence was introduced into clinical practice.[1,9,13] This sequence provided a very useful approach for disease detection based on differences in T2, and it subsequently became the mainstay of clinical diagnosis in many regions of the body. T1-weighted SE sequences also provided a method for obtaining T1-weighted images that were lower in lesion contrast and quicker than IR sequences. As a result of these developments there was less need for the IR sequence.

Magnetic resonance (MR) studies in 1980 to early 1982 involved only a single slice and were performed at low fields (0.04 to 0.15 T).[9,58] After this time there was a tendency to increase the operating field strength, which increased tissue T1 and prolonged the time required for the T1-weighted IR sequence to achieve equivalent image contrast. Multiple slice techniques were also implemented, and these required slice-selected 180-degree pulses. Whereas slice-selected 90-degree pulses were easy to design and implement, it took longer to do this with 180-degree pulses. The IR sequence, with its relatively long interval between the initial 180-degree pulse and the subsequent 90-degree pulse, was more difficult to package in a multislice format than conventional SE sequences. In addition, high lesion contrast is often

achieved with IR sequences when tissues have a low signal, and this produces a noisy appearance to the image. For these reasons the conventional T1-weighted IR pulse sequence was displaced as the principal pulse sequence used for diagnostic purposes, but it continued to have applications when highly T1-weighted contrast was desired, such as for detecting contrast enhancement[29] or in demonstrating myelination in infants[48,55] (Box 5-1).

A particular variant of the IR sequence, in which the timing of the interval between the initial inversion pulse and the following 90-degree pulse was set to null the signal from fat (which has a very short T1) and the echo time (TE) was chosen to provide very high lesion contrast, proved to be very useful in body and musculoskeletal applications.[10,90] This short inversion time IR (STIR) sequence combined fat suppression with high T1- and T2-weighted lesion contrast. In 1985, when various orthopedic, bone marrow, and oncological applications were difficult, STIR proved a valuable addition to MRI and remains in active use at the present time. It is particularly well suited to mid- and low-field applications where chemical shift (spectroscopic) techniques for fat suppression are difficult or impossible.

The capacity of the IR sequence to null fluids was demonstrated in early studies,[10,52] but this technique has been used most successfully in the form of the fluid-attenuated inversion recovery (FLAIR) sequence, where cerebrospinal fluid (CSF) is suppressed and mild or heavy T2 weighting (long TE) is used to detect lesions in the brain and spinal cord.[14,33,109]

With the further development of faster imaging techniques, such as the fast spin echo (FSE) or rapid acquisition with relaxation enhancement (RARE) sequence,[41] the rapid gradient-echo sequence[7,23,31,69] combinations of these,[26] and echo-planar imaging,[61] there has been renewed interest in the use of the IR sequence. With these sequences the time penalty associated with the IR sequence is no longer a problem. Many of the faster imaging sequences have unfavorable tissue contrast properties when used alone, and these can be improved by applying an appropriately timed inversion pulse before the rest of the sequence. In addition, there has been a considerable improvement in machine performance since the early 1980s. This improvement has included better optimization of radiofrequency pulses, reduction in eddy currents with self-shielded gradients, improved image processing, and many other features. These advances have produced better image signal-to-noise and contrast-to-noise ratios, which have particularly benefited the noisy variants of the IR sequence.

The flow effects of the IR sequence have not received the attention of those of the SE sequence, and these are now a subject of considerable interest. Blood nulling is widely used to control artifacts, IR forms of angiography are being implemented, and inversion pulses have been used to label inflowing arterial blood outside of the slice interest to provide measures of tissue perfusion.[16]

In the following section the basic form of the IR sequence is described, followed by outlines of the short TI, medium TI, and long TI sequences, as well as a discussion of flow effects and other variants of the sequence. The objective is to present an overview of the options available with the IR sequence and to explain how these are applied in clinical practice.

BASIC FORM OF THE INVERSION RECOVERY SEQUENCE

The dependence of signal intensity on proton density seen with the IR sequence, T1, and T2 can be described in mathematical terms and modeled using the Bloch equations, but for simplicity a qualitative descrip-

BOX 5-1
Some Variants of the Inversion Recovery Sequence

BIR	Balanced inversion recovery[18,117] (T1-weighted IR with TI approximately one half of TR); also known as *MDEFT* (see below)	MT-STIR	Magnetization transfer–STIR[32]
		OIL-FLAIR	Optimized, interleaved, fluid-attenuated inversion recovery[56]
DIR	Double inversion recovery;[9] also known as *STAIR* and *STIR-FLAIR* (see right)	PAIR	Precise and accurate inversion recovery[95]; method for T1 measurement
DISE	Driven inversion spin echo[12]	PARIS	Perfusion assessment by repetitive inversion of spins[39]
EPI-STAR	Echo-planar imaging[13] and signal targeting with alternating radiofrequency[14]	PIETIR	Prolonged inversion and echo-timed inversion recovery[33]; also known as *FLAIR* (see left)
EPI-FLAIR	Echo-planar imaging–FLAIR[33] (see below)	PRESTO	Preinversion segmented turbo fast low-angle shot (FLASH)[21]; unselected then selected inversion for blood nulling; PRESTO also stands for principle of echo shifting with a train of observations[104]
FAIR	Flow-sensitive alternating inversion recovery[51]		
Fast DIR	Fast double inversion recovery[4]		
Fast STIR	Fast spin-echo STIR (see right)		
Fast FLAIR	Fast spin-echo FLAIR[33] (see below)		
FIR	Fast inversion recovery[85,91] (uses T1-weighted fast spin echo or RARE)	SIR	Selective inversion recovery[71]; an arterial inflow technique
FLAIR	Fluid-attenuated inversion recovery[14]	SOS	Silicone-only scanning[70]; combines STIR (fat) and binomial (water) suppression
FLAIR-FSE	FLAIR–fast spin echo[33]	STAIR or STIR-FLAIR	Solution and tissue-attenuated inversion recovery; also know as *double inversion recovery* (DIR)[10]
FLAIR-GRASE	FLAIR–gradient and spin echo[43]		
FLAT TIRE	Fluid-attenuated turbo inversion recovery[80,89]; also known as *FLAIR* (see above)		
HIRE	High-intensity reduction[15]	SPIR	Spectral presaturation with inversion recovery[119]
IR(I)-EPI	Inversion recovery (interleaved) echo-planar imaging[61,112]	STIR	Short TI inversion recovery[9,10]
IR-FSE	Inversion recovery fast spin echo	STIR-FLAIR	Also known as *STAIR* and *DIR* (see above and right)
IR-HASTE	Inversion recovery half-Fourier single-shot turbo spin echo[45]		
IR-PREP	Inversion recovery magnetization preparation[69]	T1W IR	T1-weighted inversion recovery
IRSE	Inversion recovery spin echo	T2-FLAIR	T2-prepared FLAIR, see *DISE*[111]
LOOK-LOCKER	Inversion followed by multiple low flip-angle pulses for T1 measurement[57]; named after authors of paper	TIREX	Total inversion recovery examination
		Turbo-FLAIR	Turbo (RARE/fast spin echo) fluid-attenuated inversion recovery, see *fast FLAIR*
MDEFT	Modified driven-equilibrium Fourier transformation (T1 approximately one half of TR)[44,102]; also known as *BIR* (see above)	Turbo-FLASH	Turbo-fast low-angle shot[31]; inversion pulse followed by rapid gradient-echo sequence; also known as *IR turbo-FLASH*, see *MP-RAGE*
MIR	Multiple inversion recovery[17]		
MPIR	Multiplanar inversion recovery	Turbo-STIR	Turbo (RARE/fast spin echo) STIR (see above)
MP-RAGE	Magnetization-prepared rapid acquisition gradient echo[69]; inversion (or other pulse followed by rapid gradient echo, see *turbo-FLASH*)	ULSTIR-EPI	Ultra-short TI inversion recovery echo-planar imaging[88] (TI 5 to 40 ms)
		UNFAIR	Uninverted flow-sensitive alternating recovery[38]

tion of the sequence is used in this chapter.* The proton magnetization induced in the patient by the static magnetic field can be represented by a vector M. The component of the magnetization in the longitudinal direction (parallel with the static magnetic field) at any given time is then represented by M_z, and that in the transverse direction at the same time by M_{xy}. The effect of a 90-degree pulse is to rotate M_z into the transverse plane to become M_{xy}. This is illustrated in Figure 5-1, which shows a simple IR sequence.

After the 90-degree pulse from the previous repetition of the sequence (Figure 5-1, *A,* pulse A), M_z increases exponentially from zero with time-constant T1 (Figure 5-1, *A*), and M_{xy} decays exponentially with time-constant T2 (Figure 5-1, *B*). If the recovery period of M_z is followed by a 180-degree pulse, M_z is inverted to become $-M_z$ and recovers with a time-constant T1 but at twice the initial rate of the earlier longitudinal recovery after the 90-degree pulse (Figure 5-1, *A*). At the next 90-degree pulse (pulse B in Figure 5-1, *B*), M_z is rotated to become M_{xy}. M_{xy} then decays exponentially with time-constant T2. Using a gradient-echo data collection, signal is collected during the period (data collection [DC]) that straddles the time TE after the 90-degree pulse. The cycle is then repeated.

A composite diagram, first after M_z and then following M_{xy} after the 90-degree pulse (which followed the previous 180-degree pulse), can be used to represent the "potential signal intensity" at various stages in the sequence (Figure 5-1, *C*). The size of the received signal and ultimately the signal intensity of a voxel in the image is proportional to M_{xy} at the midpoint of the DC. M_{xy} is also proportional to the number of MR-visible protons per voxel or tissue proton density.

*References 11, 18, 19, 40, 66, 77.

The times TR (repetition time), TI, and TE are shown in Figure 5-1. TI is the inversion time, which is the time between the inverting 180-degree pulse and the following 90-degree pulse, and TE is the time from the 90-degree pulse to the echo formed during data collection. The decay of the available transverse magnetization is shown. In this and all the other diagrams in this chapter a gradient-echo data collection is used. An SE data acquisition also may be used. This method includes one or more 180-degree pulses shortly after the 90-degree pulse to refocus the transverse magnetization. The data collection is then the same as for the gradient-echo form of the sequence. TR is the duration of each cycle of the sequence (Figure 5-1).

Using Figure 5-1, *C,* as a model of the IR sequence, we can next compare the signal intensities of white matter (a tissue with a relatively short T1), gray matter (a tissue with a longer T1), and CSF (which has a very long T1) as shown in Figure 5-2. In this and subsequent sequences, M_z is plotted until the 90-degree pulse, which then rotates M_z to become M_{xy}. Thereafter, M_{xy} is plotted. The signal intensity observed in a voxel or an image is proportional to the height of M_{xy} on the graph at the time of the data collection. With the timings employed in Figure 5-2, it can be seen that the shorter T1 of white matter eventually results in a higher signal intensity than for gray matter. The very long T1 of CSF results in a low signal intensity, which may be negative as in Figure 5-2. (Negative signal intensity is darker than the zero background signal, which is gray.) The last segment of the decay converges toward zero for both gray and white matter with their respective positive signal intensities, as well as for CSF with its negative signal intensity. Display of the resultant image after phase-corrected processing (see later discussion) gives white for white matter, light gray for gray matter, and black for CSF (Figure 5-3). The signal for gray matter is slightly greater

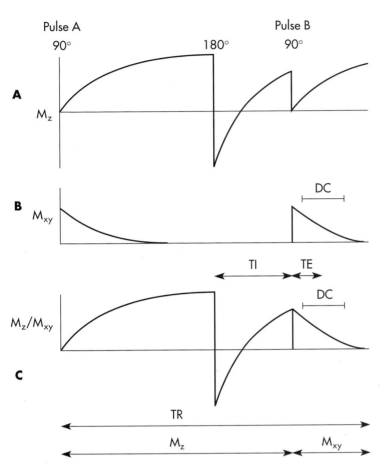

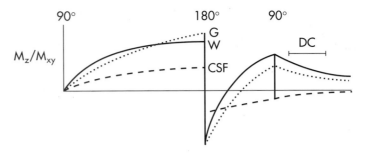

FIGURE 5-2   Changes in M_z/M_{xy} with time in the IR sequence (medium TI) for white matter *(W)*, gray matter *(G)*, and CSF using a gradient-echo data collection *(DC)*. The signal intensity on the image is proportional to the height of M_{xy} at the middle of DC. White matter is highest, followed by gray matter, and then CSF.

FIGURE 5-1   Changes in M_z **(A)** and M_{xy} **(B)** with time in the IR sequence (medium TI) using a gradient-echo data collection *(DC)*. **C** shows M_z initially and then M_{xy} in the last segment. The first 90-degree pulse, **A,** is from the previous cycle. The DC follows the second 90-degree pulse, **B.** The repetition time *(TR)* is shown.

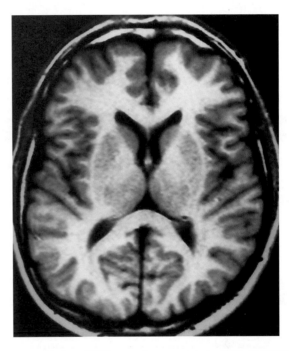

FIGURE 5-3   Medium TI IR scan of a normal brain (1 T). IR1800/30/500 (TR/TE/TI). The white matter is white, the gray matter is gray, and the CSF is black.

than that for white matter at the time of the 180-degree pulse because of its greater proton density.

A general rule is that a TR of at least 3T1 should be allowed for recovery of the longitudinal magnetization between the 90-degree pulse of the last cycle and the following 180-degree pulse of the next cycle to allow a high level of recovery of M_z, though in practice it is possible to use shorter times. Reducing TR produces a reduction in signal intensity for tissues with a long T1. There is less effect on tissues with a short T1, where TR is still greater than 3T1.

There are two types of image reconstruction available—phase corrected (where positive values of signal intensity appear positive, and negative values appear negative) and magnitude (where the magnitude of the signal is used irrespective of its sign). CSF appears dark with phase-corrected processing but may show a "rebound" with a lighter central area with magnitude processing. The signal intensities follow directly from consideration of Figure 5-2.

The 90-degree pulse in the IR sequence is always slice selected, although the 180-degree pulse(s) need not be. When the IR sequence is used to obtain an interleaved set of slices, in most cases the initial 180-degree pulse(s) is slice selected. When the 180-degree pulse is slice selected, it is possible for flowing blood to experience only part of the IR sequence, depending on where it is at the time of the inversion pulses. For example, blood flowing into a slice between the 180-degree and 90-degree pulses may miss the initial 180-degree pulse and experience only the 90-degree pulse, thus behaving as though it is being imaged with a gradient-echo sequence. Blood may then produce a high signal intensity rather than the low signal intensity, in keeping with its relatively long T1, which would be expected had it experienced a 180-degree pulse.

In initial studies the data collection was achieved with a single phase-encoding step after each 90-degree pulse (e.g., a conventional SE). More complex data acquisitions with multiple data collections that are phase encoded differently after each excitation have been employed to decrease the scan time. This image acquisition method, which is known as RARE,[41] FSE, or turbo SE, may be preceded by an inversion pulse to produce the IR variant of the sequence.

Rapid gradient-echo sequences can be used to acquire data for a whole image in 1 or 2 seconds as a comprehensive data collection. These sequences also may be preceded by an inversion pulse. The term *magnetization preparation* has been applied to the use of IR (and other pulse sequences) for this purpose. The three-dimensional, magnetization-prepared, rapid-acquisition gradient echo (3D MP-RAGE, or 3D turbo fast low-angle shot [FLASH]) has proved particularly useful in producing highly T1-weighted volume images of the brain.[7] The same approach can be used with the echo-planar imaging (EPI)[61] sequence, where the single shot form can acquire data for a single image in 40 to 400 ms.

The contrast properties described here and in the following sections apply to data collections with these faster sequences, though in slightly more complex form. For example, contrast is significantly affected by the order of the phase-encoding steps with the FSE sequence, and rapid sequences may show varying degrees of steady-state behavior. Nevertheless, with both conventional and fast forms of the IR sequence, the main determinant of contrast is usually the timing of the inversion pulse.

It is useful to consider the following three main variants of the IR sequence according to their values of TI (Table 5-1):

1. The short TI IR (STIR) sequence (e.g., TIs of 80 to 105 ms at 0.15 T)
2. The medium TI IR sequence (e.g., TIs of 200 to 800 ms at 0.15 T)
3. The long TI IR sequence (e.g., TIs of 1500 to 2500 ms at 0.15 T)

The medium T1 sequence has been described so far. Each of the variants is dealt with in the next three sections. Because tissue T1s increase with field strength, the appropriate values of TI in each group also increase with field strength (Table 5-2).[6,20] In our experience, some of the values quoted in Table 5-2 for tissues at higher fields may be on the high side.

SHORT TI INVERSION RECOVERY SEQUENCE

Values of TI discussed here are approximately 80 to 150 ms. At these times the longitudinal magnetization for all or virtually all tissues is negative when the 90-degree pulse is applied. Recovery is just beginning for most tissues. The magnetization curves can be represented as shown in Figure 5-4. When magnitude reconstruction with TI in the range of 80 to approximately 150 ms is used, an IR image of the brain appears like an SE image, although with greater gray matter–white matter contrast.

After the second 90-degree pulse the T1 contrast and the T2 contrast are additive; that is, increasing the T1 of a tissue increases the tissue's relative signal intensity and so does increasing its T2. (This is not the case in Figure 5-2, which illustrates medium values of TI.) The STIR sequence is very sensitive to changes in T1 and T2 and can be used as a screening sequence in the brain in a way similar to the SE sequences with long TEs and long TRs, such as SE 2500 to 3000/80. To reduce the signal intensity of CSF to less than that of white matter, TR can be shortened to 1000 to 1500 ms with a sequence such as IR 1000/44/100 (TR/TE/TI) (at 0.15 T).

Because many pathological lesions produce an increase in both T1 and T2, the addition of these two types of contrast with the STIR sequence produces a high net tissue contrast. This type of sequence also enables some T1-dependent decay to be substituted for the T2-dependent decay in the equivalent SE sequence. This finding may be of value where the T1 and T2 decays of the tissue differ, and it explains why the gray matter–white matter contrast of this sequence is greater than the equivalent SE sequence.

It is also possible to choose a value of TI so that the signal intensity of a particular tissue is zero at the time of the 90-degree pulse. (This occurs at a value of TI between 0.65 and 0.69 of the tissue T1 for TR greater than 3T1.) At 0.15 T, values of approximately 100 ms are suitable to eliminate the fat signal, whereas 255 ms eliminates white matter (Figure 5-5). In this situation the tissue signal is said to be nulled or

Table 5-1   Common Clinical Variants of the Inversion Recovery Sequence

DESCRIPTION	TYPICAL TI VALUES (ms)	SIGN OF LONGITUDINAL MAGNETIZATION (M_z)	STATE OF LONGITUDINAL MAGNETIZATION (M_z)	USUAL CONTRAST WEIGHTING FOR TARGET TISSUE	TISSUES AND FLUIDS WITH T1S SUITABLE FOR NULLING	EXAMPLES
Short TI	80-150	Negative	Beginning recovery	Combined T1 & T2	Fat, white matter, liver	STIR
Medium TI	200-800	Mixed negative & positive	Partially recovered	Heavy T1	Blood (CSF)	BIR, FIR, MP-RAGE
Long TI	1500-2500	Positive	Almost fully recovered	Heavy T2	CSF	FLAIR

Table 5-2   Tissue and Fluid T1 Values at Different Field Strengths

TISSUE	T1 (MS)					T2 (MS)
	0.15 T	0.25 T	0.5 T	1 T	1.5 T	
Adipose	174 ± 28	190 ± 28	214 ± 28	242 ± 28	260 ± 28	84 ± 36
White matter	354 ± 17	422 ± 17	537 ± 17	684 ± 17	787 ± 17	92 ± 36
Gray matter	453 ± 17	531 ± 17	657 ± 17	814 ± 17	922 ± 17	101 ± 13
Liver	206 ± 22	520 ± 22	325 ± 22	423 ± 22	493 ± 22	43 ± 14
Kidney	268 ± 27	418 ± 27	496 ± 27	560 ± 27	652 ± 27	58 ± 24
Muscle (skeletal)	330 ± 18	409 ± 18	548 ± 18	733 ± 18	869 ± 18	47 ± 13
Muscle (heart)	377 ± 16	454 ± 16	583 ± 16	749 ± 16	868 ± 16	57 ± 16

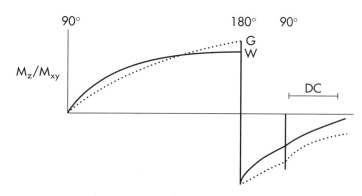

FIGURE 5-4   Changes in M_z/M_{xy} with time for fat *(F)*, white matter *(W)*, and gray matter *(G)* using a fat-suppressed STIR sequence. The signal from gray matter is greater than that from white matter. Fat gives no signal.

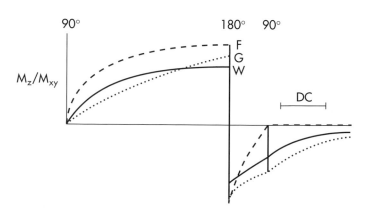

FIGURE 5-5   Changes in M_z/M_{xy} with time for fat *(F)*, white matter *(W)*, and gray matter *(G)* using a fat-suppressed STIR sequence. The signal from gray matter is greater than that from white matter. Fat gives no signal.

suppressed. Suppression of the fat signal is of particular value in imaging of the body and musculoskeletal system (Figures 5-6 and 5-7).

Faster forms of the sequence employ selective reduction in both STIR[27] and FSE (or turbo SE) data collections.[93,107] The STIR sequence is mainly used for venography and for applications in the head and neck, spine, musculoskeletal system, abdomen, and pelvis (Figures 5-8 and 5-9).* Because of difficulties in performing chemical shift–sensitive fat suppression at fields less than 1.5 T, STIR is the fat suppression technique of choice at medium and low field strengths. It has the disadvantage that it is generally insensitive to contrast enhancement un-

*References 27, 28, 30, 76, 79, 87, 90, 91, 96, 97, 113.

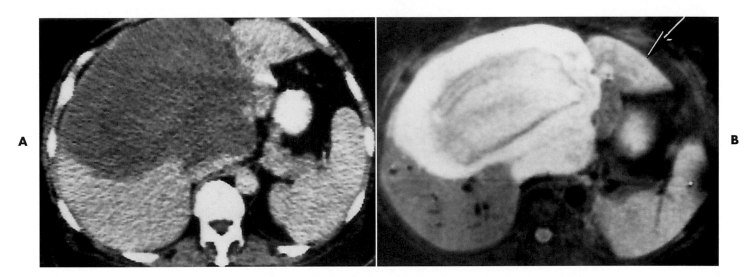

FIGURE 5-6   Giant hemangioma with left lobe atrophy (0.15 T). **A,** CT scan. **B,** STIR 1500/44/100 (TR/TE/TI) scan. The tumor is highlighted and so is the atrophic left lobe (*arrow,* in **B**).

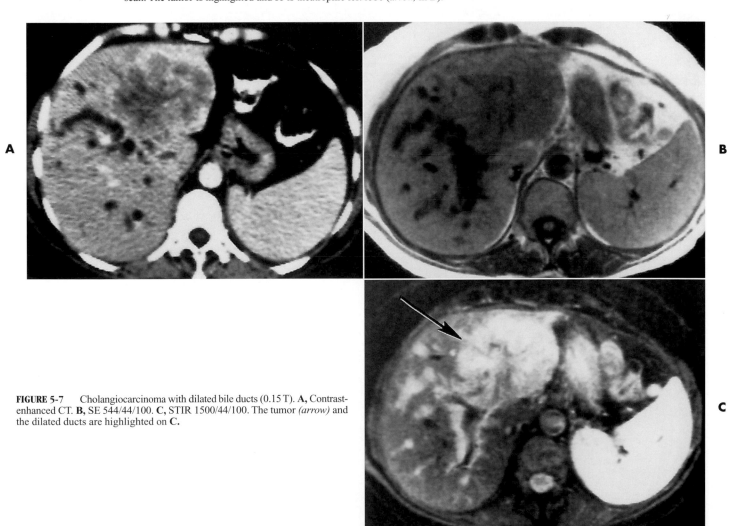

FIGURE 5-7   Cholangiocarcinoma with dilated bile ducts (0.15 T). **A,** Contrast-enhanced CT. **B,** SE 544/44/100. **C,** STIR 1500/44/100. The tumor *(arrow)* and the dilated ducts are highlighted on **C.**

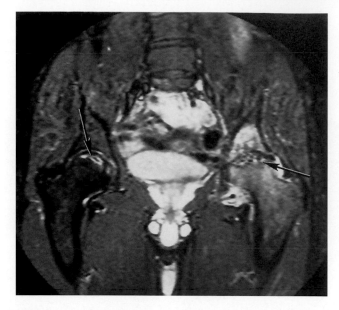

FIGURE 5-8   Bilateral avascular necrosis (1 T). Coronal STIR 2500/30/130 scan. There is increased signal involving the heads of the femurs *(arrows)* and surrounding the left acetabulum.

less TR and TI are shortened[27] or very short values of T1 are involved, as in the liver, where the STIR sequence is highly sensitive to contrast enhancement with the new hepatic contrast agent, manganese dipyridoxal diphosphate (Mn-DPDP).[36]

It is also possible to selectively null tissues other than fat or white matter, such as normal liver, and produce very high-contrast images of focal hepatic disease[54] and the bile ducts.[91] T1-related fat suppression can also be used in combination with a binomial pulse to selectively eliminate the signal from water and produce "silicone only" images of breast implants.[70]

MEDIUM TI INVERSION RECOVERY SEQUENCE

TI values under discussion here are about 200 to 800 ms. The longitudinal magnetization of the tissue(s) of interest is positive, and tissue magnetization is partially recovered. With this type of image, white matter is white, gray matter is gray, and the level of contrast between them is high (Figure 5-10). The hematoma in Figure 5-10, *A,* has a short T1 and a high signal. To obtain an image with good contrast between two tissues of different T1 values with the medium TI, long TR sequence, the rule is to choose a value of TI intermediate between the two T1s of the tissues of interest (neglecting the effects of proton density and T2). Thus satisfactory contrast (at 0.15 T) between white matter (T1 = 350 ms) and gray matter (T1 = 450 ms) is achieved with a TI of approximately 400 ms. Though contrast is high at this point, signal intensity is low, so the image appears noisier than that obtained with, for

A   **B**   **C**

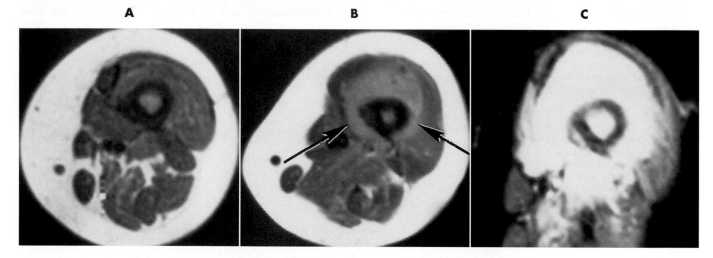

FIGURE 5-9   Osteosarcoma of the lower end of the femur (0.15 T). Transverse IR 1500/44/500 before **(A)** and after **(B)** intravenous Gd-DTPA, as well as STIR 1500/44/100 **(C)** scan. There is enhancement of the soft tissue outside the femur *(arrows in **B**)*. The abnormal areas within and outside of the bone are highlighted on **C**.

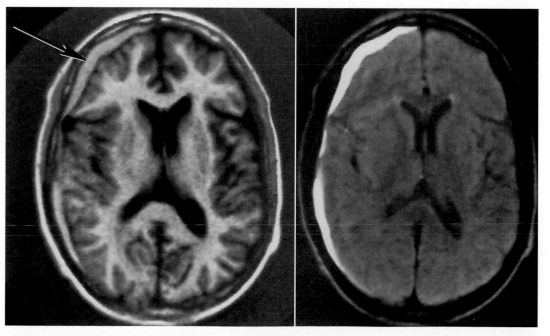

A   **B**

FIGURE 5-10   Subacute subdural hematoma (0.15 T). **A,** Transverse IR 1500/44/500 scan. **B,** SE 1500/80 scan (0.15 T). There is good gray-to-white contrast in **A**. The rim of the hematoma has a short T1 and a high signal *(arrow in **A**)*.

example, a TI of 500 ms. The TI for optimum contrast between gray matter and a tumor or an infarct (which have an increased T1) is greater than that for gray and white matter.

There are two additional modifying factors. First, the lower mobile proton density of white matter relative to gray matter results in slightly less contrast between the two tissues in medium TI sequences. Second, the T2-dependent period between the 90-degree pulse and the subsequent data collection tends to produce a reduction in net tissue contrast. This is particularly true for lesions that follow the common pattern and have an increase in both T1 and T2. The T2 decay in the last component of the sequence opposes the effect of the T1-dependent contrast developed earlier in the sequence.

The method of image acquisition and the type of data collection affect TE and thus the T2 dependence of the sequence. TE can generally be shorter with projection reconstruction than with two-dimensional Fourier transformation (2D FT) because a single vector-encoding gradient is used without the need for a previous phase-encoding gradient as with 2D FT. A gradient-echo data collection can be completed earlier than an SE data collection with the same bandwidth, although the former is more vulnerable to B_0 field inhomogeneities. In the brain (T2 approximately 90 to 100 ms) the T2 dependence of the IR sequence is not such a problem as it is in the body, where values of T2 are typically half of those in the brain (45 to 60 ms), making the same IR sequence much more T2 dependent than when it is used in the brain for the same value of TE. The use of short TE values to control this problem then becomes important.

Somewhat longer TI values are used in pediatric brain imaging for detecting myelination and subtle pathology. The brain contains increased water at this age, and high lesion contrast for ischemia and infarction is helpful in this situation (Figure 5-11).

One of the difficulties with the medium TI IR sequence is packaging it in a time-efficient manner for multislice imaging. The inversion pulse produces an additional constraint compared with an SE sequence and reduces the number of slices obtained in a given time period. More efficient packaging schemes have been described for the T1-weighted IR sequence, but a simple solution to this problem is to make TI approximately one half of TR, thus producing the balanced IR (BIR) sequence (Figures 5-12 and 5-13). This method allows time on either side of the pulses to be used efficiently for interleaving slices. The sequence is technically undemanding and produces good contrast over a wide range of T1 values. It provides superior contrast to the T1-weighted SE in similar imaging times. The sequence is also known as *modified driven-equilibrium Fourier transformation* (MDEFT), a name derived from the DEFT sequence, which has been used in both spectroscopy and imaging.[44,74,78,102,103]

Fast SE, T1-weighted approaches have been successfully implemented for the brain[63,85] and the spine.[65] The latter study used a se-

quence with a TI close to one half of TR, which was T1-weighted and also nulled CSF.

Another way around the packaging problem is the use of a 3D sequence, such as IR turbo FLASH or MP-RAGE.[69] The medium TI magnetization preparation provides high-contrast, thin-section 3D images of the brain with sensitivity to pathology comparable to that of conventional 2D, T2-weighted SE sequences but with the addition of 3D capability and sensitivity to contrast enhancement with IV gadolinium diethylene-triamine-pentaacetic acid (Gd-DTPA) (dimeglumine gadopentetate). T2-weighted 3D volumes have been difficult to achieve, and they are not sensitive to contrast enhancement, so 3D MP-RAGE (and its equivalent) has been proposed as the basic approach to imaging the brain.

The T1-weighted IR sequence is also of value in the body and shows high contrast in imaging of the liver (Figures 5-14 and 5-15). The medium TI sequence also has been used as a basis for T1 measurements.[47,57,78,95,118]

LONG TI INVERSION RECOVERY SEQUENCE

If the TI is increased to 1500 to 2500 ms, the longitudinal magnetization of most tissues (such as brain) is almost fully recovered. The signal from CSF can be nulled or largely nulled at these TIs (Figure 5-16).[14,24,33,109] With the signal from CSF reduced to zero, it is possible to use a long echo time, such as 120 to 200 ms, and develop very heavily T2-weighted contrast without problems from CSF partial volume effects and artifacts (Figure 5-17). The resultant FLAIR sequence has been used in the brain in infarction, multiple sclerosis, and other conditions* (Figures 5-18 and 5-19).

The long TI sequence is particularly useful in regions of the brain where partial volume effects from CSF cause difficulty. Its reduced gray to white matter contrast (as a result of the not quite complete recovery of the brain magnetization) provides a bland background against which lesions are readily seen (Figure 5-20).

The FLAIR sequence usually is used in heavily T2-weighted form in the brain, where most lesions are highlighted.† It is of considerable value in detecting low-contrast lesions (Figures 5-21 and 5-22). It also can be used to improve the accuracy of detecting T2 prolongation in the hippocampus in mesial temporal sclerosis.[110] The nulling of CSF maximizes the sensitivity of the sequence to changes in the T1 of CSF. This finding has been of value in detecting acute subarachnoid hemorrhage, which shortens T1 and may otherwise be difficult to visualize with MRI.[72,73] Short T2 clotted blood may not be seen so readily, however.[8]

*References 2, 3, 5, 34, 37, 43, 45, 80, 83, 98, 100, 105, 108.
†References 2, 5, 46, 82, 84, 101.

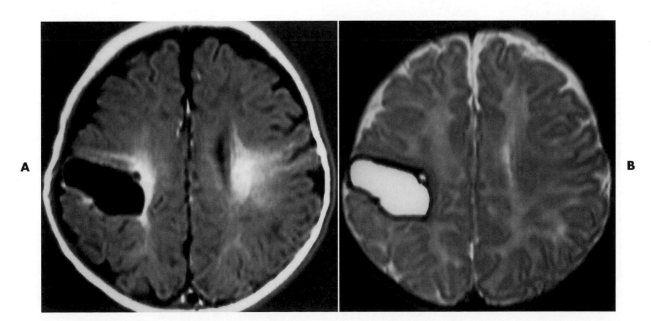

FIGURE 5-11   Hemorrhagic cyst in a 3-month-old infant. **A**, T1-weighted IR 3400/30/800 scan. **B**, SE 2700/120 scan (1 T). There is high contrast between the central myelin and surrounding brain in **A** and between the cyst and brain.

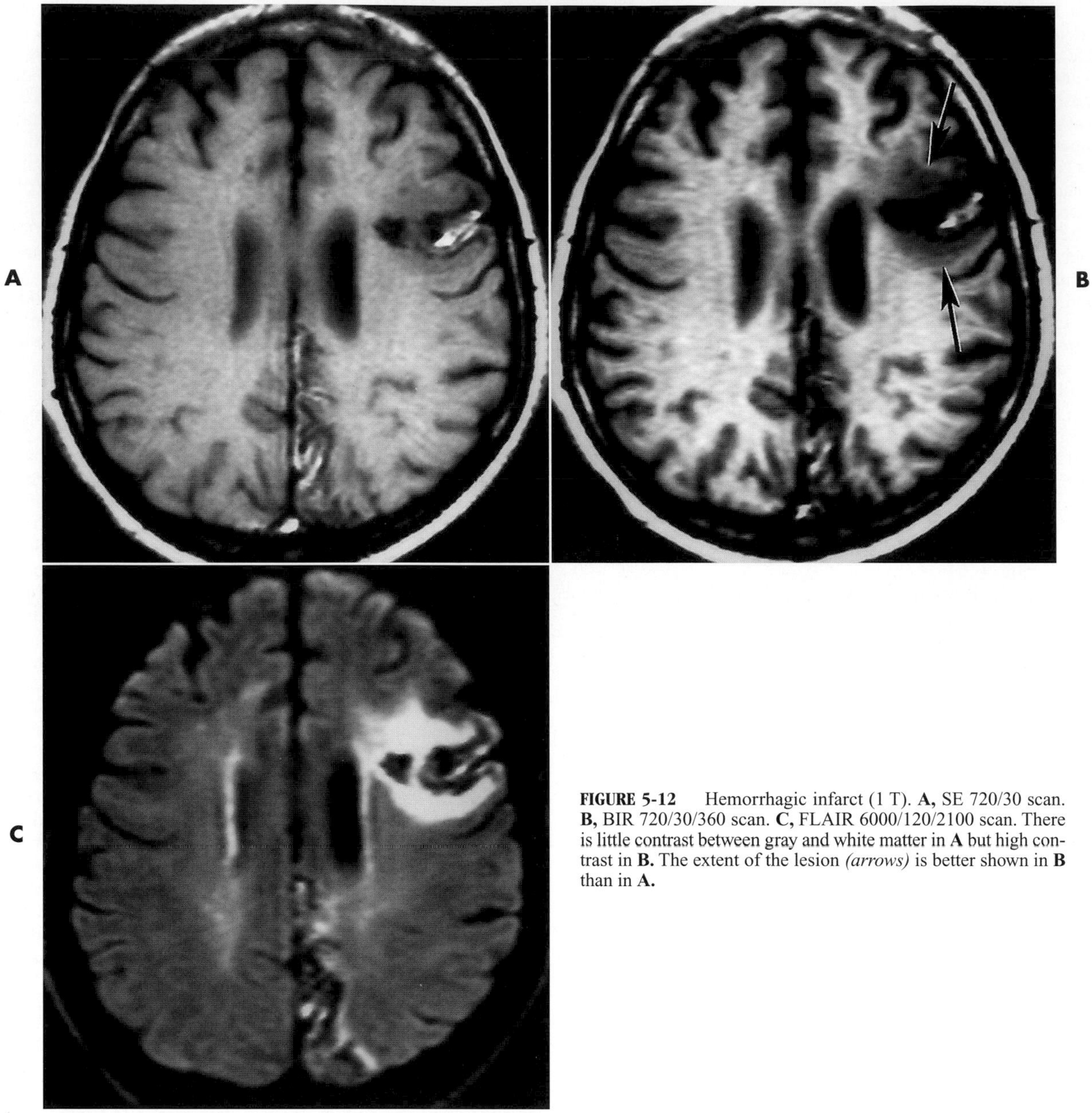

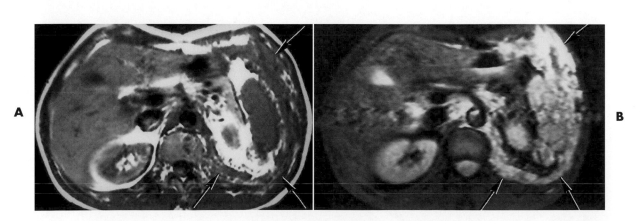

FIGURE 5-12   Hemorrhagic infarct (1 T). **A,** SE 720/30 scan. **B,** BIR 720/30/360 scan. **C,** FLAIR 6000/120/2100 scan. There is little contrast between gray and white matter in **A** but high contrast in **B.** The extent of the lesion *(arrows)* is better shown in **B** than in **A.**

FIGURE 5-13   AVM in abdominal wall. **A,** BIR 1060/30/530 scan. **B,** STIR 2580/30/120 scan (1 T). The abnormality *(arrows)* is well seen on both images.

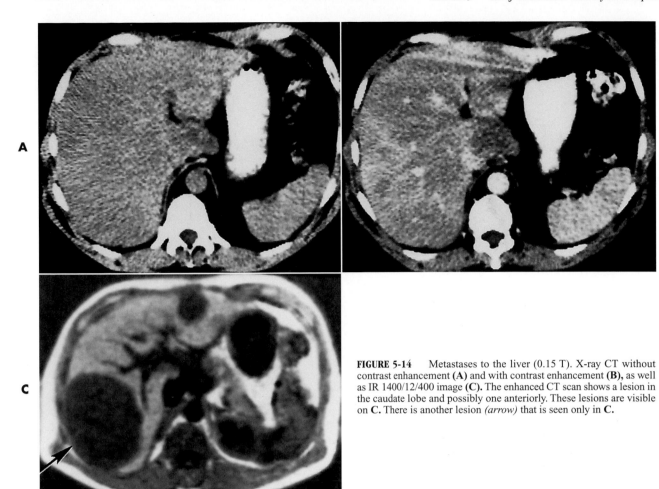

FIGURE 5-14   Metastases to the liver (0.15 T). X-ray CT without contrast enhancement **(A)** and with contrast enhancement **(B),** as well as IR 1400/12/400 image **(C).** The enhanced CT scan shows a lesion in the caudate lobe and possibly one anteriorly. These lesions are visible on **C.** There is another lesion *(arrow)* that is seen only in **C.**

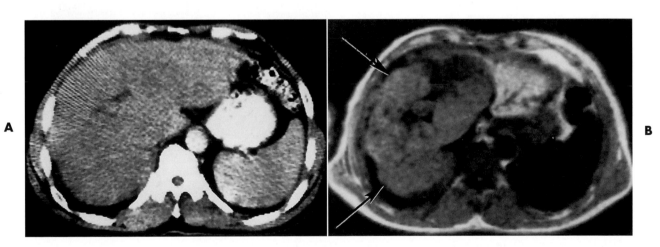

FIGURE 5-15   Hepatoma (0.15 T). **A,** X-ray CT. **B,** IR 1400/12/400. The low signal of the lesion *(arrows)* is well seen in **B.**

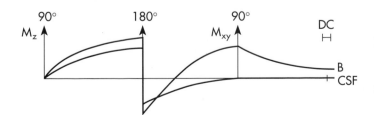

FIGURE 5-16 M_z followed by M_{xy} for brain *(B)* and CSF during FLAIR sequence. After the first 90-degree pulse, the brain recovers more quickly than the CSF. After the 180-degree pulse, the brain largely recovers, but CSF, with its long T1, only reaches zero magnetization when the second 90-degree pulse is applied. The brain signal then decays with time-constant T2, while the CSF signal remains zero.

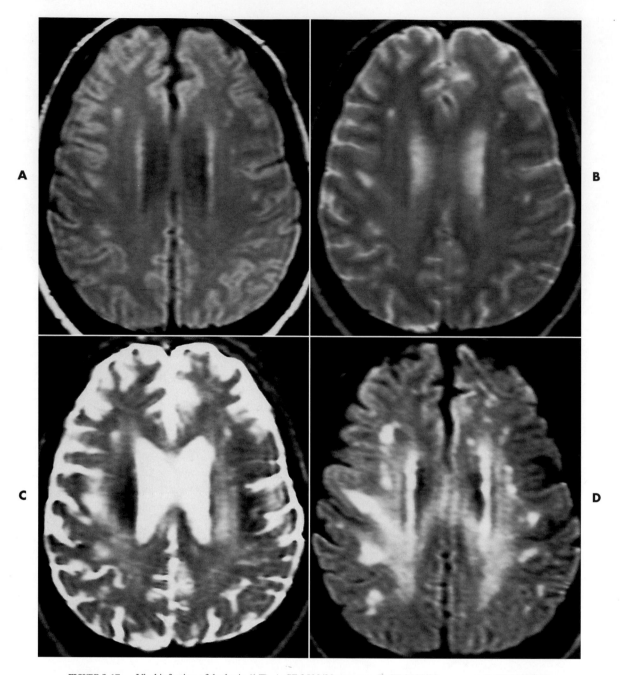

FIGURE 5-17 Viral infection of the brain (1 T). **A,** SE 2500/20 sequence **B,** SE 2500/80 sequence. **C,** SE 2500/160 sequence. **D,** FLAIR 6000/160/2100 sequence. Deep white matter and periventricular lesions are seen in **A** and **B.** Increasing TE to 160 ms in **C** increases artifact from the CSF and produces little net benefit. **D,** The FLAIR sequence at the same TE (160 ms) suppresses the CSF signal and highlights the lesions, which appear more extensive than in **A** or **B.**

One of the disadvantages of the FLAIR sequence is the fact that un-inverted CSF may flow into the slice of interest during the TI period when a slice-selected initial inversion pulse[14] is used. This effect can be reduced by increasing the width of the initial inverted slice[14] or using a non–slice-selective pulse.[109] This latter technique is the preferred approach to imaging of the spinal cord, and increased lesion sensitivity has been described when using it.[34,65,99,109] In addition, the sequence is very sensitive to intramedullary cysts and syrinxes (provided they have a very long T1)[109] (Figures 5-23 and 5-24). Results in the spine using slice-selected inversion pulses have been much less satisfactory because of CSF flow effects and poor lesion contrast.[42,50]

The imaging time may be shortened by reducing TR or the flip angle of the initial inverting pulse[2,105] or by optimizing interleaving.[49,56,75] The FLAIR technique also has been of value in diffusion weighting[25,52]

and has shown an unexpected sensitivity to contrast enhancement.[62,86] It can also be combined with fat suppression.[68]

The STIR-FLAIR, or solution and tissue-attenuated inversion recovery (STAIR), sequence combines features of the STIR and FLAIR sequences. It is also known as the *double inversion recovery sequence*[10] because it employs two 180-degree inversion pulses. It can be used to null the signal from solutions, such as CSF, urine, or bile, and tissues, such as fat, white matter, and gray matter (Figure 5-25).[4,10,81,120] It also can be used to isolate the cerebral cortex by nulling white matter and CSF (Figure 5-26).[4,69,76,81] The same principle can be applied to null the signal from fat and bile (very long T1) in the abdomen (Figure 5-27).

The STAIR sequence suffers from a low signal-to-noise ratio and is likely to have specialized applications. It may be used in combination

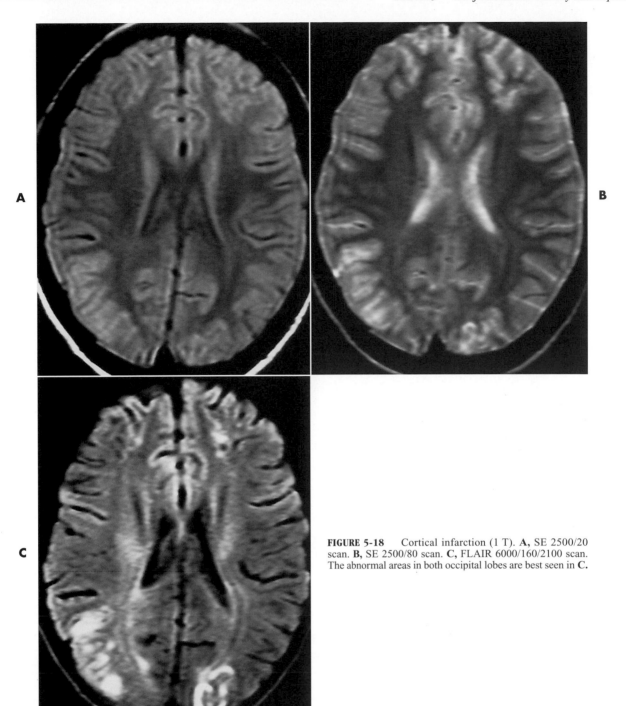

FIGURE 5-18   Cortical infarction (1 T). **A,** SE 2500/20 scan. **B,** SE 2500/80 scan. **C,** FLAIR 6000/160/2100 scan. The abnormal areas in both occipital lobes are best seen in **C.**

with subvoxel registration for following disease of the cerebral cortex over time.

FLOW EFFECTS, ANGIOGRAPHY, AND PERFUSION

Approaches are summarized in Table 5-3. Inversion pulses are frequently applied out of slice to invert the magnetization of blood flowing into the slice so that it does not give a signal. These presaturation pulses are used to suppress arterial and venous blood flow and to reduce unwanted signals arising as artifacts from moving tissues. The value of TI may be reduced if the flip angle of the inverting pulse is reduced, for example, to 120 degrees. In-slice nulling of blood may be of value in demonstrating pulmonary embolisms. It is also possible to combine a nonselective 180-degree pulse and a selective 180-degree

pulse to null blood and preserve the longitudinal magnetization in the slice of interest.[21,94]

By suppressing background tissue using magnetization transfer or multiple inversion nulling, it is possible to selectively image blood.* These techniques generally exploit the long T1 and T2 of blood rather than its flow properties and are particularly useful for slow-flowing or stationary blood.

One approach to measuring tissue perfusion is to image the brain and then apply an inversion pulse out of slice to invert the magnetization of the inflowing arterial blood and obtain a second image. The two

Text continued on p. 85

---

*References 17, 32, 38, 59, 71, 106, 114.

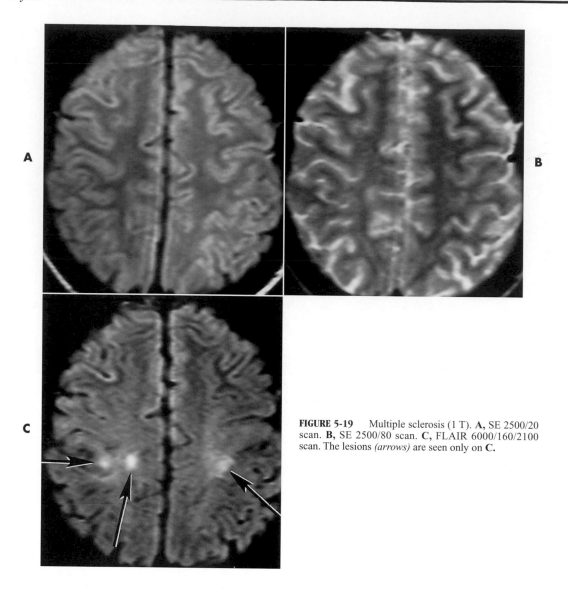

FIGURE 5-19   Multiple sclerosis (1 T). **A,** SE 2500/20 scan. **B,** SE 2500/80 scan. **C,** FLAIR 6000/160/2100 scan. The lesions *(arrows)* are seen only on **C.**

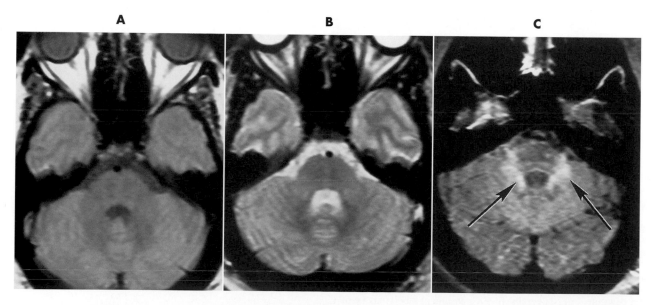

FIGURE 5-20   Sarcoidosis with bilateral seventh nerve palsy (1 T). **A,** SE 2500/20 scan. **B,** SE 2500/80 scan. **C,** FLAIR 6000/160200 scan. The abnormalities *(arrows)* are seen only on **C.**

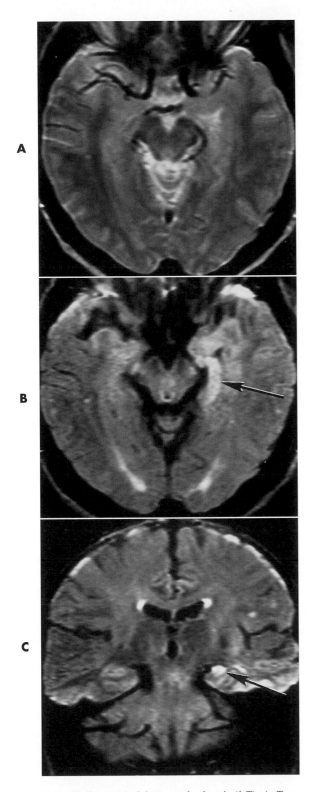

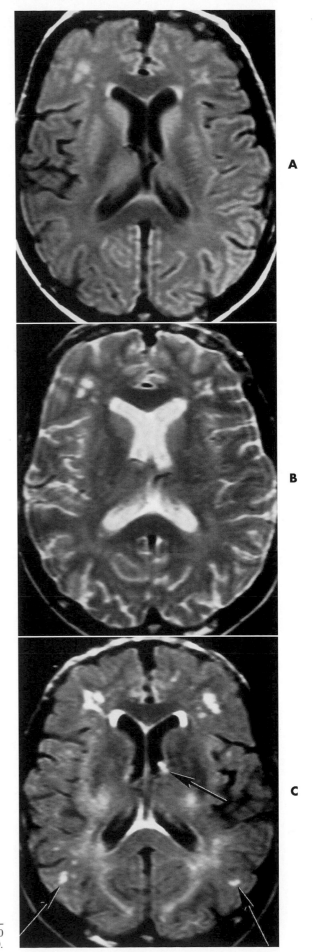

FIGURE 5-21   Epilepsy. Mesial temporal sclerosis (1 T). **A,** Transverse SE 2500/80 scan. **B,** FLAIR 6000/160/2100 scan. **C,** Coronal IR 6000/160/2100 scan. Some dilatation of the temporal horn is seen in **A.** The left hippocampus is highlighted in **B** and **C** *(arrows).*

FIGURE 5-22   Cerebral metastases (1 T). **A,** SE 2500/20 scan. **B,** SE 2500/80 scan. **C,** IR 6000/160/2100 scan. Additional lesions are seen only on **C** *(arrows).*

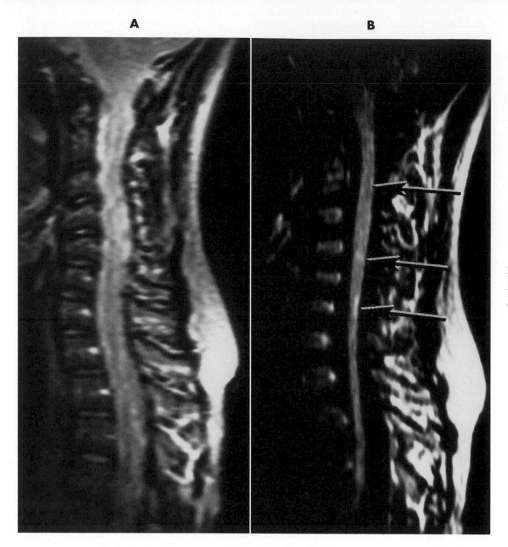

FIGURE 5-23 Multiple sclerosis (1 T). **A,** SE 2500/80 scan. **B,** IR 6000/90/2100 scan. No lesions are seen in **A,** but highlighted areas are seen in **B** *(arrows).*

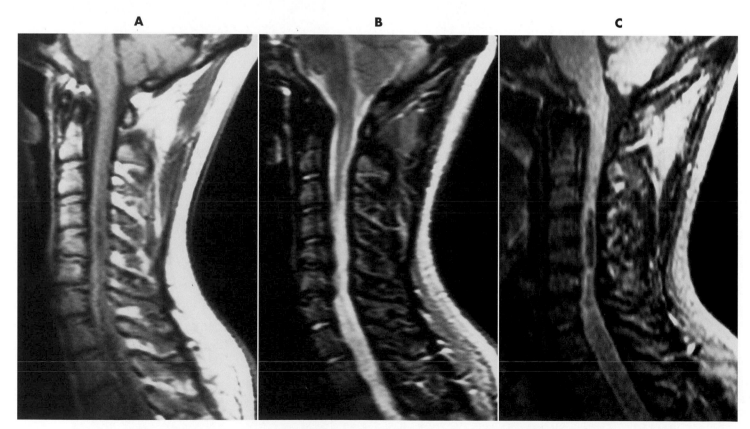

FIGURE 5-24 Syringomyelia (1 T). **A,** SE 540/20 scan. **B,** SE 2500/80 scan. **C,** FLAIR 6000/90/2100 scan. The cavity is best outlined in **C.**

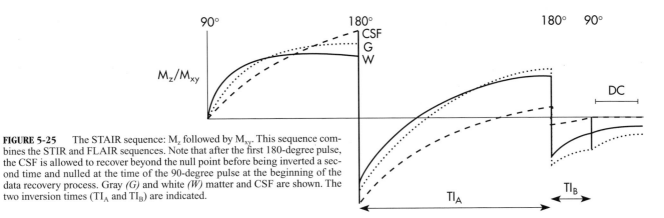

FIGURE 5-25   The STAIR sequence: M_z followed by M_{xy}. This sequence combines the STIR and FLAIR sequences. Note that after the first 180-degree pulse, the CSF is allowed to recover beyond the null point before being inverted a second time and nulled at the time of the 90-degree pulse at the beginning of the data recovery process. Gray *(G)* and white *(W)* matter and CSF are shown. The two inversion times (TI_A and TI_B) are indicated.

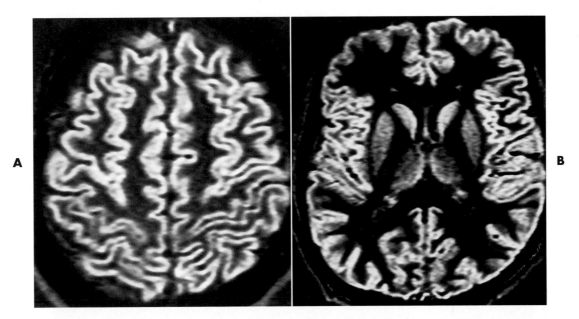

FIGURE 5-26   Normal transverse head scan (1 T). **A** and **B**, STAIR 3000/20/2300/245 ($TR/TE/TI_A/TI_B$) scans at two levels. The gray matter has been isolated and gives a high signal. The complex folding of the cortex is readily seen.

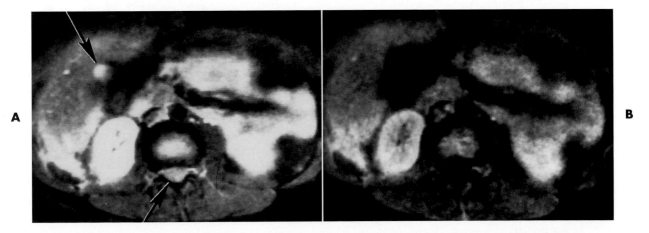

FIGURE 5-27   Liver abscess (0.15 T). **A**, Transverse STIR 1000/44/100 sequence. **B**, STAIR 3000/44/1200/100 sequence. The high signal in the posterior aspect of the liver is shown in both sequences. The gall bladder and CSF are shown in **A** *(arrows)* but are suppressed in **B**.

Table 5-3   Flow Effects, Angiography, and Perfusion

TECHNIQUE	INVERSION PULSE IN-SLICE/OUT-OF-SLICE	TISSUE/FLUID FOR WHICH SIGNAL IS REDUCED	TISSUE/FLUID SIGNAL IS OBTAINED FROM	USES
Inflow presaturation	Out Out (unselected 180-degree)	Inflowing blood Out-of-slice tissues	Tissues in slice —	General tissue presaturation Selective venous or arterial blood nulling
Presaturation and reinversion	In & out of slice, then in-slice (selected 180-degree)	Inflowing blood	Tissues in slice	Angiography, cardiac imaging; can also be combined with STIR to null fat
Selective nulling of tissue	In-slice multiple 180-degree pulses	Tissue	Blood	Arteriography & venography
Perfusion	Out-of-slice alternate inversion & noninversion	Inflowing	Tissue & blood	Brain & muscle perfusion

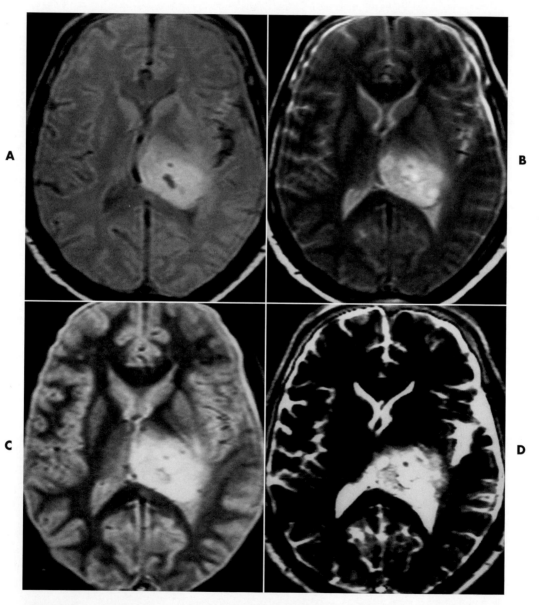

FIGURE 5-28   Thalamic glioma (1 T). **A,** Transverse SE 2500/16 scan. **B,** MT-SE 2500/16 scan. **C,** STIR 2500/16/130 scan. **D,** MT-STIR 2500/16/130 scan. MT alone drops the signal from gray and white matter more than from tumor, increasing the lesion contrast from **A** to **B. C,** the STIR sequence shows the tumor with higher contrast. **D,** The MT-STIR sequence virtually reduces the gray and white matter signal to zero, leaving only the tumor and CSF.

images can then be subtracted. The inverted spins change the brain signal as a function of the rate of blood flow, the distance the blood has traveled, the T1 of blood, the fraction of blood in the tissue, and other factors.[16] These techniques and variants of them have been applied to the brain.* There is an essential requirement to ensure that the detected signals are not caused by CSF flow. When the inversion is performed over the carotid and vertebral arteries beneath the skull base, this can be readily achieved. If it involves a comparison of slice-selected and non–slice-selected pulses in the brain, considerable care may be necessary to control or eliminate effects caused by CSF flow. Studies have also been performed on muscle.[60]

OTHER VARIANTS OF THE INVERSION RECOVERY SEQUENCE

A variant of the STIR sequence that is of interest is the spectral presaturation with IR (SPIR) sequence, which employs a frequency-selective inversion pulse to invert the magnetization of protons in fat but not that of protons in water.[119] The TI is then selected to null the fat signal, and any pulse sequence can be used subsequently to selectively image the remaining water. This sequence provides fat suppression and can be used in a heavily T1-weighted form to provide sensitivity to contrast enhancement. It has the disadvantage that it requires a high field and good shimming for successful chemical shift–selective fat suppression. Applications to date have mainly been in the spine.

Magnetization transfer (MT) also can be used with the IR sequence in angiography and other applications.[32,67] In addition, it can be used to markedly reduce the signal from gray and white matter in the brain and increase lesion contrast (Figure 5-28).

Methods have been developed for making T1 and T2 contrast additive. Whereas this is easy to achieve with the STIR sequence, with the medium TI sequence it requires the initial 180-degree pulse to be split into two 90-degree pulses, with time between to develop T2-dependent contrast.[12] T2-dependent contrast is then additive to the T1-dependent contrast that is subsequently developed. This approach is known as *driven inversion spin echo* (DISE),[12] or T2-FLAIR.[111]

Two technical developments are now being implemented: FSE data collection to shift the null points of fat and CSF[64] (because the echo time encroaches on TR) and the use of adiabatic inversion pulses to obtain more uniform signal nulling[35] (where the radiofrequency pulse power is reduced at the periphery of the transmitter coil).

Subtraction approaches have been used to selectively remove the signal from CSF,[15] and ultrashort TI values (5 to 40 ms) may be of value in increasing sensitivity to contrast enhancement.[88]

SUMMARY

Different aspects of each of the common forms of the IR sequence have been described, and a unified approach to understanding the contrast developed by each of them has been outlined. The IR sequence is versatile and can provide high tissue contrast by several different mechanisms, the most important of which are heavy T1- or T2-weighting and nulling of unwanted signals from fat, blood, or CSF.

---

*References 22, 38, 39, 57, 53, 115.

REFERENCES

1. Bailes DR, et al: NMR imaging of the brain using spin-echo sequences, Clin Rad 33:395, 1982.
2. Baratti C, et al: Partially saturated fluid attenuated inversion recovery (FLAIR) sequences in multiple sclerosis: comparison with fully relaxed FLAIR and conventional spin echo, Magn Reson Imag 13:513, 1995.
3. Barker GJ, et al: 3D fast FLAIR: a CSF nulled 3D fast spin echo pulse sequence, Proceedings of the International Society for Magnetic Resonance in Medicine (ISMRM), Fifth Annual Meeting, Vancouver, April 12-18, 1997, p. 284.
4. Bedell BJ, et al: Fast double inversion recovery sequence for white matter and CSF suppression, International Society for Magnetic Resonance in Medicine (ISMRM), Book of Abstracts, Fifth Annual Meeting, Vancouver, April 12-18, 1997, p. 667.
5. Bergin PS, et al: MRI in partial epilepsy: additional abnormalities demonstrated with the fluid attenuated inversion recovery (FLAIR) pulse sequence, J Neurol Neurosurg Psych 58:439, 1995.
6. Bottomley PA, et al: A review of normal tissue hydrogen, NMR relaxation times, and mechanisms from 1-100 MHz: dependence on tissue type, NMR frequency, temperature species, exercise and age, Med Phys 11:425, 1984.
7. Brant-Zawadzki M, et al: MP RAGE: a three-dimensional, T1-weighted gradient-echo sequence—initial experience in the brain, Radiology 182:769, 1992.
8. Busch E, et al: Are subarachnoid blood clots visible on FLAIR MRI? International Society for Magnetic Resonance in Medicine (ISMRM), Book of Abstracts, Fifth Annual Meeting, Vancouver, April 12-18, 1997, p. 625.
9. Bydder GM, et al: Clinical NMR imaging of the brain: 140 cases, Am J Roentgenol 139:215, 1982.
10. Bydder GM, et al: MRI: clinical use of the inversion-recovery sequence, J Comput Assist Tomogr 9:659, 1985.
11. Constable RT, et al: Signal to noise and contrast in fast spin echo (FSE) and inversion recovery FSE imaging, J Comput Assist Tomogr 16:41, 1992.
12. Conturo TE, et al: Cooperative T1 and T2 effects on contrast using a new driven inversion spin-echo (DISE) MRI pulse sequence, Magn Reson Med 15:397, 1990.
13. Crooks LE, et al: Nuclear magnetic resonance whole-body imager operating at 3.5 KGauss, Radiology 143:169, 1982.
14. De Coene B, et al: MR of the brain using fluid attenuated inversion recovery (FLAIR) pulse sequences, Am J Neurorad 13:1555, 1992.
15. Deimling M, et al: HIRE (high intensity reduction): a new dark fluid sequence, International Society for Magnetic Resonance in Medicine (ISMRM), Fourth Annual Meeting, New York, April 27-May 2, 1996, p. 557.
16. Detre JA, et al: Perfusion imaging, Magn Reson Med 23:37, 1992.
17. Dixon WT, et al: Multiple inversion recovery reduces static tissue signal in angiography, Magn Reson Med 18:257, 1991.
18. Droege RT, et al: A strategy for magnetic resonance imaging of the head: results of a semi-empirical model, Part I, Radiology 153:419, 1984.
19. Droege RT, et al: A strategy for magnetic resonance imaging of the head: results of a semi-empirical model, Part II, Radiology 153:425, 1984.
20. Duewell S, et al: MR imaging contrast in human brain tissue: assessment and optimization at 4T, Radiology 199:780, 1996.
21. Edelman RR, et al: Fast selective black blood MR imaging, Radiology 181:655, 1991.
22. Edelman RR, et al: Quantitative mapping of cerebral blood flow and functional localization with echoplanar MR imaging and signal targeting with alternating radio frequency, Radiology 192:513, 1994.
23. Elster AD: Gradient echo imaging: technique and acronyms, Radiology 186:1, 1992.
24. Epstein FH, et al: CSF-suppressed T2-weighted three-dimensional MP-RAGE MR imaging, J Mag Res Imag 4:463, 1995.
25. Falconer KC, et al: Cerebrospinal fluid suppressed high resolution diffusion imaging of human brain, Magn Reson Med 37:119, 1997.
26. Feinberg DA, et al: GRASE (gradient and spin echo) MR imaging: a new fast clinical imaging technique, Radiology 181:597, 1991.
27. Fleckenstein JL, et al: Fast short-tau inversion-recovery MR imaging, Radiology 179:499, 1991.
28. Goddard P, et al: Magnetic resonance imaging of the chest in infectious mononucleosis, Br J Radiol 63:138, 1990.
29. Graif M, et al: Contrast enhanced MRI of malignant brain tumors, Am J Neurorad 6:855, 1985.
30. Greco A, et al: Spin-echo and STIR MR images of sports related muscle injuries at 1.5T, J Comput Assist Tomogr 15:994, 1991.
31. Haase A, et al: FLASH imaging: rapid NMR imaging using low flip angle pulses, J Magn Reson Imag 67:258, 1986.
32. Hajnal JV, et al: Design and implementation of magnetization transfer pulses for clinical use, J Comput Assist Tomogr 16:7, 1992.
33. Hajnal JV, et al: High signal regions in normal white matter shown by heavily T2-weighted CSF nulled IR sequences, J Comput Assist Tomogr 16:506, 1992.
34. Hajnal JV, et al: MRI: spinal cord imaging with the turbo-fluid attenuated inversion recovery (FLAIR) pulse sequence, Clin Rad 50:1, 1995.
35. Hajnal JV, et al: Use of adiabatic inversion pulses with STIR and FLAIR sequences to improve signal nulling, Magn Reson Med (in press).
36. Halawaara JT, et al: MRI of focal liver lesions with Mn-DPDP: evaluation of T1-weighted SE and GRE, and STIR images at 1.0T, International Society for Magnetic Resonance in Medicine (ISMRM), Third Annual Meeting, Nice, France, April 19-25, 1995, p. 1447.
37. Hashemi RH, et al: Suspected MS: MR imaging with a thin section fast FLAIR pulse sequence(initial experience in the brain, Radiology 196:505, 1995.
38. Helpern JA, et al: Perfusion assessment by repetitive inversion of spins (PARIS), International Society for Magnetic Resonance in Medicine (ISMRM), Fifth Annual Meeting Book of Abstracts, Vancouver, April 12-18, 1997, p. 1752.
39. Helpern JA, et al: Perfusion imaging by uninverted flow sensitive attenuating inversion recovery (UNFAIR), Magn Reson Imag 15:135, 1997.
40. Henkleman RM, et al: Optimal pulse sequence for imaging hepatic metastases, Radiology 161:727, 1986.
41. Hennig J, et al: RARE imaging: a fast imaging method for clinical MR, Magn Reson Med 3:823, 1986.
42. Hittmair K, et al: Fast FLAIR imaging of the brain using fast spin echo and gradient spin echo technique, Magn Reson Imag 15:405, 1997.
43. Hittmair K, et al: Spinal cord lesions in patients with multiple sclerosis: comparison of MR pulse sequences, Am J Neurorad 17:1555, 1996.
44. Hochmann J, et al: Proton NMR of deoxyhemoglobin: use of a modified DEFT technique, Magn Reson Q 38:23, 1980.
45. Ikushima I, et al: Evaluation of intracranial lesions with inversion-recovery half-Fourier single-shot turbo spin-echo MR, Am J Neurorad 18:421, 1997.
46. Jack CR, et al: Mesial temporal sclerosis: diagnosis with fluid-attenuated inversion recovery versus spin echo MR imaging, Radiology 199:367, 1996.
47. Jezzard P, et al: MR relaxation times in human brain: measurement at 4T, Radiology 199:773, 1996.
48. Johnson MA, et al: Clinical NMR imaging of the brain in children: normal and neurologic disease, Am J Neurorad 4:1013, 1983, and Am J Roentgenol 141:1005, 1983.

49. Keller PJ, et al: A facile implementation of fast FLAIR employing inversion anticipation, International Society for Magnetic Resonance in Medicine (ISMRM), Fifth Annual Meeting, Vancouver, April 12-18, 1997, p. 676.
50. Kelper MD, et al: The low sensitivity of fluid attenuated inversion-recovery MR in the detection of multiple sclerosis of the spinal cord, Am J Neurorad 18:1035, 1997.
51. Kim SG: Quantification of relative cerebral blood flow change by flow sensitive attenuating inversion recovery (FAIR) technique: application to functional mapping, Magn Reson Med 34:293, 1995.
52. Kwong KK, et al: CSF suppressed quantitative single shot diffusion imaging, Magn Reson Med 21:157, 1991.
53. Kwong KK, et al: MR perfusion studies with T1-weighted echo planar imaging, Magn Reson Med 34:878, 1995.
54. Lehman B, et al: Signal suppression of normal liver tissue by phase-corrected inversion recovery: a screening technique, J Comput Assist Tomogr 13:650, 1989.
55. Levene MI, et al: Nuclear magnetic resonance imaging of the brain in children, Br Med J 285:774, 1982.
56. Listerud J, et al: OIL-FLAIR optimized interleaved fluid attenuated inversion recovery in 2D fast spin echo, Magn Reson Med 36:320, 1996.
57. Look DC, et al: Time saving in measurement of NMR and EPR relaxation times, Rev Sci Instrum 41:250, 1970.
58. Mallard J, et al: In vivo NMR imaging in medicine: the Aberdeen approach both physical and biological, Phil Trans R Soc Lond 289:519, 1980.
59. Mani S, Pauly J, Conolly S, et al: Background suppression with multiple inversion recovery nulling: applications to projective angiography, Magn Reson Med 37:898, 1997.
60. Mansfield P, et al: NMR imaging in biomedicine, New York, 1982, Academic Press.
61. Marro KI, et al: Skeletal muscle perfusion measurement using adiabatic inversion or arterial water, Magn Reson Med 38:40, 1997.
62. Matthews VP, et al: Gadolinium enhanced fast FLAIR imaging of the brain, American Society of NeuroRadiology (ASNR), Proceedings of 35th Annual Meeting, Toronto, May 18-22, 1997.
63. Melhem ER, et al: Fast inversion recovery MR imaging: the effect of hybrid-RARE readout on the null points of fat and CSF, American Society of NeuroRadiology (ASNR), Proceedings of 35th Annual Meeting, Toronto, May 18-22, 1997.
64. Melhem ER, et al: MR of the spine with a fast T1-weighted fluid attenuated inversion recovery sequence, Am J Neurorad 18:447, 1997.
65. Melhem ER, et al: Multislice T1-weighted hybrid-RARE in CNS imaging: assessment of magnetization transfer effects and artifacts, J Magn Reson Imag 6:903, 1996.
66. Mitchell MR, et al: Understanding basic MR pulse sequences. In Partain CL, Price RR, and Patton JA, et al, eds: Magnetic resonance imaging, ed 2, Philadelphia, 1988, WB Saunders.
67. Miyazaki M, et al: A new application of fast FLAIR with fat suppression, International Society for Magnetic Resonance in Medicine (ISMRM), Fifth Annual Meeting, Vancouver, April 12-18, 1997, p. 1159.
68. Miyazaki M, et al: Optimization of inversion pulse by means of MT effects in fast FLAIR, International Society for Magnetic Resonance in Medicine (ISMRM), Fourth Annual Meeting, New York, April 27-May 3, 1996, p. 1851.
69. Mugler JP, et al: Three dimensional magnetization-prepared rapid gradient-echo imaging (3D MP RAGE), Magn Reson Med 15:152, 1992.
70. Mukundan S, et al: MR imaging of silicone gel-filled breast implants in vivo with a method that visualizes silicone selectively, J Magn Reson Imag 3:713, 1993.
71. Nishimura D, et al: MR angiography by selective inversion recovery, Magn Reson Med 4:193, 1987.
72. Noguchi K, et al: Acute subarachnoid hemorrhage: MR imaging with fluid attenuated inversion recovery pulse sequences, Radiology 196:773, 1995.
73. Noguchi K, et al: Subacute and chronic subarachnoid hemorrhage diagnosis with fluid attenuated inversion recovery MR imaging, Radiology 203:257, 1997.
74. Norris DG, et al: The MDEFT sequence is applicable for clinical systems operating at 1T, International Society for Magnetic Resonance in Medicine (ISMRM), Book of Abstracts, Fifth Annual Meeting, Vancouver, April 12-18, 1997, p. 686.
75. Oh CH, et al: An optimized multislice acquisition sequence for inversion-recovery MR imaging, Magn Reson Imag 9:903, 1991.
76. Ohkawa S, et al: MR venography using 3D-fast STIR sequence for lower extremities, International Society for Magnetic Resonance in Medicine (ISMRM), Fourth Annual Meeting, New York, April 27-May 3, 1996, p. 738.
77. Ortendahl DA, et al: MRI parameter selection techniques. In Partain CL, Price RR, Patton JA, et al, eds: Magnetic resonance imaging, ed 2, Philadelphia, 1988, WB Saunders.
78. Pan JW, et al: High resolution neuroimaging at 4.1T, Magn Reson Imag 13:915, 1995.
79. Panish D, et al: Inversion recovery fast spin-echo MR imaging: efficacy in the evaluation of head and neck lesions, Radiology 187:421, 1993.
80. Papanikolou N, et al: Comparison between fluid attenuated turbo inversion recovery (FLAT TIRE) and conventional long repetition time spin echo (long TR CSE) in the detection of multiple sclerosis lesions, MAGMA 4(S):175, 1996.
81. Redpath TW, et al: Imaging gray brain matter with a double inversion pulse sequence to suppress CSF and white matter signals, MAGMA 2:451, 1994.
82. Riederer SJ, et al: New technical developments in magnetic resonance imaging of epilepsy, Magn Reson Imag 13:1095, 1995.
83. Rydberg JN, et al: Contrast optimization of fluid-attenuated inversion recovery (FLAIR) imaging, Magn Reson Med 34:868, 1995.
84. Rydberg JN, et al: Initial clinical experience in MR imaging of the brain with a fast fluid attenuated inversion recovery pulse sequence, Radiology 193:173, 1994.
85. Rydberg JN, et al: T1-weighted imaging of the brain using a fast inversion recovery pulse sequence, J Magn Reson Imag 6:356, 1996.
86. Sarkar S, et al: Additional characterization of tumor and stroke by contrast enhanced FLAIR compared to post-contrast spin echo MR imaging, International Society for Magnetic Resonance in Medicine (ISMRM), Fourth Annual Meeting, New York, April 27-May 3, 1996, p. 583.
87. Schnapf DJ, et al: MR venography of the lower extremities: evaluation of short inversion-time inversion recovery pulse sequences, Radiology 165(P):90, 1987.
88. Schwickert HC, et al: Quantification of liver blood volume: comparison of dynamic 3D-SPGR with a fast inversion recovery echo-planar approach (ULSTIR-EPI) and in-vitro measurements, International Society of Magnetic Resonance in Medicine (ISMRM), Book of Abstracts, Third Annual Meeting, Nice, France, August 19-25, 1995, p. 1074.
89. Sheppard SK: Personal communication, 1991.
90. Shields AF, et al: The detection of bone marrow involvement by lymphoma using magnetic resonance imaging, J Clin Oncol 5:225, 1987.
91. Shiono T, et al: MRCP with use of fast inversion recovery sequence during single breath-hold period: a clinical evaluation of 40 cases, International Society of Magnetic Resonance in Medicine (ISMRM), Book of Abstracts, Third Annual Meeting, Nice, France, August 19-25, 1995, p. 1454.
92. Smith FW, et al: Nuclear magnetic resonance tomographic imaging in liver disease, Lancet 1:963, 1981.
93. Smith RC, et al: Fast spin echo STIR imaging, J Comput Assist Tomogr 18:209, 1994.
94. Steen RG, et al: Precise and accurate measurement of proton T1 in human brain in vivo: validation and preliminary clinical application, J Magn Reson Imag 4:681, 1994.
95. Stehling MK, et al: Single shot T1- and T2-weighted magnetic resonance imaging of the heart with black blood: preliminary experience, MAGMA 4:231, 1996.
96. Stimoe GK, et al: Gadolinium DTPA enhanced MR imaging of spinal neoplasms: preliminary investigation and comparison with unenhanced spin-echo and STIR sequences, Am J Neurorad 9:839, 1988.
97. Stoller DW, et al: Marrow imaging. In Stoller DW, ed: MRI in orthopaedics and sports medicine, Philadelphia, 1993, Lippincott.
98. Takahashi J, et al: MR evaluation of tuberous sclerosis: increased sensitivity with fluid-attenuated inversion recovery and relation to severity of seizures and mental retardation, Am J Neurorad 16:1923, 1995.
99. Thomas DJ, et al: MRI: use of fluid attenuated inversion recovery (FLAIR) pulse sequences for imaging the spinal cord on MS, Lancet 341:593, 1993.
100. Tsuchiya K, et al: Fast fluid-attenuated inversion recovery MR of intracranial infections, Am J Neurorad 18:909, 1997.
101. Tsuchiya K, et al: Preliminary evaluation of fluid attenuated inversion recovery MR in the diagnosis of intracranial tumors, Am J Neurorad 17:1081, 1996.
102. Ugurbil K, et al: Imaging at high magnetic fields: initial experiences at 4T, Mag Res Q 9:259, 1993.
103. Uijen CMJ, et al: Driven-equilibrium radiofrequency pulses in NMR imaging, Magn Reson Med 1:502, 1984.
104. Van Gelderen P, et al: Three dimensional functional magnetic resonance imaging of human brain on a 1.5T scanner, Proc Natl Acad Sci USA 92:6906, 1995.
105 Wad A, et al: MR imaging of the brain with FLAIR sequences with variable prepared flip angle, Radiology 201(P):309, 1996.
106. Wang SJ, et al: Multiple-readout selective inversion recovery angiography, Magn Reson Med 17:244, 1991.
107. Weinberger E, et al: Nontraumatic pediatric musculoskeletal imaging: comparison of conventional and fast-spin-echo short inversion time inversion recovery technique, Radiology 194:721, 1995.
108. White ML, et al: Fluid attenuated inversion recovery (FLAIR) MRI of herpes encephalitis, J Comput Assist Tomogr 19:501, 1995.
109. White SJ, et al: Use of fluid attenuated inversion recovery pulse sequences for imaging of the spinal cord, Magn Reson Med 28:153, 1992.
110. Woermann FG, et al: Measurement of hippocampal T2 relaxation time: a new fast FLAIR dual echo technique, International Society for Magnetic Resonance in Medicine (ISMRM), Fifth Annual Meeting, Vancouver, April 12-18, 1997, p. 212.
111. Wong EC, et al: A T1 and T2 selective method for attenuation of signal from CSF (T2-FLAIR), International Society for Magnetic Resonance in Medicine (ISMRM), Book of Abstracts, Fifth Annual Meeting, Vancouver, April 12-18, 1997, p. 1730.
112. Worthington BS, et al: Interactive optimization of pulse sequence selection and T1 mapping in ultra high speed inversion-recovery echo planar imaging, Radiology 173:42, 1989.
113. Worthington BS, et al: Use of short TI inversion recovery sequence in evaluating carcinoma of the cervix, Radiology 161(P):279, 1986.
114. Wright GA, et al: Flow-independent magnetic resonance projection angiography, Magn Reson Med 17:125, 1991.
115. Ye FQ, et al: Perfusion imaging of the human brain at 1.5T using a single shot EPI spin tagging approach, Magn Reson Med 36:219, 1996.
116. Young IR, et al: Comparative efficiency of different pulse sequences in MR imaging, J Comput Assist Tomogr 10:271, 1986.
117. Young IR, et al: Nuclear magnetic resonance imaging of the brain in multiple sclerosis, Lancet 31:1063, 1981.
118. Young IR, et al: The design of multiple inversion recovery sequences for T1 measurement, Magn Reson Med 5:99, 1987.
119. Zee CS, et al: SPIR MRI in spinal disease, J Comput Assist Tomogr 16:356, 1992.
120. Zheng J, et al: Fast STIR-FLAIR imaging with contrast enhancement, International Society for Magnetic Resonance in Medicine (ISMRM), Book of Abstracts, Fourth Annual Meeting, New York, April 27-May 3, 1996, p. 1710.

6 Rapid Scan Techniques

Jens Frahm and Wolfgang Häenicke

 KEY POINTS

- Rapid MR techniques are based on either gradient reversal or RF refocusing.
- Gradient echoes achieve their speed by using a low flip angle and gradient reversal, resulting in a short TR.
- RF-refocused techniques (e.g., fast spin echo, turbo spin echo, and HASTE) achieve their speed by sampling multiple lines of κ space per TR.
- EPI is a very rapid gradient reversal technique that forms a complete image (i.e., samples all of κ space) during a single T2* decay (approximately 100 ms in brain tissue).

As a result of ongoing technical developments, rapid scan techniques have established themselves as indispensable for state-of-the-art clinical magnetic resonance imaging (MRI) (Box 6-1). The basic motivation for rapid scanning is the desire for short investigational times to improve throughput and patient comfort and to reduce motion-related image artifacts (thereby improving diagnostic confidence). A major breakthrough came with the introduction of low flip angle gradient-echo imaging, which inspired the development of a new class of methods yielding noninvasive insights in areas formerly believed to be incompatible with MRI. Examples include dynamic scanning, cine studies, high-resolution three-dimensional (3D) imaging, angiography, and functional brain mapping. In parallel the demand for more flexibility in pulse sequence programming stimulated significant improvements in MR hardware. This demand particularly applied to the development of actively shielded gradient systems that provide stronger magnetic field gradients, shorter switching times, variable waveforms, minimized eddy currents, and reduced noise.

Although related, the various fast-scan applications are diverse. For example, the achievement of good temporal resolution in high-speed imaging has a penalty in image quality; conversely the requirement for high spatial resolution in 3D imaging is at the expense of measuring time.

Table 6-1 classifies the different MR sequences as conventional, fast-scan, and high-speed techniques according to their typical measuring times for the acquisition of one cross-sectional image. The scan time for a Fourier image, in which a certain number of phase-encoding steps (i.e., N[S] Fourier lines) are acquired per repetition time (TR), is given by:

(EQ. 1)

$$\text{Scan time} = \text{NAC} \times \text{N(2D)} \times \text{N(3D)} \times \text{TR} / \text{N(S)}$$

where N(2D) and N(3D) are the numbers of two- and three-dimensional phase-encoding steps and NAC is the number of acquisitions. N(2D), N(3D), and NAC equal the number of accumulations desired for signal averaging. The minimum possible TR is determined by the properties of a particular MR sequence (e.g., the time required for the acquisition of a single Fourier line with a given number of data points in the frequency-encoding direction (N[1D] data samples). The actual TR, however, depends on the chosen experimental conditions. As far as imaging time is concerned, no signal averaging with NAC equal to 1 is faster than multiple accumulations, low-resolution images with N(2D) less than 256 are faster than high-resolution acquisitions, and 2D images with N(3D) equal to 1 are faster than 3D images. An additional gain in imaging speed may be achieved by segmented scanning of N(S) greater than or equal to 2 Fourier lines per TR. Such choices are user dependent and therefore do not strictly refer to a particular sequence. It is always the clinician's choice to make trade-offs between spatial resolution, signal-to-noise ratio (SNR), and imaging speed, whereas a reduction of the TR beyond a certain limit requires a change of the MR sequence.

Unless otherwise noted, images were acquired at the Biomedizinische NMR Forschungs GmbH at the Max-Planck-Institut für biophysikalische Chemie, Göttingen, Germany, using a 2 T whole-body system (Siemens Vision). We especially thank Michael L. Gyngell for his contributions to the previous edition of this chapter; Dietmar Merboldt and Gunnar Krüger for their help in preparing many imaging examples; and Joachim Graessner for providing illustrative material not available in-house. We are indebted to many colleagues who allowed us to use their results.

BOX 6-1
List of Abbreviations

1D	One dimensional	M_0	Equilibrium magnetization
2D	Two dimensional	M_z	Steady state longitudinal magnetization
3D	Three dimensional	MBEST	Modulus-blipped echo-planar single-pulse technique
α	Flip angle less than 90 degrees	MIP	Maximum-intensity projection
β	Flip angle greater than 90 degrees	MR	Magnetic resonance
γ	Magnetogyric ratio	MRA	Magnetic resonance angiography
ΔB_0	Static magnetic field inhomogeneity	MRI	Magnetic resonance imaging
Acq	Acquisition	MTC	Magnetization-transfer contrast
BOLD	Blood oxygenation level–dependent	NAC	Number of acquisitions
CBO	Cerebral blood oxygenation	N(1D)	Number of data points in the frequency-encoding direction
CE-FAST	Contrast-enhanced Fourier acquisition in the steady state	N(2D)	Number of 2D phase-encoding steps
CHESS	Chemical-shift selective	N(3D)	Number of 3D phase-encoding steps
CSF	Cerebrospinal fluid	N(S)	Number of phase-encoding steps per repetition time
CSI	Chemical-shift imaging	RARE	Rapid acquisition with relaxation enhancement
DANTE	Delay alternating with nutation for tailored excitation	RF	Radiofrequency
DEFT	Driven-equilibrium Fourier transformation	S	Signal strength
ECG	Electrocardiogram	SE	Spin echo
EPI	Echo-planar imaging	SNR	Signal-to-noise ratio
FAST	Fourier acquisition in the steady state	SSFP	Steady state free precession
FID	Free-induction decay	STE	Stimulated echo
FISP	Fast imaging with steady precession	STEAM	Stimulated-echo acquisition mode
FLASH	Fast low-angle shot	T1	Spin-lattice (longitudinal) relaxation time
FOV	Field of view	T2	Spin-spin (transverse) relaxation time
FT	Fourier transformation	T2*	Effective spin-spin relaxation time
G_x, G_y	Gradients in x and y direction	TE	Echo time
GRASE	Gradient-echo spin-echo	TI	Inversion time
GRASS	Gradient-recalled acquisition in the steady state	TM	Middle interval
IR	Inversion recovery	TOF	Time of flight
k_x, k_y	κ-Space coordinates (spatial frequencies)	TR	Repetition time

Table 6-1   Measuring Time Required for One Cross-Sectional Image in MR Sequences

MRI	MEASURING TIME
Conventional	Minutes
Fast scan	Seconds
High speed	Fractions of a second

This chapter outlines the basic principles of different classes of rapid scan techniques, demonstrates the achievable image quality and contrast, describes state-of-the-art applications, and indicates future perspectives. Because a truly comprehensive overview of all pulse sequence possibilities is beyond the scope of this text, special emphasis is given to the mainstream of clinically useful techniques.

GENERAL APPROACHES

This section describes some generally applicable approaches that reduce either the number of Fourier lines per image without compromising spatial resolution (partial Fourier and reduced field-of-view [FOV] imaging) or the number of repetition intervals by covering multiple Fourier lines per radiofrequency (RF) excitation (hybrid or segmented scanning). Both methods are independent of a particular imaging sequence and at least in principle can be combined with most MR techniques.

Partial Fourier Imaging

According to Equation 1, measuring times may be reduced by reducing the N(2D), or number of Fourier lines in a 2D, cross-sectional Fourier image. Whereas a simple reduction of N(2D) sacrifices spatial resolution (e.g., in a 192 × 256 image), partial Fourier imaging methods attempt to arrange a limited number of phase-encoding steps in such a way that the images experience a loss in SNR but not in spatial resolution.

Half-Fourier imaging,[140] the first proposal in this direction, used only about half the number of phase-encoding steps of a conventional (quadratic) image matrix. To visualize the concepts underlying half-Fourier imaging, as well as those of other fast-scan and high-speed techniques, it is helpful to introduce the concept of κ space.[134,154,194] κ Space is a representation of how raw image data are acquired (see Chapter 7). A schematic diagram of the pathways of conventional Fourier imaging through κ space is sketched in Figure 6-1, *A*. Horizontal lines along the direction k_x (Fourier lines) refer to the typically N(1D) equal to 256 data samples acquired during one "readout" acquisition period of a Fourier image. In the presence of a constant frequency-encoding "read" gradient G_x, the spatial frequency $k_x(t) = \gamma G_x t$, with γ representing the magnetogyric ratio and t the time during the acquisition period. The vertical dimension k_y of the κ space is typically sampled in N(2D) = 256 repetitive experiments, each acquiring 1 horizontal Fourier line for a particular phase-encoding gradient strength G_y. Although a variation of the gradient duration t_y is possible,[127] most implementations of Fourier imaging take advantage of the spin-warp method,[38] which steps through κ space by varying the amplitude of the phase-encoding gradient according to $k_y(G_y) = \kappa \gamma G_y t_y$. A κ space consisting of N(2D) = 256 horizontal lines with N(1D) = 256 data samples represents the raw data acquired in a typical Fourier imaging experiment with a spatial resolution of N(1D) × N(2D) or 256 × 256 pixels. An example of a corresponding spin-echo (SE) image obtained by 2D Fourier transformation (2D FT) is shown in Figure 6-2, *A*.

When fully sampled, the k_x and k_y information of κ space is redundant because positive and negative spatial frequencies are "conjugate symmetrical."[46] Thus the spatial information in either half of κ space (top or bottom, left or right) is identical, so in theory even a quarter of κ space would yield an image with the same spatial resolution.[141] Because a reduction of k_x (i.e., the duration of the acquisition period) is not very efficient in reducing imaging times, "asymmetrical" or even "fractional" echoes[115,171] have been used only in conjunction with high-speed gradient-echo imaging or to achieve extremely short echo times (TEs) for specialized applications, such as imaging flow or short T2 components. On the other hand, imaging times may be cut by a factor of 2 if only half of the data along k_y is acquired (i.e., either the positive or negative Fourier lines). The resulting half-Fourier image ex-

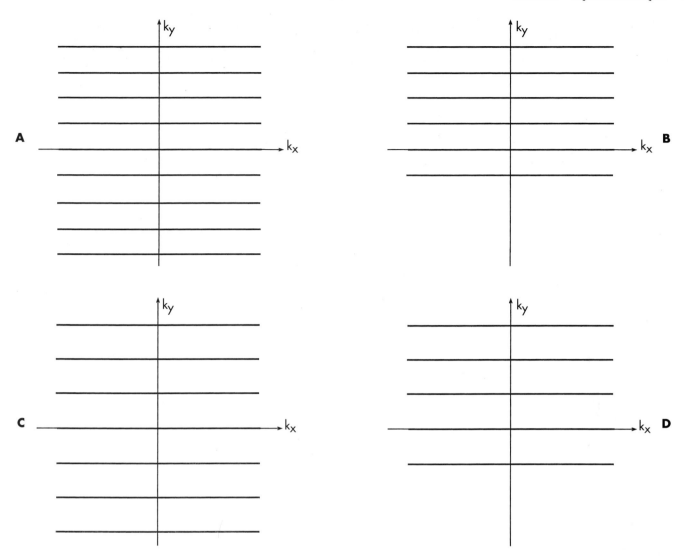

FIGURE 6-1   Schematic κ-space diagrams (image raw data) for 2D Fourier imaging **(A)**, half-Fourier imaging **(B)**, rectangular FOV imaging **(C)**, and combined rectangular FOV and half-Fourier imaging **(D)**. Whereas conventional 2D Fourier imaging consists of N(2D) = 256 Fourier lines with incremented phase-encoding gradients and N(1D) = 256 data samples acquired in the presence of a frequency-encoding "read" gradient, half-Fourier imaging requires only N(2D)/2 + 8 Fourier lines for reconstruction of an N(1D) × N(2D) image. The additional 8 Fourier lines are needed for optimization of the necessary phase correction. In rectangular FOV imaging a reduced number of Fourier lines with proportionally increased increments of the phase-encoding gradient is employed to cover a correspondingly reduced FOV without a loss in spatial resolution.

hibits a loss of SNR by about a factor of $\sqrt{2}$ but no loss in spatial resolution.

Figures 6-1, *B,* and 6-2, *B,* display a schematic representation of κ space and an SE image obtained using half-Fourier principles, respectively. Whereas full-conjugate symmetrical data acquired in conventional Fourier imaging allow magnitude reconstruction of the image, neglecting half of the data requires a phase correction that is commonly derived from the 16 central, low spatial frequencies along k_y. Thus a 256 × 256 pixel-resolution image requires the acquisition of a (128 + 8) × 256 data set to perform adequate phase corrections. Because the presence of magnetic field inhomogeneities would introduce spatially dependent phase variations, half-Fourier techniques are generally more suitable for RF-refocused (SE or stimulated-echo [STE]) imaging than for gradient-echo imaging.[142]

A more recent, commonly applied technique is reduced or rectangular FOV imaging. It is applicable to all types of MR pulse sequences and delivers conventional magnitude images. The approach restricts the dimension of the acquired data set along the phase-encoding direction to the actual size of the object to be imaged. In other words, it avoids measuring κ space data outside the object and therefore employs a matched rectangular FOV rather than the usual square FOV. As illustrated in Figure 6-1, *C,* data acquisition involves a reduced density of Fourier lines in κ space but leaves the bandwidth covering the phase-encoding dimension unchanged to keep the spatial resolution constant. This may be achieved by enhancing the strength of the incremented phase-encoding gradient so that the reduced number of steps still expands to the original size of κ space. After image reconstruction, the displayed image contains information only in the reduced central part of the matrix, with absent signal on either side. A pertinent example using three quarters of the original 256 Fourier lines (i.e., N[2D] = 192, leading to a 192 × 256 image in three quarters of the original imaging time) is shown in Figure 6-2, *C.*

Of course, a rectangular FOV and the principle of half-Fourier imaging may be combined (Figures 6-1, *D,* and 6-2, *D*). A significant reduction in measuring time thus may be achieved without too harmful a reduction in SNR, provided the original acquisition is of sufficiently high quality. This is normally the case with long-TR SE imaging.

Segmented Scanning

In all of the Fourier imaging methods discussed so far, only 1 Fourier line is acquired per RF excitation (i.e., within one repetition interval).

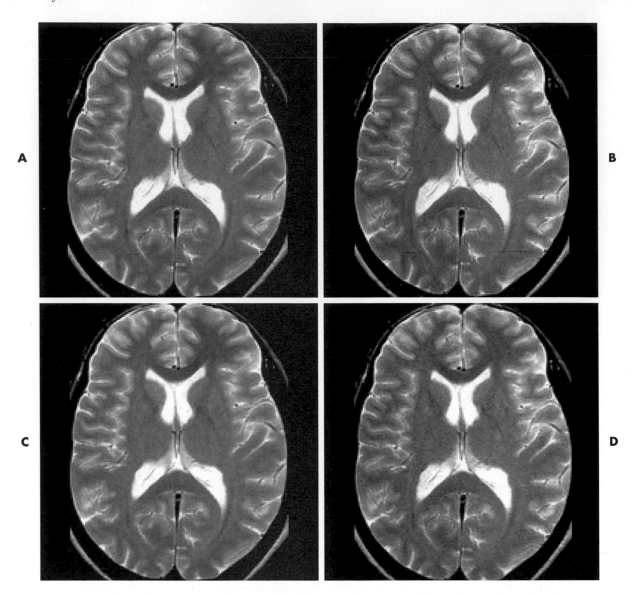

FIGURE 6-2   SE images of the human brain (2 T, TR/TE = 2500/80 ms, slice thickness of 4 mm, NAC = 1) with identical spatial resolution demonstrating the trade-off between SNR and measuring time for a 2D Fourier image (magnitude) **(A),** a half-Fourier image (real) **(B),** a rectangular FOV image (magnitude) **(C),** and a combined rectangular FOV and half-Fourier image (real) **(D).** All sequences were operated in a double-echo multislice mode. Other parameters are 256 × 256 matrix, square FOV 230 mm, measuring time = 10 min 44 sec, relative SNR = 1 **(A);** 128 × 256 matrix, square FOV 230 mm, measuring time = 5 min 44 sec, SNR = 0.71 (√0.5) **(B);** 192 × 256 matrix, rectangular FOV 172.5 × 230 mm², measuring time = 8 min 4 sec, SNR = 0.87 (√0.75) **(C);** and 96 × 256 matrix, rectangular FOV 172.5 × 230 mm², measuring time = 4 min 24 sec, SNR = 0.61 (√0.375) **(D).** For high-quality SE imaging at intermediate to high field strengths, the loss in SNR with shorter measuring times is often barely visible.

Obviously, such a strategy is not very efficient, and in most conventional MR sequences the need for a relaxation "waiting" period is therefore exploited for interleaved multislice excitations. Alternatively, multiple Fourier lines (i.e., larger regions of κ space) may be scanned within each TR interval if multiple signals can be generated and differently phase encoded to carry complementary spatial information. The corresponding imaging experiment becomes partitioned into new partial experiments, often termed *segments,* in which each segment acquires the equivalent of N(S) Fourier lines.[3,35] Such a scheme is demonstrated in Figure 6-3, *A,* for the case of N(S) = 3 and should be compared with conventional scanning as shown in Figure 6-1, *A.* Although the overall scan time of a segmented image acquisition is reduced by the factor N(S), the number of acquired echo signals is not. Thus the SNR of the resulting image is affected only as much as the differently phase-encoded echoes are attenuated by spin-lattice (longitudinal, or T1), spin-spin (transverse, or T2), or effective spin-spin (T2*) relaxation time.

The most obvious ways of generating several encodable signals per repetition interval involve the creation of multiple SEs (Figure 6-23), multiple STEs (Figure 6-26), and multiple gradient echoes (Figure 6-31). In their extreme forms as single-shot techniques with all Fourier lines encoded into a single echo train (i.e., N[S] = N[2D]), pertinent sequences have been developed and are called *rapid acquisition with relaxation enhancement* (RARE),[100] *high-speed stimulated echo acquisition mode* (STEAM),[54] and *echo-planar imaging* (EPI),[138,139] respectively.

Segmented multishot MR sequences normally acquire the raw image data in the presence of a constant frequency-encoding read gradient, as in classic Fourier imaging. Although this allows rectangular coverage of κ space and simplifies image reconstruction, it represents only one possible approach. From the historical perspective, segmented image acquisition, or data grouping, was first achieved by a slightly more complex scanning strategy—adding a sinusoidally oscillating gradient in the phase-encoding direction during data acquisition.[197] The path-

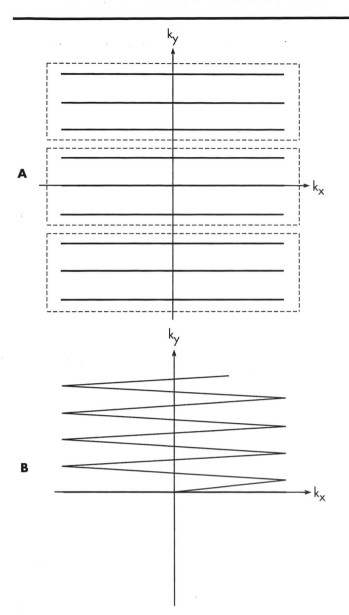

FIGURE 6-3   Schematic κ-space diagrams for segmented scanning **(A)** and original EPI **(B)**.[138,139] Segmented image acquisition in **A** attempts to reduce scan times by covering multiple Fourier lines within the same repetition interval. This may be achieved by generating several differently phase-encoded SE, STE, or gradient-echo signals. As an extreme case the original single-shot EPI technique in **B** covers half of κ space in only one sweep. The corresponding imaging sequence acquires all Fourier lines as a single train of differently phase-encoded gradient echoes. A state-of-the-art implementation that symmetrically covers the full κ space is shown in Figure 6-31, *D,* together with alternative versions of high-speed EPI in Figure 6-31, *B* and *C,* that replace the constant phase-encoding gradient with more conventional gradient pulses to sample κ space on a rectangular grid as sketched in Figure 6-31, *A.*

way in κ space corresponds to an oscillation that covers multiple Fourier lines, the number of which depends on the strength of the gradient oscillation. Experimental reduction factors of 4 have been realized (hybrid imaging).[86] Interestingly, if the oscillating amplitude is large enough to cover the whole or at least half of κ space, then a single RF excitation is sufficient for image reconstruction and no further phase-encoding gradient step is required. This concept underlies the original form of EPI.[138,139] In a corresponding κ-space diagram (Figure 6-3, *B*), only half of κ space is sampled.

Classic hybrid imaging schemes have not found general applications. Apart from the need for data interpolations because of nonrectangular sampling of κ space and phase distortions caused by chemical shift and flow phenomena, there is now effective competition from both segmented scanning with constant frequency-encoding gradients and more advanced EPI sequences. In general the concept of segmented

scanning may be used to either accelerate conventional MRI by a factor N(S) or conversely to remove artifacts or improve resolution in high-speed MRI by slowing pertinent single-shot sequences down into segmented multishot versions with N(2D) / N(S) repetitions.

LOW FLIP ANGLE GRADIENT-ECHO IMAGING

The bulk of fast-scan MRI is based on imaging sequences that combine low flip angle RF excitations and gradient-recalled echo acquisitions.[55,58,88] Typical measuring times for a single 2D FT image are seconds. The images do not exhibit a loss of spatial resolution as compared with conventional SE images or suffer from an unacceptable trade-off in SNR. Typical measuring times for rapid gradient-echo images compare favorably with the time constants of most physiological motion in humans. The only exception is the heart, in which periodicity of the motion may be exploited to synchronize the data acquisition to the electrocardiogram (ECG) signal. Such techniques provide access to functional information of blood flow and myocardial wall movements in cine MRI movie loops with an apparent temporal resolution of a few milliseconds. On the other hand, low flip angle gradient-echo images offer superior spatial resolution within classic SE scan times of a few minutes, either by large matrix cross-sectional imaging in conjunction with a rectangular FOV or by true 3D imaging.

The following section begins with a simple outline of basic MR signals and their properties in RF pulse sequences with short TRs. After a condensed analysis of respective signals and contrast, fast-scan MR sequences exploiting the free-induction decay (FID), steady state free precession–FID (SSFP-FID), and SSFP-echo are covered in detail.

Repetitive Radiofrequency Pulse Excitations

Basic Magnetic Resonance Signals. In general there are only three different types of single-quantum MR signals[93]—the FID, following a single RF pulse; the SE, created by two RF pulses; and the STE, created by three RF pulses (Figure 6-4). These signals have been used for conventional MRI with intermediate to long TRs. Under these conditions, a 90-degree RF pulse elicits the maximum signal (i.e., it excites the entire longitudinal magnetization). The resulting FID decays with T2*, comprising both natural T2 relaxation and all types of dephasing mechanisms reflecting magnetic field inhomogeneities (ΔB) according to $1/T2^* = 1/T2 + \gamma\Delta B$. For the SE sequence the maximum echo signal at TE is obtained with a 90-degree excitation pulse and a 180-degree refocusing pulse. In contrast to the FID the SE signal is independent of magnetic field inhomogeneities, and its intensity decreases with the true T2 relaxation time. Finally the maximum STE signal results from the application of three 90-degree RF pulses, provided that the transverse magnetization excited by the first RF pulse becomes completely dephased before application of the second RF pulse. This may be accomplished by a dephasing magnetic field gradient. Attenuation of the STE signal is caused by T2 relaxation during TE and T1 relaxation during the middle interval (TM); for a given TE it has only half the strength of a corresponding 90-degree–180-degree SE signal. In addition to the STE signal a three-pulse sequence creates three FID signals and up to four SE signals.[53] Spoiler gradients are necessary to eliminate overlap of the STE signal with unwanted FID and SE contributions. Of course, sequences with four or more RF pulses lead to an even larger number of FID, SE, and STE signals generated from all possible combinations of RF pulses.[119]

Magnetic Resonance Signals During Repetitive Radiofrequency Excitation. In the context of MRI, RF pulse sequences are used in a repetitive manner to acquire differently phase-encoded Fourier lines. For TRs less than or equal to T1, the spins become saturated with the RF pulses probing the steady state longitudinal magnetization determined by T1, TR, and flip angle. The corresponding FID signals are shown in Figure 6-5, *A.* For short TRs (TR ≤ T2) the situation becomes more complex, and a steady state of the longitudinal and transverse magnetization, termed *SSFP,*[18] results in the additional formation of echoes (Figure 6-5, *B*). In the schematic drawing the total signal has been partitioned into an SSFP-FID and an SSFP-echo. In practice this is achieved only by applying magnetic field gradients as required for MRI. In fact, all three MR signal types may be used for fast-scan imag-

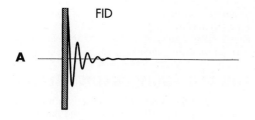

FID

A

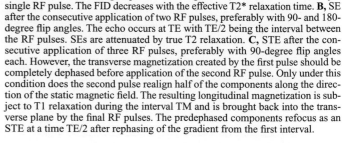

FIGURE 6-4 Basic single-quantum MR signals. **A,** FID after excitation by a single RF pulse. The FID decreases with the effective T2* relaxation time. **B,** SE after the consecutive application of two RF pulses, preferably with 90- and 180-degree flip angles. The echo occurs at TE with TE/2 being the interval between the RF pulses. SEs are attenuated by true T2 relaxation. **C,** STE after the consecutive application of three RF pulses, preferably with 90-degree flip angles each. However, the transverse magnetization created by the first pulse should be completely dephased before application of the second RF pulse. Only under this condition does the second pulse realign half of the components along the direction of the static magnetic field. The resulting longitudinal magnetization is subject to T1 relaxation during the interval TM and is brought back into the transverse plane by the final RF pulses. The predephased components refocus as an STE at a time TE/2 after rephasing of the gradient from the first interval.

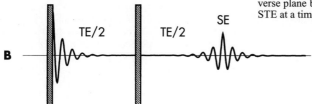

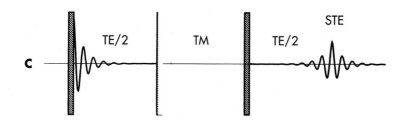

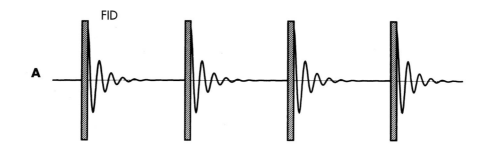

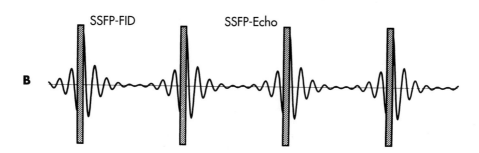

FIGURE 6-5 MR signals generated by repetitive RF pulse excitations. **A,** A steady state of the longitudinal magnetization gives rise to an FID signal (according to Equation 2). **B,** SSFP of both the longitudinal and transverse magnetization requires phase stability of the MR signal from one repetition cycle to the next and TR ≤T2. Under such conditions the signal is an SSFP-FID after the RF pulses and an SSFP-echo preceding the RF pulses (according to Equations 3 and 4, respectively). An experimental separation of the SSFP-FID and SSFP-echo as suggested in this schematic drawing may be accomplished only with magnetic field gradients. The SSFP-FID is composed of the conventional FID, as in **A,** and contributions from transverse coherences.

ing. Pertinent techniques generate a gradient-recalled echo by reversal of the frequency-encoding gradient and thereby shift the acquisition of the FID, the SSFP-FID, or the SSFP-echo signal to some time before or after the center of the RF pulses. (Their individual dependencies on T1 and T2 relaxation are the subject of the following section.) In addition, the gradient echoes of the FID, SSFP-FID, or SSFP-echo signal are sensitive to magnetic field inhomogeneities and tissue susceptibility differences in proportion to the gradient-echo time.

The SSFP-echo represents the overlap of the primary SE from the last two RF pulses and the primary STE from the last three RF pulses with all higher-order echoes that are characterized by even greater effective TEs (TE = $n \times$ TR and $n \geq 3$). This multitude of components is often referred to as *transverse coherences*.[85,119] The access to TEs longer than the actual TR renders SSFP-echo sequences attractive for the detection of disorders with prolonged T2 values. However, SSFP signals are observed only if a number of biological and experimental conditions are fulfilled, allowing the establishment of steady state transverse magnetizations. Conditions for tissue parameters (e.g., long T2 relaxation times), physiological behavior (e.g., no motion), and experimental imaging parameters (e.g., refocused phase-encoding gradients) are summarized in Table 6-2. Because all conditions must be fulfilled at the same time, gradient-echo imaging sequences based on SSFP-echo signals are primarily applicable to brain studies. In cases in which short T2 relaxation times lead to low SSFP-echo signal strengths, such as in liver and muscle, any pathological prolongation of T2 results in excellent contrast for lesion detection if motion-induced phase variations are minimal.

In general, any kind of phase instability from one repetition interval to the next precludes the generation of transverse coherences and therefore does not establish an SSFP signal. In particular this applies to rapidly moving objects (e.g., the heart) or the use of technical means, such as variable spoiler gradients or phase-incoherent RF excitations. Under these conditions, gradient-echo images of SSFP-echoes vanish, and gradient-echo images of SSFP-FID signals change into conventional gradient-echo images.

Free-Induction Decay Signal Strength. This and the following section summarize theoretical expressions for the FID, SSFP-FID, and SSFP-echo. Signal strengths are given as a function of the equilibrium magnetization (M_0), T1 and T2 relaxation times, TR, and flip angle (α). Steady state conditions are assumed, and signal alterations caused by slice-profile deformations are ignored.

If transverse coherences in low flip angle gradient-echo imaging sequences can be neglected (motion, short T2), avoided (low flip angle, long TR), or removed (spoiling), the theoretical description of the true FID signal is greatly simplified. It may be directly derived from the progressive saturation[44] behavior of the longitudinal magnetization weighted by the effective T2* decay between excitation and detection of the gradient echo.

(EQ. 2)

$$S(\text{FID}) = M_0 \sin\alpha \frac{1 - E1(TR)}{1 - E1(TR)\cos\alpha} E2^* (TE)$$

where $E1(TR) = \exp(-TR/T1)$ and $E2^*(TE) = \exp(-TE/T2^*)$, with T2* including magnetic field inhomogeneities. Practical applications

Table 6-2 Conditions for the Generation and Observation of SSFP Signals

PARAMETER	CONDITION
Tissue	Stationary spins
	No motion
	Long T2 relaxation times
Sequence	Phase-coherent RF pulses
	Constant repetition times
	Constant integral gradients
User	Short repetition times
	Medium flip angles
	No interleaved multislicing

in which the gradient-echo times are made as short as possible (E2* $\approx$ 1) result in pure T1 contrast. Low flip angles (cosα $\approx$ 1 and S[FID] $\approx$ M_0 sinα) correspond to pure spin-density contrast.

SSFP-FID and SSFP-Echo. The use of TRs shorter than T1 and T2 establishes a dynamic equilibrium in both the longitudinal and transverse magnetization components. The evolution of the transverse magnetization during each repetition interval requires a complex mathematical treatment.[85] The MR signal consists of two distinct components representing an FID type of signal (SSFP-FID), which occurs immediately after the RF pulse, and an echo type of signal (SSFP-echo), which refocuses at the end of each repetition interval at TR.

(EQ. 3)

$$S(\text{SSFP-FID}) = M_0 \sin\alpha \frac{1 - E1(TR)}{p} [u - E2(TR) \cdot v]$$

(EQ. 4)

$$S(\text{SSFP-echo}) = M_0 \sin\alpha \frac{1 - E1(TR)}{p} [E2(2TR) \cdot u - E2(TR) \cdot v]$$

The terms *u* and *v* are given by

(EQ. 5)

$$u = 1 + \sum_{m=1}^{\infty} \left(\frac{q}{2p}\right)^{2m} \binom{2m}{m}$$

(EQ. 6)

$$v = \frac{1}{2} \sum_{m=1}^{\infty} \left(\frac{q}{2p}\right)^{2m-1} \binom{2m}{m}$$

with

(EQ. 7)

$$p = 1 - E1(TR) \cos\alpha - E2^2(TR) [E1(TR) - \cos\alpha]$$

(EQ. 8)

$$q = E2(TR) [1 - E1(TR)] (1 + \cos\alpha)$$

and $\binom{n}{k}$ are binomial coefficients. The infinite summations in Equations 5 and 6 converge within 3 or 4 iterations for high flip angles (90 degrees or greater) and 50 to 100 iterations for low flip angles (10 degrees or less), depending on T1 and T2. Intuitively, SSFP signals are composites of a number of coincident contributions from FIDs and different orders of SEs and STEs. Transforming a single RF-pulse experiment (Figure 6-4, *A*) into a repetitive sequence of equidistant RF pulses can simulate the situation. For short TR values, such a sequence generates FID signals and allows mutual interaction of pairs of pulses, giving rise to SEs (Figure 6-4, *B*), as well as interaction of three pulses, giving rise to STEs (Figure 6-4, *C*). Moreover, arbitrary combinations of pulses from different TR intervals contribute to the overall SSFP signal.

E2(TR) = exp($-$ TR/T2) in Equations 3 and 4 denotes signal attenuation by true T2 relaxation. This property results from the fact that the underlying MR signals represent RF-refocused echoes and therefore provide access to T2 contrast in SSFP-echo sequences. Experimentally the SSFP-FID signal depends on the ratio of T1/T2, although an exact theoretical derivation starting from Equation 3 has not been reported. For imaging purposes the SSFP-FID and SSFP-echo signals are acquired in the form of a gradient-recalled echo, which then causes additional T2* relaxation and spin dephasing as a result of field inhomogeneities. Accordingly the SSFP signals in Equations 3 and 4 must be weighted by a factor E2*, similar to the pure FID signal in Equation 2.

If there is no transfer of transverse magnetization from one repetition interval to the next (i.e., if E2[TR] = 0), then the SSFP-echo signal (Equation 4) vanishes. Correspondingly, p = 1 $-$ E1(TR) cosα, q = 0, and u = 1, so that the SSFP-FID (Equation 3) becomes independent of transverse coherences and T2 and therefore identical to the classic saturation behavior of the FID (Equation 2). In practice there are situations in which certain regions of an image exhibit SSFP characteristics, whereas others do not (e.g., compare the distortions caused by ventricular cerebrospinal fluid [CSF] flow in Figures 6-19, *A*, and 6-21).

FLASH Imaging

This section describes the basic features, contrast, and applications of a generic fast-scan MR sequence that interrogates the longitudinal magnetization generated by a series of repetitive RF excitations.

Fast low-angle shot (FLASH)[52,55,56,88] imaging may be considered the prototype of rapid scan techniques based on low flip angle RF excitations and gradient-echo acquisitions. Schematic timing diagrams for cross-sectional imaging, nonselective 3D imaging, and slab-selective 3D imaging are shown in Figure 6-6. The FLASH technique employs RF pulses with flip angles of less than 90 degrees. Thus the available longitudinal magnetization is partitioned into an excited transverse part and a remaining longitudinal part (Figure 6-7). For example, a single RF excitation with a flip angle $\alpha = 30$ degrees rotates the magnetization vector such that the observable transverse magnetization component yields $M_z \sin\alpha$, or 50% of the available longitudinal magnetization (M_z). This component is detected as a gradient echo by reversal of the dephasing frequency-encoding read gradient. Because, on the other hand, $M_z \cos\alpha$, or 87% of the longitudinal magnetization remains untouched, an imaging sequence may proceed immediately after data acquisition without a waiting period. When starting from equilibrium, the spin system approaches a steady state (Equation 2) only after a number of excitations.

Although FLASH is compatible with projection reconstruction techniques[130] or classic Fourier imaging varying the duration of the phase-encoding gradient,[127] it is most commonly implemented in the form of spin-warp Fourier imaging,[38] with the amplitude of the phase-encoding gradient sweeping from negative to positive values (or reversed) during image acquisition (Figure 6-6, *A*). TR and TE of FLASH sequences may be as short as the existing hardware of the gradient system can realize. TE is given by the interval between the center of the RF pulse and the peak amplitude of the gradient echo.

With the advent of short TR sequences, the acquisition of 3D data sets became possible within measuring times of minutes. For example, a 3D data set of $256 \times 256 \times 128$ pixels may be obtained within a scan time of 8.2 min using TR = 15 ms, N(1D) = 256 complex data samples in the read direction, N(2D) = 256 phase-encoding steps in the second direction, N(3D) = 128 phase-encoding steps in the third direction, and NAC = 1 (Equation 1). Because of the large number of N(2D) × N(3D) RF excitations, 3D images benefit from a significant gain in SNR as compared with 2D images with only N(2D) excitations. In the general case of nonselective 3D imaging the slice-selective RF pulse in Figure 6-6, *A*, is replaced by a nonselective pulse in Figure 6-6, *B*, which excites the entire volume accessible to the RF coil. Spatial discrimination along the third dimension is achieved by means of a second phase-encoding gradient.

In most cases of 3D imaging it is advantageous to restrict the FOV in one of the phase-encoding directions. This is achieved by exciting a thick slice (slab) perpendicular to this direction, as shown in Figure 6-6, *C*.

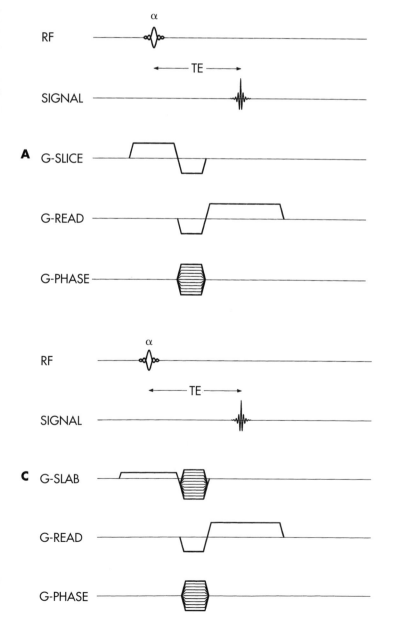

FIGURE 6-6 Schematic FLASH MR sequences for cross-sectional imaging (**A**), nonselective 3D imaging (**B**), and slab-selective 3D imaging (**C**). All FLASH sequences use low flip angle RF excitation pulses α <90 degrees *(RF)*. **A**, In cross-sectional imaging a slice-select gradient *(G-SLICE)* is used in conjunction with a frequency-selective RF pulse. The frequency-encoding read gradient *(G-READ)* creates the gradient echo *(SIGNAL)*, and a phase-encoding gradient *(G-PHASE)* performs spatial encoding in the second dimension (Figure 6-1, *A*). **B**, In nonselective 3D imaging the slice-select gradient is replaced by a second phase-encoding gradient for spatial encoding in the third dimension, and a broad-band RF pulse is used to excite the whole volume. **C**, In slab-selective 3D imaging, phase-encoding is combined with slice selection to restrict the FOV in this axis.

The 3D phase-encoding gradient covers the FOV across the selected slab by dividing it into a stack of slices (partitions). Slab-selective 3D MRI is of particular interest in studies in which only a part of the full object ought to be investigated at the highest possible spatial resolution. In such applications, aliasing in the frequency-encoding dimension is avoided by oversampling as usual. Additional aliasing in the second dimension may be eliminated by spatial presaturation.[57]

To exclude potential contributions from transverse coherences,[74] T1-weighted FLASH sequences may be complemented by additional RF[26,217,218] or gradient spoiling.[59] Inadequate spoiling leads to image ar-

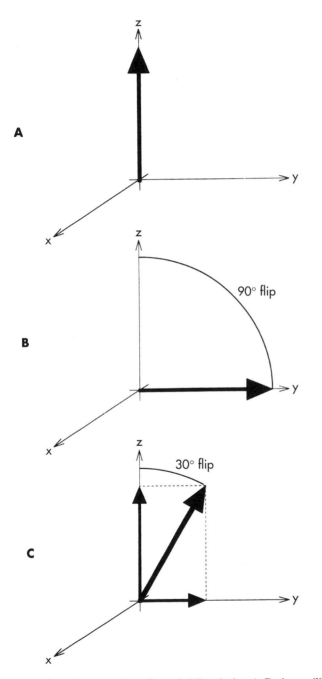

FIGURE 6-7   Principle of low flip angle RF excitation. **A,** During equilibrium the macroscopic magnetization is entirely aligned along the direction of the static magnetic field. **B,** When flipped by a 90-degree RF pulse, the available longitudinal magnetization along the z direction is completely transformed into observable transverse magnetization with no longitudinal component remaining. **C,** A flip angle α <90 degrees rotates the magnetization vector so that it splits into a transverse and a longitudinal component. The excited transverse magnetization is proportional to sin α. For α = 30 degrees this results in 50% of the available transverse magnetization, whereas the longitudinal magnetization is reduced to cos α, or 87% of its original value.

tifacts in the form of parallel bands of residually phase-encoded transverse coherences along the direction of the phase-encoding gradient.[25,185] Although gradient spoiling using an incremented gradient in the slice-selection direction after data acquisition turns out to be sufficient for cross-sectional imaging, it is less efficient in 3D applications. In general, therefore, RF-spoiling schemes are recommended. They may be adopted without a time penalty because spoiling is achieved by incoherent RF excitation, preferably by means of incremented phase differences. To avoid distortions of the acquired gradient echo, the phase of the receiver channel must be changed accordingly. RF spoiling may be simplified by refocusing the high-intensity artifacts into proper SSFP signal contributions by reversing the action of the phase-encoding gradient after data acquisition, as in SSFP-FID imaging (Figure 6-18).

Spin-Density and T1 Contrast. The contrast capabilities of FLASH MR sequences as given by Equation 2 indicate access to spin-density and T1 contrast, depending on imaging parameters. Figures 6-8 and 6-9 show the typical signal variations of FLASH images of the human brain as a function of flip angle (Figure 6-8), ranging from 10 to 70 degrees (TR = 100 ms), and TR (Figure 6-9), ranging from 20 to 400 ms (α = 30 degrees). For a given TR (Figure 6-8), T1 contrast between gray and white matter is obtained for flip angles of 40 degrees or more, whereas reversed spin-density contrast is achieved at low flip angles (10 degrees or less). For a fixed flip angle (Figure 6-9), T1 contrast at short TRs turns into spin-density contrast at long TRs.

The observed signal intensities deviate slightly from the theoretical behavior of Equation 2 as a result of slice-profile changes as a function of TR, flip angle, and RF-pulse shape.[94,214] For this reason, quantitative T1 calculations from differently T1-weighted FLASH images are difficult to achieve, although qualitative tissue contrasts are quite convincing. Similar findings hold for other sequences employing multiple slice-selective excitation (or refocusing) RF pulses, especially for SSFP imaging, in which slice profiles are even more complicated. Such problems may be avoided by using nonselective 3D imaging. Slab-selective sequences exhibit minor intensity distortions only for the outermost sections along the restricted FOV in the direction of the 3D phase-encoding gradient.

FLASH MR sequences may be advantageously applied to all parts of the body. In addition to studies of the central nervous system, abdominal imaging with and without breath-holding clearly benefits from reduced scan times.[65] Figure 6-10 shows 3 out of 19 multislice transverse images covering the entire pancreas and liver within a single breath-hold (20 sec) in a patient with recurrent pancreatic carcinoma. Much shorter measuring times are possible when using single-slice acquisitions with TRs of a few milliseconds. Such studies provide additional insights into the vasculature because single-slice gradient-echo images exhibit strong time-of-flight (TOF) signal enhancements from spins flowing perpendicular to the imaging plane (see Chapters 11, 19, and 56). In contrast, multislice acquisitions demonstrate decreased signal from flowing blood because RF excitations from neighboring sections presaturate spins in the more central slices (e.g., note the low signal from the vena cava in Figure 6-10). The effect is similar to that accomplished by additional spatial presaturation RF pulses employed for flow-suppressed imaging[57] (Figure 6-13).

Magnetic Susceptibilities. The historical reason for using SE sequences was the poor quality of early gradient-echo images, resulting from long TEs and the poor magnetic field homogeneity of the first whole-body systems. Although technological progress has reduced these problems, there are still several sources of local magnetic field distortions of either a macroscopic (intervoxel) or microscopic (intravoxel) nature. Among them are metallic implants (clips, prostheses, and crowns), paramagnetic contrast agents (including endogenous levels of deoxyhemoglobin), differences in the magnetic susceptibilities of neighboring tissues (air–tissue interfaces), and pathological tissue alterations (hemorrhage, hemosiderin, and iron deposits[183]). In all cases the inherent field gradients cause a local loss of signal in a gradient-echo image.

As indicated in Table 6-3, magnetic field inhomogeneities may alter the field (or frequency) distribution of nuclear spin moments in an image voxel in two different ways—by changing its broadness and by shifting its mean value.[71] Although details depend on the actual mechanism, such alterations generally occur in all three dimensions and

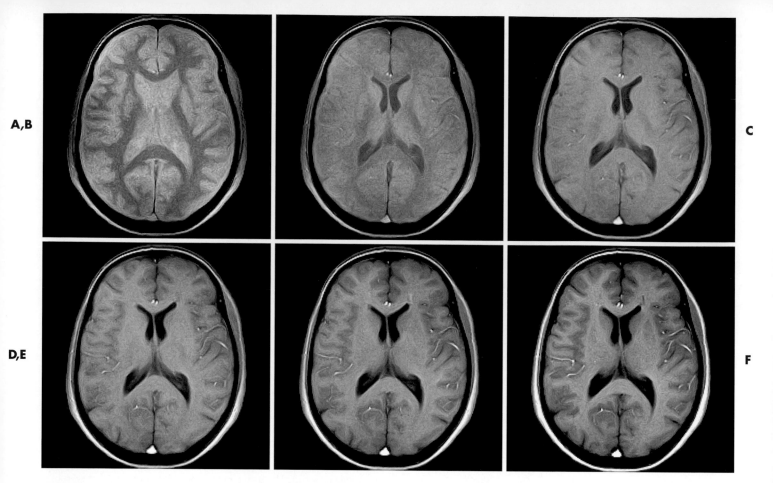

FIGURE 6-8 Spin-density and T1 contrast in gradient-echo imaging as a function of flip angle. Transverse head images (2 T, RF-spoiled FLASH, 256 × 256 matrix, FOV 230 mm, slice thickness of 4 mm, TR/TE = 100/4 ms) with flip angles of 10 degrees **(A)**, 20 degrees **(B)**, 30 degrees **(C)**, 40 degrees **(D)**, 50 degrees **(E)**, and 70 degrees **(F)**. Each image was obtained in a multislice mode within an imaging time of 26 sec (NAC = 1, for 10 degrees NAC = 2). The images are scaled individually to emphasize variations of contrast rather than signal strength.

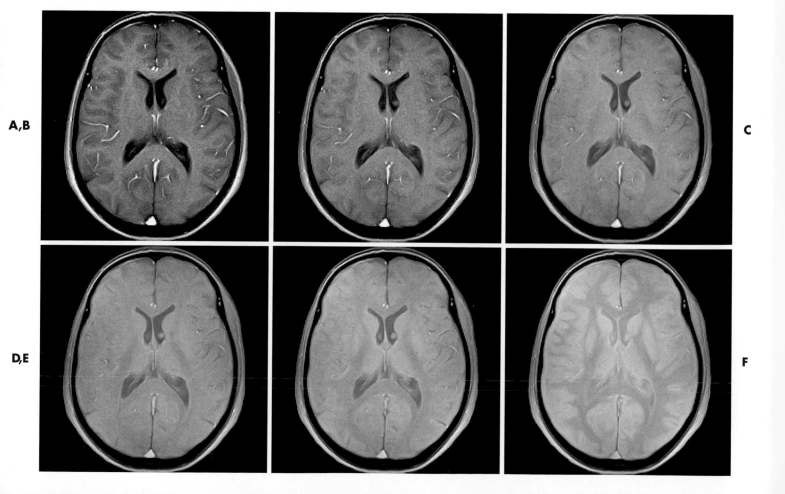

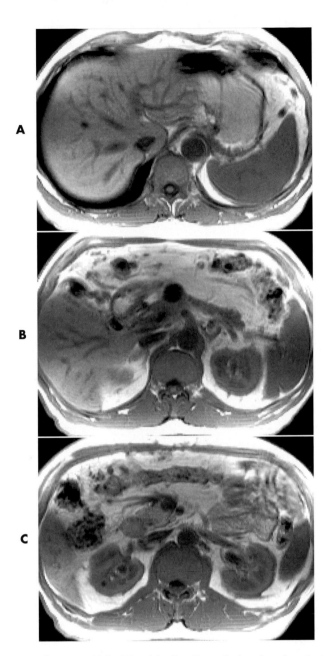

FIGURE 6-10 Multislice T1-weighted gradient-echo imaging of a patient with a recurrent pancreatic carcinoma acquired during a single breath-hold. **A** to **C,** The transverse images represent 3 out of a total of 19 sections obtained in an interleaved multislice mode within an imaging time of 20 sec (1.5 T, RF-spoiled FLASH, 140 × 256 matrix, rectangular FOV 300 × 400 mm², slice thickness of 8 mm, TR/TE = 146.1/4.1 ms, flip angle of 75 degrees, NAC = 1). (Courtesy E. Grabbe.)

therefore independently affect the imaging gradients. As far as frequency-encoding and phase-encoding gradients are concerned, intravoxel signal changes result entirely from a change in broadness of the frequency distribution. A change in mean frequency shifts the echo position in κ space and leads to distortions of the image geometry. Conversely, however, both types of distribution changes alter the MR signal

FIGURE 6-9 Spin-density and T1 contrast in gradient-echo imaging as a function of TR. Transverse head images (2 T, RF spoiled FLASH, 256 × 256 matrix, FOV 230 mm, slice thickness of 4 mm, TE = 4 ms, flip angle of 30 degrees) with TRs of 20 ms (**A**), 50 ms (**B**), 100 ms (**C**), 150 ms (**D**), 200 ms (**E**), and 400 ms (**F**). Each image was obtained in a single-slice mode (NAC = 1, for TR = 20 ms NAC = 2). The images are scaled individually to emphasize variations of contrast rather than signal strength.

Table 6-3 Influences of Magnetic Field Inhomogeneities

Magnetic field inhomogeneities change the broadness and mean of the intravoxel field (or frequency) distribution and therefore cause either signal loss or geometric distortions within a gradient-echo image, depending on the functionality of the MR gradients.

	CHANGE OF INTRAVOXEL FIELD DISTRIBUTION	
MR GRADIENT	**BROADNESS**	**MEAN**
Frequency encoding	Intravoxel dephasing (→ signal loss)	Echo shift (→ image distortion)
Phase encoding	Intravoxel dephasing (→ signal loss)	Echo shift (→ image distortion)
Slice selection	Intravoxel dephasing (→ signal loss)	Incomplete refocusing (→ signal loss)

intensity in the slice-select direction. Intravoxel dephasing is often even stronger than in the frequency-encoding and phase-encoding direction because section thickness usually surpasses in-plane voxel dimensions. A shift of the entire distribution easily may preclude most spins from rephasing because it causes a net phase offset after normal slice refocusing that further increases with TE.

The sensitive behavior of the slice-select gradient[61] to field inhomogeneities is illustrated in Figure 6-11, *A* to *C.* Imbalanced refocusing (Figure 6-11, *B* and *D*) may be overcompensated for by recalibrating the strength of the slice-select gradient (Figure 6-11, *C*) at the expense of losing all signal from unaffected regions of the image (Figure 6-11, *E* to *H*). Summation of pertinent images[61,210] yields an anatomical map apparently free from inhomogeneity artifacts (Figure 6-11, *I*). A more elegant approach arises from FT of a series of properly adjusted gradient-echo signals.[211] Although several images with different degrees of slice refocusing must be acquired, such techniques allow the acquisition of SE-like gradient-echo images in the presence of otherwise unavoidable magnetic field gradients. Geometrical distortions caused by alterations of the phase-encoding or frequency-encoding gradients are expected only in the presence of very strong (e.g., metallic clip-induced) field gradients, weak imaging gradients, or both.[63]

The imaging parameters in Figure 6-11, *D,* were deliberately chosen to degrade image quality. The observed susceptibility-induced signal losses in the vicinity of air-tissue interfaces are a linear function of the induced local gradient strength and the user-dependent (and/or system-dependent) parameters—echo time and voxel size.[215] Obviously the longer the precession time between excitation and detection, the larger the precession angle that a certain spin can acquire; the larger the voxel size of an image, the higher the probability to cancel with another spin of opposite phase within the same voxel. Moreover the use of weak slice-selection gradients for thick slices further emphasizes the relative strength of the local field distortion.

The effect of TE and slice thickness on image quality in critical locations of the human brain is demonstrated in Figure 6-12. Focal signal losses caused by spin dephasing at natural air-tissue interfaces can be almost completely avoided by means of a short TE (4 ms or less), a high pixel resolution (256 × 256 or greater) together with a matched FOV (250 mm or less), and a thin slice or 3D partition (4 mm or less). Apart from the ability to remove image artifacts and improve overall quality, high spatial resolution in addition to imaging speed and SNR is also a clinically desirable feature.

Chemical Shift. In an MR experiment, all spins have the same phase immediately after RF excitation. During the subsequent free-precession period (i.e., during evolution of the FID signal), components with different resonance frequencies, such as water and fat, precess at different rates. Accordingly these components in general exhibit different phases. The relative phase difference depends on the TE and the difference in the respective resonance frequencies (chemical shift), which for fat and water is about 3.5 parts per million of the static magnetic field. In SE or STE sequences that employ RF-refocused echoes, the dephasing effect is refocused by reversal of the precession sense. In gradient-echo imaging the sense of precession is not reversed by reversal of a gradient, so for a selected TE the phase of the water signal may be either opposite or identical to the phase of the fat component.

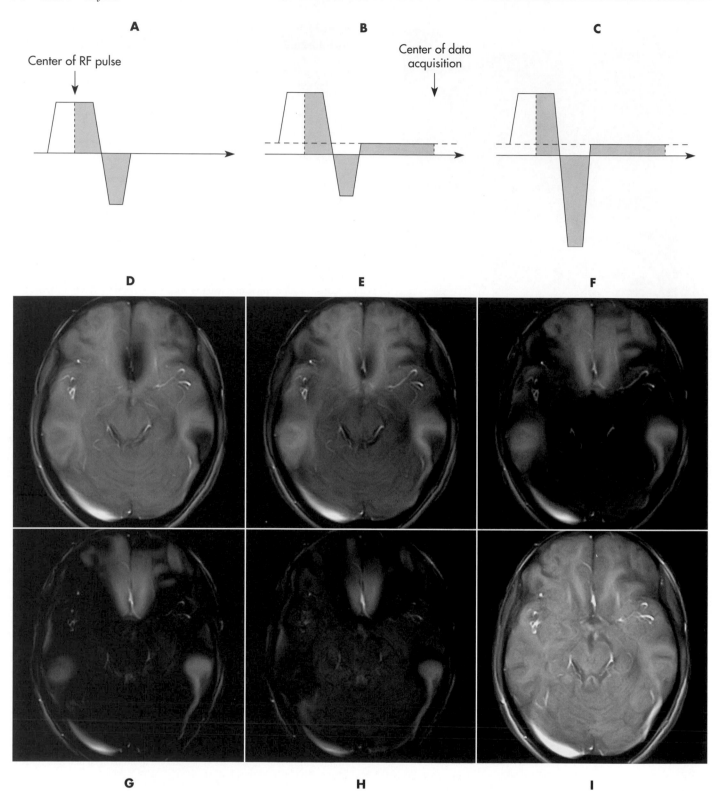

FIGURE 6-11   Field inhomogeneity effects in gradient-echo imaging of a normal volunteer. **A,** Normal refocusing of the slice-select gradient. **B,** Signal loss in the presence of a magnetic field inhomogeneity predominantly results from an imbalanced slice-select gradient. **C,** Such signal loss may be compensated for by recalibrating the refocusing part of the slice-select gradient. **D,** Transverse image with the experimental conditions chosen to emphasize susceptibility-induced signal losses in the proximity of air-filled cavities (2 T, RF-spoiled FLASH, 192 × 256 matrix, rectangular FOV 172.5 × 230 mm², slice thickness of 10 mm, TR/TE = 100/12 ms, flip angle of 70 degrees, NAC = 1). **E** to **H,** Recalibration of the refocusing part of the slice-select gradient in steps of about 10% of its normal strength recovers pertinent signal losses at the expense of all signals that are unaffected by field inhomogeneities. **I,** Sum of images **D** and **H** corrects the artifacts and shows a normal brain. All images were obtained in a single-slice mode within an imaging time of 19 sec.

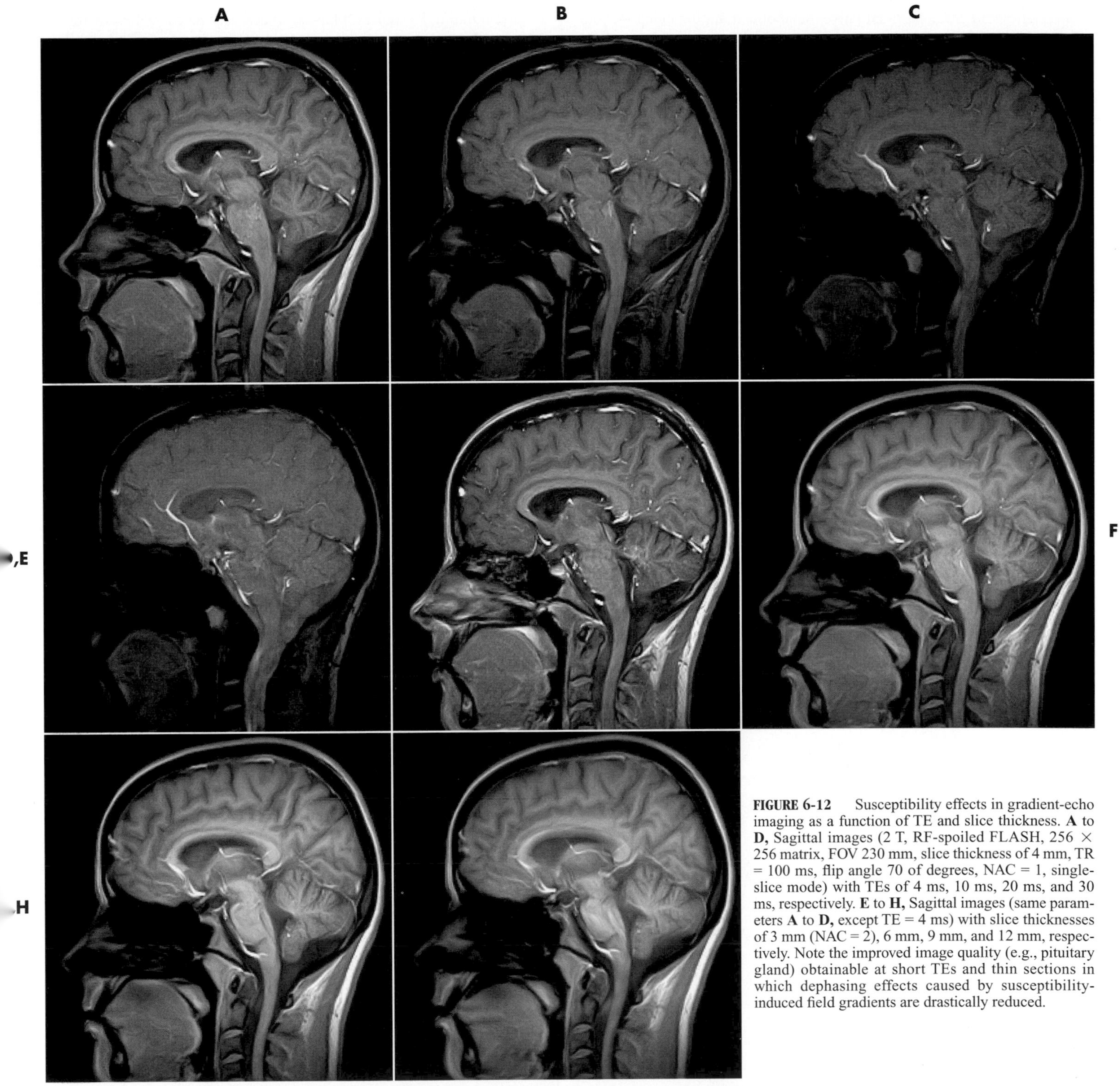

A   **B**   **C**

,E

F

H

FIGURE 6-12   Susceptibility effects in gradient-echo imaging as a function of TE and slice thickness. **A** to **D,** Sagittal images (2 T, RF-spoiled FLASH, 256 × 256 matrix, FOV 230 mm, slice thickness of 4 mm, TR = 100 ms, flip angle 70 of degrees, NAC = 1, single-slice mode) with TEs of 4 ms, 10 ms, 20 ms, and 30 ms, respectively. **E** to **H,** Sagittal images (same parameters **A** to **D,** except TE = 4 ms) with slice thicknesses of 3 mm (NAC = 2), 6 mm, 9 mm, and 12 mm, respectively. Note the improved image quality (e.g., pituitary gland) obtainable at short TEs and thin sections in which dephasing effects caused by susceptibility-induced field gradients are drastically reduced.

The superposition of the two signals results in cancellation or reinforcement of the intensity in a magnitude image whenever both types of signal contribute to the same image pixel. The situations are commonly referred to as *opposed-phase* and *in-phase conditions.*[29] Because the chemical shift is a linear function of magnetic field, TEs for destructive and constructive interference must be optimized for each field strength.

A true separation of water and fat images may be achieved by frequency-selective saturation of the unwanted component and may be applied to FLASH sequences in the same way as for conventional SE sequences.[87] A chemical shift–selective (CHESS) pulse and a subsequent gradient spoiler for dephasing of the unwanted magnetizations are easily included in the sequence before slice selection (Figure 6-6, *A*). For nonselective 3D imaging (Figure 6-6, *B*), adequate water-fat separation may be accomplished by low flip angle CHESS excitation of the desired component. For such applications the use of self-refocusing RF pulses[96,157] is recommended to avoid SNR losses caused by incomplete refocusing of diverging signal components.

In situations in which more detailed spectroscopic information is desired, FLASH principles may be combined with chemical-shift imaging (CSI). Although spectroscopic phase-encoding may be achieved by varying the gradient-echo time,[90] severe disadvantages are T2* losses with increasing TE and poor spectroscopic resolution as a result of a limited number of TE values. It is therefore preferable to use the classic CSI approach,[13,147] which retains the chemical shift information by spatial phase-encoding of a signal that is detected in the absence of a magnetic field gradient. Qualitative metabolite mapping using low flip angle CSI has been applied to phosphorus spectroscopic imaging of the brain.[200]

Flow and Angiography. Signals from flowing (or moving) spins affect rapid gradient-echo imaging sequences in two ways. First, cross-sectional images that are acquired by repetitive RF excitations commonly exhibit strong flow-related enhancement, which results from a steady inflow of spins unsaturated by preceding RF excitation pulses. Second, the images exhibit phase effects that are induced whenever transverse magnetizations are displaced to a location with a different magnetic field strength or, in other words, move in the presence of a magnetic field gradient. Whereas amplitude effects may be manipulated

by presaturating RF pulses, phase changes may be controlled by motion-compensating or encoding gradient waveforms.[75,168] Both amplitude and phase effects may be exploited for flow imaging and magnetic resonance angiography (MRA)[32,129] (see Chapters 11 and 56). The remarkable progress in this field is based on the specific features of FLASH sequences to provide particularly strong flow signals and access to rapid high-resolution 3D imaging.

Typical flow enhancements in imaging planes transverse to the major flow direction are shown in Figure 6-13. The images represent single-slice acquisitions from the neck, in which spatial presaturation of flowing spins has been accomplished by additional slab-selective RF pulses on either one or both sides of the imaging plane.[57] Single-sided flow suppression may be used to discriminate between flow directions

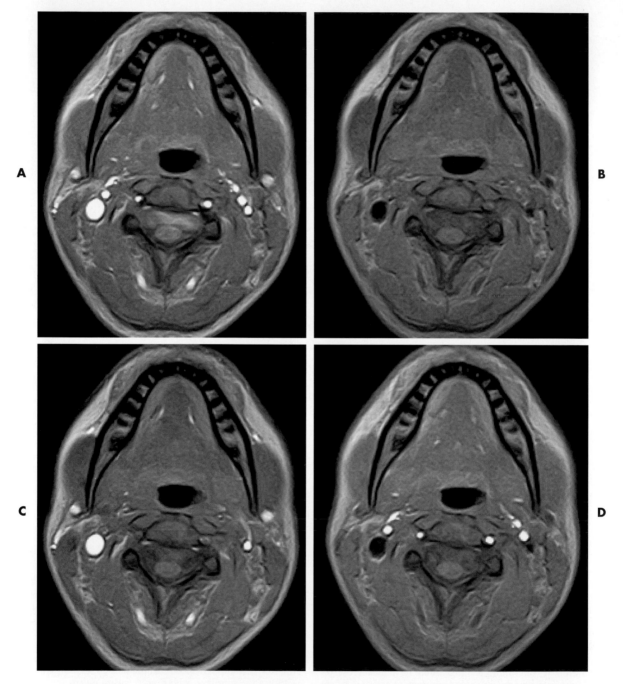

FIGURE 6-13   Flow-related enhancement in gradient-echo imaging as a result of inflow of unsaturated spins from outside the imaging volume. **A** to **D,** Transverse images of the neck (2 T, RF-spoiled FLASH, 192 × 256 matrix, rectangular FOV 150 × 200 mm², slice thickness 4 of mm, TR/TE = 50/4 ms, flip angle of 40 degrees, NAC = 2) without flow suppression in **A** and with dual-side flow suppression by spatial presaturation in **B.** Single-side flow saturation results in a selective visualization of either venous flow in **C** or arterial flow in **D.** All images were obtained in a single-slice mode to emphasize inflow phenomena.

(i.e., between arterial and venous flow). For example, when imaging in the brain, presaturation in the neck region eliminates signals that may originate from arterial flow.

Quantitative information about flow characteristics (e.g., velocity distributions) may be obtained by Fourier flow-imaging techniques[104,105,149] that acquire multiple images with incremented flow-encoding gradients. Corresponding 3D studies (two spatial dimensions, one velocity dimension) clearly benefit from the speed of low flip angle gradient-echo sequences. In fact, 2D variants (one spatial dimension, one velocity dimension) allow real-time acquisitions and quantitative evaluations of velocity profiles.[155,158]

In MRA it is sufficient to qualitatively distinguish between stationary tissue and flowing spins in an angiogram displaying only vascular structures. The maximum-intensity projection (MIP) algorithm allows transverse data to be projected into transverse, sagittal, and coronal planes. Whereas 3D applications exhibit the advantage of very small voxels and correspondingly low signal losses caused by dephasing,[129,177] MR angiograms from a series of stacked 2D flow images are particularly useful for imaging slow flow perpendicular to the orientation of the image section.[80]

Although the basic features of MRA are determined by proper choice of the imaging parameters and use of dedicated postprocessing algorithms,[43] a variety of additional means have been developed to further improve flow contrast. For example, reducing the T1 of the blood-water protons by administering a paramagnetic contrast agent may enhance vascular signals. MRA acquisitions are then based on strongly T1-weighted images with either conventional (very short TR/TE, intermediate flip angle) or magnetization-prepared (inversion recovery [IR]) subsecond FLASH sequences. Such approaches even allow for dynamic digital subtraction MRA when combined with complex image subtraction.[201] A better elimination of signals from stationary tissue may be achieved by the use of magnetization-transfer contrast (MTC).[209] MTC pulses attenuate signals from water protons in tissues with macromolecules, most likely via a dipolar exchange with immobilized hydroxy protons, whereas this mechanism fails in fluids.

More recently, flow studies have been extended from intracranial vasculature to peripheral and abdominal MRA and even to successful visualizations of coronary and pulmonary arteries. In the last case the challenges from air–tissue susceptibilities and motion are met by very short TEs and navigator echo gating.[42,125,202]

High-Resolution Imaging. Complementary to rapid scanning emphasizing imaging speed, low flip angle gradient-echo imaging may be efficiently used to improve the accessible spatial resolution in a given measuring time. For example, cross-sectional high-resolution studies of the hand can now be performed routinely with a slice thickness of 2 mm and a matrix size of 512 × 512 pixels covering an FOV of 100 mm.[15]

The considerable potential of 3D MRI is demonstrated in Figure 6-14. In brain imaging, excellent T1 contrast is obtained by RF-spoiled 3D FLASH (Figure 6-6, *B* and *C*) without being compromised by slice-profile artifacts. High SNR allows the acquisition of very thin partitions, which in Figure 6-14 results in an isotropic resolution of 1 mm. Together with a short TE (4 ms), the small voxel size effectively eliminates any image distortions (i.e., signal loss) from dephasing caused by susceptibility gradients or the presence of flow. Postprocessing options include the reconstruction of oblique or arbitrarily curved sections, as well as surface rendering or surgical planning using virtual reality.

In general, 3D MRI is of advantage for detailed imaging of complex anatomical structures as encountered, for example, in joints, spine, and brain. 3D studies of the thorax and abdomen[146] may be best performed by means of interrupted 3D gradient-echo imaging sequences,[159] in which 3D phase-encoding is performed in repetitive low angle excitations after a magnetization recovery period, whereas the 2D phase-encoding gradient is incremented with each recovery period. The pause in this 3D experiment may be used for breathing and contrast manipulations by various preparation sequences, such as IR or SE diffusion weighting. Magnetization-prepared rapid acquisitions of gradient echoes have been proposed for both 2D[52,88] and 3D FLASH.[159]

Dynamic Scanning. Depending on the desired resolution and SNR, fast-scan MRI may be used to study dynamic processes with time periods on the order of 1 sec. Low flip angle gradient-echo sequences may allow continuous monitoring of most physiological motions in humans by direct time-sequential scanning. Matching the imaging time

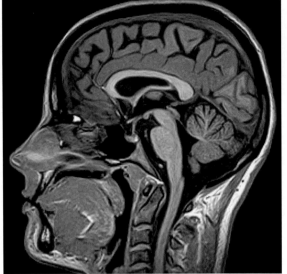

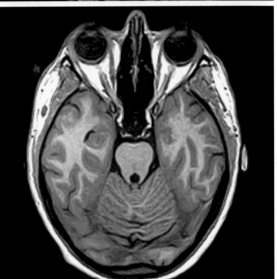

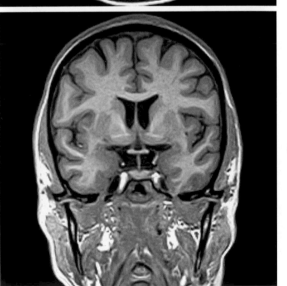

FIGURE 6-14   High-resolution 3D gradient-echo imaging of the brain of a normal volunteer (2 T, RF-spoiled FLASH, 256 × 192 × 256 matrix, rectangular FOV 192 × 256 mm² [2D] and 256-mm slab [3D], TR/TE = 15/4 ms, flip angle of 20 degrees, NAC = 1). Selected section from the original sagittal data set **(A)**; retrospective reconstructions in transverse **(B)** and coronal **(C)** orientation delineating the pituitary gland and the optic nerves. Note the absence of susceptibility artifacts as a result of the small voxel size of 1 mm³ in this isotropic-resolution scan. The imaging time was 12 min.

to the time scale of the movement yields optimum image quality in terms of spatial resolution and SNR. Thus it is generally not advisable to image faster than necessary. The user-dependent trade-off in a high-speed technique may involve choosing between a large number of limited-quality scans and a smaller number of higher-quality images. A practical compromise should attempt to balance the needs for volume coverage (multislice acquisitions) and in-plane resolution.

A typical example of dynamic scanning is the investigation of the time course of tissue contrast after injection of a paramagnetic contrast agent.[145] In gradient-echo images, two different types of contrast phenomenon have to be discriminated. First, immediately after bolus injection a paramagnetic contrast agent may lead to susceptibility-induced signal losses (i.e., T2* contrast) that are related to tissue perfusion. Early experiments conducted on rabbit kidneys and brain revealed time constants of the order of a few seconds.[89] More recently this effect found applications in stroke studies delineating areas of reduced perfusion.[10,34,49,176]

Second, in a later stage after injection of the contrast agent, shortening of the T1 relaxation times of affected tissues causes enhanced signal intensities in T1-weighted images. The dynamics of this second process may be exploited for the investigation of tumor vascularization and in particular for MR mammography.[108,120] Figure 6-15 shows data from a dynamic 3D contrast study of a patient with a breast carcinoma. Direct visualization of contrast agent uptake in consecutive frames acquired before (Figure 6-15, *A*) and after (Figure 6-15, *B*) bolus injection is facilitated in corresponding difference maps (Figure 6-15, *C*). In analogy to angiographic processing, Figure 6-15, *D*, depicts an MIP of all difference maps. Of course, such data may be displayed in arbitrary orientations.

Visualization of cardiac-related motions, such as flow of blood and CSF,[4] myocardial wall thickening, and movements of valves, may be accomplished by ECG synchronization of data acquisition and subsequent reordering of Fourier lines with respect to cardiac phase. The procedure results in a series of images that cover one full (though synthetic) cardiac cycle,[76] assuming a stable periodicity of the heartbeat. Thus quasi-real-time assessments become possible by rapid cine displays of respective image series. Considerable refinements for clinical applications of functional MR cardiology have replaced triggering to the R wave of the ECG with "retrospective" cardiac gating, in which images are acquired at a fixed repetition rate.[76,133] The 2D phase-encoding gradient is incremented only after a time slightly longer than the average heart cycle. Sorting, interpolation, and reconstruction of the images according to the individual cardiac phases is performed after the end of data acquisition by using the simultaneously recorded ECG signal. The advantages of retrospective cardiac gating are improved accuracy in the timing and removal of signal variations caused by steady state distortions that occur when a cine sequence is stopped after a fixed number of repetition cycles and restarted with the next heartbeat. Selected images out of a series of retrospectively gated cine images are shown in Figure 6-16. Additional stability against respiratory motion may be achieved with use of a diaphragmatic navigator echo.[202]

Functional Brain Mapping. Experimental work in animals first demonstrated that the level of cerebral blood oxygenation (CBO) influences the signal intensity of gradient-echo images.[163,193] Whereas oxyhemoglobin is diamagnetic, paramagnetic deoxyhemoglobin (see Chapters 58 and 70) provides endogenous image contrast as related magnetic field inhomogeneities induce a concentration-dependent dephasing of surrounding water proton spins. Thus a change in CBO that decreases the deoxyhemoglobin concentration yields an increase of the T2* and a corresponding signal rise in gradient-echo images. Acquiring the images at prolonged TEs (e.g., 20 to 40 ms) may enhance this phenomenon.

Most important, the blood oxygenation level–dependent (BOLD) contrast may be exploited for functional mapping of the human brain.[7,12,68,128,164] This is because neuronal activation is accompanied by a rise in blood flow that at least transiently "uncouples" from oxygen consumption[50] and therefore results in a venous hyperoxygenation (i.e., decreased deoxyhemoglobin). Although the temporal evolution of associated hemodynamic and metabolic correlates of a change in neural activity is not yet fully understood,[72,126] the initial signal intensity rise 2 to 5 sec after stimulus onset is easily observed and well documented in both gradient-echo and echo-planar images.

In physical terms, intravascular susceptibility changes in the human brain that are associated with activation-related changes in CBO alter both the broadness and mean of the intravoxel magnetic field or frequency distribution.[71] As discussed in Table 6-3, the slice-selection process is expected to be particularly sensitive because it is affected by both spin dephasing and incomplete slice refocusing. This consideration should be taken into account when optimizing volume coverage in CBO-sensitive functional brain mapping. For example, multislice ap-

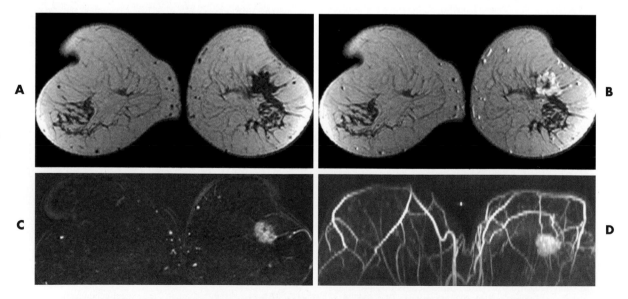

FIGURE 6-15 Dynamic contrast study of the breast using 3D gradient-echo imaging. **A** and **B,** Coronal images of a patient with a breast carcinoma; the images were selected from a series of 3D images acquired continuously every 1.5 min (1.5 T, RF-spoiled 3D FLASH, 112 × 256 × 64 matrix, rectangular FOV 160 × 320 mm² [2D] and 160-mm slab [3D], TR/TE = 11.8/5 ms, flip angle of 25 degrees, NAC = 1). **A** and **B,** Before and after administration of Gd-DTPA. **C,** Contrast agent uptake is best visualized in a difference map obtained by subtracting post-contrast and precontrast images. **D,** MIP of all difference maps in transverse orientation. (Courtesy E. Grabbe.)

proaches are likely to be preferable over 3D MRI because both the 2D and 3D phase-encoding gradients at least partially compensate for magnetic field inhomogeneities by echo shifts in data space.

In contrast to the macroscopic nature of most structurally induced susceptibility differences (e.g., at air-tissue interfaces), the deoxyhemoglobin-induced magnetic field variations around the microvasculature are microscopic in nature (e.g., less than 50 μm) and well below the size of a typical image voxel (e.g., 1 mm). This is advantageous for defining functional anatomy at high spatial resolution[69] and also helpful in reducing macroscopic susceptibility artifacts by decreasing voxel sizes. Finally, "functional contrast" also is affected by the strength and shape of the imaging gradients and is sensitive to involuntary subject motion. Often, however, the latter problem is at least partially caused by the fact that pertinent sequences are sensitive to both increases in oxygenation (i.e., reduced spin dephasing) and increases in blood flow ve-locity (i.e., reduced spin saturation). Thus suitable strategies that "desensitize" MR sequences with respect to motion and flow range from motion-compensating gradient waveforms and navigator echoes[114] (i.e., to reduce phase artifacts) to the recording of spin density–weighted gradient-echo images[70] (i.e., to eliminate spin saturation).

As demonstrated in Figure 6-17, the low flip angle approach acquires spin density–weighted rather than T1-weighted images but retains full T2* sensitivity for CBO-induced susceptibility contrast via the independently controlled gradient-echo time. Resulting activation maps exhibit focal responses without any significant contamination by motion artifacts. The observation of "activated" small veins is to be expected if they exclusively drain activated tissue and reach voxel size. Macroscopic veins that may blur topographical specificity of stimulus-related activations may be identified by an integration of color-coded activation maps and flow-sensitized anatomical images. Image overlap allows a congruent delineation of the macrovasculature (provided that the functional and morphological maps employ the same spatial resolution). In addition, the temporal and spatial characteristics of stimulus-related MR signal alterations may be exploited in defining truly activated areas by a proper choice of data analysis. For example, a pixel-by-pixel correlation[7,8,123] of signal-intensity time courses with a reference (or model) function that represents the activation protocol or its hemodynamic modulation is advantageous over time-locked averaging of images and subsequent subtraction across functional states. Such strategies eliminate any statistical signal fluctuations as a source of contrast and are most helpful when recording multiple stimulation cycles that alternate between an activated and a control state.

Although the effective temporal resolution of mapping CBO responses seems to be limited by the physiological rates of hemodynamic (and metabolic) adjustments, the merits of rapid imaging are nonetheless considerable, ranging from data acquisition in very restricted time spans to volume coverage by multislice approaches. Moreover, short imaging times allow dynamic recordings for sensitivity improvements by correlational analyses. The classic paradigm of functional neuroimaging with positron emission tomography creates one map per condition and often includes an ill-defined "resting" state. In contrast, functional neuroimaging by MRI offers unique "on-line" monitoring of the actual transition between different functional states related to external stimuli, task performance, or even intrinsic brain activity.[11]

In general, gradient-echo sequences offer the highest spatial resolution of any functional neuroimaging technique for noninvasive studies of the human brain. Apart from applications in cognitive neuroscience, foreseeable clinical applications range from monitoring pharmacological manipulations[16,124] to mapping disease-related dysfunction or reorganization after recovery from brain lesions.

SSFP-FID Imaging

Although FLASH MR sequences require only a minor modification to generate SSFP signal contributions from both the transverse and longitudinal magnetization (see conditions in Table 6-2), the resulting images give rise to completely different contrast. From a technical point of view, only the overall phase of the transverse magnetization in a FLASH sequence must be made constant from one repetition to the next.[59,83,84,205] This easily can be done by reversing the phase-encoding gradient after acquisition of the gradient echo and before application of the subsequent RF pulse. The "refocused" FLASH sequence (Figure 6-18) acquires a gradient echo of the SSFP-FID that differs from the regular FID by the inclusion of transverse coherences according to Equation 3. Basically, for a given short TR interval, tissue contrast varies from T1/T2 weighting for medium to high flip angles to spin-density contrast at low flip angles. The latter observation is similar to the contrast obtained with regular (spoiled) FLASH images at low flip angles because any absence of transverse coherences automatically transforms the SSFP-FID into a regular FID.

The contrast behavior of refocused FLASH images is demonstrated in Figure 6-19 in comparison with RF-spoiled FLASH images of the human brain. Clear differences between both sequences are obtained only at short TRs (15 ms) and intermediate to high flip angles (40 degrees). Whereas the refocused image in Figure 6-19, *A*, shows T1/T2 contrast yielding isointense gray and white matter, the corresponding spoiled image in Figure 6-19, *D*, exhibits T1 contrast between gray and white matter, as well as strong saturation of CSF signals. When the TR

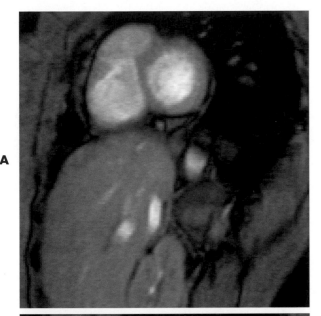

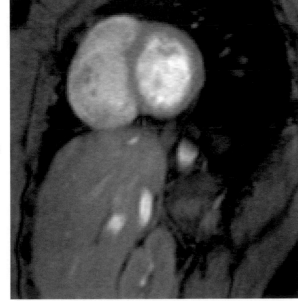

FIGURE 6-16   Cine cardiac study using retrospectively ECG-gated gradient-echo imaging. Systolic **(A)** and diastolic **(B)** frames selected from 20 consecutive images of the heart (1.5 T, refocused FLASH, 112 × 256 matrix, rectangular FOV 306 × 350 mm², slice thickness of 7 mm, TR/TE = 40/7 ms, flip angle of 25 degrees, NAC = 1, dual-slice mode) obtained in double-oblique orientation (−45 degrees sagittal to transverse, −29 degrees transverse to coronal) with a temporal resolution of 40 ms. The total imaging time was 5 min, 42 sec. (Courtesy R.D. White.)

A **B** **C**

D **E** **F**

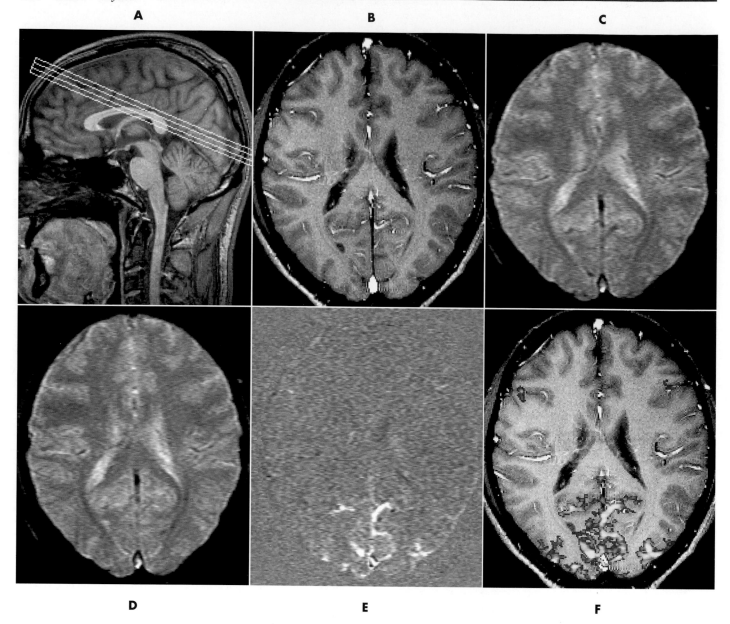

FIGURE 6-17 Functional mapping of visual stimulation using dynamic gradient-echo imaging. Definition of section orientation (2 T, RF spoiled 3D FLASH, $256 \times 256 \times 32$ mm³, partition thickness of 4 mm, TR/TE = 15/6 ms, flip angle of 20 degrees, NAC = 1) **(A)** and section anatomy and vasculature (RF-spoiled FLASH, 256×256 mm², FOV 200 mm, TR/TE = 70/6 ms, flip angle of 50 degrees, NAC = 4) **(B)** in a normal volunteer. In going from darkness **(C)** to flickerlight stimulation **(D)**, dynamic acquisitions of spin density–weighted gradient-echo images with T2* sensitivity (RF-spoiled FLASH, 96×256 matrix, rectangular FOV 150×200 mm², slice thickness of 4 mm, TR/TE = 62.5/30 ms, flip angle of 10 degrees, NAC = 1, measuring time = 6 sec) detect a focal increase in MR signal intensity (i.e., a decrease in deoxyhemoglobin) in the visual cortex. Difference map **(E)** and color-coded activation map **(F)** calculated by a pixel-by-pixel cross-correlation of image intensity time courses with a reference vector representing the repetitive stimulus protocol with six cycles of flickerlight (18 sec) and darkness (36 sec). (Modified from reference 123.)

is increased to 100 ms and the flip angle to 70 degrees, both sequences yield T1 contrast to almost the same degree. In cases in which the observable SSFP effect is further reduced by low flip angles of 10 degrees (TR = 100 ms), the two sequences yield identical spin density–weighted images (Figure 6-19, *C* and *F*). SSFP effects are also absent in the presence of motion,[73,169] such as in cardiac applications, and in tissues with short T2 relaxation times, such as muscle and liver. In these circumstances, refocused, RF-spoiled, and unspoiled FLASH images appear similar. Motion "spoiling" of the SSFP signal is demonstrated in Figure 6-19, *A,* where the expected high signal from CSF (T1/T2 ≈1) is effectively destroyed, with residual intensities giving rise to flow-related phase distortions. Furthermore, gradient-echo imaging of the SSFP-FID signal is possible only as a single-slice or 3D method because the application of slice-selection gradients from interleaved multislice acquisitions destroys steady state conditions.

SSFP-Echo Imaging

Fast-scan MR acquisitions of the SSFP-echo[84,98] are of interest because this signal type provides heavy T2 weighting. Of course the experimental conditions for gradient-echo imaging of the SSFP-echo signal are identical to those for imaging of the SSFP-FID (Table 6-2). Moreover, to derive a gradient echo from the SSFP-echo signal that refocuses on top of the RF pulses, the SSFP-echo sequence (CE-FAST)[84] depicted in Figure 6-20 employs a "time reversal" of the switches for the slice-selection and frequency-encoding gradient as compared with refocused FLASH (Figure 6-18). Because visualization of the spin-echo character of the primary echo signal requires a minimum of two RF pulse excitations, two repetition cycles are shown. Although the TEs of the overlapping SE and STE signal contributions forming the SSFP-echo are multiples of the TR, the acquired signal is a gradient echo obtained by reversal of the read gradient. It therefore exhibits the same

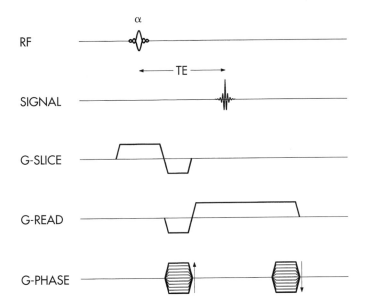

RF

α

TE

SIGNAL

G-SLICE

G-READ

G-PHASE

FIGURE 6-18   Schematic diagram for gradient-echo imaging of SSFP-FID signals (refocused FLASH). This sequence is identical to the cross-sectional FLASH sequence in Figure 6-6, *A*, complemented by an additional phase-encoding gradient that rephases the action of the first phase-encoding gradient after the gradient echo has been acquired. The procedure ensures stability of the phase of the MR signal in each repetition interval and therefore allows the development of a steady state of transverse magnetization ("transverse coherences"). Reversal of the read gradient creates a gradient echo of the SSFP-FID (compare with Figure 6-5, *B*). Nonselective and slab-selective 3D imaging versions are possible as for (spoiled) FLASH (Figure 6-6, *B* and *C*).

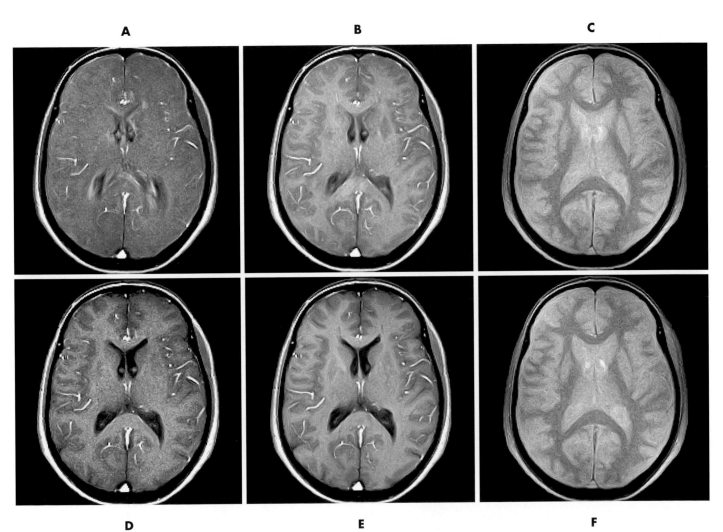

FIGURE 6-19   Spin-density, T1/T2, and T1 contrast in refocused FLASH (**A** to **C**) and RF-spoiled FLASH (**D** to **F**) images of the brain (2 T, 256 × 256 matrix, FOV 230 mm, slice thickness of 4 mm, TE = 4 ms). Parameters are TR = 15 ms, flip angle of 40 degrees, NAC = 2 (**A** and **D**); TR = 100 ms, flip angle of 70 degrees, NAC = 1 (**B** and **E**); TR = 100 ms, flip angle of 10 degrees, NAC = 2 (**C** and **F**). The influence of transverse coherences on the contrast diminishes with increasing TR, decreasing flip angle, and increasing motion. Accordingly the T1/T2 weighting in **A** clearly differs from the T1 weighting in **D**, and even slow CSF flow in the ventricles suffices to preclude the establishment of SSFP conditions, yielding motion-related phase distortions. For TR = 100 ms, high flip angles lead to very similar T1 contrast in **B** and **E**, whereas low flip angles result in identical spin-density contrast in **C** and **F**. The images are scaled individually to emphasize variations of contrast rather than signal strength.

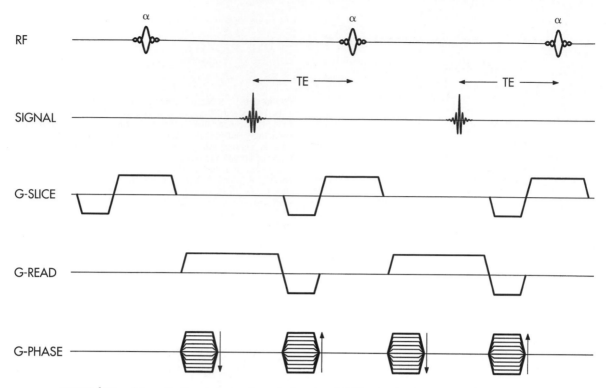

FIGURE 6-20   Schematic diagram for gradient-echo imaging of SSFP-echo signals (CE-FAST).[84] This sequence resembles the refocused FLASH sequence shown in Figure 6-18, mirrored with respect to the center of the repetition interval. Time reversal of both the slice-select and read gradient is required to create a gradient echo from the SSFP-echo (compare with Figure 6-5, *B*). The SSFP-echo represents a complicated overlap of SEs and STEs originating from arbitrary combinations of two or three RF pulses within the repetitive sequence (Equation 4). Because the underlying TEs expand over a time of the order of T2, SSFP-echo images appear heavily T2 weighted. However, these TEs must not be confused with the TE of the gradient-echo signal. As a convention, negative TE values (Figure 6-21) symbolize the fact that the gradient echo of the SSFP-echo occurs before an RF pulse, whereas gradient echoes of an FID and SSFP-FID follow some time after an RF pulse. Slab-selective and nonselective 3D imaging versions are possible in complete analogy to Figure 6-6.

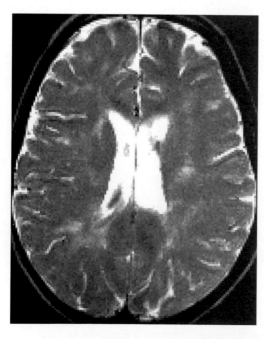

FIGURE 6-21   T2 contrast in SSFP-echo imaging. Transverse image of a patient with multiple sclerosis (2 T, CE-FAST, 256 × 256 matrix, FOV 250 mm, slice thickness of 4 mm, TR/TE = 13.8/−6 ms [Figure 6-20], flip angle of 40 degrees, NAC = 4, imaging times = 14 sec each, single-slice mode).

sensitivity to magnetic field inhomogeneities and susceptibility-induced signal losses as gradient echoes that are derived from an FID or SSFP-FID. The gradient-echo time (TE) is given as a negative value to indicate that it occurs ahead of the SSFP-echo.

According to Equation 4, contrast in SSFP-echo images is a complex function of T1 and T2. However, it turns out that relatively strong T2 weighting is available if transverse coherences are emphasized by the use of appropriate experimental conditions. Whereas low flip angles result in a drastic loss of signal strength, high flip angles cause slice profile deformations. Under conditions of intermediate flip angles, brain images exhibit little contrast between gray and white matter but strongly emphasize signals from CSF or pathological tissue alterations with prolonged T2 relaxation times. For example, Figure 6-21 shows a CE-FAST image of a patient with multiple sclerosis. A major problem for more widespread clinical use of SSFP images is their greater sensitivity to motion and even slow flow[169] compared with SE and fast-SE sequences.

Many variants of SSFP-echo sequences have been proposed. For example, Figure 6-22, *A,* shows a version that acquires both the SSFP-FID and SSFP-echo within the same TR interval and therefore results in two images.[14,131,174] The underlying sequence simply combines the gradient switches necessary for gradient-echo imaging of SSFP-FID and SSFP-echo signals (compare Figures 6-18 and 6-20). Alternatively, complete overlap of the two separate gradient-echo signals may be accomplished by shifting the respective echo positions to the center of the repetition interval as depicted in Figure 6-22, *B.* In this original fast imaging with steady precession (FISP) sequence[165] the net gradient over each repetition cycle becomes zero. Reduced flow sensitivity may be achieved by using motion-compensating gradient

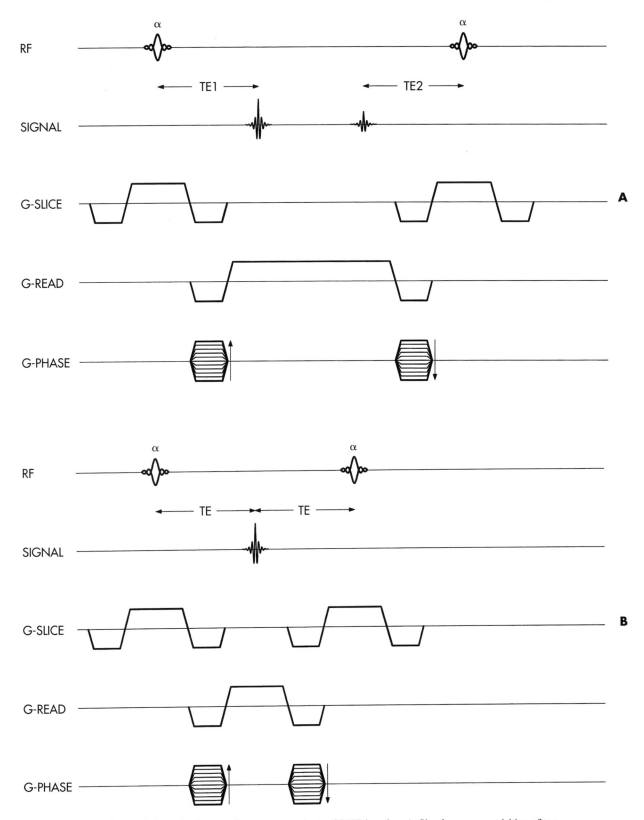

FIGURE 6-22   Schematic diagrams for sequence variants of SSFP imaging. **A,** Simultaneous acquisition of two separate gradient-echo images from the SSFP-FID and SSFP-echo signals in a single experimental run with gradient-echo times TE1 and TE2, respectively.[14,131,174] The sequence combines the gradient switches for SSFP-FID imaging and SSFP-echo imaging (compare with Figures 6-18 and 6-20). **B,** To acquire a single gradient-echo image from the overlapping gradient echoes of the SSFP-FID and SSFP-echo signals (true FISP),[165] the timing of the gradient scheme in **A** is modified such that the echo maxima coincide.

waveforms for both the frequency-encoding and slice-selection gradient in a completely symmetrical sequence.[27] Corresponding 3D implementations at high spatial resolution have promising applications in studies of fluid compartments, such as in the inner ear, where the high signals from CSF and labyrinthine fluids allow excellent delineation of pathologies.[19] A "missing pulse" SSFP-echo sequence[170,182] that acquires the true RF-refocused SSFP-echo by replacing one RF pulse with a data acquisition period has been proposed to overcome the sensitivity to magnetic field inhomogeneities. The resulting images behave like SE images with respect to inhomogeneities, chemical shifts, and flow. More generalized versions with similar properties are based on coherent and incoherent acquisitions of SE signals in the steady state.[207]

HIGH-SPEED RADIOFREQUENCY-REFOCUSED ECHO IMAGING

RF refocusing of an MR signal refers to echo formation by means of an RF pulse rather than reversal of a gradient. This section describes pertinent fast-scan and high-speed techniques that acquire SE or STE signals but (apart from some historical SE methods) do not require N(2D) repetitions of the entire sequence for recording N(2D) phase-encoding steps. Instead they differently phase-encode the individual signals of either a reduced number of segmented multiecho excitations or in the extreme case a single-shot multiecho sequence. A subsequent section deals with high-speed techniques using gradient echoes.

Spin-Echo Imaging

If measuring time were not an issue, SE Fourier imaging[39] would be the method of choice for most clinical studies. SE sequences provide contrast based on differences in spin density, T1, and T2 relaxation times and are insensitive to magnetic field inhomogeneities. This section first explains why SE sequences cannot be accelerated sufficiently by reducing the TR and then addresses more recent developments in fast-scan and high-speed SE imaging.

Short Repetition-Time Sequences.
Short TRs for rapid scanning with SE sequences result in problems that preclude simple solutions:

1. Reduction of TR leads to progressive saturation of the spins and thus low SNR. The effect primarily results from the use of 90-degree RF pulses.[40,213]
2. For TR less than T1, SE sequences exhibit significant slice-profile deformations, which are principally caused by the use of slice-selective 180-degree refocusing pulses.[51] Slice profiles are improved only by the use of nonselective 180-degree refocusing pulses at the expense of losing the multislice feature of the sequence.
3. The use of 180-degree RF pulses with TRs as short as 10 ms may cause considerable RF heating beyond the limits set by security guidelines for RF power deposition in body tissues.[132,162]

Although a few modified SE sequences have been proposed to overcome the saturation problem, none of them answers the second and third problems. An early idea for rapid SE imaging involved converting the excited transverse magnetization back into longitudinal magnetization subsequent to data acquisition. For this purpose the sequence must be complemented by a second 180-degree pulse to rephase the transverse magnetization with respect to all magnetic field gradient encodings and chemical shift effects. Then a second 90-degree pulse flips the transverse magnetization of the second echo back along the direction of the static magnetic field according to

(EQ. 9)

$$90° (x') - 180° - Acq - 180° - 90° (-x')$$

The principle of this driven-equilibrium Fourier transformation (DEFT[9]) technique was adopted for MRI[196] and may be modified by reducing the 90-degree RF pulses to lower flip angles.[41] Although the resulting images have contrast proportional to T1/T2, which is similar to SSFP techniques,[109,110] DEFT imaging with very short TRs or at high field strengths is precluded because of RF heating and slice-profile deformations.

Similar problems hold for the sequence[204]

(EQ. 10)

$$\alpha - 180° - Acq - 180°$$

in which the use of a low flip angle RF pulse (α <90 degrees) leaves a part of the longitudinal magnetization untouched. However, this magnetization cannot be used for immediate excitation and detection of a subsequent Fourier line because the 180-degree pulse of the SE sequence, in addition to refocusing the excited transverse magnetization, inverts the residual longitudinal magnetization. This magnetization has to be reinverted by a second 180-degree pulse before subsequent low flip angle excitations. Experimental images were of poor quality even when acquired with long TRs of 200 ms or more.[189] The 180-degree reinversion pulse in Equation 10 may be removed if the first excitation pulse already preinverts any residual longitudinal magnetization. This can be accomplished by using a flip angle β >90 degrees according to[173]

(EQ. 11)

$$\beta - 180° - Acq$$

Typical images with short TEs and TRs of approximately 500 ms exhibit T1 contrast. But again, fast-scan applications using TRs less than 200 ms result in slice-profile deformations and RF heating problems in the same way as the sequences in Equations 9 and 10.

Fast Spin Echoes.
If a long train of RF-refocusing pulses can be applied to create multiple SEs after an initial RF excitation pulse, then the individual echoes may be differently phase encoded to produce a data set for image reconstruction. This principle underlies the single-shot RARE imaging technique,[100] which provided the basis for the more general development of segmented fast SE (or multishot RARE[161]) sequences (see Chapter 7).

Figure 6-23, *A,* depicts a diagram for the RF pulses and gradient scheme commonly employed for the acquisition of fast-SE images. In contrast to the SE sequences described in Equations 9 to 11, this method does not attempt to reduce the TR but rather uses a very long TR value. In most clinical applications the emphasis is not on rapid scanning per se but on improved image quality, diagnostic accuracy, and overall efficiency. This may be achieved by increasing the in-plane resolution (e.g., to a 512 matrix) while maintaining conventional T2 contrast, adequate multislicing, and measuring times of several minutes. An example is shown in Figure 6-24, which compares a selected section of a double-echo multislice study at a short and long TE. In each case the images are based on five differently phase-encoded echoes per TR (and TE). The total imaging time was approximately 6 min.

A further gain in speed would require the acquisition of even more SE signals per unit time. However, the extension of the fast-SE sequence is limited by problems caused by increased RF power deposition and technical demands on gradient switching. It is therefore more effective to reduce the flip angle of the refocusing pulses (e.g., to 120 degrees) and to complement every SE signal by a preceding and following gradient echo. The resulting fast gradient-echo spin-echo (GRASE)[48,167] sequence emerges as a segmented version of the fast-SE sequence in which the Fourier lines encoded by SEs sample the central part of κ space, while the accompanying gradient echoes cover the outer positive and negative portions, respectively. The phase-encoding ordering and its influence on image quality have been specifically addressed.[117]

The example shown in Figure 6-25, *A,* represents an acquisition with 23 SE signals and 46 gradient echoes, yielding a total of 69 differently phase-encoded signals per TR. Whereas the images exhibit the same properties (long TR/TE, high matrix resolution, number of slices) as the corresponding long-TE, fast-SE image in Figure 6-24, *B,* the imaging time was reduced to only 1 min. It is also noteworthy that arbitrary combinations of gradient echoes and SEs are not possible. This is because techniques that employ gradient-echo acquisitions with interleaved κ space samplings, such as GRASE and segmented EPI,[180] suffer off-resonance image artifacts[160] from fat and tissue susceptibility differences. For example, in-phase and opposed-phase effects from intravoxel water and fat contributions, which have been described for conventional gradient-echo imaging, may give rise to image ghosting when

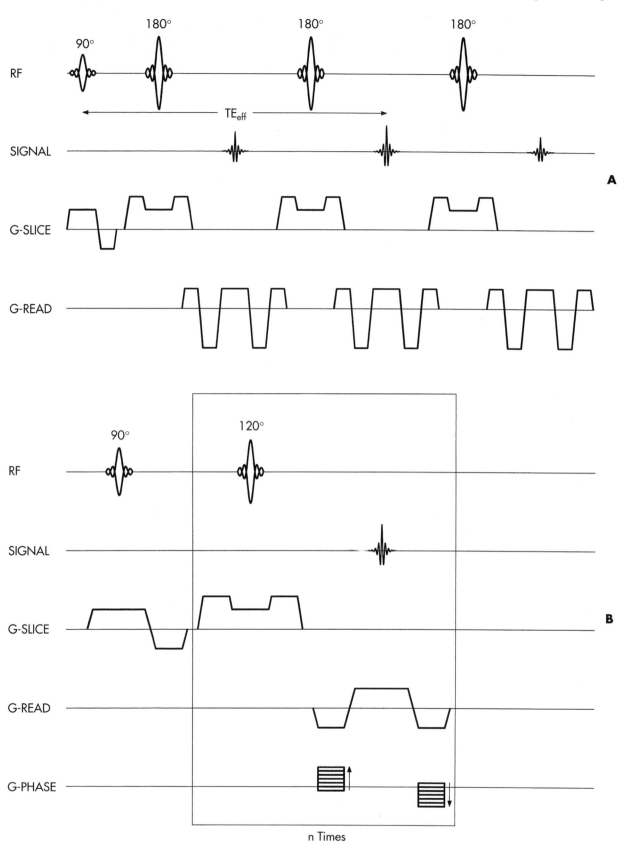

FIGURE 6-23 Schematic diagrams for fast SE imaging. **A,** The technique covers multiple Fourier lines per repetition interval by using different phase encodings for the individual echoes of a multiple SE train. The action of the phase-encoding gradient must be reversed in each echo interval as in SSFP imaging (compare with Figures 6-18, 6-20, and 6-22). **B,** In the extreme case all echoes of a single SE train are differently phase encoded and used for image reconstruction (single-shot RARE imaging).[100] In this case short acquisition times are also achieved by a combination with half-Fourier imaging (Figure 6-1, *B*) as suggested by the drawing of the phase-encoding gradient. Potential problems with RF power deposition are circumvented by reducing the flip angle of the refocusing RF pulses to 120 degrees.

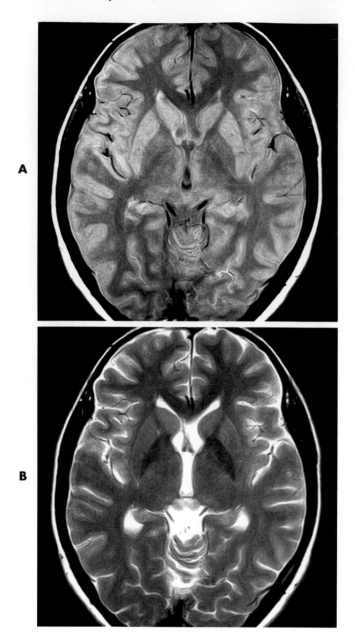

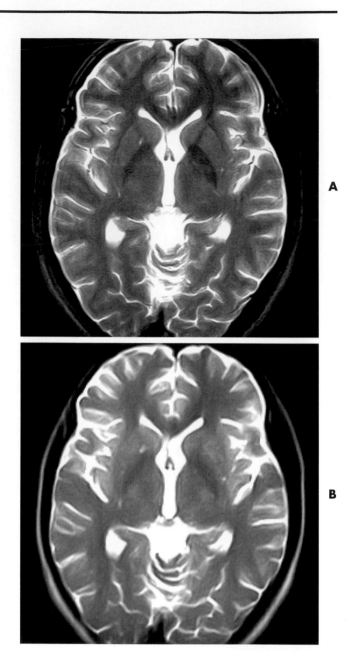

FIGURE 6-24   Spin-density contrast (TE = 16 ms) **(A)** and T2 contrast (TE = 98 ms) **(B)** in fast SE imaging using five echoes per excitation. The transverse images (2 T, fast SE, 220 × 512 matrix, rectangular FOV 156 × 250 mm², slice thickness of 5 mm, TR/TE = 2625/16-98 ms, flip angles of 90 and 180 degrees, NAC = 3) represent 1 section out of a total of 12 sections obtained in a double-echo multislice mode with an imaging time of 5 min, 53 sec.

FIGURE 6-25   A and **B**, T2 contrast fast-SE imaging with interleaved gradient echoes (GRASE) and half-Fourier single-shot RARE imaging in a section identical to that selected for Figure 6-24. **A**, The transverse image (2 T, fast SE/GE, 276 × 512 matrix, rectangular FOV 156 × 250 mm², slice thickness of 5 mm, TR/TE = 7400/115 ms, flip angles of 90 and 120 degrees, NAC = 1) represents 1 out of a total of 12 sections obtained in a multislice mode with an imaging time of 1 min, 6 sec. Data acquisition consists of 69 echoes per repetition interval (23 SEs each with a preceding and following gradient echo). **B**, The transverse image (2 T, half-Fourier single-shot RARE, 240 × 256 matrix, FOV 250 mm, slice thickness of 5 mm, TR/TE = 10.92/87 ms, flip angles of 90 and 120 degrees, NAC = 1) represents a single slice acquisition obtained within an imaging time of about 1.4 sec.

they periodically modulate Fourier lines along the phase-encoding dimension after reordering of segmented acquisitions.

Single-Shot RARE. The single-shot RARE sequence depicted in Figure 6-23, *B*, is a true high-speed sequence with measuring times of 1 sec or less. In this case all Fourier lines are recorded within a single sweep through κ space, during which tissue magnetization becomes attenuated by T2 relaxation. Thus the RARE sequence provides sufficient signal intensities only for those components that exhibit very long T2 relaxation times and therefore emphasizes fluid compartments. Although image contrast mainly is due to T2, it also depends on the order of the phase-encoding gradient steps. Moreover, convolution of the relaxation decay into the Fourier lines may affect spatial resolution as it modulates the point-spread function (i.e., the spatial definition of the image pixels) and gives rise to ringing artifacts.

Particularly at high magnetic field strengths, where high frequencies facilitate energy dissipation into the human body, the considerable

RF power deposition associated with large numbers of successive 180-degree RF pulses poses a severe problem. As indicated in Figure 6-23, B, a solution to this complication is provided by refocusing pulses with reduced flip angles.[102,103] Interestingly, reduced flip angle refocusing creates additional STEs that, when brought in line with pertinent SEs, establish an SSFP-like signal. Whereas quantitative T2 determinations using fast-SE sequences therefore require additional gradient or RF-spoiling schemes, the deliberate inclusion of SSFP signal contributions in reduced flip angle RARE sequences benefits from an apparent prolongation of the true T2 decay. It has indeed been demonstrated that SSFP-like signals may be generated within a few repetition cycles us-

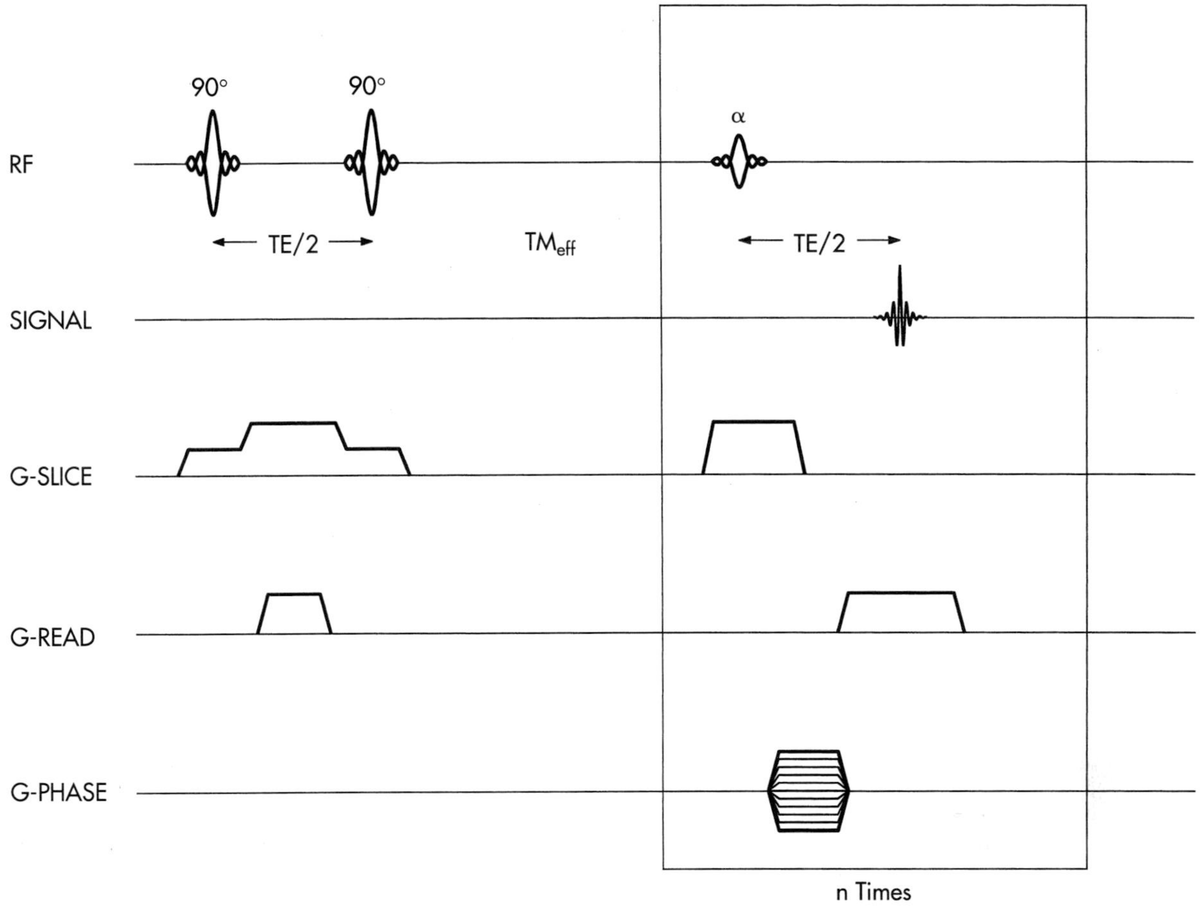

FIGURE 6-26   Schematic diagram for STEAM imaging.[54] In contrast to a conventional STEAM sequence consisting of three 90-degree RF pulses, the high-speed version replaces the final read pulse with a series of low flip angle read pulses (α <90 degrees). Together with the initial slice-selective 90-degree RF pulses, each slice-selective read pulse gives rise to an RF-refocused STE signal. For this purpose the slice-select gradient and the read gradient in each echo interval must rephase the action of the corresponding gradients in the first TE/2 interval. The individual echoes are differently phase encoded, representing the Fourier lines of the image raw data. The STE signal is attenuated by both T2 relaxation during TE and T1 relaxation during the effective middle intervals TM_{eff}.

ing intermediate to high flip angles. Accordingly, even subsecond CE-FAST images have been obtained with measuring times of 800 ms.[81] Another mechanism that contributes to fast-SE and RARE images is magnetization transfer contrast caused by off-resonance RF irradiation[209] because the slice-selective refocusing pulses span a large frequency range.

Figure 6-25, *B*, shows a single-shot half-Fourier RARE image from the same section shown in Figures 6-24 and 6-25, *A*. This 1.4-sec acquisition is of surprising quality, although careful inspection and comparison with the long-TE image of Figure 6-24, *B*, reveals artifactual manipulations of contrast borders.

High-speed applications with some compromises in image quality are therefore most useful in body parts in which they help to overcome other more severe problems, such as motion. Accordingly a main application of RARE may be in T2-weighted imaging of the abdomen.[121,186] Because T2 relaxation times in the abdomen are generally much shorter than those in the brain, segmented dual-shot half-Fourier RARE[122] has been used to improve the visibility of such tissues while still allowing for multislice coverage of large volumes during a single breath-hold. Conversely, some studies specifically exploit the extreme T2 sensitivity to "edit" images by selectively emphasizing signals from either CSF in myelographical applications[101,102] or other body fluids in urography[102] and cholangiography.

For interventional applications a further gain in speed for single-shot RARE imaging may be obtained by combining half-Fourier and rectangular FOV acquisitions as shown in Figure 6-1, *D*. Aliasing artifacts may be avoided by in-plane slab selection using the 90-degree RF excitation pulse, whereas conventional slice selection is accomplished by the RF-refocusing pulses, as in Figure 6-23, *B*.[199]

Stimulated-Echo Imaging

In addition to FID signals and SEs, STEs may be used for MRI.[53,181] The basic STEAM sequence consists of three 90-degree RF pulses (Figure 6-4, *C*) and a dephasing gradient during the first TE/2 interval, with rephasing after the third RF pulse. In an imaging context, dephasing of the exited transverse magnetization is usually ensured by the presence of the imaging gradients, whereas the design of pure slice-selective STEAM sequences for localized imaging or spectroscopy should pay special attention to this physical requirement.[60,66] Retransformation into longitudinal magnetization by the second RF pulse subjects the signal to T1 relaxation. For high-speed imaging the final 90-degree RF pulse of the basic sequence is replaced by a series of low flip angle read pulses[54] as shown in Figure 6-26. Each pulse uses only a part of the longitudinal magnetization that refocuses as an STE after another time period TE/2. In close analogy to RARE sequences the individual STE signals are differently phase encoded to cover κ space as fast as possible. However, whereas SE signals in RARE are attenuated by T2 relaxation, the individual STE signals in high-speed STEAM experience different degrees of T1 weighting in accordance with the duration of the effective middle interval TM_{eff}. Using state-of-the-art gradient hardware, both the duration of the repetitive read interval TR and the STE time may be as short as 2 to 4 ms.

In contrast to FLASH and EPI techniques, RARE and STEAM sequences acquire RF-refocused echoes rather than gradient echoes and therefore yield SE-like images with respect to inhomogeneity, susceptibility, flow, and chemical shift. In particular, cardiac applications of high-speed STEAM[67] show properties similar to gated SE images. Signals from flowing blood are completely eliminated by dephasing of the spins in the imaging gradients. ECG-triggered heart images with measuring times of 190 ms are shown in Figure 6-27, depicting the end-diastolic myocardium in a short-axis view. The flip angle for the read pulses was 12 degrees for an acquisition with 48 echoes. The clear delineation of the myocardium without interference from residual blood may be considered an advantage when compared with subsecond FLASH and EPI.

Another application of the high-speed STEAM sequence deals with diffusion imaging. Diffusion weighting is achieved through use of strong gradient pulses during the TE/2 intervals and by prolonging the duration of the first middle interval. Anisotropic diffusion has been studied in the white matter of the human brain without compromise as a result of motion artifacts.[150] A related high-speed STEAM technique has been obtained by combination with EPI. The STEAM-EPI[190] sequence employs three 90-degree RF pulses but replaces the acquisition of the single STE signal with a series of multiple gradient echoes derived therefrom. This version is completely analogous to replacement of the 90-degree–180-degree SE signal by an EPI readout module in an SE-EPI sequence (Figure 6-31, *C* and *D*).

Miscellaneous

Because steady progress in instrumentation often renders techniques of apparently limited usefulness attractive, this section briefly describes two very different concepts that may be used for rapid scanning (single-shot sequences with multiexcitation pulses and line-scan imaging).

Burst Excitations. Figure 6-28, *A*, shows a generic burst excitation sequence for cross-sectional imaging. The technique generates frequency-encoded magnetizations by an equidistant train or burst of rapidly successive, nonselective excitation pulses (e.g., with flip angles of 5 degrees) in the presence of a constant gradient.[107] Pertinent signals are refocused by a slice-selective 180-degree pulse to yield a series of temporally displaced, frequency-encoded SE signals. In this implementation, phase-encoding is accomplished by a constant gradient with a predephasing component to cover both parts of κ space.[135] The original version without predephasing sampled only half of κ space, with a trajectory similar to that of original EPI (compare with Figure 6-3, *B*). In contrast to all other techniques discussed so far, the burst approach enables high-speed imaging without the need for rapid gradient switching, so imaging times may be even less than for EPI. Complementary to the sequence shown in Figure 6-28, *A*, the 180-degree pulse may be replaced by a refocusing burst pulse after conventional 90-degree slice-selective RF excitation.

A major problem with the burst technique is its low SNR, which is caused by an inefficient use of the available magnetization of each image voxel. The application of a delay alternating with nutation for tailored excitation (DANTE) pulse[156] in the presence of a constant gradient excites only equally spaced, narrow strips of magnetization and therefore leaves larger parts of the image voxels unaffected. To improve the efficiency of burst excitations, a number of modifications have been proposed,[30] including pulse series with optimized phase modulations[195,216] and versions with frequency-shifted excitations[33] that shift the locations of successively excited strips. Such techniques are essential for all types of repeated burst excitations, such as for signal averaging, multislicing, dynamic studies, and ultrafast 3D gradient-echo imaging.[99] Of course, burst sequences also may be combined with other imaging principles, such as radial excitations for projection reconstruction imaging[116] or segmented scanning.[144]

Line Scans. Line-scan techniques, originally proposed as strategies for conventional imaging,[24,148] have recently found renewed interest for high-speed imaging. Applications include artifact-free imaging of moving objects, such as the heart; motion-insensitive studies of diffusion; and access to very high temporal resolution in real-time 1D imaging. Technically, line-scan sequences excite a line or column of a 3D object and acquire the data in the presence of a frequency-encoding read gradient. Image reconstruction by 1D FT yields an intensity profile of the column that may be arranged line-by-line in a 2D array, together with subsequent acquisitions. Line-scan approaches are compatible with gradient-echo, SE, STE, and corresponding high-speed multiecho sequences, although 2D selection of a true column of transverse magnetization requires some special consideration.

Some advantages are striking. Because the basic experiment consists of only a single excitation and acquisition followed by 1D FT, the individual lines of a line-scan image are completely independent from each other. As a consequence, an arbitrary FOV (i.e., an arbitrary number of lines) may be matched to the clinical needs and focus on an inner region of interest without folding or aliasing artifacts from outer volumes. Moreover, line-scan images are extremely robust with respect to motion artifacts because intrinsic acquisitions are in the millisecond range but mainly because no phase encoding is involved. Thus in contrast to Fourier images, line-scan images do not suffer from flow-related or motion-related phase errors that normally lead to smearing or ghosting of intensities along the second spatial dimension. Finally, line-scan approaches are most suitable for MR fluoroscopy or other real-time manipulations because image update is easy, artifact free, immediate, and continuous by replacing individual lines as soon as they have been acquired and Fourier transformed (every few milliseconds). Image update may scroll over the entire FOV, focus on selected parts, or be

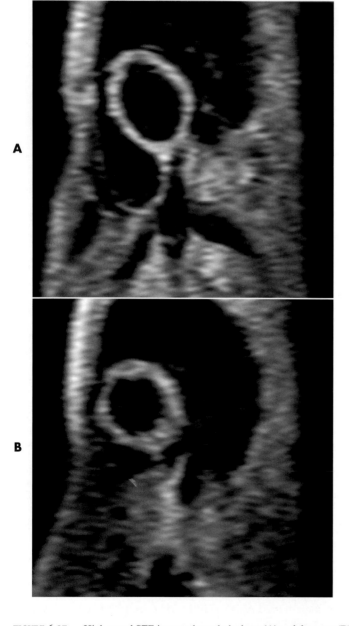

FIGURE 6-27 High-speed STE images through the base **(A)** and the apex **(B)** of the heart of a normal volunteer. Each image (2 T, high-speed STEAM, FOV 300 mm, 48 × 128 matrix, slice thickness of 8 mm, TR/TE = 3.96/4.4 ms, flip angle of 12 degrees, imaging time = 190 ms) was obtained from a single cardiac cycle (late diastole, ECG trigger) in an oblique orientation to achieve a short-axis view (−40 degrees transverse to sagittal). (Modified from reference 67.)

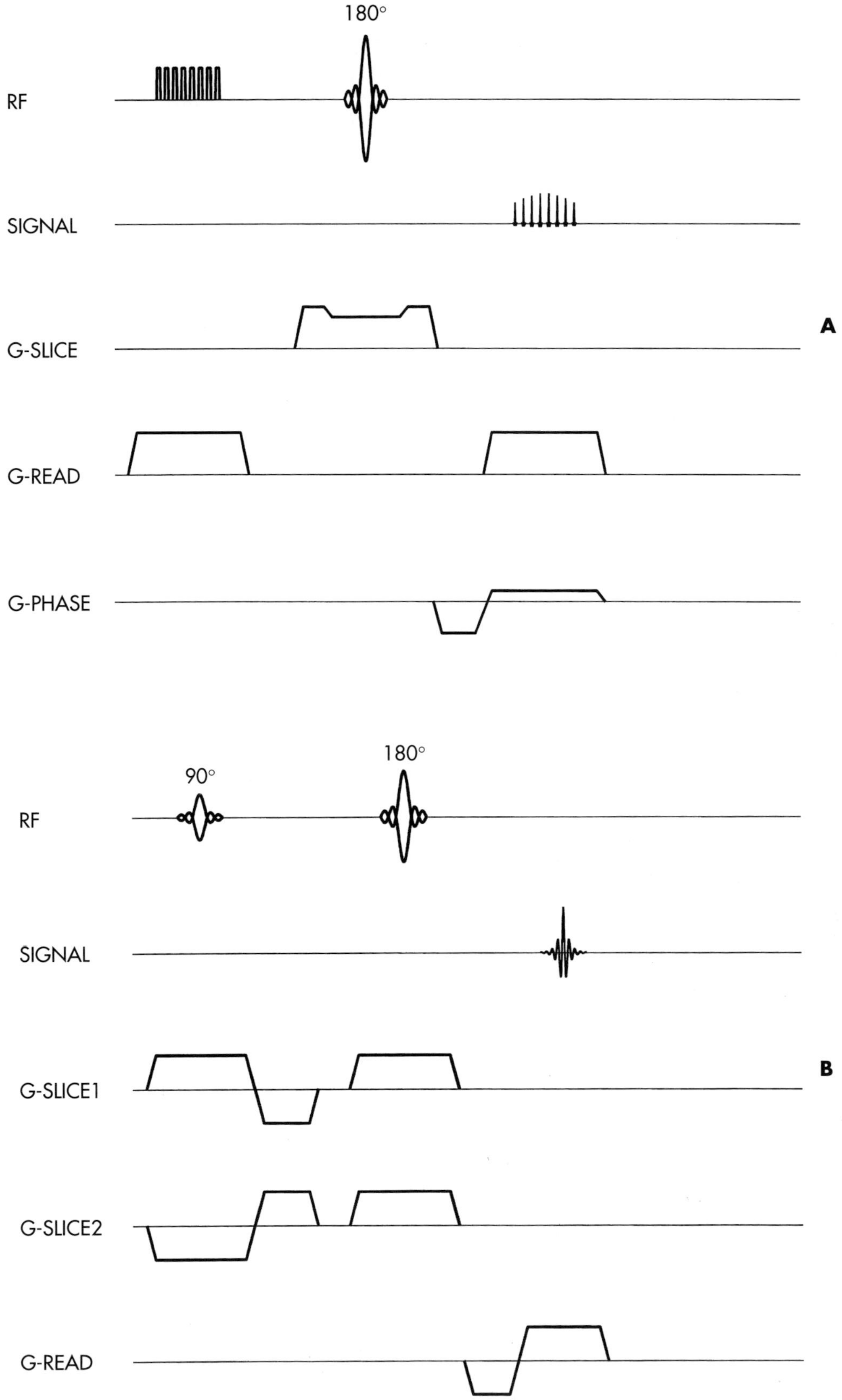

FIGURE 6-28   Schematic diagrams for high-speed imaging using a generic burst[107] excitation sequence **(A)** and slice-selective line-scan imaging **(B)**.[82] In **A** the function of the two RF pulses in the SE sequence may be interchanged so that a 180-degree refocusing burst pulse follows a conventional 90-degree slice-selective excitation pulse. In **B**, image reconstruction is achieved by arranging a series of consecutively recorded line projections obtained after 1D FT. The individual lines in this SE-based implementation exhibit cross-sections that are defined by the overlap of two tilted sections excited by the slice-selective 90-degree and 180-degree RF pulses with opposing orientations.

performed with different frequencies in different parts of the FOV. Moreover, the orientation of lines (i.e., the read gradient axis) may be adjusted parallel to the principal direction of a movement so that the corresponding anatomy or an interventional device may be tracked at optimum spatial resolution.

The simplest line-scan implementation is without slice selection (e.g., for rapid MRA using MIPs).[62] For cross-sectional line-scan imaging, Figure 6-28, *B,* shows a basic SE sequence in which the slice-selective 90-degree and 180-degree pulses result in oblique sections. The cross-section of the column is defined by the intersection of the two slices. Accordingly, subsequent excitations may move the line to a neighboring column along a perpendicular orientation without being compromised by presaturated magnetizations. Unwanted echo signals that originate from intersections of successive line-scan excitations outside the desired section must be spoiled by appropriate means.

Cross-sectional line-scan techniques have been used for single-shot cardiac imaging[2] with measuring times of 250 ms (16 lines) and for motion-insensitive diffusion imaging of the brain[82] with measuring times of within 33 sec (255 lines). Applications of slice-selective line-scan versions with orthogonal sections[153] are restricted to single-shot imaging. In a corresponding SE sequence, multiple 90-degree excitations of "time-encoded" line magnetizations are refocused by only one 180-degree RF pulse that gives rise to a respective number of SE signals defining the serial columns. The underlying pulse and gradient scheme bears some similarity to the SE-based burst sequence in Figure 6-28, *A,* with the DANTE pulse being replaced by a series of regular slice-selective RF pulses.

So far, several 1D versions of line-scan imaging have attracted attention. In these studies the second spatial dimension has been traded-off for temporal resolution or for complementary information about velocity or temperature profiles. When applied to cardiac wall motion and blood flow, such 1D applications are analogous to M-mode echocardiography. A most elegant approach is based on a low flip angle, 2D, selective-RF pulse for continuous repetitive excitations and acquisition of a flow-compensated gradient echo.[22,97] The "beam" of the resulting cylinder of transverse magnetization may be moved along arbitrary orientations to probe the myocardium, whereas the profile plots resemble an M-mode ECG. A similar technique uses a line-scan version of the β–180-degree SE sequence described in Equation 11 but with slice-selective RF pulses along orthogonal directions.[143]

HIGH-SPEED GRADIENT-ECHO IMAGING

The scan times of high-speed MR images vary from fractions of a second down to a few tens of milliseconds. In general, such imaging times are achieved by technical means and are accomplished at the expense of image quality. Typically the spatial resolution is reduced from a 256 × 256 matrix size to a 64 × 128 matrix size, and SNR penalties are compensated for by corresponding increases in absolute pixel size and slice thickness. In most cases spatial accuracy is further compromised by relaxation convolution that affects the spatial definition of the image voxel (i.e., the point-spread function). This reflects the fact that data are no longer acquired in a steady state but rather collected under conditions in which successive Fourier lines are weighted differently. This weighting is by T2 in RARE, T1 in high-speed STEAM, T2* in EPI, and dynamic saturation (or T1 or T2, depending on magnetization preparation) in subsecond FLASH. In all cases in which Fourier lines have nonuniform intensity, both the spatial resolution and image contrast are also affected by the order in which the phase-encoding steps are acquired.[112]

This section refers to high-speed imaging based on the acquisition of gradient-recalled echoes. The two basic sequences are EPI, with its single RF excitation followed by multiple refocused gradient echoes, and subsecond FLASH, with its multiple RF excitations and the acquisition of one gradient echo per repetition cycle. Hybrid sequences combining FLASH and EPI have been reported[45] but so far offer no significant advantages over the basic sequences. Segmented FLASH sequences using multiple "regular" (i.e., unipolar) gradient echoes with different phase encodings are most likely to provide the best practical compromise between speed and image quality.

Subsecond FLASH Imaging

High-speed applications of FLASH[64,91,92] are not based on a fundamental alteration of the pulse sequence diagram shown in Figure 6-6, *A,*

but attempt to "squeeze" gradient switches to shorten the sequence as much as possible. Using MRI systems with 25 mT m⁻¹ gradients, TRs of 2 to 5 ms and TEs of 1 to 3 ms can easily be achieved. Under these circumstances, T2* dephasing is kept to a minimum, so neither susceptibility artifacts nor motion artifacts are observable even from rapid blood flow in nontriggered heart images.

In contrast to conventional gradient-echo imaging, subsecond FLASH sequences acquire the data during the approach to steady state. Because the image acquisition is commonly completed before a steady state is reached, the expressions for the signal strength as given in Equation 2 are no longer valid. The available signal for imaging is much higher than expected from steady state considerations, and flip angles of up to 12 degrees may be used for 64 RF excitations.[95] Without presaturation and for very low flip angles (e.g., 5 to 8 degrees), subsecond FLASH sequences result in pure spin-density images. However, contrast may be introduced by preparing the equilibrium magnetization before high-speed imaging.[52,92,159] Typical preparations provide for inversion recovery T1 contrast, SE T2 contrast, diffusion contrast, magnetization transfer contrast,[209] CHESS presaturation for water-fat separation,[87] spatial presaturation of unwanted flow signals,[57] and tagging pulses for dynamic flow-motion monitoring.[5,6,105,106]

The spin-density, T1, and T2 contrast resulting from IR- and DEFT-preparation sequences are demonstrated in Figure 6-29, showing subsecond FLASH images of the brain. Although illustrative, the clinical value of low-resolution, high-speed images of the head remains to be determined. Prominent exceptions are diffusion-weighted scans, because high-speed acquisitions are required to effectively freeze involuntary motion. However, if even brief periods of breath-holding are possible, single-shot measurements may be replaced by segmented scanning to obtain images at conventional resolution with fewer artifacts because of reduced relaxation convolution. Other areas of application are imaging of the thorax and abdomen. Although high-speed gradient-echo sequences face competition from conventional breath-hold FLASH[65] for T1-weighted imaging (Figure 6-10) and RARE[121,122,186] for T2-weighted imaging, they clearly overcome all problems with peristaltic motion.

Because imaging times of subsecond FLASH are mainly determined by the number of phase-encoding steps and the minimum possible TR, spatial resolution can always be traded for speed to reduce scan times. Using data matrices of 48 × 128 pixels and a 10 mT m⁻¹ gradient system, single-shot images of the heart have been obtained within measuring times of about 200 ms.[21] However, in contrast to high-speed RARE and STEAM, gradient-echo signals from flowing blood have to be suppressed by spatial presaturation or IR preparation to "null" the blood signal according to its T1 relaxation time. Although the T1 discrimination sacrifices SNR of the myocardium and the long IR delays may extend into a subsequent cardiac cycle, time-sequential series of IR-FLASH images with short inversion times have been successfully employed to monitor blood flow and myocardial perfusion in real time after bolus injection of a paramagnetic contrast agent.[3,49] A demonstration of the effects is shown in Figure 6-30, depicting dynamic contrast alterations in consecutive short-axis images of a patient with myocardial infarction. A few seconds after administration of the contrast agent, sequential blood flow has high signal as a result of shortening of the blood T1 relaxation time. Myocardial perfusion is visualized at slightly later stages, with the perfusion deficit appearing as a hypointense zone of the myocardial wall.

Echo-Planar Imaging

The original EPI sequences[138,139] employed an oscillating, frequency-encoding read gradient in combination with a constant weak phase-encoding gradient. The resulting trajectory in κ space is shown in Figure 6-3, *B.* More recently, several modifications have been adopted. First, problems associated with scanning only half of κ space have been omitted by total κ space acquisitions.[178] Second, "blips" of short phase-encoding gradient pulses have been introduced as an alternative to the constant phase-encoding gradient. This modification simplifies image reconstruction because it does not require data interpolation to a rectangular grid before 2D FT.[20,31] To further perform a symmetrical coverage of all of κ space and thus allow the calculation of magnitude rather than phase images, the phase-encoding blips cumulatively compensate a large predephasing gradient pulse. Figure 6-31, *A,* outlines the κ space trajectory for this modulus-blipped echo-planar single-

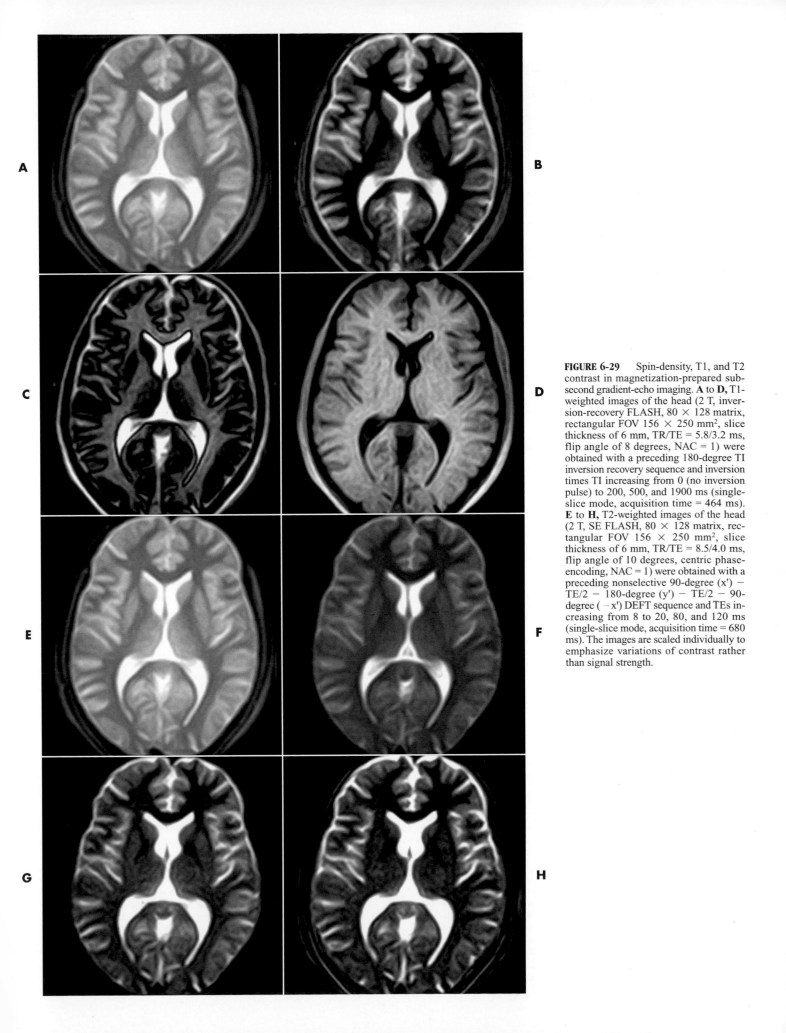

FIGURE 6-29 Spin-density, T1, and T2 contrast in magnetization-prepared subsecond gradient-echo imaging. **A to D,** T1-weighted images of the head (2 T, inversion-recovery FLASH, 80 × 128 matrix, rectangular FOV 156 × 250 mm², slice thickness of 6 mm, TR/TE = 5.8/3.2 ms, flip angle of 8 degrees, NAC = 1) were obtained with a preceding 180-degree TI inversion recovery sequence and inversion times TI increasing from 0 (no inversion pulse) to 200, 500, and 1900 ms (single-slice mode, acquisition time = 464 ms). **E to H,** T2-weighted images of the head (2 T, SE FLASH, 80 × 128 matrix, rectangular FOV 156 × 250 mm², slice thickness of 6 mm, TR/TE = 8.5/4.0 ms, flip angle of 10 degrees, centric phase-encoding, NAC = 1) were obtained with a preceding nonselective 90-degree (x') − TE/2 − 180-degree (y') − TE/2 − 90-degree (−x') DEFT sequence and TEs increasing from 8 to 20, 80, and 120 ms (single-slice mode, acquisition time = 680 ms). The images are scaled individually to emphasize variations of contrast rather than signal strength.

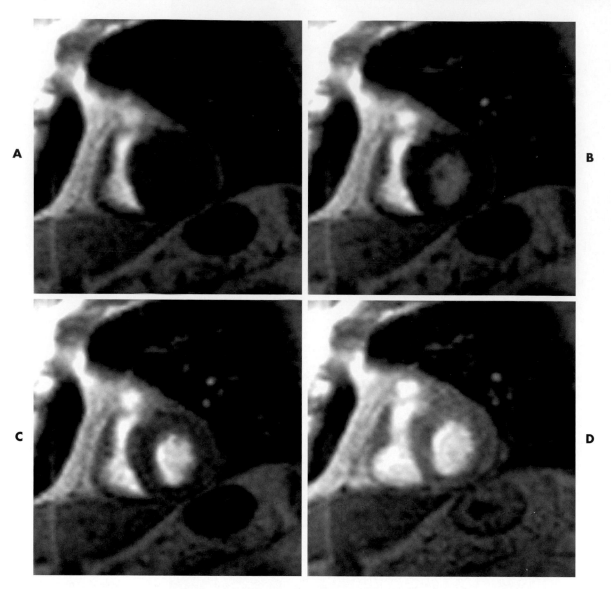

FIGURE 6-30   Dynamic subsecond gradient-echo imaging of cardiac blood flow and myocardial perfusion. **A** to **D,** Selected frames of a patient with myocardial infarction from a consecutive series of T1-weighted images after administration of Gd-DTPA (1.5 T, body-array coil, IR FLASH, 92 × 128 matrix, rectangular FOV 293 × 390 mm², slice thickness of 10 mm, TR/TE = 2.5/1.2 ms, flip angle of 8 degrees, inversion time TI = 12 ms). Individual images had a measuring time of 800 ms and were obtained in double-oblique orientation (−39 degrees coronal to sagittal, −10 degrees sagittal to transverse). Continuous acquisitions in a multislice mode (three sections) resulted in a temporal resolution of 2.4 sec. Stable localization of the section and artifact reduction from breathing were ensured by a pulmonary trigger. The perfusion defect is appreciated by a hypointense zone in image **D.** (Courtesy K.G. Bis.)

pulse technique (MBEST)[113] and also shows corresponding gradient-echo and SE-based sequence versions in Figure 6-31, *B* and *C,* respectively.[172,179] The gradient-echo signals are maximum on the central phase-encoding views (i.e., $k_y \approx 0$). For completeness, Figure 6-31, *D,* depicts an SE-based EPI sequence with constant phase-encoding also preceded by a dephasing gradient to fully cover κ space. EPI sequences with constant phase encoding have the advantage of continuous data sampling, which allows for shorter acquisition times than with blipped encoding.

The gradient-echo signals in Figure 6-31, *B,* decrease with the effective T2* relaxation time and thus lead to the well-known sensitivity of EPI to magnetic field inhomogeneities and susceptibility differences. T2* convolution may cause ringing artifacts and blurring as a result of the truncation of high spatial frequencies for short T2* components. The same holds for the SE-EPI sequences in Figure 6-31, *C* and *D.* They refocus an SE at TE but nevertheless detect a train of gradient-recalled echoes derived therefrom. Consequently these gradient echoes experience a T2* attenuation to a degree that corresponds to their distance from the SE maximum.

Apart from T2* effects, EPI sequences suffer from a number of additional problems[37] (see Chapter 7). The most prominent artifact originates from periodic intensity fluctuations of Fourier lines acquired with odd and even echoes (i.e., in opposite directions of κ space) (Figure 6-31, *A*). This problem presents itself as a ghost image in the phase-encoding dimension (similar to breathing ghosts in conventional imaging). In single-shot EPI, odd-even discontinuities are treated by a postacquisition phase correction using data from prerecorded gradient echoes without phase encoding. For example, in SE-based versions, such extra gradient reversals are most easily incorporated into the first TE/2 interval. Although echo signals with the same sign may be obtained by strong predephasing gradient lobes before each gradient echo,[47] which in effect changes EPI into a multiecho FLASH sequence, gradient demands are further increased and imaging times prolonged unless such a sequence is used in a segmented mode with multiple excitations.

Another class of artifacts stems from off-resonance effects (i.e., from signal contributions with different chemical shifts, such as fat or susceptibility-shifted water resonances that vary between in-phase and

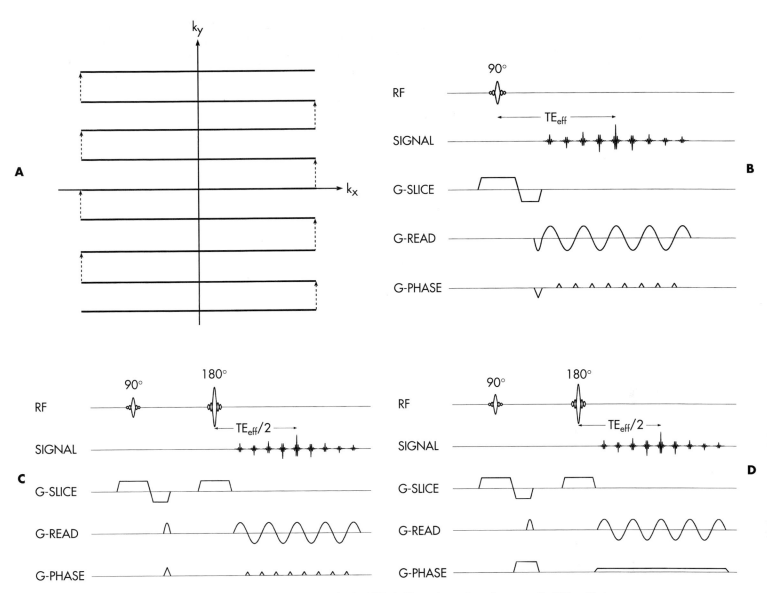

FIGURE 6-31   Schematic diagrams for single-shot EPI. **A,** The pathway through κ space for "blipped" phase-encoding versions of EPI allows data sampling on a rectangular grid as in conventional Fourier imaging. **B** and **C,** Blipped EPI sequences using either pure gradient-echo signals or gradient echoes that are derived from a RF-refocused SE. **D,** SE-EPI sequence as in **C** but with constant phase encoding. Traversal of κ space is in an oblique pattern (compare with Figure 6-3, *B*) and therefore requires data interpolation before image reconstruction by FT. In contrast to the original EPI sequence, which samples only half of κ space (compare with Figure 6-3, *B*), the more recent EPI versions shown here symmetrically cover all of κ space and thus allow magnitude image reconstruction. Phase corrections that account for positive and negative gradient echoes may be derived from gradient echoes without phase encoding.

opposed-phase conditions in sequential gradient echoes). As already discussed for GRASE sequences,[160] corresponding signal fluctuations in interleaved Fourier lines result in ghosting along the phase-encoding dimension. The off-resonance artifact is particularly strong in EPI because it uses weak phase-encoding gradients. A minimum prerequisite therefore is fat suppression, usually performed by preceding CHESS or binomial frequency-selective RF pulses. Limitations of EPI techniques are also borne out by safety concerns in relation to physiological effects reported for rapid gradient oscillations.[17,23] In this context the use of sinusoidal read gradients is preferred over trapezoidal waveforms because of reduced high-frequency components for gradient switching and subsequent reduced risk for peripheral nerve stimulation.

As far as applications are concerned, the natural primary target of a high-speed sequence should be cardiac imaging. Although early EPI studies addressed snapshot imaging of the heart,[166,187] not much work has followed. This may be explained by a better recognition of the detrimental effects on image quality from some of the aforementioned problems. More recent EPI studies have focused on the brain. Whereas

"plain" EPI might be considered superfluous because it compromises spatial resolution and SNR, exceptions are uncooperative or severely ill patients, pediatric patients, and motion-sensitive investigations, such as diffusion-weighted imaging.[191,192]

Figure 6-32 shows single-shot brain images of a patient with acute stroke; the images were acquired with an SE-EPI sequence with constant phase encoding (Figure 6-31, *D*) and different degrees of diffusion weighting up to a b factor of 1000 s mm^{-2}. Data acquisition lasted for approximately 100 ms, with the gradient echoes centered around the SE refocusing at a TE of 123 ms. Despite these very encouraging results in the upper part of the brain, the most serious problem remains the EPI-inherent sensitivity to susceptibility artifacts at the base of the skull, near the paranasal sinuses, and in the anterior orbits. Similar arguments hold for EPI images used for functional brain mapping and for dynamic brain perfusion studies after either contrast injection[10,176,188] or spatial tagging (i.e., saturation[28] or inversion[208]) of a selected blood pool.[36] A critical evaluation of pertinent TOF perfusion studies that aim at quantitative assessments of regional cerebral blood volume has recently been reported.[212]

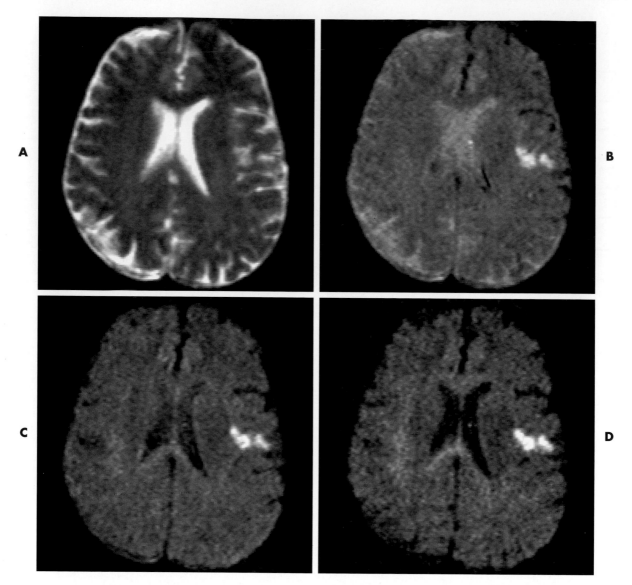

FIGURE 6-32 Diffusion contrast in diffusion-weighted EPI. **A** to **D,** Transverse images of the head (1.5 T, SE-EPI with constant phase encoding, 96 × 256 matrix, rectangular FOV 180 × 240 mm², slice thickness of 7 mm, TE = 123 ms, flip angles of 90 and 180 degrees, NAC = 1) in a patient with acute stroke and diffusion encodings increasing from no diffusion weighting **(A)** to b factors of 360 **(B),** 640 **(C),** and 1000 s mm⁻² **(D)** (single-slice mode, acquisition time about 100 ms). The images are scaled individually to emphasize variations of contrast rather than signal strength. (Courtesy R.R. Edelman.)

The major advantage of EPI is its overall efficiency in terms of data acquisition per unit time, which guarantees optimum volume coverage by multislice acquisitions. With its more widespread availability, the evaluation of high-speed EPI will be based on the achievable image quality in a clinical setting. Whereas limitations in spatial resolution may be overcome by segmented scanning, susceptibility artifacts represent an inherent problem. Whether other gradient-echo sequences (such as diffusion-prepared subsecond FLASH with very short gradient-echo times and centric phase encoding) or RF-refocused sequences (such as high-speed RARE, STEAM, or even line-scan techniques) will provide more satisfactory alternatives remains to be seen.

Spiral Scanning

In addition to projection reconstruction, Fourier imaging, and echo-planar techniques, a further class of imaging sequences relies on spiral trajectories through κ space. Spiral scanning is accomplished by combining two increasing, oscillating gradients. Figure 6-33 depicts a round spiral coverage of κ space and a gradient-echo version of a related imaging sequence using sinusoidal gradient waveforms.[1] So far, prac-tical implementations on conventional scanners frequently take advantage of interleaved techniques (i.e., segmented scanning) rather than emphasizing single-shot capabilities. The acquired κ space data must be interpolated onto a rectangular grid before 2D FT image reconstruction can be applied. Experimental variants include SE-based acquisitions analogous to SE-based EPI, as well as spirals with constant velocity or constant angular velocity with respect to density of data sampling. Square spirals[137] have the advantage of requiring only a 1D interpolation before FT. They may be obtained by a proper combination of trapezoidal (rectangular) gradient pulses of increasing amplitude (or duration) but require enhanced gradient performance. A dual-echo interleaved spiral sequence has been reported in which acquisitions spiral out from the origin during the first series of gradient echoes and spiral back in during the second series of echoes.[78] The actual application addressed T1-related and T2*-related effects of blood flow and oxygenation in functional neuroimaging.

Of course, phase corrections for odd-even echo differences and off-resonance problems with interleaved acquisitions affect spiral imaging as much as EPI. Fat contributions in spiral scanning therefore are often removed by spectral–spatial RF pulses.[151] An advantage of spiral se-

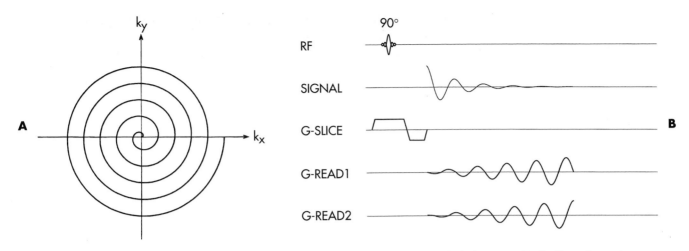

FIGURE 6-33   Rapid spiral imaging. **A,** Pathway through κ space for a round spiral sequence. **B,** Gradient-echo implementation of a corresponding imaging sequence. SE versions analogous to those obtained for EPI are possible (Figure 6-31).

quences over EPI is the circularly symmetrical T2* weighting of data points in κ space. Another interesting aspect stems from the fact that spiral acquisitions always start at the origin and end at the edge of κ space. Consequently the low spatial frequencies are only minimally affected by T2* signal attenuation. A directly related advantage is the robustness with respect to motion-induced phase errors[77] that surpasses the motional stability of EPI and outperforms 2D FT spin-warp and projection-reconstruction techniques. Motion insensitivity of spiral scanning may be explained by both the "early" acquisition of the low spatial frequencies and the inherent symmetry of the spiral gradient switches that provide for an intrinsic compensation of gradient moments by periodically returning to zero.

Although spiral scanning seemed to be of only theoretical interest for some time, more recent studies provide promising and even convincing results. A successful implementation using segmented round spirals involves imaging of the coronary arteries.[152] Figure 6-34 depicts four frames of a 16-frame, single breath-hold movie that dynamically monitors the right coronary artery of a normal subject in a right anterior oblique view. At least for segmented acquisitions, the achievable overall performance renders spiral scanning preferable to EPI.

SUMMARY AND FUTURE PERSPECTIVES

Rapid scan techniques have revolutionized the utility and potential of MRI. In particular the steady impact of low flip angle gradient-echo techniques has led to major instrumental improvements over the past decade. The present generation of whole-body MR systems is therefore capable of taking full advantage of fast-scan techniques.

Fast-scan MRI opens new areas of application, such as in the abdomen and in pediatric imaging, improves the accessible information by dynamic functional studies or 3D imaging, and increases patient tolerance and cost efficiency. However, to achieve its ultimate goal, short scan times must be translated into short investigational times. This may be accomplished by exclusively using rapid scan techniques for routine clinical examinations. Though differences in the sequence mix must reflect differences in organ systems and diseases, almost every field of application will be able to develop a basic 10-min MRI protocol. Such protocols are also a prerequisite for the clinical acceptance of additional studies, such as angiography, functional assessments, and metabolic spectroscopy.

As far as high-speed imaging is concerned, its most remarkable capabilities (e.g., measuring without breath-holding and efficient multislicing) have to justify the unavoidable loss in individual image quality and, with some techniques, the increase in costs. It is up to the medical community to exploit the new modalities and develop them further into practical clinical tools.

Most importantly, the combination of continuous scanning, real-time reconstructions, and advanced feedback strategies puts MRI on the verge of interactive imaging. Preliminary steps already have been taken and briefly are discussed in the final section. Their general real-ization will place MRI in the center of medical imaging modalities and in particular pave the way for interventional studies.

Major Rapid Scan Techniques

Table 6-4 classifies the major fast-scan MR sequences with respect to signal type and available contrast. The flexibility of pertinent studies may be further increased by interleaved or preceding contrast manipulations and the combination with contrast agents.

As an example, efficient screening of the brain may be accomplished by combining T1-weighted 3D FLASH images with T2-weighted fast-SE images. Typically, slab-selective 3D spoiled-FLASH sequences (TR = 15 ms, flip angle of 20 degrees) yield 32 images with 4-mm partition thickness covering a 150 × 200 × 128 mm³ volume with a 192 × 256 × 32 matrix in about 1.5 min (or 64 partitions in 3 min). High-resolution 3D data sets that cover the entire head with isotropic 1-mm resolution may be obtained within 12 min (Figure 6-14). Complementary, multislice dual-echo fast-SE sequences yielding both spin density– and T2-weighted images with high in-plane resolution (512 matrix) require 5 to 10 min (Figure 6-24). Shorter measuring times are possible for a more conventional resolution (256 matrix), as well as for a single-echo acquisition with more differently phase-encoded echoes per TR. An additional factor of 3 may be gained by the incorporation of two gradient echoes per SE signal in GRASE (Figure 6-25, *A*).

Interactive Imaging

The dream of real-time MRI comes close to realization with the combination of continuous scanning, on-line reconstructions, and rapid image display with feedback control. The acquisition part of a continuously measuring MR system may be based simply on a low flip angle gradient-echo sequence. The first step then is to release image reconstructions from the timing structure determined by successive acquisitions of full sets of raw image data. Assuming a conventional linear sweep through κ space, MR "fluoroscopy"[175] allows image reconstructions with a time resolution better than that required for total κ space coverage by updating calculations as soon as only a portion of κ space has been measured. The resulting set of Fourier lines is used to replace the corresponding Fourier lines from a preceding acquisition. Other more complex patterns for selective replacements during sequential acquisitions may involve partial updates of data space using "keyhole" techniques[198] that preferentially replace Fourier lines with low spatial frequencies, or image space, using wavelet encodings.[203,206] Care must be taken to avoid "hopping" of updated images caused by infrequent refreshing of the dominant low spatial frequencies.[125] For segmented EPI and spiral techniques, image update may occur with every segment. For line-scan imaging, updates are likely to occur with every line.

The development of appropriate means for providing external feedback to the MR instrument[79] has already extended fluoroscopy studies

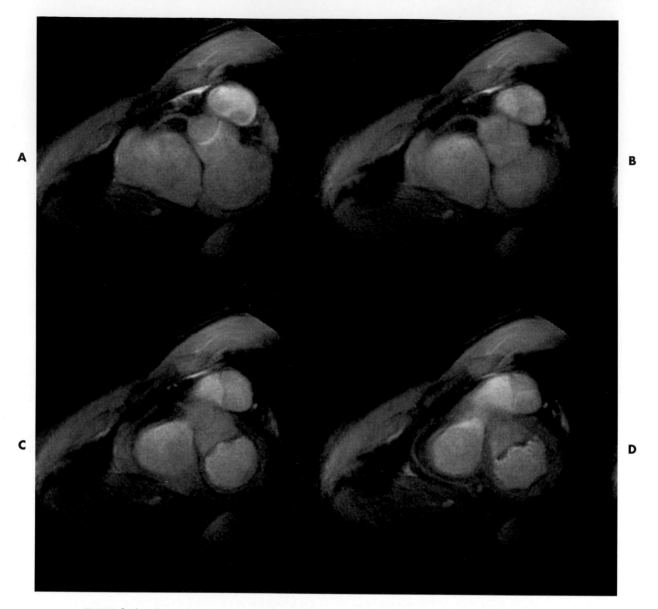

FIGURE 6-34 Dynamic coronary artery imaging using segmented spiral scanning in a single breath-hold. **A** to **D,** The double-oblique images of the right coronary artery of a normal volunteer (right anterior oblique view) represent four frames of a 16-frame movie (1.5 T, anteroposterior surface coil, 20 interleaved gradient-echo spirals, 186 × 186 matrix, FOV 200 mm, slice thickness of 10 mm, TR = 42 ms, 17.5 ms acquisition period, 15.5 ms spectral–spatial RF pulse, flip angle of 45 degrees, plethysmograph trigger). (Courtesy C.H. Meyer.)

Table 6-4 Summary of Major Rapid Scan Techniques

	SEQUENCE			
	SPOILED FLASH	**REFOCUSED FLASH**	**EPI/SPIRALS**	**FAST SE/RARE**
T1 contrast	Medium flip, short TR/TE	—	Short TR/TE	Short TR/TE
Spin density contrast	Low flip, medium TR, short TE	Low flip, medium TR, short TE	Long TR, short TE	Long TR, short TE
T1/T2 contrast	—	Medium flip, short TR/TE	—	—
T2 contrast	—	—	—	Long TR/TE
T2* contrast	Long TE	Long TE	Long TE	—
Multislicing	Interleaved	Sequential	Sequential	Interleaved

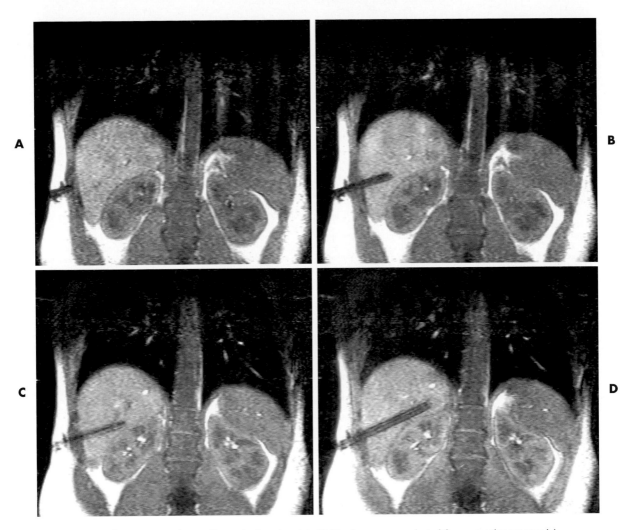

FIGURE 6-35   Interactive gradient-echo imaging. **A** to **D,** The frames were selected from a continuous acquisition of coronal images of a patient with recurrent liver tumors (0.2 T, RF-spoiled FLASH, 128 × 256 matrix, FOV 350 × 350 mm², slice thickness of 8 mm, TR/TE = 66/9 ms, flip angle of 70 degrees, NAC = 1). The series tracks the positioning of a biopsy needle. (Courtesy R.B. Lufkin.)

of dynamic processes to truly interactive imaging. Desirable features range from user-dependent manipulations, such as variations of image orientation or contrast,[111] to "self-control" via actual measurements, such as recently proposed for real-time gating with navigator echoes.[202] The potential of such imaging modes for monitoring interventional procedures that are carried out on the patient table of "open" MR systems,[184] often referred to as *interventional MRI,* is the subject of ongoing studies.[118,136] Figure 6-35 shows an example where MRI has been used to dynamically track the position of a biopsy needle. The frames were selected from a continuous acquisition of gradient-echo images of a patient with recurrent liver tumors.

REFERENCES

1. Ahn CB, Kim JH, and Cho ZH: High speed spiral-scan echo planar NMR imaging. I. IEEE Trans Med Imaging MI-5:2, 1986.
2. Ailion DC, Ganesan K, Case TA, et al: Rapid line scan techniques for artifact-free images of moving objects, Magn Reson Imaging 10:747, 1992.
3. Atkinson DJ, Burstein D, and Edelman RR: First-pass cardiac perfusion: evaluation with ultrafast MR imaging, Radiology 174:757, 1990.
4. Atlas SW, Mark AS, and Fram EK: Aqueductal stenosis: evaluation with gradient-echo rapid imaging, Radiology 169:449, 1988.
5. Axel L, and Dougherty L: MR imaging of motion with spatial modulation of magnetization, Radiology 171:841, 1989.
6. Axel L, and Dougherty L: Heart wall motion: improved method of spatial modulation of magnetization for MR imaging, Radiology 172:349,1989.
7. Bandettini PA, Wong EC, Hinks RS, et al: Time course EPI of human brain function during task activation, Magn Reson Med 25:390, 1992.
8. Bandettini PA, Jesmanowicz A, Wong EC, et al: Processing strategies for time-course data sets in functional MRI of the human brain, Magn Reson Med 30:161, 1993.
9. Becker ED, Ferretti JA, and Farrar TC: Driven equilibrium Fourier transform spectroscopy: a new method for nuclear magnetic resonance signal enhancement, J Am Chem Soc 91:7784, 1969.
10. Belliveau JW, Rosen BR, Kantor HL, et al: Functional cerebral imaging by susceptibility-contrast NMR, Magn Reson Med 14:538, 1990.
11. Biswal B, Yetkin FZ, Haughton VM, et al: Functional connectivity in the motor cortex of resting human brain using echo-planar MRI, Magn Reson Med 34:537, 1995.
12. Blamire AM, Ogawa S, Ugurbil K, et al: Dynamic mapping of the human visual cortex by high-speed magnetic resonance imaging, Proc Natl Acad Sci USA 89:11069, 1992.
13. Brown TR, Kincaid BM, and Ugurbil K: NMR chemical shift imaging in three dimensions, Proc Natl Acad Sci USA 79:3523, 1982.
14. Bruder H, Fischer H, Graumann R, et al: A new steady state imaging sequence for simultaneous acquisition of two MR images with clearly different contrast, Magn Reson Med 7:35, 1988.
15. Bruhn H, Gyngell ML, Hänicke W, et al: High-resolution FLASH MRI of the normal hand, Skeletal Radiol 20:259, 1991.
16. Bruhn H, Kleinschmidt A, Boecker H, et al: The effect of acetazolamide on regional cerebral blood oxygenation at rest and under stimulation as assessed by MRI, J Cereb Blood Flow Metab 14:742, 1994.
17. Budinger TF, Fischer H, Hentschel D, et al: Physiological effects of fast oscillating magnetic field gradients, J Comput Assist Tomogr 15:909, 1991.
18. Carr HY: Steady-state free precession in nuclear magnetic resonance, Physiol Rev 112:1693, 1958.
19. Casselman JW, Kuhweide R, Deimling M, et al: Constructive interference in steady state-3DFT MR imaging of the inner ear and cerebellopontine angle, Am J Neuroradiol 14:47, 1993.
20. Chapman B, Turner R, Ordidge RJ, et al: Real-time movie imaging from a single cardiac cycle by NMR, Magn Reson Med 5:246, 1987.
21. Chien D, Merboldt KD, Hänicke W, et al: Advances in cardiac applications of subsecond FLASH MRI, Magn Reson Imaging 8:829, 1990.
22. Cline HE, Hardy CJ, and Pearlman JD: Fast MR cardiac profiling with two-dimensional selective pulses, Magn Reson Med 17:390, 1991.

23. Cohen MS, Weisskoff RM, Rzedzian RR, et al: Sensory stimulation by time-varying magnetic fields, Magn Reson Med 14:409, 1990.

24. Crooks LE: Selective irradiation line scan techniques for NMR imaging, IEEE Trans Nucl Sci 27:1239, 1980.

25. Darrasse L, Mao L, and Saint-Jalmes H: Steady-state management in fast low-angle imaging, Society for Magnetic Resonance Medicine, Fifth Annual Meeting, Montreal, August 19-22, 1986, p. 944.

26. Darrasse L, Mao L, and Décorps M: Spoiling techniques in very fast TR imaging, Society for Magnetic Resonance Medicine, Seventh Annual Meeting, San Francisco, August 20-26, 1988, p. 611.

27. Deimling M, and Laub G: Constructive interference in steady state (CISS) for motion sensitivity reduction, Society for Magnetic Resonance Medicine, Eighth Annual Meeting, Amsterdam, August 12-18, 1989, p. 842.

28. Detre JA, Leigh JS, Williams DS, et al: Perfusion imaging, Magn Reson Med 23:37, 1992.

29. Dixon WT: Simple proton spectroscopic imaging, Radiology 153:189, 1984

30. Doran SJ, Jakob P, and Décorps M: Rapid repetition of the BURST sequence: the role of diffusion and consequences for imaging, Magn Reson Med 35:547, 1996.

31. Doyle M, Turner R, Cawley M, et al: Real-time cardiac imaging of adults at video frame rates by magnetic resonance imaging, Lancet 2:682, 1986.

32. Dumoulin CL, Souza SP, and Hart HR: Rapid scan magnetic resonance angiography, Magn Reson Med 5:238, 1987.

33. Duyn JH, van Gelderen P, Liu G, et al: Fast volume scanning with frequency-shifted BURST MRI, Magn Reson Med 32:429, 1994.

34. Edelman RR, Mattle HP, Atkinson DJ, et al: Cerebral blood-flow: assessment with dynamic contrast-enhanced T2*-weighted MR imaging at 1.5 T, Radiology 176:211, 1990.

35. Edelman RR, Wallner B, Singer A, et al: Segmented TurboFLASH: method for breath-hold MR imaging of the liver with flexible contrast, Radiology 177:515, 1990.

36. Edelman RR, Sievert B, Darby DG, et al: Qualitative mapping of cerebral blood flow and functional localization with echo-planar MR imaging and signal targeting with alternating radio frequency, Radiology 192:513, 1994.

37. Edelman RR, Wielopolski P, and Schmitt F: Echo-planar imaging, Radiology 192:600, 1994.

38. Edelstein WA, Hutchison JMS, Johnson G, et al: Spin warp NMR imaging and application to human whole-body imaging, Phys Med Biol 25:751, 1980.

39. Edelstein WA, Bottomley PA, Hart HR, et al: NMR imaging at 5.1 MHz: work in progress. In Witcofsci RL, Karstaedt N, and Partain C, eds: NMR imaging, Proceedings of an international symposium on nuclear magnetic resonance imaging, October 1-3, 1981, Winston-Salem, NC, 1982.

40. Edelstein WA, Bottomley PA, Hart HR, et al: Signal, noise, and contrast in nuclear magnetic resonance (NMR) imaging, J Comput Assist Tomogr 7:391, 1983.

41. Edelstein WA: Nuclear magnetic resonance imaging using pulse sequences combining selective excitation and driven free precession, US Patent 4,532,474, September 9, 1983.

42. Ehman RL, and Felmlee JP: Adaptive technique for high-definition MR imaging of moving structures, Radiology 173:255, 1989.

43. Ehricke HH, and Laub G: Integrated 3D display of brain anatomy and intracranial vasculature in MR imaging, J Comput Assist Tomogr 14:846, 1990.

44. Ernst RR, and Anderson WA: Application of Fourier transform spectroscopy to magnetic resonance, Rev Sci Instrum 37:93, 1966.

45. Farzaneh F, Riederer SJ, and Pelc NJ: Analysis of T2 limitations and off-resonance effects on spatial resolution and artifacts in echo-planar imaging, Magn Reson Med 14:123, 1990.

46. Feinberg DA, Hale JD, Watts JC, et al: Halving MR imaging time by conjugation: demonstration at 3.5 kG, Radiology 161:527, 1986.

47. Feinberg D, Turner R, Jakab PD, et al: Echo-planar imaging with asymmetric gradient modulation and inner-volume excitation, Magn Reson Med 13:162, 1990.

48. Feinberg DA, and Oshio K: GRASE (gradient-echo and spin-echo) MR imaging—a new fast clinical imaging technique, Radiology 181:597, 1991.

49. Finelli DA, Kiefer B, Deimling M, et al: Dynamic contrast-enhanced perfusion studies of the brain with snapshot FLASH, Radiology 173(P):42, 1989.

50. Fox PT, and Raichle ME: Focal physiological uncoupling of blood flow and oxidative metabolism during somatosensory in human subjects, Proc Natl Acad Sci USA 83:1140, 1986.

51. Frahm J, and Hänicke W: Comparative study of pulse sequences for selective excitation in NMR imaging, J Magn Reson 60:320, 1984.

52. Frahm J, Haase A, Matthaei D, et al: Hochfrequenz-Impuls- und Gradienten-Impuls-Verfahren zur Aufnahme von schnellen NMR-Tomogrammen unter Benutzung von Gradienten-Echos, German Patent 3504734, Feb 12, 1985.

53. Frahm J, Merboldt KD, Hänicke W, et al: Stimulated echo imaging, J Magn Reson 64:81, 1985.

54. Frahm J, Haase A, Matthaei D, et al: Rapid NMR imaging using stimulated echoes, J Magn Reson 65:130, 1985.

55. Frahm J, Haase A, and Matthaei D: Rapid NMR imaging of dynamic processes using the FLASH technique, Magn Reson Med 3:321, 1986.

56. Frahm J, Haase A, and Matthaei D: Rapid three-dimensional MR imaging using the FLASH technique, J Comput Assist Tomogr 10:363, 1986.

57. Frahm J, Merboldt KD, Hänicke W, et al: Flow suppression in rapid FLASH NMR images, Magn Reson Med 4:372, 1987.

58. Frahm J: Rapid FLASH NMR imaging, Naturwissenschaften 74:415, 1987.

59. Frahm J, Hänicke W, and Merboldt KD: Transverse coherence in rapid FLASH NMR imaging, J Magn Reson 72:304, 1987.

60. Frahm J, Merboldt KD, and Hänicke W: Localized proton spectroscopy using stimulated echoes, J Magn Reson 72:502, 1987.

61. Frahm J, Merboldt KD, and Hänicke W: Direct FLASH MR imaging of magnetic field inhomogeneities by gradient compensation, Magn Reson Med 6:474, 1988.

62. Frahm J, Merboldt KD, et al: Rapid line scan angiography, Magn Reson Med 7:79, 1988.

63. Frahm J, Hänicke W, Merboldt KD, et al: Metallic surgical clip-induced artifacts in rapid FLASH MR imaging, Edward Weck Inc., Research Triangle Park, NC, Technical Report #11-0000-119, 1988.

64. Frahm J, Merboldt KD, Bruhn H, et al: 0.3-Second FLASH MRI of the human heart, Magn Reson Med 13:150, 1990.

65. Frahm J: Fast-scan MRI of the abdomen. In Ferrucci JT, and Stark DD, eds: Liver imaging: current trends and new techniques, Boston, 1990, Andover Medical Publishers.

66. Frahm J, Michaelis T, Merboldt KD, et al: Improvements in localized proton NMR spectroscopy of human brain: water suppression, short echo times, and 1 ml resolution, J Magn Reson 90:464, 1990.

67. Frahm J, Hänicke W, Bruhn H, et al: High-speed STEAM MRI of the human heart, Magn Reson Med 22:133, 1991.

68. Frahm J, Bruhn H, Merboldt KD, et al: Dynamic MRI of human brain oxygenation during rest and photic stimulation, J Magn Reson Imaging 2:501, 1992.

69. Frahm J, Merboldt KD, and Hänicke W: Functional MRI of human brain activation at high spatial resolution, Magn Reson Med 29:139, 1993.

70. Frahm J, Merboldt KD, Hänicke W, et al: Brain or vein: oxygenation or flow? On signal physiology functional MRI of human brain activation, NMR Biomed 7:45, 1994.

71. Frahm J, Merboldt KD, and Hänicke W: The effects of intravoxel dephasing and incomplete slice refocusing on susceptibility contrast in gradient-echo MRI, J Magn Reson B 109:234, 1995.

72. Frahm J, Krüger G, Merboldt KD, et al: Dynamic uncoupling and recoupling of perfusion and oxidative metabolism during focal brain activation in man, Magn Reson Med 35:143, 1996.

73. Fram EK, Karis JP, Evans A, et al: Fast imaging of CSF: the effect of CSF motion, Society for Magnetic Resonance Medicine, Sixth Annual Meeting, New York, August 17-21, 1987, p. 314.

74. Freeman R, and Hill HDW: Phase and intensity anomalies in Fourier transform NMR, J Magn Reson 4:366, 1971.

75. Glover GH: Flow artifacts in MRI. I. Theory and reduction by gradient moment nulling, General Electric Co., Milwaukee, Technical Note #ASL 85-55, 1985.

76. Glover GH, and Pelc NJ: A rapid gated cine MRI technique. In Kressel HY, ed: Magnetic resonance annual, New York 1988, Raven Press.

77. Glover GH, and Lee AT: Motion artifacts in fMRI: comparison of 2DFT with PR and spiral scan methods, Magn Reson Med 33:624, 1995.

78. Glover GH, Lemieux SK, Drangova M, et al: Decomposition of inflow and blood oxygen level–dependent (BOLD) effects with dual-echo spiral gradient-recalled echo (GRE) fMRI, Magn Reson Med 35:299, 1996.

79. Gregory CD, Potter CS, and Lauterbur PC: Interactive stereoscopic MRI with the NMRScope, International Society for Magnetic Resonance in Medicine, Fourth Annual Meeting, New York, April 27-May 3, 1996, p. 1601.

80. Groen JP, de Graaf RG, and van Dijk P: MR angiography based on inflow, Society for Magnetic Resonance Medicine, Seventh Annual Meeting, San Francisco, August 20-26, 1988, p. 906.

81. Groen JP, and de Graaf RG: Contrast in sub-second gradient echo imaging, Society for Magnetic Resonance Medicine, Ninth Annual Meeting, New York, August 18-24, 1990, p. 407.

82. Gudbjartsson H, Maier SE, Mulkern RV, et al: Line scan diffusion imaging, Magn Reson Med 36:509, 1996.

83. Gyngell ML, Nayler GL, Palmer N, et al: A comparison of fast acquisition modes in MRI, Magn Reson Imaging 4:101, 1986.

84. Gyngell ML: The application of steady-state free precession in rapid 2DFT NMR imaging: FAST and CE-FAST sequences, Magn Reson Imaging 6:415, 1988.

85. Gyngell ML: The steady-state signals in short-repetition-time sequences, J Magn Reson 81:474, 1989.

86. Haacke EM, Bearden FH, Clayton JR, et al: Reduction of MR imaging time by the hybrid fast-scan technique, Radiology 158:52, 1986.

87. Haase A, Frahm J, Hänicke W, et al: ^{1}H NMR chemical-shift selective (CHESS) imaging, Phys Med Biol 30:341, 1985.

88. Haase A, Frahm J, Matthaei D, et al: FLASH imaging: rapid NMR imaging using low flip-angle pulses, J Magn Reson 67:258, 1986.

89. Haase A, Matthaei D, Hänicke W, et al: Dynamic digital subtraction imaging using fast low-angle shot movie sequences, Radiology 160:537, 1986.

90. Haase A, and Matthaei D: Spectroscopic FLASH NMR imaging (SPLASH imaging), J Magn Reson 71:550, 1987.

91. Haase A, Matthaei D, Bartkowski R, et al: Inversion recovery snapshot FLASH MR imaging, J Comput Assist Tomogr 13:1036, 1989.

92. Haase A: Snapshot FLASH MRI: applications to T1, T2, and chemical-shift imaging, Magn Reson Med 13:77, 1990.

93. Hahn EL: Spin echoes, Phys Rev 80:580, 1950.

94. Hänicke W, Merboldt KD, and Frahm J: Slice selection and T_1 contrast in FLASH NMR imaging, J Magn Reson 77:64, 1988.

95. Hänicke W, Merboldt KD, Chien D, et al: Signal strength in subsecond FLASH MR imaging: the dynamic approach to steady-state, Med Phys 17:1004, 1990.

96. Hardy CJ, Bottomley PA, O'Donnell M, et al: Optimization of two-dimensional spatially selective NMR pulses by simulated annealing, J Magn Reson 77:233, 1988.

97. Hardy CJ, Darrow RD, Nieters EJ, et al: Real-time acquisition, display and interactive graphic control of NMR cardiac profiles and images, Magn Reson Med 29:667, 1993.

98. Hawkes RC, and Patz S: Rapid Fourier imaging using steady-state free precession, Magn Reson Med 3:9, 1987.

99. Heid O, Deimling M, and Huk WJ: Ultra-rapid gradient echo imaging, Magn Reson Med 33:143, 1995.

100. Hennig J, Nauerth A, and Friedburg H: RARE imaging: a fast imaging method for clinical MR, Magn Reson Med 3:823, 1986.

101. Hennig J, Friedburg H, and Ströbel B: Rapid nontomographic approach to MR myelography without contrast agents, J Comput Assist Tomogr 10:375, 1986.

102. Hennig J, and Friedburg H: Clinical applications and methodological developments of the RARE technique, Magn Reson Imaging 6:391, 1988.

103. Hennig J: Multiecho imaging sequences with low refocusing flip angles, J Magn Reson 78:397, 1988.
104. Hennig J, Mueri M, Brunner P, et al: Quantitative flow measurement with the fast Fourier flow technique, Radiology 166:237, 1988.
105. Hennig J, Mueri M, Brunner P, et al: Fast and exact flow measurements with the fast Fourier flow technique, Magn Reson Imaging 6:369, 1988.
106. Hennig J, Ott D, Adam T, et al: Measurement of CSF flow using an interferographic MR technique based on the RARE-fast imaging sequence, Magn Reson Imaging 8:543, 1990.
107. Hennig J, and Hodapp M: Burst imaging, MAGMA 1:39, 1993.
108. Heywang SH, Wolf A, Pruss E, et al: MR imaging of the breast with Gd-DTPA: use and limitations, Radiology 171:95. 1989.
109. Hinshaw WS: Spin mapping: the application of moving gradients to NMR, Phys Lett 48A:87, 1974.
110. Hinshaw WS: Image formation by magnetic resonance: the sensitive-point method, J Appl Phys 47:3709, 1976.
111. Holsinger AE, Wright RC, Riederer SJ, et al: Real-time interactive magnetic resonance imaging, Magn Reson Med 14:547, 1990.
112. Holsinger AE, and Riederer SJ: The importance of phase-encoding order in ultra-short TR snapshot MR imaging, Magn Reson Med 16:481, 1990.
113. Howseman AM, Stehling MK, Chapman B, et al: Improvements in snapshot nuclear magnetic-resonance imaging, Br J Radiol 61:822, 1988.
114. Hu XP, and Kim SG: Reduction of signal fluctuation in functional MRI using navigator echoes, Magn Reson Med 31:495, 1994.
115. Hurst GC, Hua J, Simonetti OP, et al: Signal-to-noise, resolution, and bias function analysis of asymmetric sampling with zero-padded magnitude FT reconstruction, Magn Reson Med 27:247, 1992.
116. Jakob PM, Kober F, and Haase A: Radial BURST imaging, Magn Reson Med 36:557, 1996.
117. Johnson G, Feinberg DA, and Venkataramaran V: A comparison of phase encoding ordering schemes in T_2-weighted GRASE imaging, Magn Reson Med 36:427, 1996.
118. Jolesz FA, and Blumenfeld SM: Interventional use of magnetic resonance imaging, Magn Reson Q 10:85, 1994.
119. Kaiser R, Bartholdi E, and Ernst RR: Diffusion and field-gradient effects in NMR Fourier spectroscopy, J Chem Phys 60:2966, 1974.
120. Kaiser WA, and Zeitler E: MR imaging of the breast: fast imaging sequences with and without Gd-DTPA—preliminary-observations, Radiology 170:681, 1989.
121. Kiefer B, and Hausmann R: Fast imaging with single-shot MR imaging techniques based on turbo SE and turbo GSE, Radiology 189(P):289, 1993.
122. Kiefer B, and Kolem H: Imaging the abdomen in a single breathhold with 2-shot HASTE, Society for Magnetic Resonance, Second Annual Meeting, San Francisco, August 6-12, 1994, p. 481.
123. Kleinschmidt A, Requardt M, Merboldt KD, et al: On the use of temporal correlation coefficients for magnetic resonance mapping of functional brain activation individualized thresholds and spatial response delineation, Intern J Imag Sys Technol 6:238, 1995.
124. Kleinschmidt A, Steinmetz H, Sitzer M, et al: Magnetic resonance imaging of regional cerebral blood oxygenation changes under acetazolamide in carotid occlusive disease, Stroke 26:106, 1995.
125. Korin HW, Farzaneh F, Wright RC, et al: Compensation for effects of linear motion in MR imaging, Magn Reson Med 12:99, 1989.
126. Krüger G, Kleinschmidt A, and Frahm J: Dynamic MRI of cerebral oxygenation and flow during sustained activation of human cortex, Magn Reson Med 35:797, 1996.
127. Kumar A, Welti D, and Ernst RR: NMR Fourier zeugmatography, J Magn Reson 18:69, 1975.
128. Kwong KK, Belliveau JW, Chesler DA, et al: Dynamic magnetic resonance imaging of human brain activity during primary sensory stimulation, Proc Natl Acad Sci USA 89:5675, 1992.
129. Laub G, and Kaiser WA: MR angiography with gradient motion refocusing, J Comput Assist Tomogr 12:377, 1988.
130. Lauterbur PC: Image formation by induced local interactions: examples employing nuclear magnetic resonance, Nature 242:190, 1973.
131. Lee SY, and Cho ZH: Full utilization of the echo and FID signal in SSFP fast NMR imaging, Society for Magnetic Resonance Medicine, Sixth Annual Meeting, New York, August 17-21, 1987, p. 460.
132. Leigh JS: FDA safety guidelines for MR devices, Newsletter SMRM 20:9, 1990.
133. Lenz GW, Haacke EM, and White RD: Retrospective cardiac gating: a review of technical aspects and future directions, Magn Reson Imaging 7:445, 1989.
134. Ljunggren S: A simple graphical representation of Fourier-based imaging methods, J Magn Reson 54:338, 1983.
135. Lowe IJ, and Wysong RE: DANTE ultrafast imaging sequence (DUFIS), J Magn Reson B 101:106, 1993.
136. Lufkin RB: Interventional MR imaging, Radiology 197:16, 1995.
137. Macovski A, and Meyer C: A novel fast-scanning system, Society for Magnetic Resonance Medicine, Works-in-Progress, Fifth Annual Meeting, Montreal, August 19-22, 1986, p. 156.
138. Mansfield P: Multi-planar image formation using NMR spin echoes, J Phys C: Sol State Phys 10:L55, 1977.
139. Mansfield P, and Pykett IL: Biological and medical imaging by NMR, J Magn Reson 29:355, 1978.
140. Margosian P, and Schmitt F: Faster MR imaging methods, Proceedings of the Society of Photo-Optical Instrumentation Engineers: Medical Image Processing 593:6, 1985.
141. Margosian P: MR images from one quarter of the data: combination of half Fourier methods with a linear recursive data extrapolation, Society for Magnetic Resonance Medicine, Sixth Annual Meeting, New York, August 17-21, 1987, p. 375.
142. Margosian P, and Lenz G: Reconstruction of gradient echo MR measurements with very short TE by half Fourier methods, Society for Magnetic Resonance Medicine, Sixth Annual Meeting, New York, August 17-21, 1987, p. 446.
143. Matsuda T, Shimizu K, Sakurai T, et al: Spin-echo M-mode NMR imaging, Magn Reson Med 27:238, 1992.
144. Matsuda T, Inoue H, Hayashi K, et al: Segmented BURST imaging, International Society for Magnetic Resonance in Medicine, Fourth Annual Meeting, New York, April 27-May 3, 1996, p. 1501.
145. Matthaei D, Frahm J, Haase A, et al: Regional physiological functions depicted by sequences of rapid magnetic resonance images, Lancet 2:893, 1985.
146. Matthaei D, Frahm J, Haase A, et al: Three-dimensional FLASH MR imaging of thorax and abdomen without triggering or gating, Magn Reson Imaging 4:381, 1986.
147. Maudsley AA, Oppelt A, and Ganssen A: Rapid measurement of magnetic field distributions using nuclear magnetic resonance, Siemens Forsch Entwickl Ber 8:326, 1979.
148. Maudsley AA: Multiple-line-scanning spin density imaging, J Magn Reson 41:112, 1980.
149. Merboldt KD, Hänicke W, and Frahm J: Rapid Fourier flow imaging using FLASH sequences, Magn Reson Med Biol 1:137, 1988.
150. Merboldt KD, Hänicke W, Bruhn H, et al: Diffusion imaging of the human brain in vivo using high-speed STEAM MRI, Magn Reson Med 23:179, 1992.
151. Meyer CH, Pauly JM, Macovski A, et al: Simultaneous spatial and spectral excitation, Magn Reson Med 15:287, 1990.
152. Meyer CH, Hu BS, Nishimura DG, et al: Fast spiral coronary artery imaging, Magn Reson Med 28:202, 1992.
153. Meyer ME, and Wong EC: A time encoding method for single-shot imaging, Magn Reson Med 34:618, 1995.
154. Mezrich R: A perspective on κ-space, Radiology 195:297, 1995.
155. Möller HE, Klocke HK, Bongartz GM, et al: MR flow quantification using RACE: clinical application to the carotid arteries, J Magn Reson Imaging 6:503, 1996.
156. Morris GA, and Freeman R: Selective excitation in Fourier transform nuclear magnetic resonance, J Magn Reson 29:433, 1978.
157. Morris PG, McIntyre DJO, Rourke DE, et al: Rational approaches to the design of NMR selective pulses, NMR Biomed 2:257, 1989.
158. Mueller E, Laub G, Graumann R, et al: RACE—real time acquisition and evaluation of pulsatile blood flow on a whole body MRI unit, Society for Magnetic Resonance Medicine, Seventh Annual Meeting, San Francisco, August 20-26, 1988, p. 729.
159. Mugler III JP, and Brookeman JR: Three-dimensional magnetization-prepared rapid gradient-echo imaging (3D MP-RAGE), Magn Reson Med 15:152, 1990.
160. Mugler III JP, and Brookeman JR: Off-resonance image artifacts in interleaved-EPI and GRASE pulse sequences, Magn Reson Med 36:306, 1996.
161. Mulkern RV, Wong STS, and Winalski C, et al: Contrast manipulation and artifact assessment of 2D and 3D RARE sequences, Magn Reson Imaging 8:557, 1990.
162. National Radiological Protection Board: Revising guidance on acceptable limits of exposure during nuclear magnetic resonance clinical imaging, Br J Radiol 56:974, 1983.
163. Ogawa S, Lee TM, Kay AR, et al: Brain magnetic resonance imaging with contrast dependent on blood oxygenation, Proc Natl Acad Sci USA 87:9868, 1990.
164. Ogawa S, Tank DW, Menon R, et al: Intrinsic signal changes accompanying sensory stimulation: functional brain mapping with magnetic resonance imaging, Proc Natl Acad Sci USA 89:5951, 1992.
165. Oppelt A, Graumann R, Barfuss H, et al: FISP: a new fast MRI sequence, Electromedica 54:15, 1986.
166. Ordidge RJ, Howseman A, Coxon R, et al: Snapshot imaging at 0.5 T using echo-planar techniques, Magn Reson Med 10:227, 1989.
167. Oshio K, and Feinberg DA: GRASE (gradient- and spin-echo imaging): a novel fast MRI technique, Magn Reson Med 20:344, 1991.
168. Pattany PM, Phillips JJ, Chiu LC, et al: Motion artifact suppression technique (MAST) for MR imaging, J Comput Assist Tomogr 11:369, 1987.
169. Patz S, and Hawkes RC: The application of steady-state free precession to the study of very slow fluid flow, Magn Reson Med 3:140, 1986.
170. Patz S, Wong STS, and Roos MS: Missing pulse steady-state free precession, Magn Reson Med 10:194, 1989.
171. Provost TJ, and Hurst GC: Asymmetric sampling in 2DFT magnetic resonance imaging, Society for Magnetic Resonance Medicine, Fifth Annual Meeting, Montreal, August 19-22, 1986, p. 265.
172. Pykett IL, and Rzedzian RR: Instant images of the body by magnetic resonance, Magn Reson Med 5:563, 1987.
173. Ra JB, Hilal SK, and Cho ZH: Contrast enhancement of T_2 weighted image using non-90° flip angle, Society for Magnetic Resonance Medicine, Sixth Annual Meeting, New York, August 17-21, 1987, p. 366.
174. Redpath TW, and Jones RA: FADE: a new fast imaging sequence, Magn Reson Med 6:224, 1988.
175. Riederer SJ, Tasciyan T, Farzaneh F, et al: MR fluoroscopy: technical feasibility, Magn Reson Med 8:1, 1988.
176. Rosen BR, Belliveau JW, Vevea JM, et al: Perfusion imaging with NMR contrast agents, Magn Reson Med 14:249, 1990.
177. Ruggieri PM, Laub GA, Masaryk TJ, et al: Intracranial circulation: pulse-sequence considerations in three-dimensional (volume) MR angiography, Radiology 171:785, 1989.
178. Rzedzian R, Mansfield P, Doyle M, et al: Real-time nuclear magnetic resonance clinical imaging in pediatrics, Lancet 2:1281, 1983.
179. Rzedzian RR, and Pykett IL: Instant images of the human heart using a new, whole-body MR imaging system, Am J Roentgenol 149:245, 1987.
180. Rzedzian RR: High speed, high resolution, spin echo imaging by mosaic scan and MESH, Society for Magnetic Resonance Medicine, Sixth Annual Meeting, Works-in-Progress, New York, August 17-21, 1987, p. WIP-51.
181. Sattin W, Mareci TH, and Scott KN: Exploiting the stimulated echo in nuclear magnetic resonance imaging. I. Method, J Magn Reson 64:177, 1985.
182. Sattin W: Syncopated periodic excitation, Radiology 165(P):337, 1987.

183. Schenck JF, Mueller OM, Souza SP, et al: Iron-dependent contrast in NMR imaging of the human brain at 4.0 Tesla, Society for Magnetic Resonance Medicine Eighth Annual Meeting, Amsterdam, August 12-18, 1989, p. 9.

184. Schenck JF, Jolesz FA, Roemer PB, et al: Superconducting open-configuration MR-imaging system for image-guided therapy, Radiology 195:805, 1995.

185. Sekihara K: Steady-state magnetizations in rapid NMR imaging using small flip angles and short repetition intervals, IEEE Trans Med Imaging MI-6:157, 1987.

186. Semelka RC, Kelekis NL, Thomasson D, et al: HASTE MR imaging: description of technique and preliminary results in the abdomen, J Magn Reson Imaging 6:698, 1996.

187. Stehling MK, Howseman AM, Ordidge RJ, et al: Whole-body echo-planar MR imaging at 0.5 T, Radiology 170:257, 1989.

188. Stehling MK, Turner R, and Mansfield P: Echo-planar imaging: magnetic resonance imaging in a fraction of a second, Science 254:43, 1991.

189. Tkach JA, and Haacke EM: A comparison of fast spin echo and gradient field echo sequences, Magn Reson Imaging 6:373, 1988.

190. Turner R, von Kienlin M, Moonen CTW, et al: Single-shot localized echo-planar imaging (STEAM-EPI) at 4.7 Tesla, Magn Reson Med 14:401, 1990.

191. Turner R, and Le Bihan D: Single-shot diffusion imaging at 2.0 Tesla, J Magn Reson 86:445, 1990.

192. Turner R, Le Bihan D, Maier J, et al: Echo-planar imaging of intravoxel incoherent motion, Radiology 177:407, 1990.

193. Turner R, Le Bihan D, Moonen CTW, et al: Echo-planar time course MRI of cat brain oxygenation changes, Magn Reson Med 22:159, 1991.

194. Twieg DB: The κ-trajectory formulation of the NMR imaging process with applications in analysis and synthesis of imaging methods, Med Phys 10:610, 1983.

195. van Gelderen P, Duyn JH, and Moonen CTW: Analytical solution for phase modulation in BURST imaging with optimum sensitivity, J Magn Reson Biol 107:78, 1995.

196. van Uijen CMJ, and den Boef JH: Driven-equilibrium radiofrequency pulses in NMR imaging, Magn Reson Med 1:502, 1984.

197. van Uijen CMJ, den Boef JH, and Verschuren FJJ: Fast Fourier imaging, Magn Reson Med 2:203, 1985.

198. van Vaals JJ, Brummer ME, Dixon WT, et al: Keyhole method for accelerating imaging of contrast agent uptake, J Magn Reson Imaging 3:671, 1993.

199. van Vaals JJ, van Yperen GH, and de Boer RW: Real-time MR imaging using the LoLo (Local Look) method for interactive and interventional MR at 0.5 T and 1.5 T, Society for Magnetic Resonance, Second Annual Meeting, San Francisco, August 6-12, 1994, p. 421.

200. Vigneron DB, Nelson SJ, Murphy-Boesch J, et al: Chemical-shift imaging of human brain: axial, sagittal, and coronal P-31 metabolite images, Radiology 177:643, 1990.

201. Wang Y, Johnston DL, Breen JF, et al: Dynamic MR digital subtraction angiography using contrast enhancement, fast data acquisition, and complex subtraction, Magn Reson Med 36:551, 1996.

202. Wang Y, Rossman PJ, Grimm RC, et al: 3D MR angiography of pulmonary arteries using real-time navigator gating and magnetization preparation, Magn Reson Med 36:579, 1996.

203. Weaver JB, Xu Y, Healy DM, et al: Wavelet-encoded MR imaging, Magn Reson Med 24:275, 1992.

204. Wehrli FW: Method for rapid acquisition of NMR data, US Patent 4,587,489, Oct 7, 1983.

205. Wehrli FW: Fast-scan imaging: principles and contrast phenomenology. In Higgins CB, and Hricak H, eds: Magnetic resonance imaging of the body, New York, 1987, Raven Press.

206. Wendt M, Busch M, and Lenz G, et al: Dynamic tracking algorithm for interventional MRI using wavelet-encoding in 3D gradient-echo sequences, International Society for Magnetic Resonance in Medicine, Fourth Annual Meeting, New York, April 27-May 3, 1996, p. 49.

207. Werthner H, Krieg R, Ladebeck R, et al: COSESS and INSESS: coherent and incoherent spin echoes in the steady state, Magn Reson Med 36:294, 1996.

208. Williams DS, Detre JA, and Leigh JS, et al: Magnetic resonance imaging of perfusion using spin inversion of arterial water, Proc Natl Acad Sci USA 89:212, 1992.

209. Wolff SD, and Balaban RS: Magnetization transfer contrast (MTC) and tissue water proton relaxation in vivo, Magn Reson Med 10:135, 1989.

210. Yang QX, Dardzinski BJ, Li S, et al: Multi-gradient echo with susceptibility inhomogeneity compensation (MGESIC): demonstration of fMRI in the olfactory cortex at 3.0 T, Magn Reson Med 37:331, 1997.

211. Yang QX, Demeure RJ, Dardzinski BJ, et al: Fourier transform of multi-gradient echo with susceptibility inhomogeneity compensation (3DFT-MGESIC): improved SNR and T_2^* weighting, International Society for Magnetic Resonance in Medicine, Fifth Annual Meeting, Vancouver, April 12-18, 1997, p. 1638.

212. Ye FQ, Pekar JJ, Jezzard P, et al: Perfusion imaging of the human brain at 1.5 T using a single-shot EPI spin tagging approach, Magn Reson Med 36:219, 1996.

213. Young IR, Bryant DJ, and Payne JA: Variations in slice shape and absorption as artifacts in the determination of tissue parameters in NMR imaging, Magn Reson Med 2:355, 1985.

214. Young IR, and Payne JA: Slice-shape artifact changes with precession angle in rapid MR imaging, Magn Reson Med 5:177, 1987.

215. Young IR, Cox IJ, Bryant DJ, et al: The benefits of increasing spatial resolution as a means of reducing artifacts due to field inhomogeneities, Magn Reson Imaging 6:585, 1988.

216. Zha L, and Lowe IJ: Optimized ultra-fast imaging sequence (OUFIS), Magn Reson Med 33:377, 1995.

217. Zur Y, and Bendel P: Elimination of the steady-state transverse magnetization in short TR imaging, Society for Magnetic Resonance Medicine, Sixth Annual Meeting, New York, August 17-21, 1987, p. 440.

218. Zur Y, Stokar S, and Bendel P: An analysis of fast imaging sequences with steady state transverse magnetization refocusing, Magn Reson Med 6:175, 1988.

7 Fast Spin-Echo and Echo-Planar Imaging

William G. Bradley Jr., Dar-Yeong Chen, Dennis J. Atkinson, and Robert R. Edelman

Fast Spin Echo
    Introduction to κ Space
    Fast Spin Echo versus Conventional Spin Echo
Echo-Planar Imaging
    Echo-Planar Diffusion Imaging
    Echo-Planar Perfusion Imaging
    Echo-Planar Imaging in Stroke
    Cardiac Echo-Planar Imaging
    Abdominal Echo-Planar Imaging

✔ KEY POINTS

κ Space: A mathematical representation of an MR acquisition ("κ" comes from the constant in the Fourier transform.)
    Analog representation: A temporal stack of spin echoes from the first (bottom) to the last (top) viewed from above
    Digital representation: A matrix consisting of N_p lines of N_f points each

Single Line κ-Space Techniques
Conventional spin echo
Conventional gradient echo

Multiple Line κ-Space Techniques
Fast or turbo spin echo
GRASE
Multishot EPI

Complete κ-Space Coverage (Single Shot)
HASTE
Single-shot EPI

Spin-Echo Continuum
Conventional spin echo: (90 and 180 degrees) $\times N_p$
Fast/turbo spin echo: (90 and 180 degrees$_{ETL}$) $\times N_s$
HASTE: 90 and 180 degrees$_{Np}$

Gradient-Echo Continuum
Conventional gradient echo: (single gradient reversal) $\times N_p$
Multishot EPI: (ETL gradient reversals) $\times N_s$
Single-shot EPI: N_p gradient reversals

Key
N_p, Number of phase steps
N_f, Number of frequency steps
N_s, Number of shots, each taking time TR

Although magnetic resonance imaging (MRI) has advanced steadily since the late 1970s, every 5 or 10 years there is a quantum leap in technology. In the beginning there were only low-field (0.15 Tesla [T]) resistive magnets. In the early 1980s low-field superconducting systems were first installed. In the mid 1980s GE and Siemens introduced the first high-field systems at 1.5 T. Early whole-body gradients had a max-imum strength of 3 to 6 mT/m with rise times on the order of 1.5 to 2 ms. In the mid 1980s GE introduced shielded gradients with a maximum strength of 10 mT/m and a minimum rise time of 0.675 ms (675 μs). The first generation of high-performance systems (Siemens VISION, GE EchoSpeed, Picker EDGE, Philips ACS-NT) feature gradient strengths as high as 27 mT/m with rise times as short as 180 μs. With such gradients, scan times for a slice through the brain have fallen from 20 min to 100 ms.

To decrease acquisition time, t, using conventional gradient-echo and spin-echo (SE) techniques, the repetition time (TR), the number of phase-encoding steps (N_p), or the number of excitations (N_{ex}) can be reduced:

$$t = TR \times N_p \times N_{ex}$$

With a decrease in TR, N_p, or N_{ex}, there will be a linear decrease in scan time, t; however, other factors may be affected as well. A decrease in TR is also associated with a decrease in the amount of T2 and proton-density contrast, the number of slices, and the signal-to-noise ratio (SNR). Decreasing N_p for a fixed field of view (FOV) results in decreased spatial resolution along the phase-encoding axis. Reduction in either N_p or N_{ex} also leads to a reduction in the SNR in proportion to the square root of these quantities. In general, halving the acquisition time results in a 40% ($\sqrt{2}$) decrease in SNR.

One way to scan faster without this loss of SNR is to use gradient-echo techniques. Because these techniques have a lower flip angle, they require a much shorter TR to return to near equilibrium magnetization. Ultrafast gradient-echo techniques, such as turbo fast low-angle shot (turboFLASH) and fast spoiled gradient-recalled acquisition in the steady state (SPoiled GRass, or SPGR), allow images to be acquired in less than 1 sec. TurboFLASH imaging, for example, typically uses a TR of 7 ms and a TE of 2 ms (with partial Fourier in read or fractional echo), with a 128 × 128 matrix to acquire images in 896 ms. Unfortunately, contrast on gradient-echo techniques is limited, and they generally cannot be used to replace conventional spin-echo (CSE) techniques.

FAST SPIN ECHO

Fast spin echo (FSE) is one of the most important recent advances in MRI. It was originally called *RARE* (*r*apid *a*cquisition with *r*elaxation *e*nhancement) by Hennig when he described it in 1986.[23] Today it is more commonly called *fast spin echo* (by GE, Picker, Toshiba, and Hitachi) or *turbo spin echo* (by Siemens and Philips). For ease of discussion, we refer to it as *FSE* hereinafter.

The primary advantage of FSE is speed, without the usual concomitant loss of SNR. In CSE every time the acquisition time is reduced by 50%, the SNR is also reduced by 40%. In FSE the SNR penalty for going faster is minimal. To understand how FSE is performed and how it differs from CSE, it is useful to introduce the concepts of Fourier analysis, the Fourier transform, and κ space.[58,64]

Introduction to κ Space

The basic idea behind Fourier analysis is that any shape can be approximated by a weighted sum of sines and cosines.[64] Low-frequency sine waves describe the bulk outline, and high-frequency sine waves fill in the details. (Because these sine waves describe an object in the x-y plane, the axes have units of spatial frequency or cycles per millimeter rather than the cycles per second units of temporal frequency.)

A Fourier transform is a mathematical process that breaks any complex signal into its component frequencies (Figure 7-1, *A*). A free-

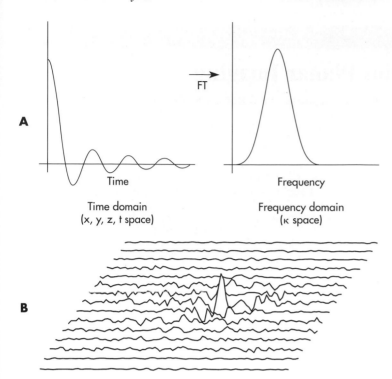

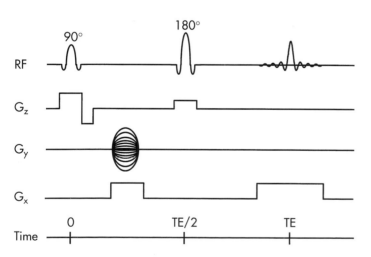

FIGURE 7-1 Fourier transform. **A,** One-dimensional Fourier transform (1D FT). The FID on the left is a plot of amplitude versus time. This signal is composed of multiple frequencies. The data can be replotted as amplitude versus frequency (on the right); the central peak being the dominant frequency in the FID. The x axis of this new representation in κ space has units of frequency (temporal frequency for spectroscopy and spatial frequency for imaging). This is the spectrum in MR spectroscopy. **B,** Temporal stack of SEs from beginning *(bottom)* to end *(top)* of acquisition.

FIGURE 7-2 SE pulse-sequence diagram (PSD). The top line demonstrates radiofrequency (RF) transmission and reception. The SE is formed after 90- and 180-degree RF pulses. The time between the 90- and 180-degree RF pulses (TE/2) is the same as the time between the 180-degree RF pulse and the SE. The slice-select gradient *(Gz)* is applied at the same time as the RF pulses so that only the desired slice is excited. The phase-encoding gradient *(Gy)* is activated after the 90-degree pulse. Each cycle through the sequence changes the phase-encoding gradient. The frequency-encoding (readout) gradient *(Gx)* is applied as the SE is read out. The initial gradient prepulse dephases the spins so that they are perfectly rephased along the x axis at the midpoint of the SE. Thus the SE is rephased in time by the 180-degree pulse and in space by the initial prepulses of G_x and G_z.

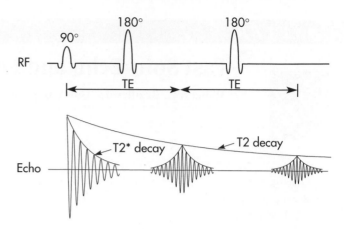

FIGURE 7-3 Conventional double SE PSD. Applying two 180-degree pulses after a 90-degree pulse produces two SEs with decreasing signal intensity as a result of T2 decay. Also shown is the T2* decay of the FID resulting from the 90-degree pulse before initial rephasing by the first 180-degree pulse. This signal usually is not acquired.

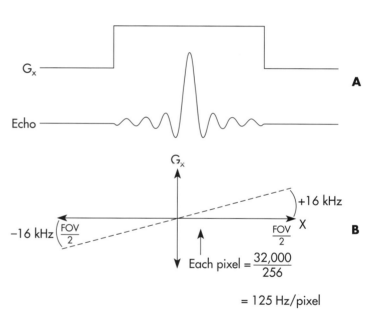

FIGURE 7-4 Frequency encoding. **A,** The readout (frequency-encoding) gradient G_x is applied during readout of the SE to provide spatial discrimination along that axis. **B,** Activating the readout gradient changes the magnetic field and thus the resonance frequency at each point along the readout axis. The maximum frequency change occurs at the borders of the FOV (i.e., FOV/2) and is known as the Nyquist frequency (16 kHz in this case). The *Nyquist frequency* is the same as the bandwidth (±16 kHz in this case). Another way to represent the bandwidth is to divide the full bandwidth (32 kHz) by the number of pixels along the readout axis (256 in this example), giving a bandwidth of 125 Hz/pixel.

induction decay (FID), which is one half of an SE, is represented as an oscillating signal of decreasing amplitude versus time. There are many frequencies included in the signal. Some are strong (high amplitude); others are weak (low amplitude). The data in the FID can also be represented as amplitude versus frequency. The FID in its original form is in the time domain (i.e., the x axis has units of time). The transformed data are in the frequency domain or κ space. The units along the x axis in κ space are in either temporal frequency (i.e., cycles per second for spectroscopy) or spatial frequency (i.e., cycles per millimeter for imaging). The κ comes from a variable in the mathematical formula for the Fourier transform. As you will see, the concept of κ space markedly simplifies the discussion of FSE and echo-planar imaging (EPI).

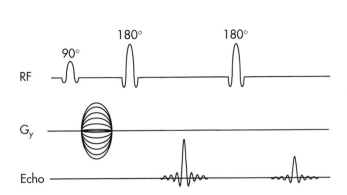

FIGURE 7-5   In a CSE image the phase-encoding gradient is applied once after the 90-degree RF pulse, regardless of the number of echoes produced (two in this example).

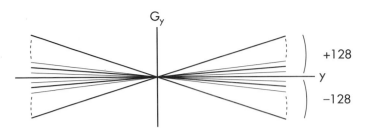

256 Phase-encoding "projections" (N_p = 256 different values of phase-encoding gradient G_y)

$$t = TR \times N_p \times N_{ex}$$

FIGURE 7-7   Phase encoding for CSE imaging. This plot of gradient strength versus position along the phase-encoding axis demonstrates the most negative values of the phase-encoding gradient (-128) passing through the weakest to the most positive ($+128$).

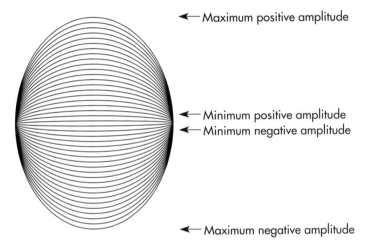

FIGURE 7-6   Phase encoding. The maximum negative amplitudes of the phase-encoding gradient are generally applied first, passing through the weakest amplitudes to the maximum positive amplitude on each cycle through the pulse sequence of a CSE image.

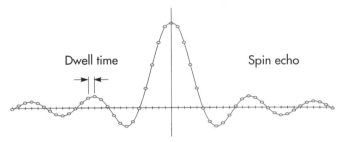

256 Readout (frequency–encoding) "projections"
(256 points digitizing along spin echo [Nyquist theorem])

Bandwidth = 1/ (Dwell time)

FIGURE 7-8   Routine frequency encoding. This plot of amplitude versus time indicates an SE *(solid black line)* digitized 256 times, thereby providing frequency discrimination of 256 points along the readout axis (according to the Nyquist theorem). The sampling interval is known as the *dwell time,* which is the inverse of the bandwidth. The sampling is performed by a piece of equipment called the *ADC,* which converts the continuous variation of voltage versus time of the SE to a stream of digits that can be handled by a digital computer.

This transformation of one axis of data is called a *one-dimensional Fourier transform* (1D FT). Transformation of two axes of data (e.g., the x and y axes of an MR image) is a two-dimensional Fourier transform (2D FT). The representation of the image data in κ space also has two axes (with units of spatial frequency), corresponding to phase (κ_y) and frequency (κ_x).

Just as there was no similarity between the shape of the FID in the time domain and its representation in the frequency domain, there is no correspondence between an MR image as we see it in x, y, or z space and its representation in κ space. In a sense the κ-space representation of an object consists of a temporal stack (Figure 7-1, *B*) of multiple (e.g., 256) SE signals viewed from above. Low spatial frequencies (e.g., 0.01/mm) are found in the center of κ space, and high spatial frequencies (0.5/mm) are found at the periphery.[58,64]

To understand more about κ space, it is useful to consider the interplay between the RF (radiofrequency) pulses and the x, y, and z gradient pulses that are needed to produce a conventional SE image. This representation is called a *pulse-sequence diagram.* Figure 7-2 shows a 90-degree RF pulse followed a time (TE/2) later by a 180-degree RF pulse. An interval TE/2 after that (i.e., time TE after the 90-degree pulse) the SE forms. For a double-echo technique, a second 180-degree pulse is added, producing a second echo (Figure 7-3). In general any number of rephasing 180-degree pulses can be added to produce a train of echoes. The only limitation to the length of such an echo train is the

T2 decay, which results in ever diminishing signal from the last echoes (Figure 7-3).

To limit RF excitation to a single slice, the 90- and 180-degree RF pulses must be applied while the slice-select gradient is activated (Figure 7-2). (For purposes of discussion we shall assume that we are producing an image in the transverse axial plane in a conventional superconducting magnet, in which case G_z is the slice-select gradient.) To obtain spatial information along the frequency-encoding, or readout, axis, another gradient (e.g., G_x) must be activated while the SE is being read out (Figures 7-2 and 7-4).

To provide spatial information along the remaining phase-encoding axis in the MR image, the phase-encoding gradient is activated once between the 90- and 180-degree pulses (Figures 7-2, 7-5, and 7-6). On each pass through the sequence (i.e., after each 90-degree pulse) the phase-encoding gradient is advanced. To distinguish 256 points along the phase-encoding axis, 256 different values of the phase-encoding gradient are required on 256 separate passes (each taking time TR) through the sequence. Typically the first pass is with the most negative value (-127) of the phase-encoding gradient followed by the next most negative up to zero (Figures 7-6 and 7-7). After zero, the phase-encoding gradient increases up to its most positive value ($+128$).

The process of reading out an SE involves converting a continuous (analog) signal to a stream of digits that can be processed by a digital computer (Figures 7-4 and 7-8). The computer hardware that performs

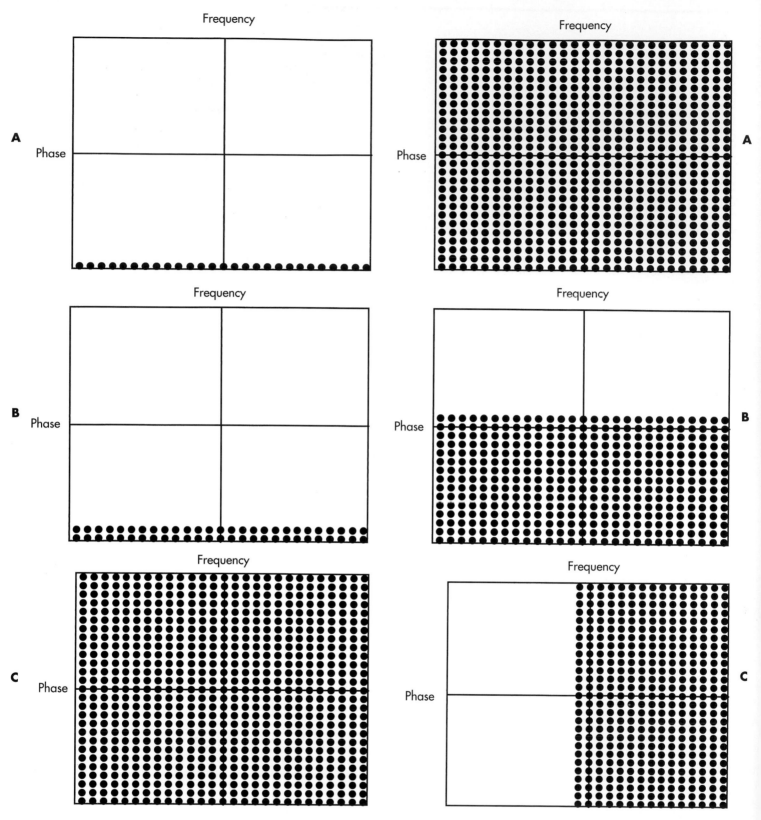

FIGURE 7-9 Conventional 256 × 256 SE representation in κ space. **A,** After sampling of the first echo after the first TR interval, 256 points fill a single line in κ space at a single value of the phase-encoding gradient. **B,** After the second TR interval, 256 additional points are produced by a single SE at another value of the phase-encoding gradient, filling another line in k space. **C,** This process continues until 256 phase encodes have been applied, filling 256 lines in κ space, completing the κ-space representation of a 256 × 256 SE image. Most of the signal and therefore most of the contrast come from the center of κ space, where the values of the phase-encoding gradient are weakest.

FIGURE 7-10 Properties of κ space. **A,** κ Space has Hermetian symmetry, which means that the top right-hand corner is symmetrical with the lower left-hand corner, and the top left-hand corner is symmetrical with the lower right-hand corner. Thus only the top half or the right half of κ space need be acquired, and the other half can be calculated. This 1 N_{ex} acquisition fills κ space completely. **B,** This *half N_{ex}* acquisition fills slightly more than the bottom half of κ space in slightly more than half the usual time for a 1 N_{ex} acquisition. This is called a *half Fourier acquisition in phase.* The advantage of this technique is that it has the spatial resolution of a 256 × 256 matrix and is acquired in half the time (with a concomitant loss of $\sqrt{2}$ in SNR). **C,** This *fractional echo* samples just over half of the right side of κ space, allowing the use of shorter TE for ultrafast gradient-echo techniques, such as turboFLASH and fast SPGR. This is also called *half Fourier in frequency* and *asymmetrical sampling of the echo.*

this task is called an *analog-to-digital converter* (ADC). To distinguish 256 frequencies along the readout axis, the ADC must sample the SE 256 times (i.e., it must produce a stream of 256 digits). The time between samplings is called the *sampling interval* or the *dwell time* (Figure 7-8). Dwell time is the primary determinant of noise in the MR image; noise is proportional to the square root of the receiver bandwidth, and the bandwidth is inversely proportional to the dwell time. Thus the longer the dwell time, the lower the noise and the greater the SNR. Prolonging the dwell time also prolongs the total echo sampling time, which is simply the product of the number of readout projections (e.g., 256) and the dwell time. As the dwell time is increased to improve SNR, the total echo sampling time begins to encroach on the 180-degree pulse, requiring that the entire echo sampling process be shifted to a later time (i.e., a longer TE) (Figure 7-5). Thus the lower bandwidth techniques at lower fields are associated with longer TE values than are typically seen at higher fields.

Each time an SE is read out along the frequency-encoding axis, 256 points are filled in κ space, corresponding to N_f (i.e., the number of points used to digitize the SE and the number of pixels along the readout axis in the image matrix) (Figure 7-9, *A*). These points are all at one spatial frequency, κ_y, along the phase-encoding axis. On the next pass through the sequence, after another 90-degree pulse during another interval TR, a second κ_y line at another spatial frequency along the phase-encoding axis is filled in κ space (Figure 7-9, *B*), and so on up to N_p κ_y lines (Figure 7-9, *C*), N_p phase steps, and N_p TR intervals.

κ Space has some interesting properties that lead to potential modifications of the basic SE sequence. For example, κ space is symmetrical. The upper right-hand corner is symmetrical with the lower left-hand corner, and the upper left-hand corner is symmetrical with the lower right-hand corner. This κ-space Hermitian symmetry reflects the physical symmetry of the SE about the midpoint at TE (Figure 7-8) and the fact that the −128 phase-encoding steps are symmetrical with the +128 phase-encoding steps (Figures 7-6 and 7-7). Because of this symmetry, it is possible to acquire half of κ space and calculate the other half.

When the bottom half of κ space is acquired (i.e., half of the phase steps), the acquisition time is halved (with a reduction of SNR by $\sqrt{2}$). This has been called a *half N_{ex}* acquisition to emphasize the halving of the acquisition time (Figure 7-10). Actually there is no such thing as a half excitation; however, truth in advertising would require that the manufacturer point out that it is one N_{ex} and 128 phase steps all in one half of κ space (rather than being centered in κ space as usual). The spatial resolution is thus the same as a 256 × 256 acquisition and not a lower-resolution 128 × 128 acquisition.

κ Space is also symmetrical about a vertical axis so that only the right half needs to be acquired; the left half can be calculated (Figure 7-10, *C*). Physically this corresponds to sampling only half of the SE. When the second half of the SE (after TE) is sampled, the first half can be ignored and the TE moved to a shorter value. This has been called a *fractional echo* and is used for fast gradient-echo techniques, such as turboFLASH and fast SPGR. The correct terms for *half N_{ex}* and *fractional echo* are *partial Fourier in phase* and *partial Fourier in frequency,* respectively. Although these partial Fourier techniques each have their advantages, they also have the disadvantage that any errors in the acquired part will propagate to the half of κ space that is calculated. Full Fourier techniques, although they include a certain redundancy, tend to self-correct many errors.

The spacing of the κ_y lines and the area occupied by κ space correspond physically to the FOV and the spatial resolution, respectively. The more closely spaced the lines, the larger the FOV. The greater the number of lines for a fixed spacing, the better the spatial resolution. This finding is discussed further in the section on EPI.

Fast Spin Echo versus Conventional Spin Echo

The essential difference between CSE and FSE is that in CSE all echoes in a train are preceded by a single value of the phase-encoding gradient (Figure 7-11), whereas in FSE each echo in the train is preceded by a different value of the phase-encoding gradient[27] (Figure 7-12). Because each value of the phase-encoding gradient corresponds to a separate line in κ space, the result is that κ space is filled that much faster. For an eight-echo train, eight lines of κ space would be filled during one TR, reducing the scan time by a factor of 8 (Figure 7-13, *A*). For a 16-echo train the acquisition time would be reduced by a factor of 16 (Figure 7-13, *B*). The only limitation on the total number

of echoes is the speed and strength of the gradients and signal remaining after T2 decay at long TE.

By sampling κ space more efficiently, FSE can afford to increase TR, the matrix (improving spatial resolution), or the number of averages (improving SNR) without unduly prolonging the acquisition time.[27] In the brain, increasing the TR to 4000 to 5000 ms decreases the T1 contribution to contrast, thereby improving gray-white differentiation on proton density–weighted and T2-weighted images (Figure 7-14). Given the need to spend more time at each slice position to acquire long echo trains, fewer slices are acquired for a given TR. A long TR is therefore desirable for contrast and necessary for coverage. The acquisition matrix can also be increased to 512 × 512 (Figure 7-15), improving spatial resolution without requiring an excessive acquisition time. FSE can use a higher TR, larger matrix, and more averages than CSE and still do it in half the time (Figure 7-16).

Several new parameters are required to describe FSE (Figure 7-12). The echo train length (ETL), or *turbo factor,* is a measure of the temporal efficiency of the sequence. It is the number of 180-degree pulses and the number of echoes. The acquisition time for CSE is the product of the TR, the number of phase-encoding steps (N_p), and the number of

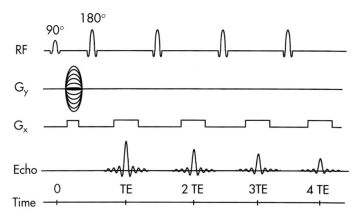

FIGURE 7-11   Conventional four–echo train SE PSD. Notice the single application of the phase-encoding gradient after the 90-degree pulse before production of four echoes that decrease in amplitude as a result of T2 decay.

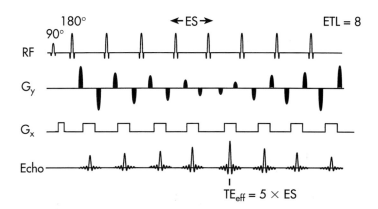

FIGURE 7-12   FSE imaging. The essential difference between CSE and FSE imaging is that in the latter each echo is preceded by a different value of the phase-encoding gradient (G_y in this example). As a result, each echo in the echo train fills a separate line in κ space. In this example the echo train length (ETL) is eight; thus eight lines of κ space are filled after a single 90-degree pulse during a single TR interval. Unlike CSE imaging, in which the echoes after the 90-degree pulse continue to decrease in amplitude as a result of T2 decay, in FSE imaging the amplitude of the echo is also determined by the magnitude of the specific phase-encoding gradient preceding it. (Weaker phase-encoding gradients result in stronger echoes.) The TE of the strongest echo thus produced is termed the *effective TE* and is equal to the product of the echo number (five in this case) and the echo spacing (ES) (i.e., the time between the 180-degree pulses or the time between the echoes produced).

Frequency

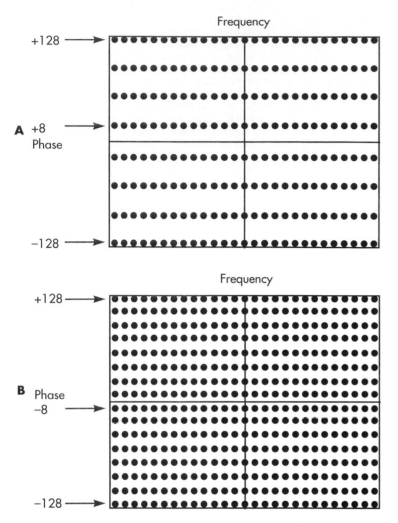

FIGURE 7-13 FSE in κ space. **A,** An eight-echo train FSE fills eight lines in κ space for each 90-degree pulse or TR interval. Thus the total acquisition time is one eighth that of a CSE. **B,** With an ETL of 16, 16 lines of κ space are filled in one TR interval, taking one sixteenth of the time of CSE.

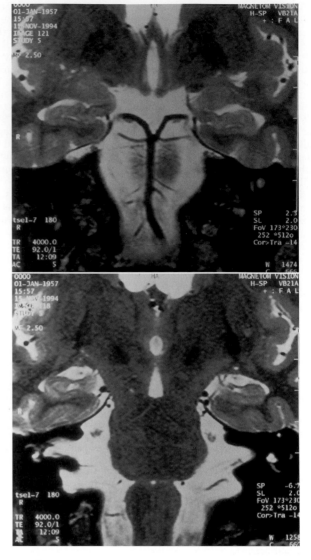

FIGURE 7-14 Long-TR capability. Using an ETL of seven, these images were acquired with a TR of 4000 ms in reasonable acquisition times, despite the relatively large matrix required to achieve 0.5-mm in-plane spatial resolution.

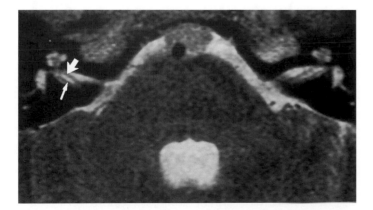

FIGURE 7-15 Large matrix acquisition. This 512 × 512 FSE image (ETL = eight) acquired through the seventh and eighth nerves clearly demonstrates the facial nerve *(large arrow)* and the superior vestibular nerve *(small arrow)* within the internal auditory canals. Also noted are the basal and secondary turns of the cochlea (located lateral to the large arrow).

excitations (N_{ex}). The acquisition time for an FSE is this number divided by the ETL.[27]

The echo spacing (ES) is the time between 180-degree pulses and the time between echoes (Figure 7-12). It is determined by the duration of the 180-degree pulses and the echo sampling time. To shorten the ES, either the duration of the 180-degreee pulse or the echo sampling time must be shortened. As the 180-degree pulses are shortened, they become less slice selective and more broad banded. Rather than exciting a rectangular pulse profile, the slice becomes less well defined (i.e., more gaussian). Cross-talk between slices increases, and the interslice gap must be increased accordingly. As the echo sampling time decreases, noise increases because of the higher bandwidth. Typical echo spacings are on the order of 16 to 20 ms at a typical high-field bandwidth of ±16 kHz (125 Hz/pixel).

The third and most important new parameter in FSE is the effective TE (TE_{eff}) because this parameter determines image contrast[27] (Figure 7-12). TE_{eff} is the TE of one of the echoes in the echo train; therefore it is an integer multiple of the ES. To understand the concept of the TE_{eff}, it is necessary to return to κ space.[58,64]

Most of the signal and therefore most of the contrast come from the center of κ space (Figure 7-1, *B*). Physically this is a result of the vary-

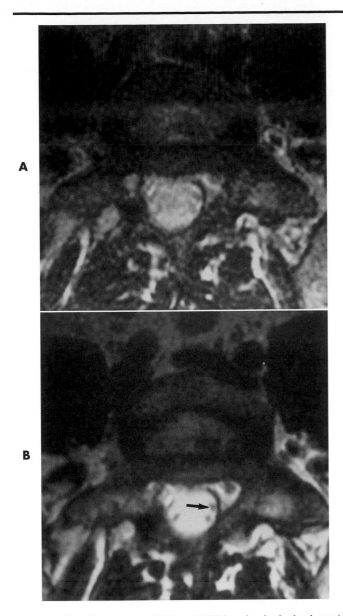

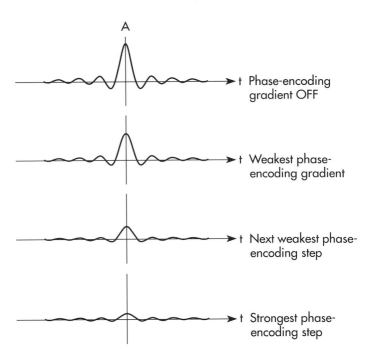

FIGURE 7-17   Signal strength versus strength of the phase-encoding gradient. With the phase-encoding gradient turned off, a strong SE is produced. As the phase-encoding gradient is increased, protons at one end of the phase-encoding axis become 180-degrees out of phase with protons at the other end, leading to phase cancellation and decreased signal. As the strength of the phase-encoding gradient is increased, more and more automatic cancellation occurs, resulting in decreasing signal amplitude. Thus the strongest signal comes from the center of κ space, where the strength of the phase-encoding gradient is weakest.

FIGURE 7-16   Comparison of CSE and FSE imaging in the lumbar spine. **A,** CSE image acquired with 192 × 256 matrix barely demonstrates nerve roots. This acquisition took 9 min, 10 sec. **B,** This FSE image clearly demonstrates the nerve roots *(arrow)*, has greater SNR than the CSE image, and was acquired in approximately one half the time (5 min, 30 sec).

ing strength of the phase-encoding gradient (Figure 7-17). In the center of κ space the phase-encoding gradient is weakest. This leads to the least dephasing along the phase-encoding axis and thus the strongest SE signal. Moving up or down from the center of κ space, the phase-encoding gradient gets stronger, causing spins at one end of the phase-encoding axis to be out of phase with spins at the other end with partial cancellation of signal. With increasing gradient strength, there is increasingly more dephasing and an increasingly weaker signal.

Contrast in an FSE sequence is determined by matching the weakest value of the phase-encoding gradient with the echo to be emphasized (Figure 7-12). The TE_{eff} is that echo preceded by the weakest value of the phase-encoding gradient,[27] resulting in the least dephasing. To minimize adverse contrast averaging, the echoes on either side of TE_{eff} are matched to the next weakest phase-encoding gradients. Those echoes with TE values farthest from TE_{eff} are assigned the strongest values of the phase-encoding gradient, thereby minimizing their overall contribution to the signal coming from the entire echo train (Figure 7-12). Given this weighted averaging of multiple echoes to form an image, FSE contrast is clearly going to be different from CSE contrast. Because the averaging of late echoes will enhance long-T2 substances, CSF tends to be relatively brighter on a proton density–

weighted FSE image than on a CSE image with the same TR and TE (Figure 7-18). Because fat makes a relatively strong contribution to early echoes in the echo train, it is relatively brighter on T2-weighted FSE images than it would be on a CSE image of the same TR and TE (Figure 7-19). Actually, adipose tissue is artifactually dark on CSE images. Adipose tissue is 50% water and 50% fat. Fat and water resonate at different frequencies. As the spins diffuse through these different magnetic environments, they get out of phase. The amount of dephasing depends on the time diffusion is allowed to occur (i.e., the time before the next rephasing 180-degree pulse is applied). The dephasing is minimized by the closely spaced 180-degree pulses in FSE, which minimize diffusion effects.[22] Thus the signal of fat on a T2-weighted FSE image is truer than on a CSE image, where it is decreased because of diffusion-mediated dephasing.

Contrast averaging is one of the limitations of FSE. It can be minimized by reducing the number of echoes averaged together. In addition to this *k-space averaging,* there are two additional differences in contrast between FSE and CSE images. The multiple, rapidly repeated 180-degree pulses leave little time for spins to dephase as they diffuse through regions with different magnetic fields. This dephasing leads to signal loss associated with so-called *magnetic susceptibility effects* on T2-weighted CSE images. In FSE images the signal loss is minimized as a result of the rephasing effects of the multiple 180-degree pulses.[27] Thus T2-weighted FSE images are relatively less sensitive to the magnetic susceptibility effects of hemorrhage (e.g., deoxyhemoglobin and hemosiderin) than T2-weighted CSE images (Figures 7-20 and 7-21).

There are also some positive features resulting from the multiple 180-degree pulses. Because they are evenly spaced, there is a natural *even echo rephasing* effect.[56] Thus CSF motion artifacts are much less severe than on non–flow-compensated, T2-weighted CSE images (Figure 7-22). In addition, the rephasing resulting from the multiple 180-degree pulses leads to less distortion from metal on FSE images (Figure 7-23).[53] Finally, FSE images are much more tolerant of a poorly shimmed magnet than CSE images (Figure 7-24).[3]

Another manifestation of the rapid, multiple 180-degree pulses is an inadvertent magnetization-transfer (MT) effect.[48] Intentional MT is

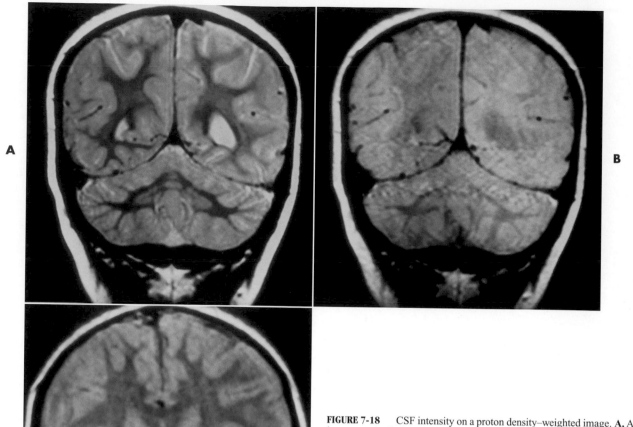

FIGURE 7-18 CSF intensity on a proton density–weighted image. **A,** An FSE image acquired with a TR of 4000 ms and minimum possible TE (17 ms at ±16 kHz bandwidth) demonstrates high-intensity CSF. **B,** CSE image (SE 3000/30) demonstrates desired CSF isointensity to brain, despite longer TE. **C,** To make the intensity of CSF equal to that of brain on an FSE image at the minimum effective TE of 17 ms, the TR could be reduced to approximately 2500 ms. This reduction adds significant undesirable T1 weighting to what should be a proton density–weighted image, particularly at high field.

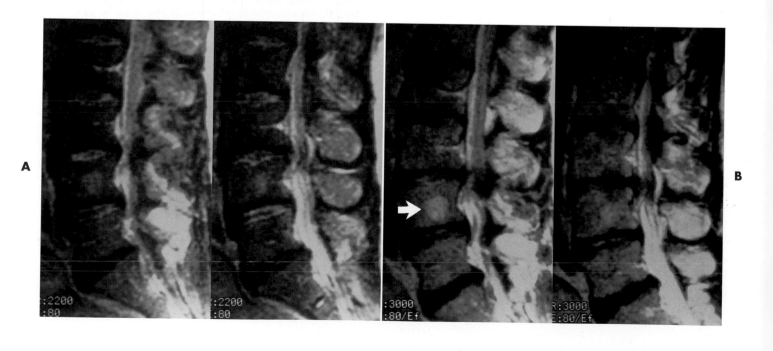

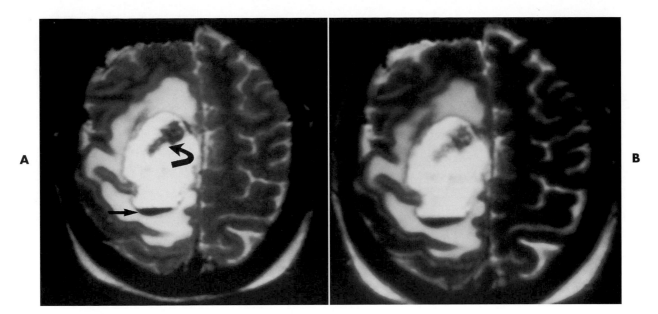

FIGURE 7-20   Relative sensitivity to magnetic susceptibility effects: CSE versus FSE imaging. **A,** CSE image demonstrates low signal in the recently postoperative tumor bed resulting from deoxyhemoglobin *(straight arrow)* and gel foam *(curved arrow)*. **B,** On the FSE image the low signal intensity from the diamagnetic susceptibility effects of the gel foam is somewhat reduced; however, the low intensity from the deoxyhemoglobin is maintained.

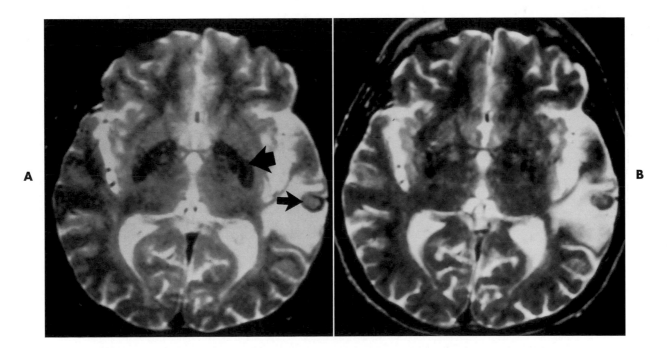

FIGURE 7-21   Sensitivity to hemosiderin. **A,** On a T2-weighted CSE image a hemosiderin ring surrounding hemorrhagic metastasis *(small arrow)* is quite noticeable, as is the magnetic susceptibility effect from the ferritin in the globus pallidus *(large arrow)*. **B,** On an FSE image the hemosiderin rim is much more subtle. The low intensity of the globus pallidus is harder to see as a result of decreased sensitivity of FSE sequences to magnetic susceptibility effects, and darker white matter is due to the natural MT effects by FSE.

FIGURE 7-19   Intensity of fat: FSE versus CSE imaging. **A,** A T2-weighted CSE image barely demonstrates a "fat island" because of relatively low signal. **B,** On a T2-weighted FSE image the intensity of the fat island is significantly increased *(arrow)*.

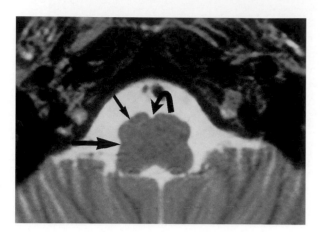

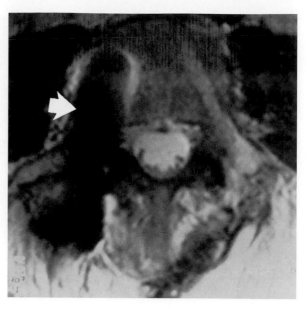

FIGURE 7-22   Natural flow compensation effect of FSE imaging. A transverse FSE image through the medulla demonstrates boundaries distinctly, including the preolivary sulcus *(small arrow),* postolivary sulcus *(large arrow),* and ventral sulcus *(curved arrow).* The apparent flow compensation in this example reflects the multiple 180-degree pulses and the even-echo rephasing effect.

FIGURE 7-23   Minimizing metallic artifacts with FSE imaging. T2-weighted FSE image through the lumbar spine demonstrates minimal distortion *(arrow)* resulting from metallic pedicle screws.

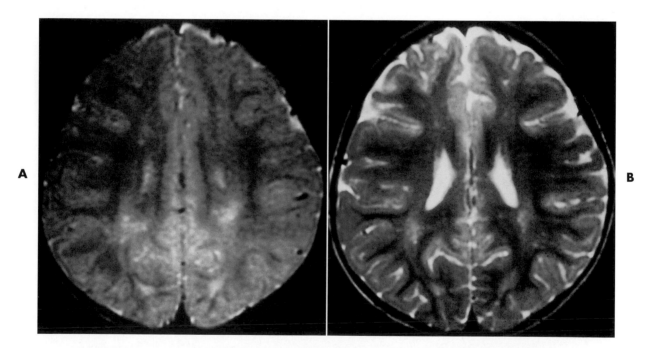

FIGURE 7-24   Benefit of FSE imaging in a poorly shimmed magnet. CSE **(A)** and FSE **(B)** images both acquired after the metallic wheel from a rolling intravenous pole somehow appeared in the bore of the magnet leading to marked B_o nonuniformity. The multiple rephasing 180-degree pulses of the FSE sequence are much more tolerant of a poorly shimmed magnet than is the CSE sequence.

produced by an off-resonance RF pulse that saturates protein-bound water in the broad peaks on either side of the narrow, bulk-phase water peak. Because the short 180-degree pulses in FSE are more broad banded, they also contain frequencies off the bulk-water resonance. Thus protein-bound water is relatively suppressed on FSE images compared with CSE images. This effect is most noticeable in the spine, where normally hydrated disks are bright on T2-weighted CSE images but somewhat darker on FSE images (Figure 7-25). Thus the contrast between normal (usually bright) disks and desiccated (usually dark) disks is diminished.

On a conventional double-SE acquisition, the first echo is free (i.e., it neither prolongs the overall acquisition time nor limits the total number of slices). In FSE, on the other hand, each 256 × 256 image requires filling a 256 × 256 matrix in κ space. Thus the time required to acquire proton density–weighted and T2-weighted FSE images is twice the time it would take to acquire either one alone (assuming the same TR, which is no longer a necessary requirement in FSE).[27]

There are three ways to acquire a double-echo image in FSE—a full echo train,[27] a split echo train,[27] and a shared-echo approach[25] (Figure 7-26). In a full echo train all echoes in the train contribute to the image

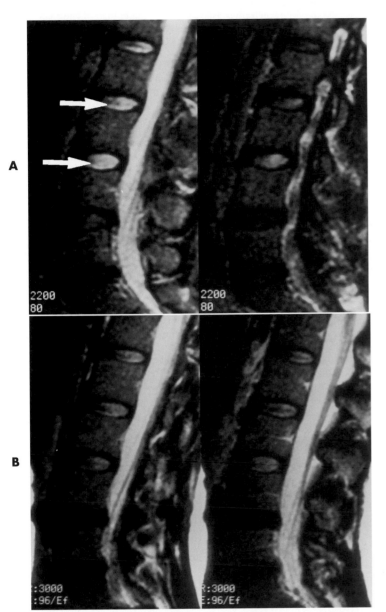

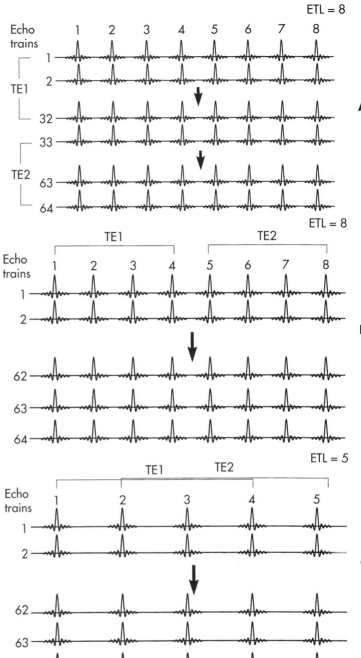

FIGURE 7-25   MT effect. Comparing the CSE image **(A)** to an FSE image **(B)**, normal intravertebral disks are bright on the T2-weighted CSE image *(arrows)*. This reflects an MT effect that is intrinsic to the FSE sequence. Specifically the protein-bound water in the normal disks is partially saturated by the off-resonance frequencies in the rapidly applied 180-degree RF pulses of which the FSE image is composed. As a result, the contrast between normal disks and dehydrated disks (at L4-5 and L5-S1) is decreased.

FIGURE 7-26   Double-echo FSE approaches. **A,** Full echo train. In this double-echo FSE technique, 256 lines in κ space are filled by 32 echo trains, each eight echoes long. Two such sequences are concatenated (i.e., applied sequentially) and thus take twice the time of a single sequence. The advantage of this approach is complete flexibility in the choice of the TE_{eff} for both sequences. The disadvantage is the greater contrast averaging (and blurring) that occurs when eight echoes are averaged together. **B,** Split echo train. In this technique the first four echoes in an eight-echo train contribute to the first TE_{eff}, and the second four echoes contribute to the second TE_{eff}. Because only four lines are filled in κ space for each echo train, a total of 64 echo trains must be acquired to fill 256 lines in κ space. The advantage of this approach is that there is less contrast averaging with four echoes (as opposed to eight with the full-echo approach). The disadvantage is restriction on the minimum TE_{eff} of the second-echo image (5 times the ES in this example). (Although not a significant restriction with an ETL of eight, it does become significant with ETLs of 16 or longer.) **C,** Shared-echo approach. In this technique the central three echoes are shared (i.e., they contribute to both echoes). For the first effective TE, the first echo is prioritized; for the second effective TE, the last is prioritized. The advantage of this approach is ETL = 8 efficiency (i.e., four lines of κ space filled for two images per pass) with a five-echo train, leading to more slices per TR. The disadvantage is some theoretical redundancy in the information.

with a particular TE_{eff} (Figure 7-26, *A*). For an ETL of 8 and a 256 × 256 image, 32 echo trains would be required (8 × 32 = 256) for each image. In a split echo train the first half of the echo train contributes to the image with the shorter TE_{eff}, and the second half of the echo train contributes to the second TE_{eff} (Figure 7-26, *B*). For an ETL of 8, only 4 echoes would be applied to each image from each train. Therefore 64 trains would be required to fill κ space (4 × 64 = 256). In a shared-echo approach[25] the first and last echoes in the train are emphasized for TE1 and TE2, respectively, and the echoes in between are shared for both images (Figure 7-26, *C*). This method has the advantage of a shorter ETL compared with a full or split echo train approach, allowing more slices to be acquired for a given TR. Because the number of slices is determined by the TR divided by the product of the ES and the ETL, a shorter ETL allows more slices. The example shown in Figure 7-26, *C,* uses an ETL of five. Four lines of κ space are filled per TR, three of which are the same for the first and second echo images. Thus there is some overlap of the information in the two images compared with the full- or split- echo train approach. Filling four echoes per pass provides the same efficiency as an 8 ETL split-echo approach (i.e., 64 echo trains total will be required to fill κ space [4 × 64 = 256]). On the other hand, the shorter ETL allows 60% more slices to be acquired in the same time.[3]

A variant of the shared-echo approach is called *keyhole imaging.*[31] In this technique, κ space is covered completely on the first image, but only the central part (approximately 20%), which provides most of the contrast, is covered on subsequent images (Figure 7-27). This method has the disadvantage that the high-frequency outer 80% of κ space is shared information; however, it has the advantage of speeding up imaging by a factor of 5. Thus keyhole imaging is useful when fast repetitive imaging of the same slice is required (e.g., for perfusion imaging).[31]

Each of these double-echo FSE techniques has advantages and disadvantages.[3] The split echo train has the disadvantage that the effective TE of the second echo is constrained (Figure 7-26, *B*). It can be no shorter than the first echo in the second half of the train. For short echo trains (i.e., those with ETLs of 8 or less) this is not a problem. However, for long echo trains (i.e., those with ETLs of 16 or larger) it could pose a limitation. For example, for an ETL of 16 and an ES of 20 ms, the minimum effective TE of the second-echo image would be 9 × 20 =

180 ms, which might be longer than desired for a T2-weighted image of the brain. This is not a problem with a full echo train because there is complete flexibility in the choice of the second TE_{eff}. An advantage of the split-echo approach, however, is that there is less contrast averaging than with the full echo train; therefore the images are sharper (Figure 7-28). In practice the split echo train is generally used for ETLs of 8 or less, and the full echo train is used for ETLs greater than 8. The shared-echo approach and keyhole imaging have the advantage of better coverage and faster scanning, respectively; however, the information in the two images is not truly unique.

Although we have thus far dealt with only traditional T2-weighted FSE techniques, a 180-degree inversion pulse can be added to create a fast inversion recovery (IR) sequence. The inversion time (TI) in fast IR can be chosen to null specific tissues based on their respective T1 values. Short TI IR sequences (e.g., fast STIR) can be used to null fat or bone marrow.[59] TI values on the order of 300 to 400 ms partially null gray matter, increasing gray-white differentiation in the brain. TI values on the order of 2000 to 2500 ms can be chosen to null cerebrospinal fluid (CSF) (e.g., fast fluid-attenuated inversion recovery [FLAIR]). Like traditional FLAIR, fast FLAIR is particularly useful to detect early parenchymal abnormalities in the brain, especially at the brain-CSF interfaces (e.g., the sulci or the periventricular region).[21] Fast FLAIR can be performed much more quickly than traditional FLAIR. For example, we have developed a fast FLAIR technique that yields 30 slices in 8 min[21] (Figure 7-29). When applied to possible multiple sclerosis (MS) patients, we reduce the slice thickness to 2 mm (to minimize partial volume effects) and scan in the sagittal plane (to visualize the undersurface of the corpus callosum) with a 50% to 100% gap (to cover all of the white matter). Using this technique, we have reported a series of 25 potential MS patients, 13 of whom had a normal diagnosis using a routine CSE 3000/30 and 80 technique. Of these patients, 43% had abnormalities on the fast FLAIR consistent with early MS[22] (Figure 7-29).

FSE can also be combined with spectral presaturation pulses (e.g., fat saturation). Fat-saturated, T2-weighted FSE is particularly useful for detecting early bone marrow abnormalities (Figure 7-30), such as

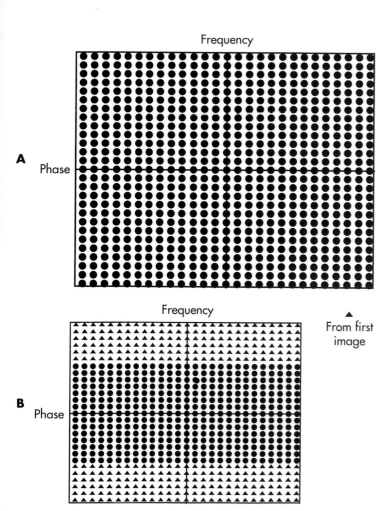

FIGURE 7-27 Keyhole imaging. **A,** On the first pass, all of κ space is filled. **B,** On subsequent passes, only the central 20% or so of κ space is filled, and the outer 80% is repeated from the first pass. This has the advantage of decreasing the acquisition time by a factor of 5 (e.g., for perfusion studies).

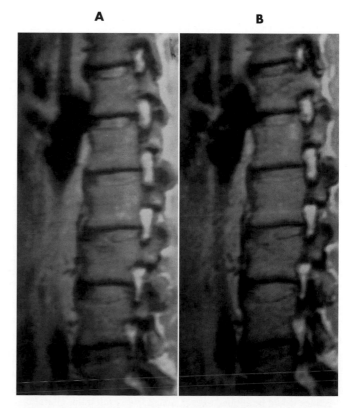

FIGURE 7-28 Comparison of full echo train (**A**) and split echo train (**B**) FSE images. Both images were acquired with ETLs of eight. The split echo train images are clearly crisper than the slightly blurred images in the full echo train acquisition.

metastases,[28] and bone marrow contusions.[29] In one series, fat-saturated, T2-weighted FSE was applied to a series of 73 knees with suspected internal derangement. It was found that 30% of the patients in this series who had ostensibly normal bone marrow on the routine 3-mm, T2-weighted CSE examination had clearly defined bone marrow contusions on the fat-saturated, T2-weighted FSE.[29] In another series of 29 patients with head and neck lesions,[31] fat-saturated, T2-weighted FSE was shown to be comparable in characterizing lesions to the "gold standard," gadolinium-enhanced, fat-saturated, T1-weighted CSE (Figure 7-31).

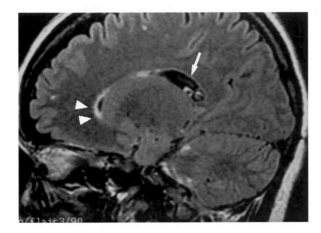

FIGURE 7-29   Fast FLAIR imaging. This 2-mm thick sagittal acquisition features the contrast of FLAIR and the speed of FSE imaging. Note the excellent gray-white differentiation and normal subependymal stripe *(arrow)*. In this patient with suspected MS, subcallosal striations are noted on the inner aspect of the corpus callosum *(arrowheads)* consistent with early diagnosis of MS. The conventional axial 5-mm SE images were normal in this patient.

3D FSE is the newest enhancement to FSE imaging.[32] In 3D FSE the slice thickness is decreased to 1 mm, comparable to the in-plane spatial resolution. With isotropic resolution a single acquisition can be reformatted into multiple planes. Whereas 3D T1-weighted gradient-echo data sets have been used for some time, for example, magnetization prepared–rapid acquisition gradient echo (MP-RAGE) from Siemens, 3D SPGR from GE, and 3D RF-spoiled Fourier acquisition in the staedy state (FAST) from Picker, 3D T2-weighted data sets have not previously been available. This is now possible with 3D FSE. A single, bright-CSF, 3D FSE acquisition can yield images in the reformatted planes (Figure 7-32) of near-comparable quality to the primary plane of acquisition. As an added bonus in the cervical spine, oblique, en face views through the neural foramina can be obtained without increasing acquisition time (Figure 7-32, *C*).

3D FSE is like 2D FSE except that the multiple slices in 2D FSE are replaced by multiple slabs, each of which is subsequently partitioned into 1-mm slices (Figure 7-33). The slab profiles are more gaussian than rectangular, partly because of the need to use extremely short RF pulses.[32] Gaussian slice profiles do not pose a serious problem on 2D (multislice) techniques because 50% gaps can be inserted between slices without sacrificing image quality. However, for 3D techniques in which perpendicular reformations are being contemplated, the slices or slabs must be contiguous. Forcing the slabs together results in cross-talk, leading to loss of signal on the edges of the slab. This is particularly prominent for long-T1 substances such as CSF. One partial solution to this problem is to increase the gap to 100% and to interleave two separate acquisitions. This approach eliminates cross-talk but runs the risk of slab misregistration as a result of patient motion between the two acquisitions (Figure 7-34). Another solution involves exciting odd slabs first and then exciting even slabs on a second pass within the same TR interval[32] (Figures 7-35 and 7-36). This method has the advantage of no misregistration and, at long enough TR, no cross-talk (Figures 7-35 and 7-36).

With the new high-performance gradient systems it is now possible to scan even faster with FSE. FSE techniques with longer echo trains,

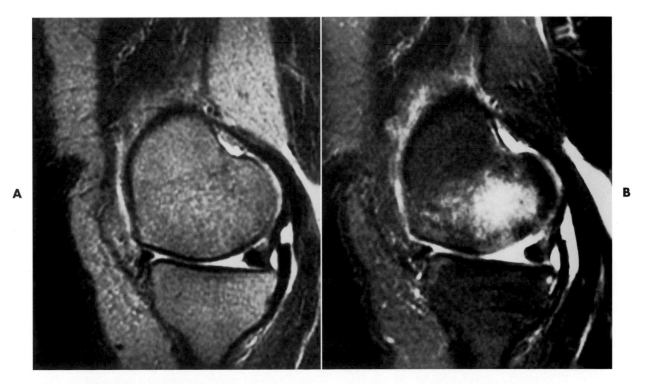

FIGURE 7-30   A 65-year-old woman had persistent knee pain approximately 2 months after arthroscopic evaluation. Further clinical evaluation demonstrated osteonecrosis. **A,** SE T2-weighted image (SE 2700/80). **B,** T2-weighted, fat-saturated FSE image (FS-FSE 4500/95). The area of osteonecrosis is poorly visualized using the conventionally T2-weighted technique. The focus and extent of osteonecrosis are readily apparent using the T2-weighted FS-FSE technique. (From reference 29.)

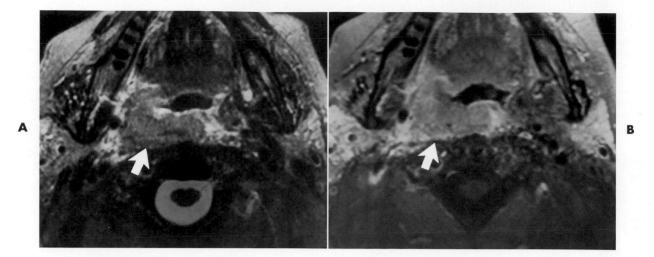

FIGURE 7-31 A 73-year-old man with squamous cell carcinoma of the tongue base. **A,** An axial, T2-weighted, fat-saturated FSE (FS-FSE 4700/108) MR image shows a right posterolateral pharyngeal mass *(arrow)* that extends across the glossotonsillar recess to involve the right posterolateral base of the tongue. Note the excellent contrast between the mass and adjacent fat and lymphoid tissue of the posterior pharyngeal wall, as well as adjacent muscle and fat of the tongue base. **B,** An axial, contrast-enhanced, T1-weighted, fat-saturated SE (FS-SE 500/16) MR image at the same level as **A** shows poorer contrast between the mass *(arrow)* and the fat of the adjacent pharyngeal wall, as well as muscle and fat at the base of the tongue. (From reference 10.)

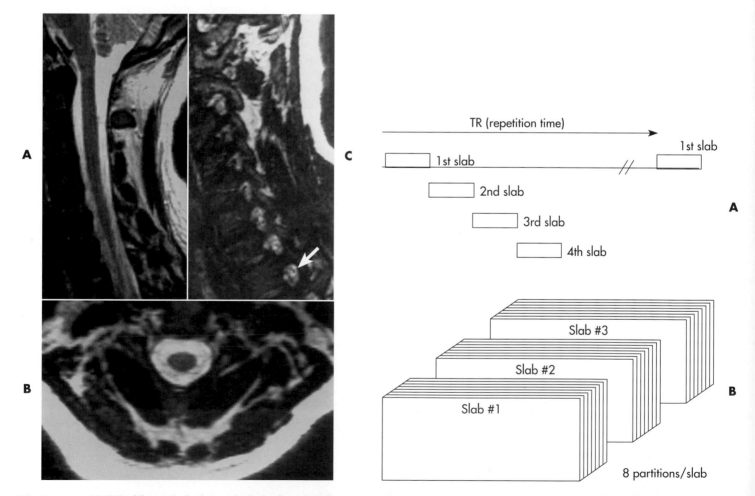

FIGURE 7-32 3D FSE of the cervical spine. **A,** Sagittal reformation of a primary axial acquisition. **B,** Primary 1-mm thick axial 3D FSE acquisition. **C,** Oblique 3D FSE reformation demonstrating neural foramina en face *(arrow).*

FIGURE 7-33 3D FSE schematic. **A,** First step: Multiple slabs are excited similar to multislice imaging. Unfortunately, these slab profiles are more gaussian than rectangular; thus there is a tendency for cross-talk. To obtain contiguous slabs, two acquisitions (with 100% gaps) can be interleaved or odd slabs can be excited, followed by even slabs, within a given acquisition. **B,** Second step: Slabs are subdivided into contiguous partitions by the second phase-encoding gradient.

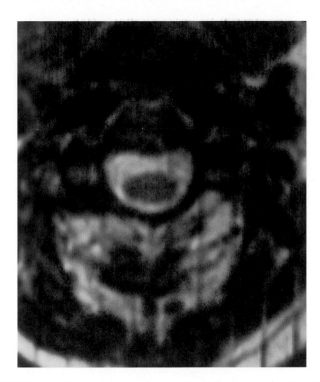

FIGURE 7-34   Misregistration artifact in 3D FSE imaging. Axial reformation of primary sagittal acquisition demonstrates misregistration artifacts caused by patient motion between two interleaved acquisitions.

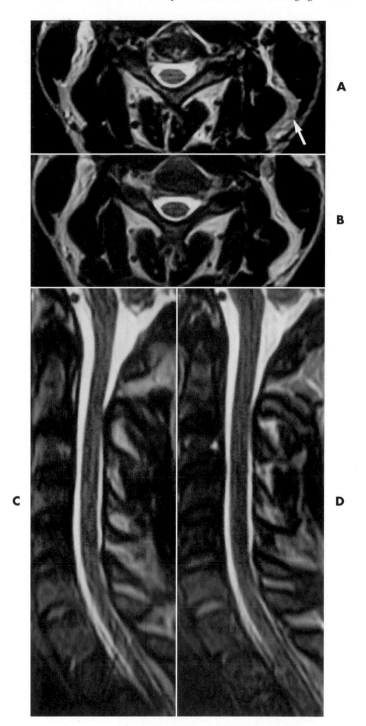

FIGURE 7-35   Nonslab interleaved 3D FSE imaging of the cervical spine. In this technique the odd slices are excited first and then the even slices are excited within the same TR interval, thereby avoiding patient-motion misregistration artifact. Axial reformations of primary coronal acquisition using TR of 8000 ms with ETL of 16 (**A**) or TR of 16,000 ms with ETL of 32 (**B**) for the same acquisition time. Note the more prominent Venetian-blind artifacts caused by saturation effects *(arrow)* in **A** than in **B.** Sagittal reformations of primary coronal acquisition using TR of 8000 ms and ETL of 16 (**C**) or TR of 16,000 ms and ETL of 32 (**D**).

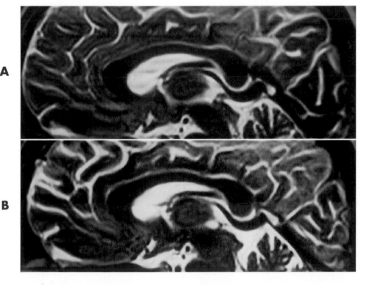

FIGURE 7-36   Nonslab interleaved 3D FSE of the brain. Comparison of sagittal reformations of primary axial acquisition using TR of 8000 ms (**A**) versus TR of 12,000 ms (**B**). The more prominent Venetian-blind artifacts in **A** reflect the saturation effects caused by cross-talk from the interleaved slabs, which are largely eliminated in **B.**

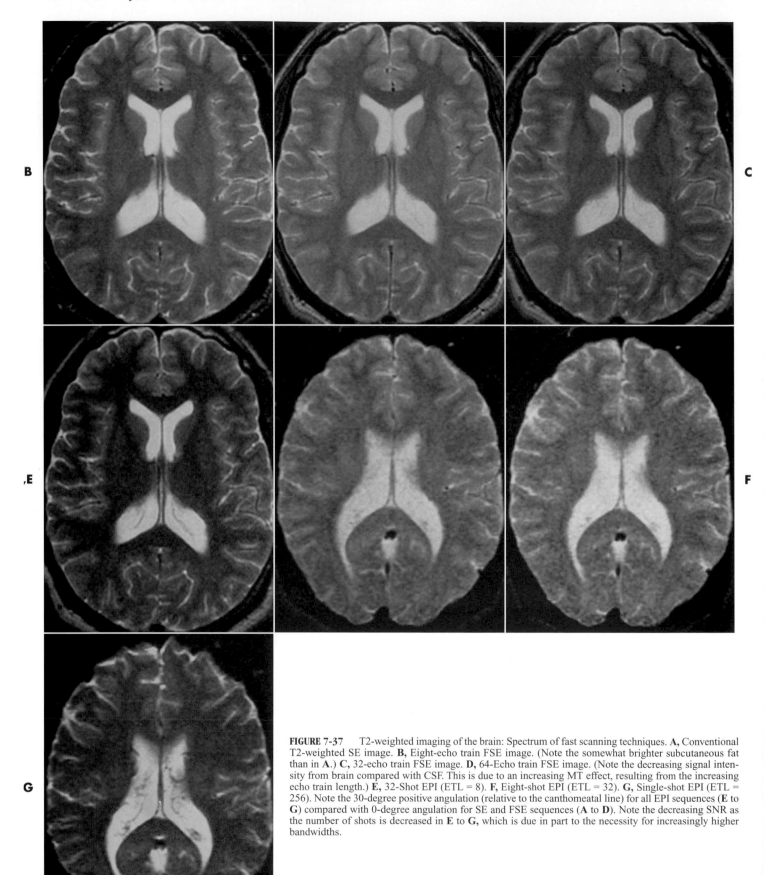

B

C

,E

F

G

FIGURE 7-37   T2-weighted imaging of the brain: Spectrum of fast scanning techniques. **A,** Conventional T2-weighted SE image. **B,** Eight-echo train FSE image. (Note the somewhat brighter subcutaneous fat than in **A.**) **C,** 32-echo train FSE image. **D,** 64-Echo train FSE image. (Note the decreasing signal intensity from brain compared with CSF. This is due to an increasing MT effect, resulting from the increasing echo train length.) **E,** 32-Shot EPI (ETL = 8). **F,** Eight-shot EPI (ETL = 32). **G,** Single-shot EPI (ETL = 256). Note the 30-degree positive angulation (relative to the canthomeatal line) for all EPI sequences (**E** to **G**) compared with 0-degree angulation for SE and FSE sequences (**A** to **D**). Note the decreasing SNR as the number of shots is decreased in **E** to **G**, which is due in part to the necessity for increasingly higher bandwidths.

such as half-Fourier single-shot turbo spin echo (HASTE), gradient spin echo[42] (GRASE, also called *turbo GSE,* or *TGSE*), multishot EPI, and single-shot EPI are all new fast scanning techniques. These techniques owe their speed to the fact that they cover multiple lines of κ space during each TR interval or shot (Figure 7-37). With increasing κ-space coverage per shot, the acquisition time is decreased in direct proportion. Unlike single-line κ-space trajectory techniques (e.g., CSE), these techniques suffer only a minimal SNR penalty with faster scanning. If it were not for T2 decay, there would be no loss of SNR at all compared with conventional κ-space trajectories. (With ultrafast techniques, such as single-shot EPI, SNR is reduced primarily because of the higher sampling bandwidths used.)

In CSE a single line of κ space is filled for each 90-degree pulse and each TR. In FSE, multiple (ETL) lines of κ space are filled per TR. In HASTE the ETL is 128 (i.e., 128 180-degree RF pulses) covering half of κ space (i.e., half N_{ex} or partial Fourier in phase). This so-called RF-EPI is extremely fast, producing images in less than 1 sec. In GRASE, some of the spin echoes in an FSE technique are replaced by gradient echoes (Figure 7-38).[42] Contrast in GRASE techniques reflects the TE_{eff} and the ratio of gradient to spin echoes.[19] In multishot EPI, all of the spin echoes are replaced by gradient echoes, but κ space is still segmented into multiple shots, each filling ETL lines in κ space. The relationship between the number of shots (N_s), the ETL, and the total number of κ_y lines in κ space (N_p) is as follows:

$$N_s \times ETL = N_p$$

In single-shot EPI, all lines of κ space are filled by multiple gradient reversals, producing multiple gradient echoes in one acquisition during a single T2* decay (i.e., $N_s = 1$ and $ETL = N_p$).

As noted earlier, κ space represents the raw data matrix before Fourier transformation into an image. The axes of κ space are κ_x (horizontal) and κ_y (vertical). The units of measurement along these axes are in spatial frequencies (cycles per millimeter). For 1-mm spatial resolution the span of spatial frequencies from the bottom to the top of κ space must be 1 cycle/mm. Thus the maximum κ_y values are ±0.5 cycles/mm (at the periphery) and 0 cycles/mm (in the center).

The κ_x data result from the readout of a single echo. The number of points along κ_x is the same as the number of points used to digitize the SE (e.g., 256) (Figure 7-8). The spacing $\Delta\kappa_x$ between the points along κ_x reflects the strength of the readout gradient and the time for which it is activated. To be more specific, the spacing (in cycles per millimeter) is such that two points at the periphery of the FOV describe the highest frequency that can be detected by the radio receiver. This is also called the *Nyquist frequency,*[64] and it is the same as the bandwidth measured in ± kilohertz.

The total number of lines κ_y is the same as the number of phase-encoding projections (N_p). The spacing $\Delta\kappa_y$ between these lines depends on the phase-encoding gradient increment (in milliTesla per meter [mT/m]) and the time (in milliseconds) for which the phase-encoding gradient is applied. In practice the time for each of the phase-encoding steps remains constant: only the gradient strength is changed. This is the distinguishing characteristic of the usual *spin-warp* technique; however, newer techniques that vary the encoding time[17] more efficiently cover κ space. The spacing $\Delta\kappa_y$ determines the FOV along the phase-encoding (y) axis. The larger the spacing, the smaller the FOV. Thus at a given matrix size, the greater the spacing between points along κ_x or the wider the separation of lines κ_y (smaller FOV), the larger the area of the κ-space trajectory. By definition:

$$\kappa_x = \gamma G_x \Delta t$$
$$\kappa_y = \gamma G_y t_y$$

where

κ_x and κ_y = Spatial frequencies (in cycles per millimeter)
γ = Gyromagnetic ratio (42.57 mHz/T for hydrogen)
G_x and G_y = Gradient strengths (in milliTesla per minute, incremental or fixed)
Δt = Dwell time (sampling interval)
t_y = Time the phase-encoding gradient is applied

From the preceding discussion it is obvious that κ space (the raw data matrix) has physical dimensions (Figure 7-39).[3] The incremental phase (or frequency) gain ($\Delta\kappa$) is the spacing between points κ_y or κ_x. The greater the spacing $\Delta\kappa$, the smaller the FOV (along either axis). The number of κ_y lines in κ space corresponds to the matrix dimension in the phase direction and, with the spacing $\Delta\kappa$ (FOV), determines the spatial resolution (Figure 7-39). In Figure 7-39, *A,* $\Delta\kappa_y$ and $\Delta\kappa_x$ are small, so the FOV is large in Figure 7-39, *B.* There are 128 κ_y lines corresponding to a 128 × 128 matrix. In Figure 7-39, *C,* $\Delta\kappa_y$ and $\Delta\kappa_x$ are twice as large, so the FOV in Figure 7-39, *D,* is half of what it is in Figure 7-39, *B.* For a 64 × 64 matrix (i.e., half of the κ_y lines), spatial resolution is the same in in Figure 7-39, *B* and *D.* In Figure 7-39, *E,* the spacing $\Delta\kappa_x$ and $\Delta\kappa_y$ are still doubled, so the FOV is still halved in Figure 7-39, *F.* Because there are now 128 Fourier lines (128 × 128 matrix), spatial resolution is doubled. Notice that the area of the κ-space trajectory in Figure 7-39, *E,* is twice that of Figure 7-39, *A* and *C.* The larger the area covered by κ space, the better the spatial resolution because a larger area could be produced by greater spacing $\Delta\kappa$ (small FOV) or by more κ_y lines (larger matrix).[3]

As discussed, the physical equivalent of the κ-space trajectory is the pulse-sequence diagram (Figure 7-11). Gradient activation is characterized by three parameters—strength, rise time, and duration (Figure 7-40). Activation of the phase-encoding gradient leads to a certain amount of marginal phase accumulation at a particular point. This depends on the integral of the gradient over time or, stated differently, the area under the gradient-versus-time curve. Whether this is accomplished by the gradient pulse in Figure 7-40, *A,* or by any of those in Figure 7-40, *B,* is inconsequential because only the area under the curve is important, and it is the same in all three. The advantage of high-performance gradients with their greater strength and faster rise times is their ability to generate the same area in less time. Regardless of how it is achieved, the area under the gradient-versus-time curve determines the κ-space trajectory and the FOV.

The simplest example to demonstrate the use of κ space is the concept of encoding along a single dimension (e.g., readout) (Figure 7-41).[54] Typically, data sampling is coordinated with this κ-space trajectory, and a series of equally spaced samples is taken. At the beginning, no gradient events have occurred, and the κ_x position is at the origin.[5] A typical readout from a gradient-echo sequence begins with activation of a negative lobe of a readout gradient G_x. This negative lobe acts to dephase spins along the read axis or move the position of κ_x off-center to the left. A positive lobe acts to rephase spins or move the κ_x trajectory to the right. As it passes through zero, spins are maximally rephased and an echo is produced.

In this example a Fourier transform of these 128 points yields a 1D projection of the object. Spacing these same 128 samples farther apart and extending the two end points (through either higher gradient amplitude or longer sampling duration) produces higher spatial resolution along this axis. If the number of samples is doubled to 256 with the same two end points maintained, the net effect is to double the range of frequencies, or bandwidth. If the gradient readout is the same and the dwell time is halved, the result is a doubling of the bandwidth and the FOV.[4]

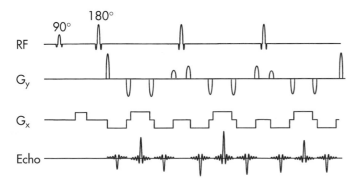

FIGURE 7-38 GRASE imaging. In this variation of FSE imaging, some of the spin echoes have been replaced by gradient echoes; hence the name *GRASE* for gradient spin echo. In this example there are two gradient echoes for each spin echo. Because there are nine echoes total (three spin echoes and six gradient echoes), the sequence is as efficient as an FSE image with an ETL of nine. However, contrast appears more like a gradient echo with increased sensitivity to magnetic susceptibility effects like hemorrhage. Also, there is less RF power deposition because there are fewer 180-degree pulses than in FSE imaging.

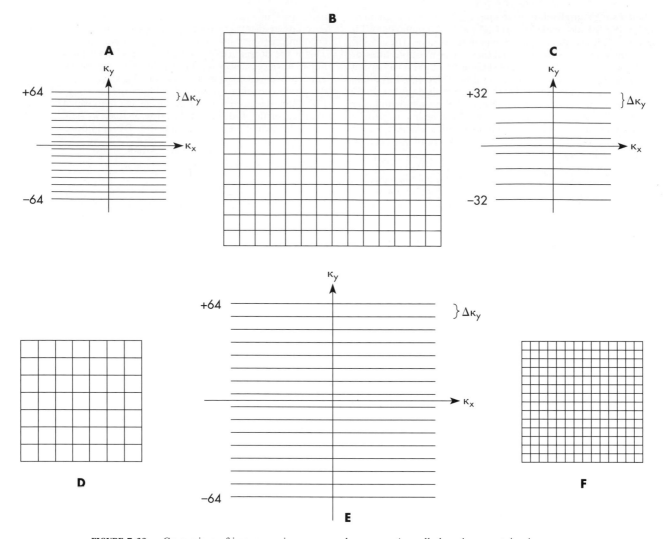

FIGURE 7-39   Comparison of image area in κ space and xy space. A small phase increment $\Delta\kappa_y$ in κ space **(A)** results in a large FOV in xy space **(B)**. The 128 lines in κ space result in a low-resolution image in xy space. The line spacing $\Delta\kappa_y$ in κ space **(C)** has been doubled, halving the FOV in xy space **(D)**. Because the number of κ space lines has been halved, the overall area of the image in κ space is unchanged. The resulting halving of both the FOV and the number of matrix elements in xy space leaves the spatial resolution unchanged. By keeping the phase increment $\Delta\kappa_y$ doubled in κ space, the FOV remains small in xy space **(F)**. By increasing the number of Fourier lines to 128 in κ space, the spatial resolution is doubled in xy space. The larger the area in κ space, the better the spatial resolution in xy space.

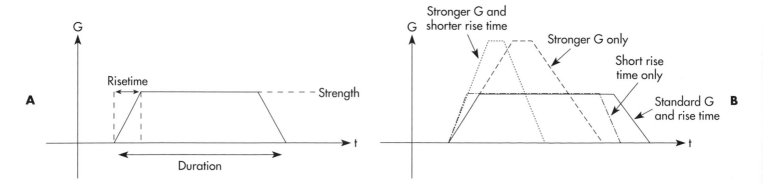

FIGURE 7-40   Gradient-performance parameters. **A,** Gradient performance can be characterized by the maximum strength (in milliTesla per meter [mT/m]) and the rise time (in milliseconds). The gradient strength (in milliTesla per meter) divided by the rise time (in milliseconds) is known as the *slew rate.* **B,** This illustrates the effect of change in gradient strength and rise times on the FOV. The area under the gradient-versus-time curve determines the incremental phase advance, which in turn determines the FOV (larger areas corresponding to smaller FOVs). High-performance gradients produce more area under the curve in less time than conventional weaker gradients.

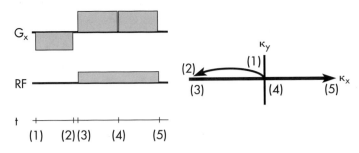

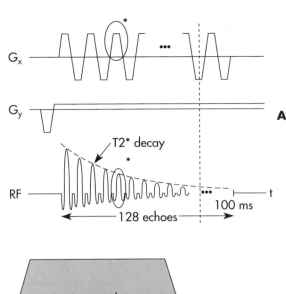

FIGURE 7-41 One-dimensional κ-space trajectory. Position 1 (before gradient activation) is in the center of κ space. Activation of negative G_x at time 1 moves to the left along κ_x to arrive at position 2. At time 3 the positive G_x is activated, moving the κ-space trajectory to the right. At time 4 the area under the positive lobe equals the area under the negative lobe, returning to the center of κ space *(4)*. Continued readout and application of the positive G_x gradient moves us to the right edge of κ space *(5)*. Moving from 3 to 5, the RF channel (ADC) is opened and 128 points are sampled, corresponding to the readout of a single GRE.

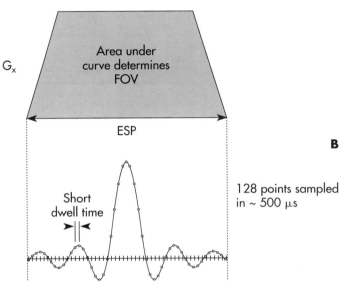

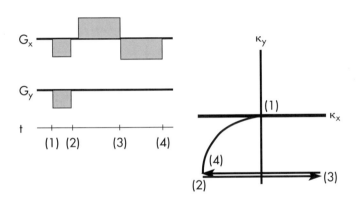

FIGURE 7-42 Two-dimensional κ-space trajectory. In this example, negative G_x and G_y lobes are activated simultaneously. The negative G_x lobe moves us to the left of the origin in κ space, and the negative G_y lobe moves us down in κ space. After the application of both gradients, we are at position 2 in the lower left-hand corner of κ space. Subsequent activation of a positive G_x moves us to the right *(3)*, during which time 128 points could be sampled during a GRE readout. When the next negative G_x lobe is applied, we move to the left in κ space, allowing readout of an additional 128 points for a second GRE.

FIGURE 7-43 EPI readout. **A,** During a single T2* decay *(bottom),* 128 gradient echoes are formed from 128 reversals of the readout gradient G_x. During this time the phase-encoding gradient is either continuously on (as shown here) or blipped in between each readout gradient reversal. **B,** Here the G_x gradient lobe and one of the gradient echoes *(asterisk in A)* are shown in greater detail, where the G_x lobe has a trapezoidal waveform. The area under the curve determines the FOV, larger areas leading to smaller FOVs. The G_x gradient lobe can also have a sinusoidal (quarter-wave) ramp. While the gradient lobe G_x is applied, a gradient echo is formed *(below)* and digitized by the ADC. To have 128 readout projections, this signal must be sampled 128 times during the echo sampling period (ESP). This necessitates extremely short dwell times (e.g., 5 μs), resulting in extremely high bandwidths (e.g., $\frac{1}{5\mu s} = 200$ kHz) for single-shot EPI.

This same analysis can be extended to two dimensions of κ space.[4] In Figure 7-42 the negative first lobe of G_x shifts the κ-space position to the left (as in the previous example). The simultaneous negative lobe G_y shifts the κ-space position downward to the lower left-hand corner. If there is no further G_y gradient application, filling of κ space will not progress upward along κ_y. As in the previous example, the next positive lobe of the x gradient causes a rightward trajectory along κ_x, during which the first echo is acquired. If there is a second negative lobe, the position in κ space will move leftward and a second echo will be produced.

The second pass would merely repeat the first pattern, albeit in the opposite direction. In practice the phase encoding gradient would be activated to move upward along κ_y. In discussing this effect, we say that the second echo is "time reversed" or filled in "backwardly" from the first.[4] Half the lines in κ space would be filled in this backward fashion. This may have the effect of introducing *N/2 ghosts* into the image if eddy current–induced phase errors are uncorrected or the timing is slightly off.[4]

ECHO-PLANAR IMAGING

From this simple example it is easy to extrapolate other methods to fill κ space via a series of gradient echoes. EPI, for example, fills κ space after a single RF pulse (i.e., in a single measurement or shot). This was dubbed *echo-planar imaging*[36] by Sir Peter Mansfield in 1977 because an entire 2D raw data set (i.e., a plane of data) could be filled during a single echo decay. To do so, the readout gradient must be reversed rapidly from maximum positive to maximum negative 128 times during a single T2* decay or there will be *T2 blurring.* This requirement limits the total readout time (T) to about 100 ms (Figure 7-43, *A*). During each G_x reversal, a gradient echo is produced (Figure 7-43, *B.* Each lobe of the readout gradient above or below the baseline corresponds to a separate κ_y line of κ space (Figure 7-44). The total number of lobes is also the number of phase-encoding steps (N_p). The area under the G_x lobe determines the FOV; larger areas correspond to smaller FOVs (Figure 7-36, *B*). Thus single-shot EPI places tremendous demands on the gradients in terms of maximum strength and minimum rise time. The rapid sampling of each gradient echo also places tremendous demands

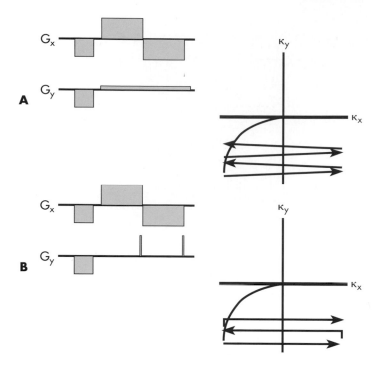

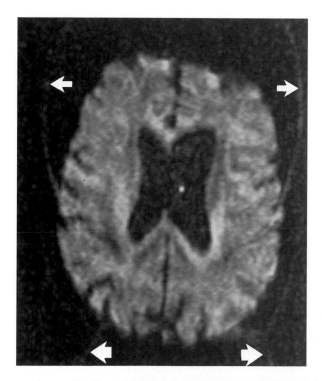

FIGURE 7-44 EPI κ-space trajectory. **A,** In the original version of EPI, initial negative G_x and G_y lobes move us to the lower left-hand corner of κ space. The G_x gradient is subsequently alternated positive and negative 128 times as the G_y gradient is left continuously on. This produces a ramped trajectory in κ space, which changes in direction as G_x is reversed. **B,** In the blipped version of EPI, the phase-encoding gradient G_y is pulsed very briefly to add a stepwise phase increment, resulting in a more Cartesian trajectory through κ space, which is easier to Fourier transform.

FIGURE 7-45 EPI artifacts. This EPI diffusion image has both chemical-shift artifact *(small arrows)* and N/2 artifact *(large arrows)*. The chemical-shift artifact is approximately one sixth of the FOV, and the N/2 artifact is approximately one half of the FOV.

on the ADC. Whereas the echo sampling time for the usual 256 × 256, ±16 kHz high-field technique is 8 ms, a typical echo sampling period (ESP) for EPI would be 500 to 700 μs (Figure 7-43, *B*).

In the original EPI method the phase-encoding gradient was kept on weakly but continuously during the entire acquisition, resulting in zigzag coverage of κ space (Figure 7-44). This led to some difficulties during Fourier transformation compared with the usual Cartesian κ-space trajectories. To rectify this situation, a stronger phase-encoding gradient is now applied very briefly when the readout gradient is zero (i.e., when the κ-space position is at either end of the $κ_x$ axis). This method is referred to as *blipped phase encoding* because the duration of the phase-encoding pulse is minimal (typically less than 200 μs). The technique is called *blipped EPI,* and the κ-space trajectory (Figure 7-44, *B*) is much more amenable to Fourier transformation.[37] In the following discussion, EPI implies *blipped EPI* unless otherwise stated.

Even with blipped EPI, phase errors may result from the multiple positive and negative passes through κ space (i.e., alternating polarity of the readout gradient). If gradient-induced eddy currents build up or if there is a slight but systematic mismatch in the timing of the odd and even echoes, a complete replica or ghost of the main image will appear along the phase-encoding axis. Because the ghosts are derived from half of the data (even or odd passes), they are called *N/2 ghosts*[4] (Figure 7-45).

As discussed, the shorter the minimum rise time and the stronger the gradient, the greater the area under the gradient-versus-time curve (Figure 7-40). This area determines the distance Δκ between points in κ space. The greater the Δκ spacing, the smaller the FOV. Thus the greater the area under the curve, the smaller the FOV (Figure 7-43, *B*).

As shown in Figure 7-46 there is a trade-off between the two determinants of spatial resolution in EPI—matrix size and FOV.[4] If half of the matrix elements are acquired during a given total readout time (T), the ESP can be doubled. This potentially doubles the area under the curve, halving the FOV (Figure 7-46). Because the matrix is also halved, spatial resolution is left unchanged, but the chance of aliasing is increased. If twice the matrix elements (N_p) during a given T are acquired, ESP will be halved, potentially halving the area under the curve if the gradients can keep up (Figure 7-46). Half the area translates to twice the FOV, again maintaining spatial resolution. This has the advantage of a lower chance of aliasing, but it puts greater demands on the gradients. In the end the only way to achieve high spatial resolution, which requires both a large number of matrix elements and a small FOV, is to use high-performance gradients.[4]

One of the problems with single-shot EPI is that any phase errors tend to propagate all the way through κ space. This is not a problem for a CSE in which the TR is long compared with T2 so that no signal and thus no phase error remains at the end of the cycle. The usual phase error in a CSE image arises from line-to-line motion over the TR interval. By comparison, there is little opportunity for involuntary or even

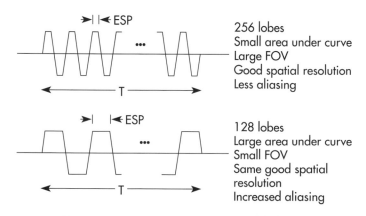

256 lobes
Small area under curve
Large FOV
Good spatial resolution
Less aliasing

128 lobes
Large area under curve
Small FOV
Same good spatial resolution
Increased aliasing

FIGURE 7-46 EPI spatial resolution. The top figure demonstrates 256 reversals of the readout gradient, producing 256 lobes and 256 phase-encoding lines. With such rapid gradient reversal, there is little area under the curve; therefore the FOV is relatively large. Alternatively the readout gradient can be reversed 128 times, producing 128 lobes and 128 phase-encoding lines with a greater area under the curve, leading to a smaller FOV. Although the spatial resolution is comparable in the two cases, there is a greater chance of aliasing in the latter scenario.

physiological motion during a typical 100 ms single-shot EPI acquisition. Instead, protons resonating at frequencies different from the main Larmor frequency tend to build up phase errors, which increase over time. Because the temporal progression is mapped along the phase-encoding axis, these errors are mismapped along the phase-encoding axis. Fat protons, for example, resonate at a frequency 220 Hz below water at 1.5 T. This results in the phase of fat protons lagging behind the phase of water protons. Because position along the phase-encoding axis is based on the phase of water protons, fat signal is mismapped, producing chemical-shift artifact (Figure 7-45). For CSE the chemical-shift artifact is along the readout axis and is predicted from the bandwidth per pixel, which is in turn derived from the EST. In EPI, chemical-shift artifact is along the phase-encoding axis because it has a much lower bandwidth than along the readout axis. The bandwidth is so low that the chemical shift is one sixth of the FOV.[57] For this reason a spectroscopic fat-saturation (fat-sat) pulse must be applied before a single-shot EPI acquisition.

Intrinsic nonuniformities in the main magnetic field (B_o) and diamagnetic susceptibility effects result in variable resonance frequencies and growing phase errors. For example, the chemical shift associated with diamagnetic susceptibility differences between air in the sinuses and tissue is estimated at 1 ppm, or about one third of the chemical shift between fat and water. Over the course of a single-shot EPI readout, the phase errors that build up lead to several centimeters of spatial mismapping.[57] Thus one of the persistent technical difficulties with EPI is distortion at the base of the brain, particularly where air in the sinuses and mastoid bones is in close proximity with brain (Figure 7-47). For this reason, axial EPI sequences may be angled +30 degrees to the canthomeatal line to avoid the paranasal sinuses.

By dividing the EPI readout into multiple shots (N_s), phase errors have less time to build up, resulting in a subsequent decrease in the diamagnetic susceptibility artifacts (Figure 7-47). This is called *multishot EPI*[5] or, because κ space is segmented into multiple acquisitions, *segmented EPI*.[14] For an eight-shot EPI acquisition at the same bandwidth as the comparable single-shot technique, there would be one eighth the phase-encoding error. Unfortunately, multishot techniques also take a lot longer than single-shot techniques; therefore they are more susceptible to motion artifacts and new artifacts arising from the potential misregistration of the multiple shots.[14]

Although multishot EPI may not be as fast as single-shot EPI, it does have certain advantages compared with FSE. For about half the time it takes to acquire an 8-ETL FSE sequence, a 16-shot, 16-ETL multishot EPI sequence has contrast much closer to CSE imaging (i.e., greater sensitivity to magnetic susceptibility effects such as hemorrhage).[14] Because each echo in FSE is produced by a 180-degree RF pulse (which takes time and increases the RF power deposition), the total time per slice and the total RF heating are greater than for multishot EPI[9] (which uses only gradient reversal to produce echoes). For this reason, more slices can be acquired per TR interval with multishot EPI than with FSE. Compared with single-shot EPI techniques, multishot methods typically have higher SNR (as a result of less T2* decay and a lower bandwidth), better spatial resolution (because of a larger matrix), and better proton density and T1 contrast (because of shorter TEs). Unfortunately, even at a large number of shots, some diamagnetic susceptibility artifact still remains at the skull base (Figure 7-47).

Contrast in single-shot and multishot EPI depends on the root sequence from which it is derived (i.e., the succession of 90- and 180-degree RF pulses) rather than the component gradient or spin echoes in the readout.[57] In this context it is useful to separate the root sequence from the signal. For example, a single 90-degree RF pulse produces an FID signal. A 180-90-180–degree combination is an IR root with an SE signal. (A 90-180–degree combination is an SE root and an SE signal.) For echo-train techniques covering multiple lines in κ space, the signal for each RF excitation (or TR) is more accurately termed a *readout module* (ETL echoes long). Thus FSE is a 90-(180)$_{ETL}$–degree readout (i.e., a 90-degree RF pulse followed by ETL 180-degree RF pulses [Figure 7-12]). IR-FSE is a 180-90-(180)$_{ETL}$–degree readout (i.e., a 180-degree followed by an FSE readout module ETL echoes long) (Figure 7-29).

In the same way, EPI can be considered a readout module, whether as a single-shot or multishot technique. For example, a 90-180–degree EPI would be an SE root with an EPI readout module (i.e., SE-EPI) (Figure

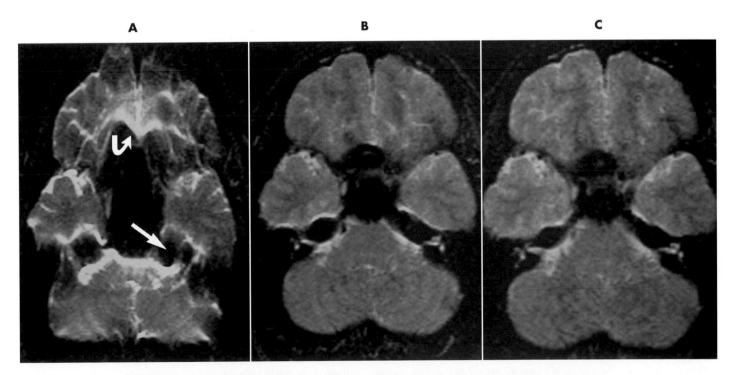

A   **B**   **C**

FIGURE 7-47   EPI susceptibility effects. **A,** Single-shot EPI demonstrates marked distortion at the skull base, including the petrous bones *(arrow)* and sphenoid sinus *(curved arrows)*. This results from differences in diamagnetic susceptibility between air and tissue. **B,** Eight-shot EPI sequence markedly reduces the geometric distortion resulting from differences in diamagnetic susceptibility. Persistent distortion is noted along the anterior margin of the temporal bones and above the sphenoid sinus. **C,** 32-shot EPI results in minor diminution in degree of susceptibility-induced distortion, although the image quality is generally inferior because of artifacts introduced in the interleaving of the 32 shots.

7-48, *A*). An RF pulse followed by an EPI readout module would be a GRE-EPI (i.e., an EPI sequence with gradient-echo contrast) (Figure 7-48, *B*). Unlike FSE, where echoes acquired with weaker values of the phase-encoding gradient (in the center of κ space) determine contrast (TE_{eff}), all of the echoes in EPI are acquired with the same value of the phase-encoding gradient. Thus contrast on SE-EPI is determined from the temporal rephasing of the 180-degree RF pulse (Figure 7-48, *A*); in GRE-EPI it is determined by the time between the negative phase-encoding gradient prepulse and the EPI readout module (Figure 7-48, *B*). Contrast in a T2-weighted EPI is very much like it is in a T2-weighted CSE (i.e., signal is determined by T2 decay, and flowing blood appears dark).[57] Contrast in a GRE-EPI sequence is T2*-weighted, which means it is perfect for performing first-pass perfusion sequences with gadolinium. Should STIR or

FLAIR contrast be desired in an EPI sequence, a 180-degree prepulse can be applied (i.e., an IR root, IR-EPI) (Figure 7-49).

Whereas contrast is determined by the root sequence, sensitivity to susceptibility effects is determined by the type of signal, gradient-echo techniques (e.g., EPI) being more sensitive than SE techniques (e.g., FSE).[57]

Echo-Planar Diffusion Imaging

Diffusion imaging is accomplished by adding diffusion-sensitizing gradient pulses on either side of the 180-degree pulse of an SE sequence, either CSE or SE-EPI (Figure 7-50). The sensitivity to diffusion effects is proportional to the duration of these extra gradient pulses and to their

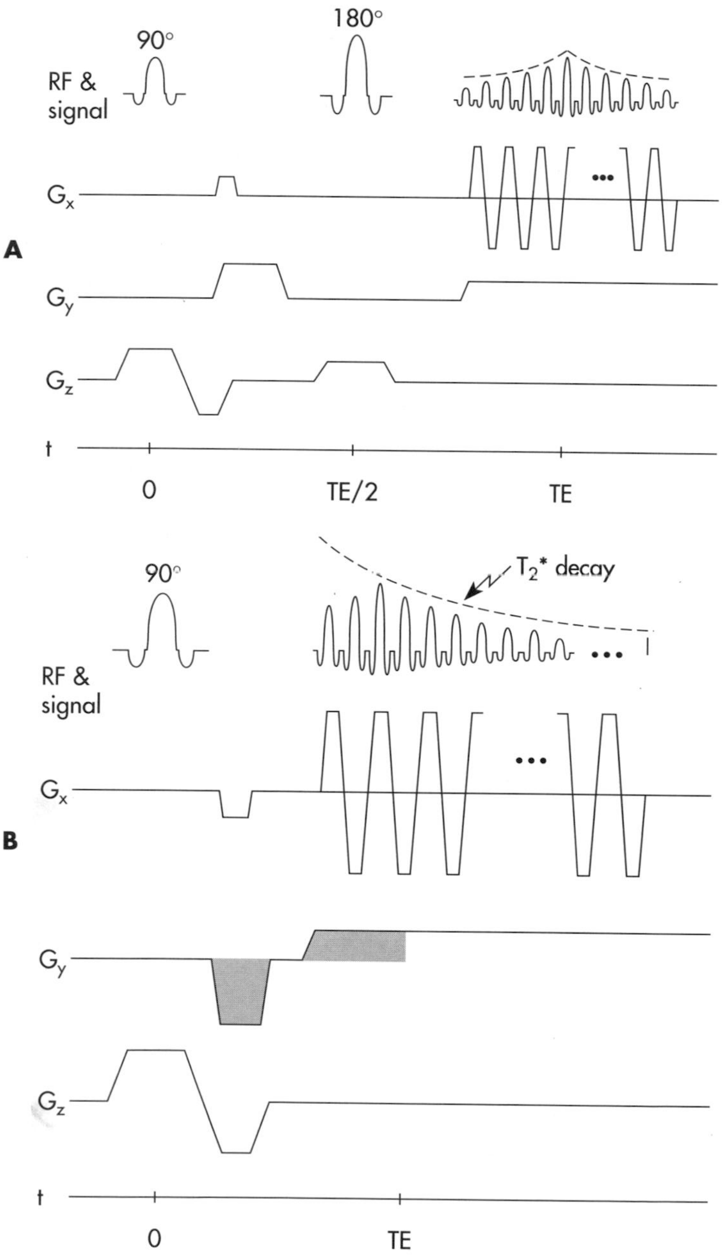

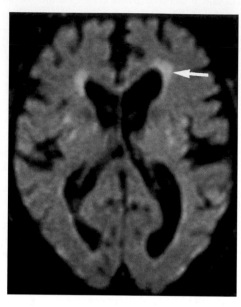

FIGURE 7-49 IR-SE-EPI. Using a TI of 3000 ms and an effectively infinite TR, this single-shot EPI-FLAIR image demonstrates effective nulling of CSF with good T2 weighting, showing bright interstitial edema *(arrow)*.

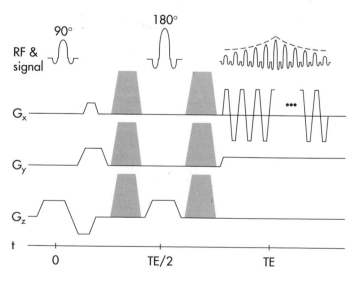

FIGURE 7-48 EPI PSDs. **A,** SE-EPI is generated by slice-selective 90- and 180-degree pulses followed by an EPI readout. Rapid reversal of the readout gradient G_x fills κ space during a single SE readout. The peak of the SE occurs at time TE when the area under the G_y curve (or the sum of individual blips) equals the area under the initial G_y prepulse. **B,** A GRE-EPI sequence is formed from an initial 90-degree (or smaller) RF pulse with rapid reversal of the G_x gradient filling κ space during a single FID. The TE is defined by the time when the shaded area under the second G_y pulse equals the shaded area of the prepulse. (Note the rephasing under the dashed T2* decay curve at the top.)

FIGURE 7-50 Echo-planar diffusion imaging is performed by adding additional gradient pulses *(shaded area)* on either side of the 180-degree pulse. The sensitivity to diffusion (b value) is determined by the amplitude, separation, and duration of these extra gradient pulses.

temporal separation[11]; it is also proportional to the square of the gradient strength. Therefore, all other factors being equal, increasing gradient strengths and shortening rise times lead to improved sensitivity to diffusion.

Diffusion is the process of random, thermal motions of molecules (brownian motion). These motions occur on a microscopic scale (i.e., on the order of tenths or hundredths of a millimeter per second). To sensitize the MR acquisition to detect these small motions, large gradients are applied across the imaging field. As water molecules traverse these field gradients, they experience a phase change dependent on their direction and velocity. Viewed as local groups of spins, these phase changes can act to constructively combine and retain signal or destructively combine and reduce signal. Signal loss is related to the product of

the apparent diffusion coefficient of the tissue and the b value of the sequence, which is determined by the amplitude, duration, and spacing of the additional gradient pulses (expressed in seconds per millimeter squared, or sec/mm^2).

In echo-planar diffusion imaging of the brain, two or more acquisitions must be made (Figure 7-44). First, a baseline SE-EPI image is made with the diffusion-sensitizing gradient off (i.e., b = 0), establishing a reference image. Next, a diffusion-sensitized image is taken using a b value in the range of 1000 sec/mm.^{2} Although such high b values are more sensitive to diffusion changes, they also have decreased SNRs (e.g., a b value of 1000 reduces the SNR by a factor of 10).

Typically the following four sequences are acquired: a b = 0 baseline image (Figure 7-51, *A*) and then three b = 1000 images, sensitizing

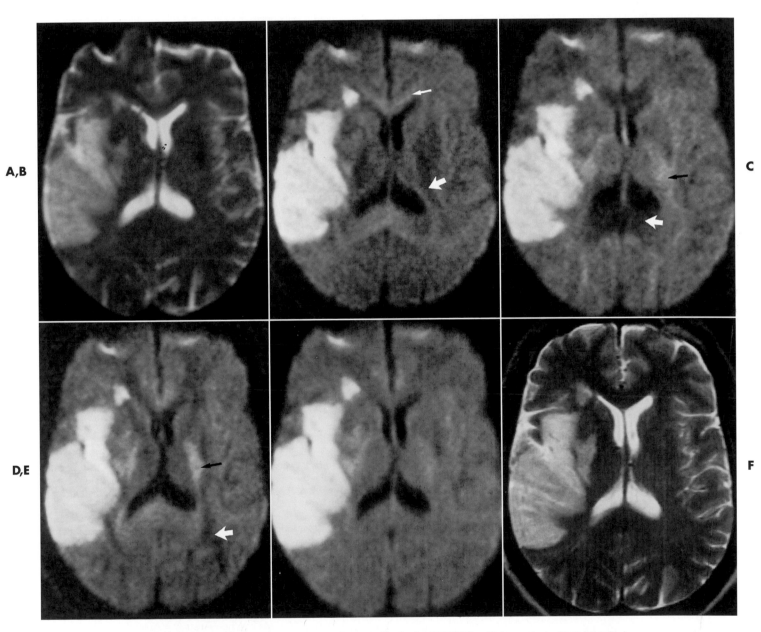

FIGURE 7-51   Subacute infarct 1-week postictus. **A,** Single-shot SE-EPI (b = 0) demonstrates hyperintensity in the right MCA distribution 1 week after infarction. **B** to **D,** Diffusion-weighted SE-EPI show marked hyperintensity in the right MCA distribution. Diffusion sensitization has been applied along the slice-select z axis in **B,** the readout (side-to-side, or x) axis in **C,** and the phase-encoding (top to bottom, or y) axis in **D.** White matter tracts running parallel to the direction of the diffusion-sensitizing gradient appear dark (e.g., the posterior limb of the internal capsules in **B,** the genu and splenium of the corpus callosum in **C,** and the major and minor forceps in **D** *[large arrow]*). White matter tracts running perpendicular to the diffusion-sensitizing gradient appear bright (e.g., the genu and splenium of the corpus callosum in **B** and the posterior limbs of the internal capsules in **C** and **D** *[small arrow]*). **E,** On the trace image, only the infarct is bright, the anisotropic effects of white matter diffusion having been averaged out. **F,** T2-weighted image demonstrating subacute left MCA infarct.

along each (x, y, and z) axis (Figure 7-51, *B* to *D*).[50] In each diffusion image, white matter tracts running parallel to the gradient turn dark and white matter tracts running perpendicular to the gradient turn bright, reflecting the preferred diffusion direction of water along the axons. Because this bright signal can potentially simulate pathology (i.e., ischemic lesions), lesions must be assessed on all three diffusion images to accurately diagnose pathology. Alternatively a *trace* image can be acquired, showing the average diffusion changes along the three axes and effectively averaging out these anisotropic white matter effects[43] (Figure 7-51, *E*). *Anisotropy* means that a property, like diffusion, depends on the direction or axis of measurement. Because the x, y, and z axes of the MR scanner are never perfectly parallel to the white matter tracts at every point in the image, it may be necessary to calculate a *diffusion tensor*[43] (Figure 7-52). Although this requires that seven (instead of four) separate images be acquired and postprocessed, with attendant potential for misregistration, it provides the pure apparent diffusion coefficient for each pixel (called the *principal eigenvalue*) along the true axis of diffusion (called the *eigenvector*), which is a different vector combination of the x, y, and z axes of the scanner at each point in the image (Figure 7-52).

Echo-Planar Perfusion Imaging

Perfusion, or blood flow to the brain, can also be assessed with EPI by monitoring the first-pass effect of an exogenous contrast agent (e.g., gadolinium) (Figure 7-53). Early studies performed using T1-weighted sequences in combination with intravenous injection of gadolinium showed limited signal change caused by T1 shortening. An alternate strategy is to use T2*-weighted EPI sequences and measure susceptibility changes caused by the passage of the paramagnetic contrast agent[30] (Figure 7-53). Large macromolecules, such as gadolinium, do not cross the blood-brain barrier and remain as a relatively compact bolus while passing through the intracerebral vasculature. As this bolus traverses the vascular bed, it changes the intravascular signal and dephases spins outside the lumen in the nearby tissues. This long-range, extravascular phenomenon has the beneficial effect of increasing the potential volume of tissue signal changes.

The transient drop in the signal intensity caused by the passage of the gadolinium bolus provides indirect evidence of the state of perfu-sion of the tissue. From these data, relative cerebral blood volume (rCBV) and mean transit time (MTT) maps can be generated[50] (Figure 7-53). The sensitivity to perfusion in vessels of a particular size depends on the specific EPI sequence used. Performing echo-planar perfusion imaging with an SE technique (SE-EPI) (Figure 7-48, *A*) provides sensitivity to the microcirculation alone, and a GRE-EPI sequence (Figure 7-48, *B*) provides sensitivity to both the microcirculation and the capillary circulation.

Echo-Planar Imaging in Stroke

Normal perfusion to the brain is about 50 ml of blood/min/100 g of brain.[20] As the cerebral blood flow (CBF) drops below about one third of normal (i.e., 17 ml/min/100 g of brain) reversible ischemic changes begin to occur.[21] Initially, function ceases as synaptic transmission fails. At 20% of normal CBF, ATP levels fall, the sodium-potassium pump fails, and the cells begin to swell. This is known as *cytotoxic edema.* It is associated with decreased water diffusion and high signal on echo-planar diffusion images (Figure 7-54), which may not be visible on routine T2-weighted images. Cytotoxic edema per se is reversible if treated quickly enough (Figure 7-55). If the blood supply is reestablished (e.g., through thrombolysis), these cells can return to normal (Figure 7-55). On the other hand, if the ischemia is sufficiently severe or prolonged, the cells may go on to irreversible infarction (Figures 7-55 to 7-56). Infarction leads to cell rupture, vasogenic edema, and high signal on conventional T2-weighted images. In early infarcts there is still a population of swollen, reversibly ischemic, cytotoxic cells. Thus early infarcts are also positive on echo-planar diffusion images (Figures 7-55 and 7-56). Therefore a positive echo-planar diffusion study does not guarantee that irreversible infarction has not already occurred.

With impaired blood supply to the brain, the echo-planar perfusion study initially becomes positive, followed by the echo-planar diffusion study as the blood supply approaches 10 ml/min/100 g of tissue (Figure 7-54). If the echo-planar perfusion and diffusion defects are matched at the time of the initial presentation, the infarct is unlikely to worsen.[50] A diffusion defect smaller than the perfusion defect defines an *ischemic penumbra* that is at risk for extension of the infarct (Figure 7-54). Unless the brain recruits collateral blood supply or neuroprotective agents or thrombolytics are administered, several weeks later the completed infarct is more likely to be the size of the initial perfusion defect than that of the initial diffusion defect (Figure 7-55).

Figures 7-55 to 7-57 demonstrate the spectrum of echo-planar diffusion and perfusion abnormalities in acute middle cerebral artery (MCA) infarction. Figure 7-55 illustrates an MCA embolus that resided only briefly in the proximal MCA (M1 segment) before breaking up

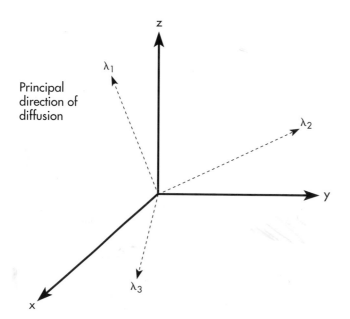

FIGURE 7-52   Relationship of diffusion eigenvector to axes of MR imager. The x, y, and z axes of the gradients in the MR scanner have no relationship to the orientation of the white matter tracts in a particular pixel. This is a problem because the measured apparent diffusion coefficient along a particular axis depends on the specific reference frame of the magnet. To obviate this problem, a tensor can be acquired. This calculates the principal axis of diffusion (the eigenvector λ_1) and the apparent diffusion coefficient along it (eigenvalue), which is no longer dependent on the coordinate system of the magnet.

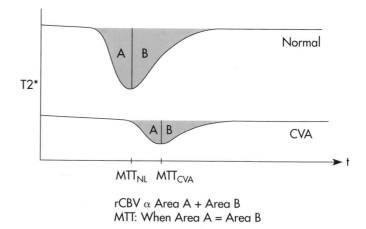

FIGURE 7-53   Echo-planar perfusion imaging. As a gadolinium bolus passes through the brain, it causes T2* shortening and loss of signal. The area under these curves (top, normal; bottom, stroke) is proportional to the rCBV, which is greater in normal areas than in perfusion-challenged stroke areas. The MTT is the midpoint of these curves, defined as the time when the area to the right of the MTT equals the area to the left. The MTT is typically prolonged in strokes because of the longer pathway via collateral channels.

and passing downstream. Initially the T2-weighted images (Figure 7-55, *A* and *B*) were essentially normal and the MTT maps of the echo-planar perfusion study showed slow collateral flow throughout the entire MCA territory (Figure 7-55, *F*). Because collateral supply was poorer proximally than distally, only the basal ganglia (supplied by the lenticulostriate arteries arising from the M1 segment) experienced a sufficient perfusion deficit to develop cytotoxic edema (Figure 4-55, *C* and *D*). Because the embolus broke up quickly and blood supply was reestablished, this edema was reversible. One week later the basal ganglia re-

turned to normal on diffusion images (Figure 7-55, *H*). Distal portions of the MCA distribution, however, were subjected to persistently decreased blood supply, leading subsequently to cytotoxic edema (Figure 7-55, *H*) and infarction (Figure 7-55, *K*). Coincident with the clearing of the basal ganglia or internal capsule cytotoxic edema, this patient's motor function improved significantly during the first week (NIH stroke scale rating improving from 11 to 3).

Figure 7-56 illustrates a more severe or persistent MCA occlusion in which the M1 embolus resided long enough to cause irreversible in-

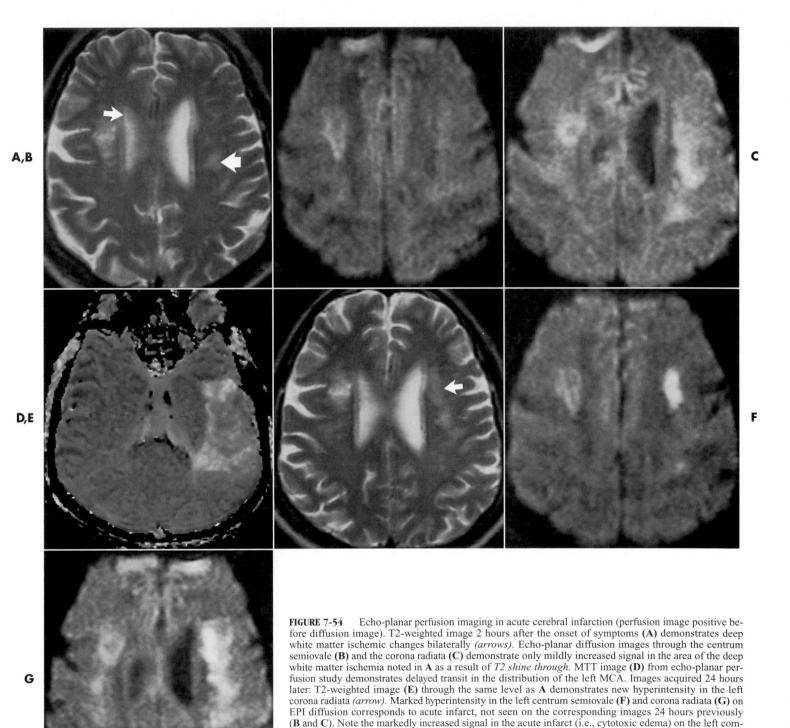

FIGURE 7-54   Echo-planar perfusion imaging in acute cerebral infarction (perfusion image positive before diffusion image). T2-weighted image 2 hours after the onset of symptoms **(A)** demonstrates deep white matter ischemic changes bilaterally *(arrows)*. Echo-planar diffusion images through the centrum semiovale **(B)** and the corona radiata **(C)** demonstrate only mildly increased signal in the area of the deep white matter ischemia noted in **A** as a result of *T2 shine through*. MTT image **(D)** from echo-planar perfusion study demonstrates delayed transit in the distribution of the left MCA. Images acquired 24 hours later: T2-weighted image **(E)** through the same level as **A** demonstrates new hyperintensity in the left corona radiata *(arrow)*. Marked hyperintensity in the left centrum semiovale **(F)** and corona radiata **(G)** on EPI diffusion corresponds to acute infarct, not seen on the corresponding images 24 hours previously **(B** and **C)**. Note the markedly increased signal in the acute infarct (i.e., cytotoxic edema) on the left compared with chronic ischemic changes on the right.

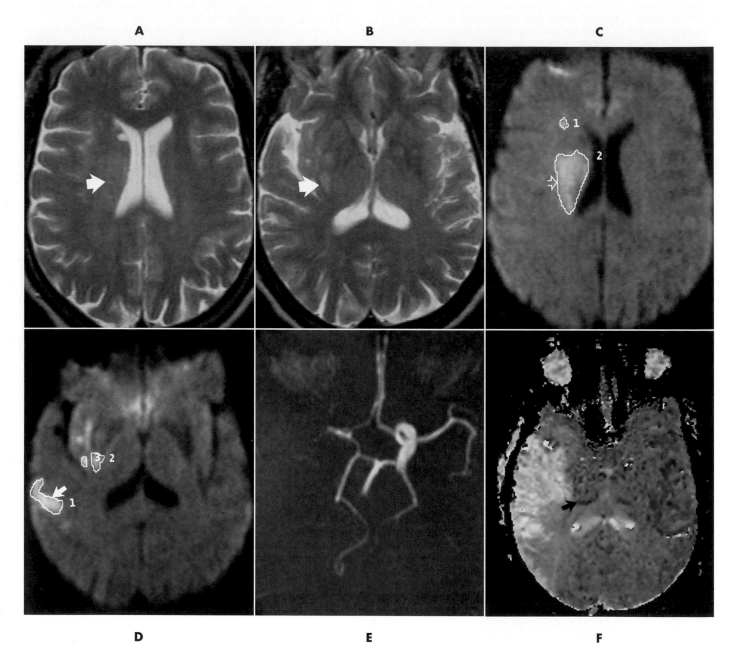

FIGURE 7-55   Acute MCA infarct with short transit time of embolus in M1 segment, leading to reversible cyto-toxic edema. **A** and **B,** Four hours postictus: T2-weighted images demonstrate subtle abnormalities in the right basal ganglia *(arrows).* **C** and **D,** Echo-planar diffusion images (b = 1000) demonstrate impaired diffusion in the right basal ganglia *(open arrow)* and, to a lesser extent, in the right temporal lobe *(solid arrow).* **E,** MRA demonstrates complete occlusion of the right MCA in the mid-M1 segment. **F,** MTT map from echo-planar perfusion study demonstrates increased transit time (i.e., slow flow in the MCA distribution with sparing of the basal ganglia), which has slightly decreased signal *(arrow)* because of early hyperemia.

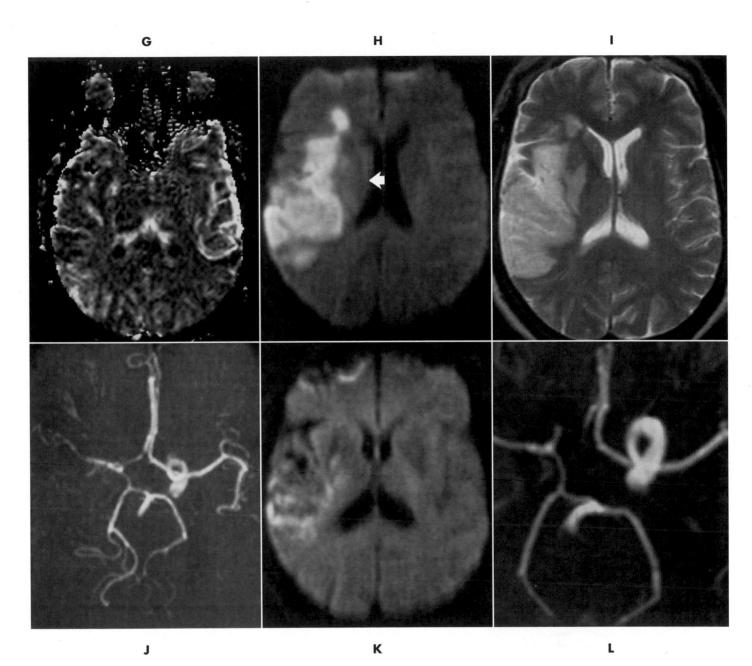

FIGURE 7-55, cont'd   G, rCBV map from echo-planar perfusion study is normal in the right MCA distribution.
H, One week postictus: echo-planar diffusion study now shows normal signal in the right basal ganglia *(solid arrow),* indicating reversal of previous cytotoxic edema. This correlated with improved motor function clinically. The remainder of the right MCA distribution now demonstrates impaired diffusion (i.e., cytotoxic edema and infarction). **I,** T2-weighted image demonstrates matching abnormality. **J,** MRA demonstrates partial recanalization of the M1 segment but not the more distal portions of the MCA. These findings are consistent with an embolus that lodged briefly in the M1 segment (leading to cytotoxic edema in the basal ganglia) with rapid breakup and infarction of the more distal portions of the MCA downstream. **K,** Twelve weeks postictus: T2-weighted single-shot EPI demonstrates encephalomalacia and gliosis in the right MCA distribution with relative sparing of the basal ganglia. **L,** MRA demonstrates that the right MCA is almost completely reconstituted 12 weeks postictus.

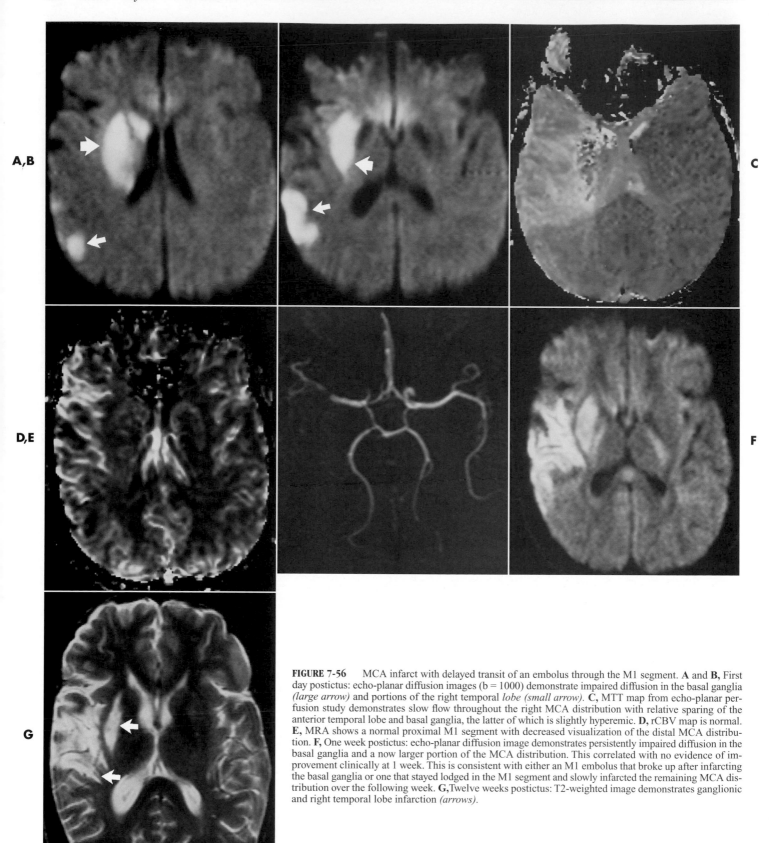

FIGURE 7-56   MCA infarct with delayed transit of an embolus through the M1 segment. **A** and **B,** First day postictus: echo-planar diffusion images (b = 1000) demonstrate impaired diffusion in the basal ganglia *(large arrow)* and portions of the right temporal *lobe (small arrow).* **C,** MTT map from echo-planar perfusion study demonstrates slow flow throughout the right MCA distribution with relative sparing of the anterior temporal lobe and basal ganglia, the latter of which is slightly hyperemic. **D,** rCBV map is normal. **E,** MRA shows a normal proximal M1 segment with decreased visualization of the distal MCA distribution. **F,** One week postictus: echo-planar diffusion image demonstrates persistently impaired diffusion in the basal ganglia and a now larger portion of the MCA distribution. This correlated with no evidence of improvement clinically at 1 week. This is consistent with either an M1 embolus that broke up after infarcting the basal ganglia or one that stayed lodged in the M1 segment and slowly infarcted the remaining MCA distribution over the following week. **G,**Twelve weeks postictus: T2-weighted image demonstrates ganglionic and right temporal lobe infarction *(arrows).*

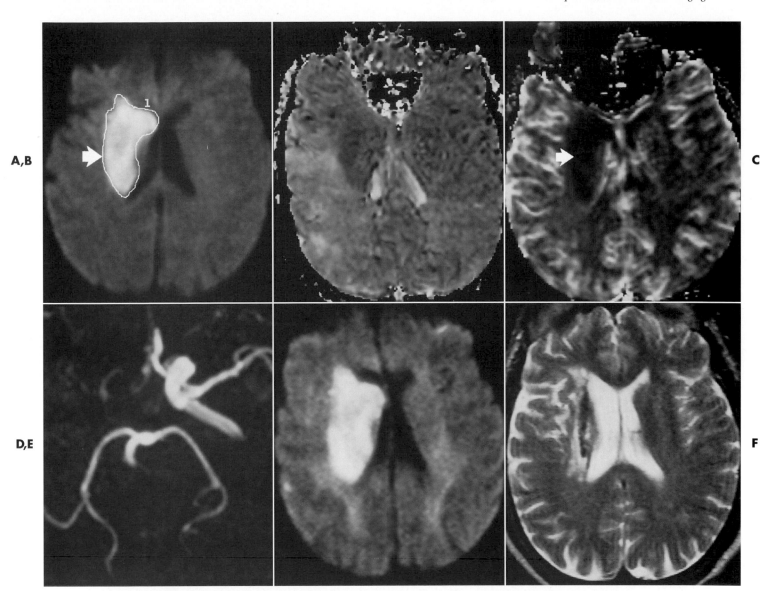

FIGURE 7-57   MCA infarct resulting from persistent occlusion of an M1 segment by an embolus. **A,** First day postictus: echo-planar diffusion image (b = 1000) demonstrates cytotoxic edema in the right basal ganglia *(arrow).* **B,** An MTT map from an echo-planar perfusion study demonstrates delayed perfusion in the right MCA distribution. **C,** rCBV map from an echo-planar perfusion study demonstrates decreased blood volume in the right basal ganglia *(arrow).* **D,** MRA demonstrates complete occlusion of the right internal carotid artery. **E,** Five days postictus: diffusion defect in the right basal ganglia is unchanged without any new abnormality in the remainder of the right MCA territory. This would suggest that the embolus stayed in the M1 segment without breaking up. Clinically the patient was unimproved at this time. **F,** Twelve weeks postictus: hemosiderin is noted in a right basal ganglia infarct secondary to petechial hemorrhage. Such hemorrhage appears to be associated with more severe ischemia or infarction with decreased initial rCBVs.

farction in the basal ganglia. This patient's motor function did not improve after 1 week. Delayed infarction in the more distal MCA territory could reflect decreased flow or delayed breakup of the embolus before floating downstream.

Figure 7-57 demonstrates a more profound infarct of the basal ganglia with delayed petechial hemorrhage. Unlike the cases in Figures 7-55 and 7-56 where the initial rCBV was normal, in this case it is markedly reduced in the basal ganglia. This could reflect a larger M1 embolus or poorer collateral blood supply to the basal ganglia. This patient did not improve clinically at 1 week. Although petechial hemorrhage is often noted in subacute infarcts, these cases would suggest that only those with a decreased rCBV actually bleed.

It has recently[65] been suggested that the mismatch between the size of the abnormalities on echo-planar perfusion and diffusion imaging rather than the duration of symptoms be used as the criterion for thrombolysis. In the extreme case of an acute stroke with a positive perfusion defect and normal diffusion study, thrombolytics should be given. If a diffusion defect is present but is still smaller than the perfusion defect, thrombolytics may still be helpful but at an increased risk of bleeding. The chance of bleeding with thrombolytics increases further as the perfusion to the brain decreases; thus patients with less than 35% of the normal rCBV on the perfusion study probably should not get thrombolytics.[65] In this case other neuroprotective agents (e.g., Citicoline or Cerestat) may be indicated.

Echo-planar perfusion methods also have been used clinically to assess neoplasm vascularity, distinguish recurrent tumor from radiation necrosis, and delineate hypervascularity associated with an epileptic focus or hypovascularity with a migraine attack.

Cardiac Echo-Planar Imaging

In general the field of cardiac MRI has been rapidly expanding over the last few years. Faster MR scanners and sequences along with a better understanding of underlying basic techniques have made it possible to image first-pass contrast uptake studies (i.e., perfusion),[1] cine wall motion,[39] and systolic wall thickening.[2] It is possible to produce T1, T2, or T2*contrast with bright or dark blood,[6] to quantitate flow, and to visualize coronary arteries.[34] All of these techniques can be performed with conventional MR scanners, and all can be performed within one breath-holding period. It is against this ongoing evolution of cardiac-imaging techniques that echo-planar applications in the heart are being assessed.

EPI's strength lies in its ability to image the heart extremely rapidly[46,52,55] (Figure 7-58). Clinically this feature is beneficial because EPI avoids the reliance either on ECG-synchronized acquisitions over multiple beats or on any patient cooperation for breath-holding. This makes the technique potentially useful for pediatric studies of congenital anomalies[7] and dysrhythmia cases in which a weak or erratic signal precludes ECG synchronization[8] (Figure 7-59). Conventional imaging using turboFLASH can demonstrate this first-pass effect, but it is limited by compromises in either spatial coverage or temporal resolution (i.e., increasing the number of slices decreases temporal resolution).[24,35]

The area in which EPI of the heart may show the most promise is in producing a rapid series of images at multiple levels of the beating myocardium.[8] Gradient-echo techniques cannot produce multislice, high-resolution images without sacrificing temporal resolution, nor can they acquire images rapidly without sacrificing slices or spatial resolution. EPI, by producing images every 32 to 200 ms, avoids these compromises and makes available a time–versus–signal intensity series of the entire heart during the first pass of the contrast agent. In general the contrast of gradient echo–echo-planar images (GRE-EPI) is T2*-weighted. With this contrast after the rapid injection of a gadolinium chelate, EPI shows well-perfused areas as local transitory signal drops.[60] Alternately the EPI contrast can be modified with an inversion pulse (to add T1 weighting) and an SE-EPI readout that reduces some of the susceptibility effects of EPI.[13] The IR-SE-EPI method is a somewhat longer imaging method than T2*-weighted GRE-EPI (because the TI = 900 ms); however, it is adequate to allow depiction of rapid contrast changes. Spatial and temporal resolution with this method is sufficient to distinguish perfusion of the various subregions (subendocardial, midcardial, and subepicardial) of the left ventricular myocardium.

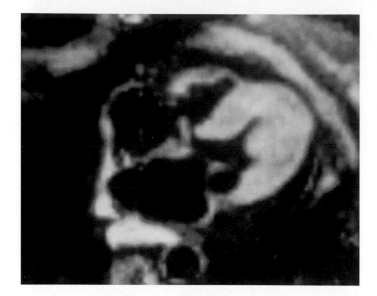

FIGURE 7-58   Single-shot SE EPI of the heart stops cardiac action.

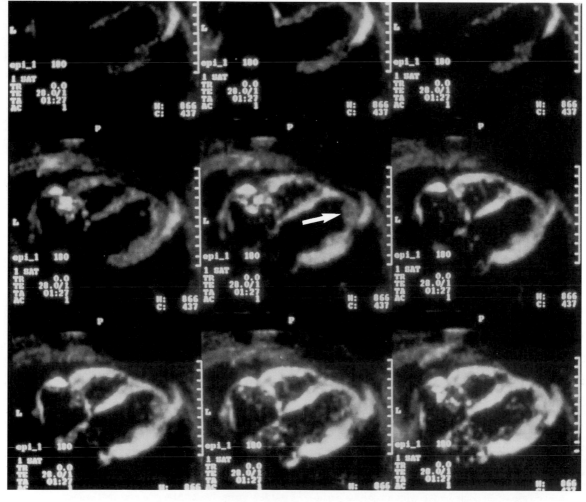

FIGURE 7-59   Serial IR-EPI postgadolinium images in a patient with LAD stenosis showing apical hypoperfusion *(arrow)*.

Similar to EPI in the brain, a rapid single-shot data acquisition of the heart allows for diffusion sensitization. Diffusion imaging of the heart is attractive in that it may provide information about ischemic changes at a cellular level and may lead to better understanding of the development and significance of muscle-fiber orientation. One study[14] demonstrated this diffusional anisotropy using EPI in combination with a stimulated-echo preparation to eliminate the substantial nearby chamber signal.[15]

There are numerous technical challenges associated with using EPI to visualize the beating heart, especially when attempting to produce fine spatial detail or gradient-induced diffusion weighting. For diffusion imaging, strong sensitizing gradients must be applied quickly to avoid gross motion and flow artifact. For imaging of the myocardium, locally pulsatile 3D flow may cause phase artifact that produces ghosting and smearing of the heart. "Black blood" imaging, with an SE preparation or a combination of invert-revert pulses,[12] can be used to re-

duce the flowing blood signal and improve image quality. Imaging of fine detail, especially during systole, is complicated by motion during the encoding of higher spatial features, resulting in blurring. Fat suppression, which is essential for EPI, is difficult in the heart because the local shim (and homogeneity) varies throughout the cardiac cycle. A lack of consistent fat suppression can also complicate visualization of coronary arteries, in which nearby pericardial signal blends with the bright blood signal.[34] Multishot EPI may be more useful for these applications in the heart as a result of a number of factors, including reduced susceptibility to fat-water misregistration[61] (Figure 7-60).

Abdominal Echo-Planar Imaging

Within the limit of one breath-hold, substantial progress has been made over the years with routine MRI of the abdomen.[16,33,49,51] Fast gradient-echo sequences with high flip angles have become routine for T1-weighted studies. GRASE, with its faster imaging potential, may prove beneficial in the abdomen.[18] For T2-weighted studies the rapid gradient-echo methods have not proved to be as useful. T2-weighted EPI[44,45] is a rapid technique that can scan the entire liver in as little as 2 sec (Figure 7-61). Saini et al[47] found that adequate T2-weighted, single-shot EPI examinations of focal hepatic lesions can be made, although the SNR and contrast must be optimized based on echo times (Figure 7-62). Single-shot EPI has difficulty imaging diamagnetic distortion from the bowel air–tissue interface and may have imperfect fat suppression because of respiratory motion and other air-tissue interfaces. HASTE[40] has demonstrated some advantages in this regard (Figure 7-63). Multishot EPI sequences have contrast comparable to that of CSE images, making the technique a potential replacement for conventional T2-weighted SE imaging of the liver. Given the rapid speed of acquisition,

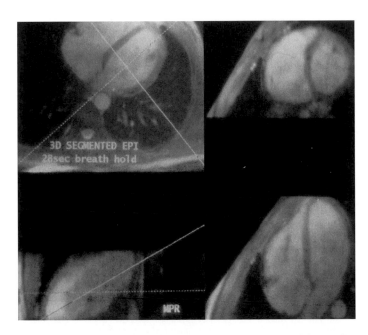

FIGURE 7-60   Breath-hold multishot 3D EPI of heart with multiplanar reformations. (Courtesy P. Wielopolski, Boston.)

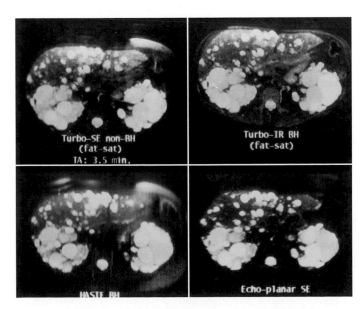

FIGURE 7-61   Sequence comparison, polycystic kidneys.

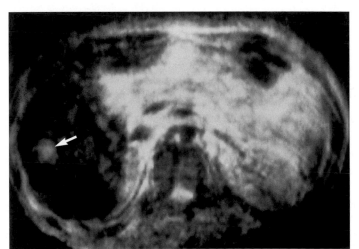
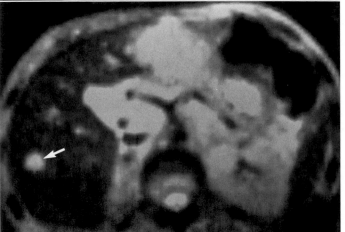

FIGURE 7-62   Cavernous hemangioma of the liver *(arrow).* **A,** A 13-min T2-weighted SE image showing motion artifact. **B,** A 200-ms T2-weighted SE EPI.

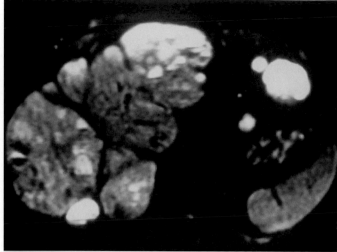

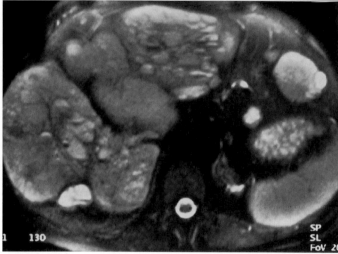

FIGURE 7-63   Neuroendocrine liver metastasis. **A,** STIR-EPI demonstrates central diamagnetic susceptibility signal loss caused by air in the stomach and bowel. **B,** HASTE gives a much better image because of decreased sensitivity to susceptibility effects.

single-shot EPI may prove useful in the assessment of diffusion[41] and perfusion[62,63] of abdominal organs, as well as visualization of flow in major vessels. With single-shot EPI, fetal anatomy has been observed with detail sufficient to identify anomalies.[38]

REFERENCES

1. Atkinson DJ, Burstein D, and Edelmann RR: First pass cardiac perfusion: evaluation with ultrafast MR imaging: preliminary observations, Radiology 174:757, 1990.
2. Atkinson DJ, and Edelman RR: Cineangiography of the heart in a single breath-hold with a segmented turboFLASH sequence, Radiology 178:359, 1991.
3. Bradley WG: Fast spin echo. In Bradley WG, and Bydder GM, eds: Advanced MR imaging techniques, London, 1997,Martin Dunitz.
4. Bradley WG, Chen D-Y, and Atkinson DJ: Using high performance gradients. In Bradley WG, and Bydder GM, eds: Advanced MR imaging techniques, London, 1997, Martin Dunitz.
5. Butts K, et al: Interleaved echo-planar imaging on a standard MRI system, Magn Reson Med 31:67, 1994.
6. Chien D, Goldman A, and Edelman RR: High speed black blood imaging of vessel stenosis in the presence of pulsatile flow, J Magn Reson Imaging 2:437, 1992.
7. Chrispin A, Small P, Rutter N, et al: Echo-planar imaging of normal and abnormal connections of the great vessels, Pediatr Radiol 16:289, 1986.
8. Davis CP, et al: Normal heart: evaluation with echo-planar MR imaging, Radiology 191:691, 1994.
9. DeLaPaz RL: Echo-planar imaging, Radiographics 14:1045, 1994.
10. Dubin MD, et al: Conspicuity of tumors of the head and neck on fat suppressed MR images: T2-weighted fast spin echo versus contrast enhanced T1-weighted conventional spin echo sequences, Am J Roentgenol 164:1213, 1995.
11. Ebisu T, et al: Hemorrhagic and nonhemorrhagic stroke: diagnosis with diffusion-weighted and T2-weighted echo-planar MR imaging, Radiology 203:823, 1997.
12. Edelman RR, Chien D, and Kim D: Fast selective black blood imaging, Radiology 181:655, 1991.
13. Edelman RR, and Li W: Contrast enhanced echo-planar MR imaging of myocardial perfusion: preliminary study in humans, Radiology 190:771, 1994.
14. Edelman RR, Wielopolski R, and Schmitt F: Echo-planar imaging, Radiology 192:600, 1994.
15. Edelman RR, et al: In vivo measurement of water diffusion in the human heart, Magn Res Med 32:L423, 1994.
16. Edelman RR, et al: Segmented turboFLASH: a method for breath-hold MR imaging of the liver with flexible contrast, Radiology 177:515, 1990.
17. Feinberg DA: MRI with variable encoding time (VET), Magn Reson Med 38:7, 1997.
18. Feinberg DA, Kiefer B, and Johnson G: GRASE imaging improves spatial resolution in single shot imaging, Magn Reson Med 33:529, 1995.
19. Feinberg DA, and Oshio K: GRASE (gradient- and spin-echo) MR imaging: a new fast clinical imaging technique, Radiology 181:597, 1991.
20. Ginsberg MD: The new language of cerebral ischemia, Am J Neuroradiol 18:1435, 1997.
21. Hashemi RH, et al: Suspected multiple sclerosis: MR imaging with a thin-section fast FLAIR pulse sequence, Radiology 196:505, 1995.
22. Henkelman RM, et al: Why fat is bright in RARE and fast spin echo imaging, J Magn Reson Imaging 2:533, 1992.
23. Hennig J, Nauerth A, and Friedburg H: RARE imaging: a fast imaging method for clinical MR, Magn Reson Med 3:823, 1986.
24. Higgins CB, et al: Measurement of blood flow and perfusion in the cardiovascular system, Invest Radiol 27(Suppl 2):S66, 1992.
25. Johnson BA, et al: Evaluation of shared-view acquisition using repeated echoes (SHARE): a dual echo fast spin echo MR technique, Am J Neuroradiol 15:667, 1994.
27. Jolesz RA, and Jones KM: Fast spin echo imaging of the brain, Top Magn Reson Imaging 5:1, 1993.
28. Jones KM, et al: Fast spin echo MR in the detection of vertebral metastases: comparison of three sequences, Am J Neuroradiol 15:401, 1994.
29. Kapelov SR, et al: Bone contusions of the knee: increased lesion detection with fast spin echo MR imaging with spectroscopic fat saturation, Radiology 189:901, 1993.
30. Kucharczyk J, et al: Echo-planar perfusion sensitive MR imaging of acute cerebral ischemia, Radiology 188:711, 1993.
31. Kucharczyk W, et al: Detection of pituitary microadenomas: comparison of dynamic keyhole fast spin echo, unenhanced, and conventional contrast-enhanced MR imaging, Am J Roentgenol 163:671, 1994.
32. Loncur M, et al: Non-slab interleaved 3D fast spin echo imaging of the brain and spine, Book of abstracts, Fourth Annual Meeting ISMRM, New York, April 27-May 3, 1996.
33. Low RN, et al: Fast spin echo MR imaging of the abdomen: contrast optimization and artifact reduction, J Magn Reson Imaging 4:637, 1994.
34. Manning WJ, Li W, and Edelman RR: A preliminary report comparing magnetic resonance coronary angiography with conventional angiography, N Engl J Med 328:828, 1993.
35. Manning WJ, et al: First pass NMR imaging studies using gadolinium-DTPA in patients with coronary artery disease, J Am Coll Cardiol 18:959, 1991.
36. Mansfield P: Multi-planar image formation using NMR spin echoes, J Phys Chem 10:L55, 1977.
37. Mansfield P, and Pykett IL: Biological and medical imaging by NMR, J Magn Reson 29:355, 1978.
38. Mansfield P, et al: Echo-planar imaging of the human fetus at 0.5 T, Br J Radiol 63:833, 1990.
39. McVeigh ER, and Atalar E: Cardiac tagging with breath-held cine MRI, Magn Reson Med 28:318, 1992.
40. Miyazaki T, et al: MR cholangiopancreatography using HASTE (half-Fourier acquisition single shot turbo spin echo) sequences, Am J Roentgenol 166:1297, 1996.
41. Mueller MF, et al: Abdominal diffusion mapping with use of a whole body echo-planar system, Radiology 190:475, 1994.
42. Oshio K, and Feinberg DA: GRASE (gradient- and spin-echo) imaging: a novel fast MRI technique, Magn Reson Med 20:344, 1991.
43. Pierpaoli C, et al: Diffusion tensor MR imaging of the human brain, Radiology 201:637, 1996.
44. Reimer P, et al: Clinical application of abdominal echo-planar imaging (EPI): optimization using a retrofitted EPI system, J Comput Assist Tomogr 18:673, 1994.

45. Reimer P, et al: Initial feasibility studies using single shot EPI for the detection of focal liver lesions, Magn Reson Med 32:733, 1994.
46. Rzedzian RR, and Pykett IL: Instant images of the human heart using a new, whole body MR imaging system, Am J Roentgenol 149:245, 1987.
47. Saini S, et al: Echo-planar MR imaging of the liver in patients with focal hepatic lesions: quantitative analysis of images made with various pulse sequences, Am J Roentgenol 163:1389, 1994.
48. Santyr GE: Magnetization transfer effect in multislice MR imaging, Magn Reson Imaging 11:521, 1993.
49. Semelka RC, et al: T1-weighted sequences for MR imaging of the liver: comparison of three techniques for single breath-held, whole volume acquisition at 1.0 and 1.5 T, Radiology 180:629, 1991.
50. Sorensen AG, et al: Hyperacute stroke: evaluation with combined multi section diffusion weighted and hemodynamically weighted echo-planar imaging, Radiology 199:1996.
51. Stark DD, Fahlvik AK, and Klaveness J: Abdominal imaging, J Magn Reson Imaging 3:285, 1993.
52. Stehling MK, Turner R, and Mansfield P: Echo-planar imaging: MRI in a fraction of a second, Science 254:43, 1991.
53. Tartaglino LM, et al: Metallic artifacts on MR images of the postoperative spine: reduction with fast spin echo techniques, Radiology 190:565, 1994.
54. Twieg DB: The k-trajectory formulation of the NMR imaging process with applications in analysis and synthesis of imaging methods, Med Phys 10:610, 1983.
55. Unterweger M, et al: Cardiac volumetry: comparison of echo-planar and conventional cine-MR data acquisition strategies, Invest Radiol 29:994, 1994.
56. Waluch V, and Bradley WG: NMR even echo rephasing in slow laminar flow, J Comput Assist Tomogr 8:594, 1984.
57. Weber DM: Echo-planar imaging: monograph, Milwaukee, 1993, GE Medical Systems.
58. Wehrli FW: Principles of magnetic resonance. In Stark DD, and Bradley WG, editors: Magnetic resonance imaging, ed 2, St Louis, 1992, Mosby.
59. Weinberger E, et al: Nontraumatic pediatric musculoskeletal MR imaging: comparison of conventional and fast spin echo short inversion time inversion recovery technique, Radiology 194:721, 1995.
60. Wendland MF, et al: Echo-planar MR imaging of normal and ischemic myocardium with gadolinium injection, Radiology 186:535, 1993.
61. Wetter DR, et al: Cardiac echo-planar MR imaging: comparison single and multi-shot techniques, Radiology 194:765, 1995.
62. Wielopolski PA, et al: Breath-hold 3D STAR angiography of the renal arteries using segmented echo-planar imaging, Magn Reson Med 32:433, 1995.
63. Wolf GL, et al: Measurement of renal transit of Gd-DTPA with echo-planar imaging, J Magn Reson Imaging 4:365, 1994.
64. Wood ML: Fourier imaging. In Stark DD, and Bradley WG, eds: Magnetic resonance imaging, ed 2, St Louis, 1992, Mosby.
65. Yuh WTC: Cerebral infarction: current status of imaging and future directions, Radiology 205(P):62, 1997.

8 Fat and Water Signal Separation Methods

Jerzy Szumowski and Jack H. Simon

Fat Signal in Magnetic Resonance Images
   Chemical Shift
   Proton Density
   Relaxation Times
   Strong Signal
Fat Signal Artifacts in Magnetic Resonance Images
   Chemical-Shift Misregistration Artifacts
   Frequency-encoding axis
   Slice-selection axis
   Phase-encoding axis
   Phase-Cancellation Intensity Artifacts
   Motion Artifacts
Fat and Water Signal-Separation Methods
   T1 Relaxation Methods
   Chemical-Shift Methods
   Selective excitation chemical-shift imaging
   SELECTIVE EXCITATION OF FAT
   SELECTIVE EXCITATION OF WATER
   Phase-sensitive methods
   2-POINT DIXON
   3-POINT DIXON
Practical Implementations of the Phase-Sensitive Methods
   Phase Unwrapping
   Data Acquisition Time
   Fast Spin Echo
   Gradient-Echo Sequences
   Mid Fields
Review of Clinical Applications
   T1-Weighted Contrast
   T1-Weighted Imaging with Paramagnetic Contrast
   T2-Weighted Contrast
   Gradient-Echo Opposed-Phase Imaging
   Chemical Specificity
   Quantitative chemical-shift imaging
   Optimization of Clinical Technique
Summary

 KEY POINTS

- Fat and water can be separated on the basis of differences in their T1 relaxation times or resonance frequencies.
- STIR sequences null the signal from fat based on its T1 relaxation time.
- Preliminary spectral saturation pulses can be used to null either fat (FatSat) or water (WaterSat) based on differences in resonance frequencies.
- The difference in resonance frequencies between fat and water causes them to precess at different rates following an initial 90-degree (or other nutating) RF pulse. Thus, although fat and water are in phase when they start to precess, they become 180 degrees out of phase at a certain TE after the 90-degree pulse and, at twice that TE, they regain phase coherence.
- By adding or subtracting the in-phase and out-of-phase images, "water only" or "fat only" images can be generated (Dixon technique).

Suppression of fat signal in magnetic resonance (MR) images extends the dynamic range of tissue contrast, eliminates the strong interfering signal of fat on T1-weighted postgadolinium (Gd) images, removes chemical-shift artifacts, and decreases motion-related ghost

artifacts.[1] These advantages helped establish a proven, decade-long record of clinical diagnostic applications for fat-suppression magnetic resonance imaging (MRI) methods.[27,44,52] Indications for these methods, frequently called *chemical-shjift imaging (CSI) methods,** have been demonstrated in many reports describing enhanced diagnostic content of fat-suppressed images.[112,127] Clinical indications have been reported for sites throughout the body, including the head and neck,[50,130] orbits,[5,55,66,106] breast,[41,58,61,98] heart,[15] spine,[9,12,37,60,120] abdomen,[81,82,87,104] liver,[52,82,102,116] prostate,[128] pelvis,[103,117] kidney,[83,101] shoulder,[35,93] hip,[80] knee,[49,133] muscle,[57,85] and bone marrow.[18,89,96,113,132] Moreover, the importance of fat suppression is further amplified by the growing use of fast spin-echo (SE) sequences, proliferation of low-field scanners, and emergence of echo-planar imaging (EPI), in which artifact-free image reconstruction is essential.[22,100,143]

The fat-suppression approach increases the conspicuity of many pathological processes and is diagnostically very valuable, providing that uniform and adequate suppression of fat signal can be achieved in routine clinical imaging (Figures 8-1 and 8-2). Reports describing clinical applications and presenting the many potential advantages of fat-suppressed MRI also emphasize the challenge of obtaining uniform fat-signal suppression and point to the potential confusion caused by inadequately performed imaging procedures.[4,82,117,138] A recent assessment of fat-suppression technology available at 1.5 Tesla (T) fields concluded that despite the existence of well-accepted clinical applications for fat-suppressed MRI, many radiologists are reluctant to use the method because it tends to generate poor-quality images that are sometimes diagnostically confusing[32] (Figure 8-3). This problem is even more troublesome at mid and low fields, where current commercial techniques generally fail to deliver adequate fat suppression. These and similar effects lead many radiologists to avoid the fat-suppression technique altogether.[32]

The authors gratefully acknowledge Frederick Keller, MD, and the Radiology Department at OHSU for their continuing support. We are indebted to Steve Quinn, MD; Don Mitchell, MD; Graeme Bydder, MD; and Vincent Ho, MD; for useful discussion, suggestions, and encouragement. Special thanks go to Ellen Pelker for her excellent assistance in manuscript preparation and to Bernard Coombs, MD, PhD, and William Coshow, MSc, for their instrumental role in developing phase-sensitive methods and their help in acquiring the images presented in this chapter.

*CSI can be defined as an MRI technique that provides spectral resolution and some degree of spatial localization or anatomic resolution.[68] This broad definition has come to include a variety of techniques, ranging from fat and water separation to localized proton (^{1}H) or phosphorous (^{31}P) spectroscopy with data presentation in an image format (spectroscopic imaging). For example, the fat and water signal-separation methods are characterized by a spatial resolution comparable to conventional MRI yet still providing chemical-shift information.

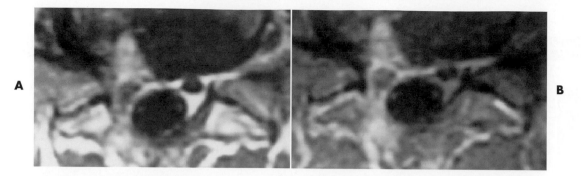

FIGURE 8-1   Epidural fibrosis. Fat-suppression imaging combined with gadolinium-contrast imaging of postoperative lumbar spine. **A,** On the conventional T1-weighted post-contrast-enhanced image, the contribution of scar and its boundaries are uncertain. Fat suppression achieved using commercially available frequency-selective pulse.**B,** On the post-contrast-enhanced fat-suppression series, epidural fibrosis (right ventral sac surrounding root sleeve) is hyperintense to vessels and normal fat in left ventral space.

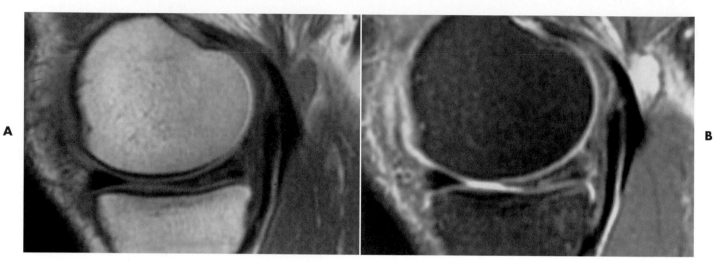

FIGURE 8-2   Meniscal tear. Proton-density, SE sagittal images of the left knee in a 62-year-old man. **A,** Without fat suppression, marrow fat and adjacent adipose tissue are hyperintense or bright. **B,** With fat saturation, the marrow fat and adjacent adipose tissue appear hypointense. Note the tear in the posterior horn of the medial meniscus and the incidental Baker's cyst. (Courtesy Drs. Paul Russ and Donna Callen.)

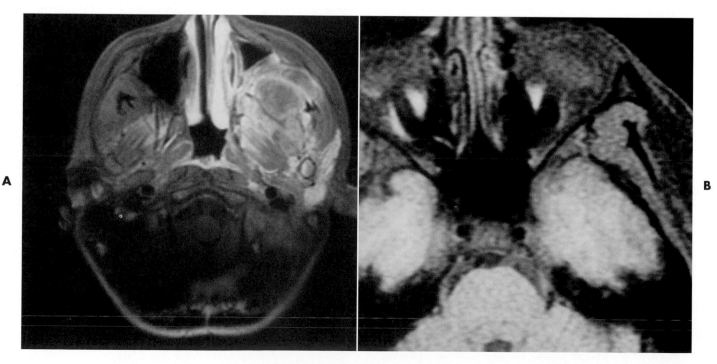

FIGURE 8-3   Magnetic field inhomogeneities. **A,** Spatial variation of fat-signal suppression and artifactual elimination of water signal. **B,** Gadolinium-enhanced image of the orbits shows susceptibility changes at air-tissue interfaces create areas of unsuppressed fat signal, which may mimic an enhancing lesion.[33] (From reference 123.)

At present there appears to be serious disparity between the scope of potential diagnostic benefits of a fat suppression approach and the breadth of actual clinical use. Fortunately, this disparity has created a renewed research interest in fat-suppression technology and provided an impetus for the development of reliable fat-suppression methods. In this chapter we review the relevant features of MRI fat signal, the current techniques for fat suppression, general clinical advantages of fat-suppressed MRI, the disadvantages of currently used techniques, and the benefits of the new forthcoming methodology.

FAT SIGNAL IN MAGNETIC RESONANCE IMAGES

In conventional in vivo ^{1}H MRI the major contribution to the detectable MR signal originates from water protons and from methylene protons in triglycerides ($[-CH_2-]_n$), with much smaller contributions from less abundant lipid protons, such as terminal methyl $[-CH_3]$ or vinyl [HC=CH] groups.[29] Because of the predominance of methylene protons, fat is often characterized by a single signal component resonating at a frequency 3.5 parts per million (ppm), downfield from the water resonance. This effect is called the *chemical shift*.[1,127]

Chemical Shift

At a given field strength B_0, nuclei resonate at frequency γ_0, described by the Larmor equation as follows:

(EQ. 1)

$$v_0 = \gamma\, B_0$$

where γ is the gyromagnetic ratio, a constant for a given nucleus (γ = 42.576 million hertz per Tesla [MHz/T] for protons).[1]

This equation implies a unique linear relationship between field strength and resonance frequency. However, electrons surrounding the nucleus and electrons from adjacent or nearby atoms alter the local magnetic field (Figure 8-4), resulting in a specific alteration in resonance frequency δv, called the *chemical shift*.

(EQ. 2)

$$\delta v = \sigma v_0$$

where σ is the dimensionless shielding constant.

The shielding constant ($\sigma = B_{loc}/B_0$) is typically on the order of a few parts per million relative to the strength of the external magnetic field B_0 and varies with the position of the nucleus in the molecule. Resulting resonance frequencies of different nuclei are customarily displayed relative to highly shielded reference nuclei, whose reference frequency is set to 0 ppm (e.g., tetramethylsilane).[10] Using this convenient scale, which is independent of magnetic field strength B_0, water [$-OH$] protons resonate at 4.7 ppm and methylene $[-CH_2-]_n$ protons of fatty acids at 1.2 ppm.[141]

On the other hand, the frequency shift of the resonance lines, measured in frequency units, depends on the magnetic field B_0 and increases with the operational frequency of the MR scanner. At 1.5 T, where γ_0 is 63.89 MHz, the chemical shift between water and fat methylene protons is approximately 225 Hz (3.5 ppm × 64 MHz = 225 Hz), whereas at 0.35 T the chemical-shift difference is only 52 Hz. This chemical shift provides a basis for distinguishing the contribution of chemically distinct protons in both spectroscopy and CSI.

Proton Density

Proton density is a nuclear magnetic resonance (NMR) term that refers to the number of MR-detectable protons in a volume of tissue. In conventional in vivo ^{1}H MRI the major contribution to the detectable MR signal originates from two sources—tissue water, present in a concentration less than or equal to 55 moles per liter of tissue, and fat protons. The relative ratio of fat to water in normal tissues, as determined by analytical chemistry methods, shows considerable variation, which depends on the tissue or organ of origin. For example, subcutaneous fat has a fat content (percent of fat by wet weight) of 77%, whereas lean skeletal muscle and liver have a fat content in the range of 5% to 10% wet weight. The fat-to-water ratios vary in healthy individuals as a result of factors such as diet and also vary as a result of pathological conditions. Skeletal-muscle fat content increases with muscular atrophy, and liver fat content increases up to 40% to 50% with fatty infiltration of the liver.[2]

Although in MRI fat is often thought of as a single signal component, the detectable signal is a composite of a larger number of distinct chemical contributions. These include the major contribution from protons in the methylene group $[-CH_2-]_n$, which are a component of long-chain fatty acids. These fatty-acid residues form the side chains of the triglyceride molecule. Smaller contributions from less abundant fatty protons include the terminal methyl $[-CH_3]$ and vinyl $[-HC=CH-]$ groups, also found in fatty acids, and the choline $[N-(CH_3)_2]$-derived signal, principally from phosphatidyl choline.[2,29,72,73]

Hydrogen protons associated with metabolites, such as lactate, and N-acetyl aspartate (NAA) also may contribute to the MR signal but are present in millimolar concentrations, a factor of 10^{-4} to 10^{-5} relative to water. The low concentration of the metabolites and less abundant fatty protons preclude their observation by standard MRI methods. They can be detected, however, using spectroscopic methods that suppress the dominant water or fat signals.[11,76,142]

Relaxation Times

A high concentration of protons is a necessary but insufficient requirement to ensure their detection by MRI. Myelin lipids, for example, make up as much as 70% of the dry weight of brain, yet the majority of the protons in these lipids do not contribute directly to the MR signal in normal brain images. This is because most of the lipid in myelin is "immobile" within highly structured membranes, with a characteristic very short T2 relaxation time on the order of microseconds (10^{-3} times shorter than the T2 of other lipids).[36] These very short T2 times preclude the observation of the lipid signals by MR methods. Spins with a sufficiently long T2 that are observable by MRI are by convention referred to as *mobile protons*.[17]

The MR signal intensity from a volume element of tissue reflects the water and lipid proton concentrations and the respective spin-lattice and spin-spin relaxation properties for the two components. Human fat is characterized by spin-lattice relaxation times (T1) that are short compared with those of other tissues. Representative values for the T1 of fat may be 280 ms at 1.5 T and 200 ms at 0.5 T. Spin-spin relaxation times (T2) for fat have been reported in the range of 50 to 170 ms, depending on the method of measurement and tissue origin[14,62,74] (Table 8-1).

Strong Signal

The short T1, combined with intermediate T2 for fat, results in a bright fat signal on most clinically relevant SE pulse sequences, regardless of

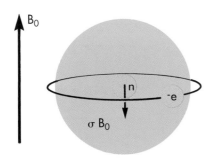

$$B = B_0 - \sigma B_0 = B_0\,(1 - \sigma)$$

FIGURE 8-4   Origin of the chemical shift. Electrons *(-e)* of an atom precess around the direction of the external magnetic field *(B₀)*. This spinning motion of electrons produces an additional local magnetic field *(σB₀)*, experienced by the nucleus *(n)*, with the shielding constant σ specific to the molecular structure. The effective field B experienced by the nucleus differs from that of the external field B_0 by the amount σB_0. The resulting alteration of the resonance frequency δv ($\delta v = \gamma \sigma B_0$), called the *chemical shift*, provides a mechanism for separating the contribution of chemically different nuclei to the MR spectrum.

the repetition time/echo time (TR/TE) combination.[127] The dominance of the fat signal is especially strong for T1-weighted sequences, where it can be a major source of contrast (Figure 8-5). Such a strong signal of fat in the SE sequences can be fully explained using a simple model based on fat relaxation times. However, this approach cannot explain the phenomenon of unusually bright fat signal on T2-weighted fast SE images. As fast SEs are used increasingly to obtain T2-weighted images in times much shorter than those for standard SE sequences, the increased signal of fat has attracted a great deal of attention.[23] The origin of the increased signal of fat on T2-weighted images has been ascribed to a lengthening of the apparent T2 of fat by diffusion, exchange effects, and stimulated echoes, in addition to the removal of scalar-coupling-mediated modulation of echo amplitude in the echo train of fast SE sequences.[146]

Occasionally the bright fat signal might be diagnostically useful; in imaging the neck, for example, fat planes can be helpful in assessing lymphadenopathy. But more often a strong fat signal can obscure the often subtle contrast between tissues of interest. Elimination of the strong fat signal component of the images allows for more efficient use of the full dynamic range of the gray scale for image filming and display of images on the MR monitor. In addition, the elimination of fat signal from an image increases tissue contrast, providing a more effective display of pathology (Figure 8-6), as is further discussed later in this chapter.

FAT SIGNAL ARTIFACTS IN MAGNETIC RESONANCE IMAGES

The combination of both fat and water protons within the tissue of interest and the generally strong signal from fat can cause problems in conventional MRI. These problems include chemical-shift spatial mis-

Table 8-1   Tissue Parameters at 1.5 Tesla

TISSUE	T1 (ms)	T2 (ms)	PROTON DENSITY (RELATIVE)
Cerebrospinal fluid	3000	2200	1.00
Vertebral bone marrow	554	50	0.80
Vertebral disk	934	90	0.80
Spinal cord	700	90	0.75
Gray matter	955	95	0.90
White matter	585	85	0.75
Fat	284	50	0.90
Muscle	758	45	0.75
Tumor	1300	150	1.00

From reference 42.

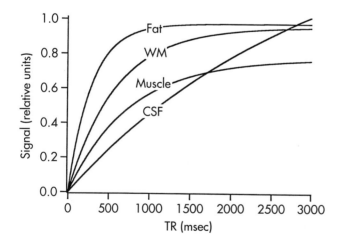

FIGURE 8-5   Relative MR signal intensities of various tissues as a function of repetition time (TR). Data were calculated based on the equation for an SE sequence,[55] using the relaxation times and proton-density values from Table 8-1 and based on an echo delay time (TE) of 20 ms. Note the dominance of the fat signal under these imaging conditions. *WM,* White matter; *CSF,* cerebrospinal fluid.

registration artifacts (CSMAs) in the frequency, slice, and phase directions and a variety of intensity and motion artifacts.

Chemical-Shift Misregistration Artifacts

In conventional two-dimensional (2D) spin-warp MRI,[31] an image is created through the selection of a slice and the spatial encoding of signals from this slice in the phase and frequency directions, followed by Fourier transformation of the raw data. By virtue of chemical shift, in each of these steps fat and water magnetizations behave differently and are mapped differently in the final image.

The frequency (chemical) shift between water and fat resonances can appear in an image as a spatial mismapping of the two components. The magnitude (distance) of spatial shift depends on the specific combination of imaging factors, including strength of the magnetic field, bandwidth of the slice-selective pulses, strength of the magnetic field gradients, data-sampling bandwidth, and voxel dimensions. These spatial misrepresentations, the so-called CSMAs, are easily visualized and best understood in the frequency-encoding direction.[8,26,114] Less generally understood and appreciated is the occurrence of CSMA in the slice-select direction[40,56,59,92,139] and in the phase-encoding direction in EPI.[22,76,99]

Frequency-Encoding Axis. During data acquisition, the MR signal is acquired in the presence of a frequency-encoding gradient. This frequency-encoding gradient G_x (also called the *readout gradient*) forces water-proton spins located at a position X_w along the frequency-encoding axis to precess with a frequency v_w, which is linearly dependent on position as follows:

(EQ. 3)

$$v_w = \gamma G_x X_w$$

The precessional frequency of fat spins v_f originating at an identical position differs by the chemical shift δv between the water and fat resonances. Because the major spectral component $[-CH2-]_n$ of the fat protons resonates at a lower frequency than water, the fat spins precess less rapidly than water spins by the chemical shift δv.

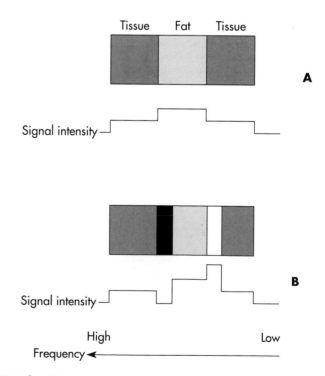

FIGURE 8-6   CSMAs in the frequency-encoding direction. A typical anatomical pattern is demonstrated in which fatty tissue is "sandwiched" between more waterlike tissues. **A,** In the absence of CSMA the signal-intensity pattern would appear as shown by signal-intensity profile. **B,** In the reconstructed image, which includes the effect of CSMA, fat is artifactually shifted along the frequency axis toward the position of decreased frequency, leaving a dark band (empty-appearing voxels) on one side and a bright band of increased signal in voxels on the other side, as a result of superimposition of fat and water signals.

(EQ. 4)

$$v_F = \gamma G_x X_w - \delta v$$

After Fourier transformation, fat in an image is mapped into an apparent position X_F.

(EQ. 5)

$$X_F = (v_w - \delta v)/\gamma G_x$$

The resultant mismapping Δx, the CSMA from the original spatial position of the fat spins, is therefore given by

(EQ. 6)

$$\Delta x = X_w - X_F = \delta v/\gamma G_x$$

From Equation 6 we can see that the CSMA magnitude increases with the chemical shift and therefore with magnetic field strength B_0 but becomes smaller when the readout gradient is increased. These dependencies must be taken into consideration as we attempt to influence the signal-to-noise ratio (SNR) in images by optimizing the bandwidth of data acquisition or by imaging in higher field strengths.[24,64,81,108] To demonstrate this relationship, Equation 6 can be rewritten using imaging parameters that are normally accessible to the MR-scanner operator. The field of view in the frequency direction FOV_x, the bandwidth BW of data acquisition, and the readout gradient G_x are related through the following formula:

(EQ. 7)

$$BW = \gamma FOV_x G_x$$

FOV in turn can be expressed as a product of the number of pixels N_x in the frequency direction and the pixel size dx:

(EQ. 8)

$$FOV = N_x dx$$

Finally, the formula for CSMA measured in pixels ($\Delta x/dx$) can be rewritten using these basic imaging parameters, as follows:

(EQ. 9)

$$\Delta x/dx = (\delta v/BW)N_x$$

For example, using typical technical factors BW = 32 kHz and N_x = 256 on a system operating at 1.5 T, CSMA results in a 1.8-pixel displacement of fat relative to water. At the same bandwidth but at a field strength of 0.35 T, the CSMA would be only a small fraction of a pixel and would not be detected (Figure 8-9).

Because the SNR in MRI depends inversely on the square root of the data acquisition bandwidth BW[53,54,137]:

(EQ. 10)

$$SNR \sim 1/(BW)1/2$$

SNR can therefore be improved by a decrease in bandwidth. Such a decrease, however, would result in an increase in CSMA. Halving the bandwidth to achieve a $\sqrt{2}$ improvement in SNR would double the CSMA to a more noticeable 3.6 pixels on the 1.5 T system.

CSMAs are most apparent at fat—water interfaces, which are common throughout the body.[5,25,111,116] These artifacts appear as low- or high-intensity bands that occur parallel to the interface (Figures 8-6 and 8-7), with fat displaced in the frequency-encoding direction toward the lower frequencies when the system frequency is set to water. Bandwidth reduction to achieve increased SNR (at constant scan time) or to reduce scan time must be balanced against the potential disadvantages of increased CSMAs—a reduction in resolution and a requirement for an increased echo delay time.[33,53,137] The last two factors may be clinically insignificant.[34,64,108] However, CSMA can be a limiting factor in reduced-bandwidth MRI, particularly in lipid-rich regions. Studies of the orbit,[106] the abdomen, and the pelvis[81,104] suggest possible advantages of combining fat-signal suppression and reduced-bandwidth techniques. By combining these two methods, images can be acquired using reduced bandwidth for improved SNR and CSI for accuracy of detail and preferred contrast patterns without CSMA limitations.

Slice-Selection Axis. The 2D spin-warp MRI process is initiated with a limited-bandwidth, radiofrequency (RF) excitation pulse executed in the presence of a slice-selection gradient G_z. As a result of chemical shift δv, spatial mismapping of fat protons occurs in the slice-selection direction, analogous to the CSMA γx in the frequency-encoding direction (Figure 8-8). The difference Δz of spatial locations of fat and water slices is given by:

(EQ. 11)

$$\Delta z = \delta v/\gamma G_z$$

Because a slice thickness dz depends on the bandwidth of the excitation pulse bw and strength of the slice-selection gradient G_z,

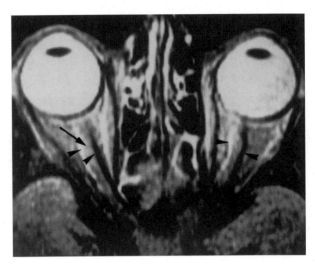

FIGURE 8-7   CSMA in the frequency-encoding direction. SE 2000/80 axial image of the orbits acquired with 16 kHz bandwidth. Upon image reconstruction, fat signal is shifted toward the patient's right side. This shift results in superimposition of the signal on one side of the optical nerve and lack of the signal on the other side. Note large CSMA (3.6 pixels) as a result of the lower-than-standard bandwidth (BW) of data acquisition.

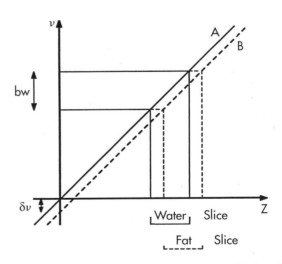

FIGURE 8-8   CSMA in the slice-selection direction. An application of a slice-selection G_z gradient causes a distribution of resonance frequencies along the slice-selection axis. In this gradient field, water protons precess at frequency v_w = $\gamma G_z z$, indicated by line A. Fat protons precess at frequency $v_F = \gamma G_z Z - \delta v$, line B. The RF excitation pulse with the limited bandwidth (bw) applied in the presence of the slice-select gradient excites a specific range of frequencies giving rise to a "water" slice along the z axis. The range of excited frequencies is the same for fat protons; however, these correspond to a position shifted along the slice axis, giving rise to a different (shifted) "fat" slice. The magnitude of the shift is inversely proportional to the pulse bandwidth (bw). Note that slopes of lines A and B are the same because they are determined by γG_z, and this results in the same slice thickness dz = bw/(γG_z) for both chemical species.

(EQ. 12)

$$dz = bw/\gamma G_z$$

Therefore CSMA in the slice-selection direction, measured in units of slice thickness, can be rewritten using these imaging parameters as follows:

(EQ. 13)

$$\Delta z/dz = \delta v/bw$$

For example, at 1.5 T, where the chemical shift is 225 Hz, and a typical slice-select RF pulse excitation bandwidth bw is 1250 Hz, the displacement in the slice-selection direction Δz is only 18% of the slice thickness dz (Figure 8-9). The CSMA offset in the slice direction is relatively small under these conditions, and its appearance in images is less obvious than CSMA in the frequency-encoding direction. Only a couple of clinical manifestations of this effect have been described, such as misregistration of calvarial fatty marrow mimicking bilateral sub-

dural hematomas in upper and lower renal poles and CSMA mimicking a low-signal mass in the renal hilum.[56,139] Because this artifact is common in the abdomen and occasionally mimics a pathological condition, awareness of its occurrence and appearance should help avoid confusing it with disease.

Phase-Encoding Axis. There is no observable CSMA in the phase-encoding direction in spin-warp imaging, for reasons that may not be immediately obvious. The purpose of phase encoding is to differentiate spins along the phase-encoding y axis. In the standard spin-warp data acquisition method, phase encoding is accomplished by exposing spins to the phase-encoding gradient Gy for a given time T. In the presence of this gradient the rate of spin precession is altered such that at the end of the period T, spins will have acquired phase, which depends on their location along the y axis (i.e., the spin-warp method of spatial encoding).[31] The collection of each line of raw data is separated by one repetition period TR, and the strength of the gradient is changed gradually for each phase-encoding step, providing a unique accumulation of phase for a given position (Figure 8-10).

In each step of spin-warp imaging the phase acquired by fatty protons differs from water protons in the same location as a result of the effect of chemical shift δv. The resulting extra phase of fat spins (δvT) relative to water is not cumulative, however, but is the same for each phase-encoding step yielding the same phase-encoding differences for each location along the y axis for both species. Because the phase difference is the actual data taken into account by Fourier transformation in this direction, no misregistration in the phase-encoding direction occurs in the spin-warp image.[127]

The method of spatial encoding in the phase direction is different in the EPI technique,[22,31,75,144] where all lines of raw data are acquired immediately after the RF excitation. In this method, data generation is very rapid and requires a high data-sampling bandwidth on the order of hundreds of kilohertz. Because of this high bandwidth, CSMA in the frequency-encoding direction is negligible, as can be seen in Equation 9. However, the effective bandwidth of data acquisition in a phase-encoding direction is very low, and this effect gives rise to a large chemical-shift artifact in this direction.

This effect can be demonstrated using an example of an actual implementation of the echo-planar method. In this acquisition technique, each line of 128 (N_x) raw data points is acquired in 500 μs so that the nominal bandwidth per pixel (BW/N_x) is approximately 2000 Hz.[22,31,144] Because this bandwidth far exceeds the fat and water chemical shift of 225 Hz at 1.5 T, spatial misregistration is not apparent in the images along the readout axis. The total scan time for this sequence is a multiple of N_y (the number of phase-encoding steps, e.g., 64) and the time re-

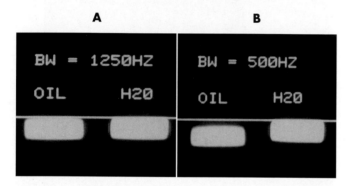

FIGURE 8-9   CSMA in the slice-selection direction. The effect of CSMA in this direction can be demonstrated by imaging the signal intensities through the thickness of the slice (slice-profile imaging). Vials containing oil and water were imaged at 1.5 T, with a modified pulse sequence in which the readout gradient is applied in the slice-selection direction, which results in an image of the slice profile. In these images the vertical axis is in the slice-seleciton direction, and the horizontal axis is in the phase-encoding direction. The images were acquired using the nominal 1250 Hz bandwidth (BW) for the RF pulse in **A** and a modified bandwidth to 500 Hz in **B**. According to Equation 13 the CSMA is 18% and 45% of the slice thickness in **A** and **B**, respectively. The horizontal white line is for reference only. Note a shift in the position of the oil slice relative to water, particularly in **B**.

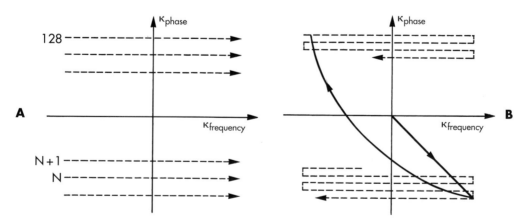

FIGURE 8-10   κ-Space trajectory. The term κ *space* is often used to describe an array of MRI raw data. The space is filled by the data during signal acquisition. The actual method of filling the κ space is called the κ-*space trajectory.* MRI spatial-encoding schemes can be characterized by their trajectories. **A,** 2D spin-warp imaging: κ-space trajectory. In this method each line of the raw data set is collected after the sequence TR. The phase acquired in the N+1 phase-encoding step is independent of the phase acquired in the previous step *(N)*, and therefore phase advances caused by the chemical shift do not accumulate in this scan. **B,** 2D EPI: κ-space trajectory. In this method the MR raw data space is traversed in a rasterlike pattern. All the spatial encoding, including phase and frequency, is performed in one scan after a single RF pulse. Phase encoding for each line in the κ space immediately follows the previous one. Phase advances caused by the chemical-shift differences are therefore cumulative, as opposed to in the spin-warp method. This phase evolution results in a large chemical-shift artifact, which can be eliminated only by using fat-suppression techniques. The creation of the CSMA in the phase-encoding direction also can be understood by considering the bandwidth of data acquisition relative to the chemical-shift difference, as indicated in the text. (Courtesy Dr. Mark Cohen.)

quired to collect a single row of data totals 32 ms (500 μs × 64). Because the bandwidth of data acquisition is inversely proportional to total scan time, the effective bandwidth of data acquisition per pixel in the phase-encoding direction is only 31 Hz (1/32 ms/64). This is much smaller than the chemical shift, and as indicated by Equation 9 the CSMA in EPIs can be severe, extending for approximately eight pixels in the phase-encoding direction. The size of the chemical-shift artifact in the phase-encoding direction makes fat suppression a prerequisite for artifact-free EPI reconstruction.[22]

Phase-Cancellation Intensity Artifacts

After an RF excitation, fat and water magnetizaitons precess at different frequencies in the transverse plane, and the magnetization vectors periodically point in parallel and antiparallel (in-phase and opposed-phase) directions. Immediately after the excitation pulse, both the water and fat magnetizations are aligned in-phase and begin precessing with a frequency difference equal to the chemical shift δν. The phase (angle) θ, measured in radians, between magnetization vectors changes as the time t from the excitation pulse progresses, according to the following equation:

(EQ. 14)

$$\Phi = 2 \pi \delta v \, t$$

If the time t is chosen such that $t = 1/(2\delta v)$, then Φ equals π and the magnetization vectors point in opposite directions (opposed-phase effect). At a time 2T ($2T = 1/\delta v$), the vectors complete a full cycle ($\Phi = 2\pi$) and point in the same direction again (in-phase effect). These in-phase and opposed-phase alignments continue to cycle, resulting in multiple in-phase and opposed-phase effects in time (Figure 8-11, *A*).

The signal intensity for a given voxel is the sum of all the contributing components. The effect of adding fat and water vectors, which precess with different frequencies, is an oscillatory behavior in the resulting signal. The signal has its maximum (W + F) when spins are aligned and its minimum (W − F) when they are in opposed phase. In addition, in the presence of magnetic inhomogeneities each component magnetization decays with the time constant $T2^{*}$[140,141] (Figure 8-11, *B*).

This type of signal behavior can be observed in images acquired using gradient-echo sequences. In these sequences a single RF excitation pulse is used, and the signal is acquired at time TE after the excitation. The signal for voxels containing fat and water oscillates as a function of TE with a superimposed $T2^{*}$ decay.[42,140] The periodic behavior of the signal in this simple two-component system ([-OH] and [-CH₂-]ₙ protons) can be calculated from the single chemical shift δv. The period of oscillation (=1/δv) is 4.4 ms and becomes correspondingly longer at lower magnetic fields. Additional oscillations of the signal in gradient-echo sequences can occur as a result of the chemical shift between several fat species[140] (e.g., vinyl versus methylene protons, with a chemical-shift difference of 4.1 ppm).

Note that the signal oscillations of adipose tissue, typical for the gradient-echo methods, are not seen when SE sequences are used because of the 180-degree refocusing pulse incorporated for the SE formation. In this case the 180-degree pulse corrects for both field inhomogeneity and chemical-shift effects (Figure 8-12).

Motion Artifacts

Motion artifacts occur in MR images in the phase direction as a result of an object's motion in any spatial direction. These "ghost" artifacts are proportional to the signal intensity in the tissue of origin.[147] Respiratory motion artifacts are dependent on the proton signal from the chest or abdominal wall, where fat is commonly the dominant source of signal. Apparently, motion artifacts are more severe at higher field strength and have been responsible in part for limitations in high-field body MRI. Several methods have been developed to eliminate or at least limit these motion effects.[148] These include gating techniques with triggering synchronized to cardiac or respiratory motion, reordering of phase encoding, different averaging schemes, and very fast imaging techniques. Another potential approach aimed at eliminating the source of the arti-

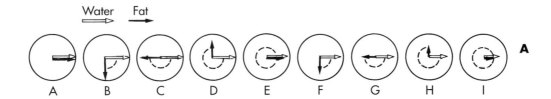

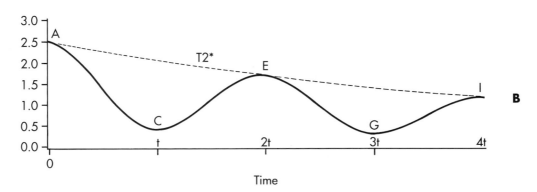

FIGURE 8-11   Phase-contrast effects. Immediately after a slice-selective RF pulses, fat and water magnetizations become aligned (in phase) in the rotating frame of reference and begin an independent precession. If the frequency of the reference frame coincides with that of the water resonance, the water magnetization appears static and the fat magnetization precesses with a frequency of the chemical shift δv. This precession causes periodic alignment (in phase) and disalignment (opposed phase) of water and fat magnetization vectors (*A* through *I*) in **A.** The period of this process is given by 1/δv and depends on the field strength of the MR system. Spins will align every 4.4 and 13.2 ms at 1.5 and 0.5 T, respectively. At any given time after the initial RF pulse, the two magnetizations present in the voxel will add vectorially, with the magnitude of the resulting vector changing as a function of time. **B,** The component magnetizations also will be decaying as a result of T2* processes. Superimposition of these two effects will result in the oscillatorily decaying signal intensity, the effect of which can be observed in gradient-echo sequences.

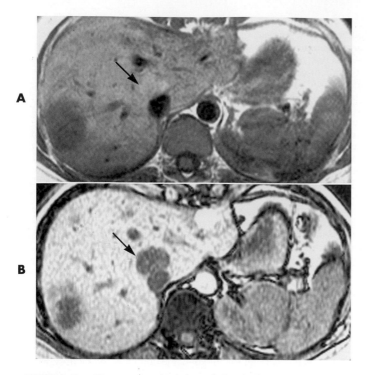

FIGURE 8-12 Phase-contrast intensity variations in the gradient-echo images. Hepatic adenoma *(arrow)*, which is subtle on T1-weighted SE 400/11 image **(A)**, is depicted with greater clarity on breath-hold opposed-phase gradient - echo 170/2.2 image at 1.5 T **(B)**. (Courtesy Dr. D. Mitchell.)

factual signal is fat-suppression sequences. Sequences that eliminate the strong fat signal potentially decrease the intensity of ghost artifacts typically encountered in conventional SE MRI.[19,81,137]

FAT AND WATER SIGNAL-SEPARATION METHODS

The effects described earlier have stimulated the development of fat-suppression pulse sequences. Although a large number of methods that use a variety of mechanisms to achieve this goal have been proposed, only a few are used in commercial imaging sequences. These methods can be divided into two basic groups based on whether they exploit chemical-shift difference (CSI methods) or differences in T1 relaxation rates (inversion recovery methods) (Figure 8-13).

T1 Relaxation Methods

The short TI inversion recovery (STIR) sequence has been advocated for fat suppression for mid-field and low-field MR scanners, in which methods based on chemical shift are more limited.[90,118] In the STIR sequence the time, TI, between the initial 180-degree inverting pulse and the slice-selective 90-degree pulse is adjusted such that longitudinal fat magnetization vanishes in the SE signal. In another approach, called *selective inversion recovery* (SPIR), the inverting pulse is made frequency selective, so only fat magnetization is selectively inverted at the beginning of the sequence. The additive effect of T1 and T2 contrast in the inversion-recovery approach, combined with fat suppression, can result in excellent tissue contrast. This sequence also can be used to null motion-induced ghosting from the abdominal wall or other fat sources.

The STIR method is insensitive to B_0 field inhomogeneity but depends on B_1 uniformity and is sensitive to relaxation time distributions. Although the STIR sequence provides generally excellent fat-signal suppression,[6,19] it is relatively restrictive in the choice of imaging parameters because TI must be set to null the fat signal and cannot be manipulated to optimize other tissue contrast. The STIR sequence has limited utility in conjunction with paramagnetic contrast agents because the mechanism responsible for fat-signal suppression also eliminates signal contributions from enhancing lesions,[111] creating the so-called negative enhancement effect (Figure 8-14). For an application with con-

trast agents, a better choice is the SPIR sequence because the fat-selective inversion pulse does not affect water-based signals.[86]

The STIR sequence typically is applied with a long repetition time (2 to 3 sec) and provides a limited number of slices compared with SE sequences with the same repetition time. This approach, however, is gaining utility at high fields now that fast SE methods provide a means to achieve shorter imaging times.

Chemical-Shift Methods

Methods that take advantage of differences between the resonance frequencies of water and methylene protons are frequently called *CSI methods*. These methods do not have the pulse-sequence parameter restrictions of the STIR method and therefore are applicable to most pulse sequences. CSI methods are divided into two distinct categories—selective excitation methods and phase-sensitive or phase-contrast methods.

Selective Excitation Chemical-Shift Imaging. These methods are based on narrow-bandwidth, frequency-selective pulses, which typically are applied in the absence of any gradient to either excite or saturate a specific chemical species.[7,30,41,44,45,63]

Two types of frequency-selective techniques for fat and water signal separation were developed primarily to create images based only on the water signal.

1. Selective excitation of the fat magnetization before the imaging sequence. In this approach fat is excited first, and its signal is eliminated before image data acquisition.
2. Selective excitation of the water magnetization to create an image formed by water only, designed such that unexcited fat magnetization does not contribute to the final image.

Selective excitation of fat. A selective-excitation pulse sequence begins with a frequency-selective pulse that rotates the fat magnetization 90 degrees into the transverse xy plane, as first implemented in the chemical-shift selective (CHESS) sequence.[44] Immediate application of a spoiling gradient disperses these transverse magnetizations such that the net transverse magnetization is averaged to zero. The unexcited water magnetization remains in the z axis and is subsequently used for imaging in the conventional pulse sequence, providing water-only images (Figure 8-13).

The frequency-selective excitation techniques may differ by the design of the narrow-bandwidth excitation pulse. A number of approaches to selective pulse design have been proposed.[77,121] A common design involves limited bandwidth sinc, gaussian, or binomial pulses for selective excitation centered on the fat resonance. Pulse length is typically in the range of 8 to 16 ms, with a frequency bandwidth of approximately 100 to 200 Hz. A pulse bandwidth is chosen to overlap the fat-resonance line width. Depending on the manufacturer of MRI hardware, these pulses are called *CHESS, FATSAT,* or *CHEMSAT.* Because of simplicity of implementation, selective-excitation fat-signal suppression methods have been used in all forms of MRI sequences, including SE, gradient echo, and echo planar. These pulses are considered standard pulses implemented on every MRI scanner.*

Selective excitation of water. A different approach for elimination of the fat signal based on the selective excitation of the water resonance, such as implemented in the three-dimensional (3D) gradient-echo sequence, is called *fast adiabatic trajectory in steady state* (3D-FATS).[47,48] A pair of adiabatic RF pulses is designed to leave the fat magnetization longitudinal while maintaining a transverse xy component for water. This sequence is unique in that no spatially selective slab selection is employed and spatial selectivity in slice direction is limited by spatial RF characteristics of an RF coil. This approach has been recommended primarily for 3D breast imaging in a single breast.

Another elegant approach to selective water-resonance excitation involves a numerical design of pulses that are simultaneously spatially and spectrally selective. These pulses are applied in the presence of a varying magnetic gradient with a variable phase and the magnitude of an RF pulse. This pulse design has found a primary application in EPI and spiral imaging.[79]

The effectiveness of all chemical-shift methods is highly dependent on inhomogeneities of the magnetic field.[123] These inhomo-

---

*References 22, 41, 43, 97, 136, 140.

Selective excitation

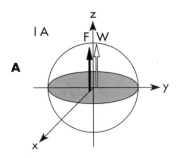 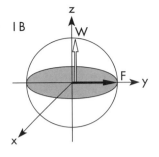

Phase control

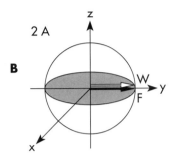 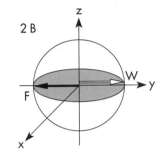

Inversion recovery

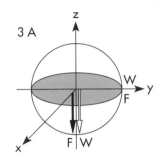 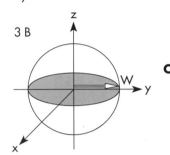

FIGURE 8-13 Fat-suppression methods. Frequency-selective (**A**) and phase-sensitive (**B**) methods explore the chemical-shift difference between fat and water resonances to create the fat-signal-suppression effect or to separate fat and water signals. In the frequency-selective method, fat magnetization is selectively rotated into the transverse plane and dispersed by a strong gradient before the imaging sequence to create a water-only image. In the phase-sensitive method, precession difference of fat and water magnetizations is used to separate fat and water signals into in-phase and opposed-phase intermediate image data, which after processing provide water-only and fat-only separated images. Inversion recovery method (STIR) (**C**) takes advantage of T1 relaxation time differences between fat and other tissues. The fat and water magnetizations are inverted by a 180-degree pulse at the beginning of the sequence and are allowed to recover according to their T1 relaxation times. At the instant when the z component of fat magnetization is zero, the rest of the imaging sequence is applied, providing a water-only image.

geneities result from imperfections of the magnet and magnetic field variations in the patient caused by the differences in magnetic susceptibility of tissue and air. If distribution of the magnetic field over an FOV of an image is substantially smaller than the chemical-shift difference $\delta\nu$ between water resonance and the main resonance peak of triglyceride in fat, then in general a standard fat-suppression method would provide adequate fat-signal suppression. If, however, this condition is not met, fat-signal suppression is incomplete and, moreover, it is accompanied by water-signal suppression as illustrated in Figures 8-3 and 8-15. In addition the effectiveness of these methods depends on the spatial uniformity of the RF field B_1. To improve the performance of selective-excitation methods, several new pulses have been proposed, including a design of spatial-spectral pulses with variable carrier frequency.[91] These new pulses improve the degree of fat suppression in specific clinical applications where field inhomogeneities are modest.

Phase-Sensitive Methods

2-point Dixon. One early phase-sensitive method proposed by Sepponen et al[105] consisted of the acquisition of a series of SE images with spectral information encoded in each image. This approach required very long acquisition times, making it impractical for clinical applications. In 1984 Dixon[27] proposed a method, technically similar to that described by Sepponen et al, that can be used to acquire high–spatial resolution MR images in a practical scan time while retaining a degree of spectral resolution. In this approach only two proton-spectral components—$[-CH_2-]_n$ of fat and $[-OH]$ of water—are targeted for signal separation.

The original method[27] employed an acquisition of a pair of images, called the *2-point Dixon method* (2PD), with fat and water magnetizations aligned in-phase in the first and opposed-phase in the second image. The first image was a conventional SE acquisition with normal timing of the 180-degree pulse, which resulted in fat and water spins aligned (in-phase) at the time TE of the signal readout. The second image of the Dixon pair (called the *opposed-phase, out-of-phase,* or *phase-contrst image*) was created using the same pulse sequence with modification of the timing of the 180-degree refocusing pulse. This adjustment is such that relative to water, the fat magnetization is 180 degrees out of phase at the time TE of the signal readout. The correct timing offset τ of the 180-degree pulse to create an opposed-phase image can be determined by the equation

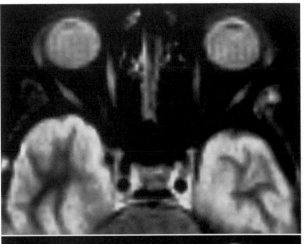

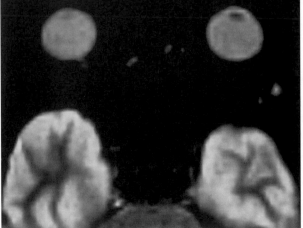

FIGURE 8-14 Negative enhancement effect on postcontrast STIR. Precontrast STIR (**A**) and postcontrast STIR (**B**) images of the orbits. Note that the signal intensity of normal enhanced structures, such as the extraocular muscles, lacrimal glands, and cavernous sinus, decreases after administration of Gd-DTPA. Enhancing lesions show the same effect (not shown).

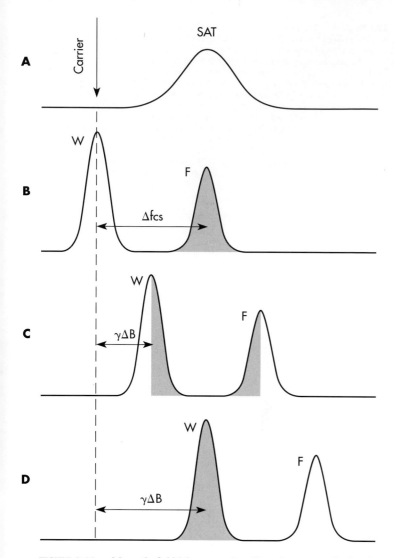

FIGURE 8-15   Magnetic field inhomogeneity affects frequency-selective fat suppression. **A,** Frequency-selective pulse (SAT) of limited bandwidth, typically in the range of 2 to 3 ppm, is tuned so that the carrier frequency of an imager matches the water-resonance peak *(W)*, and the pulse is frequency offset by a chemical-shift difference δv of 3.5 ppm to coincide with the fat resonance *(F)*, as shown in **B.** If the magnetic field is highly homogeneous, this pulse is capable of rotating all fat magnetization (indicated by the shaded area in **B**) into the transverse plane, where it is dispersed by a strong gradient-preceding imaging sequence. **C,** Magnetic field inhomogeneity γΔB offsets the resonance frequencies, an effect that may lead to partial suppression of both fat and water signals. **D,** Even larger magnetic field inhomogeneity may cause suppression of water signal instead of fat signal. (From reference 123.)

(EQ. 15)

$$\tau = 1/(4*\delta v)$$

Because chemical shift measured in hertz is proportional to the strength of the magnetic field B_0, the time offset τ is inversely related to field strength. For example, the time to offset a 180-degree pulse to achieve an opposed-phase effect is only 1.1 ms at 1.5 T but increases to 4.8 ms at 0.35 T.

By addition or subtraction of these images, either "water" or "fat" images could be displayed. To eliminate phase errors, algebraic operation was commonly performed on magnitude-calculated images. This approach eliminated sensitivity to phase errors, but because only the magnitude of the difference in fat and water intensities was displayed, the voxel intensity could not determine whether an area contained mostly water or fat—a serious drawback of the method. Despite these disadvantages the 2PD method demonstrated the diagnostic potential of fat and water signal separation and served as a starting point in the development of other phase-sensitive methods.[71,112,121,125,126,129]

A popular method of fat and water CSI involves using the Dixon approach to generate opposed-phase (phase-contrast) SE images.[5,67,70,87] This effect can be achieved with only a single excitation. The opposed-phase images are characterized by decreased signal at tissue boundaries where fat and water interface. For these voxels, where fat and water would have equal signal contributions, the subtraction of vector magnetizations, which occurs in the opposed-phase image, will result in nulling of the signal.

A one-excitation variant of the method, which combines a binomial pulse with opposed-phase data acquisition, has also been described.[12,20] This method allows for elimination of the signal originating in the minor fat resonances (such as vinyl protons), which are in close proximity to water resonance and cannot be eliminated by chemical-shift-based methods.

3-point Dixon. A data acquisition method that can potentially solve the problems with field inhomogeneity inherent in the frequency-selective and 2PD methods was first suggested by Dixon[28] and later implemented with various data processing schemes by several researchers.* This data collection method is based on a 3-point Dixon (3PD) acquisition scheme. This scheme consists of collecting three separate image data sets by means of a shifted, refocusing 180-degree RF pulse in an SE sequence.[39,71,123] Timing changes in the pulse sequence create a phase difference between fat and water magnetizations. A shift of the 180-degree pulse by τ causes fat magnetization to precess by an additional phase Φ at echo time relative to water magnetization, given by $\Phi = 2\pi\ \delta v\ 2\tau$. Knowing the chemical shift δv between fat and water, the fat and water phase difference 6 can therefore be set to any preselected value. A recent analysis demonstrated that values of Φ equal to 0, π, and 2π radians in the three images, respectively, creates a convenient optimum set,[38] as depicted in Figure 8-16. In addition to chemical shift, the phase in these images depends on overall magnetic field inhomogeneity ΔB, so the signal of an image in a 3PD sequence where the 180-degree pulse is time shifted by τ can therefore be described as follows:

(EQ. 16)

$$S = [W + F \exp(i\Phi)] \exp [I (\Theta_0 + \Theta)]$$

F and W = Fat and water signal intensities
$\Phi = 4\pi\ \delta v\ \tau$ = A phase shift caused by fat and water chemical shift δv
$\Theta = \gamma\ \Delta B\ \tau$ = A phase shift caused by the magnetic field inhomogeneity and susceptibility-induced magnetic field changes ΔB
γ = Magnetogyric ratio
Θ_0 = A constant for a given pixel, which includes effects of spatial inhomogeneity of the RF field, sequence mistuning, and digital signal processing

Selecting the appropriate value of τ in 3PD sequences yields three images, where 6 assumes values of 0, π, and 2π radians. At the field of 1.5 T these τ ($\tau = \Phi/4\pi\ \delta v$) values are 0 ms, 1.1 ms, and 2.2 ms. Signals acquired at those τ values and denoted S_0, S_π, and $S_{2\pi}$ can be described as follows:

(EQ. 17)

$$S_0 = [W + F] \exp[i\ \Theta_0]$$

(EQ. 18)

$$S_\pi = [W - F] \exp[i (\Theta_0 + \Theta)]$$

(EQ. 19)

$$S_{2\pi} = [W + F] \exp[i (\Theta_0 + 2\Theta)]$$

If the inhomogeneity ΔB would be negligibly small, then the Θ term could be neglected and the 2PD acquisition method, consisting of acquiring S_0 and S_π images, would be sufficient to calculate fat and water signal intensities. This can be illustrated by assuming Θ = 0 in Equations 17 and 18. Simple algebraic addition of S_0 and S_π would provide water signal, whereas subtraction of these two would provide fat signal

*References 13, 21, 38, 39, 43, 71, 88, 123, 124, 149.

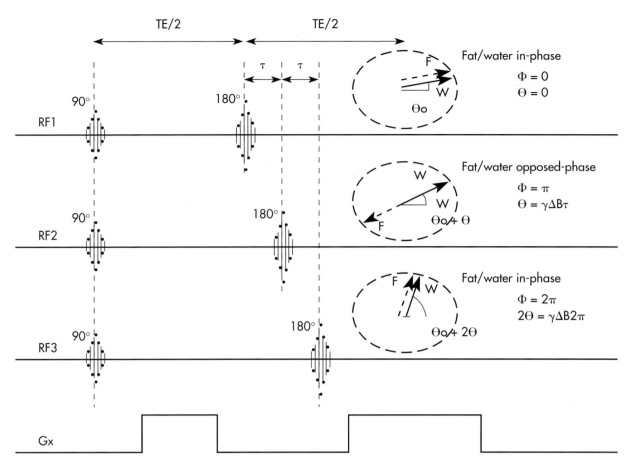

FIGURE 8-16   3PD data acquisition method. Three consecutive raw data images are acquired with timing changes to a 180-degree pulse. Slice-selection and phase-encoding gradients are not shown. To create a fat *(F)* and water *(W)* opposed-phase image, a time shift τ of the 180-degree pulse is calculated from the relationship ($6\ 4\pi\ \delta\nu\ \tau$). Because the fat and water chemical shift is 3.5 ppm (225 Hz in a 1.5 T field), the appropriate τ is 1.1 ms. The in-phase 2π image is created by doubling time τ to 2.2 ms. Additional phase shifts of magnetization vectors are the result of magnetic field inhomogeneity ΔB (Θ) and system tuning (Θ_0). (From reference 123.)

on a per-pixel basis. In this limit of very small field inhomogeneities an even simpler approach, called *Chopper,* that avoids explicit algebraic data processing has been described.[126]

On the other hand, if the limit of a very small inhomogeneity condition does not apply, a set of three images (3PD) must be acquired to provide additional information necessary to calculate Θ. Processing of the 3PD data set then involves subtracting the phases of $S_{2\pi}$ and S_0 data to obtain 2Θ, finding the Θ, and correcting a phase of S_π data by the angle Θ to obtain $S_\pi{}'$.

(EQ. 20)

$$\arg (S_{2\pi}) - \arg (S_0) = 2\Theta$$

(EQ. 21)

$$2\Theta/2 = \Theta$$

(EQ. 22)

$$\arg (S_\pi{}') = \arg (S_\pi) - \Theta$$

(EQ. 23)

$$S_\pi{}' = [W - F]\ \exp[i\ \Theta_0]$$

from Equations 17 and 23, F and W signal intensities could be calculated now by simple subtraction or addition.

This seemingly simple approach would generate properly reconstructed fat and water images, provided there are no 2π wraps in 2Θ phase data. However, if larger magnetic field inhomogeneities ($\gamma\ \Delta B\ \tau$

$\geq 4\pi\ \delta\nu\ \tau$) are present, then 2Θ will contain 2π jumps that must be unwrapped before Equation 21 for F and W intensity calculation. Note that the actual value of Θ is irrelevant in this procedure because the final images are presented after magnitude calculation. Also, because the magnitude of S_2 data is not used in the 3PD approach, there is some loss of SNR per unit acquisition time, as has previously been discussed.[38]

PRACTICAL IMPLEMENTATIONS OF THE PHASE-SENSITIVE METHODS

Although an SE 3PD method has the potential to provide an ultimate solution to fat and water signal separation in MR images, actual data acquisition and data processing schemes face a formidable challenge for practical implementation. These implementations include a phase unwrapping and a shortening of acquisition times, implementation for other widely used sequences, such as fast SE and gradient-echo, and implementations in lower fields. Currently it is a very active area of research aimed at the development of a robust fat-suppression method.

Phase Unwrapping

The effect of field inhomogeneity is an additional precession of magnetization vectors with subsequent contribution to phase changes in 3PD images. Precession of magnetization vectors is detected and recorded in the cartesian coordinate frame. The phase of the magnetization can then be calculated with the polar transformation, using an arc-tangent function. This function, however, determines a phase with module 2π, and therefore phases of, for example, Θ and $\Theta \pm 2\pi$ are not separable based on this polar transformation. Knowledge of the exact phase value in 3PD images, however, is critical for unequivocal assignment of fat and water signals on a per-pixel basis, and it therefore necessitates an application of a phase-unwrapping procedure. The effects of neglecting the unwrapping of the phase are demonstrated in Figure 8-17, where severe signal-intensity artifacts are shown.

To address the problem of phase unwrapping, several methods have been proposed, each with its own strengths and weaknesses.[13,39,51,88] One method uses phase gradients in an opposed-phase image to correct for phase wrapping, working from the center of an image outward in a one-dimensional (1D) fashion for every line of the image.[13] This algorithm, however, is very sensitive to a presence of noise on the unwrapping path, which can influence and mislead an unwrapping process. Other methods use parametric algorithms for phase unwrapping, employing an approximation based on 2D polynomial functions to map phase evolution in 3PD images.[39,88] This approximation works fairly well if the only source of field inhomogeneities is the magnet's moderate field imperfections. It fails, however, if magnetic field and susceptibility changes cause large local phase evolutions that the polynomial model cannot adequately describe. To aid in the reconstruction process, a polynomial-fit routine has been supplemented by a second pass through the data using a linear prediction algorithm.[39,88]

An alternative approach for phase unwrapping has been developed based on a nonparametric algorithm using a 2D region-growing approach, which tracks phase evolution in 3PD images and if necessary unwraps 2π jumps in phase-map images.[123] In the first step of this algorithm a signal level that corresponds to an image noise in an S_0 image is selected, and all pixels below this threshold value are flagged in 3PD images to be excluded in consecutive steps of processing. A seed point in the 2Θ image is then chosen, and a region is grown by deriv-

ing a phase of neighboring pixels using a preselected condition for the phase difference $\Delta\Psi$ between these pixels. If a larger than $\Delta\Psi$ difference is detected, then the phase of the pixel is unwrapped by adding or subtracting 2π. If the resulting pixel phase meets the $\Delta\Psi$ condition, it is added to a stack, as illustrated in Figure 8-18. Otherwise it retains its phase value and is not added to the stack. The region continues to grow by putting pixels that meet the phase difference condition on the stack and using them as new seed points. The unwrapped 2Θ phase data are consecutively used to calculate fat and water signal components on a per-pixel basis using the method prescribed in the previous section. A typical value of $\Delta\Psi$, in the range of $\pi/8$ to $\pi/4$, was used in the set of clinical images evaluated in the clinical study.[123,124]

The 3PD data-processing algorithm creates four output images—a standard SE image, a fat-suppression (water-only) image, a water-suppression (fat-only) image, and a phase-map Θ image (Figure 8-19). The Θ image depicts an actual spatial distribution of magnetic field inhomogeneities, whereas the 2Θ image is an intermediate image in the process of calculating the final output images. Before unwrapping, the 2Θ phase values are in the range of $-\pi$ to $+\pi$, with sharp transitions indicating 2π jumps. After unwrapping, the 2Θ image covers a range of phases, depending on how many wraps were in the original 2Θ image. In terms of field inhomogeneity ΔB, each consecutive wrap in the 2Θ image corresponds to a 3.5-ppm change of the magnetic field.

Images with fat-signal suppression acquired using a 3PD sequence and processed using a region-growing algorithm provide high degrees of fat-signal suppression and exhibit an excellent spatial uniformity of fat-signal suppression. This approach eliminates the effects of the field inhomogeneities that trouble the conventional sequence. The absolute SNR in 3PD images is increased relative to FATSAT images, whereas

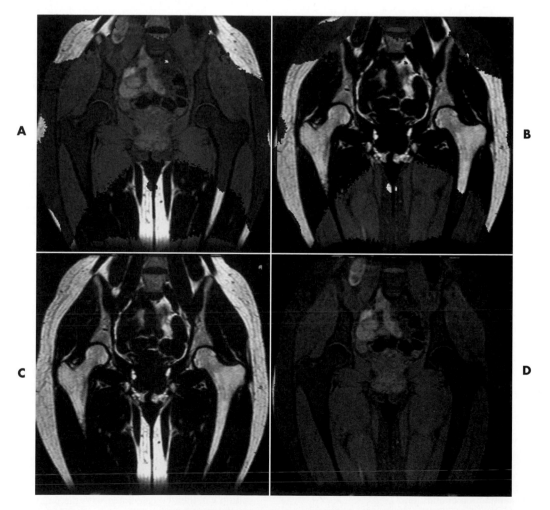

FIGURE 8-17   Phase-unwrapping effects. Reconstruction of 3PD image data without *(top)* and with *(bottom)* phase unwrapping using the region-growing algorithm: water images *(left)* and fat images *(right)*. Note the correct fat and water signal separation, but the incorrect assignment of signals into respective images with phase unwrapping is not performed. (From reference 122.)

the SNR per unit time is decreased as a result of longer acquisition times. The most critical differences between the images are in the degree and spatial uniformity of fat-signal suppression. FATSAT images exhibit fat suppression that ranges from very good suppression to no suppression and corresponding water signal elimination, whereas 3PD images exhibit uniform suppression of 85% to 95% of fat signal, depending on anatomy.[123,124] An example of the output images is shown in Figure 8-20, where axial images of the breast are demonstrated. Uniform fat-suppression can be appreciated through the entire large FOV using the processing algorithm. For comparison a standard fat suppression image employing a frequency-selective pulse also is presented. Note that fat signal is not adequately suppressed in this routine scan.

A problem of reliable phase unwrapping as applied to SE 3PD images currently forms a topic of very active research. Several new algorithms emerged at the International Society for Magnetic Resonance in Medicine annual meetings in 1995 and 1996, where special sessions were organized devoted to fat and water signal-separation methods. The most promising novel methods for phase unwrapping use Poisson formulation,[115] binary analysis,[3] and high-order polynomial fitting.[69]

Data Acquisition Time

A fundamental disadvantage of the 3PD acquisition scheme is the need to perform multiple data acquisitions. Three unknown variables, namely the water signal, the fat signal, and the local field inhomogeneity, determine the signal behavior for each pixel. Therefore it appears that three independent measurements are necessary to determine these unknown quantities for the separation of fat and water signal components.[38,71] The need for three acquisitions results in longer scan times than used for the standard frequency-selective method. Using this scheme, a typical T1-weighted image with TR = 600 ms and 192 phase

encodings requires an acquisition time of almost 6 min. These times become unacceptably long for density- and T2-weighted imaging.

The acquisition of 3PD phase-sensitive data can be shortened, however, by the use of multiple echoes for fat and water signal encoding.[65,124,145,149] In the method implemented recently, two closely spaced SEs are used to speed up the acquisition.[124] Depending on the repetition time and the time to the first echo, the double-echo 3PD can be used for T1-, density-, and T2-weighted imaging modes. Although four complex images are acquired, it is appropriate to label this method a 3PD method because three unknown variables—the fat signal, the water signal, and the field inhomogeneity map—are of interest. In the broader sense, however, as more imaging schemes that use a variety of mechanisms to sensitize data to fat and water phase are being proposed, they are becoming known as *phase-sensitive (PS) methods.*

Other strategies to shorten the imaging time also have been proposed. A recent study[24] shows that three data points are not, in general, necessary to separate fat and water signal components. In this method only 0 and π SE image data are acquired, and a phase map is extracted from the gradient of a phase in the π image using the region-growing phase unwrapping. In another two-acquisition approach the phase shifts between the magnetization vectors are $\pi/2$ and π^3, and the image data are processed based on a binary choice between fat and water signals, supported by elaborate region-growing algorithm.

The reconstruction of the final images using the double-echo approach for T1- and density-weighted imaging does not introduce additional errors compared with single-echo acquisition.[124] For T2-weighted imaging, however, where the SNR is lower, random phase mismapping may introduce errors in the fat and water signal assignments. An improvement to T2-weighted fat-suppression imaging would be to reverse the order of echo acquisition. In this approach the first echoes of each excitation would provide phase-map data, whereas late echoes would be

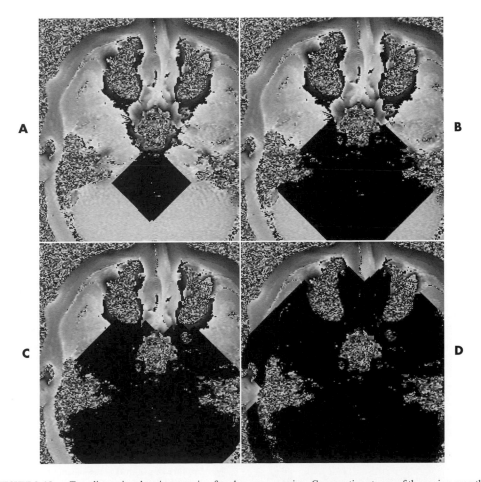

FIGURE 8-18   Two-dimensional region growing for phase unwrapping. Consecutive stages of the region growth from a seed point, marked in black, are shown in **A** through **D.** Note the capability of this method to outflank areas of noise without losing consistency for phase unwrapping. (From reference 122.)

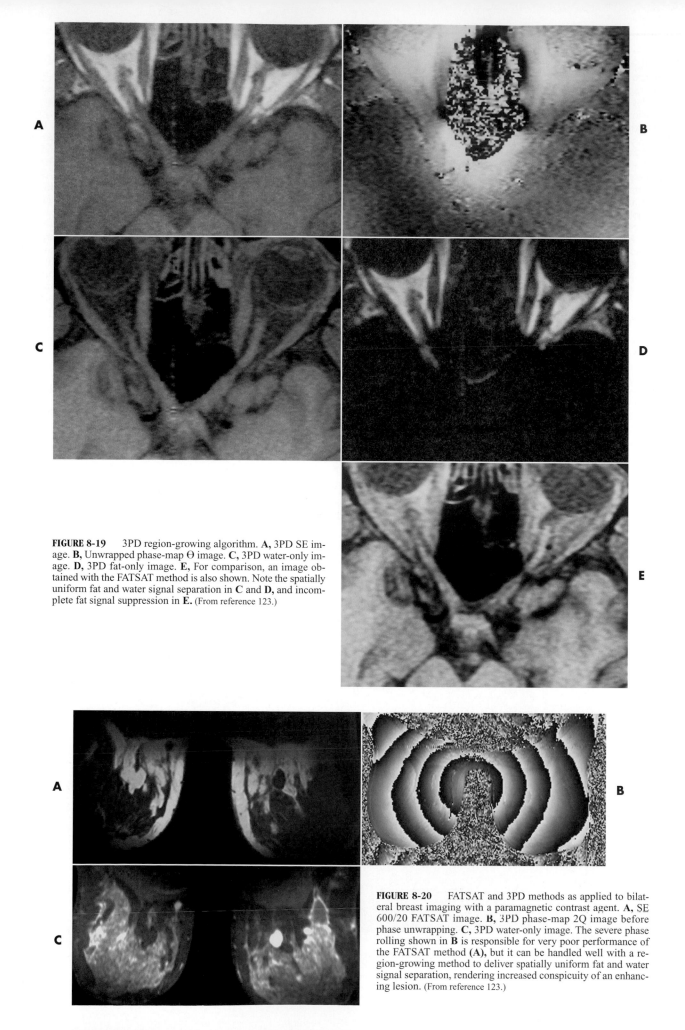

FIGURE 8-19   3PD region-growing algorithm. **A,** 3PD SE image. **B,** Unwrapped phase-map Θ image. **C,** 3PD water-only image. **D,** 3PD fat-only image. **E,** For comparison, an image obtained with the FATSAT method is also shown. Note the spatially uniform fat and water signal separation in **C** and **D,** and incomplete fat signal suppression in **E.** (From reference 123.)

FIGURE 8-20   FATSAT and 3PD methods as applied to bilateral breast imaging with a paramagnetic contrast agent. **A,** SE 600/20 FATSAT image. **B,** 3PD phase-map 2Q image before phase unwrapping. **C,** 3PD water-only image. The severe phase rolling shown in **B** is responsible for very poor performance of the FATSAT method **(A),** but it can be handled well with a region-growing method to deliver spatially uniform fat and water signal separation, rendering increased conspicuity of an enhancing lesion. (From reference 123.)

used to create fat and water magnitude images with contrast based on T2-weighting (Figures 8-21 and 8-22).

Fast Spin Echo

Obtaining a 3PD data set using a fast spin-echo (FSE) sequence requires a distinct approach to phase-sensitive imaging. The usual shift of 180-degree pulses in FSE sequences may create stimulated echoes to the detriment of image quality. A solution to this problem lies in a different design of the pulse sequence. Instead of temporal changes to the 180-degree refocusing pulses, temporal change of readout gradients delivers the required magnetization phase offsets without affecting the balance between primary and stimulated echoes. Shifting the readout gradient by a time $\Delta t = 1/(\delta \nu)$ separates the Hahn and gradient echoes by π radians. This method using a $(-\pi, 0, \text{or } \pi)$ phase-sensitive scheme has recently been described.[46]

Lumbar spine images that use a $(0, \pi, \text{or } 2\pi)$ acquisition scheme, reconstructed with use of the region-growing phase-unwrapping algorithm, are shown in Figure 8-23. Excellent fat and water signal separation is demonstrated using this approach; however, the extended time necessary to obtain π and 2π images substantially increases echo-time separation in the phase-sensitive FSE sequence as compared with the standard FSE sequence. This increased echo-time separation may cause a blurring or edge-enhancement artifact.

An alternative method for fat suppression in FSE imaging has recently been proposed.[23] This method uses J-coupling modulation of proton resonances in lipid molecules to its advantage. Two images are acquired with different echo-train lengths and echo-time separation but with the same effective echo time. Simple algebraic manipulation of the images allows separation of fat and water signal. The main advantage of the method is that it does not depend on B_0 field homogeneity. Images that have been presented using this technique, however, do not display a high degree of fat-signal elimination.

Gradient-Echo Sequences

The phase-sensitive fat-suppression approach also can be incorporated into gradient-echo sequences. In gradient-echo methods, where echoes are formed by gradient reversal, any phase evolution originating from chemical-shift effect is not refocused as in the case of SE sequences.[127,140] Instead, fat and water signals exhibit a phase modulation in proportion to the echo delay time TE, as described earlier (Figure 8-11). This effect provides a convenient vehicle for phase-sensitive imaging and, moreover, is equally applicable to 2D and 3D data acquisitions.[125]

Because these images have been acquired for three excitations, an acquisition time is still a problem. Multiple gradient echoes, however, could be used for the shortening of acquisition time. Several variants

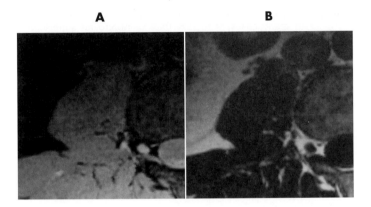

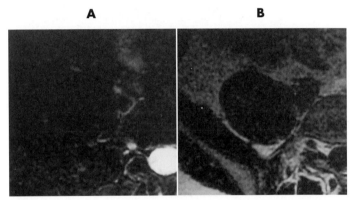

FIGURE 8-21   Double-echo phase-sensitive imaging. SE density-weighted (1800/17) lumbar spine images in an axial plane. **A,** Water-only image. **B,** Fat-only image. Excellent separation of fat and water signal components is demonstrated.

FIGURE 8-23   FSE phase-sensitive imaging. FSE 4000/108 image of a lumbar spine in an axial plane. **A,** Water-only image. **B,** Fat-only image. Note a very strong signal of fat despite a long TE time.

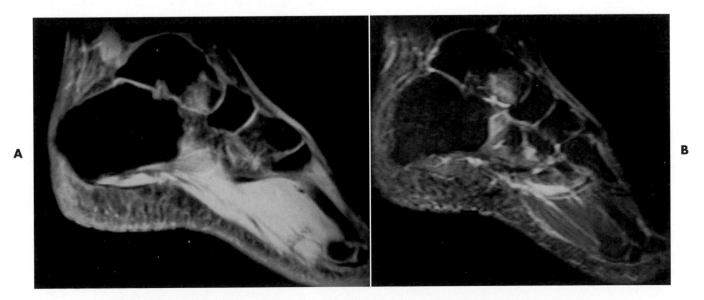

FIGURE 8-22   Double-echo phase-sensitive imaging. 600/20 SE **(A)** and 2000/80 SE **(B)** images of a foot in sagittal plane. Water-only images demonstrate the effectiveness of a phase-sensitive double-echo acquisition combined with region-growing reconstruction.

are possible, for example, a double-echo, double excitation phase-encoding scheme analogous to that described earlier, or a three-echo sequence providing 0, π, and 2π data sets in one excitation.

Mid Fields

Clinical applications of chemical-shift fat-signal suppression has been the topic of extensive research, conducted predominantly at high (greater than 1.5 T) fields. Although CSMA is less of a problem with lower-field scanners, all other general advantages of fat-suppression MRI are still applicable to systems operating in lower field strength. These systems frequently have reduced field homogeneity in comparison to higher-priced, high-field, superconductive magnets. Therefore the problems with the performance of standard frequency-selective excitation methods often may be more severe on these systems. This also explains the paucity of clinical literature evaluating diagnostic applications of chemical-shift fat-suppression methods at lower fields.

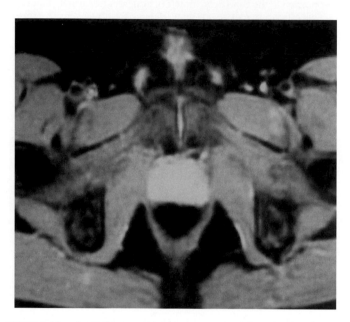

FIGURE 8-24   0.5 T phase-sensitive imaging. SE 800/25 image of the body in the axial plane. Double-echo approach was used to acquire data, and region-growing method was used to process image. Excellent suppression of fat signal demonstrates that the method functions effectively in lower fields and for large FOVs used in this image.

Clearly a technique capable of providing good and reliable fat and water signal separation would be extremely valuable for a rapidly growing number of lower-field systems in clinical use.

A phase-sensitive approach potentially can solve the problems encountered when frequency-selective pulses are used on lower-field scanners in a fashion similar to that described earlier. Two examples of such phase-sensitive acquisitions combined with region-growing processing in the body using a 0.5 T scanner are shown in Figure 8-24. A spatially uniform fat-signal suppression is demonstrated despite a large (48-cm) FOV and large phase rolling caused by field inhomogeneity. There are, however, additional obstacles for practical implementation of this approach on the lower-field scanners. As pointed out, the timing offsets in pulse sequence to achieve fat and water phase sensitivity are inversely proportional to the chemical-shift difference δν. Therefore the corresponding time shifts are 3 times longer at a 0.5 T field as compared with a 1.5 T field. This limitation may cause additional blurring and signal loss in a phase-sensitive approach to fat suppression.

REVIEW OF CLINICAL APPLICATIONS

Since publication of the last edition,[127] fat-suppression (or water-suppression) sequences have become standard commercial products, principally as CHESS-like methods based on frequency-selective pulses (FATSAT, CHEMSAT, etc.), the fat-frequency-SPIR method, and the STIR pulse sequence. Fat-suppression pulses or spectral-spatial excitation pulses also have been incorporated into early releases of EPI sequences. Although these standard pulse sequences represented compromises in many cases, with less than complete fat suppression typically achievable (particularly distant from the magnet isocenter), they nevertheless are included in routine clinical protocols. It can be anticipated that refinements in methodologies, as described earlier, should expand indications for fat-suppression imaging and improve the diagnostic yield.

So far in this chapter we have discussed some general advantages of fat-signal suppression that include elimination of CSMA, applicability to narrow bandwidth imaging, and an extension of the dynamic range of image display. Fat suppression also provides an increase in edge definition of solid organs and mass lesions, improved visualization of organs surrounded by fat, and increased signal from organs with a high aqueous-protein content. This section describes some other specific applications and advantages of fat-suppression MRI.

T1-Weighted Contrast

Fat signal strongly dominates T1-weighted images. Elimination of the fat-signal component in a T1-weighted image therefore reduces the overall image contrast-to-noise ratio. However, the contrast-to-noise ra-

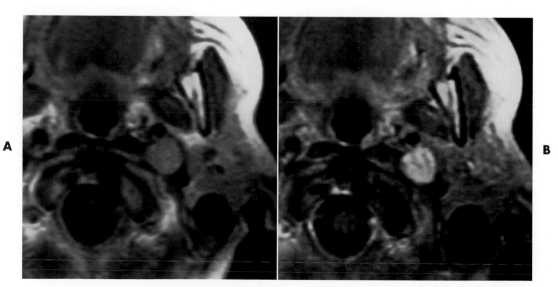

FIGURE 8-25   Chemodectoma. **A** and **B,** Fat-suppressed, gadolinium-enhanced T1-weighted images. Left-sided mass splays apart the internal and external carotid arteries.

tio within the diagnostically relevant water-signal component is preserved.[127] The elimination of lipid signal may be advantageous for T1 sequences because it can alter tissue-contrast relationships, improving the delineation of pathology. This also increases edge definition in tissues, organs, and mass lesions.[83,103,104,111] With the T1-weighted gradient-echo sequences that are used in MR angiography, fat suppression is useful because fat may overwhelm the signal from flowing blood on maximum-intensity projection displays, causing image artifacts.[16]

T1-Weighted Imaging with Paramagnetic Contrast

Fat-suppression MRI plays a critical role in conjunction with the application of paramagnetic contrast agents because tissue contrast may actually decrease when the paramagnetic contrast agents are used.

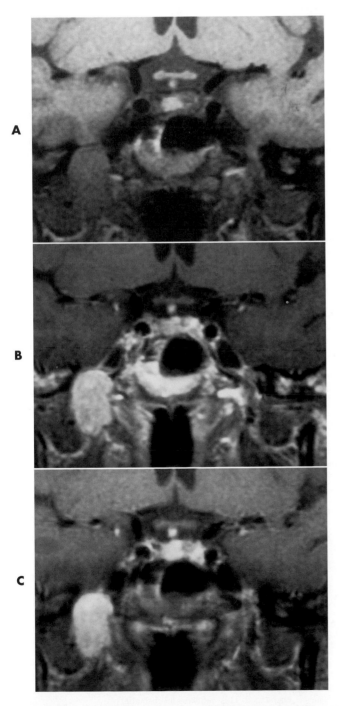

FIGURE 8-26   Schwannoma. Fat-suppressed, gadolinium-enhanced image of the skull base. Conventional precontrast **(A)**, postcontrast **(B)**, and fat-suppressed post-contrast-enhanced images **(C)** show a homogeneously enhancing mass along the undersurface of the right foramen ovale.

These agents have proved advantageous in applications in the central nervous system, where lipid is present in relatively immobile forms (principally as membranes) and does not produce a detectable MR signal. In regions of the body that are rich in mobile lipids, paramagnetic contrast enhancement may result in suboptimal contrast patterns. Here, enhanced lesions may become isointense with fat because of overlapping relaxation times for enhanced lesion and fat. For example, enhancing tumor within the orbit, bone marrow, or breast may be undetectable using a conventional T1-weighted SE pulse sequence.* In addition, fat suppression allows for quantitative assessment of the enhancement pattern, which may be useful in the diagnosis of optic neuritis.[111] Specificity also can be improved by this approach, in the context of certain clinical scenarios (e.g., hypervascularity of increased rate of enhancement on dynamic series, implying neoplasm in breast imaging and inflammation or infection in evaluation of limb infections) or in scarring versus recurrent tumor on postoperative spine imaging[12,84,101,103] (Figures 8-25 and 8-26). Alternatives to CSI mechanisms for fat suppression in paramagnetic-enhanced MRI are available. These alternatives include the SPIR method[86] (Figure 8-27) and image subtraction.[119] The most straightforward method is direct image subtraction. This method may be useful in selected cases but requires postprocessing and is highly sensitive to movement between acquisitions, which results in misregistration artifacts.

T2-Weighted Contrast

T2-weighted images can be obtained by SE, gradient-echo, or FSE sequences. Although fat signal for gradient-echo T2-weighted images is usually low because of T2* processes, the fat-signal intensity becomes significant for SE images and dominant for FSE images[23,127] (Figure 8-28). When a T2-weighted sequence is used specifically to detect ab-

*References 55, 98, 103, 107, 110, 122, 129.

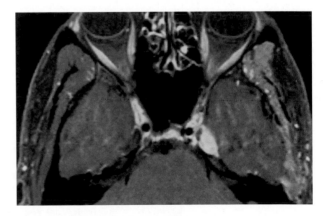

FIGURE 8-27   SPIR fat suppression. SE 669/20 SPIR shows enhancing left posterior parasellar mass. Homogeneous fat suppression is achieved in the orbit and subcutaneous fatty tissues. Unlike STIR imaging, the SPIR method is compatible with gadolinium enhancement because the lipid-selective inversion pulse does not destroy the signal of paramagnetic-relaxed (enhanced) water. (Courtesy E. Sandberg.)

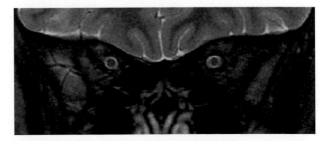

FIGURE 8-28   Optic nerve. Fat-suppressed T2-weighted FSE. Normal optic nerve is clearly defined against hyperintense cerebrospinal fluid. SE 4500/80, 3-mm slice with 512 × 384 matrix.

normalities based on the increased T2 of water,[102] a significant fat signal may mask a pathological increase in water T2 relaxation time. For example, the elevated signal of a meniscal tear may be poorly visualized against the strong signal from nearby bone marrow on T2-weighted sequences[95,133] (Figure 8-29). Because of residual T2-weighted contrast or effects of J-coupling in FSE images, density-weighted images also can benefit from fat suppression.[95]

Gradient-Echo Opposed-Phase Imaging

Opposed-phase gradient-echo images can be obtained by simply choosing an echo time such that fat and water magnetizaitons are aligned antiparallel. This approach has been found useful in the liver for diagnosis of fatty infiltration or fatty tumors, in the adrenal glands for distinction between benign and malignant masses, and in the bone marrow for detection of hypercellularity or metastases[83,94,135] (Figure 8-30). The method is simple to implement, and it does not depend on field inhomogeneities. Nevertheless it should be used with caution, especially

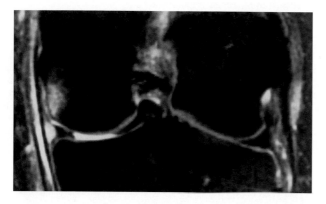

FIGURE 8-29   Bone contusion. Fat-suppressed T2-weighted FSE. Normal marrow appears hypointense. Medial femoral condyle bone bruise shows increased signal. Edema along the posterior aspect of the medial collateral ligament is bright. Medial meniscus bucket-handle fragment lies in the intercondylar notch. (Courtesy P. Russ.)

when applied with contrast agents, because the signal intensity of some fatty tissue may actually decrease on the opposed-phase images, as recently described.[84]

Chemical Specificity

The CSI methods can be used to determine or clarify the nature of ambiguous signal observed in an image. For example, on T1-weighted SE images, methemoglobin, melanin, or melanin-associated paramagnetics can all appear as indistinguishable high-intensity signal[127] (Figure 8-31). Fat-suppression CSI can improve the interpretability of such images. This approach has been helpful in clarifying the nature of the high signal observed routinely in the posterior pituitary gland, which was initially believed to be a fat resonance but was subsequently shown to be a water-based resonance[78] (Figure 8-32). This application of fat suppression is also used as a method to provide more specific information, such as for the detection of characteristic cholesterol within adrenal adenomas, which militates against the diagnosis of adrenal metastases.

Quantitative Chemical-Shift Imaging.   The CSI methods allow for quantitative assessment of fat and water content and relaxation time of each component in an image.[89] For example, quantitative CSI can be used to measure marrow response to therapy in neoplastic[96] and other infiltrative diseases, such as Gaucher's disease.[104] In addition, fat suppression allows for quantitative assessment of the enhancement pattern, as may be useful in the diagnosis of optic neuritis[109] and determination of relative fat and water content in the evaluation of fatty liver.[52,84]

Optimization of Clinical Technique

Apart from using the optimum fat-suppression pulse sequences, improved clinical fat-suppression imaging can be achieved by following some simple principles. These principles include optimization of main field homogeneity by placing the area of interest near magnet isocenter, by applying local shim methods either in a defined (limited) region of interest or at least within a slice, and by minimizing magnetic-susceptibility-induced artifacts at tissue surface–air junctions. For example, water (saline) bags can be placed locally over the body surface of interest. Minimization of these artifacts will be even more efficient using commercially available bags containing tissuelike susceptibility agents placed over the area of interest. Many of these products have the

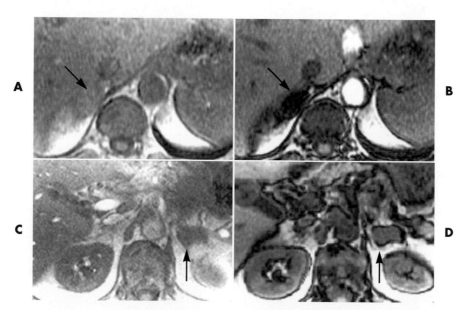

FIGURE 8-30   **A,** Gradient-echo 120/4.2/90 image, in-phase at 1.5 T, shows a right adrenal mass that is isointense to liver and hyperintense to spleen. **B,** Gradient-echo 105/2.3/90 image, opposed-phase at 1.5 T, shows the right adrenal as a signal void, and relative signal intensity of other tissues is unchanged. This indicates a substantial lipid content. Diagnosis was adenoma. **C,** Gradient-echo 120/4.2/90 in-phase image in a different patient shows a left adrenal mass that is less intense than liver and isointense to kidney and spleen. **D,** Gradient-echo 120/2.3/90 opposed-phase image shows no change in signal intensity relative to other tissues, indicating absence of lipid. Diagnosis was metastatic gastric adenocarcinoma. (Courtesy D. Mitchell.)

advantage of having no MR-detectable signal because they are perfluorocarbon rather than water based.

SUMMARY

The decade-long search for more reliable fat and water signal-separation methods has greatly intensified in recent years. Several very interesting methods have been proposed, specifically for processing 3PD image data and for more general phase-sensitive sequences. These methods include region growing,[123,124] the Poisson method,[115] binary searches,[3] and higher-order polynomials phase-map fitting,[69] and appear to be very promising for the routine application of fat-suppression MRI in clinical settings. The methods provide spatially uniform fat and water signal separation and allow for a simultaneous display of fat-only, water-only, and combined images.

Substantial progress in the fat and water signal-separation methodology is reported and reviewed in this chapter. New or refined clinical indications also are reviewed elsewhere in this text.[104,111,129] Future developments in this area are likely to occur via refinements in the technology, particularly in the development of robust phase-unwrapping algorithms, 2D and 3D gradient-echo sequences, FSE sequences, EPI, and implementations in the lower magnetic fields.

REFERENCES

1. Abragam A: The principles of nuclear magnetism, Oxford, England, 1961, Oxford University Press.
2. Alpers PH, and Isselbacher KJ: Fatty liver: biochemical and clinical aspects. In Schiff L, ed: Diseases of the liver, ed 4, Philadelphia, 1975. Lippincott.
3. An L, and Xiang Q: Quadrature 2-point water-fat imaging. In International Society for Magnetic Resonance in Medicine, 1996, New York.
4. Anzai Y, et al: Fat suppression failure artifacts simulating pathology on frequency-selective fat-suppression MR images of the head and neck, Am J Roentgenol 13(3): 879, 1992.
5. Atlas SW, et al: Orbital lesions: proton spectroscopic phase dependent contrast MR imaging, Radiology 164(2):510, 1987.
6. Atlas SW, et al: STIR MR imaging of the orbit, Am J Neuroradiol 9:969, 1988.
7. Axel L, and Dougherty L: Chemical shift selective resonance imaging of two line spectra by selective saturation, J Magn Reson Imaging 66:194, 1986.
8. Babcock EE, et al: Edge artifacts in MR images: chemical shift effect, J Comput Assist Tomogr 9:252, 1985.
9. Baker LL, et al: Benign versus pathologic compression fractures of vertebral bodies: assessment with conventional spin-echo, chemical shift and STIR MR imaging, Radiology 174(2):495, 1990.
10. Becker ED: High resolution NMR: theory and chemical applications, ed 2, New York, 1980, Academic Press.
11. Behar KL, et al: High resolution 1H NMR study of cerebral hypoxia in vivo,Proc Natl Acad Sci 80:4945, 1983.
12. Bobman SA, et al: Postoperative lumbar spine: contrast enhanced chemical shift MR imaging, Radiology 179(2):557, 1991.

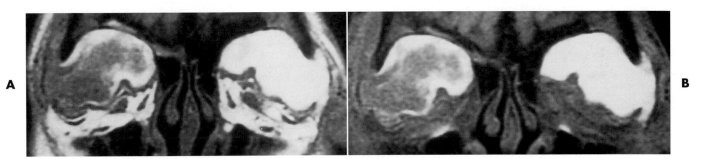

FIGURE 8-31   Hemorrhage. **A,** Conventional T1-weighted image shows homogeneous superior left orbital methemoglobin collection inseparable from inferior orbit fat. Right orbit mixed-intensity collection shows aging of hemorrhage. **B,** Fat suppression distinguishes left intraorbital fat from blood.

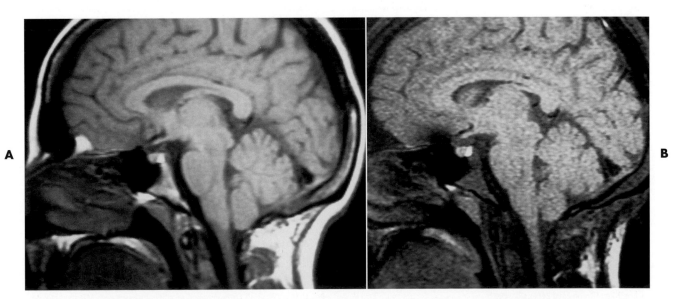

FIGURE 8-32   Study of the normal posterior pituitary gland by CSI. Conventional 5-mm SE image **(A)** compared with 3-mm fat-suppressed images **(B),** using the hybrid method for suppression. The bright signal characteristics of the posterior lobe of the pituitary gland do not lose signal intensity after lipid suppression. Note the increased magnetic susceptibility artifact in the fat-suppressed image.

13. Borrello JA, et al: Chemical shift-based true water and fat images: regional phase correction of modified spin-echo MR images, Radiology 164(2):531, 1987.
14. Bottomley PA, et al: A review of normal tissue hydrogen NMR relaxation times and relaxation mechanisms from 1-100 MHz: dependence on tissue type, NMR frequency, temperature, species, excision, and age, Med Phys 11(4):425,1984.
15. Bouchard A, et al: Visualization of altered myocardial lipids by 1H NMR chemical-shift imaging following ischemic insult, Magn Reson Med 17(2):379, 1991.
16. Bradley WG: Flow phenomena. In Stark DD, and Bradley Jr, WG, eds: Magnetic resonance imaging, vol 1, ed 3, St Louis, 1998, Mosby.
17. Brant-Zawadzki M: Magnetic resonance imaging principles: the bare necessities. In Norman D, ed: Magnetic resonance imaging of the central nervous system, Philadelphia 1987, Raven Press.
18. Buxton RB, et al: Quantitative proton chemical-shift imaging, Magn Reson Med 3(6):881,1986.
19. Bydder GM, et al: MR imaging of the liver using short T1 inversion recovery sequences, J Comput Assist Tomogr 9:1084, 1985.
20. Chan TW, Listerud J, and Kressel HY: Combined chemical-shift and phase-selective imaging for fat suppression: theory and initial clinical experience, Radiology 181(1):41, 1991.
21. Cho ZH, and Park HW: NMR chemical-shift imaging: principles and applications in advances in magnetic resonance imaging. In Ablex FE, ed: vol 1, 1989.
22. Cohen MS: Ultra-fast MRI, Magn Reson Imaging 8(S):171, 1990
23. Constable RT, Smith RC, and Gore JC: Coupled-spin fast spin-echo MR imaging, J Magn Reson Imaging 3(3):547, 1993.
24. Coombs B, et al: Two-point Dixon technique for water-fat decomposition with B0 inhomogeneity correction. In International Society for Magnetic Resonance in Medicine, 10th Annual meeting, Book of abstracts, Nice, France, 1995.
25. Daniels DL, et al: MR imaging of the optic nerve and sheath: correcting the chemical shift misregistration effect, Am J Neuroradiol 7:249, 1986.
26. Dick BW, et al: The effect of chemical shift misrepresentation on cortical bone thickness on MR imaging, Am J Radiol 151:537, 1988.
27. Dixon WT: Simple proton spectroscopic imaging, Radiology 153(1):189, 1984.
28. Dixon WT, and Lee JK: Separate water and fat MR images, Radiology 157:551, 1985.
29. Dooms G, et al: MR imaging of fat, Radiology 158:51, 1986.
30. Dumoulin CL: A method for chemical-shift selective imaging, Magn Reson Med 2:583, 1985.
31. Edelstein WA, et al: Spin-warp NMR imaging and applications to human whole body imaging, Phys Med Biol 25:751, 1980.
32. Egerter DE: Innovations tackle fat suppression problems, J Magn Reson 15, 1993.
33. Enzmann D, and Augustyn GT: Improved MR images of the brain with use of a gated, flow-compensated, variable bandwidth pulse sequence, Radiology 172:777, 1993.
34. Foster T, et al: Applications of variable bandwidth imaging at 1.5 T. In Society for Magnetic Resonance Imaging, 7th Annual Meeting, San Francisco 1988.
35. Fritz RC, and Stoller DW: Fat-suppression MR arthrography of the shoulder, Radiology 185:614, 1992.
36. Fullerton GD, and Cameron IL: Relaxation of biological tissues. In Wehrli FW, Shaw D, and Kneeland JB, eds: Biomedical magnetic resonance imaging: principles, methodology and applications, New York, 1988, VCH Publishers.
37. Georgy A, and Hesselink JR: Evaluation of fat suppression in contrast-enhanced MR of neoplastic and inflammatory spine disease, Am J Neuroradiol 15:409, 1994.
38. Glover GH: Multipoint Dixon technique for water and fat proton susceptibility imaging, J Magn Reson Imaging 1:521, 1991.
39. Glover GH, and Schneider E: Three-point Dixon technique for true water/fat decomposition with B0 inhomogeneity correction, J Magn Reson Med 18(2):371, 1991.
40. Gomori JM, et al: Fat suppression by section-select gradient reversal on spin-echo MR imaging, Radiology 168:493, 1988.
41. Guilfoyle DN, and Mansfield P: Chemical-shift imaging, Magn Reson Med 2:469, 1985.
42. Haacke EM: Image behavior: resolution, signal-to-noise, contrast and artifacts. In Modic MT, Masaryk TJ, and Ross JS, eds: Magnetic resonance imaging of the spine, St Louis, 1989, Mosby.
43. Haacke EM, et al: The separation of water and lipid components in the presence of field inhomogeneities, Rev Magn Reson Med 1:123, 1986.
44. Haase A, et al: 1H NMR chemical shift selective (CHESS) imaging, Phys Med Biol 30(4):341, 1985.
45. Hall LD, Sukumar S, and Talagala SL: Chemical shift resolved tomography using frequency-selective excitation and suppression of specific resonances, J Magn Reson Imaging 56:275, 1984.
46. Hardy PA, Hinks RS, and Tkach JA: Separation of fat and water in fast spin echo MR imaging with the three point Dixon technique, J Magn Reson Imaging 5:181, 1995.
47. Harms SE, et al: Fat-suppressed three-dimensional MR imaging of the breast, Radiographics 13(2):247, 1993.
48. Harms SE, Flamig DP, and Griffey RH: New MR pulse sequence: fat-suppressed steady state, Radiology 177:270, 1990.
49. Harned EM, et al: Bone marrow findings on MR images of the knee: accentuation by fat suppression, J Magn Reson Imaging 8(1):27, 1990.
50. Haughton YM, et al: Sensitivity of Gd-DTPA-enhanced MR imaging of benign extraaxial tumors, Radiology 166(3):829, 1988.
51. Hedley M, and Rosenfeld D: A new two-dimensional phase unwrapping algorithm for MRI images, Magn Reson Med 24(1):177, 1992.
52. Heiken M, Lee HKT, and Dixon WT: Fatty infiltration of the liver: evaluation by proton spectroscopic imaging, Radiology 157(2):707, 1985.
53. Hendrick RE: Sampling time effects on signal-to-noise and contrast-to-noise ratios in spin-echo MRI, Magn Reson Imaging 5:31, 1987.
54. Hendrick RE: Image contrast and noise. In Stark DD, and Bradley WG Jr, eds: Magnetic resonance imaging, vol 1, ed 3, St Louis, 1998, Mosby.
55. Hendrix LE, et al: MR imaging of optic nerve lesions: value of gadopentetate dimeglumine and fat-suppression technique, Am J Neuroradiol 155(4):849, 1990.
56. Henkelman RM, Bronskill M, et al: Artifacts in magnetic resonance images, Rev Magn Reson Med 2(1), 1987.
57. Hernandez RJ, et al: Fat-suppressed MR imaging of myositis, Radiology 182(1):217, 1992.
58. Heywang SW: MR imaging of the breast with Gd-DTPA, Radiology 171:95, 1989.
59. Hinks RS, and Quencer RM: Multislice chemical shift imaging by slice-selection gradient reversal, Magn Reson Imaging 6(S1):22, 1988.
60. Jones KM, et al: Fast spin-echo MR in the detection of vertebral metastases: comparison of three sequences, Am J Neuroradiol 15:40, 1994.
61. Kaiser WA, and Zeitler E: MR imaging of the breast: fast imaging sequences with and without Gd-DTPA: preliminary observations, Radiology 170(3):681, 1989.
62. Kamman RL, et al: Multi-exponential relaxation analysis with MR imaging and NMR spectroscopy using fat-water systems, Magn Reson Imaging 5:381, 1987.
63. Keller PJ, Hunter WW, and Schmalbrock P: Multisection fat-water imaging with chemical shift selective presaturation, Radiology 164(2):539, 1987.
64. Ketonen L, et al: Comparison of default and reduced bandwidth MR imaging of the spine at 1.5T, Am J Neuroradiol 11(9):9, 1990.
65. Kunz D: Double pulse echoes: a novel approach for fat-water separation in magnetic resonance imaging, Magn Reson Med 3:639, 1986.
66. Lee DH, et al: Optic neuritis and orbital lesions: lipid-suppressed chemical shift MR imaging, Radiology 179(2):543, 1991.
67. Lee JKT, et al: Fatty infiltration of the liver: demonstration by proton spectroscopic imaging, Radiology 153:195, 1985.
68. Levy TL, et al: Glossary. In Stark DD, and Bradley Jr, WG, eds: Magnetic resonance imaging, St Louis, 1988, Mosby.
69. Liang ZP: A new algorithm for obtaining unwrapped phase images. In International Society for Magnetic Resonance in Medicine, Annual Meeting, Book of abstracts, Nice, France, 1995.
70. Listerud J, et al: Combined echo offset (Dixon) and line volume chemical shift imaging as a clinical imaging protocol, Radiology 173:288, 1988.
71. Lodes CC, et al: Proton MR chemical shift imaging using double and triple phase contrast acquisition methods, J Comput Assist Tomogr 13(5):855, 1989.
72. Luyten PR: Proton spectroscopy of the human brain. In Society for Magnetic Resonance in Medicine, 8th Annual Meeting, Amsterdam, 1989.
73. Luyten PR, et al: Metabolic imaging of patients with intracranial tumors: H-1 MR spectroscopic imaging and PET, Radiology 176:791, 1990.
74. Luyten PR, Anderson CM, and Den Hollander JA: IH NMR relaxation measurements of human tissues in situ by spatially resolved spectroscopy, Magn Reson Med 4:431, 1987.
75. Mansfield P: Multi-planar image formation using NMR spin echoes, J Physics C 10:L55, 1977.
76. Mansfield P: Spatial mapping of the chemical shift in NMR, Magn Reson Med 1:370, 1984.
77. Mao J, Yan H, and Bidgood WD Jr: Fat suppression with an improved selective presaturation pulse, Magn Reson Imaging 10(1):49, 1992.
78. Mark LP: Sources of high intensity within the posterior pituitary fossa studied with fat suppression techniques, Am J Neuroradiol 10:892, 1989.
79. Meyer CH, et al: Simultaneous spatial and spectral selective excitation, Magn Reson Med 15(2):287, 1990.
80. Mitchell DG, et al: Chemical shift MR imaging of the femoral head: an in vitro study of normal hips and hips with avascular necrosis, Am J Roentgenol 148(6):1159, 1987.
81. Mitchell DG, et al: Sampling bandwidth and fat suppression: effects on long TR/TE MR imaging of the abdomen and pelvis at 1.5, Am J Roentgenol 153:419, 1989.
82. Mitchell DG, et al: Liver and pancreas: improved spin-echo T1 contrast by shorter echo time and fat suppression at 1.5T, Radiology 178(1):67-71, 1991.
83. Mitchell DM, et al: Benign adrenocortical masses: diagnosis with chemical shift MR imaging, Radiology 185:345, 1992.
84. Mitchell DG, et al: MR images: paradoxical suppression of signal intensity by paramagnetic contrast agents, Radiology 198:351, 1996.
85. Morrison WB, et al: Diagnosis of osteomyelitis: utility of fat-suppressed contrast-enhanced MR imaging, Radiology 189(1):251, 1993.
86. Oh CH, Hilal SK, and Cho ZH: Selective partial inversion recovery (SPIR) in steady state for selective saturation MRI. In Society for Magnetic Resonance in Medicine, 7th Annual Meeting, San Francisco, 1988.
87. Paling MR, Brookeman JR, and Mugler JP: Tumor detection with phase-contrast imaging: an evaluation of clinical potential, Radiology 162:199, 1987.
88. Pohjonen JA, and Castren EA: Automatic phase image correction for CSI. In Society for Magnetic Resonance in Medicine, 11th Annual Meeting, San Francisco, 1991.
89. Poon CS, et al: Fat/water quantitation and differential relaxation time measurement using chemical shift imaging technique, Magn Reson Imaging 7(4):369, 1989.
90. Porter BA: Low field, STIR advance MRI in clinical oncology, Diagn Imaging 11:222, 1988.
91. Purdy DE, Thomassson DM, and Finn JP: Variable-frequency spectral-spatial water excitation pulses. In International Society for Magnetic Resonance in Medicine, 3rd Annual Meeting, Nice, France, 1995.
92. Quencer RM, et al: Improved orbital MR imaging with section selection gradient reversal technique, Radiology 169:311, 1988.
93. Quinn SF, et al: Rotator cuff tendon tears: evaluation with fat-suppressed MR imaging with arthroscopic correlation in 100 patients, Radiology 195:497, 1995.
94. Reinig JW, et al: Differentiation of adrenal masses with MR imaging: comparison of techniques, Radiology 192:41, 1994.
95. Rose PM, et al: Chondromalacia patellae: fat suppressed MR imaging, Radiology 193(2):437, 1994.
96. Rosen BR: Hematologic bone marrow disorders: quantitative chemical shift MR imaging, Radiology 169(3):799, 1988.
97. Rosen BR, Wedeen VJ, and Brady TJ: Selective saturation NMR imaging, J Comput Assist Tomogr 8:813, 1984.

98. Rubens D, et al: Gadopentetate dimeglumine—enhanced chemical shift MR imaging of the breast: an improvement in lesion visualization, Am J Roentgenol 157(2):267, 1991.
99. Rzedzian RR: An instant technique for real time MR imaging, Radiology 161(P):333, 1986.
100. Saini S, et al: Forty-millisecond MR imaging of the abdomen at 2.0 T, Radiology 173(1):111, 1989.
101. Semelka RC, et al: Combined gadolinium-enhanced and fat-saturation MR imaging of renal masses, Radiology 178(3):803, 1991.
102. Semelka RC, et al: Focal liver disease: comparison of dynamic contrast-enhanced CT and T2-weighted fat-suppressed, FLASH and dynamic gadolinium enhanced MR imaging at 1.5T, Radiology 184:687, 1992.
103. Semelka RC, et al: Primary ovarian cancer: prospective comparison of contrast-enhanced CT and pre- and postcontrast fat-suppressed MR imaging, with histologic correlation, J Magn Reson Imaging 3:99, 1993.
104. Semelka RC, and Shoenut JP: MRI of the abdomen with CT correlation, Philadelphia, 1993. Raven Press.
105. Sepponen RE, Sipponen JT, and Tanttu JI: A method for chemical shift imaging: demonstration of bone marrow involvement with proton chemical shift imaging, J Comput Assist Tomogr 8:585, 1984.
106. Simon J, et al: Fat-suppression MR imaging of the orbit, Am J Neuroradiol 9(5):961, 1988.
107. Simon J, and Szumowski J: Chemical shift imaging with paramagnetic contrast material enhancement for improved lesion depiction, Radiology 171(2):539, 1989.
108. Simon JH, et al: Reduced bandwidth magnetic resonance imaging of the head at 1.5T, Radiology 172:771, 1989.
109. Simon JH, et al: Quantitative contrast-enhanced MR imaging of the optic nerve, Acta Radiol 35:526, 1994.
110. Simon JH, et al: The application of lipid suppression sequences in paramagnetic-enhanced MRI. In Dinger JC, ed: Contrast media in MRI, 1990, Medicom.
111. Simon JH, and Rubinstein D: Contrast-enhanced fat-suppression neuroimaging, Neuroimaging Clin N Am 4(1):153, 1994.
112. Simon JH, and Szumowski J: Proton (fat/water) chemical shift imaging in medical magnetic resonance imaging: current status, Invest Radiol 27:865, 1992.
113. Smith SR, et al: Bone marrow disorders: characterization with quantitative MR imaging, Radiology 172:805, 1989.
114. Soila KP, Viamonte Jr M, and Starewicz PM: Chemical shift misregistration effect in magnetic resonance imaging, Radiology 153(3):819, 1984.
115. Song SM, et al: Phase unwrapping of MR phase images using Poisson equation, IEEE Trans Imaging Proc 4:667, 1995.
116. Stark DD, et al: Liver metastases: detection by phase-contrast MR imaging, Radiology 158(2):327, 1986.
117. Stevens SK, Hricak H, and Campos Z: Teratomas versus cystic hemorrhagic adnexal lesions: differentiation with proton-selective fat-saturation MR imaging, Radiology 186(2):481, 1993.
118. Stimac GK, Porter BA, and Olson DO, et al: Gadolinium-DTPA-enhanced MR imaging of spinal neoplasms: preliminary investigation and comparison with an enhanced spin-echo and STIR sequences, Am J Neuroradiol 9:839, 1988.
119. Suto Y, et al: Subtracted synthetic images in Gd-DTPA enhanced MR, J Comput Assist Tomogr 13:925, 1989.
120. Sze G, et al: Gadolinium-DTPA in the evaluation of intradural, extramedullary spinal disease, Am J Roentgenol 150(4):911, 1988.
121. Szumowski J, et al: Hybrid methods of chemical-shift imaging, Magn Reson Med 9(3):379, 1989.
122. Szumowski J, et al: A chemical shift imaging strategy for paramagnetic contrast-enhanced MRI in tissue characterization in MRI imaging, Berlin, 1990, Springer-Verlag.
123. Szumowski J, et al: Phase unwrapping in the three-point-Dixon method for fat suppression MR imaging, Radiology 192:555, 1994.
124. Szumowski J, et al: Double-echo three-point-Dixon method for fat suppression MR, Magn Reson Med 34:120, 1995.
125. Szumowski J, and Plewes D: Fat suppression in the time domain in fast MR imaging, Magn Reson Med, 8(3):345, 1988.
126. Szumowski J, and Plewes DB: Separation of lipid and water MR imaging signals by chopper averaging in the time domain, Radiology 165(1):247, 1987.
127. Szumowski J, and Simon JH: Proton chemical shift imaging in magnetic resonance imaging. In Stark DD, and Bradley Jr WG, eds: Magnetic resonance imaging, vol 1, ed 2, St Louis, 1992, Mosby.
128. Tamler B, et al: Prostatic MR imaging performed with the three-point Dixon technique, Radiology 179(1):43, 1991.
129. Tien RD: Fat-suppression MR imaging in neuroradiology: techniques and clinical applications, Am J Roentgenol 158(2):369, 1992.
130. Tien RD, et al: Improved detection and delineation of head and neck lesions with fat suppression spin-echo MR imaging, Am J Neuroradiol 12(1):19, 1991.
131. Tien RD, et al: Intra- and paraorbital lesions: value of fat-suppression MR imaging with paramagnetic contrast enhancement, Am J Neuroradiol 12(2):245, 1991.
132. Totterman S, et al: Chemical shift imaging in the evaluation of leukemia. In Society for Magnetic Resonance in Medicine, 8th Annual Meeting, Amsterdam, 1989.
133. Totterman S, et al: MR fat suppression technique in the evaluation of normal structures of the knee, J Comput Assist Tomogr 13(3):473, 1989.
134. Totterman S, et al: Magnetic resonance imaging of pelvic and femoral bone marrow in normal adults and patients with acute leukemia, Radiographics 13(2):247, 1993.
135. Tsushima Y, Ishizaka H, and Matsumoto M: Differentiation of adrenal masses with MR imaging: comparison of techniques, Radiology 186:705, 1993.
136. Twieg DB, et al: Multiple-output chemical shift imaging (MOCSI): a practical technique for rapid spectroscopic imaging, Magn Reson Med 12:64, 1990.
137. Vinitski S, et al: Effect of the sampling rate on magnetic resonance imaging, Magn Reson Med 5:278, 1987.
138. Vogl TJ, et al: Improved visualization and delineation of lesions of the head and neck with fat-suppressed MR imaging. In Radiological Society of North America, Chicago, 1994.
139. Wachsberg RH, et al: Chemical shift artifact along the slice-select axis. In Society for Magnetic Resonance in Medicine, 7th Annual Meeting, San Francisco, 1988.
140. Wehrli FW: In Fast scan magnetic resonance: principles and applications, New York, 1991, Raven Press.
141. Wehrli FW, et al: Chemical shift induced amplitude modulations in images obtained with gradient refocusing, Magn Reson Imaging 5:157, 1987.
142. Weiner MW: MR spectroscopic imaging approaches clinical realm, Diagn Imaging 12:48, 1989.
143. Weiskoff RM: Improved hard-pulse sequences of frequency selective presaturation in magnetic resonance, J Magn Reson 86:170, 1990.
144. Weiskoff RM, Dalcanton J, and Cohen MS: High resolution 64 msec instant images of the head, Magn Reson Imaging 8(S1):92, 1990.
145. Williams SCR, Horsfield MA, and Hall LD: True water and fat MR imaging with use of multiple-echo acquisition, Radiology 173:249, 1989.
146. Williamson DS, et al: Coherence transfer by isotropic mixing in Carr-Purcell-Meiboom-Gill imaging: implications for the bright fat phenomenon in fast spin-echo imaging, Magn Reson Med 35:506, 1996.
147. Wood BP, et al: MR imaging artifacts form periodic motion, Med Phys 12:143, 1985.
148. Wood ML, Runge VM, and Henkelman R: Overcoming motion in abdominal MRI imaging, Am J Roentgenol 150:513, 1988.
149. Yeung HN, and Kormos DW: Separation of true and water images by correcting magnetic field inhomogeneity in situ, Radiology 159(3):783, 1986.

9 Spectroscopy

Gerald B. Matson and Michael W. Weiner

✓ KEY POINTS

- MRS is a diagnostic MR technique that distinguishes various metabolites on the basis of their slightly different chemical shifts or resonance frequencies.
- The pattern of metabolite ratios often provides clinically relevant information contributing to the noninvasive diagnostic process.
- MRS can be performed using a range of nuclei (e.g., hydrogen-1, phosphorus-31, carbon-13, and fluorine-19) on a single voxel or on an entire organ (chemical-shift imaging).

Magnetic resonance spectroscopy (MRS) is the only noninvasive technique capable of measuring chemicals within the body. The rapid proliferation of whole-body magnetic resonance imaging (MRI) magnets, with the potential for MRS, throughout the United States and Europe has heightened interest in the development of MRS as a technique for clinical diagnosis.

Although MRI and MRS are based on similar fundamental principles, many important differences exist between these two techniques. For the clinician the major difference is that MRI produces a visual image, whereas MRS obtains chemical information that may be expressed as numerical values. The distinction between MRI and MRS has now

The authors gratefully acknowledge the assistance of Dr. D.J. Meyerhoff in preparation of the section on human brain tumors.

been blurred by the development of magnetic resonance spectroscopic imaging (MRSI), which provides metabolic information in an imaging format. For the physicist the fundamental difference between the techniques is that the MRI is obtained from the water-proton signal acquired in the presence of a magnetic field gradient, whereas the MRS signals are acquired from metabolites at much lower concentrations and usually in the absence of a field gradient.

This chapter presents a brief overview of MRS and MRSI in vivo, including physical principles, and animal and clinical applications. In this edition the discussion concerning clinical applications and MRSI has been expanded. Several detailed reviews of MRS have been published[104,182,259,455,501]; additional references to review articles and important original publications are given in the text. This chapter does not represent a detailed review of the entire field, but it does provide representative examples.

FUNDAMENTAL PRINCIPLES

The frequency of the nuclear magnetic resonance (NMR) signal is determined by the following two factors: (1) the gyromagnetic ratio, an intrinsic property of the nucleus under question (Table 9-1), and (2) the intensity of the magnetic field at the site of the nucleus. The observed (Larmor) frequency of a particular nucleus is proportional to the intensity of the magnetic field at the site of the nucleus.

This magnetic field is largely determined by the external magnetic field (B_0) applied by the magnet. However, the magnetic field detected

Table 9-1 Properties of Nuclei Important to In Vivo MRS

NUCLEUS	SPIN QUANTUM NUMBER	NATURAL ABUNDANCE (%)	GYROMAGNETIC RATIO (MHz/TESLA)	RESONANCE FREQUENCY (MHz) AT 1.5 TESLA
^{1}H	½	100	42.6	63.9
^{19}F	½	100	40.1	60.1
^{31}P	½	100	17.2	25.9
^{7}Li	3/2	92.6	16.5	24.8
^{23}Na	3/2	100	11.3	16.9
^{13}C	½	1.1	10.7	16.1
^{2}H	1	0.016	6.5	9.8
^{15}N	½	0.36	4.3	6.5
^{14}N	1	99.6	3.1	4.6
^{39}K	3/2	93.1	2.0	3.0

by the nucleus is also a function of the electrons immediately surrounding the nucleus, as well as electrons of adjacent atoms. This interaction of the electrons with the external field to alter the field at the site of the nucleus is termed the *chemical shift*. Therefore at a given external field, every chemically distinct nucleus of a given species resonates at a slightly different frequency, resulting in different NMR frequencies and separate peaks in the NMR spectrum (see later discussion).

This property of chemical shift allows the spectroscopist to detect a wide variety of individual protons on a given protein, different phosphates on adenosine triphosphate (ATP), or many different carbons of metabolic intermediates. Additional information may be available from the multiplicity of the resonance, in which the resonance exists as a pattern of resonances (e.g., a doublet or a triplet). The pattern is related to interactions with a neighboring nuclear spin and is known as *J coupling* or *spin-spin coupling*. Irradiating the neighboring spin giving rise to the J coupling collapses the multiplet pattern to a single resonance line, confirming the identification of the neighbor giving rise to the J coupling. Further complexities, such as spin-spin coupling related to multiple neighbors and structural interpretations, are ignored in this brief overview. In general, MRI does not use chemical-shift information and often seeks to suppress it, although MR techniques for separate detection of water and fat signals are used.[155,413,435] To take advantage of the information provided by the very small changes in the NMR frequency produced by the chemical shift, it is vital that the external magnetic field be extremely homogeneous.

Small alterations or imperfections in the homogeneity of B_0 result in differing frequencies over the sample for the same chemical species. This causes broadened MRS resonance peaks so that the individual peaks caused by different chemical species are no longer distinguishable.

The need for excellent magnetic field homogeneity for MRS can cause difficulties in applying the magnetic field gradient techniques of MRI to MRS. The principal problem is that, even after the field gradients are turned off, eddy currents persist, spoiling the homogeneity of the main field. However, improved magnet and gradient designs, including self-shielding gradients, have alleviated this difficulty, and there is now considerable ongoing work in combining the spatial information provided by MRI with chemical information produced by MRS using MRSI.[81,344-346,534]

As in all modern NMR experiments, the MRS technique requires brief pulses of radiofrequency (RF) energy (B_1) to excite the nuclei followed by a period of signal acquisition. The acquired signal is the free-induction decay (FID), and this information is Fourier transformed to produce a spectrum. Alternatively a pair of RF pulses, spaced by an interval designated TE/2, can be used to form an echo of the FID beginning at time TE (a spin-echo experiment).

For chemicals in solution the spectrum consists of a series of relatively narrow peaks, the areas of which are proportional to the number of nuclei detected, provided that the experiment is repeated slowly enough (at time intervals TR) to allow full recovery of magnetization between excitations. The horizontal axis (abscissa) of a spectrum represents resonance frequency. Many different MR field strengths are used for MRS; therefore the abscissa is usually depicted as parts per million (ppm), representing a small frequency span proportional to the total resonance frequency used for the experiment.

The sharpness of each peak, or linewidth, is affected by several factors.

1. The homogeneity of the external magnetic field (Optimizing the homogeneity of the field over the sample volume is termed *shimming the field.*)
2. Magnetic field inhomogeneities (magnetic susceptibility gradients) within the sample (A nonhomogeneous sample can distort field homogeneity causing broadening of the peaks.)
3. The transverse relaxation time (T2) (see Chapters 1 and 3) (The longer the T2, the narrower the line. Many factors cause shortening of T2, including interaction with macromolecules, the viscosity of the environment, and the presence of paramagnetic substances.)

In general, MRS seeks to detect signals that are much weaker than those obtained for proton (^{1}H) MRI. Therefore the MRS experiment is repeated many times, with the resulting signals summed in computer memory to obtain an acceptable level of signal with respect to noise. Several minutes are usually required to collect a single MRS spectrum, so the data obtained represent an average of the signals acquired during the time of acquisition. Each RF pulse causes a perturbation of the nuclear spin system, so a short delay is normally provided after signal acquisition and before the next pulse to allow the spins to return toward equilibrium. This return to equilibrium is usually exponential with a longitudinal time constant (T1), which may vary from a small fraction of a second to several seconds. If the delay is relatively short, the spectrum is not obtained under "fully relaxed conditions" and is partially "saturated," resulting in reduced signal levels.

Analysis of MR spectra usually includes calculation of the following features:

1. Center of the resonance frequency for the peak in question, which is usually provided in reference to some internal or external standard with a resonance frequency that remains relatively invariant
2. Peak height
3. Linewidth at half height, which indicates the sharpness of the peak
4. Peak area, which represents the total area encompassed by the peak and is proportional to the concentration of the species producing the peak, provided that the experiment was repeated slowly (i.e., under fully relaxed conditions)
5. Peak shape, which may be lorentzian, gaussian, or some combination of the two; and whether the peak is symmetrical or asymmetrical
6. Multiplicity of the resonance, caused by spin-spin coupling, so that the resonance may be composed of several peaks (e.g., a doublet or a triplet)

Conventions and nomenclature used in displaying MR spectra include the following:

Upfield is to the right (representing lower frequencies), and downfield is to the left.

Upfield resonances are said to be shielded, and downfield resonances deshielded.

Chemical shift in parts per million is positive going to the left, the zero point being set by the resonance frequency of a particular compound.

- Tetramethylsilane (TMS) is used for ^{1}H (making H_2O at room temperature close to 4.8 ppm).
- TMS is also used for carbon 13 (^{13}C) spectra, whereas phosphocreatine is typically used for the reference with in vivo phosphorus 31 (^{31}P) spectra.

Instrumentation

The instrumentation for MRI is discussed in detail in Chapter 2. The instrumentation for MRS is essentially the same as for MRI in that a magnet, RF synthesizer, amplifier, RF receiver, and computer are required. However, several differences exist between the instrumentation necessary for MRI and MRS.

First, magnetic field B_0 homogeneity must be much greater for MRS so that chemical shift information is not lost. For typical MRS experiments, inhomogeneity in B_0 must be less than 0.1 ppm over the region of interest. Second, magnetic field gradient coils are not required for MRS, although they are necessary for implementation of most spatial localization techniques (see later discussion). Third, the ability to generate a broad range of frequencies is necessary to allow study of various nuclei with very different resonant frequencies (a so-called broadbanded spectrometer). Although MRS does not require image-processing equipment, computer hardware and software are required for display of spectra, calculation of chemical-shift frequency, measurement of peak areas, and other data manipulation.

For proton MRS the coils used are the same as those used for MRI. As in MRI the use of array coils[452] provides improved sensitivity for tissue close to the surface.[221,375] For nuclei other than protons, special coils are required that tune to the nuclear frequency of interest. In addition, for proton decoupling (see later discussion), double-tuned coils are required. A variety of $^{31}P/^{1}H$ double-tuned birdcage designs are now available.*

LOCALIZATION TECHNIQUES

The interpretation of MRS results is greatly facilitated if the volume of tissue giving rise to the signals is localized so as to correspond to a limited volume of interest (VOI). In general, localization requires the use of magnetic field gradients in either the B_0 field, as in imaging, or the B_1 (RF) field. The imposition of a B_0 gradient for localization brings with it the problem of eddy currents; these currents are induced in the magnet's conductive structures during the gradient switching, and they produce transient inhomogeneities in the B_0 field. These eddy currents can persist beyond the duration of the applied gradient to spoil the homogeneity of the external field during signal acquisition. However, the advent of self-shielding gradient coils[329,533] promises to greatly alleviate the eddy-current difficulties.

The following discussion follows (roughly) the historical development of localization methods; thus some methods no longer in use are briefly reviewed.

Surface Coils

The use of a surface coil, which basically consists of a circle of wire, affords rough localization in that metabolites in tissue close to the coil are detected with good sensitivity and metabolites far from the coil are not detected.[2] Thus the spatial localization afforded by the surface coil depends primarily on the size of the coil. Some additional spatial selectivity can be achieved by simply varying the length of the pulse. A relatively short pulse detects sample close to the surface. As the pulse length (or power) is increased, deeper portions of the sample are detected.

Surface Spoiling

Several methods using surface coils have been demonstrated to eliminate signals from the surface of the tissue but preserve the signals from deeper layers of the tissue. One method makes use of a grid of wire carrying current to spoil the homogeneity of the external field close to the grid[113,114]; other methods use a sheet of immobilized ferrite[195] or a paramagnetic liquid[326] to accomplish this same effect.

Surface Coil B_1-Gradient Methods

The use of B_1 gradients for localization avoids problems of rapid switching of B_0 gradients and the concomitant problem of eddy currents. Because surface coils generate B_1 fields that have an inherent gradient (inhomogeneous field), many of the B_1-gradient techniques are designed around the use of surface coils, even though the resulting B_1 gradient is nonlinear. Finally, it is possible to use a combination of gradient techniques to achieve localization.

A number of pulse sequences have been developed to obtain signals from the sample region experiencing a small range of B_1 field strength.* Thus the sampled region is bounded by curved surface coil B_1 isocontours (surface over which the B_1 field is a constant), and control of the size of the sampled region is limited.

Another, more advanced technique that uses the surface coil B_1 inhomogeneity is known as the *surface coil rotating-frame experiment*[193,218] and was based on an imaging method developed by Hoult.[242] The surface coil rotating-frame experiment generates a suite of data files, each of which is acquired with a larger (incremented) observation pulse. Because the resulting signal amplitudes are a function of position within the sample, two-dimensional Fourier transformation (2D FT) of the data sets produces a one-dimensional (1D) metabolite map where sequential spectra represent greater distance from the surface coil (Figure 9-1). Quite a number of variations on the surface coil rotating-frame experiment have appeared.†

Perhaps the greatest difficulty with the surface coil B_1-gradient methods is that the surface coil B_1 isocontours curve back to the plane of the surface coil; therefore it is difficult to avoid contamination of the VOI by signals from surface layers of tissue. Multiple coil configurations can alleviate this problem of surface contamination.[49,514] However, the use of multiple coils requires that coil-decoupling techniques be incorporated so that the current in one of the coils does not induce current in an adjacent coil.

B_0-Gradient Methods

Static field gradients. Use of a static magnetic field that was homogeneous over only a small volume to achieve localization was first demonstrated by Damadian[135,136] for imaging and later by Oxford Research Systems for spectroscopy.[202,203] Although this approach has been

---

*References 168, 257, 332, 377, 442, 531.

*References 45, 46, 48, 50, 485-487, 535.
†References 49, 56, 192, 194, 273, 274, 352, 418, 450, 514.

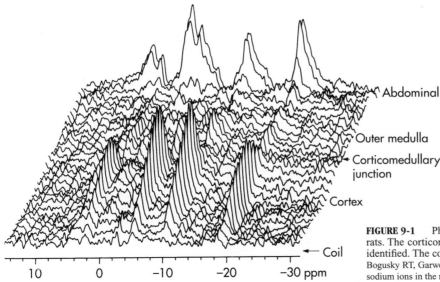

FIGURE 9-1 Phosphorus metabolite map of exteriorized kidney from normal rats. The corticomedullary junction and the abdominal wall of the rat are also identified. The cortex contains the greatest amount of ATP in the kidney. (From Bogusky RT, Garwood, M, Matson GB, et al: Localization of phosphorus metabolites and sodium ions in the rat kidney, Magn Reson Med 3:251, 1986.)

used to obtain ^{31}P spectra of human brain and liver,[514] the technique has proved to be difficult and its use has been limited.

Slice-Selective B_0-Gradient Techniques

Slice selection. The slice-selective B_0-gradient methods referred to in this section rely on frequency-selective RF pulses applied during the application of a B_0 gradient. The gradient is used to produce a spread of NMR frequencies across the sample. By exciting spins over a limited frequency range, the frequency-selective RF pulse excites only a slice of the sample. This is the same principle used for slice selection in conventional MRI. An early example of 1D localization achieved by slice selection was the depth-resolved surface spectroscopy (DRESS) technique.[64,69,71,73] However, if the length of the refocusing gradient lobe was not sufficiently short compared with the T2 of the desired signal, significant signal was lost and sensitivity reduced.

Three-Dimensional Localization

The use of slice selection for three-dimensional (3D) localization of a VOI is depicted in Figure 9-2. The large cube represents the sample, and successive excitation of three orthogonal slices results in signal from the volume represented by the intersection of the slices (the VOI). The number of localization methods developed over the last dozen or so years, along with their variations, are too numerous to list here. However, four methods for 3D localization have emerged as the most viable for use in people, and the majority of localized spectra from human beings are now obtained by either surface coil localization or one (or a combination) of the four methods described here.

STEAM. The stimulated-echo acquisition mode (STEAM) experiment was first demonstrated as a viable localization method for proton spectroscopy of the human brain by Frahm et al[173] and was rapidly taken up by other groups.[170,171,371,479] As shown in Figure 9-3, *A*, the STEAM sequence consists of three 90-degree selective pulses, each applied in the presence of an orthogonal gradient to excite a slice. Because these are 90-degree pulses, gradient refocusing lobes must be used. The resulting signal is from the VOI defined by the intersection of the orthogonal slices as depicted by Figure 9-2. Although the STEAM sequence is both simple and robust, it suffers from the fact that a stimulated echo at time TE and TM (Figure 9-3, *A*) is produced, yielding only half of the possible signal from the VOI. Also, although it can be used advantageously for short TE times, it still is not well suited for observation of nuclei with short T2 values, such as ^{31}P, because of the time required for application of the gradient refocusing lobes.

PRESS. The point-resolved spectroscopy (PRESS) localization experiment consists of a 90-180-180–degree pulse sequence (Figure 9-3, *B*), with each pulse applied in the presence of an orthogonal gradient[62,411] so that the final echo comes from the intersection of the planes

as depicted in Figure 9-2. Unlike STEAM, the PRESS sequence retains the full signal. A disadvantage of PRESS is that it cannot be performed down to TE values as short as those used in the STEAM sequence (compare Figure 9-3, *A* and *B*) and thus is not so advantageous for observation of proton metabolites with more rapidly decaying signals. At present, most human brain spectroscopy experiments conducted at short TE times (approximately 40 ms or less) are conducted with STEAM, whereas longer TE experiments are typically conducted with PRESS.

Image-selected in vivo spectroscopy. The image-selected in vivo spectroscopy (ISIS) experiment also uses frequency-selective pulses in the presence of orthogonal gradients. However, the selective pulses are inversion pulses and a fourth, nonselective pulse is applied for observation of the signal (Figure 9-4). A series of eight acquisitions, with different combinations of inversion pulses, is required to achieve the localization of the VOI defined by the intersection of the orthogonal slices.[412] Because the signal is received immediately after the final RF pulse, there is minimal loss from T2 relaxation, and ISIS has proved to be a particularly effective localization experiment for observation of nuclei with short T2 values, such as ^{31}P. The availability of frequency-selective pulses with immunity to B_1 inhomogeneity[310,320] has made ISIS an important localization experiment for use with surface coils, in which the B_1 field is inherently inhomogeneous.[2] In addition, improvements to the basic experiment have been suggested,[127] including improvements designed for rapid repetition with coils producing inhomogeneous B_1 fields.[310,320]

Magnetic resonance spectroscopic imaging. In general, the term *magnetic resonance spectroscopic imaging (MRSI)* refers to techniques in which the spatial information is encoded by switched gradients in the B_0 field (spatial encoding). The number of encodings required is equal to the desired number of pixels in the final spectroscopic image. The encoded data have become known as κ-space data, and the data are processed by Fourier transformation to provide a visual image based on an NMR signal at a specific chemical shift or range of chemical shifts.[81,344] For example, the intent is to produce an image that reflects the distribution of a particular metabolite, such as N-acetyl aspartate (NAA). For a patient who has had a stroke, such an image is expected to show the region of infarcted tissue in the brain (Figure 9-5).[249] The spatial encoding in spectroscopic imaging is accomplished by B_0 phase-encoding gradient steps as used in conventional MRI (Figure 9-6). However, to preserve the chemical-shift information, the data in spectroscopic imaging methods are collected in the absence of a (readout) gradient; this is in contrast to the usual MRI methods in which a readout gradient is used to obtain spatial information in one of the dimensions.

The term *chemical-shift imaging (CSI)* was originally applied to spectroscopic imaging methods. However, MRI methods that provide

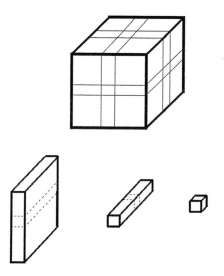

FIGURE 9-2 Schematic illustration shows how sequential excitation of orthogonal slices can define a VOI. The VOI is defined by the intersection of the three slices.

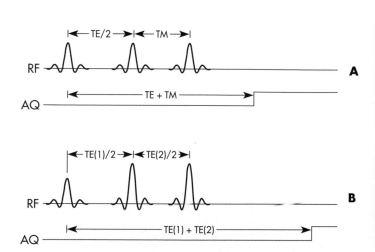

FIGURE 9-3 **A,** The STEAM sequence acquires the stimulated echo at time TE + TM. **B,** The PRESS sequence acquires the SE at TE1 + TE2.

separate images of water and fat by use of a readout gradient[75,155,413,435] are also designated CSI; therefore the term MRSI is used here to distinguish between these two kinds of experiments.

Because the concentration of metabolites in tissue is typically more than three orders of magnitude less than that of the protons in the tissue water, high-resolution MRSI of metabolite signals with resolution comparable to MRI is not feasible. Complicating this issue is the fact that the other nuclei of interest in MRS are considerably less sensitive than protons. On the other hand, sodium ions exist at relatively high concentrations, exceeding 100 mmol/L in many body fluids, so that low-resolution images of sodium ion are possible.[96,150,237,374]

Haselgrove et al[222] and Maudsley et al[346] provided early demonstrations that MRSI methods may be used to observe distributions of metabolites in tissue. Because of the difficulty in obtaining signals from metabolites in low concentration, the volume of tissue over which the metabolite signals are observed in MRS is made much larger than the voxel size in MRI. The minimum voxel size in MRS or MRSI is typically several milliliters or even larger.

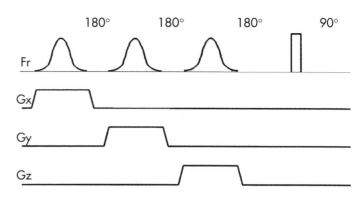

FIGURE 9-4   The ISIS experiment uses selective inversion pulses in the presence of orthogonal gradients, followed by an acquisition (90-degree) pulse. A series of eight different acquisitions is required to achieve localization.

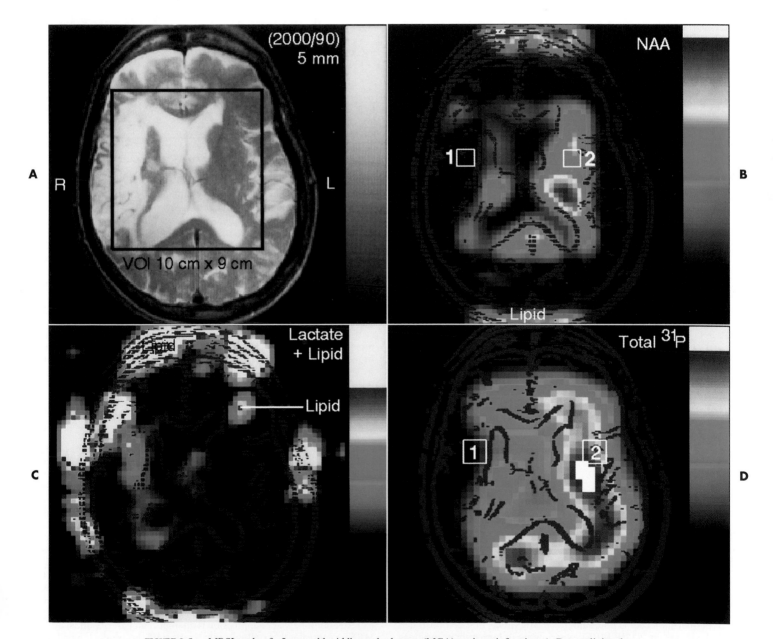

FIGURE 9-5   MRSI study of a 2-year-old middle cerebral artery (MCA) territory infarction. **A,** Box outlining the VOI selected for ^{1}H MRSI. **B,** NAA metabolite map with high-pass filtered MR image superposed in red, showing NAA deficit within the infarct. **C,** Lactate (plus lipid) metabolite map. Lactate is indicated within the infarct, and lipid signals (identified from spectra, not shown) are seen around the skull. **D,** Total ^{31}P metabolite map with high-pass filtered MR image superposed in red, showing metabolite deficits within the infarct.

Continued

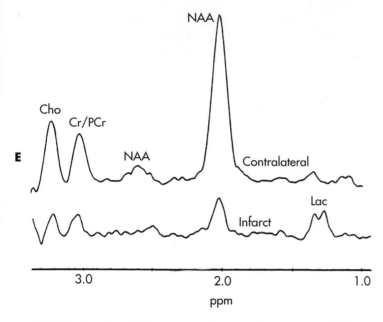

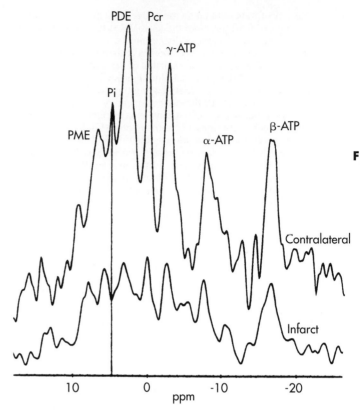

FIGURE 9-5, cont'd **E**, ^{1}H spectra from the regions indicated in **B**. **F**, ^{31}P spectra from the regions indicated in **D**. (From reference 249.)

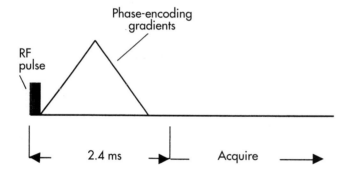

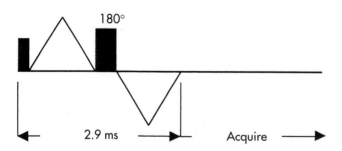

FIGURE 9-6 Timing diagrams for free-induction decay **(A)** and SE **(B)** MRSI acquisitions. For simplicity, only gradients along a single axis are depicted. (From Maudsley AA, Twieg DB, Sappey-Marinier D, et al: Magn Reson Med 14:415, 1990.)

In human subjects the potential of ^{31}P MRSI was first demonstrated by Bailes et al[24] in 1D ^{31}P MRSI experiments in human liver, whereas the potential for ^{1}H MRSI in human subjects was first demonstrated by Segebarth et al[479] in 2D ^{1}H experiments in human brain.

The MRSI approach has a number of advantages. The efficiency of data collection is much increased, so data over many volumes are ob-

tained in a time period comparable with that used for a single-volume method; the data may be displayed in an image format and in a spectral format, and the region (or regions) of interest do not have to be identified before initiating the study. In spite of these advantages, some difficulties remain. The volumes are not as sharply delineated as in single-volume methods,[347] and there are difficulties in quantitation of the metabolite levels. Nevertheless, the many advantages of the MRSI method have led to increased use of MRSI for examination of metabolite levels in human beings. In addition, it has recently been demonstrated that echo-planar (fast) MRI methods can be extended to apply to MRSI, yielding echo-planar spectroscopic imaging (EPSI).[4,353,427]

Finally, the use of B_0-gradient pulses to encode the spatial information is not an essential feature of MRSI methods. For instance, rotating frame methods may be considered 1D applications of MRSI methods. In addition, the spatial information may be encoded longitudinally through frequency-selective RF pulses.[58,343] The flexibility and increased information content of the MRSI approach ensure that this method will attain increased importance as the field of clinical MRS matures.

Combination Experiments. Many practical experiments are actually combinations of experiments. For instance, the use of outer-volume suppression pulses[127] has been suggested in the use of ISIS to lessen contamination from signals outside of the VOI. In addition, 2D ISIS experiments have been used successfully in conjunction with rotating-frame experiments to provide improved localization of ^{31}P signals in dog hearts (FLAX-ISIS[448] and related methods[230]). Most proton ^{1}H MRSI experiments in human brain are also combination experiments in that the region over which the MRSI is to be performed is first localized by a STEAM or PRESS sequence. This enables the strong lipid signals originating from subcutaneous tissue adjacent to the scalp, which would otherwise interfere with metabolite resonances, to be avoided. Outer-volume suppression pulses also may be incorporated to minimize contamination of spectra by these strong lipid signals. In addition, water suppression is an important part of almost all ^{1}H MRSI experiments to allow visualization of the much lower-level metabolite signals. An example of a 3D ^{1}H MRSI experiment using PRESS for localization and incorporating water and outer-volume suppression pulses is provided in Figure 9-7.[158] Additional variations and refinements of MRSI experiments include sampling over a spherical

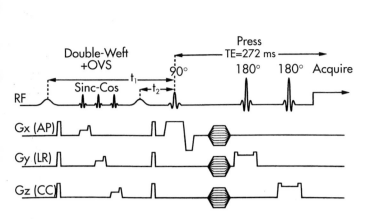

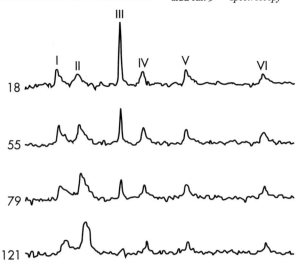

FIGURE 9-7   Timing diagram for a 3D ^{1}H MRSI experiment. The first section consists of a double–water elimination by Fourier transformation (WEFT) sequence for water suppression; t_1 and t_2 indicate inversion delay times. Three sinc-cosine *(SINC-COS)* outer volume-suppression pulses are placed between the WEFT water suppression pulses. The second section contains the PRESS VOI selection, together with the MRSI phase-encoding gradients. (From reference 158.)

FIGURE 9-8 ^{31}P MR spectrum of an intact muscle from the hind leg of a rat recorded at 129 MHz. Peak assignments: *I*, Sugar phosphate and phospholipid; *II*, inorganic phosphate (Pi); *III*, phosphocreatine (PCr); *IV*, γ-ATP; *V*, α-ATP; *VI*, β-ATP. The times are the midpoints of the 50-scan spectral accumulations (referred to excision time as zero). As the experiment progressed, PCr (peak III) gradually fell and Pi (peak II) rose. Ultimately, ATP (peaks IV, V, and VI) also fell. (From reference 243.)

extent of κ space[160] with use of multiple echos for improved data collection efficiency[160] and multiple-slice experiments[159] to improve the coverage of tissue. Other MRSI κ-space strategies include the use of hexagonal κ-space sampling,[475] and methods for reduction of the lipid truncation artifacts in MRSI experiments.[223]

Other Experiments.   Numerous additional experiments have been proposed for localized spectroscopy. Although the techniques previously discussed appear to be the most useful and practical at the current stage of MRS technology, some of the experiments omitted for discussion may become important for MRS in human beings in the future. Among those omitted are several that rely on rapidly switched gradients, others that feature nonoptimal sensitivity, and still others that have yet to be demonstrated in tissue samples. The recent advent of improved switching of B_0 gradients with minimal eddy currents (i.e., self-shielding gradients) can be expected to improve the performance of some of the experiments already discussed and may open the door to additional localization techniques.

Quantitation.   The quantitation of metabolites in terms of concentrations is important to avoid the ambiguities inherent in measurement of metabolite ratios (lack of certainty in which metabolite levels are changing), to facilitate distinctions between normal and diseased tissues, and for comparison of results from different laboratories. In general, quantitation must rely on replication of the localization experiment on a vessel containing a solution of known concentration (a phantom), with corrections for coil loading and differences in relaxation times T1 and T2 between the phantom and tissue metabolite resonances. Any inhomogeneities in the RF (B_1) field also must be taken into account. In some cases an intermediate resonance from sample in a vial attached to the coil may be used to relate the in vivo experiment to the phantom experiment.

For quantitation of ^{1}H resonances the tissue water may be used as an internal standard, thus avoiding a separate experiment on a phantom. However, a number of potential pitfalls exist, including (1) knowledge of the water content of the tissue, (2) measurement of the water signal with appropriate corrections for tissue water T1 and T2, (3) avoidance of cerebrospinal fluid (CSF) water signal, and (4) use of proper concentration units.[296,297] Despite these potential pitfalls, the water signal is widely used for quantitation of ^{1}H resonances in brain (see later discussion on normal brain).

For quantitation of resonances other than protons, it is difficult to avoid the replication of the localization experiment on a phantom of known concentration; in principle this replication must be repeated each

time some parameter of the localization experiment is altered. However, it has been demonstrated that the replication can be avoided for an ISIS ^{31}P experiment by careful computer simulation of the experiment, including correction of the B_1 inhomogeneities.[334]

CLINICAL AND RESEARCH APPLICATIONS
Development of In Vivo Spectroscopy

Since the initial development of NMR,[401,434] investigators have recognized that noninvasive measurement of tissue chemicals was possible with this technique. Early experiments demonstrated that water protons in living tissue could be detected.[410,490] Several investigators used ^{1}H NMR to investigate the properties of tissue water.[40,129,220] The protons of pure water in free solution have long T1 and T2 relaxation times. In contrast the relaxation times of tissue water are considerably shorter, suggesting to some that this water was "bound" (i.e., having severely restricted motion). This led to considerable investigation and debate, although it is currently thought that most tissue water is free in solution and only a small fraction is transiently immobilized by macromolecules (see Chapter 3). A very important observation was made in the early 1970s by Damadian,[134] who found that the relaxation times of protons in malignant tissues were longer than those of nonmalignant tissues. He suggested that this represented a qualitative difference between normal and malignant cells and that MR could be used to diagnose malignancy.

A major impetus to in vivo application of MRS was the demonstration that signals from various phosphates involved with energy metabolism could be detected from within intact red blood cells[229,370] and muscle.[243] Figure 9-8 depicts ^{31}P NMR spectra from the classic article by Hoult et al.[243] This observation encouraged numerous investigators to study various aspects of energy metabolism in isolated cells,[8,382,503,542] perfused organs,* and organs in vivo.[2,211,293,305] Lauterbur's demonstration that visual images could be produced by the MRI technique[309] and Damadian's first human image using the FONAR technique[135] prophetically pointed the way for the development of MR technology for clinical investigation and clinical diagnosis.

Intermediary Metabolism

Because MRS detects chemicals involved in metabolism, intermediary metabolism is briefly reviewed. Figure 9-9 depicts the major metabolic

---

*References 1, 3, 25, 190, 238, 258, 350, 436, 467.

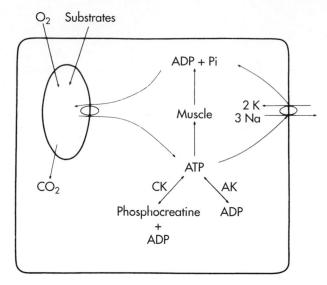

FIGURE 9-9 High-energy phosphate reactions within the cell. *ADP,* Adenosine diphosphate; *ATP,* adenosine triphosphate; *AK,* adenylate kinase; *CK,* creatine kinase; *Pi,* inorganic phosphate. (From reference 294.)

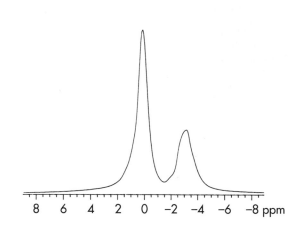

FIGURE 9-10 ¹H NMR spectrum of human adductor pollicus muscle obtained at 85 MHz with a single acquisition. The large peak centered at 0 ppm is the water proton line, and the smaller peak at −3.3 ppm is caused by lipid protons.

pathways for biological energy production and the cellular work functions that use energy for ion transport, muscle contraction, and biosynthesis. In the living tissues of higher animals, energy is largely generated by oxidation. Long-term storage of energy occurs in the forms of glycogen, carbohydrates, and long-chain fatty acids. Glycogen can be converted to glucose, which is oxidized to lactate by anaerobic glycolysis. In oxygen-breathing animals, lactate production occurs when the oxidation of glucose exceeds the capacity of the citric acid cycle to oxidize pyruvate. For example, vigorous muscular exercise is associated with glycogen breakdown and lactate production.

The mitochondria of cells contain enzymes of the citric acid cycle that convert pyruvate to carbon dioxide and produce reduced nicotinamide adenine dinucleotide (NADH). The NADH is oxidized by the electron transport chain to NAD⁺ plus water, energizing the production of ATP by oxidative phosphorylation. The ATP is used for biological work, such as muscle contraction and ion transport. ATP is transported out of the mitochondria by the adenine nucleotide translocase in exchange for adenosine diphosphate (ADP). Cytosolic ATP is used by the actinomycin ATPase for muscular contraction and by the sodium-potassium ATPase for active transport of sodium and potassium ions across the plasma membrane and for the biosynthesis of carbohydrates (gluconeogenesis), lipids (lipogenesis), proteins, and nucleic acids.

Phosphocreatine (PCr) is a high-energy storage compound. The enzyme creatine kinase (CK) catalyzes an equilibrium reaction between PCr and ATP:

(EQ. 1)

$$PCr + ADP + H^+ \xleftarrow{\;CK\;} ATP + Cr$$

When ATP is abundant, PCr is synthesized and remains in the cell as a high-energy phosphate reservoir. When ATP hydrolysis is stimulated and ADP is produced, PCr is converted to ATP plus creatine (Cr), thus maintaining ATP levels. In tissues in which CK is abundant (i.e., muscle and nerve), the reaction is maintained close to equilibrium. Furthermore, when the concentrations of PCr, ATP, Cr, and pH are measured, the concentration of the important metabolic regulator ADP can be calculated. Examination of this reaction also demonstrates that the balance of reactants of CK is influenced by the concentration of H⁺. For example, acidosis shifts the equilibrium to the right. Similarly a decrease of PCr produces alkalosis.

Another important enzyme, adenylate kinase (AK), catalyzes interconversion between ATP, ADP, and adenosine monophosphate (AMP):

(EQ. 2)

$$2ADP \xleftarrow{\;AK\;} ATP + AMP$$

This enzyme also serves to maintain ATP levels, keeping ADP concentrations low. Therefore if ATP is broken down to ADP, AK generates

AMP. The AMP is further broken down to either inosine monophosphate (by the enzyme AMP deaminase) or adenosine (by 5′-nucleotidase), which is a potent vasodilator. Further breakdown of these adenine nucleotides leads to the production of urate.

In conditions in which insufficient oxygen is provided to cells (e.g., anoxia or ischemia), the breakdown of ATP for cell work exceeds the production of ATP by oxidative phosphorylation. This produces a rise of ADP, which stimulates glycolysis, accelerating lactate formation. If CK and PCr are present, PCr hydrolysis maintains ATP and ADP concentrations. When PCr is exhausted, ATP begins to fall. Hydrolysis of PCr and ATP produces increased concentrations of inorganic phosphate (Pi). Therefore anoxia, ischemia, or cell death produces breakdown of high-energy phosphates (PCr and ATP), a rise in Pi, and lactic acid production, leading to a fall of pH.

By a fortuitous coincidence, MRS can detect many important compounds in these pathways. The MRS of ³¹P detects ATP, PCr, and Pi, in which chemical shift is an indicator of tissue pH. The MRS of ¹H can be used to measure lactate and other compounds (see later discussion).

MRS detects ¹³C (not ¹²C), which is only 1.1% naturally abundant. Naturally abundant ¹³C NMR signals can be detected from tissue glycogen and some lipids. The MRS of ¹³C can be used to detect a wide variety of other compounds through use of ¹³C-labeled metabolites.

Information From In Vivo Spectroscopy

Hydrogen 1

The proton (nucleus of hydrogen 1, or ¹H) is the most abundant nucleus in the body. The first NMR experiments were performed on protons, and observation of this nucleus serves as the basis for MRI. Figure 9-10 demonstrates a ¹H NMR spectrum of human muscle. A very large peak for water protons is seen. In addition, resonances for tissue lipids appear on the right, at a chemical shift of −3.3 ppm from water, with lipids resonating at a lower frequency than water. It is also possible to observe protons of tissue metabolites present at much lower concentrations by so-called water-suppression techniques, which eliminate the water signal by saturation or by selective excitation of the nonwater region.*

Figure 9-11 shows a ¹H spectrum of the rat brain in vivo accompanied by a ¹H spectrum of brain extract. The major peak is from NAA; this compound is found solely in the central nervous system (CNS) and largely in neurons and not glial cells.† Therefore NAA has been used widely as a marker of neuron density and viability.¹⁴³,⁴⁵⁵ Neurodegenerative diseases that cause neuronal loss (e.g., Alzheimer's disease [AD], epilepsy, and ischemia) are frequently associated with prolifera-

---

*References 21, 63, 79, 241, 512, 532.
†References 52, 288, 366, 368, 508, 515.

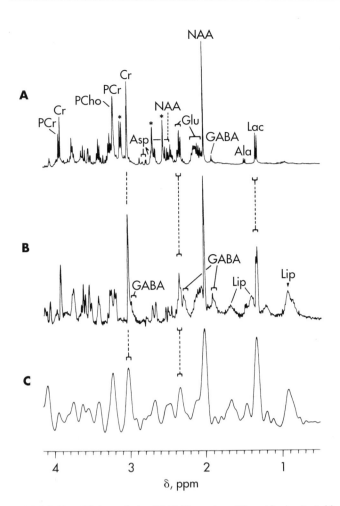

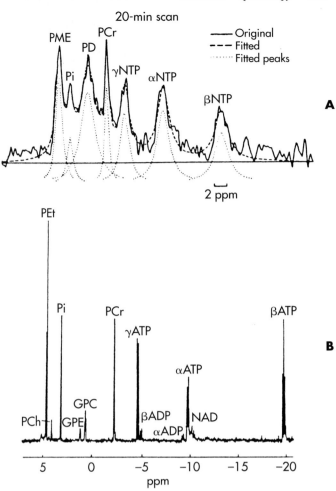

FIGURE 9-11 High-resolution ¹H NMR spectra of the rat brain. **A,** Acid extract of the in situ frozen brain of a rat breathing 20% oxygen and 80% nitric oxide. The extracts and lyophilized brain powder were suspended in 0.38 ml of 0.1 mmol/l phosphate buffer in ²H₂O (pH 7.2). *PCho,* Phosphocholine; *PCr,* phosphocreatine; *Cr,* creatine; *GABA,* γ-aminobutyric acid; *Asp,* aspartate; *Glu,* γ-glutamate; NAA, N-acetyl aspartate; *Ala,* alanine; *Lac,* lactate; *Lip,* lipid; *, added ethylenediamine tetraacetic acid (EDTA). **B,** ¹H NMR spectrum of excised brain tissue from a decapitated rat. A small amount of ²H₂O was added with the tissue, and the magnetic field was shimmed on the deuterium (²H) resonance. The H₂O signal was suppressed by a saturating RF field that was centered on the resonance for 2 sec during each scan cycle. **C,** In vivo ¹H spectrum of the posthypoxic rat brain obtained with a surface coil. Total time for spectrum was 2.3 min (sum of 32 FIDs). Resolution was enhanced by gaussian multiplication of the FID after removal of broad components by the convolution difference method. (From Behar KL, den Hollander JA, Stromski ME, et al: High resolution ¹H NMR study of cerebral hypoxia in vivo, Proc Natl Acad Sci U S A 80:4945, 1984.)

FIGURE 9-12 **A,** ³¹P NMR spectrum of a 17-day-old puppy brain. *PME,* Phosphomonoesters; *Pi,* inorganic phosphate; *PD,* phosphodiesters; *PCr,* phosphocreatine; γ-*NTP,* α-*NTP,* and β-NTP, respectively, γ, α, and β-phosphate of nucleotide triphosphates, largely ATP. The fitted peaks are shifted down for display. **B,** ³¹P NMR spectrum of puppy brain extract. Assignment of peaks in the PME region made in accordance with experimental results. *PEt,* Phosphorylethanolamine; *PCh,* phosphorylcholine; *GPC,* glycerophosphorylcholine; *GPE,* glycerophosphorylethanolamine. (From reference 217.)

tion of glia (gliosis), which to some extent replace the space occupied by the lost neurons. Therefore gliosis attenuates the atrophy that would have been produced by neuron loss. Measurements of NAA are expected to be a more sensitive marker of neuron loss than atrophy. The ¹H MRS spectra also show a peak for Cr. (This peak represents the sum of Cr and PCr and does not indicate the energy state of the cell.) The peak marked choline (Cho) represents the sum of all visible Cho metabolites, especially phosphocholine. Lactate also may be detected; lactate concentrations in muscle are rapidly increased by muscular exercise, and lactate levels in muscle and other tissues are increased by ischemia and hypoxia (Figure 9-11). A variety of other metabolites, including *myo*-inositol (mI), the amino acids glutamine and glutamate, and neurotransmitter substances, such as γ-aminobutyric acid (GABA), also may be detected.

One problem with ¹H MRS is that the large lipid peak can obscure some of the metabolite resonances. Thus ¹H MRS techniques have been applied primarily to brain, where there is little detectable lipid (except in some tumors and certain degenerative diseases, such as stroke and multiple sclerosis, where mobile lipids may be detected, presumably as

a consequence of membrane breakdown or infiltration by inflammatory cells). However, there are large amounts of lipid in subcutaneous tissue, and signals from this lipid pool and from cellular macromolecules may contaminate spectra obtained from brain when obtained at short TEs. In principle it is possible to achieve separation of signals from macromolecules from the much smaller metabolite molecules on the basis of T1 differences.[44] Application of ¹H MRS to other tissues that contain lipid is more difficult. Spectral editing techniques, which improve the selectivity of ¹H MRS for peaks that exhibit spin coupling, also have been developed,[462,464] including methods relying on multiple-quantum (MQ) pathways.[558]

Phosphorus 31

Figure 9-12, *A,* depicts the important features of an in vivo ³¹P MRS spectrum. Figure 9-12, *B,* depicts a high-resolution spectrum of acid-extracted tissue, demonstrating with certainty the assignments of each peak. On the right in Figure 9-12, *A,* are peaks for the three phosphates of ATP—α, β, and γ. The α- and β-phosphates of ADP overlap with the α- and γ-phosphates of ATP; however, because concentrations of ADP are kept so low, almost no ADP is detectable in healthy tissue by ³¹P MRS in vivo. The β peak of ATP is frequently used to assess ATP concentration because no other peak overlaps with it, and the baseline is relatively flat in this region. The peak for PCr is to the left of γ-ATP. Further to the left is a peak for phosphodiesters (PDEs) largely composed (in brain) of glycerol phosphocholine and phosphoethanolamine. The significance of peaks in this spectral region has been reviewed elsewhere.[88,102,103]

The Pi peak is important because it represents the sum of visible monobasic and dibasic inorganic phosphates, which are in rapid exchange. The chemical shift of this peak represents a weighted mean of these two species. Changes in pH alter the balance between monobasic and dibasic phosphate, thus producing a change in the chemical shift of the Pi peak. Acidosis shifts the Pi peak to the right, whereas alkalosis shifts the peak to the left. Changes in the chemical shift of Pi, usually referenced to PCr, can be used to noninvasively estimate intracellular pH. Several problems occur with this approach and have been extensively discussed. For instance, factors other than pH, especially ionic strength and magnesium (Mg^{+2}) ions, affect the chemical shift. Nevertheless, comparison of pH measured by other techniques with NMR measurements demonstrates that this is a valid approach to measure intracellular pH.[398]

The last peak on the left is composed of phosphomonoesters (PMEs). This peak contains several compounds[197,217] but is usually made up of phosphocholine, phosphoethanolamine, and a small contribution from sugar phosphates. The composition of this peak depends on the metabolic state of the cell. This peak is increased in some malignant tissues,[32,330] suggesting alterations of lipid membrane metabolism.

ATP complexed with Mg^{+2} is the most important substrate for metabolic reactions. The binding of Mg^{+2} to ATP alters the chemical shift of the β and γ peaks. Several investigators have used this property to estimate the ratio of free and Mg^{+2}-bound ATP in the cell. If an equilibrium constant for the binding of Mg^{+2} to ATP is assumed, concentration of free Mg^{+2} may be estimated. This technique has been used to investigate Mg^{+2} metabolism in red blood cells,[214] perfused heart,[562] and other tissues.[215,216,546] The Mg^{+2} concentration also has been estimated from the T2 of PCr.[120]

Magnetization-transfer measurements of metabolite exchange. In addition to measuring the steady state concentrations of metabolites, magnetization-transfer tecniques may be used to measure various exchange reactions (reviewed elsewhere).[12,294,536] In principle these techniques involve magnetic labeling of one or several peaks and subsequently observing the chemical transfer of the label to other peaks. In saturation transfer or inversion transfer, one peak is selectively saturated (the net magnetization eliminated) or inverted (receives a 180-degree pulse); the reduced intensity of other observed peaks (and the measured T1 of these peaks) allows the rate of the reaction to be measured. In 2D NMR, resonances are labeled and then observed after a period during which chemical exchange can take place.[29,191,261,291]

Magnetization-transfer techniques have been used to study the rate of exchange catalyzed by the enzyme CK in muscle, perfused heart, and brain.* In addition, the steady state synthesis of ATP has been studied in several tissues by saturation transfer.†

Nuclear magnetic resonance "visible" and "invisible" metabolites. Conventional high-resolution NMR techniques detect only highly mobile species. If the mobility is restricted because of binding to macromolecules or membranes, T2 is markedly shortened and the signals become broad, reducing peak height and signal-to-noise ratio (SNR). So-called solid state techniques[351] may be used to detect these broad resonances, but generally these methods have not been applied to biological studies. If the mobility of an observed species is severely restricted, the signal will be lost as a result of broadening of the resonance.

Several investigators have performed experiments comparing ^{31}P NMR spectra of various organs with the spectra of extracted tissues. In general, almost all the ATP and PCr that is detected in the extract is seen in vivo. In contrast, large amounts of Pi and ADP are not detected in vivo. These findings suggest that these metabolites are bound or located in a compartment that prevents them from being detected. It has been suggested that the location of ADP and Pi in mitochondria might render them invisible to the conventional NMR experiment. This could be caused by the presence of paramagnetic materials in mitochondria, by binding, or by the high viscosity of intramitochondrial water restricting mobility of metabolites in this organelle.

Proton decoupling and nuclear Overhauser effect. Many ^{31}P phosphate resonances are slightly broadened at 1.5 Tesla (T) because of

residual J couplings to protons (of the order of 10 Hz). These couplings can be removed by proton decoupling (irradiation at the ^{1}H frequency), which sharpens the resonance lines to improve SNR. Further SNR improvement can arise from saturation of the proton signals as a result of the nuclear Overhauser effect (NOE). This effect does not depend on J couplings but arises in relation to the magnetic dipole-dipole interactions between ^{1}H and ^{31}P nuclei. The advantages of proton decoupling for ^{31}P MRS have been demonstrated in brain,[199,318] heart,[318] and tumors.[386]

Carbon 13

The naturally abundant nucleus of carbon is ^{12}C, which is not detected by MRI. However, ^{13}C is detected and has been used extensively in high-resolution NMR studies. If sufficient ^{13}C label is added through a labeled compound to an in vivo system, some of the subsequent metabolism of the compound label can be detected by following the label by NMR. Several investigators have used this approach to assess regulation of various metabolic pathways.[123,387,502] This approach is demonstrated in Figure 9-13. In addition, the 1.1% naturally abundant ^{13}C signals in glycogen have been detected in vivo.[507] Despite the high molecular weight of this molecule, the carbons have sufficient mobility

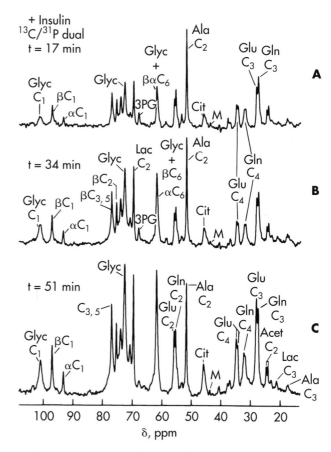

FIGURE 9-13 ^{31}C NMR spectra of isolated perfused rat liver at 35 ± 1° C. **A,** Spectrum of liver experiment measured intermittently during the period 17 to 33 min after the addition of 9 mmol/L (2-^{13}C) pyruvate, 7.3 mmol/L (1,2-^{13}C) ethanol, and 3.6 mmol/L NH_4Cl; 7 nmol insulin was present in the perfusate). Substrate and insulin were maintained at or near these levels. **B** and **C,** Spectra accumulated intermittently during the periods 34 to 50 min and 51 to 67 min, respectively, after addition of substrate and insulin. A spectrum of the ^{13}C natural-abundance background of this liver was accumulated under identical conditions before the substrate was added. For clarity of presentation this background spectrum was subtracted from each of the spectra shown. The labeled ^{13}C NMR peaks in these spectra include those caused by the α- and β-anomers of D-glucose—β-C-l, α-C-1-β-C-6, and α-C-6. The peaks labeled *Glyc* result from glycogen. Other abbreviations are as follows: *3PG,* 3-phospho-D-glycerate; *Ala* C_2, alanine C-2; *Cit,* citrate-CH_2; *M,* malate C-3; *Glu* C_3, glutamate C-3; *Gln* C_3, glutamate C-3; *Lac* C_2, lactate C-2; *Acet* C_2, acetate C-2. (From Cohen SM: J Biol Chem 258:14294, 1983.)

to enable detection by MRS, as illustrated by Figure 9-14. This subject has been reviewed[507] and has considerable promise for investigating various aspects of intermediary metabolism. Shulman and co-workers have developed ^{13}C NMR techniques for measurement of metabolic pathways* in subjects, including humans.[22,263-265,497] An important application of this approach was demonstrated in studies aimed at determining whether there was a defect in glycogen synthesis in subjects with non–insulin-dependent diabetes.[499] Figure 9-15 shows the incremental glycogen content in muscle as a function of time in diabetic and nondiabetic subjects. As shown, the diabetic subjects demonstrated a prolonged lag before the onset of muscle glycogen synthesis, and the mean rate of glycogen synthesis was less than half that of normal subjects. The authors concluded that defects in muscle glycogen synthesis play a dominant role in the insulin resistance observed in subjects with non–insulin-dependent diabetes.

Proton decoupling and proton observation. The ^{13}C atoms with directly bonded protons have large J couplings (approximately 150 Hz)

---

*References 10, 42, 47, 95, 121-126, 151, 152, 308, 387, 389, 463, 498, 502, 507.

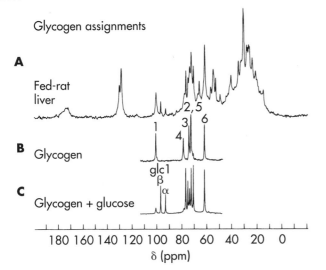

FIGURE 9-14 Proton-decoupled ^{13}C natural-abundance NMR spectra. **A,** The excised liver (wet weight 12.7 g) from a 374-g rat given free access to food. **B,** Solution of rabbit liver glycogen (200 mg/ml) in ^2H_2O. **C,** Mixture of glycogen with α-D- and β-D-glucose. These spectra show the assignments for the ^{13}C resonances from glycogen C_1-C_6, where C_1 is the anomeric carbon. (From reference 507.)

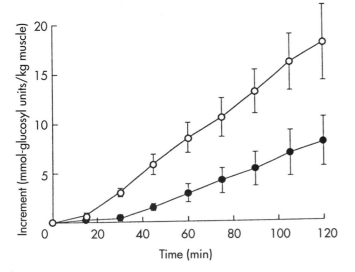

FIGURE 9-15 Time course for mean incremental changes in muscle glycogen concentration from baseline in normal subjects *(open circles)* and subjects with non–insulin-dependent diabetes *(solid circles)*. (From reference 499.)

and, without proton decoupling to collapse these couplings and improve SNR (see previous discussion), would be observed as multiplets. Thus most ^{13}C in vivo experiments are conducted with proton decoupling.* Other methods for dealing with these couplings are also available for in vivo experiments.[47] Potentially, one of the most powerful methods uses the existence of the J couplings to observe the presence of the ^{13}C resonances with improved sensitivity through the ^1H signal.[463,465]

Sodium 23 and Potassium 39
Sodium is the major extracellular cation, and potassium is the major intracellular cation. The activity of the sodium-potassium–activated ATPase located in the cell membrane maintains large gradients of these cations. Both sodium and potassium can be detected by MRS. They are quadrupolar nuclei (nuclear spin quantum number greater than ½), which means that the nuclear orientation can be influenced by local electric field gradients (such as that created by a chemical bond). This sensitivity to electric field gradients makes quadrupolar nuclei extremely sensitive to transient immobilization, which in turn produces broadening of the signal.

The MRS of ^{23}Na has been used to investigate the regulation of intracellular sodium in several tissues. Early investigations of tissue ^{23}Na indicated that only about 40% of the signal was detected, apparently as a result of quadripolar broadening of the signal.[325] Initially this was interpreted to suggest that much of the intracellular sodium was "bound," although it was later demonstrated that only a tiny fraction of sodium is transiently immobilized, leading to quadripolar broadening of the signal.[51,118,260,496] In addition, ^{23}Na MRI has been used to produce sodium images of the CNS[237] and other tissues.[96,150,374] Factors that inhibit the activity of the sodium pump result in increased levels of intracellular sodium, which enhances the intensity of the ^{23}Na image. However, changes in ^{23}Na signal intensity always must be interpreted with caution because they may represent variations of the quadripolar broadening effect rather than true changes of sodium concentration. Moreover, the observed signal represents extracellular, as well as intracellular, sodium.

Representative potassium 39 (^{39}K) NMR spectra are shown in Figure 9-16. Although the ^{39}K nucleus has a low gyromagnetic ratio, the abundance of potassium within cells and the short relaxation times (which allow rapid pulsing) permit detection of ^{39}K signals within a relatively short period in a high-field magnet system.[85,130] It has been demonstrated that potassium infusion and depletion produce changes in the ^{39}K NMR signal that are proportional to changes in total tissue potassium.[6] Therefore ^{39}K MRS may be used noninvasively to measure alterations of K^+ homeostasis in animals and patients, perhaps to determine effects of diuretics and other alterations.

Fluorine 19 and Lithium 7
Almost no naturally abundant ^{19}F exists in vivo. Therefore MR of this nucleus is performed by exogenous addition of various fluorine-containing compounds. The MRS of ^{19}F has been used to study anesthetic metabolism in vivo,[563-566] as illustrated by Figure 9-17, to monitor the pH of lymphocytes,[153] and to measure levels of fluorinated anticancer[348,482,506,560] and antipsychotic drugs.

The MRS of ^7Li has been used to detect brain Li in patients treated for bipolar disorder[200,289,290,446] and could be used to monitor Li levels.

Nitrogen 14 and 15
Both the ^{14}N and ^{15}N nuclei of nitrogen can be detected by MRS; ^{14}N is the naturally abundant species.[31] The natural abundance of ^{15}N is very low; thus ^{15}N-labeling studies may be performed to study nitrogen flux. So far there has been very little application of this finding to in vivo NMR. However, ^{14}N studies of the kidney have demonstrated peaks for urea, ammonium, and several other nitrogen-containing compounds (Figure 9-18).[31]

APPLICATIONS
Muscle

Animal and Ex Vivo Studies
The MRS of muscle has recently been reviewed.[282,283,359,365] The first use of MRS to detect metabolite concentrations in intact tissue was performed on excised muscle.[243] Since that time, ^{31}P MRS has been used

---

*References 212, 213, 266, 429, 498, 500.

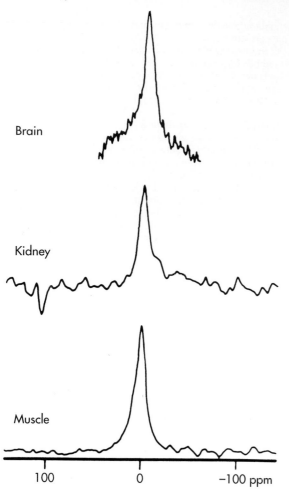

Brain

Kidney

Muscle

100   0   -100 ppm

FIGURE 9-16   [39]K MR spectra of in vivo rat thigh muscle, kidney, and brain. The spectra were obtained with 1000 accumulations using a 90-degree pulse and 0.3-sec delay between acquisitions, with 30-Hz line broadening applied before Fourier transformation. (From reference 6.)

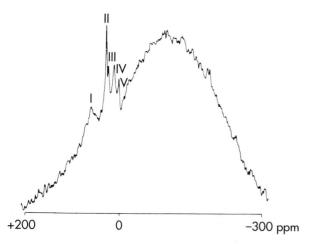

+200   0   -300 ppm

FIGURE 9-18   [14]N MR spectrum of in vivo rat kidney. *Peak I,* urea; *peak II,* trimethylamines; *peaks III* and *IV,* amino acids; *peak V,* ammonium (NH$_4^+$). (From reference 31.)

extensively to investigate muscle physiology, metabolic control, and the effects of disease.* Muscle is an excellent tissue with which to work because, compared with most internal organs, it is relatively homogeneous. However, muscle contains connective tissue, adipose tissue, and different fiber types, which may severely complicate data interpretation.

*References 35, 138-140, 162, 186, 440, 516.

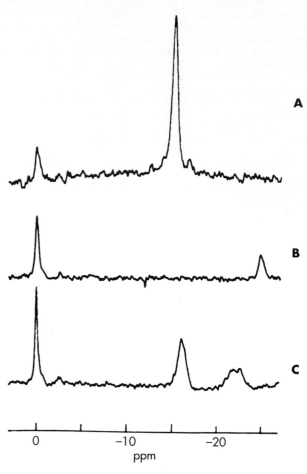

A

B

C

0   -10   -20 ppm

FIGURE 9-17   [19]F MR spectra of halothane **(A)**, methoxyflurane **(B)**, and isoflurane **(C)**. Each animal was premedicated with ketamine (50 mg/kg) and xylazine (5 mg/kg), intubated, and positioned in the magnet. Subsequently the rabbit was connected to an anesthesia machine, and a background spectrum was taken before administration of the inhalation agent (1% halothane for 30 min, 1.5% methoxyflurane for 80 min, or 1% isoflurane for 40 min). Spectra were acquired on an Oxford Research Systems TMR-32 spectrometer with a surface coil (3.5 cm in diameter) placed on the frontal bones midway between the eyes. Chemical shifts are reported relative to an external standard of 2.5% C$_2$Br$_2$F$_4$ in CHCl$_3$ (contained in a sealed 4-mm sphere) with Å 0.2-ppm accuracy. (From reference 566.)

Many ^{31}P MRS studies have demonstrated that muscular contraction produces a rapid drop of PCr, a rise of Pi, and an acid shift of the Pi peak. The ATP peaks are usually (but not always) unchanged until PCr is virtually depleted; this observation is consistent with a single pool of CK and its reactants. Dawson et al[138-140] performed a series of experiments that quantitated the concentrations of high-energy phosphates in perfused frog muscle and correlated the force of contraction with the levels of various high-energy phosphates. Figure 9-19 presents some results from these studies. Many other investigators also have used ^{31}P MRS to study the metabolism and pH of animal muscle.[87,89,227,570] In addition, ^{31}P NMR saturation transfer techniques have been used to investigate the kinetics of the reaction catalyzed by CK in vivo.[400]

Clinical Studies

Investigation of human muscle metabolism by ^{31}P MRS was pioneered by groups in Oxford[16,106,437,459,517] and Philadelphia.[108,109,555] These experiments involved placement of a surface coil over a muscle of the arm or leg, followed by the acquisition of MRS data during observation of control ^{31}P MR spectra. Muscle energy metabolism is subsequently perturbed by an exercise protocol, which might include the application of a tourniquet to produce ischemia, followed by recovery. In normal subjects, exercise induces rapid depletion of PCr, whereas

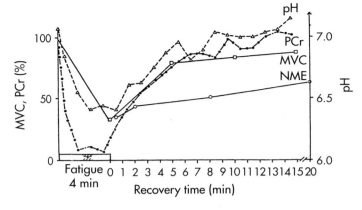

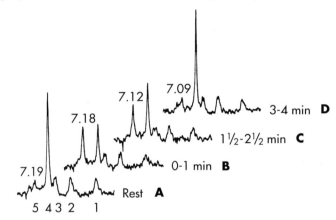

FIGURE 9-20 Exercise (4-min duration) and recovery effects on maximum voluntary contraction *(MVC)*, PCr, pH, and neuromuscular efficiency *(NME)*. MVC is defined as force-integrated EMG at maximum force. Exercise causes lowering of all parameters. During recovery, pH, PCr, and MVC recovered rapidly, whereas NME recovered much more slowly.

FIGURE 9-21 ^{31}P MR spectra in a patient, showing the effects of aerobic exercise. The first spectrum (**A**) was recorded at rest before exercise; subsequent spectra (**B** to **D**) were recorded during the periods shown, in which 0 min corresponds to the start of exercise. Exercise was maintained from 0 to 1 min, and aerobic recovery followed. The signals are assigned as follows: *1, 2,* and *3,* the α, and γ-phosphates of ATP; *4,* phosphocreatine *(PCr)*; *5,* inorganic phosphate *(Pi)*. The pH values were determined from the frequency separation of the Pi and PCr signals. (From reference 459.)

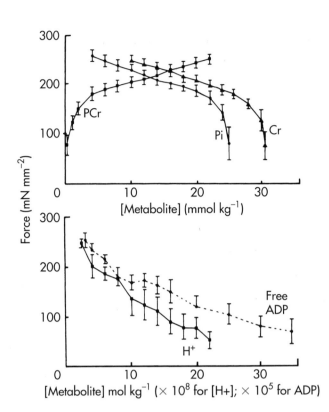

FIGURE 9-19 Force developed as a function of metabolite levels: averaged results of six frog experiments. Spectra were accumulated for 5-min periods if the muscles were stimulated for 1 sec every 60 sec or 5 sec every 5 min, and for 2-min periods if the stimulation was for 1 sec every 20 sec. The force developed at particular metabolite levels was obtained by linear interpolation between the data points so as to obtain the standard errors shown by the vertical bars. (From reference 139.)

ATP concentrations are unchanged or only partially reduced. A thorough study of normal subjects was reported by Taylor et al.[516] In all cases exercise produced an initial rapid decrease in PCr, with a corresponding rise in Pi and a fall in pH. The fact that recovery of initial metabolite levels began as soon as exercise ceased was interpreted to mean that glycolysis was switched off as soon as exercise stopped.

^{31}P MRS has been used extensively to investigate the relationship between work and steady state oxidative phosphorylation in human muscle. Chance's group has studied human muscle by MRS in a wide variety of diseases and conditions. For moderate exercise a linear relationship between the work rate and the Pi/PCr ratio was found, suggesting that ADP levels regulated oxygen consumption.[108,110,554] Miller et al[364] simultaneously measured oxygen, electromyogram (EMG), and ^{31}P MRS signals in normal subjects during exercise and recovery to investigate the metabolic correlates of fatigue. Figure 9-20 depicts the changes in maximum force and metabolite levels measured by MRS during a 4-min maximally sustained contraction and the subsequent recovery period. In general, changes in force correlated with changes in both PCr and pH. Subsequent studies used varying degrees of intermittent muscular contraction to produce various steady states of fatigue. During recovery from fatiguing exercise, muscle force was closely correlated with metabolic recovery. These experiments demonstrated that loss of maximum force (i.e., fatigue) best correlated with accumulation of total Pi or $H_2PO_4^-$ rather than with changes of H^+.[364,365]

MRS has been used to investigate metabolic derangements in a variety of clinical myopathies. Ross et al[459] first used ^{31}P MRS to characterize McArdle's syndrome as shown in Figure 9-21; they found that the usual decrease of pH produced by exercise did not occur. The lack of acidification was attributed to the inhibition of glycogenolysis associated with the absence of phosphorylase, which characterizes McArdle's syndrome. Other investigators have used MRS to study glycogen storage diseases,[106,108] mitochondrial myopathies,[186,437,439] muscular dystrophies,[390] neuropathies, and systemic disorders.[438] Patients with Duchenne's dystrophy[390] have been found to have a signal in the phosphodiester region similar to that noted in dystrophic chicken muscles.[88,102] In a study of a patient with a severe defect in complex III of the electron transport chain (Figure 9-22), the resting PCr/Pi ratio was extremely low.[163] Treatment of this patient with menadione (vitamin K$_3$) and ascorbate (vitamin C) produced a 25-fold increase of the recovery rate relative to the pretherapy value.

Muscular exercise in patients with congestive heart failure produced more rapid depletion of PCr and greater acidosis than in control subjects, suggesting impairment of muscle metabolism.* Blood flow was not reduced in these patients, suggesting that metabolic abnormalities

---

*References 7, 327, 328, 331, 441, 554, 559.

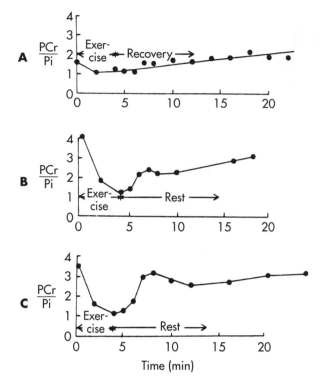

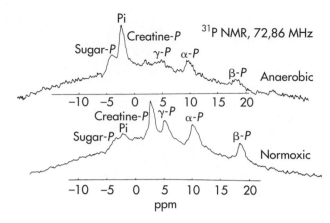

FIGURE 9-23 ^{31}P MR spectra of the normoxic and anaerobic in situ mouse head performed at room temperature with 2000 scans each at 0.4 sec/scan. (From reference 111.)

FIGURE 9-22 **A,** Pretreatment exercise evaluation of a patient with a defect in complex III of the electron transport chain, illustrating an initial PCr/Pi value of 1.7, an exercise level of 1.0, and a recovery extending over 20 min. **B** and **C,** Exercise evaluation after therapy with menadione and ascorbate, showing a higher resting PCr/Pi and faster recovery kinetics. **B,** Right arm. **C,** Left arm. (From reference 163.)

within the muscle contribute to the symptoms of fatigue and exercise intolerance in heart failure.[20,331,554] Alterations in the muscle have been detected by MRS in patients with Duchenne's muscular dystrophy[208,390,571] and myotonic dystrophy.[518] In patients with multiple sclerosis compared with control subjects, PCr is decreased during electrical stimulation, indicating greater muscle fatigability that was associated with an impaired metabolic capacity.[284] During voluntary exercise in patients with multiple sclerosis,[284] postpolio syndrome,[488] and amyotrophic lateral sclerosis,[489] the fall of PCr and pH was less than that expected from the fall in force, indicating that activation failure, rather than metabolic inhibition, was a significant cause of muscle fatigue.

Brain

Animal Studies

Noninvasive investigation of brain metabolism is an important area for MRS.[430,455] Chance et al[111] first obtained ^{31}P MRS spectra from an anesthetized mouse placed in an NMR tube, within a conventional NMR spectrometer. Figure 9-23 shows that anoxia reversibly produced PCr depletion. Another early method used a surface coil to obtain ^{31}P MRS spectra from the brain of a living rat.[2] The PCr/ATP ratio was 1.9, which is considerably greater than that obtained from chemical assay of freeze-clamped samples but considerably lower than that of resting muscle. This suggests the possibility that continued electric activity of the brain produces a lower steady state PCr/ATP ratio, although the concentration of brain cell Cr also may limit PCr levels.

Other researchers have used surface coils and ^{31}P MRS to investigate various aspects of brain metabolism. Phosphodiester peaks are prominent in the brains of adult animals, consisting of glycerol-3-phosphorylcholine, glycerol-3-phosphorylethanolamine, and other metabolites.[72,131,197,430] Studies of neonates have shown that these phosphodiester signals are lower and the phosphomonoester peaks are higher, perhaps representing alterations of certain lipid components in developing brains.[91,201,217,529,572]

Prolonged ischemia of the brain produces brain infarction or stroke, and MRS has been used extensively to study brain ischemia in animal

models. Thulborn et al[526,527] were the first to study the effects of ischemia produced by carotid occlusion. Ischemia (stroke) produced the expected loss of PCr and ATP, a rise in Pi, and acidification. Subsequently, other investigators have studied experimental stroke models using ^{31}P MRS. In addition, the effects of ischemia, hypoxia, and status epilepticus on brain metabolism have been studied in rabbits.[380,381] Hypoglycemia caused depletion of both PCr and ATP similar to the effects of ischemia.[131] The changes were reversible after the administration of glucose. Hypoxia and seizures also produced similar changes in high-energy phosphates. It is not surprising that the injection of cyanide produced a loss of brain high-energy phosphates and acidification similar to the effects of ischemia.[119]

In investigation of seizures, it was found that chemically induced status epilepticus produced a 50% decrease in the PCr/Pi ratio, with a drop of intracellular pH (pHi) from 7.1 to 6.8.[419] Calculations using the equilibrium constant for the CK reaction suggested that intracellular acidosis was responsible for most of the PCr reduction. Subsequent ^{1}H MRS studies have shown that a marked rise in brain lactate occurs, which is presumably responsible for much of the acidosis.[43] The use of ^{13}C-labeled glucose has demonstrated that the prolonged elevation of brain lactate that follows cessation of seizures is caused by continued production of lactate and not sequestration in an inaccessible metabolic pool.[465]

In analogy with previous ^{31}P MR saturation-transfer measurements in muscle, Shoubridge et al used ^{31}P NMR saturation transfer to measure the rate of ATP synthesis in rat,[495] rabbit,[144] and monkey[373] brains. The measured forward and reverse rates of CK were approximately equal. Exchange between the γ- and β-phosphate of ATP was also detected, complicating the analysis. 2D NMR saturation-transfer studies of brain also demonstrated equal forward and reverse fluxes but did not detect γ-/β-ATP exchange.[29] This difference may represent fundamental differences between the saturation transfer (a continuous-labeling technique) and 2D NMR (a pulse-labeling technique).[291,292]

MRS of ^{13}C has been used in brain studies on animals.[34,64,151] These studies demonstrate the carbon resonances of lactate, glutamine, and glutamate. Hypoxia caused an increase in the ^{13}C lactate signal, whereas the amino acids also rose steadily. Methods with improved sensitivity (^{13}C decouple and ^{1}H observe) have been used to estimate the flux through the metabolic pathways of glycolysis (i.e., glucose to lactate) and the citric acid cycle (i.e., glucose to glutamate). However, derivation of metabolic rates from ^{13}C flux measurement is dependent on the validity of several assumptions that have not been thoroughly tested. Nevertheless, these experiments demonstrated the potential feasibility of ^{13}C labeling studies for clinical use.

The application of ^{1}H MRS to investigate metabolism requires the use of water-suppression techniques.[41,43,464] Most ^{1}H MRS studies were performed on the brain because brain lacks the mobile lipid that interferes with certain metabolite resonances. As discussed, hypoxia produces a reversible rise in lactate. Hypoglycemic encephalopathy produces a decrease in glutamate and an increase in aspartate.[41] For spins exhibiting spin-spin coupling (multiplet structure), specialized MRS experiments (spectral editing experiments) can elicit signal from only the desired multiplet. Spectral editing techniques are useful for obtaining the methyl signal from lactate,[464] which is a doublet.

In recent years, MRS and spectroscopic imaging studies have been performed on animal brain to investigate a variety of disease models, including ischemia,[205] epilepsy,[161] brain tumors,[445,458] and others.[141]

Clinical Studies

The major clinical use of MRS is for studies of the brain. When the first edition of this book was written, there were only two published clinical studies of human brain; for the second edition there were about 50; and now there are hundreds. This subject is also reviewed in Chapter 72. The rapid increase in the use of MRS for clinical studies is the result of the proliferation of high-field magnets that are capable of MRS and the development of clinically usable image-guided MRS techniques. The brain is particularly suitable for MRS and MRSI studies because the head can be immobilized, brain tissue is close to the surface, and there are virtually no detectable lipid signals within brain parenchyma that contaminate ^{1}H MRS spectra. Because of the large number of publications, it is impossible to provide a detailed review of the entire MRS literature; therefore important examples are discussed with an emphasis on possible clinical applications. At present, most but not all (see Chapter 72), scientists in the field consider the use of MRS and MRSI for routine clinical evaluation to be uncertain. However, clinical applications are promising in a few areas, such as epilepsy, AD, brain tumors, and possibly other types of cancer; these and other areas are discussed in the following sections.

Normal Adult Brain

The first MRS studies of adult brain were performed by Bottomley et al[69] and Radda and co-workers.[408] Luyten et al reported both ^{31}P MR (ISIS) spectra[319,320] and [1]H (SPARS) spectra.[322] Following those initial results, Frahm et al[172] and den Hollander, Luyten, and their colleagues[545] reported the use of stimulated-echo techniques to obtain localized, high-resolution ^{1}H MRS spectra from human brain in vivo. Spectra showed NAA, glutamate, glutamine, aspartate, Cr, Cho, and mI. Differences in spectra have been noted between gray and white matter and between different regions of the brain.* A number of reported methods for estimating absolute metabolite concentrations of ^{1}H and ^{31}P metabolites using an external standard or water as an internal standard now exist.† Relaxation times (T1 and T2) for the various metabolites were also reported in a number of the studies referenced earlier.

Alzheimer's Disease

AD produces a slowly progressive loss of cognitive function. It is the most common dementia and is very difficult to diagnose during life. ^{1}H MRS studies of AD in brain in vitro showed decreased NAA levels.[369] Single-voxel ^{1}H MRS‡ and ^{1}H MRSI[360] have shown that NAA is reduced in the frontoparietal and temporal lobes and hippocampus.[267] Ross et al[363,367,494] reported increased mI in AD (Figure 9-24), but increased mI may occur in other conditions as well and may not be completely specific for AD.[84] Increased Cho levels have been reported,[112] but this result has not been found by other investigators.[363,367] Mackay et al[323] reported that NAA decreases are independent of tissue changes and that MRI and MRSI provide complementary information for diagnosis. Recently, investigators in our laboratory have shown decreased NAA levels in the hippocampus of patients with AD[474] and in patients with mild cognitive impairments who are at risk of developing AD. Our use of a newly developed multislice ^{1}H MRSI technique allows sampling of multiple brain regions, which appears to provide better discrimination between patients with AD and control subjects. Ross and co-workers[455] have suggested that MRS provides sufficient diagnostic information to be used in the routine assessment of dementia. However, until the reports of high diagnostic sensitivity and specificity are replicated in large numbers of patients, it seems prudent to consider MRS in the clinical investigation stage for assessment of dementia.

^{31}P MRS studies of AD have shown increased frontal lobe phosphomonoesters, with decreasing phosphomonoesters as the disease progresses, and increased phosphodiesters in late disease.[420,421] Decreased PCr and Pi were also found.[132,509] The lack of these findings previously[376] possibly may have been related to different localization techniques.

Brain Tumors

^{31}P and ^{1}H MRS have yielded a plethora of data and a striking diversity of metabolic patterns in tumors of the brain. Initially, single-volume localization techniques were used until it became clear that metabolic heterogeneity and often small tumor sizes favored the use of spectroscopic imaging techniques. ^{1}H MRSI has been especially helpful in assessing metabolic heterogeneity and regional metabolic variations associated with brain neoplasms.[321] Using ^{1}H MRSI, spatial resolutions of less than 0.5 ml have been achieved using phased-array surface coils and special data-reconstruction routines.[375] However, with most articles on tumor MRS, care has to be taken in the interpretation of these spectra because of the possible contribution of surrounding tissue to the "tumor" spectrum. More comprehensive treatments of tumor studies by MRS are available in the recent literature.[38,383,384] Tumors generally yield abnormal spectra, with the most commonly reported abnormalities being an alkaline pH (measured by ^{31}P MRS), increased Cho and phosphomonoester (PME), increased lactate as a result of anaerobic glycolysis, decreased NAA (or complete absence of NAA because of the nonneuronal origin of many brain tumors), and decreased Cr and PCr because of the compromised energy state of tumor tissue (or lack of Cr and PCr in brain tumor metastases). The Cho is generally increased in the solid regions of tumors, with decreased Cho in the central portion. Much of the Cho increase is likely to come from breakdown products of membrane phospholipids as a result of rapid cell turnover; thus necrotic areas show reduced Cho signal. Altered tumor metabolism, however, also may be a source of Cho changes. Furthermore, tumors appear to be characterized by prolonged metabolite T1 and T2 relaxation times.[246,444,543] An example of a ^{1}H MRSI data set from an anaplastic astrocytoma is shown in Figure 9-25.

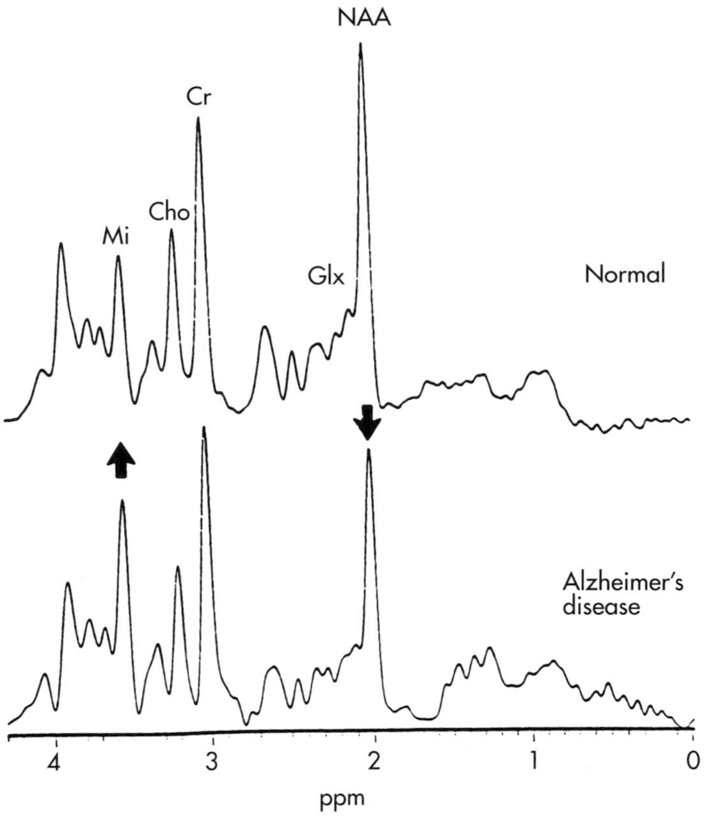

FIGURE 9-24 ^{1}H MR spectra from the occipital cortex (gray matter) of a patient with probable Alzheimer's disease compared with an age-related normal subject. Peaks are scaled to creatine *(Cr)* and provide a relative measure of concentration of individual metabolites. (From reference 455.)

---

*References 153, 170, 174, 234, 316, 520, 521.
†References 39, 65, 86, 90, 116, 235, 252, 296, 297, 306, 333, 362, 415, 433, 460, 510, 528.
‡References 84, 112, 267, 317, 363, 367, 421, 491, 494.

Studies of malignant gliomas reveal a broad variety of metabolic alterations compared with uninfiltrated control tissue; the most consistent findings are high levels of Cho[82,181] and lactate[82] and an alkaline pH.[226,407] Alkaline pH is commonly observed in the presence of high levels of lactate. Tumors with high lactate levels also had increased glucose metabolism by fluorodeoxyglucose (FDG) positron emission tomography (PET).[232] ^{1}H MRS studies of meningiomas have found a decrease or absence of Cr plus PCr and NAA, with a prominent Cho peak,[82,543] and aspartate, taurine, and alanine also have been found.[36,414]

^{31}P MRS studies showed decreased concentrations of all brain tumor metabolites relative to control brain, reflecting loss of viable tissue.[248] PDE tends to be decreased in high-grade gliomas[226] and low-grade astrocytomas.[13] ^{31}P MRS of meningiomas revealed decreased PDE, a tendency for decreased PCr, increased PME, and alkaline pH,[13,224,226] which is consistent with ^{1}H MRS findings as described earlier.

Brain tumors have been studied before, during, and after chemotherapy or radiotherapy.* Malignant degeneration has been correlated with increasing Cho, whereas clinical improvement of gliomas parallels Cho decreases.[181] Cho is decreased in chronic radiation necrosis, suggesting a potential discriminator between radiation necrosis and tumor tissue.[181] A patient with non-Hodgkin's lymphoma was studied serially by ^{1}H MRSI[54] (Figure 9-26). During the course of radiation therapy, Cho and lipid signal decreased, whereas NAA and Cr levels returned to normal in the tumor region. Arnold et al[17,18] reported transient decreases in PCr and PDE and pH changes after intraarterial and intravenous 1,3-bis-(2-chloroethyl)-1-nitrosurea for treatment of astrocytomas and glioblastomas. Although the detection of changes in metabolite concentrations

during cancer treatment is readily observable by in vivo MRS, tumor- or treatment-specific changes have yet to be identified in studies with a large number of well-defined patients. Only those studies will show whether MRS will be able to guide treatment of intracranial tumors.

None of the individual metabolic characteristics of brain tumors determined by in vivo MRS are specific to cancer. Brain tumor spectra almost always differ from spectra obtained from controls, whereas intraindividual spectral differences of a single tumor in various locations are often greater than differences between spectra from tumors of different histological sources. Recent findings suggest that malignancy may be differentiated on the basis of low NAA and normal or elevated Cho, low Cr, and high lactate.[181,384,455] There is conflicting evidence, however, whether high-grade tumors can be distinguished from their low-grade counterparts. Whereas Negendank et al[384] and Arnold et al[19] find high lactate levels in high- versus low-grade glial tumors, Herholtz et al[232] and Kugel et al[299] did not find a significant correlation between tumor grade and lactate levels. Thus lactate does not appear to be of prognostic value in tumor management. The relationship of Cho levels and tumor grading also remains an area of discussion.[181] A recent article suggests that a statistically determined linear combination of metabolic parameters from short-TE ^{1}H MRS is useful in distinguishing between control tissue and low- and high-grade tumors.[219] The final evaluation of the diagnostic and prognostic value of in vivo brain tumor MRS awaits the completion of well-designed prospective trials in large patient populations.

Apart from these clinical trials, future work[384] will focus on correlation of in vivo MR spectroscopic findings with histopathological findings,[298] with in vitro analysis of the same tumor tissue,[196,298,417,543] and with results from tumor-cell cultures[295] and animal-tumor models.[457]

*References 18, 54, 224, 225, 312, 429, 478, 525.

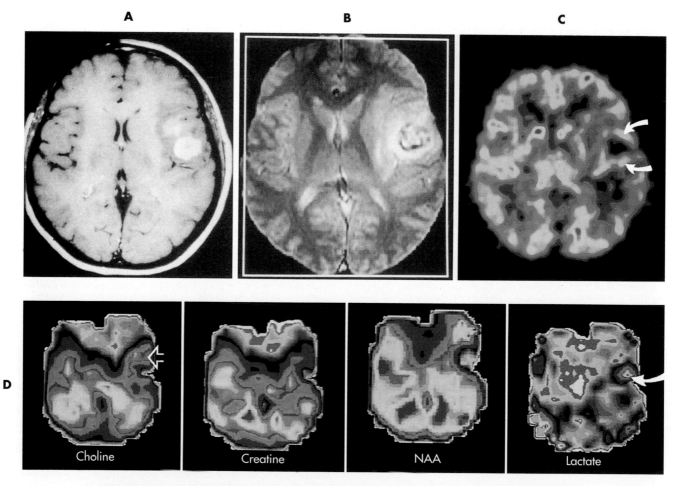

FIGURE 9-25 Images obtained in a 44-year-old woman with an anaplastic astrocytoma. **A,** Gadolinium-enhanced T1-weighted image showing enhancing lesion in the left temporal lobe and insula. **B,** Multiplanar GRE localization image. **C,** Axial FDG PET scan. Hypometabolic areas are bluish-green; hypermetabolic areas are yellowish-red. A rim of hypermetabolic tissue *(arrows)* surrounds the hypometabolic core. **D,** ^{1}H MRSI metabolite maps for Cho, Cr, NAA, and lactate. Low-intensity areas are grayish-blue; higher-intensity areas are yellowish-red. Deficits are apparent for Cho, Cr, and NAA, and lactate is elevated in the core. (From reference 181.)

Early correlative studies have confirmed in vivo findings described previously, but they also have yielded information that could not be obtained by in vivo MRS of human brain tumors alone. For example, it has been shown that high-grade astrocytomas accumulate lipids in necrotic tissue.[298] Of more far-reaching consequences for the interpretation of in vivo tumor spectra are findings in human brain tumor cell cultures that suggest that lactate and Cho changes could reflect secondary metabolic changes, such as hypoxia and necrosis, rather than tumor characteristics.[295]

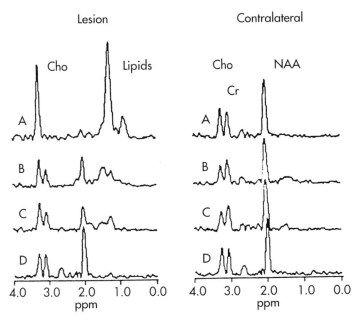

FIGURE 9-26   ¹H MR spectra from a non-Hodgkin's lymphoma lesion center *(left)* and from the contralateral hemisphere *(right)* in four consecutive studies (**A** to **D**). The studies were obtained before radiation therapy **(A)**, during radiation therapy **(B)**, after therapy **(C)**, and at follow-up (33 months) **(D)**. Calibration was accomplished with the assumption that the NAA signal from the contralateral hemisphere did not change. (From reference 54.)

Epilepsy

³¹P MRS single-voxel[247] imaging and MRSI[187,250] showed that the region of the seizure focus in temporal lobe epilepsy[247,250] and frontal lobe epilepsy[187] is more alkaline than the contralateral brain region. Tissue alkalosis could be a result of the severe acidosis that occurs during seizure activity. Alternatively, because alkalosis increases seizure frequency, this increased pH may be a clue to the pathogenesis of epileptic seizures. Changes in the PCr/Pi ratio that lateralize the focus, without changes in pH, also have been reported in temporal lobe epilepsy.[117,303]

A major potential clinical application of MRS is use of ¹H MRSI for seizure-focus lateralization in temporal lobe epilepsy, which has been demonstrated in dozens of reports from different institutions. After the initial report of reduced NAA in the ipsilateral hippocampus,[336] subsequent work found a 21% reduction of NAA in the ipsilateral hippocampus and correctly lateralized the focus in all cases studied.[251] This essential finding has been replicated repeatedly (Figure 9-27).* NAA/Cr is also reduced in the ipsilateral frontal lobe in patients with frontal lobe epilepsy.[188] In temporal lobe epilepsy NAA/(Cr + Cho) appears to be the best metabolite measurement for seizure-focus localization.[164] Reduced NAA on the contralateral hippocampus was reported in many cases of unilateral temporal lobe epilepsy, suggesting contralateral disease, which seemed to predict outcome after surgical removal of the seizure focus. Finally, some patients with epilepsy showed ipsilateral reduction of NAA without hippocampal atrophy.[164] This is consistent with gliosis masking neuron loss and suggests that NAA is a more sensitive marker of hippocampal disease than is atrophy. In conclusion, ¹H MRS and MRSI provide clinically useful information for the presurgical evaluation of temporal lobe epilepsy. Decreased NAA levels lateralize the seizure focus even when there is no hippocampal atrophy. The presence of contralateral disease seems to predict a poor surgical outcome in subjects without ipsilateral hippocampal atrophy. Although more studies are needed, ¹H MRSI is rapidly becoming a clinical tool that provides information assisting clinical management.

Multiple Sclerosis

It is not too surprising that NAA is reduced in multiple sclerosis (MS) plaques.† However, Arnold et al[15,340] and others[236,453] have sug-

---

*References 76, 97-101, 128, 164, 183, 233, 311, 313, 391, 544.
†References 14, 15, 307, 340, 416, 561.

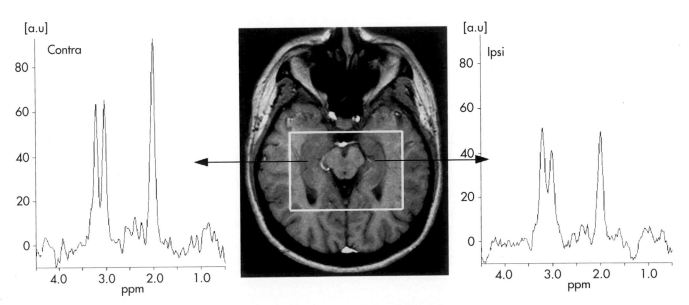

FIGURE 9-27   ¹H MRSI results of a patient with temporal lobe epilepsy. *Center,* Transverse FLASH localizer image angulated parallel to the long axis of the hippocampus, with PRESS box indicated in white. *Left,* Contralateral *(Contra)* spectrum from the indicated region. *Right,* Ipsilateral *(Ipsi)* spectrum from the indicated region showing decreased NAA.

gested that a variety of metabolic changes might help differentiate acute early-MS plaques, which are primarily characterized by edema and perhaps some demyelination, from chronic plaques, which represent neuron loss and gliosis. There have been numerous clinical MRS and MRSI studies of MS plaque.* In some cases NAA reduction within plaques is reversible,[143] suggesting that this change represents a metabolic or T1 change rather than irreversible neuronal injury. Many investigators have observed increased Cho/Cr in MS plaques. This change has been suggested to indicate alterations in the myelin-containing membranes. Acute active-MS plaques, characterized by gadolinium enhancement, often show increased lactate, mobile lipids,[137,307,561] and so-called marker peaks in the 2.1 to 2.6 ppm region.[210] Diminished magnetization-transfer ratios (measured by magnetization-transfer MRI) correlate with increased marker peaks.[210] Most investigators believe that the NMR-visible lipids probably represent products of myelin breakdown. The observation of lactate, lipid, and marker peaks suggests that MRS may be able to distinguish between acute (potentially reversible) and chronic (irreversible) MS plaques. An MRS study of MS in children did not show elevated lactate or lipid levels.[83]

Husted et al[253] reported that regions of so-called normal-appearing white matter in MS showed decreased NAA/Cr, probably as a result of increased Cr and decreased total ^{31}P signals. The major ^{31}P change was a 35% decrease in the phospholipid broad component on the ^{31}P MR spectrum[254] (Figure 9-28), possibly as a result of reduced myelin phospholipid concentration or altered relaxation times.

Prematurity and Birth Asphyxia

The topic of prematurity and birth asphyxia has been reviewed elsewhere.[23,447] Before the availability of high-field, whole-body magnets, clinical MRS studies on brain were performed on infants by using small magnets. The first ^{31}P clinical studies were performed on the brains of premature infants who were 44 hours to 17 days old.[26] The ^{31}P spectra of normal infant brains showed a large PME peak initially thought to be ribose 5-phosphate but later suggested to be caused by phosphoethanolamine.[240] An intense PME resonance in human infants also was observed and suggested to be caused by phosphorylcholine and phosphorylethanolamine with only a small contribution from sugar phosphates.[572] The PME/PDE ratio was shown to decrease during the first 6 months of life.[57] During the same period, the PCr/ATP ratio significantly increased. In addition, the NAD region under the α-ATP peak varied with age. Several investigators have shown that birth asphyxia, complications of premature birth, birth trauma, and other insults during

---

*References 142, 179, 262, 341, 378, 522.

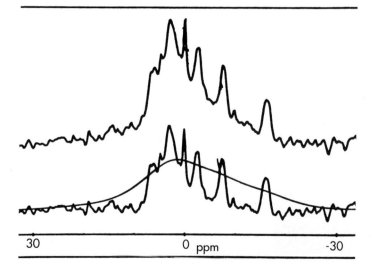

FIGURE 9-28 ^{31}P MRSI results from a patient with MS. *Top,* Phosphorus spectrum from a single MRSI voxel with the phospholipid broad component included. *Bottom,* Identical spectrum with the phospholipid broad component removed by convolution difference. The computer-simulated fit of the filtered broad component is superimposed on the spectrum. The amount of broad component was found to be approximately 35% less in patients with MS. (From reference 254.)

infancy produce detectable changes in brain metabolism. On the first day of life, brain spectra from birth-asphyxiated infants were no different from those of normal infants. From the second to ninth days after birth, the PCr/Pi ratio significantly decreased in the asphyxiated infants compared with control subjects. The latency of the change of PCr/Pi suggested the possibility of early treatment before irreversible metabolic damage develops. Ratios of PCr/Pi below 0.8 were associated with a very poor prognosis for survival. It was also shown that the PCr/Pi ratio increased as the patient's clinical condition improved, and treatment with intravenous mannitol caused a rapid increase in the PCr/Pi ratio in several cases.[91] In a longitudinal study after birth asphyxia, there was a relationship between the minimum brain PCr/Pi and the severity of adverse outcomes.[461] Another report showed that brain Pi/ATP below the normal range predicted adverse outcome after asphyxia with a positive predictive value of 88%, sensitivity of 96%, and specificity of 88%.[372] Lactate/NAA ratios were much higher in brains of infants after perinatal hypoxia ischemia[92]; decreased NAA also may convey a poor prognosis.[447] Although many reports suggest that MRS is useful to evaluate the condition of the infant brain, there are no signs that this approach has gained any widespread clinical acceptance.

Psychiatric Diseases

In schizophrenia, numerous changes in ^{31}P metabolites have been found,[180,557] including increased PCr/ATP and PCr/Pi ratios in the right temporal lobe,[93,149] together with decreased left frontal PME,[147] higher PDE and lower PCr in the frontal lobes,[146-148] and decreased ATP in the basal ganglia.[145] In bipolar disorder, changes in frontal and temporal lobe PME,[147] as well as increased PME,[275-277] have been reported. MRS also has been used to assess lithium levels during treatment of bipolar disorder.[200,289,290]

Stroke

Initial studies of stroke were performed with ^{31}P MRS.[551] Most recent studies of stroke have used ^{1}H MRS or MRSI because of the ability to measure NAA, lactate, and Cho metabolites (Figure 9-5). Studies of patients with stroke almost always show loss of NAA and increased lactate in the infarcted region.* Lactate increase and NAA reduction correlate with clinical measures of disability and functional outcome.[204] One MR study of a patient with a 2-day-old infarct showed a nonspecific inhomogeneous signal intensity in the area of the stroke.[304] Computed tomography (CT) showed a small region of hypointensity, but neither CT nor MRI identified areas of cell death or edema or areas at risk of infarction. MRS demonstrated total loss of NAA signal in regions that appeared only slightly abnormal on MRI and normal on CT. This finding suggested that the region was affected by irrecoverable cell death. A CT scan obtained 2 months later showed signal consistent with tissue loss in those regions that had shown NAA loss 2 days after stroke onset. Using multislice ^{1}H MRSI, Barker et al[37] also showed decreased NAA in the stroke core, but they also noted increased lactate without significant decrease of NAA in the peripheral region, suggesting an ischemic penumbra.

Acute infarcts show elevated lactate levels. Elevated Cho has been correlated with pathological findings of macrophage infiltration. Increased Cho signal in the infarcted region is also thought to represent membrane degradation and demyelination. In contrast, regions of low-grade ischemia are characterized by increased lactate and unchanged levels of NAA and Cho. Chronic strokes often show increased lactate, which is accompanied by an alkaline pH.[249]

Other Brain Disorders

Use of MRS for assessment of metabolic encephalopathies is reviewed in Chapter 72. Welch and colleagues[552,553] found that brain free magnesium levels were low during a migraine attack without a change in pH, suggesting that decreased brain magnesium may be involved in migraine. MRS also has been used to investigate changes in brain metabolism associated with substance abuse,[324,361] cerebellar degeneration,[519] and childhood ataxia.[522] Still other brain diseases have been investigated but with relatively small patient populations.

Pritchard et al[431] and Sappey-Marinier et al[468] have observed increased concentrations of lactate in the brain of human subjects during

---

*References 204, 228, 244, 249, 304, 432, 469, 550.

photic stimulation. This observation is consistent with PET observations of increased glucose uptake in regions of the brain associated with enhanced neuronal activity. The observation of increased lactate concentrations is consistent with the concept that glycolysis is activated to a greater extent than is oxidative metabolism. Conceivably the approach of measuring tissue lactate may be useful for mapping various types of mental activity.

Heart

Animal Studies

The ^{31}P NMR spectrum of the heart in vivo is similar to that of muscle, except that the PCr concentration is less, compared with Pi and ATP. This probably occurs because the heart is actively contracting, resulting in a lower steady state PCr/ATP ratio (and higher ADP) than resting skeletal muscle. Heart spectra of some animals show phosphodiesters. In addition, ^{31}P MRS of the heart in situ detects 2,3-diphosphoglycerate (2,3-DPG) in red blood cells, which are abundant in chamber blood. Therefore interpretation of the Pi-PME region in vivo is difficult. Several investigators have shown that localization techniques can be used to obtain spectra from the subepicardium and subendocardium of animal heart, without contamination of signal from 2,3-DPG of cardiac-chamber blood.

Investigation of the metabolic factors that regulate myocardial contraction has been the subject of considerable interest since pioneering studies in Oxford[184,189] and Baltimore.[239,258] Most of this work has used the isolated perfused rat or rabbit heart,[157] but several investigators have studied the heart in situ in the rat,[211,292,293] guinea pig,[387,388] cat,[314,513] and dog.[30,59,71,314] MRS spectra and studies of the heart have been reviewed in detail elsewhere.[255]

Living-animal studies used acutely placed MR coils around the heart of an open-chest animal, such as a rat[211] or guinea pig,[387] or used a chronically implanted coil.[293] A "catheter coil" was developed to obtain spectra from the endocardium of the right ventricle.[268] ^{31}P spectra have been reported from the hearts of cats,[513] and the DRESS technique was used to record MR spectra from the surface of dogs with experimental myocardial ischemia.[71]

Magnetization-transfer techniques have been used to quantitate the rate of metabolic exchange catalyzed by the CK reaction* or the rate of ATP synthesis.[285,337] The effects of changing work load, substrates, and inotropic agents have also been investigated.[157,342] The rate of the CK reaction seems to be closely related to the metabolic rate.[53] Several investigators have found that the "forward" unidirectional rate of CK (i.e., the synthesis of ATP) appears to be greater than the "reverse" rate (i.e., the synthesis of PCr). This difference has been attributed to metabolite compartmentation and various competing reactions.†

The ability to measure exchange rates by magnetization-transfer experiments raises the possibility that changes in cardiac metabolism produced by altering workload or ischemia may produce detectable variations of exchange rates without altering steady state concentrations. However, magnetization-transfer techniques require considerably more sensitivity because they are "subtraction" techniques that compare one spectrum (a control) with a second spectrum (with a particular resonance saturated). Subtraction techniques require stability of the sample and the spectrometer and greater sensitivity because noise is added in the subtraction procedure.

An intriguing experiment was reported by Fossel et al,[169] who performed gated ^{31}P NMR spectroscopy of the perfused rat heart (Figure 9-29). They found that the concentrations of high-energy phosphates PCr and ATP were significantly lower during systole than in diastole, whereas the concentration of Pi was higher in systole than in diastole. This observation is supported by that of Wikman-Coffelt et al[556] in the perfused heart and by Toyo-Oka et al[530] in vivo. In contrast, Koretsky[292] performed similar experiments using the heart in situ and was unable to find cyclical changes. Similarly, Katz et al[279] found no cyclical changes in the normal or paced dog heart. Nevertheless, Fossel's observations[169] suggest that when the substrate delivery (e.g., glucose perfusion of the heart) or oxygenation of the heart is limited (e.g., during ischemia), cyclical changes of high-energy phosphates may occur. Therefore this finding could become a sensitive index of cardiac ischemia.

*References 80, 256, 287, 292, 338, 339, 541.
†References 80, 291, 292, 294, 338, 400, 541.

In contrast to the studies of Fossel et al,[169] studies have shown that the high-energy phosphates of the right ventricular septum of dog heart, monitored with a catheter coil, did not change despite wide variations of workload.* The interpretation was that myocardial respiration was not regulated solely by ADP but also might also be controlled by substrate use and the oxidation-reduction state. These observations have stimulated considerable work. Because the catheter-coil technique also obtained contaminating ^{31}P NMR signals from red blood cells, studies were performed using a coil placed on the left ventricle in dogs in which whole blood was replaced with the fluorochemical perfusion blood substitute (oxipherol). Under these conditions the intracellular inorganic phosphate (Pi = 0.8 μmol/g wet weight) and intracellular pH could be unambiguously determined. Myocardial work was increased by electrical pacing and epinephrine and phenylephrine infusions. Despite a greater than threefold increase of oxygen consumption, these protocols produced insignificant or only slight changes in myocardial ATP, Pi, PCr, calculated intracellular free-magnesium concentration, ADP, and pH. Subsequent studies showed that ^{31}P NMR spectra gated to various portions of the cardiac cycle with 50-ms time resolution revealed no changes in ATP, ADP, or Pi during the course of the cardiac cycle. Finally, paced tachycardia associated with increased coronary sinus flow and oxygen consumption had no significant transient or sustained effect on the PCr/ATP ratio. However, when the coronary flow response to tachycardia was insufficient, ischemia was produced and PCr was quickly depleted. Similar studies on newborn lambs showed decreased PCr/ATP ratios and increases in calculated ADP and intracellular Pi in contrast to mature sheep in which there were no significant changes. These results suggested that cytosolic ATP hydrolysis products may be more important in the regulation of myocardial energy metabolism in the infant than in the adult.

The regulation of myocardial respiration also has been studied with the isolated perfused-heart model.† When the exogenous carbon source was varied, neither the ATP/ADP ratio, phosphorylation potential, or cytosolic ADP level was found to be uniquely related to oxygen consumption. Rather, exogenous carbon sources had a marked effect on the oxygen consumption of the heart. When the heart was perfused with octanoate or pyruvate, oxygen consumption was linearly dependent on ATP, with apparent Michaelis-Menten constant (K_m) values in the range previously observed in isolated mitochondria. The authors concluded

*References 27, 28, 30, 269, 278, 279, 425.
†References 177, 178, 422, 536, 538, 539, 541.

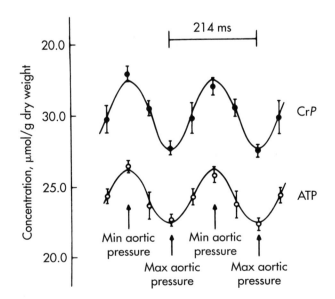

FIGURE 9-29 ATP and PCr concentrations during different phases of the cardiac cycle in isolated, working rat hearts perfused at an aortic pressure of 150/90-cm H_2O and supplied with 11 mmol/L glucose in Krebs-Henseleit bicarbonate buffer. Error bars are standard errors of the mean (SEM). Data were acquired by gating the acquisition RF pulse to the cardiac cycle. (From reference 169.)

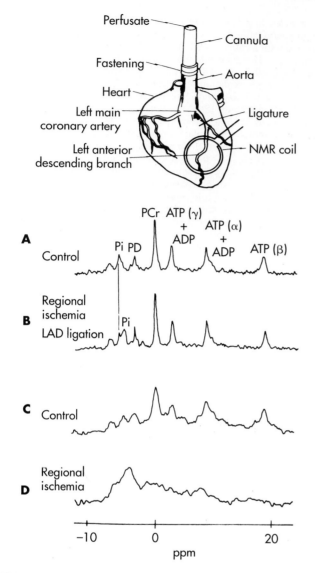

FIGURE 9-30   Diagram of a perfused heart showing the location of the ligature used in producing a localized ischemic area in the left ventricle of the rabbit. For surface-coil experiments a small coil was positioned approximately as depicted. **A,** A 5-min spectrum from an entire, well-perfused heart. The spectrum was obtained with a conventional NMR probe. **B,** Spectrum obtained as in **A,** after ligation of the left anterior descending (LAD) coronary artery. **C,** Spectrum of the left ventricular area of a well-perfused heart with a surface coil of 8 mm inner diameter (compare with **A**). **D,** Spectrum obtained as in **C** but for the 25-min period immediately after LAD ligation, with the surface coil placed on the surface of the heart below the ligature (compare with **B**). Chemical shifts are indicated relative to the PCr resonance. In **A** and **C** the intracellular pH is—7.1; in **B** the apparent pH of the ischemic region is—6.4, and in **D** it is—6.15. These pH values were determined from the chemical shifts of the Pi peaks relative to the PCr peak. Peak assignments: *Pi,* inorganic phosphate; *PD,* phosphodiester; *PCr,* phosphocreatine; *ATP,* adenosine triphosphate; and *ADP,* adenosine diphosphate. (From reference 399.)

that the heart is not "near equilibrium" and that both phosphates and carbon sources exert kinetic control on mitochondrial respiration.

Localization methods (FLAX-ISIS[448] and related methods[230]) have been used to acquire localized spectra from various zones in the heart.[231,448,449,540,573] In the normal canine myocardium the PCr level and PCr/ATP ratio were significantly lower than in the subendocardium and subepicardium. ATP levels were constant in all zones. Both the PCr level and the PCr/ATP ratio were unaltered in relationship to the phase of the cardiac cycle or a fourfold increase in workload. The α-ADP was relatively higher in the subendocardium than in the subepicardium. The Fourier series window-localization technique[192] also has been used in porcine myocardium to obtain spectra from the epicardium and endocardium.[198] Moderate ischemia caused a decrease in the PCr/ATP ratio only in the endocardium.[198]

Cardiac Ischemia

One important use of ^{31}P MRS has been investigation of the metabolic effects of cardiac ischemia. Acute coronary occlusion of the heart in vivo produces a rapid fall of PCr followed by depletion of ATP.[71,513] In almost all instances complete ischemia produces rapid cessation (within seconds) of myocardial contraction, accompanied by a progressive fall in PCr, a rise in Pi, and acidification, which occurs within minutes.[184,189,258] In most cases ATP concentrations remain stable until PCr is depleted. Cessation of ventricular contraction occurs so rapidly that it is difficult to attribute this to changes in high-energy phosphates or pH. Regional ischemia produced by coronary occlusion also has been studied by using a small surface coil over the rabbit ventricle[399] (Figure 9-30). The investigators found significant myocardial protection with verapamil or chlorpromazine. Other investigators have studied the role of adenine nucleotide depletion by adding metabolic precursors and observing changes in the ^{31}P NMR spectra.

Studies have been performed to investigate the relationship of phosphorus metabolites to alterations of contractile function and coronary blood flow in the pig heart.[470,472,473,476,477] During periods of partial steady state coronary occlusion[471,472] or brief periods of total coronary occlusion,[476,477] decreases in PCr and increases in Pi levels roughly paralleled decreases in contractile function. Changes in pH had a less well-defined relationship to alterations of contraction. After release of a brief period of coronary occlusion, the reactive hyperemia of coronary blood flow persisted considerably beyond the period of time necessary to restore phosphorus metabolites to control values, suggesting that reactive hyperemia was regulated by a mechanism independent of PCr, Pi, and pH. The effects of ischemia also have been investigated in perfused and intact canine hearts.* In perfused hearts, ischemia altered the mode of respiratory regulation, from non-ATP control to an ADP/Pi–controlled domain. After an ischemia-reperfusion insult, the K_m for the relationship between oxygen consumption and ADP was reduced. Finally, the postischemic oxidative capacity was significantly reduced. With ^{31}P NMR saturation techniques,† these investigators suggested that ischemia caused mitochondrial uncoupling. This effect might be related to the toxic effects associated with fatty-acid exposure.

The effects of regional ischemia and reperfusion have been studied in the intact rabbit heart.[280,281] The use of calcium channel blockers provided a protective effect on mitochondrial high-energy phosphates during regional ischemia and reperfusion. ^{1}H MRS has been used to evaluate changes in myocardial lipid metabolism associated with ischemia.[166,423,443] These experiments demonstrated that 15 min of myocardial ischemia followed by reperfusion produced a significant increase in the NMR-detectable lipid content. This finding might be useful in the assessment of ischemic damage in humans. Finally, Canby et al[94] demonstrated significant changes in myocardial allografts in transplanted rat hearts. PCr/ATP and PCr/Pi ratios decreased, and there was an initial alkaline shift followed by acidosis. These results suggested that transplant rejection may produce changes in phosphorus metabolism and pH, which might be useful for clinical assessment of cardiac transplants.

Clinical Studies

Clinical MRS studies of the heart are difficult, largely because of motion. Almost all clinical MRS studies of the heart have involved ^{31}P MRS. Although it would be interesting to obtain ^{1}H MR spectra from heart, little success has been reported, probably because of the large lipid signal that obscures other metabolites.

A number of studies have shown that ^{31}P MR spectra can be obtained from hearts of healthy subjects and patients with various cardiac diseases.‡ Bottomley et al[61] reported extensive experience with use of the DRESS technique to obtain ^{31}P NMR spectra from normal human heart. Bottomley et al[70] obtained ^{31}P MR spectra from hearts of patients with anterior myocardial infarction. During the immediate postinfarct period, there were significant reductions in the PCr/Pi ratio and elevations of the Pi/ATP ratio. No changes in the metabolite contents during the cardiac cycle were observed. Blackledge et al[55,56] used the rotating-frame technique to obtain spectra from normal human heart. Several other investigators have used the ISIS approach to obtain human-heart

*References 285, 286, 449, 466, 540, 574.
†References 285, 286, 449, 536, 537, 539, 541.
‡References 60, 66-68, 70, 74, 221, 318, 320.

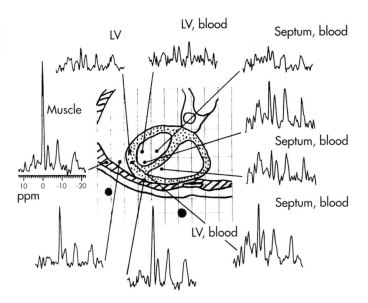

FIGURE 9-31   Tracing of 1-cm thick transaxial scout image of human heart, with MRSI grid overlaid, and optimally combined (from array coil) spectra from various voxels displayed. Voxel size is 2×4 cm3. The 31P spectra (at 1.5 T) are displayed from the various voxels as indicated. (From reference 221.)

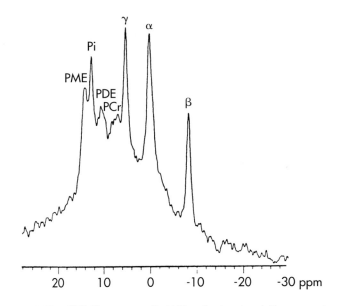

FIGURE 9-32 ^{31}P MR spectrum of rat kidney in vivo. Acquisition parameters: 90-degree pulse, 2-sec delay, 128 acquisitions. α, β, and γ, Three phosphates of ATP; *PCr,* phosphocreatine; *PDE,* phosphodiesters; *Pi,* inorganic phosphate; *PME,* phosphomonoesters.

spectra.[320,335,471,473] Bottomley et al reported a quantitative approach for MRSI of human heart.[68]

Weiss et al[549] used isometric hand-grip exercise to increase cardiac workload while performing spatially localized ^{31}P MRS in human subjects.[549] The [PCr]/[ATP] ratio decreased in the patients with coronary artery disease, implying inadequate myocardial perfusion for the increased demand; there was no change in control subjects. In patients with coronary bypass grafting, there was no change in the [PCr]/[ATP] ratio with exercise. Therefore surgical revascularization of the myocardium reversed the energetic defect.

Yabe et al[568] also used ^{31}P MRS with hand-grip exercise and compared the results with standard thallium 201 perfusion imaging. In patients with perfusion defects detected by thallium scans, the [PCr]/[ATP] ratio was low and did not change during exercise. Patients with reversible defects showed near-normal [PCr]/[ATP] ratios at rest, but there were decreases during exercise. Recently, Yabe et al[567] used ^{31}P MRSI measurements to improve the localization to the myocardium and found that myocardial segments that were viable but possibly ischemic (reversible defects according to thallium scans) manifested normal [PCr]/[ATP] ratios and normal ATP content but moderately depressed PCr content, whereas nonviable (i.e., infarcted) myocardium demonstrated reductions in both ATP and PCr content.

For the reasons already enumerated, the amount of useful clinical information that is derived from cardiac MRS is disappointingly small. Increased phosphodiesters have been reported in cardiomyopathies,[471] but the significance of this finding is unclear. The difficulty of obtaining high-quality ^{31}P spectra from human heart tissue is exemplified in Figure 9-31.

Kidney, Bowel, Prostate, and Testicle

Animal Studies

A typical ^{31}P NMR spectrum of a rat kidney in vivo is shown in Figure 9-32. The first MRS studies of kidney were performed by Sehr et al,[480,481] who extirpated kidneys from rats and rapidly cooled them to preserve high-energy phosphates. Subsequently a metabolically and physiologically stable perfused-kidney preparation was developed for MRS.[456] This technique demonstrated that ^{31}P MRS could be used to measure renal pHi.[436] Acidification of the perfusion medium produced acidification of pHi, but pHi fell only 0.04 pH unit for each 0.1 unit of the medium.

^{31}P MRS has been used to investigate the hypothesis that renal pHi may be an important signal for the regulation of renal ammoniagenesis.[5,293] Various acid-base disturbances were used to alter renal ammoniagenesis. Acute metabolic acidosis lowered the renal pHi level from 7.35 to 7.16. Chronic metabolic acidosis lowered pHi to 7.26. Dietary

potassium depletion, which produces adaptive stimulation of renal ammoniagenesis, greatly lowered the level to 7.0. Acute respiratory acidosis also lowered the renal pHi level. In contrast to these disorders, chronic respiratory acidosis did not alter the renal pHi level; however, it also did not stimulate renal ammoniagenesis. Therefore these findings suggest that the renal pHi level is an important determinant of and may be the primary signal for renal ammoniagenesis.

Magnetization-transfer techniques (discussed previously) were used to study the rate of ATP synthesis in the perfused kidney.[176] The ratio of ATP synthesis to oxygen consumption was found to be 3.0, which is consistent with previous work with isolated mitochondria. Magnetization-transfer studies of the kidney in vivo found a lower ATP/oxygen ratio.[175,293] Magnetization transfer, oxygen consumption, and sodium reabsorption were measured simultaneously.[493] The ATP/oxygen ratio was 0.8, considerably less than that expected. Marked variations of sodium transport (produced by the hormone atrial natriuretic factor) failed to produce parallel changes of ATP turnover. A major problem with these techniques is the relatively low SNR of the Pi peak, making accurate saturation-transfer measurements of ATP synthesis difficult. Furthermore, the heterogeneous cell population of the kidney hampers interpretation of these results. These findings emphasize the difficulty of obtaining interpretable information from ^{31}P NMR saturation-transfer studies of tissues in situ.

The metabolic health of an organ is indicated by its metabolic reserve, or ability to perform organ functions at an increased rate or under an increased load. Observation of the response of renal high-energy phosphates to fructose loading is useful to monitor the metabolic reserve of the kidney. The sugar fructose is rapidly taken up by the renal cortex and phosphorylated to fructose-1-phosphate. This action is associated with depletion of cellular Pi and ATP. Studies that compared the responses of kidney and liver with fructose infusion demonstrated that the liver is more sensitive to the effects of fructose than is the kidney.[293]

The first studies using MRS to investigate metabolic changes during acute renal failure were reported by Sehr et al.[480] Acute ischemia of the perfused kidney produced rapid hydrolysis of ATP and a fall in renal pHi. Several models of acute renal failure produced by shock, ischemia, noradrenaline infusion, and various nephrotoxins have been studied.[107] Prolonged hypertension, ischemia, or noradrenaline caused a fall in ATP, a rise in Pi, and tissue acidosis. In contrast, acute renal failure produced by injections of uranyl nitrate, folate, or mercuric chloride had no effect on the NMR spectrum. These results suggest that the nephrotoxic renal failure caused by these agents may be produced by mechanisms other than tissue acidosis or ATP depletion. These findings raise the possibility that ^{31}P MRS might be useful to distinguish nephrotoxic from ischemic renal failure.

Recovery from ischemic renal failure also has been investigated (Figure 9-33).[504,505] Improved recovery in renal function followed infusion of magnesium (Mg) ATP.[505] Similar to the functional response, Mg ATP infusions accelerated the recovery of the high-energy phosphates of the kidney.

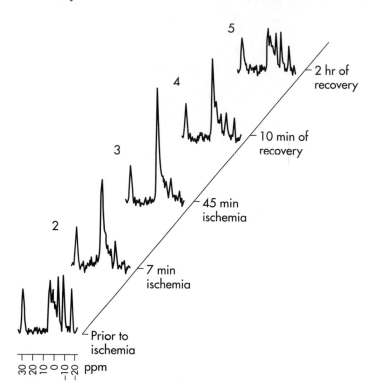

FIGURE 9-33   [31]P MR spectra obtained from a rat kidney in vivo during the course of acute ischemia. Scan obtained before ischemic insult is used as the control value for comparison of changes in β-ATP peak and chemical shift of Pi during and after ischemia. (From Shine NR, Adam WR, Xuan JA, et al: NMR studies of renal metabolism: regulation of renal function by ATP and pH, Ann N Y Acad Sci 508:99, 1987.)

Sehr et al[480] first suggested that ^{31}P MRS could be used to evaluate high-energy phosphate metabolism and pH of the transplanted kidney. Chan et al[105] reported experiments of human kidneys flushed with cold solutions and stored. Detectable ATP signals were noted for as long as 32 hours after preservation. Kidneys flushed with citrate buffer had better preservation of renal pH than kidneys flushed with unbuffered solutions. In addition, the use of ^{31}P MRS for assessment of renal transplant viability has been reported.[424] The investigators believed that the PME/Pi ratio was a predictor of posttransplant functional recovery. These preliminary results suggest that ^{31}P MRS may be useful to investigate a variety of techniques to improve renal preservation and predict renal viability.

Karczmar et al[272] obtained ^{31}P MRS spectra of the small and large intestine. Despite the presence of liquid and gaseous luminal contents, resolvable peaks were obtained. Bowel contains considerable PCr, as might be expected because of smooth muscle. A solenoidal coil was constructed to accommodate loops of intestine. The homogeneous B_1 field of this coil permitted SEs and measurement of T2.

Clinical Studies

Clinical studies of kidney, prostate, and testicle have recently been reviewed in detail.[548] The viability of kidneys undergoing hypothermic storage for transplantation was studied using ^{31}P MRS.[77,78] The presence of ATP was associated with good posttransplant function, and it was suggested that MRS provides a better correlation with renal function after transplantation than do other methods. Renal transplants undergoing rejection show elevated PDE/PME and Pi/ATP ratios, and these ratios have high sensitivity and specificity for predicting rejection.[209] ^{1}H MRS shows that normal prostate and prostatic hypertrophy contain high levels of citrate, whereas prostate cancers have reduced citrate.[523] Kurhanewicz et al[302] have recently demonstrated ^{1}H single-voxel imaging and ^{1}H MRSI[301] of the human prostate with very small voxels; the results show decreased or absent citrate in cancerous areas (Figure 9-34).

^{31}P MRS detects increased PME in prostate cancers, and the PME is decreased after therapy.[300,524] ^{31}P MRS of human testicles shows decreased PME/ATP ratios and reduced PME/PDE ratios in patients with primary testicular failure.[115]

Liver

Animal Studies

Although the liver is the major organ concerned with maintaining metabolic homeostasis, it has received relatively little study by MRS. ^{31}P MRS spectra of liver in vivo are shown in Figure 9-35. Similar to

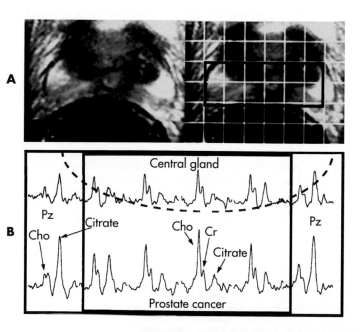

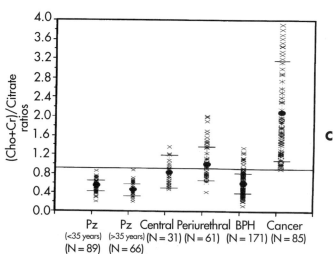

FIGURE 9-34   **A** and **B**, Axial T2 image and corresponding ^{1}H spectra from a 3D MRSI data set acquired from the prostate of a patient with stage 3 (T3) carcinoma of the prostate. Cancer is identified metabolically by lowered citrate and higher Cho levels compared with the surrounding regions of normal peripheral zone *(Pz)*. **C**, Plot of individual *(Xs)* and mean *(circles)* (Cr + Cho)/citrate ratios for regions of prostate cancer, benign prostatic hyperplasia (BPH), and normal peripheral zone in volunteers and patients. The metabolite ratio distinguishes regions of prostate cancer from normal peripheral zone *(Pz)*. (From reference 301.)

the kidney, in the liver, no PCr is present, providing a useful unique characteristic of signals from this tissue. It has been suggested that the T1 relaxation times of liver phosphates are quite short perhaps because of the presence of iron or other paramagnetics. As in the fructose-loading experiments described previously in the kidney, fructose infusion has been used to explore the metabolic reserve in the liver. ^{31}P MRS has been used with the implanted-coil technique to demonstrate that fructose infusion induces a rapid rise of the PMEs accompanied by depletion of ATP and Pi (Figure 9-35).[293] Similar studies have been reported in human subjects.[402]

Sillerud and Shulman[507] used ^{13}C MRS to investigate rat liver glycogen metabolism. They demonstrated that 100% of liver glycogen was visible despite the expectation that the correlation time of this macromolecule might be rather long. They demonstrated infusion of ^{13}C glucose–labeled glycogen in the expected position. Infusion of glucagon produced rapid glycogenolysis.

Clinical Studies

The earliest studies of human liver were performed by Styles et al.[514] Oberhaensli et al[403-406] reported studies of adult livers. The first spectra of human livers were obtained in two infants by means of a small-bore magnet.[330] Ban et al[33] reported slight increases in PME but otherwise no significant differences between healthy subjects and patients with cirrhosis. Meyerhoff et al[355,356,358] reported studies with alcoholic hepatitis, alcoholic cirrhosis, and viral hepatitis. Hepatic metabolite ratios were not significantly different between alcoholic liver disease and normal liver; however, absolute hepatic concentrations were decreased 25% to 46% in alcoholic hepatitis and 13% in 50% in alcoholic cirrhosis. Finally, hepatic intracellular pH was more acidic in alcoholic cirrhosis and more alkaline in alcoholic hepatitis.

Oberhaensli et al[402,409] demonstrated the effects of intravenous fructose injections on human liver metabolites. Patients with fructose intolerance show a marked sensitivity to the ATP-depletion effects of fructose loading. Furthermore, heterozygous relatives of these patients also demonstrate increased sensitivity to the metabolic effects of fructose, accompanied by a rise of uric acid production. The increased urate produced was attributed to the increased rate of ATP breakdown.

Malignancy

Animal Studies

Reviews of in vivo MRS in the study of cancer have been published.[9,271,457] Since the original work of Damadian[134] demonstrating that ^{1}H MR relaxation times were prolonged in malignant tissue, there has been considerable interest in the use of various aspects of MR for the investigation of malignancy.

Many investigators have studied high-energy phosphate metabolism of dispersed tumor cells by ^{31}P MRS.[216,382] Others also have shown considerable interest in MRS studies of experimental tumors implanted in laboratory animals. Resonances for ATP, Pi, and PME and smaller phosphodiester resonances with no detectable PCr were found in the Walker-256 carcinosarcoma.[207] Intracellular pH was similar to that of normal tissues, and glucose infusion did not affect pH. Glucose infusion caused a selective decrease of the pHi of radiation-induced fibrosarcoma (RIF-1) tumors,[167] suggesting that glucose infusion may selectively sensitize tumor cells to hyperthermia.

Depending on the age and size of the tumor, different ^{31}P MR spectra may be observed. Figure 9-36 shows the changes of a MOPC-104E myeloma during an 11-day growth period. Fifteen days after implantation, intense ATP and PCr peaks were noted. Intracellular pH was 7.1, suggesting that the tumor was reasonably well vascularized and predominantly aerobic. Three days later, the spectra showed a dramatic decrease in PCr, an increase in Pi, and little change in ATP. The authors suggested that these changes were caused by a decrease in vascularization and an increase in the proportion of hypoxic cells in the tumor. Once PCr was depleted, further tumor growth was accompanied by a decrease of ATP and growth of Pi and PME peaks. [31]P MR spectra of human tumors grown in athymic mice appear to be similar to those of

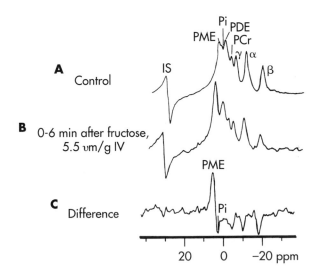

FIGURE 9-35 **A,** Control ^{31}P MR spectrum of rat liver. **B,** Spectrum obtained 6 min after fructose loading. **C, B** minus **A.** The assignments of the signals are indicated in the figure. *IS,* Internal standard; *PME,* phosphomonoesters; *PDE,* phosphodiester; *Pi;* inorganic phosphate; α, β, and γ, ATP resonances.

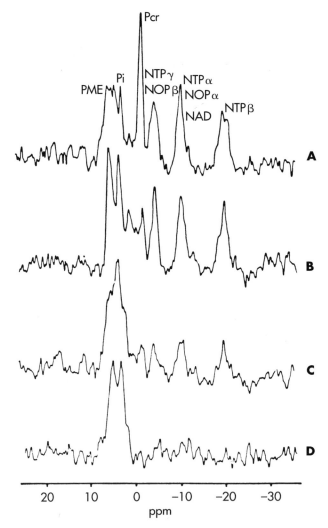

FIGURE 9-36 ^{31}P MR spectra of a growing, untreated subcutaneously implanted (1 _ 10[6] cells) MOPC-l04E myeloma, in vivo, 80.96 MHz. An unshielded surface coil probe was used. The tumor was monitored at day 0 (baseline), pH 7.1 **(A);** day 3, pH 6.9 **(B);** day 7, pH 6.6 **(C);** and day 11, pH not determined **(D).** (From Evanochko WT, Ng TC, and Glickson JP: Applications of in vivo NMR spectroscopy to cancer, *Magn Reson Med* 1:508, 1984.)

mouse tumors, particularly RIF-1. These preliminary findings suggest that the observations of experimental tumors may have direct relevance to the clinical situation.

Ng et al[392] first demonstrated that ^{31}P MRS can detect a rapid response to chemotherapy. Figure 9-37 shows a series of spectra of a MOPC-104E myeloma after administration of a curative dose of cyclophosphamide. Before therapy, the PCr peak was smaller than the ATP peaks, but following therapy, the PCr peak rose. These changes appear to be the inverse of those that occur during untreated tumor growth. The authors did not provide a mechanistic explanation for the increase in PCr. The spectral changes became evident before any decrease in tumor size was detected.

The effects of cyclophosphamide on ^{31}P MRS of brain tumors have been reported.[379] The spectral responses were rapid and strikingly different from those observed by Ng. ATP decreased rapidly and eventually disappeared, accompanied by an increase in Pi, suggesting cell ischemia or death. The effects of radiation and hyperthermia on experimental tumors also have been reported.[165,315] In addition, the effect of the lymphokine tumor necrosis factor (TNF) on the phosphate metabolism of mouse tumors has been reported.[492] Within 90 min of TNF injection, PCr and ATP began to fall, whereas Pi rose.

Thus many different animal experiments repeatedly show rapid spectral changes in response to treatment.[245,349,451,511] These results suggest that MRS may be used to monitor the effects of therapy, perhaps providing an early predictor of whether a particular treatment will be effective.

Clinical Studies

Studies of brain tumors and prostate cancer already have been discussed. The first demonstration that NMR could be used to investigate tumor metabolism in man was the report of Griffiths et al[206] demonstrating abnormal ^{31}P MR spectra of an alveolar rhabdomyosarcoma located on the dorsum of a hand. In the study of a massive hepatic infiltration of an adrenal neuroblastoma in a small child,[330] the ^{31}P MR spectra showed a high PME peak, most likely consisting of phosphoethanolamine and phosphocholine. Initially, when radiation and chemotherapy were begun, there was no response and the PME continued to rise. Subsequently a fall of PME preceded a clinical response.

Many studies of human and animal tumors show increased PME levels. To determine the metabolic mechanism of this alteration, the composition of human breast cancer cells has been investigated in vitro.[133] Results assigned the PME peak of these cells to phosphocholine and phosphoethanolamine and the PDE peaks to glycerophosphocholine and glycerophosphoethanolamine. Furthermore, the pathways producing these metabolites were defined. The PMEs were shown to be products of Cho and ethanolamine kinase (the first step in phospholipid synthesis), and the PDEs were substrates of glycerophosphocholine and phosphodiesterase (the last step in phospholipid metabolism).

Various studies have used ^{31}P and ^{19}F MRS to evaluate human tumors and their response to therapy. In a report on a non-Hodgkin's lymphoma,[396] transient elevation of PCr, decrease of PDE, and increase in intracellular pH were found within 3 hours after radiotherapy. Long-term changes indicated that the decrease in PDE was most sensitive in response to radiation therapy. Investigators have also studied 35 human cancers, including 13 squamous cell carcinomas of the head and neck, 8 Hodgkin's lymphomas, 6 non-Hodgkin's lymphomas, 4 carcinomas of the breast, and a number of miscellaneous tumors.[394,395] Most of the neoplasms had normal to slightly alkaline pH before radiation therapy. During treatment, pH remained near neutral to alkaline or increased. The authors concluded that most tumor cells and neoplasms are well oxygenated and only a negligible fraction are chronically hypoxic. They

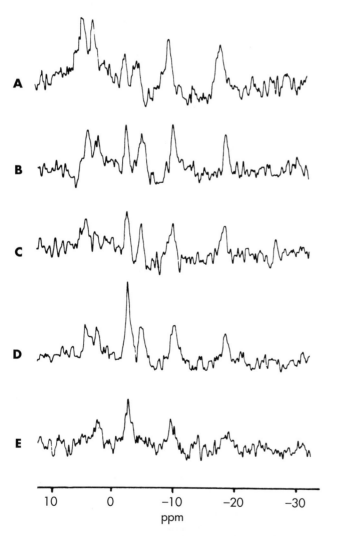

FIGURE 9-37 ^{31}P MR spectra of a MOPC-104E myeloma (1×10^6 cells implanted) before treatment with cyclophosphamide, in vivo, 80.96 MHz. Treatment, pH 7.3 **(A)**; 17 hours, pH 7.3 **(B)**; 38 hours, pH not determined **(C)**; 46 hours, pH 7.4 **(D)**; and 60 hours, pH 7.4 **(E)**. Spectra were obtained using the unshielded surface-coil probe. Spectral assignments are shown in Figure 9-36. (From Evanochko WT, Ng TC, and Glickson JP: NMR studies of renal metabolism: regulation of renal function by ATP and pH, Magn Reson Med 1:508, 1984.)

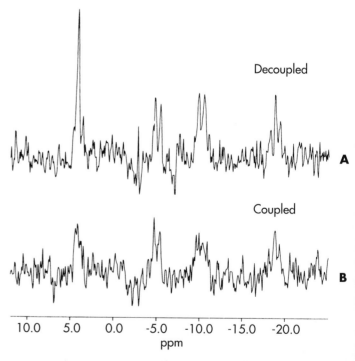

FIGURE 9-38 ^{1}H decoupling and NOE enhancement effects on the ^{31}P MR in vivo spectrum localized to the lymph node of a patient with a lymph node lymphoma. **A**, ^{31}P spectrum acquired with ^{1}H decoupling and NOE enhancement. **B**, ^{31}P spectrum without ^{1}H decoupling or NOE enhancement. (From reference 385.)

also found that the total mobile phosphate content of breast carcinomas was 2 to 3 times higher than that of normal breast tissue but that the metabolite profiles of normal and cancerous breast are generally similar.[393] After treatment of breast cancer, the PME/ATP ratio decreased and pH fluctuated at a value greater than 7. The PDE/ATP ratio also diminished in response to therapy.

In a ^{31}P MRS study of malignant tumors of bone, tumors had increased Pi levels and an unusual peak of PME consistent with excessive glycolysis.[454] Intracellular pH was normal in 12 bone tumors but acidic in a single soft tissue sarcoma. Metabolic response was frequently observed during chemotherapy. Treatment produced an increase in Pi and loss of ATP and PME. Tumor regression was indicated by a loss of all abnormal metabolites. Tumor relapse was accompanied by reappearance of abnormalities in the ^{31}P MR spectrum. Another ^{31}P MRS study followed patients with soft tissue sarcomas treated with combined local hyperthermia and fractionated radiation therapy followed by surgical resection.[154] The pretherapy tumor pH correlated positively, and changes of pH, PCr/Pi, ATP/Pi, and PME correlated negatively with the percentage of tumor necrosis on the surgical specimen. Various sarcomas, carcinomas, lymphomas, adenomas, and benign lesions had increased PME, PDE, and Pi, whereas PCr was lower in comparison to adjacent muscle tissue.[385,547] In nearly all cases pH showed a slight alkaline shift. Existence of necrotic regions, detected by MRI, was paralleled by an increase in Pi. Tumor growth was characterized by increased concentrations of PME. Treatment of a lymphoma and squamous cell carcinoma demonstrated metabolic changes that correlated with clinical response. Although only a few benign tumors were studied, there was no reliable difference between benign and malignant neoplasms. Bone tumors were found to have high ATP and Pi and low PCr, whereas PME and PDE were not elevated.[397] Slight changes were observed in one tumor after chemotherapy. In a ^{31}P MRS study of 23 patients with cancer,[483] the response of 5 patients was monitored in a long-term follow-up study. Tumors showed increased Pi, PME, and PDE with reduced PCr, and ATP was normal. Tumor treatment particularly affected the Pi/PCr ratio. Tumor treatment caused a fall in PCr/Pi and a rise in the sum of PCr plus Pi.

Increased PME/ATP ratios have been reported in tumors outside the brain; PME/ATP was higher in lymphomas than in other cancers.[270] After therapy, tumor response was usually accompanied by a diminishing PME/ATP ratio, but PME/ATP did not always parallel or precede changes of tumor size. Chemoembolization of liver tumors caused marked loss of ATP and transient increase of Pi, indicating response to therapy.[357] One of the most definitive studies in this field was performed by Dewhirst et al,[154] who found that ^{31}P MRS of sarcomas helped to predict the extent of necrosis after radiation therapy.

The metabolism of fluorinated chemotherapeutic agents has been monitored in experimental animals[564,566] and patients.[482,560] ^{19}F MRS liver spectra were obtained in eight patients after intraarterial 5-fluorouracil (5-FU) chemotherapy for liver tumors.[482] ^{19}F MRS allowed monitoring of the parent compound and its major catabolite, α-fluoro β-alanine (FBAL). Time constants for the kinetics of 5-FU were 8 to 75 min, whereas the time constants for the buildup of FBAL were 15 to 50 min. These studies demonstrated the feasibility of short-term monitoring of 5-FU metabolites.

Unfortunately, at present it is difficult to say whether MRS has a clinical role in assessing cancer outside the brain (brain tumor diagnosis and therapy management were discussed previously). There are considerable animal and clinical data demonstrating that cancer therapy causes detectable changes in spectra and that these changes may precede morphological changes detected by MRI or other imaging techniques. However, most studies are anecdotal and involve a limited number of cases. A controlled, multicenter clinical trial currently is under way to evaluate the use of MRS in the management of several types of cancer. The results of this study should help determine the clinical role of MRS in this area. Obviously a major problem is that most cancers are quite small (e.g., approximately 1 cm in diameter or less, which is close to the limit of spatial resolution, especially for ^{31}P MRS). Once tumors become large enough for detection by MRS, they already may be incurable or untreatable. However, the sensitivity of ^{31}P MRS is aided by proton decoupling, which improves the SNR through the NOE and also can improve resolution by removal of proton J coupling to some of the phosphorus resonances (Figure 9-38). Therefore there is much more work to be done in the future to develop improved techniques and ob-

tain sufficient clinical data to determine the role of MRS in cancer diagnosis and treatment.

VALUE OF MAGNETIC RESONANCE SPECTROSCOPY FOR CLINICAL DIAGNOSIS

Although there is considerable enthusiasm for the use of MRS and MRSI for clinical research and growing optimism about their application for clinical diagnosis, there are two different views concerning the current status of MRS and MRSI as practical and useful tools for clinical management.

A conservative view (held by the authors of this chapter) is that spectroscopy is still largely an investigational tool. This view holds that MRS has clinical value only if it provides the clinician information that has a beneficial influence on patient management (i.e., outcome is improved). MRS does appear to have particular clinical value for seizure-focus lateralization in temporal lobe epilepsy, although this should be further substantiated in a large longitudinal study. Recent studies suggest that MRS may provide useful presurgical information for brain-tumor diagnosis and may assist treatment of brain tumors by identifying regions of necrosis and tumor regrowth, but this assertion must also be replicated. MRS may have value for diagnosis of AD and stroke evaluation, but existing data on these diseases should be replicated with longitudinal studies. The many other neurological conditions discussed earlier are certainly worthy of clinical investigation with MRS, but the practical value of this research in terms of improved patient outcome appears uncertain.

In Chapter 72, Ernst and Ross make the interesting case that MRS as currently used has a number of direct clinical applications. They present convincing evidence that MRS offers added information to MRI and that the MRS result is often abnormal when the MRI result is normal. For example, 20% of MRI-negative HIV-positive patients have MRS abnormalities; MRI-negative adrenoleukodystrophy subjects have MRS changes; in subjects recovering from drowning, MRS identified 5 of 5 with good outcome and 11 of 12 with poor outcome; in temporal lobe epilepsy, MRS successfully lateralizes before surgery or invasive electroencephalography. Ross and Michaelis[455] have reported a three-center trial that demonstrates that the "added value" of MRS is between 21% and 28%. In summary, some investigators believe that MRS has practical value for the management of selected cases.

Despite the differences between these two positions, there is general agreement that the clinical applications of MRS and MRSI are growing as the techniques are improved, the manufacturers provide more user-friendly MRS packages, and more clinical studies are reported that demonstrate the value of MRS data for patient care. Finally, the economics of the health care marketplace, especially as managed care increasingly dominates US health care, also will affect the availability of expensive technologies, such as MRS, for clinical diagnosis; it is likely that the health maintenance organization will pay for MRS only if clinical-outcome studies demonstrate a reasonable cost benefit, which should be an objective of future MRS (and MRI) studies.

FUTURE DEVELOPMENTS

The unique ability of MRS to monitor body chemistry seems to ensure an important role for this technology in clinical investigation and medical diagnosis. The major technical problem to overcome is sensitivity. MR signals are extremely weak, and the SNR of spectra acquired at 1.5 to 2.0 T is barely adequate. There are many ways to improve the sensitivity of this approach, but the most straightforward method is by increasing magnet field strength. This method will result in increased cost because of the more expensive magnets, as well as the need for increased shielding. Development of improved MR localization techniques is expected, especially as the problems associated with eddy currents are reduced by use of shielded gradients. The major advantages of single-voxel techniques are high definition of spatial resolution and ease in obtaining short-TE spectra. MRSI (or CSI) techniques, which use phase encoding, provide much more information about spatial resolution than do "single-point" techniques but have reduced precision of spatial resolution as a result of the point-spread function. Furthermore, MRSI of the brain currently is complicated by lipid contamination, which makes acquisition of short-TE spectra even more difficult. ^{1}H MRSI outside the brain is extremely difficult because of lipid contamination, and few ^{1}H MRS spectra outside the brain have been reported. Nevertheless, for clinical use it is expected that MRSI techniques, including those acquiring multiple slices[159] and full cortex, will increasingly become the standard because many more regions can be sampled and metabolite images can be generated. The ultimate goal in this area is the development of short-TE MRSI techniques[426] that obtain signal from small voxels throughout the entire field of view; perhaps echo-planar MRSI[4,427] will help accomplish this objective.

Despite the problems, the unique ability of MRS to noninvasively measure a wide variety of metabolites in the human body guarantees this technology a permanent place in the armamentarium of tools for basic biochemical research, clinical investigation, and diagnosis of human disease.

REFERENCES

1. Ackerman JJH, Bore PJ, Gadian DG, et al: NMR studies of metabolism in perfused organs, Philos Trans R Soc Lond B 289:425, 1980.
2. Ackerman JJH, Grove TH, Wong GG, et al: Mapping of metabolites in whole animals by ^{31}P NMR using surface coils, Nature 283:167, 1980.
3. Ackerman JJH, Lowry M, Radda GK, et al: The role of intrarenal pH in regulation of ammoniagenesis: ^{31}P NMR studies of the isolated perfused rat kidney, J Physiol 319:65, 1981.
4. Adalsteinsson E, Irarrazabal P, Spielman DM, et al: Three-dimensional spectroscopic imaging with time-varying gradients, Magn Reson Med 33:461, 1995.
5. Adam WR, Koretsky AP, and Weiner MW: Measurement of renal intracellular pH in rats in vivo using ^{31}P NMR: effects of acidosis and K$^+$ depletion, Am J Physiol 251:F904, 1986.
6. Adam WR, Koretsky AP, and Weiner MW: Measurement of tissue potassium in vivo using ^{39}K nuclear magnetic resonance, Biophys J 51:265, 1987.
7. Adamopoulos S, and Coats AJ: Peripheral abnormalities in chronic heart failure, Postgrad Med J 67(Suppl 1):S74, 1991.
8. Agris P, and Campbell ID: Proton NMR studies of intact friend leukemia cells, Science 216:1325, 1982.
9. Aiken NR, McGovern KA, Ng CE, et al: ^{31}P NMR spectroscopic studies of the effects of cyclophosphamide on perfused RIF-1 tumor cells, Magn Reson Med 31:241, 1994.
10. Alger JR, Behar KL, Rothman DL, et al: Natural-abundance carbon-13 NMR measurement of hepatic glycogen in the living rabbit, J Magn Reson 56:334, 1984.
11. Alger JR, den Hollander JA, and Shulman RG: In vivo phosphorus-31 nuclear magnetic resonance saturation transfer studies of adenosine-triphosphatase kinetics in *Saccharomyces cerevisiae*, Biochemistry 21:2957, 1982.
12. Alger JR, and Shulman RG: NMR studies of enzymatic rates in vitro and in vivo by magnetization transfer, Q Rev Biophys 17:83, 1984.
13. Arnold DL, Emrich JF, Shoubridge EA, et al: Characterization of astrocytomas, meningiomas, and pituitary adenomas by phosphorus magnetic resonance spectroscopy, J Neurosurg 74:447, 1991.
14. Arnold DL, Matthews PM, Francis G, et al: Proton magnetic resonance spectroscopy of human brain in vivo in the evaluation of multiple sclerosis: assessment of the load of disease, Magn Reson Med 14:154, 1990.
15. Arnold DL, Matthews PM, Francis GS, et al: Proton magnetic resonance spectroscopic imaging for metabolic characterization of demyelinating plaques, Ann Neurol 31:235, 1992.
16. Arnold DL, Matthews PM, and Radda GK: Metabolic recovery after exercise and the assessment of mitochondrial function in vivo in human skeletal muscle by means of ^{31}P NMR, Magn Reson Med 1:307, 1984.
17. Arnold DL, Shoubridge EA, Emrich J, et al: Early metabolic changes following chemotherapy of human gliomas in vivo demonstrated by phosphorus magnetic resonance spectroscopy, Invest Radiol 24:958, 1989.
18. Arnold DL, Shoubridge EA, Feindel W, et al: Metabolic changes in cerebral gliomas within hours of treatment with intra-arterial BCNU demonstrated by phosphorus magnetic resonance spectroscopy, Can J Neurol Sci 14:570, 1987.
19. Arnold DL, Shoubridge EA, Villemure JG, et al: Proton and phosphorus magnetic resonance spectroscopy of human astrocytomas in vivo: preliminary observations on tumor grading, NMR Biomed 3:184, 1990.
20. Arnolda L, Conway M, Dolecki M, et al: Skeletal muscle metabolism in heart failure: a ^{31}P nuclear magnetic resonance spectroscopy study of leg muscle, Clin Sci 79:583, 1990.
21. Arus C, and Barany M: ^{1}H NMR of intact tissues at 11.1T, J Magn Reson 57:519, 1984.
22. Avison MJ, Rothman DL, Nadel E, et al: Detection of human muscle glycogen by natural abundance ^{13}C NMR, Proc Natl Acad Sci U S A 85:1634, 1988.
23. Azzopardi D, and Edwards D: Magnetic resonance spectroscopy in neonates, Curr Opin Neurol 8:145, 1995.
24. Bailes DR, Bryant DJ, Bydder GM, et al: Localized phosphorus-31 NMR spectroscopy of normal and pathological human organs in vivo using phase-encoding techniques, J Magn Reson 74:158, 1987.
25. Bailey IA, Gadian DG, Matthews PM, et al: Studies of metabolism in the isolated, perfused rat heart using NMR, FEBS Lett 123:315, 1981.
26. Bailey IA, Seymour AML, and Radda GK: A ^{31}P-NMR study of the effects of reflow on the ischemic rat heart, Biochim Biophys Acta 637:1, 1981.
27. Balaban RS: NMR spectroscopy of the heart. I. Concepts Magn Reson 1:15, 1989.
28. Balaban RS, and Heineman FW: Control of mitochondrial respiration in the heart in vivo, Mol Cell Biochem 89:191, 1989.
29. Balaban RS, Kantor HL, and Ferretti JH: In vivo flux between phosphocreatine and adenosine triphosphate determined by two-dimensional phosphorous NMR, J Biol Chem 258:127, 1983.
30. Balaban RS, Kantor HL, Katz LA, et al: Relation between work and phosphate metabolite in the in vivo paced mammalian heart, Science 232:1121, 1986.
31. Balaban RS, and Knepper MA: Nitrogen-14 nuclear magnetic resonance spectroscopy of mammalian tissues, Am J Physiol 245:C439, 1983.
32. Baleriaux D, Arnold DA, Segebarth C, et al: ^{31}P MR evaluation of human brain tumor response to therapy. In Book of Abstracts, Society of Magnetic Resonance in Medicine 1:41, 1986 (abstract).
33. Ban N, Moriyasu F, Tamada T, et al: In vivo P-31 MR spectroscopic studies of liver in normal adults and cirrhotic patients, RSNA 1:340, 1986 (abstract).
34. Barany M, Arus C, and Chang YC: Natural-abundance carbon-13 NMR of brain, Magn Reson Med 2:289, 1985.
35. Barany M, Barany K, Burt CT, et al: Structural changes in myosin during contraction and the state of ADP in the intact frog muscle, J Supramol Struct 3:125, 1975.
36. Barany M, Langer BG, Glick RP, et al: In vivo H-1 spectroscopy in humans at 1.5 T1, Radiology 167:839, 1988.
37. Barker PB, Gillard JH, van Zijl PC, et al: Acute stroke: evaluation with serial proton MR spectroscopic imaging, Radiology 192:723, 1994.
38. Barker PB, Glickson JD, and Bryan RN: In vivo magnetic resonance spectroscopy of human brain tumors, Top Magn Reson Imaging 5:32, 1993.
39. Barker PB, Soher BJ, Blackband SJ, et al: Quantitation of proton SMR spectra of the human brain using tissue water as an internal concentration reference, NMR Biomed 6:89, 1993.
40. Beall PT, Hazelwood CF, and Rao PN: Nuclear magnetic resonance patterns of intracellular water as a function of HeLa cell cycle, Science 192:904, 1976.
41. Behar KL, den Hollander JA, Petroff OAC, et al: The effect of hypoglycemic encephalopathy upon amino acids, high energy phosphates, and a pH$_i$ in the rat brain in vivo: detection by sequential ^{1}H and ^{31}P NMR spectroscopy, J Neurochem 44:1045, 1985.
42. Behar KL, Petroff OAC, Prichard JW, et al: Detection of metabolites in rabbit brain by carbon-13 NMR spectroscopy, Magn Reson Med 3:911, 1986.
43. Behar KL, Rothman DL, Shulman RG, et al: Detection of cerebral lactate in vivo during hypoxemia by ^{1}H NMR at relatively low field strengths (1.9 tesla), Proc Natl Acad Sci U S A 81:2517, 1984.
44. Behar KL, Rothman DL, Spencer DD, et al: Analysis of macromolecule resonances in ^{1}H NMR spectra of human brain, Magn Reson Med 32:294, 1994.
45. Bendall MR: Surface coils and depth resolution using the spatial variation of radiofrequency field. In James TL, and Margulis AR, eds: Biomedical magnetic resonance, San Francisco, 1986, Radiology Research and Education Foundation.
46. Bendall MR, and Aue WP: Experimental verification of depth pulses applied with surface coils, J Magn Reson 54:149, 1983.
47. Bendall MR, den Hollander JA, Arias-Mendoza F, et al: Application of multipulse NMR to observe ^{13}C-labeled metabolites in biological systems, Magn Reson Med 2:56, 1985.
48. Bendall MR, and Gordon RE: Depth and refocusing pulses designed for multipulse NMR with surface coils, J Magn Reson 53:365, 1983.
49. Bendall MR, McKendry JM, Cresshull ID, et al: Active detune switch for complete sensitive volume localization in in vivo spectroscopy using multiple RF coils and depth pulses, J Magn Reson 60:473, 1984.
50. Bendall MR, and Pegg DT: Theoretical description of depth pulse sequences on and off resonance, including improvements and extensions thereof, Magn Reson Med 2:91, 1985.
51. Berendsen HJL, and Edzes HT: The observation and general interpretation of sodium magnetic resonance in biological material, Ann N Y Acad Sci 204:459, 1973.
52. Birken DL, and Oldendorf WH: N-acetyl-L-aspartic acid: a literature review of a compound prominent in ^{1}H-NMR spectroscopic studies of brain, Neurosci Biobehav Rev 13:23, 1989.
53. Bittl JA, and Ingwall JS: Reaction rates of creatine kinase and ATP synthesis in the isolated rat heart, J Biol Chem 260:3512, 1985.
54. Bizzi A, Movsas B, Tedeschi G, et al: Response of non-Hodgkin lymphoma to radiation therapy: early and long-term assessment with H-1 MR spectroscopic imaging, Radiology 194:271, 1995.
55. Blackledge MJ, Oberhaensli RD, Styles P, et al: Measurement of in vivo ^{31}P relaxation rates and spectral editing in human organs using rotating-frame depth selection, J Magn Reson 71:331, 1987.
56. Blackledge MJ, Rajagopalan B, Oberhaensli RD, et al: Quantitative studies of human cardiac metabolism by ^{31}P rotating-frame NMR, Proc Natl Acad Sci U S A 84:4283, 1987.
57. Boesch D, Gruetter R, Martin E, et al: Variations in the in vivo P-31 MR spectra of the developing human brain during postnatal life, Radiology 172:197, 1989.
58. Bolinger L, and Leigh JS: Hadamard spectroscopic imaging (HSI) for multivolume localization, J Magn Reson 80:162, 1988.
59. Bore PJ, Chan L, Gadian DG, et al: Noninvasive pH, measurements of human tissue using ^{31}P NMR. In Nuccitelli R, and Deamer DW, eds: Intracellular pH: its measurement, regulation and utilization in cellular functions, New York, 1982, Alan R. Liss.
60. Bottomley PA: Noninvasive studies of high-energy phosphate metabolism in human heart by depth resolved ^{31}P NMR spectroscopy, Science 299:769, 1985.
61. Bottomley PA: Noninvasive study of high-energy metabolism in human heart by depth-resolved ^{31}P NMR spectroscopy, Science 229:769, 1985.
62. Bottomley PA: Spatial localization in NMR spectroscopy in vivo, Ann N Y Acad Sci 508:333, 1987.
63. Bottomley PA, Edelstein WA, Foster TH, et al: In vivo solvent-suppressed localized hydrogen nuclear magnetic resonance spectroscopy: a window to metabolism? Proc Natl Acad Sci U S A 82:2148, 1985.
64. Bottomley PA, Foster TB, and Darrow RD: Depth-resolved surface coil spectroscopy (DRESS) for in vivo ^{1}H, ^{31}P, and ^{13}C NMR, J Magn Reson 59:338, 1984.
65. Bottomley PA, and Hardy CJ: Rapid, reliable in vivo assays of human phosphate metabolites by nuclear magnetic resonance, Clin Chem 35:392, 1989.
66. Bottomley PA, and Hardy CJ: Proton Overhauser enhancements in human cardiac phosphorus NMR spectroscopy at 1.5 T, Magn Reson Med 24:384, 1992.

67. Bottomley PA, and Hardy CJ: Mapping creatine kinase reaction rates in human brain and heart with 4 Tesla saturation transfer ^{31}P NMR, J Magn Reson 99:443, 1992.
68. Bottomley PA, Hardy CJ, and Roemer PB: Phosphate metabolite imaging and concentration measurements in human heart by nuclear magnetic resonance, Magn Reson Med 14:425, 1990.
69. Bottomley PA, Hart HA, and Edelstein WA: Anatomy and metabolism of the normal human brain studied by magnetic resonance at 1.5 Tesla, Radiology 150:441, 1984.
70. Bottomley PA, Herfkens RJ, Smith LS, et al: Altered phosphate metabolism in myocardial infarction: P-31 MR spectroscopy, Radiology 165:703, 1987.
71. Bottomley PA, Herfkens RJ, Smith LS, et al: Noninvasive detection and monitoring of regional myocardial ischemia in situ using depth-resolved phosphorus-31 NMR spectroscopy, Proc Natl Acad Sci U S A 82:8747, 1985.
72. Bottomley PA, Kogure K, Namon R, et al: Cerebral energy metabolism in rats studied by phosphorus nuclear magnetic resonance using surface coils, Magn Reson Imaging 1:81, 1982.
73. Bottomley PA, Smith LS, Leue WM, et al: Slice-interleaved depth-resolved surface-coil spectroscopy (SLIT DRESS) for rapid ^{31}P NMR in vivo, J Magn Reson 64:347, 1985.
74. Bottomley PA, Weiss RG, Hardy CJ, et al: Myocardial high-energy phosphate metabolism and allograft rejection in patients with heart transplants, Radiology 181:67, 1991.
75. Brateman L: Chemical shift imaging: a review, Am J Radiol 146:971, 1986.
76. Breiter SN, Arroyo S, Mathews VP, et al: Proton MR spectroscopy in patients with seizure disorders, Am J Neuroradiol 15:373, 1994.
77. Bretan PN Jr, Baldwin N, Novick AC, et al: Pretransplant assessment of renal viability by phosphorus-31 magnetic resonance spectroscopy: clinical experience in 40 recipient patients, Transplantation 48:48, 1989.
78. Bretan PN Jr, Vigneron DB, Hricak H, et al: Assessment of clinical renal preservation by phosphorus-31 magnetic resonance spectroscopy, J Urol 137:146, 1987.
79. Brindle KM, and Campbell ID: ^{1}Hydrogen nuclear magnetic resonance studies of cells and tissues. In James TL, and Margulis AR, eds: Biomedical magnetic resonance, San Francisco, 1984, Radiology Research and Education Foundation.
80. Brown TR, Gadian DG, Garlick PB, et al: Creatine kinase activities in skeletal and cardiac muscle measured by saturation transfer NMR. In Dutton L, Leigh J, and Scarpa A, eds: Alcoholism (NY), New York, 1978, Academic Press.
81. Brown TR, Kincaid BM, and Ugurbil K: NMR chemical shift imaging in three dimensions, Proc Natl Acad Sci U S A 79:3523, 1982.
82. Bruhn H, Frahm J, Gyngell ML, et al: Noninvasive differentiation of tumors with use of localized H-1 MR spectroscopy in vivo: initial experience in patients with cerebral tumors, Radiology 172:541, 1989.
83. Bruhn H, Frahm J, Merboldt KD, et al: Multiple sclerosis in children: cerebral metabolic alterations monitored by localized proton magnetic resonance spectroscopy in vivo, Ann Neurol 32:140, 1992.
84. Bruhn H, Weber T, Thorwirth V, et al: In-vivo monitoring of neuronal loss in Creutzfeldt-Jakob disease by proton magnetic resonance spectroscopy, Lancet 337:1610, 1991.
85. Bryant RG: Potassium-39 nuclear magnetic resonance, Biochem Biophys Res Commun 40:1162, 1970.
86. Buchli R, Duc CO, Martin E, et al: Assessment of absolute metabolite concentrations in human tissue by ^{31}P MRS in vivo. I. Cerebrum, cerebellum, cerebral gray and white matter, Magn Reson Med 32:447, 1994.
87. Burt CT, Glonek T, and Barany M: Analysis of phosphate metabolites, the intracellular pH, and the state of adenosine triphosphate in intact muscle by phosphorus nuclear magnetic resonance, J Biol Chem 251:2584, 1976.
88. Burt CT, Glonek T, and Barany M: Phosphorus-31 nuclear magnetic resonance detection of unexpected phosphodiesters in muscle, Biochemistry 15:4850, 1977.
89. Busby SJW, Gadian DG, Radda GK, et al: Phosphorus nuclear magnetic resonance studies of compartmentation in muscle, Biochem J 170:103, 1978.
90. Cady EB, and Azzopardi D: Absolute quantitation of neonatal brain spectra acquired with surface coil localization, NMR Biomed 2:305, 1989.
91. Cady EB, Costello AM, Dawson MJ, et al: Non-invasive investigation of cerebral metabolism in newborn infants by phosphorus nuclear magnetic resonance spectroscopy, Lancet 1:1059, 1983.
92. Cady EB, Lorek A, Penrice J, et al: ^{1}H magnetic resonance spectroscopy of the brains of normal infants and after perinatal hypoxia-ischemia, MAGMA 2:353, 1994.
93. Calabrese G, Deicken RF, Fein G, et al: ^{31}Phosphorus magnetic resonance spectroscopy of the temporal lobes in schizophrenia, Biol Psychiatry 32:26, 1992.
94. Canby RC, Evanochko WT, Barret LV, et al: Monitoring the bioenergetics of cardiac allograft rejection using in vivo nuclear magnetic resonance spectroscopy, J Am Coll Cardiol 9:1067, 1988.
95. Canioni P, Alger JR, and Shulman RG: Natural-abundance carbon-13 nuclear magnetic resonance of liver and adipose tissue of the living rat, Biochemistry 22:4974, 1983.
96. Cannon PJ, Maudsley A, Hilal SK, et al: NMR imaging of Na-23 in myocardium following coronary artery occlusion and reperfusion, Circulation 68:III-177, 1983.
97. Cendes F, Andermann F, Dubeau F, et al: Proton magnetic resonance spectroscopic images and MRI volumetric studies for lateralization of temporal lobe epilepsy, Magn Reson Imaging 13:1187, 1995.
98. Cendes F, Andermann F, Dubeau F, et al: MR spectroscopic imaging improves the localization of the epileptogenic lesion in patients with temporal lobe epilepsy, Neurology 45:A403, 1995 (abstract).
99. Cendes F, Andermann F, Preul MC, et al: Lateralization of temporal lobe epilepsy based on regional metabolic abnormalities in proton magnetic resonance spectroscopic images, Ann Neurol 35:211, 1994.
100. Cendes F, Cook MJ, Watson C, et al: Frequency and characteristics of dual pathology in patients with lesional epilepsy, Neurology 45:2058, 1995.
101. Cendes F, Stanley JA, Dubeau F, et al: Proton magnetic resonance spectroscopic imaging for discrimination of absence and complex partial seizures, Ann Neurol 41:74, 1997.
102. Chalovich JM, Burt CT, Cohen SM, et al: Identification of an unknown P-31 nuclear magnetic resonance from dystrophic chicken as 1-serine ethanolamine phosphodiester, Arch Biochem Biophys 182:683, 1977.
103. Chalovich JM, Burt CT, Danon MJ, et al: Phosphodiesters in muscular dystrophies, Ann N Y Acad Sci 317:649, 1979.
104. Chan L: The current status of magnetic resonance spectroscopy—basic and clinical aspects, West J Med 143:773, 1985.
105. Chan L, French ME, Gadian DG, et al: Study of human kidneys prior to transplantation by phosphorous nuclear magnetic resonance. In Pegg DE, Jacobsen IA, and Halasz NA, eds: Organ preservation: basic and applied, Boston, 1982, MIT Press.
106. Chan L, Gadian DG, Radda GK, et al: In vivo investigation of phosphorylase deficiency using ^{31}P NMRS, Int Congr Neuromusc Dis 5:81, 1982.
107. Chan L, Ledingham JGG, Dixon JA, et al: Acute renal failure: a proposed mechanism based upon ^{31}P nuclear magnetic resonance studies in the rat. In Eliahou N, ed: Acute renal failure, London, 1982, John Libbey.
108. Chance B, Eleff S, Bank W, et al: ^{31}P NMR studies of control of mitochondrial function in phosphofructokinase-deficient human skeletal muscle, Proc Natl Acad Sci U S A 79:7714, 1982.
109. Chance B, Eleff S, Leigh JS, et al: Mitochondrial regulation of phosphocreatine/inorganic phosphate ratios in exercising human muscle: a gated ^{31}P NMR study, Proc Natl Acad Sci U S A 78:6714, 1981.
110. Chance B, Eleff S, Leigh JSJ, et al: Mitochondrial regulation of phosphocreatine/inorganic phosphate ratios in exercising human muscle: a gated ^{31}P NMR study, Proc Natl Acad Sci U S A 78:6714, 1981.
111. Chance B, Nakase Y, Bond M, et al: Detection of ^{31}P nuclear magnetic resonance signals in brain by in vivo and freeze-trapped assays, Proc Natl Acad Sci U S A 75:4925, 1978.
112. Charles HC, Boyko OB, Lazeyrad FS, et al: Metabolic brain mapping in Alzheimer's disease using high resolution proton spectroscopy. In Proceedings of the Society of Magnetic Resonance in Medicine, p. 228, 1993 (abstract).
113. Chen W, and Ackerman JJH: Surface-coil spin-echo localization in vivo via inhomogeneous surface-spoiling magnetic gradient, J Magn Reson 82:655, 1989.
114. Chen W, and Ackerman JJH: Surface coil single-pulse localization in vivo via inhomogeneous surface spoiling magnetic gradient, NMR Biomed 4:205, 1989.
115. Chew WM, Hricak H, McClure RD, et al: In vivo human testicular function assessed with P-31 MR spectroscopy, Radiology 177:743, 1990.
116. Christiansen P, Henriksen O, Stubgaard M, et al: In vivo quantification of brain metabolites by ^{1}H-MRS using water as an internal standard, Magn Reson Imaging 10:107, 1992.
117. Chu WJ, Hetherington HP, Kuzniecky RI, et al: Is the intracellular pH different from normal in the epileptic focus of epilepsy patients? In Proceedings of the Society of Magnetic Resonance, p. 142, 1995 (abstract).
118. Civan MM, and Shporer M: NMR of sodium-23 and potassium-39 in biological systems, In Berliner LJ, and Reuben J, eds: Biological magnetic resonance, vol I, New York, 1978, Plenum Press.
119. Cohen RD, Henderson RM, Iles RA, et al: The technique and uses of intracellular pH measurements. In Porter R, and Lawrenson G, eds: Anonymous metabolic acidosis, London, 1982, Pitman Books.
120. Cohen SM, and Burt CT: ^{31}P nuclear magnetic relaxation studies of phosphocreatine in intact muscle: determination of intracellular free magnesium, Proc Natl Acad Sci U S A 74:4271, 1977.
121. Cohen SM, Glynn P, and Shulman RG: ^{13}C NMR study of gluconeogenesis from labeled alanine in hepatocytes from euthyroid and hyperthyroid rats, Proc Natl Acad Sci U S A 78:60, 1981.
122. Cohen SM, Ogawa S, and Shulman RG: A ^{13}C NMR study of gluconeogenesis in isolated rat liver cells, Front Biol Energ 2:1357, 1978.
123. Cohen SM, Ogawa S, and Shulman RG: ^{13}C NMR studies of gluconeogenesis in rat liver cells: utilization of labeled glycerol by cells from euthyroid and hyperthyroid rats, Proc Natl Acad Sci U S A 76:4808, 1979.
124. Cohen SM, Rognstad R, Shulman RG, et al: A comparison of ^{13}C nuclear magnetic resonance and 14C tracer studies of hepatic metabolism, J Biol Chem 256:3428, 1981.
125. Cohen SM, and Shulman RG: ^{13}C NMR studies of gluconeogenesis in rat liver suspensions and perfused mouse livers, Philos Trans R Soc Lond B 289:407, 1980.
126. Cohen SM, Shulman RG, and McLaughlin AC: Effects of ethanol on alanine metabolism in perfused mouse liver studied by ^{13}C NMR, Proc Natl Acad Sci U S A 76:4808, 1979.
127. Connelly A, Counsell C, Lohman JAB, et al: Outer volume suppressed image related in vivo spectroscopy (OSIRIS), a high-sensitivity localization technique, J Magn Reson 78:519, 1988.
128. Connelly A, Jackson GD, Duncan JS, et al: Magnetic resonance spectroscopy in temporal lobe epilepsy, Neurology 44:1411, 1994.
129. Cooke R, and Wien R: The state of water in muscle tissue as determined by proton nuclear magnetic resonance, Biophys J 11:1002, 1971.
130. Cope FW, and Damadian R: Cell potassium by ^{39}K spin-echo nuclear magnetic resonance, Nature 228:76, 1970.
131. Cox DWG, Morris PG, Feeney J, et al: ^{31}P-NMR studies on cerebral energy metabolism under conditions of hypoglycemia and hypoxia in vitro, Biochem J 212:365, 1983.
132. Cuenod CA, Kaplan DB, Michot JL, et al: Phospholipid abnormalities in early Alzheimer's disease: in vivo phosphorus 31 magnetic resonance spectroscopy, Arch Neurol 52:89, 1995.
133. Daly PF, Lyon RC, Faustino PJ, et al: Phospholipid metabolism in cancer cells monitored by ^{31}P NMR spectroscopy, J Biol Chem 262:14875, 1987.
134. Damadian R: Tumor detection by nuclear magnetic resonance, Science 171:1151, 1971.

135. Damadian R, Goldsmith M, and Minkoff L: FONAR image of the live human body, Physiol Chem Phys Med NMR 9:97, 1977.

136. Damadian RV, Minkoff L, Goldsmith M, et al: Tumor imaging in a live animal by field focusing NMR (FONAR), Physiol Chem Phys Med NMR 8:61, 1976.

137. Davie CA, Hawkins CP, Barker GJ, et al: Serial proton magnetic resonance spectroscopy in acute multiple sclerosis lesions, Brain 117:49, 1994.

138. Dawson MJ, Gadian DG, and Wilkie DR: Contraction and recovery of living muscle studied by ^{31}P nuclear magnetic resonance, J Physiol (Lond) 267:703, 1977.

139. Dawson MJ, Gadian DG, and Wilkie DR: Muscular fatigue investigated by phosphorus nuclear magnetic resonance, Nature 274:861, 1978.

140. Dawson MJ, Gadian DG, and Wilkie DR: Mechanical relaxation rate and metabolism studied in fatiguing muscle by phosphorous nuclear magnetic resonance, J Physiol (Lond) 299:465, 1980.

141. De Graaf AA, Deutz NE, Bosman DK, et al: The use of in vivo proton NMR to study the effects of hyperammonemia in the rat cerebral cortex, NMR Biomed 4:31, 1991.

142. De Stefano N, Matthews PM, Antel JP, et al: Chemical pathology of acute demyelinating lesions and its correlation with disability, Ann Neurol 38:901, 1995.

143. De Stefano N, Matthews PM, and Arnold DL: Reversible decreases in N-acetyl aspartate after acute brain injury, Magn Reson Med 34:721, 1995.

144. Degani H, Alger JR, Shulman RG, et al: ^{31}P magnetization transfer studies of creatine kinase kinetics in living rabbit brain, Magn Reson Med 5:1, 1987.

145. Deicken RF, Calabrese G, Merrin EL, et al: Basal ganglia phosphorous metabolism in chronic schizophrenia, Am J Psychiatry 152:126, 1995.

146. Deicken RF, Calabrese G, Merrin EL, et al: 31 phosphorus magnetic resonance spectroscopy of the frontal and parietal lobes in chronic schizophrenia, Biol Psychiatry 36:503, 1994.

147. Deicken RF, Fein G, and Weiner MW: Abnormal frontal lobe phosphorous metabolism in bipolar disorder, Am J Psychiatry 152:915, 1995.

148. Deicken RF, Merrin EL, Floyd TC, et al: Correlation between left frontal phospholipids and Wisconsin Card Sort Test performance in schizophrenia, Schizophr Res 14:177, 1995.

149. Deicken RF, Weiner MW, and Fein G: Decreased temporal lobe phosphomonoesters in bipolar disorder, J Affect Disord 33:195, 1995.

150. Delayre JL, Ingwall JS, Malloy CR, et al: Gated sodium-23 nuclear magnetic resonance images of an isolated perfused working rat heart, Science 212:935, 1981.

151. den Hollander JA, Behar KL, and Shulman RG: Use of double-tuned surface coils for the application of ^{13}C NMR to brain metabolism, J Magn Reson 57:311, 1984.

152. den Hollander JA, Ugurbil K, and Shulman RG: ^{31}P and ^{13}C NMR studies of intermediates of aerobic and anaerobic glycolysis in *Saccharomyces cerevisiae,* Biochemistry 25:212, 1986.

153. Deutsch C, Taylor JS, and Wilson DF: Regulation of intracellular pH by human peripheral blood lymphocytes as measured by ^{19}F NMR, Proc Natl Acad Sci U S A 79:7944, 1982.

154. Dewhirst MD, Sostman HD, Leopold KA, et al: Soft tissue sarcomas: MR imaging and MR spectroscopy for prognosis and therapy monitoring, Radiology 174:847, 1990.

155. Dixon WT: Simple proton spectroscopy imaging, Radiology 153:189, 1984.

156. Doyle TJ, Bedell BJ, and Narayana PA: Relative concentrations of proton MR visible neurochemicals in gray and white matter in human brain, Magn Reson Med 33:755, 1995.

157. Dube GP, Schwartz A, Gadian DG, et al: The relationship between pressure development induced by inotropic agents and high-energy phosphate compounds in the Langendorff perfused rat heart: a phosphorus-31 NMR study. In Cohen JS, ed: Noninvasive probes of tissue metabolism, New York, 1982, John Wiley & Sons.

158. Duijn JH, Matson GB, Maudsley AA, et al: 3D phase encoding ^{1}H spectroscopic imaging of human brain, Magn Reson Imaging 10:315, 1992.

159. Duyn JH, Gillen J, Sobering G, et al: Multisection proton MR spectroscopic imaging of the brain, Radiology 188:277, 1993.

160. Duyn JH, and Moonen CTW: Fast proton spectroscopic imaging of human brain using multiple spin-echoes, Magn Reson Med 30:409, 1993.

161. Ebisu T, Rooney WD, Graham SH, et al: N-acetyl aspartate as an in vivo marker of neuronal viability in kainate-induced status epilepticus: ^{1}H magnetic resonance spectroscopic imaging, J Cereb Blood Flow Metab 14:373, 1994.

162. Edwards RHT, Wilkie DR, Dawson JM, et al: Clinical use of nuclear magnetic resonance in the investigation of myopathy, Lancet 1:725, 1982.

163. Eleff S, Kennaway NG, Buist NR, et al: ^{31}P NMR study of improvement in oxidative phosphorylation by vitamins K3 and C in a patient with a defect in electron transport at complex III in skeletal muscle, Proc Natl Acad Sci U S A 81:3529, 1984.

164. Ende G, Laxer KD, Knowlton R, et al: Quantitative ^{1}H SI shows bilateral metabolite changes in unilateral TLE patients with and without hippocampal atrophy. In Proceedings of the Society of Magnetic Resonance, p. 144, 1995 (abstract).

165. Evanochko WT, Ng TC, Lilly MB, et al: In vivo ^{31}P NMR study of the metabolism of murine mammary 16/C adenocarcinoma and its response to chemotherapy, x-radiation and hyperthermia, Proc Natl Acad Sci U S A 80:334, 1983.

166. Evanochko WT, Reeves RC, Sakai TT, et al: Proton NMR spectroscopy in myocardial ischemic insult, Magn Reson Med 5:23, 1987.

167. Evelhoch JL, Sapareto SA, Jick DEL, et al: In vivo metabolic effects of hyperglycemia in murine radiation-induced fibrosarcoma: a ^{31}P NMR investigation, Proc Natl Acad Sci U S A 81:6496, 1984.

168. Fitzsimmons JR, Beck BL, and Brooker HR: Double resonance quadrature birdcage, Magn Reson Med 30:107, 1993.

169. Fossel ET, Morgan HE, and Ingwall JS: Measurements of changes in high-energy phosphates in the cardiac cycle by using ^{31}P nuclear magnetic resonance, Proc Natl Acad Sci U S A 77:3654, 1980.

170. Frahm J, Bruhn H, Gyngell ML, et al: Localized proton NMR spectroscopy in different regions of the human brain in vivo: relaxation times and concentrations of cerebral metabolites, Magn Reson Med 11:47, 1989.

171. Frahm J, Bruhn H, Gyngell ML, et al: Localized high-resolution proton NMR spectroscopy using stimulated echoes: initial applications to human brain in vivo, Magn Reson Med 9:79, 1989.

172. Frahm J, Merboldt KD, and Hanicke W: Localized proton spectroscopy: new steps using stimulated echoes, Proceedings of the Society of Magnetic Resonance in Medicine, Works in Progress, p. 158, 1986 (abstract).

173. Frahm J, Merboldt KD, and Hanicke W: Localized proton spectroscopy using stimulated echoes, J Magn Reson 72:502, 1987.

174. Frahm J, Michaelis T, Merboldt KD, et al: Localized NMR spectroscopy in vivo: progress and problems, NMR Biomed 2:188, 1989.

175. Freeman D, Chan L, Yahaya H, et al: Magnetic resonance spectroscopy for the determination of renal metabolic rate in vivo, Kidney Int 30:35, 1986.

176. Freeman DS, Bartlett S, Radda GK, et al: Energetics of sodium transport in the kidney saturation transfer ^{31}P-NMR, Biochim Biophys Acta 762:325, 1983.

177. From AH, Zimmer SD, Michurski SP, et al: Regulation of the oxidative phosphorylation rate in the intact cell, Biochemistry 29:3731, 1990.

178. From AHL, Petein MA, Michurski SP, et al: ^{31}P studies of respiratory regulation in the intact myocardium, FEBS Lett 206:257, 1988.

179. Fu L, Matthews PM, De Stefano N, et al: Imaging axonal damage of normal appearing white matter in multiple sclerosis, Brain 1998 (in press).

180. Fujimoto T, Nakano T, Takano T, et al: Study of chronic schizophrenics using ^{31}P magnetic resonance chemical shift imaging, Acta Psychiatr Scand 86:455, 1992.

181. Fulham MJ, Bizzi A, Dietz MJ, et al: Mapping of brain tumor metabolites with proton MR spectroscopic imaging: clinical relevance, Radiology 185:675, 1992.

182. Gadian DG: Nuclear magnetic resonance and its applications to living systems, Oxford, 1992, Clarendon Press.

183. Gadian DG, Connelly A, Duncan JS, et al: ^{1}H magnetic resonance spectroscopy in the investigation of intractable epilepsy, Acta Neurol Scand Suppl 152:116, 1994.

184. Gadian DG, Hoult DI, Radda GK, et al: Phosphorus nuclear magnetic resonance studies on normoxic and ischemic cardiac tissue, Proc Natl Acad Sci U S A 73:4446, 1976.

185. Gadian DG, Radda GK, Brown TR, et al: The activity of creatine kinase in frog skeletal muscle studied by saturation-transfer nuclear magnetic resonance, Biochem J 194:215, 1981.

186. Gadian DG, Radda GK, Ross BD, et al: Examination of a myopathy by phosphorus nuclear magnetic resonance, Lancet 2:774, 1981.

187. Garcia PA, Laxer KD, van der Grond J, et al: ^{31}P magnetic resonance spectroscopic imaging in patients with frontal lobe epilepsy, Ann Neurol 35:217, 1994.

188. Garcia PA, Laxer KD, van der Grond J, et al: Proton magnetic resonance spectroscopic imaging in patients with frontal lobe epilepsy, Ann Neurol 37:279, 1995.

189. Garlick PB, Radda GK, and Seeley PJ: Studies of acidosis in the ischemic heart by phosphorus nuclear magnetic resonance, Biochem J 184.547, 1979.

190. Garlick PB, Radda GK, Seeley PJ, et al: Phosphorus NMR studies on perfused heart, Biochem Biophys Res Commun 74:1256, 1977.

191. Garlick PB, and Turner CJ: The application of phosphorous two-dimensional NMR exchange spectroscopy to cardiac metabolism, J Magn Reson 51:536, 1983.

192. Garwood M, Schleich T, Bendall MR, et al: Improved Fourier series windows for localization in in vivo NMR spectroscopy, J Magn Reson 65:510, 1985.

193. Garwood M, Schleich T, Matson GB, et al: Spatial localization of tissue metabolites by phosphorous-31 NMR rotating frame zeugmatography, J Magn Reson 60:268, 1984.

194. Garwood M, Schleich T, Ross BD, et al: A modified rotating frame experiment based on a Fourier series window function: application to in vivo spatially localized NMR spectroscopy, J Magn Reson 65:239, 1985.

195. Geoffrion Y, Rydzy M, Butler KW, et al: The use of immobilized ferrite to enhance the depth selectivity of in vivo surface coil NMR spectroscopy, NMR Biomed 1:107, 1988.

196. Gill SS, Thomas DG, and Van BN: Proton MR spectroscopy of intracranial tumors: in vivo and in vitro studies, J Comput Assist Tomogr 14:497, 1990.

197. Glonek T, Kopp S J, Kot E, et al: P-31 nuclear magnetic resonance analysis of brain: the perchloric acid extract spectrum, J Neurochem 39:1210, 1982.

198. Gober J, Schaefer S, Camacho SA, et al: Epicardial and endocardial localized ^{31}P magnetic resonance spectroscopy: evidence for metabolic heterogeneity during regional ischemia, Magn Reson Med 13:204, 1990.

199. Gonen O, Hu J, Murphy-Boesch J, et al: Dual interleaved ^{1}H and proton-ecoupled-^{31}P in vivo chemical shift imaging of human brain, Magn Reson Med 32:104, 1994.

200. Gonzalez RG, Guimaraes AR, Sachs GS, et al: Measurement of human brain lithium in vivo by MR spectroscopy, Am J Neuroradiol 14:1027, 1993.

201. Gonzalez-Mendez R, McNeill A, Gregory GA, et al: Effects of hypoxic hypoxia on cerebral phosphate metabolites and pH in the anesthetized infant rabbit, J Cereb Blood Flow Metab 5:512, 1985.

202. Gordon RE, Hanley PE, and Shaw D: Topical magnetic resonance, Prog NMR Spect 15:1, 1982.

203. Gordon RE, Hanley PE, Shaw D, et al: Localization of metabolites in animals using ^{31}P topical magnetic resonance, Nature 287:367, 1980.

204. Graham GD, Kalvach P, Blamire AM, et al: Clinical correlates of proton magnetic resonance spectroscopy findings after acute cerebral infarction, Stroke 26:225, 1995.

205. Graham SH, Meyerhoff DJ, Bayne L, et al: Magnetic resonance spectroscopy of N-acetylaspartate in hypoxic-ischemic encephalopathy, Ann Neurol 35:490, 1994.

206. Griffiths JR, Cady E, Edwards RHT, et al: ^{31}P-NMR studies of a human tumour in situ, Lancet 1:1435, 1983.

207. Griffiths JR, Stevens AN, Iles RA, et al: ^{31}P-NMR investigation of solid tumours in the living rat, Biosci Rep 1:319, 1981.

208. Griffiths RD, Cady EB, Edwards RH, et al: Muscle energy metabolism in Duchenne dystrophy studied by ^{31}P-NMR: controlled trials show no effect of allopurinol or ribose, Muscle Nerve 8:760, 1985.

209. Grist TM, Charles HC, and Sostman HD: 1990 ARRS Executive Council Award: renal transplant rejection: diagnosis with ^{31}P MR spectroscopy, Am J Roentgenol 156:105, 1991.

210. Grossman RI, Lenkinski RE, Ramer KN, et al: MR proton spectroscopy in multiple sclerosis, Am J Neuroradiol 13:1535, 1992.

211. Grove TH, Ackerman JJH, Radda GK, et al: Analysis of rat heart in vivo by phosphorus nuclear magnetic resonance, Proc Natl Acad Sci U S A 77:299, 1980.

212. Gruetter R, Magnusson I, Rothman DL, et al: Validation of ^{13}C NMR measurements of liver glycogen in vivo, Magn Reson Med 31:583, 1994.

213. Gruetter R, Rothman DL, Novotny EJ, et al: Localized ^{13}C NMR spectroscopy of myoinositol in the human brain in vivo, Magn Reson Med 25:204, 1992.

214. Gupta RK, Gupta P, Yushok WD, et al: On the noninvasive measurement of intracellular free magnesium by ^{31}P NMR spectroscopy, Physiol Chem Phys 15:265, 1983.

215. Gupta RK, and Moore RD: ^{31}P NMR studies of intracellular free Mg^{2+} in intact frog skeletal muscle, J Biol Chem 255:3987, 1980.

216. Gupta RK, and Yushok WD: Noninvasive ^{31}P NMR probes of free Mg^{2+}, MgATP, and MgADP in intact Ehrlich ascites tumor cells, Proc Natl Acad Sci U S A 77:2487, 1980.

217. Gyulai L, Bolinger L, Leigh JSJ, et al: Phosphorylethanolamine—the major constituent of the phosphomonoester peak observed by ^{31}P-NMR on developing dog brain, FEBS Lett 178:137, 1984.

218. Haase A, Malloy CR, and Radda GK: Spatial localization of high resolution ^{31}P spectra with a surface coil, J Magn Reson 55:164, 1983.

219. Hagberg G, Burlina AP, Mader I, et al: In vivo proton MR spectroscopy of human gliomas: definition of metabolic coordinates for multi-dimensional classification, Magn Reson Med 34:242, 1995.

220. Hansen JR: Pulsed NMR study of water mobility and brain tissue, Nature 230:482, 1971.

221. Hardy CJ, Bottomley PA, Rohling KW, et al: An NMR phased array for human cardiac ^{31}P spectroscopy, Magn Reson Med 28:54, 1992.

222. Haselgrove JC, Subramanian VH, Leigh JS, et al: In vivo one-dimensional imaging of phosphorus metabolites by phosphorus-31 nuclear magnetic resonance, Science 220:1170, 1983.

223. Haupt CI, Schuff N, Weiner MW, et al: Removal of lipid artifacts in ^{1}H spectroscopic imaging by data extrapolation, Magn Reson Med 35:678, 1996.

224. Heindel W, Bunke J, Glathe S, et al: Combined ^{1}H MR imaging and localized ^{31}P spectroscopy of intracranial tumors in 43 patients, J Comput Assist Tomogr 12:907, 1988.

225. Heindel W, Bunke J, Steinbrich W, et al: Human brain tumors: evaluation by image-guided localized P-31 MR spectroscopy. In Book of Abstracts, Society of Magnetic Resonance in Medicine, 1:153, 1987 (abstract).

226. Heiss WD, Heindel W, Herholz K, et al: Positron emission tomography of fluorine-18-deoxyglucose and image-guided phosphorus-31 magnetic resonance spectroscopy in brain tumors, J Nucl Med 31:302, 1990.

227. Hellstrand P, and Vogel HJ: Phosphagens and intracellular pH in intact rabbit smooth muscle studied by ^{31}P NMR, Am J Physiol 248:C320, 1985.

228. Helpern JA, Vande Linde AM, Welch KM, et al: Acute elevation and recovery of intracellular [Mg2+] following human focal cerebral ischemia, Neurology 43:1577, 1993.

229. Henderson TO, Costello AJR, and Omachi A: Phosphate metabolism in intact erythrocytes: determination phosphorus-31 nuclear magnetic resonance spectroscopy, Proc Natl Acad Sci U S A 71:2487, 1974.

230. Hendrich K, Merkle H, Weisdorf S, et al: Phase-modulated rotating-frame spectroscopic localization using an adiabatic plane-rotation pulse and a single surface coil, J Magn Reson 92:258, 1991.

231. Hendrich K, Xu Y, Kim S-G, et al: Surface coil cardiac tagging and ^{31}P spectroscopic localization with B_1-insensitive adiabatic pulses, Magn Reson Med 31:541, 1994.

232. Herholz K, Heindel W, Luyten PR, et al: In vivo imaging of glucose consumption and lactate concentration in human gliomas, Ann Neurol 31:319, 1992.

233. Hetherington H, Kuzniecky R, Pan J, et al: Proton nuclear magnetic resonance spectroscopic imaging of human temporal lobe epilepsy at 4.1 T, Ann Neurol 38:396, 1995.

234. Hetherington HP, Mason GF, Pan JW, et al: Evaluation of cerebral gray and white matter metabolite differences by spectroscopic imaging at 4.1 T, Magn Reson Med 32:565, 1994.

235. Hetherington HP, Pan JW, Mason GF, et al: Quantitative ^{1}H spectroscopic imaging of human brain at 4.1 T using image segmentation, Magn Reson Med 36:21, 1996.

236. Hiehle JF, Lenkinski RE, Grossman RI, et al: Correlation of spectroscopy and magnetization transfer imaging in the evaluation of demyelinating lesions and normal appearing white matter in multiple sclerosis, Magn Reson Med 32:285, 1994.

237. Hilal SK, Maudsley AA, Simon HE, et al: In vivo NMR imaging of tissue sodium in the intact cat before and after acute cerebral stroke, Am J Neuroradiol 4:245, 1983.

238. Hollis DP: Nuclear magnetic resonance studies of cancer and heart disease, Bull Magn Reson 1:27, 1979.

239. Hollis DP, Nunnally RL, Jacobus WE, et al: Detection of regional ischemia in perfused beating hearts by phosphorus nuclear magnetic resonance, Biochem Biophys Res Commun 75:1086, 1977.

240. Hope PL, Cady EB, Tofts PS, et al: Cerebral energy metabolism studied with phosphorus NMR spectroscopy in normal and birth-asphyxiated infants, Lancet 2:366, 1984.

241. Hore PJ: Solvent suppression in Fourier transform nuclear magnetic resonance, J Magn Reson 55:283, 1983.

242. Hoult DI: Rotating frame zeugmatography, J Magn Reson 33:183, 1979.

243. Hoult DI, Busby SJW, Gadian DG, et al: Observations of tissue metabolites using phosphorus 31 nuclear magnetic resonance, Nature 252:285, 1974.

244. Howe FA, Maxwell RJ, Saunders DE, et al: Proton spectroscopy in vivo, Magn Reson Q 9:31, 1993.

245. Howe FA, Robinson SP, and Griffiths JR: Modification of tumour perfusion and oxygenation monitored by gradient recalled echo MRI and ^{31}P MRS, NMR Biomed 9:208, 1996.

246. Hubesch B, Sappey-Marinier D, Hodes JE, et al: Increased 31-P T1 relaxation times in human brain tumor. In Book of Abstracts, Society of Magnetic Resonance in Medicine, p. 64, 1988 (abstract).

247. Hubesch B, Sappey-Marinier D, Laxer KD, et al: Alkalosis in seizure foci of temporal lobe epilepsy. In Book of Abstracts, Society of Magnetic Resonance in Medicine, p. 448, 1989 (abstract).

248. Hubesch B, Sappey-Marinier D, Roth K, et al: ^{31}P NMR spectroscopy of normal human brain and brain tumors, Radiology 174:401, 1990.

249. Hugg JW, Duijn JH, Matson GB, et al: Elevated lactate and alkalosis in chronic human brain infarction observed by ^{1}H and ^{31}P spectroscopic imaging (MRSI), J Cereb Blood Flow Metab 12:734, 1992.

250. Hugg JW, Laxer KD, Matson GB, et al: Lateralization of human focal epilepsy by ^{31}P magnetic resonance spectroscopic imaging, Neurology 43:2011, 1993.

251. Hugg JW, Laxer KD, Matson GB, et al: Neuron loss localizes human temporal lobe epilepsy by in vivo proton magnetic resonance spectroscopic imaging, Ann Neurol 34:788, 1993.

252. Husted CA, Duijn JH, Matson GB, et al: Molar quantitation of in vivo proton metabolites in human brain with 3D magnetic resonance spectroscopic imaging, Magn Reson Imaging 12:661, 1994.

253. Husted CA, Goodin DS, Hugg JW, et al: Biochemical alterations in multiple sclerosis lesions and normal-appearing white matter detected by in vivo ^{31}P and ^{1}H spectroscopic imaging, Ann Neurol 36:157, 1994.

254. Husted CA, Matson GB, Adams DA, et al: In vivo detection of myelin phospholipids in multiple sclerosis with phosphorus magnetic resonance spectroscopic imaging, Ann Neurol 36:239, 1994.

255. Ingwall JS: Phosphorus nuclear magnetic resonance spectroscopy of cardiac and skeletal muscles, Am J Physiol 242:H729, 1982.

256. Ingwall JS, Kobayashi K, and Bittl JA: Measurement of flux through the creatine kinase reaction in the intact rat heart: ^{31}P NMR studies, Biophys J 41:1a, 1983 (abstract).

257. Isaac G, Schnall MD, Lenkinski RE, et al: A design for a double-tuned birdcage coil for use in an integrated MRI/MRS examination, J Magn Reson 89:41, 1990.

258. Jacobus WE, Taylor IV GJ, Hollis DP, et al: Phosphorus nuclear magnetic resonance of perfused working rat hearts, Nature 265:756, 1977.

259. James TL, and Margulis AR: Biomedical magnetic resonance. In James TL, and Margulis AR, eds: Biomedical magnetic resonance, San Francisco, 1984, Radiology Research and Education Foundation (editorial).

260. James TL, and Noggle JH: ^{23}Na nuclear magnetic resonance relaxation studies of sodium ion interaction with soluble RNA, Proc Natl Acad Sci U S A 62:644, 1969.

261. Jeener J, Meier EH, Bachmann P, et al: Investigation of exchange processes by two-dimensional NMR spectroscopy, J Chem Phys 71:4546, 1979.

262. Johnston W, Karpati G, Carpenter S, et al: Late-onset mitochondrial myopathy, Ann Neurol 37:16, 1995.

263. Jue T: Two for one: simultaneously winnowing the ^{13}C-^{1}H and ^{12}C-^{1}H signals using only ^{1}H pulses, J Magn Reson 73:524, 1987.

264. Jue T, Lohman JAB, Ordidge RJ, et al: Natural abundance ^{13}C NMR spectrum of glycogen in humans, Magn Reson Med 5:377, 1987.

265. Jue T, Rothman DL, Shulman GI, et al: Direct observation of glycogen synthesis in human muscle with ^{13}C NMR, Proc Natl Acad Sci U S A 86:4489, 1989.

266. Jue T, Rothman DL, Tavitian BA, et al: Natural-abundance ^{13}C NMR study of glycogen repletion in human liver and muscle, Proc Natl Acad Sci U S A 86:1439, 1989.

267. Jungling FD, Wakhloo AK, Stadtmuller G, et al: Localized ^{1}H-spectroscopy in the hippocampus of normals and patients with Alzheimer's disease. In Proceedings of the Society of Magnetic Resonance in Medicine, p. 1555, 1992 (abstract).

268. Kantor HL, Briggs RW, and Balaban RS: In vivo ^{31}P nuclear magnetic resonance measurements in canine heart using a catheter-coil, Circ Res 55:261, 1984.

269. Kantor HL, Briggs RW, Metz KR, et al: Gated in vivo examination of cardiac metabolites with ^{31}P nuclear magnetic resonance, Am J Physiol 251:H171, 1986.

270. Karczmar GS, Meyerhoff DJ, Boska MD, et al: ^{31}P Spectroscopy study of response of superficial human tumors to therapy, Radiology 17:149, 1990.

271. Karczmar GS, Meyerhoff DJ, Speder A, et al: Response of tumors to therapy studied by magnetic resonance, Invest Radiol 24:1020, 1989.

272. Karczmar GS, Tavares NJ, and Weiner MW: A ^{31}P NMR study of the GI tract: effect of fructose loading and measurement of transverse relaxation times, Magn Reson Med 9:8, 1989.

273. Karczmar GS, Weiner MW, and Matson GB: Detection of residual Z magnetization: application to the surface coil rotating frame experiment, J Magn Reson 71:360, 1987.

274. Karczmar GS, Weiner MW, and Matson GB: Improvement of the rotating frame experiment by detection of residual Z magnetization: a ^{31}P MRS study of a Meth-A sarcoma, NMR Biomed 1988.

275. Kato T, Shioiri T, Takahashi S, et al: Measurement of brain phosphoinositide metabolism in bipolar patients using in vivo ^{31}P-MRS, J Affect Disord 22:185, 1991.

276. Kato T, Takahashi S, Shioiri T, et al: Brain phosphorous metabolism in depressive disorders detected by phosphorus-31 magnetic resonance spectroscopy, J Affect Disord 26:223, 1992.

277. Kato T, Takahashi S, Shioiri T, et al: Alterations in brain phosphorous metabolism in bipolar disorder detected by in vivo ^{31}P and ^{7}Li magnetic resonance spectroscopy, J Affect Disord 27:53, 1993.

278. Katz LA, Swain JA, Portman MA, et al: Intracellular pH and inorganic phosphate content of heart in vivo: a ^{31}P NMR study, Am J Physiol 255:H189, 1988.

279. Katz LA, Swain JA, Portman MA, et al: Relation between phosphate metabolites and oxygen consumption of heart in vivo, Am J Physiol 256:H265, 1989.

280. Kavanaugh KM, Aisen AM, Fechner KP, et al: Regional metabolism during coronary occlusion, reperfusion, and reocclusion using phosphorus-31 nuclear magnetic resonance spectroscopy in the intact rabbit, Am Heart J 117:53, 1989.

281. Kavanaugh KM, Aisen AM, Fechner KP, et al: Effects of diltiazem on phosphate metabolism in ischemic and reperfused myocardium using phosphorus 31 nuclear magnetic resonance spectroscopy in vivo, Am Heart J 118:1210, 1989.

282. Kent-Braun JA, Miller RG, and Weiner MW: Magnetic resonance spectroscopy studies of human muscle, Radiol Clin North Am 32:313, 1994.

283. Kent-Braun JA, Miller RG, and Weiner MW: Human skeletal muscle metabolism in health and disease: utility of magnetic resonance spectroscopy. In Holloszy JO, ed: Exercise and sport sciences reviews, Baltimore, 1995, Williams & Wilkins.

284. Kent-Braun JA, Sharma KR, Weiner MW, et al: Effects of exercise on muscle activation and metabolism in multiple sclerosis, Muscle Nerve 17:1162, 1994.

285. Kingsley-Hickman P, Sako EY, Andreone PA, et al: Phosphorus-31 NMR measurement of ATP synthesis rate in perfused intact rat hearts, FEBS Lett 198:159, 1986.

286. Kingsley-Hickman PB, Sako EY, Ugurbil K, et al: ^{31}P NMR measurement of mitochondrial uncoupling in isolated rat hearts, J Biol Chem 265:1545, 1990.

287. Kobayashi K, Fossel E, and Ingwall J: Analysis of the creatine kinase reaction in the isolated perfused rat heart using P-31 NMR saturation transfer, Biophys J 37:123a, 1982 (abstract).

288. Koller KJ, Zaczek R, and Coyle JT: N-acetyl-aspartyl-glutamate: regional levels in rat brain and the effects of brain lesions as determined by a new HPLC method, J Neurochem 43:1136, 1984.

289. Komoroski RA, Newton JE, Sprigg JR, et al: In vivo ^{7}Li nuclear magnetic resonance study of lithium pharmacokinetics and chemical shift imaging in psychiatric patients, Psychiatry Res 50:67, 1993.

290. Komoroski RA, Newton JE, Walker E, et al: In vivo NMR spectroscopy of lithium-7 in humans, Magn Reson Med 15:347, 1990.

291. Koretsky AP, Basus VJ, James TL, et al: Detection of exchange reactions involving small metabolite pools using NMR magnetization transfer techniques: relevance to subcellular compartmentation of creatine kinase, Magn Reson Med 2:586, 1985.

292. Koretsky AP, Wang S, Klein MP, et al: ^{31}P NMR saturation transfer measurements of phosphorus exchange reactions in rat heart and kidney in situ, Biochemistry 25:77, 1986.

293. Koretsky AP, Wang S, Murphy-Boesch J, et al: ^{31}P NMR spectroscopy of rat organs, in situ, using chronically implanted radiofrequency coils, Proc Natl Acad Sci U S A 80:7491, 1983.

294. Koretsky AP, and Weiner MW: ^{31}Phosphorous nuclear magnetic resonance magnetization transfer measurement of exchange reactions in vivo. In James T, and Margulis A, eds: Biomedical magnetic resonance, San Francisco, 1984, Radiology Research and Education Foundation.

295. Kotitschke K, Jung H, Nekolla S, et al: High-resolution one- and two-dimensional ^{1}H MRS of human brain tumor and normal glial cells, NMR Biomed 7:111, 1994.

296. Kreis R, Ernst T, and Ross BD: Development of the human brain: In vivo quantification of metabolite and water content with proton magnetic resonance spectroscopy, Magn Reson Med 30:424, 1993.

297. Kreis R, Ernst T, and Ross BD: Absolute quantitation of water and metabolites in the human brain. II. Metabolite concentrations, J Magn Reson 102:9, 1993.

298. Kuesel AC, Sutherland GR, Halliday W, et al: ^{1}H MRS of high grade astrocytomas: mobile lipid accumulation in necrotic tissue, NMR Biomed 7:149, 1994.

299. Kugel H, Heindel W, Ernestus RI, et al: Human brain tumors: spectral patterns detected with localized H-1 MR spectroscopy, Radiology 183:701, 1992.

300. Kurhanewicz J, Thomas A, Jajodia P, et al: ^{31}P spectroscopy of the human prostate gland in vivo using a transrectal probe, Magn Reson Med 22:404, 1991.

301. Kurhanewicz J, Vigneron DB, Hricak H, et al: Three-dimensional ^{1}H spectroscopic imaging of the in situ human prostate at high spatial (0.24 to 0.7 cm^3) resolution, Radiology 198:795, 1996.

302. Kurhanewicz J, Vigneron DB, Nelson SJ, et al: Citrate as an in vivo marker to discriminate prostate cancer from benign prostatic hyperplasia and normal prostate peripheral zone: detection via localized proton spectroscopy, Urology 45:459, 1995.

303. Kuzniecky R, Elgavish GA, Hetherington HP, et al: In vivo ^{31}P nuclear magnetic resonance spectroscopy of human temporal lobe epilepsy, Neurology 42:1586, 1992.

304. Lanfermann H, Kugel H, Heindel W, et al: Metabolic changes in acute and subacute cerebral infarctions: findings at proton MR spectroscopic imaging, Radiology 196:203, 1995.

305. Laptook AR, Corbett RJT, Uauy R, et al: Use of ^{31}P magnetic resonance spectroscopy to characterize evolving brain damage after perinatal asphyxia, Neurology 39:709, 1989.

306. Lara RS, Matson GB, Hugg JW, et al: Quantitation of in vivo phosphorus metabolites in human brain with magnetic resonance spectroscopic imaging (MRSI), Magn Reson Imaging 11:273, 1993.

307. Larsson HBW, Christiansen P, Jensen M, et al: Localized in vivo proton spectroscopy in the brain of patients with multiple sclerosis, Magn Reson Med 22:23, 1991.

308. Laughlin MR, Petit WA, Dizon JM, et al: NMR measurements of in vivo myocardial glycogen metabolism, J Biol Chem 263:2285, 1988.

309. Lauterbur PC: Image formation by induced local interactions: examples employing nuclear magnetic resonance, Nature 242:190, 1973.

310. Lawry TJ, Karczmar GS, Weiner MW, et al: Computer simulation of MRS localization techniques: an analysis of ISIS, Magn Reson Med 9:299, 1989.

311. Layer G, Traber F, Muller-Lisse U, et al: "Spectroscopic imaging." Eine neue MR-Technik in der Diagnostik von Anfallsleiden? Radiologe 33:178, 1993.

312. Lazareff JA, Olmstead C, Bockhorst KH, et al: Proton magnetic resonance spectroscopic imaging of pediatric low-grade astrocytomas, Childs Nerv Syst 12:130, 1996.

313. Li LM, Cendes F, Watson C, et al: Surgical treatment of patients with single and dual pathology: relevance of lesion and of hippocampal atrophy to seizure outcome, Neurology 48:437, 1997.

314. Ligeti L, Osbakken M, Urbanics R, et al: Species differences in cardiac metabolism as measured by ^{31}P NMR. In Book of Abstracts, Society of Magnetic Resonance in Medicine 1:504, 1985 (abstract).

315. Lilly MB, Katholi CR, and Ng TC: Direct relationship between high-energy phosphate content and blood flow in thermally treated murine tumors, J Natl Cancer Inst 75:885, 1985.

316. Lim KO, and Spielman DM: Estimating NAA in cortical gray matter with applications for measuring changes due to aging, Magn Reson Med 37:372, 1997.

317. Longo R, Giorgini A, Magnaldi S, et al: Alzheimer's disease histologically proven studied by MRI and MRS: two cases, Magn Reson Imaging 11:1209, 1993.

318. Luyten PR, Bruntink G, Sloff FM, et al: Broadband proton decoupling in human ^{31}P NMR spectroscopy, NMR Biomed 1:177, 1989.

319. Luyten PR, Groen JP, Arnold DA, et al: ^{31}P MR localized spectroscopy of the human brain in situ at 1.5 Tesla. In Book of Abstracts, Society of Magnetic Resonance in Medicine, p. 1083, 1986 (abstract).

320. Luyten PR, Groen JP, Vermeulen JWAH, et al: Experimental approaches to image localized human ^{31}P NMR spectroscopy, Magn Reson Med 11:1, 1989.

321. Luyten PR, Marien AJH, Heindel W, et al: Metabolic imaging of patients with intracranial tumors: H-1 MR spectroscopic imaging and PET, Radiology 176:791, 1990.

322. Luyten PR, Marien AJH, Sijtsma B, et al: Solvent-suppressed spatially resolved spectroscopy: an approach to high-resolution NMR on a whole-body MR system, J Magn Reson 67:148, 1986.

323. MacKay S, Ezekiel F, Di Sciafani V, et al: Combining MRI segmentation and ^{1}H MR spectroscopic imaging in the study of Alzheimer's disease, subcortical ischemic vascular dementia and elderly control, Radiology 198:537, 1996.

324. MacKay S, Meyerhoff DJ, Dillon WP, et al: Alteration of brain phospholipid metabolites in cocaine-dependent polysubstance abusers, Biol Psychiatry 34:261, 1993.

325. Magnusson JR, and Magnusson NS: NMR studies of sodium and potassium in various biological tissues, Ann N Y Acad Sci 204:297, 1973.

326. Malloy CR, Lange RA, Klein DL, et al: Spatial localization of NMR signal with a passive surface gradient, J Magn Reson 80:364, 1988.

327. Mancini DM, Coyle E, Coggan A, et al: Contribution of intrinsic skeletal muscle changes to ^{31}P NMR skeletal muscle metabolic abnormalities in patients with chronic heart failure, Circulation 80:1338, 1989.

328. Mancini DM, Ferraro N, Tuchler M, et al: Detection of abnormal calf muscle metabolism in patients with heart failure using phosphorus-31 nuclear magnetic resonance, Am J Cardiol 62:1234, 1988.

329. Mansfield P, and Chapman B: Active magnetic screening of gradient coils in NMR imaging, J Magn Reson 66:573, 1986.

330. Maris J, Evans A, McLaughlin A, et al: ^{31}P NMR spectroscopic investigation of human neuroblastoma in situ, N Engl J Med 312:1500, 1985.

331. Massie BM, Conway M, Rajagopalan B, et al: Skeletal muscle metabolism during exercise under ischemic conditions in congestive heart failure: evidence for abnormalities unrelated to blood flow, Circulation 78:320, 1988.

332. Matson GB, and Hill TC: A practical double-tuned ^{1}H/^{31}P quadrature birdcage head coil optimized for ^{31}P operation. In Proceedings of the Society of Magnetic Resonance, p. 963, 1995 (abstract).

333. Matson GB, Lara RL, Hugg JW, et al: Molar quantitation of ^{31}P metabolites in human brain: magnetic resonance spectroscopic imaging (MRSI). In Book of Abstracts, Society of Magnetic Resonance in Medicine 1:465, 1991 (abstract).

334. Matson GB, Meyerhoff DJ, Lawry TJ, et al: Use of computer simulations for quantitation of ^{31}P ISIS MRS results, NMR Biomed 6:215, 1993.

335. Matson GB, Twieg DB, Karczmar GS, et al: Image-guided surface coil ^{31}P MRS of human liver, heart, and kidney, Radiology 169:541, 1988.

336. Matthews PM, Andermann F, and Arnold DL: A proton magnetic resonance spectroscopy study of focal epilepsy in humans, Neurology 40:985, 1990.

337. Matthews PM, Bland JL, Gadian DG, et al: The steady-state rate of ATP synthesis in the perfused rat heart measured by ^{31}P NMR saturation transfer, Biochem Biophys Res Commun 103:1052, 1981.

338. Matthews PM, Bland JL, Gadian DG, et al: A ^{31}P-NMR saturation transfer study of the regulation of creatine kinase in rat heart, Biochim Biophys Acta 721:312, 1982.

339. Matthews PM, Bland JL, and Styles P: The temperature dependence of creatine kinase fluxes in the rat heart, Biochim Biophys Acta 763:140, 1983.

340. Matthews PM, Francis G, Antel J, et al: Proton magnetic resonance spectroscopy for metabolic characterization of plaques in multiple sclerosis, Neurology 41:1251, 1991.

341. Matthews PM, Pioro E, Narayanan S, et al: Assessment of lesion pathology in multiple sclerosis using quantitative MRI morphometry and magnetic resonance spectroscopy, Brain 119:715, 1996.

342. Matthews PM, Williams SR, Seymour A-M, et al: A ^{31}P NMR study of some metabolic and functional effects of the inotropic agents epinephrine and ouabain, and the ionophore R02-2985(X537A) in the isolated, perfused rat heart, Biochim Biophys Acta 720:163, 1982.

343. Maudsley AA: Sensitivity in Fourier imaging, J Magn Reson 68:363, 1986.

344. Maudsley AA, Hilal AK, Perman WH, et al: Spatially resolved high-resolution spectroscopy by "four-dimensional" NMR, J Magn Reson 51:147, 1983.

345. Maudsley AA, and Hilal SK: Field inhomogeneity correction and data processing for spectroscopic imaging, Magn Reson Med 2:1984.

346. Maudsley AA, Hilial SK, Simon HE, et al: In vivo MR spectroscopic imaging with P-31, Radiology 153:745, 1984.

347. Maudsley AA, Matson GB, Hugg JW, et al: Reduced phase encoding in spectroscopic imaging, Magn Reson Med 31:645, 1994.

348. Maxwell RJ, Workman P, and Griffiths JR: Demonstration of tumor-selective retention of fluorinated nitroimidazole probes by ^{19}F magnetic resonance spectroscopy in vivo, Int J Radiat Oncol Biol Phys 16:925, 1988.

349. McCoy CL, Parkins CS, Chaplin DJ, et al: The effect of blood flow modification on intra- and extracellular pH measured by ^{31}P magnetic resonance spectroscopy in murine tumours, Br J Cancer 72:905, 1995.

350. McLaughlin AC, Takeda H, and Chance B: P-31 NMR studies on perfused mouse liver. In Dutton PL, Leigh JS, and Scarpa A, eds: Frontiers of biological energetics, vol II, New York, 1978, Academic Press.

351. Mehring M: Principles of high-resolution NMR in solids, ed 2, Berlin, 1983, Springer-Verlag.

352. Metz KR, and Briggs RW: Spatial localization of NMR spectra using Fourier series analysis, J Magn Reson 64:172, 1985.

353. Metzger G, and Hu X: Application of interlaced Fourier transform to echo-planar spectroscopic imaging, J Magn Reson 125:166, 1997.

354. Meyer RA, Kushmerick MJ, and Brown TR: Application of ^{31}P-NMR spectroscopy to the study of striated muscle metabolism, Am J Physiol 242:C1, 1982.
355. Meyerhoff DJ, Boska MD, Thomas A, et al: Alcoholic liver disease: quantitative image-guided ^{31}P magnetic resonance spectroscopy, Radiology 173:393, 1990.
356. Meyerhoff DJ, Karczmar GS, Matson GB, et al: Noninvasive quantitation of human liver metabolites using image-guided ^{31}P magnetic resonance spectroscopy, NMR Biomed 3:17, 1989.
357. Meyerhoff DJ, Karczmar GS, Venook AP, et al: Effects of chemoembolization on human hepatic cancers monitored by ^{31}P ISIS spectroscopy. In Book of Abstracts, Society of Magnetic Resonance in Medicine, p. 318, 1990 (abstract).
358. Meyerhoff DJ, Karczmar GS, and Weiner MW: Abnormalities of the liver evaluated by ^{31}P MRS, Invest Radiol 24:980, 1989.
359. Meyerhoff DJ, Kent-Braun JA, Schwartz G, et al: Magnetic resonance spectroscopy. In Higgins CB, Hricak H, and Helms CA, eds: Magnetic resonance imaging of the body, ed 3, vol 3, New York, 1995, Raven Press.
360. Meyerhoff DJ, MacKay S, Constans JM, et al: Axonal injury and membrane alterations in Alzheimer's disease suggested by in vivo proton magnetic resonance spectroscopic imaging, Ann Neurol 36:40, 1994.
361. Meyerhoff DJ, MacKay S, Sappey-Marinier D, et al: Effects of chronic alcohol abuse and HIV infection on brain phosphorus metabolites, Alcohol Clin Exp Res 19:685, 1995.
362. Michaelis T, Bruhn H, Gyngell W, et al: Quantification of cerebral metabolites in man: results using short-echo time localized proton MRS. In Book of Abstracts, Society of Magnetic Resonance in Medicine, 1:387, 1991 (abstract).
363. Miller BL, Moats RA, Shonk T, et al: Alzheimer disease: depiction of increased cerebral myo-inositol with proton MR spectroscopy, Radiology 187:433, 1993.
364. Miller RG, Giannini D, Milner-Brown HS, et al: Effects of fatiguing exercise on high energy phosphates, force, and EMG: evidence for three phases of recovery, Muscle Nerve 10:810, 1987.
365. Miller RG, Kent-Braun JA, Sharma KR, et al: Mechanisms of human muscle fatigue: quantitating the contribution of metabolic factors and activation impairment. in Gandevia S, Enoka R, McComas A, et al, eds: Neural and neuromuscular aspects of muscle fatigue, New York, 1995, Plenum.
366. Miyake M, Kakimoto Y, and Sorimachi M: A gas chromatographic method for the determination of N-acetyl-L-aspartic acid, N-acetyl-alpha-aspartylglutamic acid and beta-citryl-L-glutamic acid and their distributions in the brain and other organs of various species of animals, J Neurochem 36:804, 1981.
367. Moats RA, Ernst T, Shonk TK, et al: Abnormal cerebral metabolite concentrations in patients with probable Alzheimer disease, Magn Reson Med 32:110, 1994.
368. Moffett JR, Namboodiri MA, Cangro CB, et al: Immunohistochemical localization of N-acetylaspartate in rat brain, Neuroreport 2:131, 1991.
369. Mohanakrishnan P, Fowler AH, Vonsattel JP, et al: An in vitro ^{1}H nuclear magnetic resonance study of the temporoparietal cortex of Alzheimer brains, Exp Brain Res 102:503, 1995.
370. Moon RB, and Richards JH: Determination of intracellular pH by ^{31}P magnetic resonance, J Biol Chem 248:7276, 1973.
371. Moonen CTW, von Kienlin M, Van Zijl PCM, et al: Comparison of single-shot localization methods (STEAM and PRESS) for in vivo proton NMR spectroscopy, NMR Biomed 2:201, 1989.
372. Moorcraft J, Bolas NM, Ives NK, et al: Global and depth resolved phosphorus magnetic resonance spectroscopy to predict outcome after birth asphyxia, Arch Dis Child 66:1119, 1991.
373. Mora BN, Narasimhan PT, and Ross BD: ^{31}P magnetization transfer studies in the monkey brain, Magn Reson Med 26:100, 1992.
374. Moseley ME, Chew WM, and James TL: ^{23}Sodium magnetic resonance imaging. In James TL, and Margulis AR, eds: Biomedical magnetic resonance, San Francisco, 1984, Radiology Research and Education Foundation.
375. Moyher SE, Nelson SJ, Wald LL, et al: High spatial resolution MRS and segmented MRI to study NAA in cortical grey matter and white matter of the human brain. In Proceedings of the Society of Magnetic Resonance, p. 332, 1995 (abstract).
376. Murphy DG, Bottomley PA, Salerno JA, et al: An in vivo study of phosphorus and glucose metabolism in Alzheimer's disease using magnetic resonance spectroscopy and PET, Arch Gen Psychiatry 50:341, 1993.
377. Murphy-Boesch J, Srinivasan R, and Brown T: A dual tuned four-ring birdcage for ^{1}H decoupled ^{31}P spectroscopy of the human head at 1.5 Tesla. In Book of Abstracts, Society of Magnetic Resonance in Medicine, p. 717, 1991 (abstract).
378. Narayanan S, Fu L, Pioro E, et al: Imaging of axonal damage in multiple sclerosis: spatial distribution of magnetic resonance imaging lesions, Ann Neurol 41:385, 1997.
379. Naruse S, Hirakawa K, Horikawa Y, et al: Measurements of in vivo ^{31}P NMR spectra in neuroectodermal tumors for the evaluation of the effects of chemotherapy, Cancer Res 45:2429, 1985.
380. Naruse S, Horikawa Y, Tanaka C, et al: Measurements of in vivo energy metabolism in experimental cerebral ischemia using ^{31}P-NMR for the evaluation of protective effects of perfluorochemicals and glycerol, Neurol Res 6:169, 1984.
381. Naruse S, Takada S, Koizuka I, et al: In vivo ^{31}P NMR studies on experimental cerebral infarction, Jpn J Physiol 33:19, 1983.
382. Navon G, Navon R, Schulman RG, et al: Phosphate metabolites in lymphoid, Friend erythroleukemia, and HeLa cells observed by high resolution ^{31}P nuclear magnetic resonance, Proc Natl Acad Sci U S A 75:891, 1978.
383. Negendank W: Studies of human tumors by MRS: a review, NMR Biomed 5:303, 1992.
384. Negendank WG, Brown TR, Evelhoch JL, et al: Proceedings of a National Cancer Institute workshop: MR spectroscopy and tumor cell biology, Radiology 185:875, 1992.
385. Negendank WG, Crowley MG, Ryan JR, et al: Bone and soft-tissue lesions: diagnosis with combined H-1 MR imaging and P-31 MR spectroscopy, Radiology 173:181, 1989.
386. Negendank WG, Padavic-Shaller KA, Li CW, et al: Metabolic characterization of human non-Hodgkin's lymphomas in vivo with the use of proton-decoupled phosphorus magnetic resonance spectroscopy, Cancer Res 55:3286, 1995.
387. Neurohr KJ, Barret EJ, and Shulman RG: In vivo carbon-13 nuclear magnetic resonance studies of heart metabolism, Proc Natl Acad Sci U S A 80:1603, 1983.
388. Neurohr KJ, Gollin G, Barrett EJ, et al: In vivo ^{31}P-NMR studies of myocardial high energy phosphate metabolism during anoxia and recovery, FEBS Lett 159:207, 1983.
389. Neurohr KJ, Gollin G, Neurohr JM, et al: Carbon-13 nuclear magnetic resonance studies of myocardial glycogen metabolism in live guinea pigs, Biochemistry 23:5029, 1984.
390. Newman RJ, Bore PJ, Chan L, et al: Nuclear magnetic resonance studies of forearm muscle in Duchenne dystrophy, Br Med J 284:1072, 1982.
391. Ng TC, Comair YG, Xue M, et al: Temporal lobe epilepsy: presurgical localization with proton chemical shift imaging, Radiology 193:465, 1994.
392. Ng TC, Evanochko WT, Hiramoto RN, et al: ^{31}P NMR spectroscopy of in vivo tumors, J Magn Reson 49:271, 1982.
393. Ng TC, Grundfest S, Vijayakumar S, et al: Therapeutic response of breast carcinoma monitored by ^{31}P MRS in situ, Magn Reson Med 10:125, 1989.
394. Ng TC, Majors AW, and Meany TF: In vivo MR spectroscopy of human subjects with a 1.4-T whole-body MR imager, Radiology 158:517, 1986.
395. Ng TC, Majors AW, Vijayakumar S, et al: Human neoplasm pH and response to radiation therapy: P-31 MR spectroscopy studies in situ, Radiology 170:875, 1989.
396. Ng TC, Vijayakumar S, Majors AW, et al: Response of a non-Hodgkin lymphoma to ^{60}Co therapy monitored by ^{31}P MRS in situ, Int J Radiat Oncol Biol Phys 13:1545, 1987.
397. Nidecker AC, Muller S, Aue WP, et al: Extremity bone tumors: evaluation by P-31 MR spectroscopy, Radiology 157:167, 1985.
398. Nuccitelli R, Webb DJ, Lagier ST, et al: ^{31}P NMR reveals increased intracellular pH after fertilization in *Xenopus* eggs, Proc Natl Acad Sci U S A 78:4421, 1981.
399. Nunnally RL, and Bottomley PA: Assessment of pharmacological treatment of myocardial infarction by phosphorus-31 NMR with surface coils, Science 211:177, 1981.
400. Nunnally RL, and Hollis DP: ATP compartmentation in living hearts: a ^{31}P NMR saturation transfer study, Biochemistry 18:3642, 1979.
401. Nussbaum GH, Purdy J, Granda C, et al: Use of the Clinac-35 for tissue activation in noninvasive measurement of capillary blood flow, Med Phys 10:487, 1983.
402. Oberhaensli R, Galloway G, Taylor D, et al: Noninvasive assessment of hepatic fructose metabolism in human by ^{31}P-NMR spectroscopy, Clin Sci 68:48, 1985.
403. Oberhaensli R, Rajagopalan B, Galloway GJ, et al: Study of human liver disease with P-31 magnetic resonance spectroscopy, Gut 31:463, 1990.
404. Oberhaensli RD, Galloway GJ, Hilton-Jones D, et al: The study of human organs by phosphorus-31 topical magnetic resonance spectroscopy, Br J Radiol 60:367, 1987.
405. Oberhaensli RD, Galloway GJ, Taylor DJ, et al: Assessment of human liver metabolism by phosphorus-31 magnetic resonance spectroscopy, Br J Radiol 59:695, 1986.
406. Oberhaensli RD, Galloway GJ, Taylor DJ, et al: First year of experience with P-31 magnetic resonance studies of human liver, Magn Reson Imaging 4:413, 1986.
407. Oberhaensli RD, Hilton-Jones D, Bore PJ, et al: Biochemical investigation of human tumors in vivo with phosphorus-31 magnetic resonance spectroscopy, Lancet 5:8, 1986.
408. Oberhaensli RD, Hilton-Jones D, Bore PJ, et al: P-31 magnetic resonance studies of human brain at 2 T, Magn Reson Imaging 4:417, 1986.
409. Oberhaensli RD, Rajagopalan B, Taylor DJ, et al: Study of hereditary fructose intolerance by use of ^{31}P magnetic resonance spectroscopy, Lancet 24:931, 1987.
410. Odeblad E, and Lindstrom G: Some preliminary observations on the proton magnetic resonance in biologic samples, Acta Radiol 43:469, 1955.
411. Ordidge RJ, Bendall MR, Gordon RE, et al: Volume selection for in-vivo biological spectroscopy. In Govil G, Khetrapal CL, and Saran A, eds: Magnetic resonance in biology and medicine, New Dehli, 1985, Tata McGraw-Hill.
412. Ordidge RJ, Connelly A, and Lohman JAB: Image-selected in vivo spectroscopy (ISIS): a new technique for spatially selective NMR spectroscopy, J Magn Reson 66:283, 1986.
413. Ordidge RJ, and Van de Vyver FL: Separate water and fat MR images, Radiology 157:551, 1985.
414. Ott D, Ernst T, and Henning J: Clinical value of ^{1}H spectroscopy of brain tumors. In Book of Abstracts, Society of Magnetic Resonance in Medicine, p. 105, 1990 (abstract).
415. Pan JW, Hetherington HP, Hamm JR, et al: Quantitation of metabolites by ^{1}H NMR, Magn Reson Med 20:48, 1991.
416. Pan JW, Hetherington HP, Vaughan JT, et al: Evaluation of multiple sclerosis by ^{1}H spectroscopic imaging at 4.1 T, Magn Reson Med 36:72, 1996.
417. Peeling J, and Sutherland G: High-resolution ^{1}H NMR spectroscopy studies of extracts of human cerebral neoplasms, Magn Reson Med 24:123, 1992.
418. Pekar J, Leigh JSJ, and Chance B: Harmonically analyzed sensitivity profile: a novel approach to depth pulses for surface coils, J Magn Reson 64:115, 1985.
419. Petroff OAC, Prichard JW, Behar KL, et al: In vivo phosphorus nuclear magnetic resonance spectroscopy in status epilepticus, Ann Neurol 16:169, 1984.
420. Pettegrew JW, Moossy J, Withers G, et al: ^{31}P nuclear magnetic resonance study of the brain in Alzheimer's disease, J Neuropathol Exp Neurol 47:235, 1988.
421. Pettegrew JW, Panchalingam K, Klunk WE, et al: Alterations of cerebral metabolism in probable Alzheimer's disease: a preliminary study, Neurobiol Aging 15:117, 1994.
422. Plateau P, and Gueron M: Exchangeable proton NMR without base-line distortion, using new strong-pulse sequences, J Am Chem Soc 104:7310, 1982.
423. Pohost GM, Reeves RC, and Evanochko WT: Nuclear magnetic resonance: potential clinical relevance to the cardiovascular system, Circulation 72:I-VIII, 1985.
424. Pomer S, Hull WE, and Rohl L: Assessment of renal viability for transplantation by high field ^{31}P NMR, Transplant Proc 20:899, 1988
425. Portman MA, Heineman FW, and Balaban RS: Developmental changes in the relation between phosphate metabolites and oxygen consumption in the sheep heart in vivo, J Clin Invest 83:456, 1989.

426. Posse S, Schuknecht B, Smith ME, et al: Short echo time proton MR spectroscopic imaging, J Comput Assist Tomogr 17:1, 1993.

427. Posse S, Tedeschi G, Risinger R, et al: High speed ^{1}H spectroscopic imaging in human brain by echo planar spatial-spectral encoding, Magn Reson Med 33:34, 1995.

428. Preul MC, Caramanos Z, Collins DL, et al: Accurate, noninvasive diagnosis of human brain tumors by using proton magnetic resonance spectroscopy, Natl Med 2:323, 1996.

429. Price TB, Rothman DL, Avison MJ, et al: ^{13}C-NMR measurements of muscle glycogen during low-intensity exercise, J Appl Physiol 70:1836, 1991.

430. Prichard JW, and Shulman RG: NMR spectroscopy of brain metabolism in vivo, Annu Rev Neurosci 9:61, 1986.

431. Pritchard J, Rothman D, Novotry E, et al: Photic stimulation raises lactate in human visual cortex. In Book of Abstracts, Society of Magnetic Resonance in Medicine, p. 1071, 1989 (abstract).

432. Pritchard JW: The ischemic penumbra in stroke: prospects for analysis by nuclear magnetic resonance spectroscopy. In Waxman SG, ed: Molecular and cellular approaches to the treatment of neurological disease, New York, 1993, Raven Press.

433. Provencher SW: Estimation of metabolite concentrations from localized in vivo proton NMR spectra, Magn Reson Med 30:672, 1993.

434. Purcell EM, Torrey HC, and Pound RV: Resonance absorption by nuclear magnetic moments in solids, Phys Rev 69:37, 1946.

435. Pykett IL, and Rosen BR: Nuclear magnetic resonance: in vivo proton chemical shift imaging, Radiology 149:197, 1983.

436. Radda GK, Ackerman JJH, Bore P, et al: P-31 NMR studies on kidney intracellular pH in acute renal acidosis, Int J Biochem 12:277, 1980.

437. Radda GK, Bore PJ, Gadian DG, et al: ^{31}P NMR examination of two patients with NADH-CoQ reductase deficiency, Nature 295:608, 1982.

438. Radda GK, Bore PJ, and Rajagopalan B: Clinical aspects of NMR spectroscopy, Br Med Bull 40:155, 1983.

439. Radda GK, Taylor DJ, and Arnold DL: Investigation of human mitochondrial myopathies by phosphorus magnetic resonance spectroscopy, Biochem Soc Trans 13:654, 1985.

440. Radda GK, Taylor DJ, Styles P, et al: Exercised-induced ATP depletion in normal human muscle, Soc Magn Reson Med 1:286, 1983.

441. Rajagopalan B, Conway MA, Massie B, et al: Alterations of skeletal muscle metabolism in humans studied by phosphorus 31 magnetic resonance spectroscopy in congestive heart failure, Am J Cardiol 62:53E, 1988.

442. Rath AR: Design and performance of a double-tuned bird-cage coil, J Magn Reson 86:488, 1990.

443. Reeves RC, Evanochko WT, Canby RC, et al: Demonstration of increased myocardial lipid with postischemic dysfunction ("myocardial stunning") by proton nuclear magnetic resonance spectroscopy, J Am Coll Cardiol 13:739, 1989.

444. Remy C, Albrand JP, Benabid AL, et al: In vivo ^{31}P nuclear magnetic resonance studies of T1 and T2 relaxation times in rat brain and in rat brain tumors implanted into nude mice, Magn Reson Med 4:144, 1987.

445. Remy C, Arus C, Ziegler A, et al: In vivo, ex vivo, and in vitro one- and two-dimensional nuclear magnetic resonance spectroscopy of an intracerebral glioma in rat brain: assignment of resonances, J Neurochem 62:166, 1994.

446. Renshaw PJ, and Wicklund S: In vivo measurement of lithium in humans by nuclear magnetic resonance spectroscopy, Biol Psychiatry 23:465, 1988.

447. Reynolds EO, McCormick DC, Roth SC, et al: New non-invasive methods for the investigation of cerebral oxidative metabolism and hemodynamics in newborn infants, Ann Med 23:681, 1991.

448. Robitaille PM, Merkle H, Lew B, et al: Transmural high energy phosphate distribution and response to alterations in workload in the normal canine myocardium as studied with spatially localized ^{31}P NMR spectroscopy, Magn Reson Med 16:91, 1990.

449. Robitaille PM, Merkle H, Sako E, et al: The measurement of ATP synthesis rates by ^{31}P NMR spectroscopy in the intact myocardium in vivo, Magn Reson Med 15:8, 1990.

450. Robitaille PM, Merkle H, Sublett E, et al: Spectroscopic imaging and spatial localization using adiabatic pulses and applications to detect transmural metabolite distribution to canine heart, Magn Reson Med 10:14, 1989.

451. Rodrigues LM, Maxwell RJ, McSheehy PM, et al: In vivo detection of ifosfamide by ^{31}P-MRS in rat tumours: increased uptake and cytotoxicity induced by carbogen breathing in GH3 prolactinomas, Br J Cancer 75:62, 1997.

452. Roemer PB, Edelstein WA, Hayes CE, et al: The NMR phased array, Magn Reson Med 16:192, 1990.

453. Roser W, Hagberg G, Mader I, et al: Proton MRS of gadolinium-enhancing MS plaques and metabolic changes in normal-appearing white matter, Magn Reson Med 33:811, 1995.

454. Ross B, Helsper JT, Cox J, et al: Osteosarcoma and other neoplasms of bone, Arch Surg 122:1464, 1987.

455. Ross B, and Michaelis T: Clinical applications of magnetic resonance spectroscopy, Magn Reson Q 10:191, 1994.

456. Ross B, Smith M, Marshall V, et al: Monitoring response to chemotherapy of intact human tumors by ^{31}P nuclear magnetic resonance, Lancet 1:641, 1984.

457. Ross BD, Chenevert TL, Kim B, et al: Magnetic resonance imaging and spectroscopy: Application to experimental neuro-oncology, Q Magn Res Biol Med 1:89, 1994.

458. Ross BD, Merkle H, Hendrich K, et al: Spatially localized in vivo ^{1}H magnetic resonance spectroscopy of an intracerebral rat glioma, Magn Reson Med 23:96, 1992.

459. Ross BD, Radda GK, Gadian DG, et al: Examination of a case of suspected McArdle's syndrome by ^{31}P nuclear magnetic resonance, N Engl J Med 304:1338, 1981.

460. Roth K, Hubesch B, Meyerhoff DJ, et al: Non-invasive quantitation of phosphorus metabolites in human tissue by NMR spectroscopy, J Magn Reson 81:299, 1989.

461. Roth SC, Edwards AD, Cady EB, et al: Relation between cerebral oxidative metabolism following birth asphyxia, and neurodevelopmental outcome and brain growth at one year, Dev Med Child Neurol 34:285, 1992.

462. Rothman DL, Arias-Mendoza F, Shulman GI, et al: A pulse sequence for simplifying hydrogen NMR spectra of biological tissues, J Magn Reson 60:430, 1984.

463. Rothman DL, Behar KL, Hetherington HP, et al: ^{1}H-observe/^{13}C-decouple spectroscopic measurements of lactate and glutamate in the rat brain in vivo, Proc Natl Acad Sci U S A 82:1633, 1985.

464. Rothman DL, Behar KL, Hetherington HP, et al: Homonuclear ^{1}H double resonance difference spectroscopy of the rat brain in vivo, Proc Natl Acad Sci U S A 81:6330, 1984.

465. Rothman DL, Howseman AM, Graham GD, et al: Localized proton NMR observation of [3-13C]lactate in stroke after [1-13C]glucose infusion, Magn Reson Med 21:302, 1991.

466. Sako EY, Kingsley-Hickman PB, From AHL, et al: ATP synthesis kinetics and mitochondrial function on the postischemic myocardium as studied by ^{31}P NMR, J Biol Chem 263:10600, 1988.

467. Salhany JM, Pieper GM, Wu S, et al: P-31 nuclear magnetic resonance measurement of cardiac pH in perfused guinea-pig hearts, J Mol Cell Cardiol 11:601, 1979.

468. Sappey-Marinier D, Calabrese G, Fein G, et al: Effect of photic stimulation on human visual cortex, lactate and phosphates using ^{1}H and ^{31}P magnetic resonance spectroscopy, J Cereb Blood Flow Metab 12:584, 1992.

469. Saunders DE, Howe FA, van den Boogaart A, et al: Continuing ischemic damage after acute middle cerebral artery infarction in humans demonstrated by short-echo proton spectroscopy, Stroke 26:1007, 1995.

470. Schaefer S, Camacho SA, Gober JR, et al: Response of myocardial metabolites to graded regional ischemia: ^{31}P NMR spectroscopy of porcine myocardium in vivo, Circ Res 64:968, 1989.

471. Schaefer S, Gober JR, Schwartz GS, et al: In vivo phosphorus-31 spectroscopic imaging in patients with global myocardial disease, Am J Cardiol 65:1154, 1990.

472. Schaefer S, Schwartz G, Gober JR, et al: Relationship between myocardial metabolites and contractile abnormalities during graded regional ischemia: ^{31}P NMR studies of porcine myocardium in vivo, J Clin Invest 85:706, 1990.

473. Schaefer S, Schwartz GS, Gober JR, et al: Magnetic resonance spectroscopy: evaluation of ischemic heart disease, Invest Radiol 24:969, 1989.

474. Schnall MD, Lenkinski R, and Milestone B: Localized ^{1}H spectroscopy of the human prostate in-vivo. In Book of Abstracts, Society of Magnetic Resonance in Medicine, p. 288, 1990 (abstract).

475. Schuff N, Ehrhardt JC, and Weiner MW: Efficient data acquisition for 2D spectroscopic imaging using hexagonal κ-space sampling. In Proceedings of the Society of Magnetic Resonance, p. 1176, 1994 (abstract).

476. Schwartz G, Schaefer S, Meyerhoff DJ, et al: The dynamic relationship between myocardial contractility and energy metabolism during and following brief coronary occlusion in the pig, Circ Res 67:490, 1990.

477. Schwartz GS, Schaefer S, Gober J, et al: Myocardial high energy phosphates in reactive hyperemia: high temporal resolution NMR, Am J Physiol 259:H1190, 1990.

478. Segebarth C, Baleriaux D, Arnold DL, et al: Image-guided localized ^{31}P MR spectroscopy of human brain tumors in situ: effect of treatment, Radiology 165:215, 1987.

479. Segebarth CM, Baleriaux DF, Luyten PR, et al: Detection of metabolic heterogeneity of human intracranial tumors in vivo by ^{1}H NMR spectroscopic imaging, Magn Reson Med 13:62, 1990.

480. Sehr PA, Bore PJ, Papatheofanis J, et al: Nondestructive measurement of metabolites and tissue pH in the kidney by ^{31}P nuclear magnetic resonance, Br J Exp Pathol 60:632, 1979.

481. Sehr PA, Radda GK, Bore PJ, et al: A model kidney transplant studied by phosphorous nuclear magnetic resonance, Biochem Biophys Res Commun 77:195, 1977.

482. Semmler W, Bachert-Baumann P, Guckel F, et al: Real-time follow-up of 5-fluorouracil metabolism in the liver of tumor patients by means of F-19 MR spectroscopy, Radiology 174:141, 1990.

483. Semmler W, Gademann G, Bachert-Baumann P, et al: Monitoring human tumor response to therapy by means of P-31 MR spectroscopy, Radiology 166:533, 1988.

484. Seymour AL, Keough JM, and Radda GK: Phosphorus-31 nuclear magnetic resonance studies of enzyme kinetics in perfused hearts from thyroidectomized rats, Biochem Soc Trans 11:376, 1983.

485. Shaka AJ, and Freeman R: Spatially selective radiofrequency pulses, J Magn Reson 59:169, 1984.

486. Shaka AJ, and Freeman R: Spatially selective pulse sequences: elimination of harmonic responses, J Magn Reson 62:340, 1985.

487. Shaka AJ, Keeler J, Smith MB, et al: Spatial localization of NMR signals in an inhomogeneous radiofrequency field, J Magn Reson 61:175, 1985.

488. Sharma KR, Kent-Braun J, Mynhier MA, et al: Excessive muscular fatigue in the postpoliomyelitis syndrome, Neurology 44:642, 1994.

489. Sharma KR, Kent-Braun JA, Majumdar S, et al: Physiology of fatigue in amyotrophic lateral sclerosis, Neurology 45:733, 1995.

490. Shaw TM, and Elsken RH: Nuclear magnetic resonance absorption in hygroscopic materials, J Chem Phys 18:1113, 1950.

491. Shiino A, Matsuda M, Morikawa S, et al: Proton magnetic resonance spectroscopy with dementia, Surg Neurol 39:143, 1993.

492. Shine N, Palladino M, Deisseroth A, et al: Effects of tumor necrosis factor on high-energy phosphates of an experimental mouse tumor, RSNA 161:340, 1986 (abstract).

493. Shine N, Xuan A, and Weiner MW: ^{31}P NMR studies of ATP concentrations and Pi ATP exchange in the rat kidney in vivo: effects of inhibiting and stimulating renal metabolism, Magn Reson Med 14:445, 1990.

494. Shonk TK, Moats RA, Gifford P, et al: Probable Alzheimer disease: diagnosis with proton MR spectroscopy, Radiology 195:65, 1995.

495. Shoubridge EA, Briggs RW, Radda GK: ^{31}P NMR saturation transfer measurements of the steady state rates of creatine kinase and ATP synthetase in the rat brain, FEBS Lett 140:288, 1982.

496. Shporer M, and Civan MM: State of water and alkali cations within the intracellular fluids: the contribution of NMR spectroscopy, Curr Top Membr Transport 9:1, 1977.

497. Shulman GI, Cline G, Schumann WC, et al: Quantitative comparison of the pathways of hepatic glycogen repletion in fed and fasted man, Am J Physiol 259:E335, 1990.
498. Shulman GI, Rothman DL, Chung Y, et al: ^{13}C NMR studies of glycogen turnover in the perfused rat liver, J Biol Chem 263:5027, 1988.
499. Shulman GI, Rothman DL, Jue T, et al: Quantitation of muscle glycogen synthesis in normal subjects and subjects with non-insulin-dependent diabetes by ^{13}C nuclear magnetic resonance spectroscopy, N Engl J Med 322:223, 1990.
500. Shulman GI, Rothman DL, Jue T, et al: Quantitation of muscle glycogen synthesis in normal subjects and subjects with non-insulin-dependent diabetes by ^{13}C nuclear magnetic resonance spectroscopy, N Engl J Med 322:223, 1990.
501. Shulman RG, ed: Biological applications of magnetic resonance, New York, 1979, Academic Press.
502. Shulman RG: Simultaneous ^{13}C and ^{31}P NMR studies of perfused rat liver, J Biol Chem 258:14294, 1983.
503. Shulman RG, Brown TR, Ugurbil K, et al: Cellular applications of ^{31}P and ^{13}C nuclear magnetic resonance, Science 205:160, 1979.
504. Siegel NJ, Avison MJ, Reilly HF, et al: Enhanced recovery of renal ATP with postischemic infusion of ATP-MgCl2 determined by ^{31}P-NMR, Am J Physiol 245:F530, 1983.
505. Siegel NJ, Glazier WB, Chaudry IH, et al: Enhanced recovery from acute renal failure by the postischemic infusion of adenine nucleotides and magnesium chloride in rats, Kidney Int 17:338, 1980.
506. Sijens PE, Huang YM, Baldwin NJ, et al: ^{19}F magnetic resonance spectroscopy studies of the metabolism of 5-fluorouracil in murine RIF-1 tumors and liver, Cancer Res 51:1384, 1991.
507. Sillerud LO, and Shulman RG: Structure and metabolism of mammalian liver glycogen monitored by carbon-13 nuclear magnetic resonance, Biochemistry 22:1087, 1983.
508. Simmons ML, Frondoza CG, and Coyle JT: Immunocytochemical localization of N-acetyl-aspartate with monoclonal antibodies, Neuroscience 45:37, 1991.
509. Smith CD, Pettigrew LC, Avison MJ, et al: Frontal lobe phosphorus metabolism and neuropsychological function in aging and in Alzheimer's disease, Ann Neurol 38:194, 1995.
510. Soher BJ, van Zijl PC, Duyn JH, et al: Quantitative proton MR spectroscopic imaging of the human brain, Magn Reson Med 35:356, 1996.
511. Soto GE, Zhu Z, Evelhoch JL, et al: Tumor ^{31}P NMR pH measurements in vivo: a comparison of inorganic phosphate and intracellular 2-deoxyglucose-6-phosphate as pH NMR indicators in murine radiation-induced fibrosarcoma-1, Magn Reson Med 36:698, 1996.
512. Starcuk Z, and Sklenar V: New hard pulse sequences for the solvent signal suppression in Fourier-transform NMR, J Magn Reson 61:567, 1985.
513. Stein PD, Goldstein S, Sabbah HN, et al: In vivo evaluation of intracellular pH and high-energy phosphate metabolites during regional myocardial ischemia in cats using ^{31}P nuclear magnetic resonance, Magn Reson Med 3:262, 1986.
514. Styles P, Scott CA, and Radda GK: A method for localizing high resolution NMR spectra from human subjects, Magn Reson Med 2:402, 1985.
515. Tallan HH, Moore S, and Stein WH: N-acetyl-l-aspartic acid in brain, J Biol Chem 219:257, 1956.
516. Taylor DJ, Bore PJ, Styles P, et al: Bioenergetics of intact human muscle: a ^{31}P nuclear magnetic resonance study, Mol Biol Med 1:77, 1983.
517. Taylor DJ, Crowe M, Bore PJ, et al: Examination of the energetics of aging skeletal muscle using nuclear magnetic resonance, Gerontology 30:2, 1984.
518. Taylor DJ, Kemp GJ, Woods CG, et al: Skeletal muscle bioenergetics in myotonic dystrophy, J Neurol Sci 116:193, 1993.
519. Tedeschi G, Bertolino A, Massaquoi SG, et al: Proton magnetic resonance spectroscopic imaging in patients with cerebellar degeneration, Ann Neurol 39:71, 1996.
520. Tedeschi G, Bertolino A, Righini A, et al: Brain regional distribution pattern of metabolite signal intensities in young adults by proton magnetic resonance spectroscopic imaging, Neurology 45:1384, 1995.
521. Tedeschi G, Righini A, Bizzi A, et al: Cerebral white matter in the centrum semiovale exhibits a larger N-acetyl signal than does gray matter in long echo time ^{1}H-magnetic resonance spectroscopic imaging, Magn Reson Med 33:127, 1995.
522. Tedeschi G, Schiffmann R, Barton NW, et al: Proton magnetic resonance spectroscopic imaging in childhood ataxia with diffuse central nervous system hypomyelination, Neurology 45:1526, 1995.
523. Thomas MA, Narayan P, Kurhanewicz J, et al: ^{1}H MR spectroscopy of normal and malignant human prostates in vivo, J Magn Reson 87:610, 1990.
524. Thomas MA, Narayan P, Kurhanewicz P, et al: Detection of phosphorus metabolites in human prostates with a transrectal ^{31}P NMR probe, J Magn Reson 99:377, 1992.
525. Thomsen C, Jensen KE, Achten E, et al: In vivo magnetic resonance imaging and ^{31}P spectroscopy of large human brain tumors at 1.5 Tesla, Acta Radiol 29:77, 1988.
526. Thulborn KR, du Boulay G, and Radda GK: In vivo non-invasive measurements of energy metabolism and pH by ^{31}P NMR in experimental stroke correlated with cerebral edema, J Cereb Blood Flow Metab 1:580, 1981.
527. Thulborn KR, du Boulay GH, Duchen LW, et al: A ^{31}P nuclear magnetic resonance in vivo study of cerebral ischemia in the gerbil, J Cereb Blood Flow Metab 2:299, 1982.
528. Tofts PS: The non-invasive measurement of absolute metabolite concentrations in vivo using surface coil NMR spectroscopy, J Magn Reson 80:84, 1988.
529. Tofts PS, and Wilkie DR: Noninvasive investigation of cerebral metabolism in newborn infants by phosphorus nuclear magnetic resonance spectroscopy, Lancet 2:1059, 1983.
530. Toyo-Oka T, Nagayama K, Umeda M, et al: Rhythmic change of myocardial phosphate metabolite content in cardiac cycle observed by depth-selected and EKG-gated in vivo ^{31}P NMR spectroscopy in a whole animal, Biochem Biophys Res Commun 135:808, 1986.
531. Tropp J, and Sugiura S: A dual-tuned probe and multiband receiver front end for X-nucleus spectroscopy with proton scout imaging in vivo, Magn Reson Med 11:405, 1989.
532. Turner DL: Binomial solvent suppression, J Magn Reson 54:146, 1983.
533. Turner R: Minimum inductance coils, J Phys E: Sci Instrum 21:948, 1988.
534. Twieg DB, Meyerhoff DJ, Hubesch B, et al: Localized phosphorus-31 MRS in humans by spectroscopic imaging, Magn Reson Med 12:291, 1989.
535. Tycko R, Pines A: Spatial localization of NMR signals by narrowband inversion, J Magn Reson 60:156, 1984.
536. Ugurbil K: Magnetization transfer measurements of creatine kinase and ATPase rates in intact hearts, Circulation 72:IV94, 1985.
537. Ugurbil K: Magnetization transfer measurements of creatine kinase and ATPase rates in intact hearts, Circulation 72:95, 1988.
538. Ugurbil K, Kingsley-Hickman PB, Sako EY, et al: ^{31}P NMR studies of the kinetics and regulation of oxidative phosphorylation in the intact myocardium, Ann N Y Acad Sci 508:265, 1988.
539. Ugurbil K, Maidan RR, Petein M, et al: NMR measurements of myocardial CK rates by multiple saturation transfer, Circulation 70(Suppl):II-84, 1984 (abstract).
540. Ugurbil K, Merkle H, Robitaille PM, et al: Metabolic consequences of coronary stenosis: transmurally heterogeneous myocardial ischemia studied by spatially localized ^{31}P NMR spectroscopy, NMR Biomed 2:317, 1989.
541. Ugurbil K, Petein M, Maidan R, et al: Measurement of an individual rate constant in the presence of multiple exchanges: application to myocardial creatine kinase reaction, Biochemistry 25:100, 1986.
542. Ugurbil K, Shulman RG, and Brown TR: High resolution ^{31}P and ^{13}C nuclear magnetic resonance studies of *Escherichia coli* cells in vivo. In Shulman RG, ed: Biological applications of magnetic resonance, New York, 1979, Academic Press
543. Usenius JP, Kauppinen RA, Vainio PA, et al: Quantitative metabolite patterns of human brain tumors: detection by ^{1}H NMR spectroscopy in vivo and in vitro, J Comput Assist Tomogr 18:705, 1994.
544. Vainio P, Usenius JP, Vapalahti M, et al: Reduced N-acetylaspartate concentration in temporal lobe epilepsy by quantitative ^{1}H MRS in vivo, Neuroreport 5:1733, 1994.
545. Van Rijen PC, Luyten PR, van der Sprenkel JW, et al: ^{1}H and ^{31}P NMR measurement of cerebral lactate, high-energy phosphate levels, and pH in humans during voluntary hyperventilation: associated EEG, capnographic, and Doppler findings, Magn Reson Med 10:182, 1989.
546. Vink R, McIntosh TK, Demediuk P, et al: Decline in intracellular free Mg^{2+} is associated with irreversible tissue injury after brain trauma, J Biol Chem 263:757, 1988.
547. Vogl T, Peer F, Schedel H, et al: ^{31}P spectroscopy of head and neck tumors—surface coil technique, Magn Reson Imaging 7:425, 1989.
548. Weiner MW: Kidney, prostate, testicle and uterus of humans. In Grant DM, Harris RK, eds: NMR encyclopedia, New York, 1995, John Wiley & Sons.
549. Weiss RG, Bottomley PA, Hardy CJ, et al: Regional myocardial metabolism of high-energy phosphates during isometric exercise in patients with coronary artery disease, N Engl J Med 323:1593, 1990.
550. Welch KM, Levine SR, Martin G, et al: Magnetic resonance spectroscopy in cerebral ischemia, Neurol Clin 10:1, 1992.
551. Welch KMA, Gross B, Licht J, et al: Magnetic resonance spectroscopy of neurologic diseases, Curr Neurol 8:295, 1988.
552. Welch KMA, Levine SR, D'Andrea G, et al: Brain pH in migraine: an in vivo phosphorus-31 magnetic resonance spectroscopy study, Cephalalgia 8:273, 1988.
553. Welch KMA, Levine SR, D'Andrea G, et al: Preliminary observations on brain energy metabolism in migraine studied by in vivo phosphorus 31 NMR spectroscopy, Neurology 39:538, 1989.
554. Wiener DH, Fink LI, Maris J, et al: Abnormal skeletal muscle bioenergetics during exercise in patients with heart failure: role of reduced muscle blood flow, Circulation 73:1127, 1986.
555. Wiener DH, Maris J, Chance B, et al: Detection of skeletal muscle hypoperfusion during exercise using phosphorus-31 nuclear magnetic resonance spectroscopy, J Am Coll Cardiol 7:793, 1986.
556. Wikman-Coffelt J, Sievers R, Coffelt RJ, et al: The cardiac cycle: regulation and energy oscillations, Am J Physiol 245:H354, 1983.
557. Williamson P, Drost D, Stanley J, et al: Localized phosphorus 31 magnetic resonance spectroscopy in chronic schizophrenic patients and normal controls, Arch Gen Psychiatry 48:578, 1991.
558. Wilman AH, and Allen PS: In vivo NMR detection strategies for γ-aminobutyric acid, utilizing proton spectroscopy and coherence-pathway filtering with gradients, J Magn Reson 101B:2:165, 1993.
559. Wilson JR, Fink L, Maris J, et al: Evaluation of skeletal muscle energy metabolism in patients with heart failure using gated phosphorus 31 NMR, Circulation 71:57, 1985.
560. Wolf W, Albright MJ, Silver MS, et al: Fluorine-19 NMR spectroscopic studies of the metabolism of 5-fluorouracil in the liver of patients undergoing chemotherapy, Magn Reson Imaging 5:165, 1987.
561. Wolinsky JS, Narayana PA, and Fenstermacher MJ: Proton magnetic resonance spectroscopy in multiple sclerosis, Neurology 40:1764, 1990.
562. Wu ST, Pieper GM, Salhany JM, et al: Measurement of free magnesium in perfused and ischemic arrested heart muscle: a quantitative ^{31}P NMR and multiequilibria analysis, Biochemistry 20:7399, 1981.
563. Wyrwicz AM, Conboy CB, Nichols BG, et al: In vivo ^{19}F-NMR study of halothane distribution in brain, Biochim Biophys Acta 929:271, 1987.
564. Wyrwicz AM, Conboy CB, Ryback KR, et al: In vivo fluorine-19 NMR study of isoflurane elimination from brain, Biochim Biophys Acta 927:86, 1987.
565. Wyrwicz AM, Li Y, Schofield JC, et al: Multiple environments of fluorinated anesthetics in intact tissues observed with ^{19}F NMR spectroscopy, FEBS Lett 162:334, 1983.
566. Wyrwicz AM, Pszenny MH, Schofield JC, et al: Noninvasive observations of fluorinated anesthetics in rabbit brain by fluorine-19 nuclear magnetic resonance, Science 222:428, 1983.
567. Yabe T, Mitsunami K, Inubushi T, et al: Quantitative measurements of cardiac phosphorus metabolites in coronary artery disease by ^{31}P magnetic resonance spectroscopy, Circulation 92:15, 1995.

568. Yabe T, Mitsunami K, Okada M, et al: Detection of myocardial ischemia by ^{31}P magnetic resonance spectroscopy during handgrip exercise, Circulation 89:1709, 1994.

569. Yahaya H, Chan L, Freeman D, et al: Renal metabolic rate by ^{31}P saturation transfer NMR in hypotension in vivo, Clin Sci 66:35, 1984.

570. Yoshizaki K, Nishikawa H, Yamada S, et al: Intracellular pH measurement in frog muscle by means of ^{31}P nuclear magnetic resonance, Jpn J Physiol 29:211, 1979.

571. Younkin DP, Berman P, Sladky J, et al: ^{31}P NMR studies in Duchenne muscular dystrophy: age-related metabolic changes, Neurology 37:165, 1987.

572. Younkin DP, Delivoria-Papadopoulos M, Leonard JC, et al: Unique aspects of human newborn cerebral metabolism evaluated with phosphorus nuclear magnetic resonance spectroscopy, Ann Neurol 16:581, 1984.

573. Zhang J, Path G, Chepuri V, et al: Responses of myocardial high energy phosphates and wall thickening to prolonged regional hypoperfusion induced by subtotal coronary stenosis, Magn Reson Med 30:28, 1993.

574. Zimmer SD, Ugurbil K, Michurski S, et al: Alterations in oxidative function and respiratory regulation in the post-ischemic myocardium, J Biol Chem 21:12402, 1989.

10 Artifacts

Michael L. Wood and R. Mark Henkelman

KEY POINTS

Common Causes of MR Artifacts

- Patient motion
  Gross movement
  Physiological movement
    Cardiac
    Respiratory
    Flowing blood
- Other patient factors
  Susceptibility effects
  Chemical shift
  Metallic artifact
  Shear

- MR hardware
  Mechanical vibration
  Poorly shimmed magnet
  Moving nearby metallic objects
  Inhomogeneous RF coil
- MR software
  Wraparound (aliasing)
  Truncation
  Cross talk
- MR enclosure
  RF leak
  Noisy lights

The word *artifact* denotes an object produced by human workmanship. Artifacts do not correspond to that which is imaged but arise instead from the imaging technique. The apparent information in an artifact is misleading and could possibly lead to an incorrect medical diagnosis. It is impossible to eliminate every artifact from magnetic resonance (MR) images, and new artifacts emerge regularly from new imaging techniques.

This work was supported by the Medical Research Council of Canada, the National Cancer Institute of Canada, and General Electric Medical Systems, Canada. The input of many outstanding graduate students and colleagues is gratefully acknowledged. Dr. Richard Ehman of the Mayo Clinic contributed to the section on ghosts in an earlier edition of this book.

In this chapter artifacts are grouped according to their visual appearance. The first discussion is on ghost artifacts because they are so common. Discussions on wraparound artifacts, ripples, lines, false contours, shading, and finally geometrical distortion follow. Possible causes of each artifact are listed, and several are developed in more detail, including methods to suppress the artifact. Only generic artifacts from standard pulse sequences on typical magnetic resonance imaging (MRI) systems are included in this chapter; thus the examples shown are in no way a disparagement of any commercial equipment. Artifacts from malfunctioning equipment have generally been left out of this chapter. Bizarre images are possible when an MRI system malfunctions, but such problems fall more into the domain of the MRI system manufacturer or service organization. Other chapters elaborate on certain artifacts, such as flow effects (Chapter 11) and chemical-shift misregistration (Chapter 8). Furthermore, many other reviews of artifacts complement this chapter.[1,3,31]

GHOSTS
Possible Causes

Ghosts are replicas of something in the image. They are undesirable because they can mask or mimic lesions. There are many sources of ghosts, including repeated motion, mechanical vibration, temporal variation of receiver coil sensitivity, fluctuations of magnetic field, imbalance of quadrature channels, and stimulated echoes. Often the source of a ghost can be deduced from its symmetry (mirror image, multiple ghosts of only moving anatomy, etc.). Motion is the most common source of ghosts, so it is described in the most detail.

Modulation of Phase-Encoding Direction of κ Space

The magnetization arising from the various volume elements (voxels) into which an MR image is partitioned is a vector, which has a magnitude and a direction specified by a phase angle. The magnetization must be measured hundreds of times to accumulate enough data for an MR image (see Chapter 1). Any process that inadvertently changes the magnitude or the phase of the magnetization from a voxel, thereby disrupting the Fourier-transform relationship between κ space and the image, can cause ghost artifacts.[45,84] Typical disruptions in conventional Fourier imaging are not rapid enough to affect the κ_x direction; however, they can modulate the κ_y direction of κ space because it is filled by phase encoding using different echoes (see Chapter 1). Consequently, typical disruptions affect only the phase-encoding direction of an MR image. The severity of the ghosts depends on the amplitude of the κ-space samples acquired during the disturbance.[50] Incidentally, three-dimensional (3D) MR images have two phase-encoding directions, and ghosts propagate along both.[78]

Motion

Motion remains one of the most significant technical problems for MRI, and in many MR examinations, motion limits image quality more than the inevitable random noise. Motion causes blurring and a pattern of ghosts along the phase-encoding direction.[25,64,78] Swapping the frequency-encoding and phase-encoding directions rotates the direction of propagation of the ghosts by 90 degrees. Because the direction for phase encoding influences the overlap of ghosts with other structures, the preferred choice depends on the anatomical site and the orientation of the slice. Motion in any direction can cause ghosts in MR images (Figure 10-1).

The ghosts in Figure 10-1 are characteristic of conventional Fourier imaging.[42] Motion during fast spin-echo (FSE) imaging also causes ghosts, but their characteristics are more complicated.[51] Motion during other imaging techniques, such as projection reconstruction, does not generate ghosts.[20] However, such specialized techniques are beyond the scope of this chapter.

Various physiological motions and body movements, the most problematic of which are blood flow, cerebrospinal fluid (CSF) pulsation, respiratory motion, and cardiac motion, degrade MR images. Blood flow can cause intense ghosts and inconsistent image intensity within vessels, which can mimic dissections and thrombi or mask pathology.[13] Body movements, such as nodding of the head or shifting of position, are encountered frequently during MRI of uncomfortable or disoriented

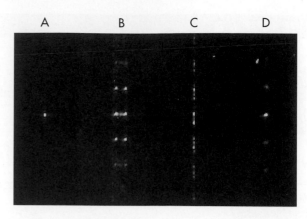

FIGURE 10-1   Four separate MR images of an oil drop illustrating that periodic motion in any direction generates ghosts in the phase-encoding direction. The blurring of the drop identifies the direction of motion. Only part of each image is shown.

patients, including infants and children. Even the slightest head movements are problematic for functional MRI.[28] Breathing is the main problem for abdominal MRI because it causes the liver, spleen, pancreas, and kidneys to move craniocaudally and anteroposteriorly.[39] The amplitude, period, and pattern of respiratory motion vary considerably among individuals.

Motion During Echo Formation
Contribution to Ghosts

The phase, $\Phi(TE)$, that accumulates after a radiofrequency (RF) pulse at time t = 0 until the center of an echo at time TE, which is important in spatial encoding, is given by the following equation:

(EQ. 1)

$$\Phi(TE) = \gamma \int_0^{TE} \mathbf{r}(t) \cdot \mathbf{G}(t)dt$$

where γ is the gyromagnetic ratio and $\mathbf{r}(t)$ and $\mathbf{G}(t)$ represent the time-dependent position of the spins and the gradient-waveform vector, respectively. Movement during the application of the gradient pulses used for spatial encoding makes the phase of the magnetization different from what it would have been without motion. Phase shifts induced by motion during TE present three problems for MR images—ghosts, intravoxel phase dispersion, and spatial misregistration.[13] Ghosts arise from velocity changes during different TE intervals. Intravoxel phase dispersion, which arises when a distribution of velocities exists within a voxel, cancels the net magnetization within the voxel and leads to lower image intensity. Misregistration of flowing blood within a vessel can occur when the vessel courses obliquely within a slice because frequency encoding and phase encoding are separated by a few milliseconds. The artifact is called an *oblique-flow artifact,* and it is classified with artifacts that generate false contours.[44,57]

Gradient Moments

Equation 10-1 can be computed more readily if one gradient waveform is considered at a time and the position along the direction of this gradient is approximated by a Taylor series. In this case Equation 10-1 reduces to the following:

$$\Phi(TE) = \gamma \left[r_0 \int_0^{TE} G(t)dt + v_0 \int_0^{TE} t\, G(t)dt + \left(\frac{1}{2}\right) a_0 \int_0^{TE} t^2\, G(t)dt + ... \right]$$

The symbols r_0, v_0, and a_0 represent the position, velocity, and acceleration, respectively at time t = 0. The integrals in Equation 10-2 are defined as the zeroth, first, and second moments of G(t). Two identical pulses in a gradient waveform contribute equally to the zeroth moment, but the later pulse has greater influence on higher-order moments. Fig-

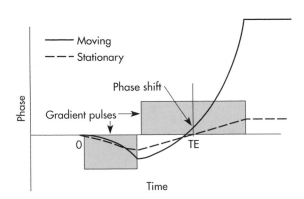

FIGURE 10-2   Phase shift at time TE, as a result of motion during application of gradient pulses. The phase of the magnetization from a stationary structure and one moving at constant velocity along the frequency-encoding direction are shown for a two-pulse gradient waveform used for frequency encoding in a gradient-echo pulse sequence. The gradient waveform is designed to yield an echo midway through the second pulse, at which time (TE) the cumulative time integral or area vanishes. Motion makes the phase of the magnetization at TE nonzero. (From reference 76.)

ure 10-2 shows a motion-induced phase shift. Assuming that the time between the two pulses is negligible, motion of constant velocity, v_0, makes Φ(TE) nonzero by the amount $(1/4)\,\gamma\,G\,v_0\,TE$.[2] Larger phase shifts occur for faster motion or longer TE.

Gradient-moment nulling. Motion-induced phase shifts can be reduced by configuring a gradient waveform to make its first and possibly higher moments vanish at TE.[22,58] This procedure is called *gradient-moment nulling (GMN), motion-artifact–suppression technique, flow compensation, gradient-motion rephasing, gradient-moment compensation,* and other names.[77] According to Equation 10-2, first-order nulling, in which the first moment of a gradient waveform becomes zero, prevents motion of constant velocity from time t = 0 to TE from shifting the magnetization's phase (Figure 10-2).

In implementing GMN, one or more pulses must be added to the gradient waveform before the echo is sampled. Unfortunately, this prolongs the minimum TE. Usually GMN is applied to the frequency-encoding and slice-selection gradient waveforms, but occasionally it is incorporated into the phase-encoding gradient waveform to eliminate oblique-flow artifacts. Once GMN has been incorporated into a pulse sequence, its use is simple and it does not prolong patient preparation or data acquisition. It applies to all types of motion and all pulse sequences. Figure 10-3 shows a typical example of GMN. A gratuitous GMN called *even-echo rephasing* is sometimes encountered in images from a second echo (see Chapter 13).

Usually GMN increases the intensity of blood vessels in images by reducing the amount of intravoxel dephasing.[13] This effect is modulated by time-of-flight effects. In spin-echo (SE) images the effect of GMN on vessel intensity can be unpredictable but not in gradient-echo images because the measured magnetization remains unchanged even if spins move out of the slice after excitation.

Displacement Between Acquisition of κ-Space Samples

Contribution to Ghosts

The amount of movement during data acquisition affects the intensity of ghosts. Greater displacement causes more modulation of κ space. In conventional Fourier imaging, substantial displacement can occur within TR, and this can be controlled by several methods, including restraining, triggering, rapid imaging, prospective gating, retrospective gating, and adaptive correction.

Rapid imaging. Images acquired rapidly enough can capture anatomical structures while they are essentially stationary. Rapidly acquired MR images tend to have lower quality, although techniques continue to improve (see Chapters 6 through 9).

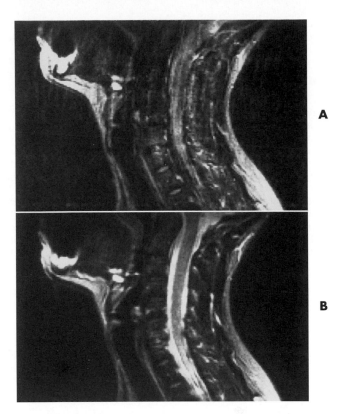

FIGURE 10-3   Demonstration of GMN for reducing ghosts from CSF pulsation in an MR image of the cervical spine. **A,** First-order GMN in both the slice-selection and frequency-encoding directions was not used. **B,** First-order GMN was used in this image. All other imaging conditions were the same for both images, including TR/TE = 3000/100, 1 T magnetic field strength, anteroposterior phase-encoding direction, 5-mm slice thickness, 300-mm FOV, 256 phase-encoding steps, and no averaging of data. (From reference 61.)

Prospective gating. Prospective gating allows data acquisition to proceed when the displacement does not exceed a predetermined limit.[60] Otherwise, data are rejected, and data acquisition is repeated until the displacement becomes acceptable. Gating prolongs data acquisition but not as much if only the most extreme displacements are rejected or if gating is used for only a fraction of data acquisition.[80] Gating relies on measurements of displacement, typically provided by a transducer, although MR signals also can be used to monitor position.[48,62,82] The use of a transducer prolongs patient preparation and adds complexity to the imaging technique. Gating has been used to overcome respiratory motion for MRI of the abdomen and thorax, but because of the limitations outlined earlier, it has not been used much in the last decade. However, there is renewed interest in gating for rapid imaging with controlled breathing and navigator echoes to monitor position.[73]

Triggering. Data acquisition can be triggered to a specific phase of a repetitive motion.[43] Triggering has been used effectively for imaging of the heart, blood vessels, and the spine, in which the pulsatile flow of CSF causes ghosts. These movements are periodic and are correlated with the electrocardiogram or a peripheral pulse, which can be monitored and used as the data-acquisition trigger. Triggering reduces ghosts and blurring to the extent that the data for each image are acquired at the same phase of a periodic motion. An irregular trigger makes TR vary, which itself causes ghosts.[59,79]

Retrospective gating. Retrospective gating monitors a signal correlated to motion and uses it later to sort the data measurements into groups acquired approximately at the same time relative to this signal.[21,46] Cardiac imaging is the most well-known application of retrospective gating.

Adaptive correction. Gross patient movements and the craniocaudal respiratory motions of abdominal organs are amenable to an adaptive correction of κ space, which basically locks the frame of reference of the reconstruction process onto the moving frame.[12] This process requires detailed information about the motion, which can be extracted from navigator echoes interleaved with the echoes used for imaging (Figure 10-4). Many variations on adaptive correction have been advanced.[30,33,37,40,81]

Motion of Highly Intense Structures

Contribution to Ghosts

The intensity of any ghost is proportional to the intensity of the moving anatomical structure that created it.[80] Reducing the intensity of a moving structure is feasible only if that structure does not need to be imaged. Several methods for reducing the intensity of certain anatomical structures have been advanced, including spatial presaturation, spectral presaturation, short TI inversion recovery (STIR), and surface coils. The most important methods are explained here, beginning with spatial presaturation, which is the most widely used. The STIR technique is described in Chapter 5.[6]

Spatial presaturation. In spatial presaturation one or more selective RF pulses are added to the imaging sequence to reduce the longitudinal magnetization in specific locations before the RF excitation pulse.[11,15,56] Spatial presaturation can affect a strip in any orientation and is compatible with most pulse sequences and imaging hardware. The addition of selective RF pulses reduces the maximum number of interleaved slices or the minimum TR and also increases the power deposited during data acquisition.

Presaturation is used to suppress blood-flow artifacts and ghosts from movement of highly intense structures within the imaging plane. Flow artifacts tend to be most severe with short TR/TE sequences, where inflowing unsaturated blood is very bright compared with adjacent tissues.[72] In these situations presaturation is effective, as illustrated

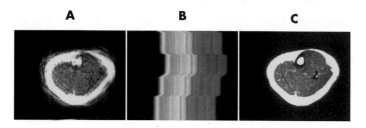

A   **B**   **C**

FIGURE 10-4   Demonstration of adaptive correction for motion. **A,** Image of the calf of a volunteer instructed to move the leg in the transverse plane occasionally during imaging. **B,** Information about the transverse position of the leg provided by a navigator echo. The vertical dimension represents time. Each horizontal row represents the projection of the cross-section of the leg along the left-right direction. **C,** Image corrected for translation based on information provided by navigator echoes in **B.**

schematically in Figure 10-5. Presaturation also improves the reliability of MRI for identifying subtle intravascular pathology. Figure 10-6 demonstrates how presaturation can reduce the intensity of moving structures within the field of view (FOV).

Spectral presaturation. The objective of spectral presaturation is to reduce the intensity of either fat or water, based on their characteristically different Larmor frequencies (225 Hz at 1.5 Tesla [T]). The RF pulse for presaturating fat at 1.5 T requires a frequency about 225 Hz less than the RF pulse for generating an MR signal from water. The attributes and limitations of spectral presaturation are similar to those of spatial presaturation; however, spectral presaturation requires a homogeneous magnetic field.

Repeated Motion

Contribution to Ghosts

It is repetitive motion that causes ghosts in MR images. Although few motions in the body are strictly periodic, sometimes one frequency dominates, resulting in a well-defined pattern of ghosts. The separation between ghosts depends on the frequency of motion and the time between data for different κ_y. As a result of aliasing, which is described later, ghosts that would extend beyond the FOV are folded back into MR images from the opposite side. Moreover, the ghosts are represented by complex numbers, with the phase depending on the phase of motion. The properties described here are the focus of several methods to suppress ghosts, including averaging, pseudogating, ordered phase encoding, and ghost interference. For example, pseudogating uses aliasing to superimpose all of the ghosts back on the moving structure or at a distance of one half of the FOV from the moving structure.[23,79] Averaging and ordered phase encoding are described in the following sections.

Averaging. Multiple sets of data can be averaged to reduce random noise and ghosts. The number of repetitions is called the *number of signal averages (NSA), acquisitions, data sets, averages, excitations, or repetitions.*[77] If the motion is in a different phase for the repeated data, ghosts corresponding to each data set have a different phase, and averaging causes some cancellation.[79] This concept is also exploited in the ghost-interference method.[32,83]

Averaging is easy to use, versatile, and reasonably effective at suppressing ghosts. However, averaging prolongs data acquisition by the factor NSA, making it more practical for shorter TRs.[69] Attempts at making averaging less time consuming have been proposed, such as repeating only part of the data.[79] It is difficult to suppress ghosts completely by averaging because the intensity of ghosts generally decreases only as $(NSA)^{1/2}$, as shown in Figure 10-7.[69]

Ordered phase encoding. Ordered phase encoding (OPE) alters the sequence in which the different κ_y are acquired to cause displacement and modulate κ space monotonically rather than periodically (Fig-

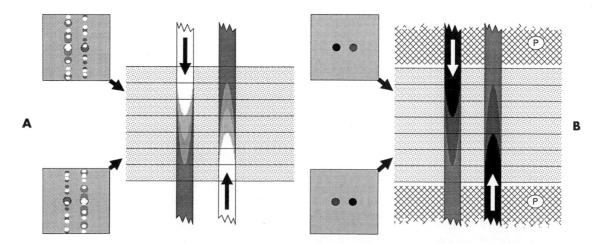

A   **B**

FIGURE 10-5   The principle behind spatial presaturation for suppressing flow artifacts and improving depiction of vascular anatomy. Two vessels pass through a stack of seven slices. The appearance of vessels in images obtained from two of these slices is shown on the left. **A,** Without spatial presaturation, the vessels have high intensity, especially in slices close to the site of inflow. Pulsatile flow causes view-to-view variations in the phase and modulus of signals received from the vessels, resulting in flow artifacts. **B,** Spatial presaturation outside the stack of slices (*crosshatched areas, P*) cause inflowing blood to have lower intensity.

ure 10-8).[2,25,38,80] Before the start of data acquisition, OPE requires information about the pattern of motion. Before each RF excitation, the position is measured to choose which particular value of κ_y to acquire. By eliminating the periodicity from the modulation of κ space, OPE

suppresses ghosts, although it leaves images blurred (Figure 10-9). A different reordering scheme for translation along the phase-encoding direction simply attempts to reduce the errors caused by motion, and it reduces both ghosts and blurring.[50]

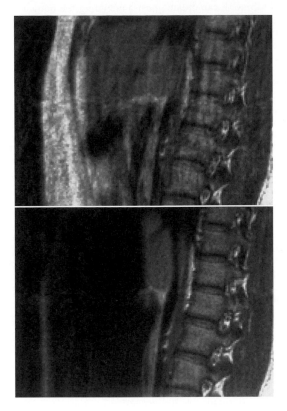

FIGURE 10-6   Demonstration of spatial presaturation on a sagittal MR image of the spine. The body coil was used as a transmitter and a receiver. The images were produced by an SE technique with TR/TE = 650/20. The only difference in the technique was that a 100-mm thick presaturation slab was positioned anteriorly in the second image. Presaturation reduced the intensity in the abdomen tenfold, thereby reducing the intensity of ghosts over the spine.

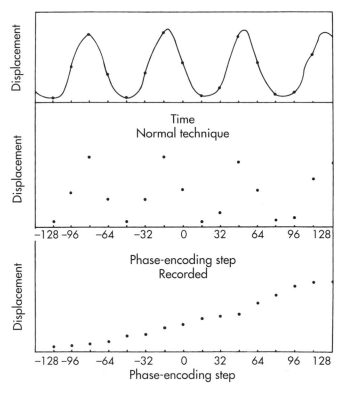

FIGURE 10-8   Mechanism of OPE. The curve represents the position of the chest during breathing, and the points demarcate times when data for a few values of κ_y are sampled. If the different κ_y are acquired in the normal linear order, these displacements are also repetitive in κ_y. The reordering scheme makes these displacements monotonic in κ_y.

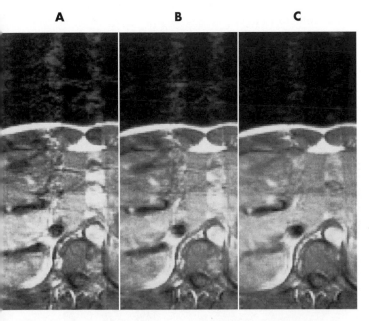

FIGURE 10-7   Demonstration of averaging for reducing ghosts. **A** to **C,** Images from 1, 2, or 4 sets of κ-space data acquired at 1 T using an SE pulse sequence with TR/TE = 1000/28, 256 phase-encoding steps, and 10-mm slice thickness. The intensity of ghosts in a region ventral to the abdomen was 95, 65, and 48 in **A, B,** and **C,** respectively.

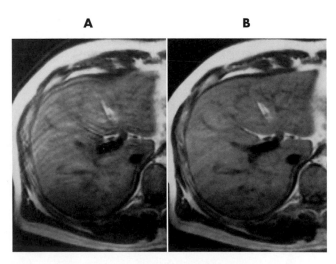

FIGURE 10-9   Reduction of ghosts by OPE demonstrated by transverse SE image of the upper abdomen (TR/TE = 450/20) without **(A)** and with **(B)** OPE.

Combination of Methods for Suppressing Motion Artifacts

Many methods to control motion artifacts have been advanced, although none are always completely effective. Table 10-1 summarizes the main attributes and deficiencies of the most important methods. All of these methods suppress ghosts, but some also prolong the imaging time, require extra preparation, dictate the choice of TR (which affects contrast), or reduce blurring. Most of the methods to control motion artifacts are not mutually exclusive so they can be combined for greater artifact suppression. For example, spatial presaturation used with cardiac gating improves the flow void in the cardiac chambers, thereby increasing the contrast with the adjacent myocardium. Spatial presaturation combined with OPE is especially useful for short TR/TE SE imaging of the abdomen and thorax (Figure 10-10).

The best methods to combine depend on the anatomical region, pulse sequence, MRI system, and personal preferences. In gradient-echo images at essentially every anatomical site, GMN is recommended for reducing flow artifacts. Spatial presaturation can be combined with GMN for increased effectiveness. In SE images with short TR and TE, spatial presaturation reduces flow artifacts. Ordered phase encoding is effective at suppressing ghosts from the high-intensity fat on the abdominal wall. However, GMN is not recommended because motion-induced phase shifts at short TE are small and because GMN can obscure vascular structures in SE images.[54] In long TE SE images of most anatomical sites, except where clear depiction of patent vessels is needed, GMN is recommended for suppressing ghosts and intravoxel dephasing. Spatial presaturation can be added to prevent increased flow artifacts.

Table 10-1   Attributes and Deficiencies of Motion-Artifact Reduction Methods

METHOD	TIME PENALTY	EXTRA PREPARATION	AFFECTS TR	LESS BLURRING
GMN	0	0	0	0
Restraining	0	+	0	+
Rapid imaging	0	0	+	+
Triggering	+	+	+	+
Prospective gating	+	+	+	+
Retrospective gating	0	+	+	+
Adaptive correction	0	0	0	+
Spatial presat	0	0	0	0
Spectral presat	0	+	0	0
Averaging	+	0	0	0
Pseudogating	+	0	+	0
OPE	0	0	0	0
Ghost interference	+	0	0	0

0, No; *+,* yes; *GMN,* gradient-moment nulling; *OPE,* ordered phase encoding; *presat,* presaturation; *TR,* repetition time.

Equipment Instabilities

Mechanical Vibration

Any repetitive disturbance that changes the amplitude or phase of MR signals can introduce ghosts into MR images. Many sources of mechanical vibration can create ghosts, including the patient table and even the building. The patient table can vibrate in response to the gradient pulses during data acquisition. Conditions that cause loud noise during data acquisition, such as thin slices, a small FOV, and short TR, make the patient table vibrate more.

Fluctuations of Magnetic Field

Repetitive movements of ferromagnetic objects close enough to perturb the magnetic field can cause ghosts in MR images (Figure 10-11). To eliminate these ghosts, the cause of the fluctuating magnetic field must be identified and removed.[17] A more subtle effect is encountered in functional MRI.[33] Namely, magnetic-susceptibility fluctuations in response to chest expansion during breathing alter the magnetic field in the brain, shifting the phase of κ-space data derived from gradient echoes, thereby creating ghosts.

Temporal Variation of Receiver Coil Sensitivity

Motion artifacts can arise if the electrical characteristics of the receiver coil change repeatedly. Regular breathing modulates the electrical loading of a body coil sufficiently for the effect to be used as a respiratory-motion monitor. Typical knee coils have a detachable top that can be dislodged during imaging, thereby causing ghosts.

Quadrature Imbalance

Ghosts that are a 180-degree rotation of the image about the center arise when the two quadrature receiver channels are amplified differently or are not exactly 90 degrees out of phase (Figure 10-12). The imbalance should be adjusted by a service engineer. This artifact does not occur in state-of-the-art MRI systems with digital transceivers, which sample signals in a single sideband mode at an intermediate frequency using only one amplifier and an analog-to-digital (ADC) converter. The intermediate-frequency signal is sampled rapidly, and the real and imaginary channels are generated digitally, which eliminates the possibility of any imbalance. Imbalance between the real and imaginary components of the transmitter can cause a ghost by exciting an additional slice at the same distance from the center of the MRI system but on the other side. Again, in state-of-the-art MRI systems, direct digital control of the transmitter eliminates this artifact.

Stimulated Echoes

A ghost reflected about the middle of the phase-encoding direction of a second-echo image is caused by stimulated echoes (Figure 10-13). Stimulated echoes are possible whenever there are three or more RF pulses, such as in multislice or multiecho imaging. The ghosts can be eliminated by using crusher gradients.[10] There have been interesting attempts to use the magnetization from stimulated echoes, but it is difficult to control.

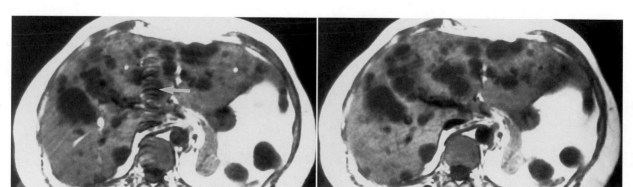

FIGURE 10-10   Combination of spatial presaturation and OPE for more effective suppression of ghosts. **A,** Image of patient with polycystic liver disease, acquired using OPE. Flow artifacts from the inferior vena cava interfere with the left lobe of the liver. **B,** Image obtained with both presaturation and OPE has diminished motion artifact. (From reference 13.)

WRAPAROUND
Possible Causes

Wraparound describes a class of artifacts in which structures, for several possible reasons, but mainly aliasing, appear to be in the wrong location in an MR image.

Aliasing

Aliasing is a phenomenon whereby the samples from a high-frequency signal cannot be distinguished from the samples of a much lower-frequency signal.[4] Aliasing makes a structure that is located beyond the FOV appear to be wrapped around from the other side of an MR image (Figure 10-14). Aliasing can occur in each direction of an MR image. Incidentally, aliasing is also the reason wagon wheels in western movies sometimes appear to rotate backward.

Nyquist sampling theorem. A continuous signal can be represented completely by a series of discrete samples, provided that the signal contains no frequencies beyond a certain limit, called the *Nyquist frequency*. At least two equally spaced samples must be acquired within

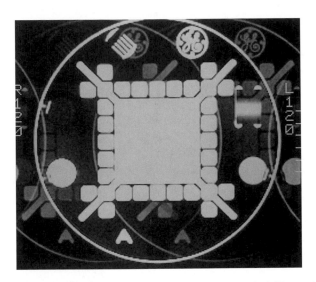

FIGURE 10-11   Ghosts from periodic changes in the magnetic field caused by a slightly ferromagnetic piston in a cryopump near the magnet.

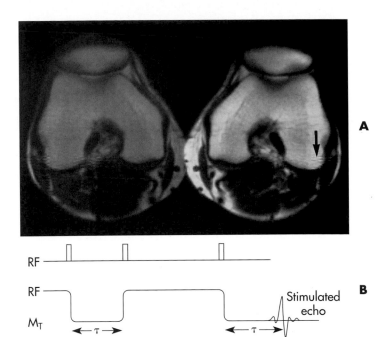

FIGURE 10-13   **A,** Ghost attributed to a stimulated echo. The ghost is inverted about the center in the phase-encoding direction (left to right). The image was made from a second echo. The horizontal striations are a zipper artifact, which can be eliminated by crusher gradients. **B,** Mechanism for stimulated echoes. Stimulated echoes can occur whenever three RF excitation pulses act on a spin system. The first RF pulse tips some longitudinal magnetization (M_L) into the transverse plane (M_T). A second RF pulse transforms this transverse magnetization into the longitudinal direction (M_L), where it remains until a third RF pulse tips it back into the transverse plane (M_T) again. A stimulated echo appears after a time (π) equal to the time between the first two RF pulses.

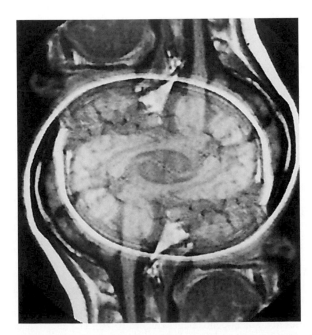

FIGURE 10-12   Ghost attributed to unbalanced real and imaginary channels in receiver section of MRI system. The imaginary channel failed so that only the real part of κ space was recorded, which forced the image to be symmetrical about the center of the FOV.

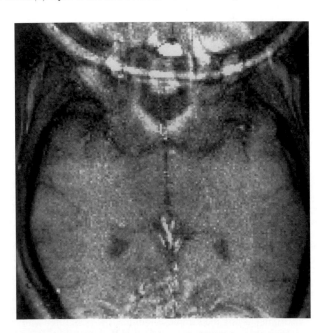

FIGURE 10-14   Wraparound of anatomy located outside the FOV along the phase-encoding direction. The wraparound was caused by aliasing.

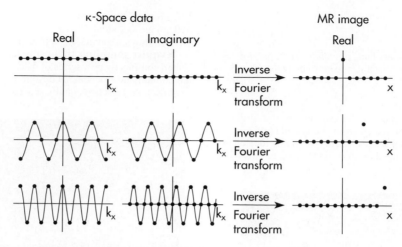

FIGURE 10-15 Mechanism of aliasing illustrated for frequency encoding. The diagram is an extension of Figure 1-27 showing hypothetical MR signals from a point at the following x coordinates: (a) 0, (b) FOV/ 2, and (c) 3 * FOV/4. The signal from region c is sampled three times in two cycles, which is not enough. These samples appear to belong to a lower-frequency signal. The inverse Fourier transform incorrectly identifies the x coordinate as FOV/4. This mistake is called *aliasing*.

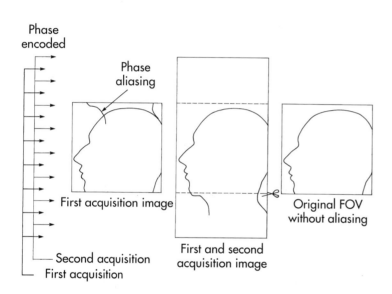

FIGURE 10-16 Extension of FOV to avoid aliasing. A second set of phase-encoding steps is interleaved with the set required to encode the specified FOV. This doubles the time for data acquisition, but it also doubles the FOV and increases the SNR by $2^{1/2}$, similar to data averaging. The extended portion of the FOV is discarded.

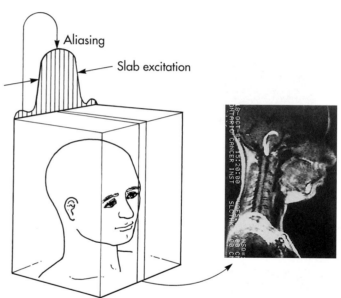

FIGURE 10-17 Aliasing in the slice-selection direction of a 3D volume MR image. The RF pulse excited magnetization according to the slice profile shown on top. This slice profile included structures beyond the desired volume, such as the ear and shoulder, which consequently were aliased back into the image.

the time that it takes for the highest-frequency component to complete one cycle. If the highest frequency is 10 kHz, two samples must be acquired at least every 100 μs. If an MR signal contains frequency components higher than the Nyquist frequency, these components are falsified by sampling and appear to originate from a lower-frequency signal (Figure 10-15). The falsified frequency equals the true frequency subtracted from the Nyquist frequency. Thus the falsified frequency is opposite in sign to the true frequency, and the corresponding structure is wrapped around from the other side of the frequency spectrum or FOV in MRI.

Frequency-encoding direction. Aliasing usually is not a problem for frequency encoding because MR signals from beyond the FOV can be eliminated by low-pass filtering using a cut-off frequency matched to the FOV. However, this filter can cause shading near the edges of the FOV. A simple solution is to double the FOV by sampling each echo twice as often, passing the samples though a low-pass filter with a cut-off frequency corresponding to an FOV slightly larger than desired, and finally extracting the desired image from the center of the extended FOV.

Phase-encoding direction. Aliasing in the phase-encoding direction is problematic because extending the FOV along this direction prolongs data acquisition. The FOV is extended by acquiring a second set of data having κ_y values between the first set (Figure 10-16). Acquisition of the second set of data doubles the imaging time, although it improves the signal-to-noise ratio (SNR) by $2^{1/2}$, similar to averaging.

Slice-selection direction. Aliasing in the slice-selection direction can occur in 3D volume imaging in which a wide slab is excited and subsequently partitioned into slices by phase encoding (see Chapter 1). Any MR signals from part of the slab beyond the range that is encoded will be aliased (Figure 10-17). Possible solutions are to ensure that essentially all of the slab is partitioned into slices or to use spatial presaturation to suppress the undesired MR signals. Nevertheless, it is usually necessary to discard a few slices at each end.

Aliasing can accentuate the effects of magnetic field inhomogeneities in gradient-echo images (Figure 10-18). The interference pattern arises from aliased anatomy in an inhomogeneous magnetic field, which gives the associated magnetization a different phase from the anatomy on which it becomes superimposed.

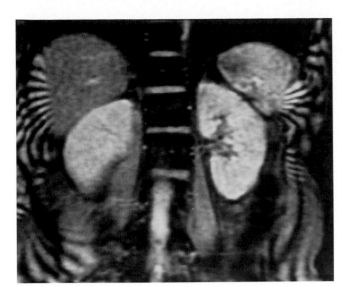

FIGURE 10-18   Moiré fringes as a side-effect of aliasing in a gradient-echo MR image.

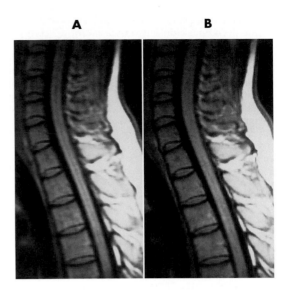

FIGURE 10-20   Truncation artifacts mimicking syringomyelia. **A,** Sagittal image of the cervical spine of a normal volunteer. The dark stripe is not pathology but actually a truncation artifact in the phase-encoding (horizontal) direction. **B,** Image of the same patient acquired under the same conditions except with twice as many phase-encoding steps. The dark stripe has essentially disappeared.

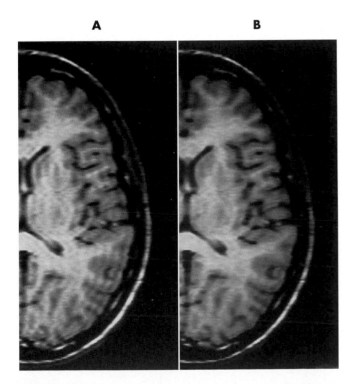

FIGURE 10-19   Truncation artifacts and their suppression. **A,** Head image acquired using only 96 phase-encoding steps in the left-right direction and reconstructed with a standard zero-filled inverse Fourier transform. **B,** Image from the same κ-space data after extrapolating the missing high-frequency data. The truncation artifacts have been diminished without blurring.

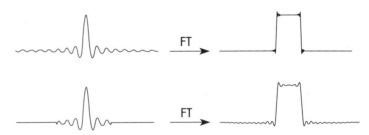

FIGURE 10-21   Mechanism for truncation artifacts. Fourier transforming truncated data causes ripples near sharp edges. The two curves on the left are sinc functions of different length. The bottom curve is only a short segment of the sinc function. Its Fourier transform is a rectangular pulse with ripples, which are the truncation artifacts. The top sinc curve is longer than the lower curve, and the ripples in its Fourier transform are less extensive.

RIPPLES
Possible Causes

Ripples propagating away from abrupt edges in MR images are common and arise from various causes, including truncation of κ-space data and short-lived eddy currents.

Truncation of κ-Space Data

The most common ripples in MR images are truncation artifacts (also called *edge,* or *Gibbs', ringing*) (Figure 10-19). Each ripple spans two pixels. Truncation artifacts can be particularly misleading in long, narrow structures, such as the spinal cord or intervertebral disks (Figure 10-20).[5] One solution is to acquire another image at higher resolution.

Truncation artifacts arise from failure to sample high spatial frequencies for an MR image (Figure 10-21). Thus the artifacts are more conspicuous in lower-resolution images and along the phase-encoding direction. Spatial resolution along this direction often is sacrificed to save time, and unlike data for frequency encoding, data for the phase-encoding direction do not decay naturally. The inverse Fourier transform, which converts the data to an MR image, assumes that all spatial frequencies higher than that measured are zero. The discontinuity between the measured data at low frequencies and the assumed zero values at higher frequencies can be eliminated by filtering, but the blurring that results is usually unacceptable.

Many methods have been proposed to overcome truncation artifacts essentially by extrapolating the measured data into the missing high-

Common Magnetic Field Strength in Different Locations

An apparent wraparound artifact can occur in a two-dimensional Fourier transformation (2D FT) image when structures outside the imaged slice are excited by an RF pulse. This can occur, for example, when the z gradient has the same value at the hips as a slice in the abdomen, with both areas within a large (body) RF coil. Such artifacts are rare and can be difficult to identify. The solution is to avoid conditions whereby MR signals from structures well beyond the slice can be detected.

frequency region. Extrapolation schemes include linear prediction with singular value decomposition, maximum entropy,[52] autoregressive-moving average,[67] and constrained reconstruction.[24] Each scheme uses a different model for the data, and some even attempt to provide higher resolution. All of the schemes are computationally intensive, and so far none has demonstrated clear superiority.[47] Maximum-entropy methods have been ineffective.[8] The method used for Figure 10-19, *B,* attempts to extrapolate only the high spatial frequencies that contribute to predominant edges.[9] First, a median filter is applied to suppress truncation artifacts until only the major edges remain. Then, high-frequency data corresponding to edges in the filtered image are extrapolated and grafted smoothly onto the measured data. As shown, this method eliminates truncation artifacts while preserving spatial resolution.

STRAIGHT LINES
Possible Causes

Several kinds of artifacts are straight lines through MR images, including RF interference, RF feedthrough, stimulated echoes, and spike in κ space.

Radiofrequency Interference

Radio waves from various sources outside an MRI system can cause a characteristic pattern of straight lines (Figure 10-22). Normally the RF shielding prevents external radio waves from contaminating an MR image. However, RF interference is possible from sources inside the magnet, such as monitoring devices and even a flickering light bulb (Figure 10-22).

Stimulated Echoes

A zipperlike artifact, with alternating bright and dark pixels in a line propagating along the frequency-encoding direction, is caused by stimulated echoes that have avoided phase encoding (Figure 10-23). This artifact can occur if phase encoding occurs between the second and third RF pulses of a particular sequence. Longitudinal magnetization that is tipped into the transverse plane by the third RF pulse will not have experienced this phase encoding and so will be assigned to a line passing through the center of the phase-encoding direction in the image.

Zipper artifacts can be eliminated by spoiler gradients arranged in a special pattern to ensure that every possible stimulated echo is removed from each data-sampling interval.[10] An alternative approach is to cycle the phase of subsequent RF excitation pulses to push the zipper to the boundary of the image, where it can be ignored or removed. All zipper artifacts and, moreover, all artifacts arising from stimulated echoes are less severe if the slice profile closely resembles the ideal rectangle. Nonideal slice profiles also lead to slice interference and degraded image contrast.[41]

Spike in κ Space

A pattern of regularly spaced lines across an MR image (Figure 10-24) arises from a spike in κ space. The frequency and orientation of the pattern depend on the κ-space point affected. If several data points are corrupted, a more complicated pattern of lines results. Such spikes can be detected and repaired automatically, although it is not routine on commercial MRI systems.[16] Electrostatic discharges in blankets can cause κ-space spikes, which can be prevented by increasing the humidity.

FALSE CONTOURS
Possible Causes

Several phenomena give rise to false contours in MR images, including misregistration from chemical shift, interference from chemical shift, inverted longitudinal magnetization, shear, and oblique flow. These contours might be aesthetically pleasing, but they really are artifacts.

Misregistration From Chemical Shift

Chemical shift refers to a range of Larmor frequencies, depending on the molecular environment. The Larmor frequency for magnetization from a watery tissue, such as muscle, is about 3.5 ppm greater than that for protons on the saturated hydrocarbons in adipose tissue. A 3.5 ppm chemical shift changes the Larmor frequency by about 225 Hz at 1.5 T ($3.5 \times 10^{-6} \times 42.576$ MHz/T $\times$ 1.5 T). Magnetic resonance spectroscopy owes its existence to the chemical shift. However, chemical shifts are a nuisance for MRI because they cause tissues with different chemical shifts to be displaced in images.[34,68] A solution is to use spectral presaturation.

Along the frequency-encoding direction, where spatial information is encoded into the Larmor frequency, chemical shift causes misregistration between adipose and watery tissue. Bright or dark contours between lipid and watery tissues arise (Figure 10-25). The width of these

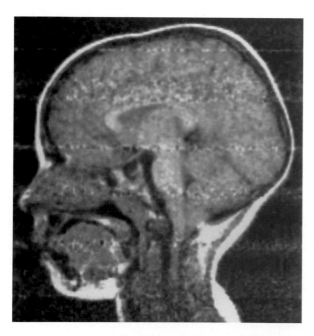

FIGURE 10-22   Lines at certain positions along the frequency-encoding direction (craniocaudal) attributed to RF interference from a flickering light bulb.

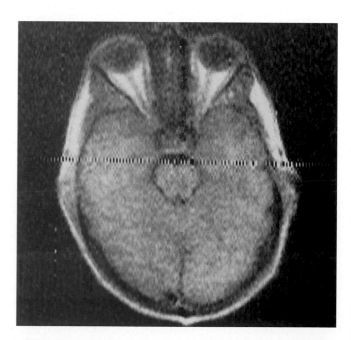

FIGURE 10-23   Zipper artifact caused by a stimulated echo. The zipper has alternately bright and dark pixels along the frequency-encoding direction (horizontal) through the center of the image.

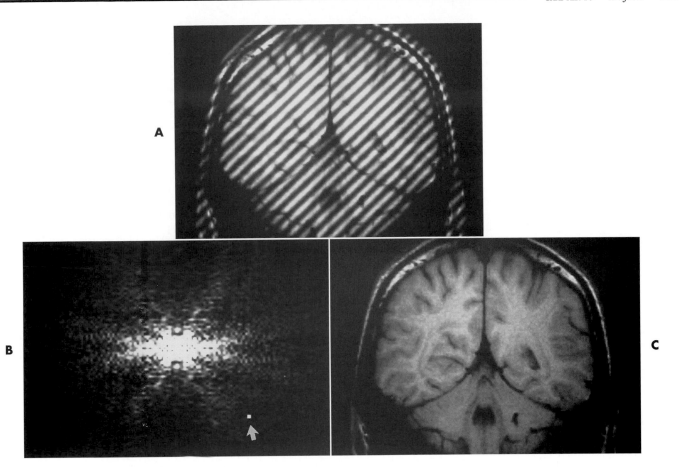

FIGURE 10-24   Pattern of lines caused by a spike in κ space. **A,** Image with lines. **B,** Corresponding κ space. **C,** Image resulting after removal of κ-space spike.

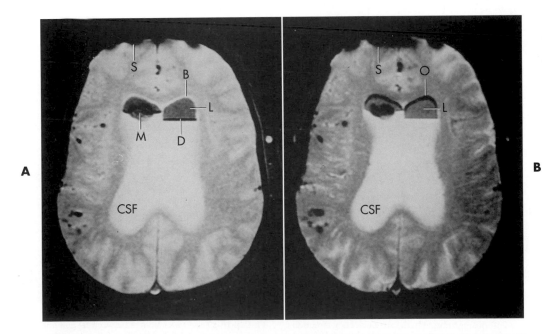

FIGURE 10-25   Chemical-shift misregistration between lipid and CSF in the lateral ventricles. **A,** Note the bright boundary *(B)* caused by lipid-rich fluid *(L)* shifted anteriorly so that the apparent location of its MR signals overlaps with those from brain tissue. The dark interface *(D)* confirms that the cysts contain lipid. Also note the solid mass *(M)* within the cysts and the shading caused by changes in magnetic susceptibility *(S)* near the frontal sinuses. **B,** Image of the same slice with the polarity of the frequency-encoding gradient inverted so that the magnetic field increases anteriorly. Now the boundary between the cysts and the brain tissue is dark and the dark interface in **A** is brighter. (Courtesy W. Kelly).

contours reflects the amount of spatial misregistration. Chemical shifts cause more spatial misregistration in low-bandwidth images. The 225 Hz chemical shift at 1.5 T displaces water and fat by 5.8 pixels or 1.1 pixel if the bandwidth across a 256-pixel FOV is 10 kHz or 50 kHz, respectively. Chemical-shift misregistration can be helpful in interpreting images when the chemical composition of a certain structure is ambiguous (Figure 10-25).

Chemical-shift misregistration also occurs along the slice-selection direction. A particular RF pulse affects adipose tissue in a slightly different location than watery tissue because of the chemical shift. The offset would be 18% of the slice thickness for a single-lobed, sinc-shaped RF pulse of 3.2 ms duration at 1.5 T. As illustrated in Figure 10-26, bone marrow from the skull can appear as a bright contour resembling a subdural hematoma. Inverting the polarity of the slice-selection gradient alters this contour, confirming its chemical-shift origin. The offset between slices of adipose tissue and water can be exploited to suppress adipose tissue. If the Larmor frequency for water is chosen for reference and the polarity of the slice-selection gradient is reversed between the 90-degree and 180-degree RF pulses, only part of the slice of adipose tissue will be refocused by the 180-degree pulse.

Interference From Chemical Shift

Compared with the magnetization from adipose tissue, the magnetization from water, which precesses approximately 225 Hz faster at 1.5 T, completes an extra revolution every 4.5 ms. At 0.5 T it takes 3 times longer for the extra revolution. At TE times that are multiples of 4.5 ms at 1.5 T, magnetization from water and adipose tissue is in phase. The magnetization from these chemically different tissues is 180 degrees out of phase at TE times halfway between the special in-phase TE times. If such an out-of-phase TE is chosen for a gradient-echo image, the magnetization in regions containing a mixture of water and adipose tissue tends to cancel, leaving dark contours[75] (Figure 10-27). These contours can be avoided by choosing an in-phase TE or an SE technique.

Inverted Longitudinal Magnetization

Inversion-recovery pulse sequences begin by inverting the net magnetization. After a prearranged time called the *inversion time* (TI), the usual RF excitation pulse is applied. For any TI chosen, there might be tissues having a special T1 equal to TI/ln2 (equal to 1.44 TI), for which the longitudinal magnetization is momentarily zero. Such tissues will have zero image intensity. At the time of the RF excitation pulse, the longitudinal magnetization for tissues with longer or shorter T1 values is negative or positive, respectively. Partial-volume effects create a dark contour between these tissues, as shown in Figure 10-28. The contours are absent in images that display the real component of complex-valued pixels, although such images require phase correction.[55]

Shear

Dark contours can appear in magnitude images as a result of the intravoxel dephasing caused by shear between two organs (Figure 10-29).[74] GMN, which was introduced in an earlier section, can eliminate the contour.

SHADING
Possible Causes

Shading occurs for many reasons, including overflow of ADC, steady state transverse magnetization, imperfect slice profile, coupling of the receiver coil with the transmitter, eddy currents and RF attenuation, and magnetic field inhomogeneities in steady state free precession pulse sequences.[66] For example, eddy currents and RF attenuation combine to make one side of the spine brighter in transverse images acquired using

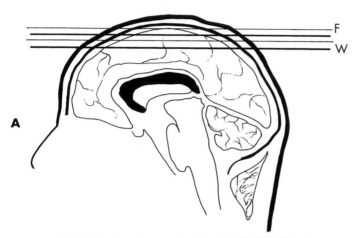

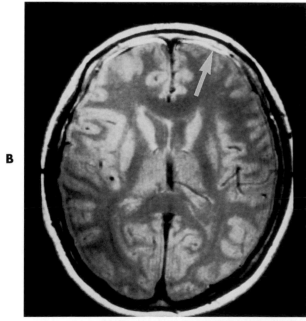

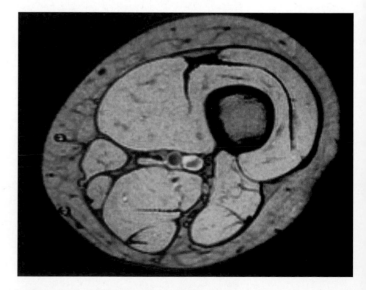

FIGURE 10-26 Chemical-shift misregistration in the slice-selection direction. **A,** Mechanism, showing the magnetic field strength increasing inferiorly, which results in misregistered slices of fat *(F)* and water *(W).* The fat consists of the subcutaneous fat and the fat in the marrow but is not visible in the brain itself. **B,** Chemical-shift misregistration in the slice-selection and frequency-encoding directions (anteroposterior) shows bright fat superimposed on the brain *(arrow).* This artifact would mimic a subdural hematoma in a short TR/TE image. (Courtesy W. Kelly).

FIGURE 10-27 Dark contours between fat and muscle in a gradient-echo MR image acquired at 1.5 T with TE = 6.8 ms, at which time magnetization from lipid and water are 180 degrees out of phase.

a surface coil as a receiver. They also create a pattern of shading when the coil is linearly polarized.[18] In the interest of brevity, only the first three aforementioned artifacts are detailed.

Overflow of Analog-to-Digital Converter

Images with distorted contrast and a halo blending into the background occur when samples from MR signals exceed the range of the ADC converter. Samples that overflow the ADC converter wraparound (Figure 10-30). It is possible to correct the data automatically.[35] The usual solution is to reacquire the image with less amplification for the MR signals. However, the signals must be amplified enough to avoid quantization errors, especially for 3D images, for which the data have a very large dynamic range.

Steady State Transverse Magnetization

When TR is short compared with T2, a steady state transverse magnetization can exist before each RF excitation pulse in a gradient-echo pulse sequence.[27] The steady state magnetization is particularly strong for fluids such as CSF, for which T2 is comparable to T1. A prerequisite for steady state is that the net phase accumulation between each RF pulse be the same. The phase-encoding gradient violates this condition, depending on the location along the phase-encoding direction. Near the center, where phase-encoding gradients cause small phase shifts, a steady state can endure. As a result, short TR gradient-echo images can exhibit a bright band at the center of the phase-encoding direction (Figure 10-31).[19] The contrast within this band reflects steady-state mag-

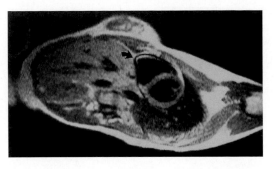

FIGURE 10-29   Dark contour caused by shear in an oblique image of the heart. Data for the image were acquired immediately after the QRS complex, during which there is substantial shear between the epicardium and pericardium. The dark contour *(arrow)* could be mistaken for the pericardium. (From reference 31.)

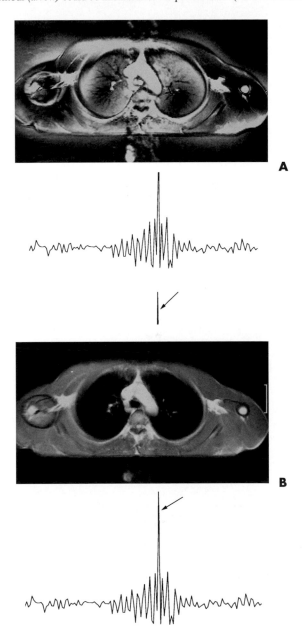

FIGURE 10-30   Shading artifact caused by overflow of ADC in the receiver section of an MRI system. **A,** One of the echoes from κ space showing that the peak exceeded the range of the ADC and was therefore assigned a negative value *(arrow)*. **B,** Retrospective correction of the data or rescanning the patient with more receiver attenuation corrects the artifact.

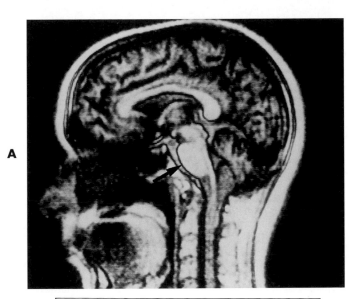

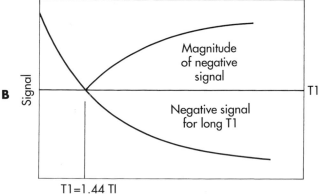

FIGURE 10-28   **A,** Dark contours in a magnitude image from an inversion-recovery pulse sequence. These contours join pixels for which the longitudinal magnetization was passing zero at the time of RF excitation. This occurs for pixels in which T1 = 1.44 TI (inversion time). **B,** The contours divide tissues with shorter and longer T1. (From reference 31.)

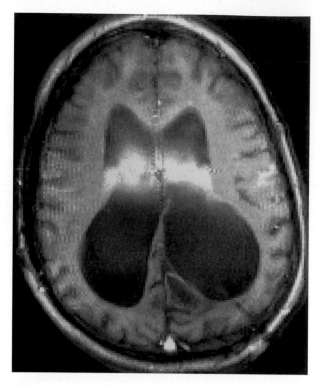

FIGURE 10-31   Bright band caused by incomplete spoiling of steady state transverse magnetization in a short TR gradient-echo MR image. The band is in the center of the phase-encoding direction, where the characteristically small incremental phase shifts fail to disrupt the steady state.

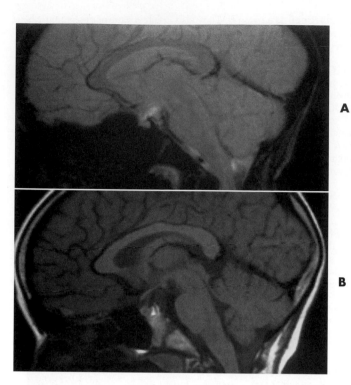

FIGURE 10-33   Comparison of distortion caused by abrupt changes in magnetic susceptibility in gradient-echo (A) and SE (B) MR images. The same imaging parameters were used, including TR/TE = 500/30. As expected, A shows more signal loss, particularly near the nasal sinuses and in the bone marrow, where trabecular bone degrades the magnetic field. The distortion in A is so severe that the normal structure of the pituitary gland cannot be discerned.

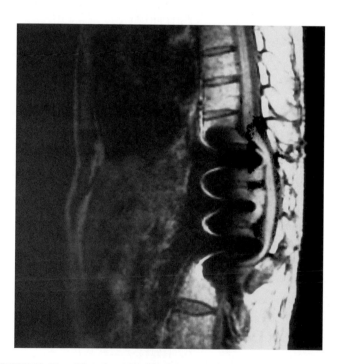

FIGURE 10-32   Distortion caused by ferromagnetic Harrington rod. The bony spinal canal and spinal cord are normal in this patient, but the apparent posterior displacement of the end is an artifact.

the frequency synthesizer and the transverse magnetization in such a way that a phase shift between the two increases linearly after each RF pulse.[86] Spoiler gradients have proved to be less effective at spoiling the transverse magnetization.

Imperfect Slice Profiles

Imperfect slice profiles degrade the quality of MR images acquired as multiple slices in an interleaved fashion. Slice interference reduces the contrast or SNR, depending on whether TR is long or short compared with T1.[41] The actual cause of the degradation is the inevitable side lobes and transition region in the slice profile (see Chapter 1). The nonideal nature of a typical slice profile also affects the uniformity of slices acquired by 3D Fourier imaging. An artifact characterized by slightly different intensity in even- and odd-numbered slices also is attributed to side lobes of the slice profile; because of the location of these side lobes, the fluctuations do not necessarily diminish as the slice separation increases.

GEOMETRICAL DISTORTION
Possible Causes

The shape and position of structures emitting MR signals are inferred from the frequency of the signals. The frequency, in turn, depends on the magnetic field strength. Various processes that distort the magnetic field strength also distort the geometry of MR images. General causes of geometrical distortion include inhomogeneous magnetic field, ferromagnetic materials, spatial variations in magnetic susceptibility, and nonlinear magnetic field gradients.

Ferromagnetic Materials

Magnetic field perturbations induced by ferromagnetic materials in the bore of the magnet or by the patient are usually severe but well localized.[65] Near the inhomogeneity, MR signals are shifted to higher or lower frequencies so the image is warped away from the inhomogeneity in the frequency-encoding direction, leaving a void with a bright crescent rim (Figure 10-32).[49]

netization. Elsewhere in the image the contrast is influenced less by the steady state. It is possible to rephase the phase-encoding gradient after sampling each echo, in which case the contrast in the image tends to resemble that in the central band. Conversely, spoiling the steady state magnetization creates contrast that is largely uninfluenced by the steady state. The preferred approach for spoiling is to adjust the phase between

Spatial Variations in Magnetic Susceptibility

Magnetic susceptibility describes the manner and amount by which a material becomes magnetized in a magnetic field. The intrinsic magnetic susceptibility of bone and other tissues differs from that of air by less than 10 ppm, but this small difference is enough to cause signal loss and distortion at the boundary of tissues with different susceptibility. Gradient-echo images are affected much more than SE images because SE images refocus the dephasing from magnetic field inhomogeneities (Figure 10-33).* The signal loss in gradient-echo images is reduced at higher spatial resolution.[26,85]

SUMMARY

Artifacts in MR images assume many different forms—ghosts, wraparounds, ripples, straight lines, false contours, shading, and geometrical distortion. Ghosts, especially those caused by motion, are the most prevalent. These ghosts persist despite enormous "ghost-busting" efforts during the past 15 years. Similar to the choice of pulse sequences, decisions for suppressing ghosts need to be reconsidered periodically, based on growing experience and new technology. The ability to recognize the appearance of the various classes of artifacts is a major step in avoiding misinterpretation. Perhaps the most important reason to understand the cause of artifacts is to motivate the development of methods to overcome these artifacts. The suppression of every possible artifact in every possible MR image is a worthwhile albeit elusive goal.

*References 7, 14, 26, 29, 36, 49, 53, 63, 71.

REFERENCES

1. Arena L, Morehouse HT, and Safix J: MR imaging artifacts that simulate disease: how to recognize and eliminate them, Radiographics 15:1373, 1995.
2. Bailes DR, Gilderdale DJ, Bydder GM, et al: Respiratory ordering of phase encoding (ROPE): a method for reducing respiratory motion artifacts in MR imaging, J Comput Assist Tomogr 9:835, 1985.
3. Bellon EM, Haacke EM, Coleman PE, et al: MR artifacts: a review, Am J Roentgenol 147:1271, 1986.
4. Bracewell RN: The Fourier transform and its applications, New York, 1978, McGraw-Hill.
5. Bronskill MJ, McVeigh ER, Kucharczyk W, et al: Syrinx-like artifacts on MR images of the spinal cord, Radiology 166:485, 1988.
6. Bydder GM, and Young IR: MR imaging: clinical use of the inversion recovery sequence, J Comput Assist Tomogr 9:659, 1985.
7. Cho ZH, and Ro YM: Reduction of susceptibility artifact in gradient-echo imaging, Magn Reson Med 23:193, 1992.
8. Constable RT, and Henkelman RM: Why MEM does not work in MR image reconstruction, Magn Reson Med 14:12, 1990.
9. Constable RT, and Henkelman RM: Data extrapolation for truncation artifact removal, Magn Reson Med 17:108, 1991.
10. Crawley AP, and Henkelman RM: A stimulated echo artifact from slice interference in MRI, Med Phys 14:842, 1987.
11. Edelman RR, Atkinson DJ, Silver MS, et al: FRODO pulse sequences: a new means of eliminating motion, flow, and wraparound artifacts, Radiology 166:231, 1988.
12. Ehman RL, and Felmlee JP: Adaptive technique for high-definition MR imaging of moving structures, Radiology 173:255, 1989.
13. Ehman RL, and Felmlee JP: Flow artifact reduction in MRI: a review of the role of gradient moment nulling and spatial presaturation, Magn Reson Med 14:293, 1990.
14. Elster AD: Sellar susceptibility artifacts: theory and implications, Am J Neuroradiol 14:129, 1992.
15. Felmlee JP, and Ehman RL: Spatial presaturation: a method for suppressing flow artifacts and improving depiction of vascular anatomy in MR imaging, Radiology 164:559, 1987.
16. Foo TKF, Grigsby NS, Mitchell JD, and Slayman BE: SNORE: spike noise removal and detection, IEEE Trans Med Imag 13:133, 1994.
17. Foo TKF, and Hayes CE: Phase-correction method for reduction of Bo instability artifacts, J Magn Reson Imag 3:676, 1993.
18. Foo TKF, Hayes CE, and Kang Y-W: Reduction of RF penetration effects in high field imaging, Magn Reson Med 23:287, 1992.
19. Frahm J, Hänicke W, and Merboldt K-D: Transverse coherences in rapid FLASH NMR imaging, J Magn Reson 72:307-314, 1987.
20. Glover GH, and Pauly JM: Projection reconstruction techniques for reduction of motion effects in MRI, Magn Reson Med 28:275, 1992.
21. Glover GH, and Pelc NJ: A rapid-gated cine MRI technique, Magn Reson Annual 299, 1988.
22. Haacke EM, and Lenz GW: Improving image quality in the presence of motion by using rephasing gradients, Am J Roentgenol 148:1251, 1987.
23. Haacke EM, Lenz GW, and Nelson AD: Pseudogating: elimination of periodic motion artifacts in magnetic resonance imaging without gating, Magn Reson Med 4:162, 1987.
24. Haacke EM, Liang ZP, and Izen SH: Constrained reconstruction: a superesolution, optimal signal-to-noise alternative to the Fourier transform in magnetic resonance imaging, Med Phys 16:388, 1989.
25. Haacke EM, and Patrick JL: Reducing motion artifacts in two-dimensional Fourier transform imaging, Magn Reson Imag 4:359, 1986.
26. Haacke EM, Tkach JA, and Parrish TB: Reduction of T2 dephasing in gradient field-echo imaging, Radiology 170:457, 1989.
27. Haase A, Frahm J, Matthaei W, et al: FLASH imaging: rapid NMR imaging using low flip-angle pulses, J Magn Reson 67:258, 1986.
28. Hajnal JV, Myers R, Oatridge A, et al: Artifacts due to stimulus correlated motion in functional imaging of the brain, Magn Reson Med 31:283, 1994.
29. Haramati N, Penrod B, Staron RB, et al: Surgical sutures: MR artifacts and sequence dependence, J Magn Reson Imag 4:209, 1994.
30. Hedley M, and Yan H: Motion artifact suppression: a review of post-processing techniques, Magn Reson Imag 10:627, 1992.
31. Henkelman RM, and Bronskill MJ: Artifacts in magnetic resonance imaging, Revs Magn Reson Med 2:1, 1987.
32. Hinks RS, Xiang Q-S, and Henkelman RM: Ghost phase cancellation with phase-encoding gradient modulation, J Magn Reson Imag 3:777, 1993.
33. Hu X, and Kim S-G: Reduction of signal fluctuation in functional MRI using navigator echoes, Magn Reson Med 31:495, 1994.
34. Ishizaka H, Tomiyoshi K, and Matsumoto M: MR quantification of bone marrow cellularity: use of chemical-shift misregistration artifact, Am J Roentgenol 160:572, 1993.
35. Jackson J, Macovski A, and Nishimura D: Low-frequency restoration, Magn Reson Med 11:248, 1989.
36. Kim JK, Kucharczyk W, and Henkelman RM: Cavernous hemangiomas: dipolar susceptibility artifacts at MR imaging, Radiology 187:735, 1993.
37. Korin HW, Farzaneh F, Wright RC, et al: Compensation for the effects of linear motion in MR imaging, Magn Reson Med 12:99, 1989.
38. Korin HW, Riederer SJ, Bampton AEH, et al: Altered phase-encoding order for reduced sensitivity to motion in three-dimensional MR imaging, J Magn Reson Imag 2:687, 1992.
39. Korin HW, Felmlee JP, Riederer SJ, and Ehman RL: Respiratory kinematics of the upper abdominal organs: a quantitative study, Magn Reson Med 23:172, 1992.
40. Korin HW, Felmlee JP, Riederer SJ, et al: Spatial-frequency-tuned markers and adaptive correction for rotational motion, Magn Reson Med 33:663, 1995.
41. Kucharczyk W, Crawley AP, Kelly WM, et al: Effect of multislice interference on image contrast in T2- and T1-weighted images, AJNR 9:443, 1988.
42. Kumar A, Welti D, and Ernst RR: NMR Fourier zeugmatography, J Magn Reson 18:69, 1975.
43. Lanzer P, Barta C, Botuinik EH, et al: ECG-synchronized cardiac MR imaging: method and evaluation, Radiology 155:681, 1985.
44. Larson TC, Kelly WM, Ehman RL, and Wehrli FW: Spatial misregistration of vascular flow during MR imaging of the CNS: cause and clinical significance, Am J Roentgenol 155:1117, 1990.
45. Lauzon ML, and Rutt BK: Generalized κ-space analysis and correction of motion effects in MR imaging, Magn Reson Med 30:438, 1993.
46. Lenz GW, Haacke EM, and White RD: Retrospective cardiac gating: a review of technical aspects and future directions, Magn Reson Imag 7:445, 1989.
47. Liang Z-P, et al: Constrained reconstruction methods in MR imaging, Res Magn Reson Med 4:67, 1992.
48. Liu YL, Riederer SJ, Rossman PH, et al: A monitoring, feedback, and triggering system for reproducible breath-hold MR imaging, Magn Reson Med 30:507, 1993.
49. Ludeke KM, Roschmann P, and Tischler R: Susceptibility artifacts in NMR imaging, Magn Reson Imag 3:329, 1985.
50. Macgowan CK, and Wood ML: Phase-encode reordering to minimize errors caused by motion, Magn Reson Med 35:391, 1996.
51. Madore B, and Henkelman RM: Motion artifacts in fast spin-echo imaging, J Magn Reson Imag 4:577, 1994.
52. Martin JF: The maximum entropy method in NMR, J Magn Reson 65:291, 1985.
53. McCarty M, and Gedroyc WMW: Surgical clip artifact mimicking arterial stenosis: problem with magnetic resonance angiography, Clin Radiol 48:232, 1993.
54. Mitchell DG, Vinitski S, Burk DL, et al: Motion artifact reduction in MR imaging of the abdomen: gradient moment nulling versus respiratory-sorted phase-encoding, Radiology 169:155, 1988.
55. Moran PR, Kumar NJ, and Karstaedt N: Tissue contrast enhancement: image reconstruction algorithm and selection of T1 in inversion recovery MRI, Magn Reson Imag 4:229, 1986.
56. Mugler JP III, and Brookeman JR: Design of pulse sequences employing spatial presaturation for the suppression of flow artifacts, Magn Reson Med 33:201, 1992.
57. Nishimura DG, Jackson JI, and Pauly JM: On the nature and reduction of the displacement artifact in flow images, Magn Reson Med 22:481, 1991.
58. Pattany PM, Phillips J, Chiu LC, et al: Motion artifact suppression technique (MAST) for MR imaging, J Comput Assist Tomogr 11:369, 1987.
59. Rogers WJ Jr, and Shapiro EP: Effect of RR interval variation on image quality in gated, two-dimensional, Fourier MR imaging, Radiology 186:883, 1993.
60. Runge VM, Clanton J, Partain CL, et al: Respiratory gating in magnetic resonance imaging at 0.5 Tesla, Radiology 151:521-523, 1984.
61. Runge VM, Wood ML, Kauffman DM, et al: The straight and narrow path to good head and spine MR imaging, Radiographics 8:507, 1988.
62. Sachs TS, Meyer CH, Hu BS, et al: Real-time motion detection in spiral MRI using navigators, Magn Reson Med 32:639, 1994.
63. Sakurai K, Fujita N, Harada K, et al: Magnetic susceptibility artifact in spin-echo MR imaging of the pituitary gland, Am J Neuroradiol 13:1301, 1992.

64. Schultz CL, Alfidi RJ, Nelson AD, et al: Effect of motion on two-dimensional Fourier transformation magnetic resonance images, Radiology 152:117, 1984.

65. Shellock FG, Mink JH, and Curtin S: MR imaging and metallic implants for anterior cruciate ligament reconstruction: assessment of ferromagnetism and artifact, J Magn Reson Imag 2:225, 1992.

66. Simmons A, Tofts PS, and Barker GJ: Sources of intensity nonuniformity in spin echo images at 1.5 T, Magn Reson Med 32:121, 1994.

67. Smith MR, Nichols ST, Henkelman RM, and Wood ML: Application of autoregressive modelling in magnetic resonance imaging to remove noise and truncation artifacts, Magn Reson Imag 4:257, 1986.

68. Soila KP, Viamonte M Jr, and Starewicz PM: Chemical shift misregistration effect in magnetic resonance imaging, Radiology 153:819, 1984.

69. Stark DD, Wittenburg J, Edelman RR, et al: Detection of hepatic metastases: analysis of pulse sequence performance in MR imaging, Radiology 159:365, 1986.

70. Sumanaweera T, Glover G, Song S, et al: Quantifying MRI geometric distortion in tissue, Magn Reson Med 31:40, 1994.

71. Tartaglino LM, Flanders AE, Vinitski S, and Friedman DP: Metallic artifacts on MR images of the postoperative spine: reduction with fast spin-echo techniques, Radiology 190:565, 1994.

72. Tasciyan TA, and Mitchell DG: Pulsatile flow artifacts in fast magnetization-prepared sequences, J Magn Reson Imag 4:217, 1994.

73. Wang Y, Rossman PJ, Grimm RC, et al: Navigator-echo-based real-time respiratory gating and triggering for reduction of respiration effects in three-dimensional coronary MR angiography, Radiology 198:55, 1996.

74. Wedeen VJ, Weisskoff RM, and Poncelet BP: MRI signal void due to in-plane motion is all-or-none, Magn Reson Med 32:116, 1994.

75. Wehrli FW, Perkins TG, Shimakawa A, and Roberts F: Chemical shift-induced amplitude modulations in images obtained with gradient refocusing, Magn Reson Imag 5:157, 1987.

76. Wood ML: Respiratory artifacts: mechanism and control. In Encyclopedia of nuclear magnetic resonance, New York, 1996, John Wiley & Sons.

77. Wood ML, Bronskill MJ, Mulkern RV, and Santyr GE: Physical MR desktop data, J Magn Reson Imag 3(S):19,1994.

78. Wood ML, and Henkelman RM: MR image artifacts from periodic motion, Med Phys 12:143, 1985.

79. Wood ML, and Henkelman RM: Suppression of respiratory motion artifacts in magnetic resonance imaging, Med Phys 13:794, 1986.

80. Wood ML, and Henkelman RM: The magnetic field dependence of the breathing artifact, Magn Reson Imag 4:387, 1986.

81. Wood ML, Stanchev PL, and Shivji MJ: Planar-motion correction using κ-space data acquired by Fourier MR imaging, J Magn Reson Imag 5:57, 1995.

82. Wu Fu Z, Wang Y, Grimm RC, et al: Orbital navigator echoes for motion measurements in magnetic resonance imaging, Magn Reson Med 34:753, 1995.

83. Xiang QS, Bronskill MJ, and Henkelman RM: Two-point interference method for suppression of ghost artifacts due to motion, J Magn Reson Imag 3:900, 1993.

84. Xiang QS, and Henkelman RM: κ-Space description for MR imaging of dynamic objects, Magn Reson Med 29:422, 1993.

85. Young IR, Cos IJ, and Bryant DJ, et al: The benefits of increasing spatial resolution as a means of reducing artifacts due to field inhomogeneities, Magn Reson Imag 6:585, 1988.

86. Zur Y, Wood ML, and Neuringer LJ: Spoiling of transverse magnetization in steady-state sequences, Magn Reson Med 21:251, 1991.

CHAPTER

11 Flow Phenomena

William G. Bradley, Jr.

Physiological Motion
    Signal of Stagnant Blood
    Types of Motion
    Reynolds Number
    Laminar Flow
    Turbulence
    Vascular Flow Characteristics
Normal Appearance of Flowing Blood
    High-Velocity Signal Loss
    Turbulence
    Dephasing
    Even-Echo Rephasing
    Stagnation
    Diastolic Pseudogating
    Flow-Related Enhancement
Combined Flow Phenomena
    Flow Artifacts and Flow-Compensation Techniques
    Distinguishing Thrombus from Slow Flow
Cerebrospinal Fluid Flow

 KEY POINTS

- Motion can lead to a signal increase (flow-related enhancement, even-echo rephasing, or diastolic pseudogating) or a signal decrease (high-velocity signal loss, first-echo dephasing, or turbulence) of flowing blood or cerebrospinal fluid.
- Pulsatile flow can lead to artifacts ("ghosts"), which might simulate disease.
- High-intensity flow artifacts can be eliminated by spatial presaturation pulses or by gradient-moment nulling (flow compensation).

Few aspects of magnetic resonance imaging (MRI) are as potentially confusing as the effect of motion on the MR image. Although the MR image is anatomically similar to the image produced by x-ray computed tomography (CT), the MR appearance of flowing blood or cerebrospinal fluid (CSF) has no correlate in CT. Flowing blood can appear bright or dark, depending on the velocity.* To a first approximation, rapidly flowing arterial blood appears dark (creating a "flow void"), and slowly flowing venous blood appears bright[20] (Figure 11-1). However, this appearance is greatly influenced by factors related to the imaging sequence and the MR imager itself. As discussed later in this chapter, the signal from flowing blood depends on the type of sequence (i.e., conventional or fast spin echo [FSE] or gradient echo), the position of the slice containing the vessel relative to the rest of the multislice imaging volume,[11] the repetition time (TR), the echo time (TE), the number of echoes, the slice thickness, and the use of various gradient-moment nulling (i.e., flow-compensation) techniques.[19,26-28,32]

---

*References 2, 7, 11, 20, 21, 36, 44, 45, 59, 60, 63.

PHYSIOLOGICAL MOTION
Signal of Stagnant Blood

Before the effects of physiological motion on the MR intensity of flowing blood or CSF are discussed, it is important to establish a baseline: what would the signal intensity be without motion? Stagnant blood and CSF have MR signal characteristics based on their proton density, T1, and T2 values. As discussed in Chapter 3, T1 values depend on field strength; however, the value is on the order of 1000 ms for stagnant unclotted blood at field strengths routinely used for MRI. The T2 value of unclotted blood is approximately 150 ms. These characteristics result in relatively high signal intensity for stagnant blood on the proton density–weighted and T2-weighted images routinely used for imaging the brain (see Chapter 58). CSF is essentially pure water and has a T1 time of 2.7 sec and a T2 time approaching 2.7 sec as the TE (and the effects of autodiffusion) are minimized.

Types of Motion

Several levels of physiological motion from microscopic diffusion to macroscopic bulk flow affect the MR image. Simple diffusion as a result of random brownian motion of molecules in the presence of a magnetic field gradient leads to dephasing and therefore signal loss.[40-41] Such losses are increased when imaging is performed with stronger gradients or longer TEs on conventional spin-echo (SE) images. The losses are minimized on FSE images as a result of the rephasing effects of the multiple 180-degree pulses. This phenomenon has been exploited to provide images in which contrast depends strongly on diffusion[17,39,41,46,47] (Figure 11-2) (see Chapter 66).

Reynolds Number

The characteristics of steady flow in tubes are described by the Reynolds relationship.[5] The Reynolds number *(Re)* is dimensionless—it has no units. The Reynolds number depends on the velocity (expressed in centimeters per second) as well as the vascular diameter (expressed in centimeters) and the viscosity (expressed in centipoise, grams per centimeter-seconds) and the density (expressed in grams per cubic centimeter) of the fluid[5,12]:

(EQ. 1)

$$Re = \frac{Density \times Velocity \times Tube\ diameter}{Viscosity}$$

For Reynolds numbers less than 2100, flow is laminar; for Reynolds numbers greater than 2100, it is turbulent. It should be stressed that this approximation applies only to steady flow in smooth-walled tubes. Any irregularity of the wall (e.g., related to atherosclerotic plaquing), vascular branching, or pulsatility disturbs the laminar flow, leading to flow "separation," vortexes, and turbulence.

Laminar Flow

"Laminar" flow arises from the shearing forces between the outer wall and the fluid, leading to concentric shells or "laminae" with the same velocity. The fluid at the wall has zero velocity; this is known as the *boundary layer.*[5] The fluid in the center has the highest velocity. The velocity profile in laminar flow is given by the following equation:

(EQ. 2)

$$V(r) = V_{max} (1 - r^2/R^2)$$

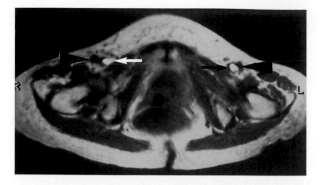

FIGURE 11-1   Flow-related enhancement and high-velocity signal loss. Increased signal in slowly flowing blood in the femoral veins *(arrow)* is caused by unsaturated protons entering the section. The absence of signal from the adjacent femoral arteries *(arrowhead)* reflects a loss of signal as a result of turbulence, dephasing, and high-velocity signal loss (i.e., time-of-flight losses) (SE 500/30).

where
V(r) = Velocity at radial position r (measuring from the center)
V_{max} = Maximum velocity in the center
R = Radius

Equation 2 describes a parabolic velocity profile, as shown in Figure 11-3, *A.* By integrating the velocity over the tube lumen, it can be shown that the average velocity is the highest velocity divided by 2.[5]

Turbulence

Turbulence develops as the velocity increases or flow otherwise becomes disturbed. *Turbulence* is defined as the random motion of fluid elements. "Plug" flow is an idealized type of turbulent flow in which the velocity across the lumen is constant; that is, the velocity profile is flat (Figure 11-3, *B*).

Vascular Flow Characteristics

Arterial flow is regularly irregular, being faster during mechanical systole than during mechanical diastole when flow may be absent or even

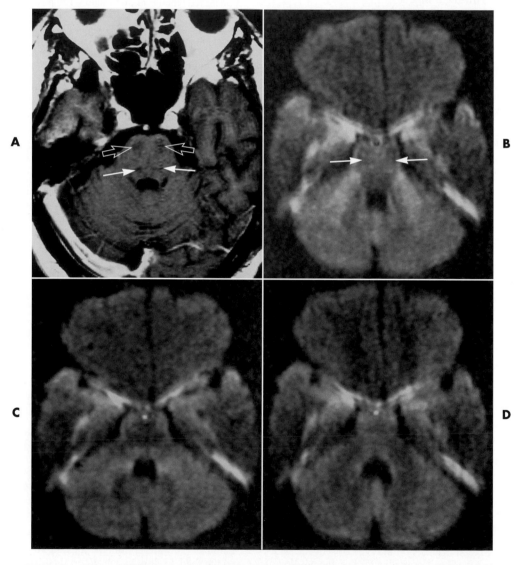

FIGURE 11-2   Effect of diffusion on the signal intensity of corticospinal tracts. T1-weighted axial image **(A)** through the pons demonstrates low signal intensity in the corticospinal tracts *(open arrows)* and medial lemnisci *(arrows).* (Because these tracts are composed of white matter, high signal on a T1-weighted image would be expected.) The observed low signal is caused by diffusion-mediated dephasing along the axons of these fiber tracts. Single-shot diffusion image (b = 1000) with diffusion sensitization through the plane **(B),** from side to side **(C),** and from front to back **(D).** The low signal corresponding to the corticospinal tracts *(arrows)* in **B,** which is not seen in the other two diffusion images, clearly establishes through-plane diffusion as the cause of signal loss on the T1-weighted images.

retrograde. Peak and average velocities for major arteries are shown in Table 11-1. Venous flow tends to be less pulsatile than the flow in arteries, although it is susceptible to respiratory variation and Valsalva maneuvers.

The MR intensity of the blood in arteries reflects its average motion during the cardiac cycle. CSF flow in the brain depends (to a first approximation) on systolic arterial inflow and thus also mirrors flow in arteries. Since most MRI is performed without cardiac gating, the signal intensity of flowing blood or CSF reflects the average motion throughout the cardiac cycle during acquisition of, for example, 512 separate SEs[13] (256 phase steps × 2 excitations). This averaging is weighted by the strength of the phase-encoding gradient for the particular acquisition, weaker gradients contributing more signal than stronger gradients (see Chapter 7).

With vascular stenosis, the velocity is increased. According to the Bernoulli equation,[5] the volumetric flow rate (in milliliters per second) must be the same on both sides of a stenosis (Figure 11-4). The volumetric flow rate is the product of the average velocity (V) and the cross-sectional area (A). Thus for two points (1 and 2) with radii r_1 and r_2 on either side of a stenosis:

(EQ. 3)
$$V_1A_1 = V_2A_2$$

(EQ. 4)
$$V_1r^2_1 = V_2r^2_2$$

Thus if a stenosis halves the radius (which quarters the cross-sectional area), the velocity increases by a factor of 4.

When flowing blood or CSF expands into a larger lumen, a Venturi (nozzle) effect can lead to turbulence downstream and therefore signal loss.[5] When a vessel expands (e.g., poststenotic dilatation), the previously parallel streams separate and vortexes (with reverse flow) may form. This flow separation may be seen, for example, when CSF flows out of the narrow aqueduct into the wider fourth ventricle (Figure 11-5). Expanding flow from the common carotid artery into the larger

Table 11-1   Peak Velocities in Arteries

ARTERY	PEAK VELOCITY (CM/SEC)
Aorta	140 ± 40
External iliac	119 ± 21
Common femoral	114 ± 24
Superficial femoral	90 ± 13
Popliteal	69 ± 13
Common carotid	100 ± 20
Internal carotid	100 ± 20
Vertebral*	36 ± 9
Basilar*	42 ± 10

Data from DeWitt LD, and Wechsler LR: Transcranial Doppler, Stroke 19(7):915, 1988.
*Data from Jager, Ricketts, and Strandness DE Jr: Duplex scanning for the evaluation of lower limb arterial disease. In Bernstein EF, ed: Noninvasive diagnostic techniques in vascular disease, St Louis, 1985, Mosby.

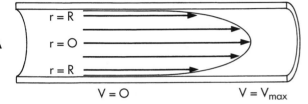
Laminar flow generating parabolic profile
$$V = V_{max}(1-r^2/R^2)$$
$$V_{ave} = V_{max}/2$$

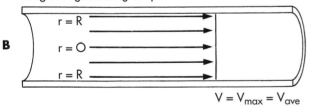
Plug flow generating flat profile

FIGURE 11-3   Flow profiles. **A,** Parabolic flow profile seen in laminar flow. The maximum velocity occurs in the center of the stream. The velocity is zero at the boundary with the vascular wall. **B,** Flat flow profile caused by rapid plug flow. In this idealized circumstance, all fluid elements move at the same velocity.

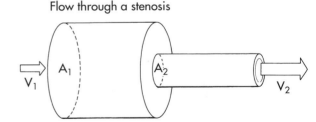
Flow through a stenosis
Bernoulli equation: $A_1V_1 = A_2V_2$

FIGURE 11-4   The Bernoulli relationship. According to the Bernoulli equation, volumetric flow (in cubic centimeters per second) must be the same at all positions in a vessel of variable diameter. The volumetric flow rate is the product of the linear velocity (in centimeters per second) and the cross-sectional area of the vessel (in squared centimeters). Thus the velocity in the larger-diameter portion of the tube (V_1) is lower than the velocity in the smaller-diameter portion of the tube (V_2).

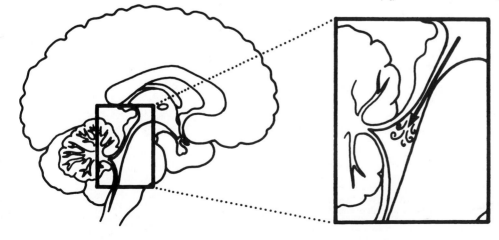

FIGURE 11-5   CSF flow through the aqueduct and the upper fourth ventricle. The velocity of CSF pulsating through the aqueduct is higher than elsewhere in the ventricular system because of the smaller cross-sectional area. As the CSF stream expands into the upper fourth ventricle, turbulence occurs because of a Venturi (nozzle) effect.

carotid bulb is also characterized by flow separation and vortex formation (Figure 11-6), which may lead to signal loss on conventional MR
images as well as on MR angiograms.

NORMAL APPEARANCE OF FLOWING BLOOD

The appearance of flowing blood can be discussed on the basis of a signal increase or decrease. Three independent factors result in decreased
signal intensity of flowing blood: high velocity, turbulence,[12] and dephasing.[61,62] These collectively lead to the flow void (i.e., signal loss

caused by rapid flow), which permits normal vessels (Figure 11-7) and
vascular malformations (Figure 11-8) to be identified. Similarly, lack of
an expected flow void may be indicative of slow flow or thrombosis.

Three independent factors also result in increased signal intensity:
flow-related enhancement (FRE),[11] even-echo rephasing,[63] and diastolic
pseudogating.[11] These phenomena result in increased signal that can be
mistaken for pathological conditions. Although these phenomena are
independent and are described separately, in practice they are almost
always found in various combinations.

The appearance of flowing blood or CSF can also be discussed on

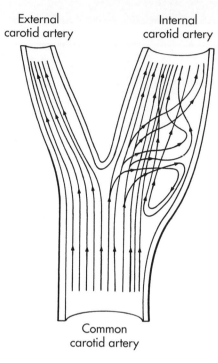

FIGURE 11-6   Flow separation at the carotid bifurcation. The flow-separation
zone and reverse flow are noted at the carotid bulb. This complex motion can result in signal loss on routine MR images and MR angiograms. (Modified from
Motomiya M, Karino T: Flow patterns in the human carotid artery bifurcation, stroke 15:50,
1984.)

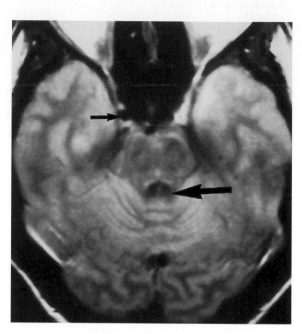

FIGURE 11-7   Flow voids. Proton density–weighted axial section through the
cavernous sinus demonstrates a normal flow void in the patent right internal
carotid *(small arrow)* and in the upper fourth ventricle *(large arrow)* caused by
the rapid motion of blood and CSF, respectively. No flow is seen in the thrombosed left internal carotid artery (SE 3000/22).

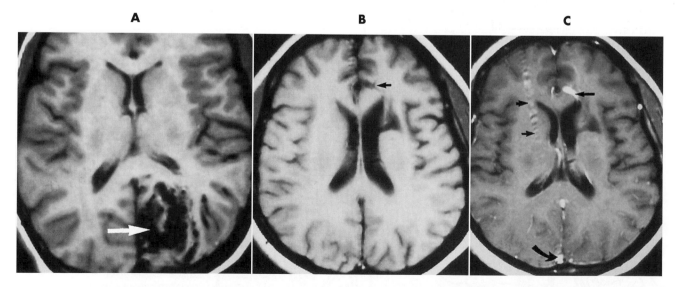

FIGURE 11-8   Vascular malformations. **A,** Axial section demonstrates characteristic arterial and venous flow
voids in an arteriovenous malformation *(arrow)* on this T1-weighted image (SE 600/15). **B,** Abnormal flow void
noted in a venous angioma anterior to the left frontal horn *(arrow)* (SE 600/15). **C,** After the administration of
gadolinium, the slowly flowing blood in the venous angioma enhances *(larger arrow),* but the more rapidly flowing blood in the pericallosal artery just medial to it does not. Note the increased flow artifacts *(smaller arrows)* arising from the torcular Herophili *(curved arrow)* as a result of contrast enhancement on this non–flow-compensated
image (SE 600/15).

the basis of the various flow phenomena involved.[11] Most flow effects are derived from the influence of simple motion (i.e., so-called time-of-flight [TOF] effects) and motion-induced phase changes on the signal intensity of the stagnant fluid. TOF effects can lead to signal loss (high-velocity signal loss or TOF losses) or signal gain (FRE or entry phenomenon). Motion-induced phase changes can be reversible (first-echo dephasing and even-echo rephasing) or irreversible (turbulence). Increased signal can also be seen in unclotted blood if it is stagnant or if it is just not moving at the time of acquisition (see later discussion of diastolic pseudogating).

High-Velocity Signal Loss

Producing a conventional SE signal involves exposing a group of protons to both 90- and 180-degree radiofrequency (RF) pulses. In the multislice techniques typically used today, these pulses are slice selective; that is, only the protons in a well-defined slice are exposed to the RF pulses. High-velocity or TOF loss[11] (Figure 11-9) occurs when protons do not remain within the selected slice long enough to acquire the 90- and 180-degree pulses required to form a conventional SE. Similarly, some signal is lost in an FSE image if the individual spins are not exposed to all the 180-degree pulses in the echo train. This is difficult to demonstrate in practice, however, because of the even-echo rephasing effects of those 180-degree pulses (see following text).

The magnitude of the high-velocity signal loss is a linear function of velocity (Figure 11-10) and reflects the relative proportions of two populations of protons: those that are within the slice for the appropriate RF pulses and those that are not.[12] The latter can be further divided into protons that flow into the upstream side of the slice (not having been exposed to the initial 90-degree pulse) and those that flow out of the slice before the 180-degree pulse. The time between these two pulses is called the *interpulse interval (TE/2)*. If one follows the course of all protons that were in the slice at the time of the initial 90-degree pulse, each will have moved a distance *(V[TE/2])* during time *TE/2*. Those protons moving a distance equal to one slice thickness *(Δz)* or more will return no signal. The fraction of protons that are exposed to the initial 90-degree pulse and then flow out of the slice is expressed as follows:

(EQ. 5)

$$\frac{V(TE/2)}{\Delta z}$$

The fraction of protons that remain within the slice until the next 180-degree pulse is:

(EQ. 6)

$$1 - \frac{V(TE/2)}{\Delta z}$$

Because the MR signal is proportional to the number of protons remaining within the slice, it is also proportional to this ratio. For velocities greater than 2Δz/TE, the signal intensity is zero. Also, protons leaving the slice after the 180-degree pulse still return a signal as if they were within the slice at the time of the SE (unless further activation of the slice-select gradient occurs). In Figure 11-10, theoretical MR signal intensity is plotted as a function of velocity.

Turbulence

High velocity and *turbulence* are not equivalent terms. Laminar flow can be maintained at high velocity in small-diameter tubes.[5] On the other hand, turbulence can occur at low velocities in larger-diameter tubes. Turbulence is present when randomly fluctuating velocity components are found in both the axial and the nonaxial directions[12] (Figure 11-11). This random motion produces dephasing and thus signal loss.

The velocity profile (the variation in velocity across the vessel) is flatter for plug flow (which is an idealized form of turbulent flow) than for laminar flow where the velocity profile is parabolic[5] (Figure 11-3). Several flow regions can be defined for flow rates in transition between laminar flow and turbulent flow in a tube[12] (Figure 11-12). Fully developed turbulence is present in the central core. Laminar flow is present in a thin sublayer at the boundary with the tube. In between, a buffer zone separates the turbulent core from the laminar sublayer. Curiously, the magnitude of the randomly fluctuating velocity components—the intensity of turbulence—is greatest in this buffer zone.[14]

As an approximation, the onset of turbulence can be predicted by use of Reynolds number.[5] For Reynolds numbers less than 2100, laminar flow is generally present; for numbers greater than 2100, turbulent

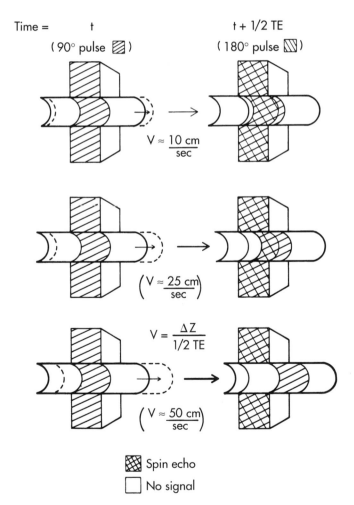

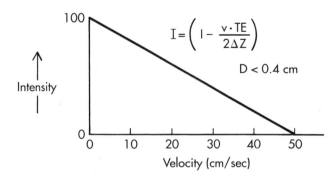

FIGURE 11-9 High-velocity (TOF) signal loss. Protons must acquire both 90- and 180-degree pulses to generate SE *(crosshatch)*. Protons that acquire the 90-degree pulse and then leave the section before acquiring the 180-degree pulse emit no signal. Protons flowing into the section after the selective 90-degree pulse also emit no signal.

FIGURE 11-10 High-velocity signal loss. The predicted intraluminal intensity *(I)* is plotted as a function of velocity *(v)*. This figure illustrates the linear relationship predicted between signal intensity and velocity for a fixed slice thickness (Δz = 7 mm) and echo-delay time (TE = 28 ms), ignoring dephasing effects and turbulence.

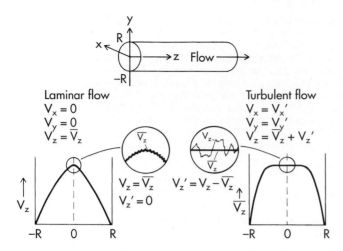

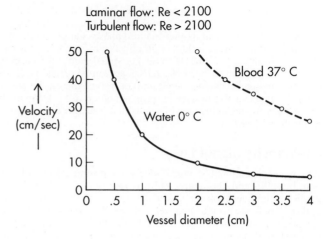

FIGURE 11-11   Comparison of laminar and turbulent flow. For flow in a tube of radius R in the axial *z* direction, the velocity components in the nonaxial directions (V_x and V_y) are zero during laminar flow. Actual velocity in the axial direction (V_z) is equal to the time-smoothed mean ($\overline{V}_z$). In turbulent flow, fluctuating velocity components are present (indicated by superscript primes [e.g., V'_x]).

FIGURE 11-13   Reynolds relationship (see also Equation 1) is shown and the velocity of the onset of the turbulence is plotted for different vascular diameters for blood and water. Velocities below the curve represent laminar flow, whereas those above are turbulent. Note that turbulence occurs at lower velocities in larger-diameter vessels and that blood, with its greater viscosity, can maintain laminar flow at higher velocities than water.

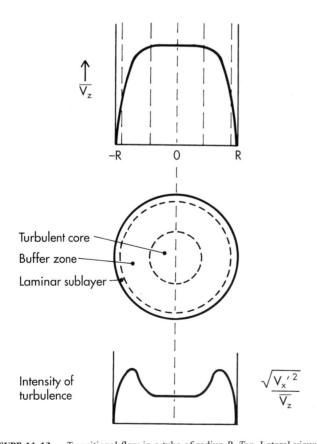

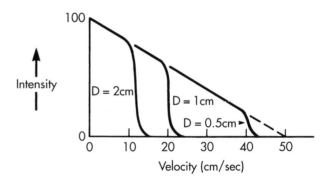

FIGURE 11-14   Additive effects of turbulence and high-velocity signal loss. Loss of signal intensity in addition to that caused by TOF effects is noted because of the onset of turbulence. Note that turbulence (and therefore signal loss) occurs at lower velocities for larger-diameter vessels, whereas laminar flow is maintained at higher velocities for smaller-diameter vessels. *D,* Tube diameter.

FIGURE 11-12   Transitional flow in a tube of radius *R. Top,* Lateral view: A flattened flow profile of the time-smoothed mean velocity ($\overline{V}_z$) is shown. *Middle,* Axial view: The turbulent core, buffer zone, and laminar sublayer are demonstrated. *Bottom,* Lateral projection: The intensity of the turbulence is plotted as a function of the radial position. The magnitude of the fluctuating velocity component, $\dfrac{\sqrt{V'^2_x}}{\overline{V}_z}$ (i.e., intensity of turbulence), is greatest in the transitional (buffer) zone.

flow is present. The lowest velocity at which turbulence occurs is plotted as a function of vessel diameter in Figure 11-13 for water and blood. It should be emphasized that this is an approximation and applies only to steady flow in smooth-walled tubes that do not branch.[5,12] Endothelial roughening caused by atherosclerosis, vascular branching, and the acceleration and deceleration that accompany pulsatile flow all contribute to turbulent or disturbed flow in arteries at velocities lower than predicted by the Reynolds number.[48] When the effect of turbulence is added to the signal loss expected from high velocity, the flow void is seen earlier for larger-diameter vessels[5,12] (Figure 11-14). The Reynolds relationship may have clinical relevance for certain classes of patients (e.g., those with sickle cell anemia). When patients with sickle cell anemia are first admitted in crisis, they are often anemic with low blood viscosity and elevated Reynolds numbers. This may lead to turbulence and signal loss in areas of curved flow (i.e., the carotid siphons) on MR angiograms. Turbulence in turn leads to signal loss and apparent stenosis in these known target areas for intimal hyperplasia.[6,43] Thus anemia per se can lead to pseudostenosis in the distal internal carotid arteries (Figure 11-15) as a result of the decreased viscosity and increased velocity that increase turbulence.[24]

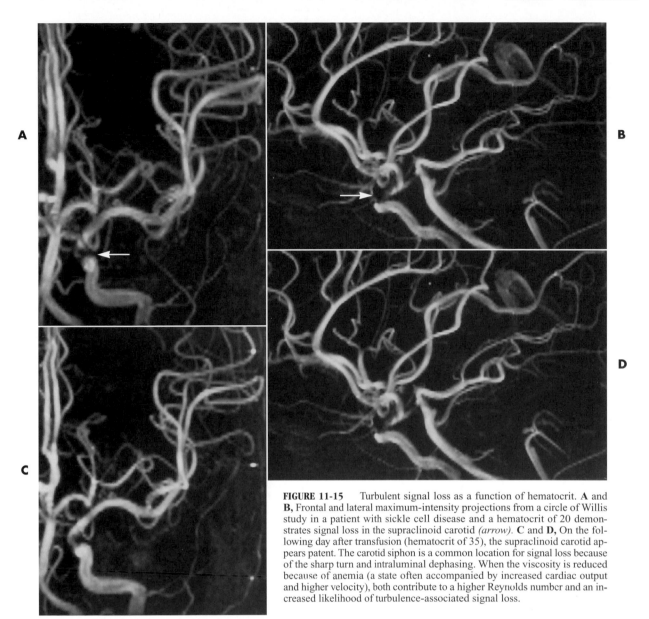

FIGURE 11-15   Turbulent signal loss as a function of hematocrit. **A** and **B,** Frontal and lateral maximum-intensity projections from a circle of Willis study in a patient with sickle cell disease and a hematocrit of 20 demonstrates signal loss in the supraclinoid carotid *(arrow).* **C** and **D,** On the following day after transfusion (hematocrit of 35), the supraclinoid carotid appears patent. The carotid siphon is a common location for signal loss because of the sharp turn and intraluminal dephasing. When the viscosity is reduced because of anemia (a state often accompanied by increased cardiac output and higher velocity), both contribute to a higher Reynolds number and an increased likelihood of turbulence-associated signal loss.

Dephasing

Laminar flow into a magnetic field gradient produces dephasing and therefore signal loss on the first and any other odd echoes in a multi-echo train.[61-63] Dephasing results when all the protons in the voxel do not move at the same velocity through a magnetic field gradient and thus precess at different frequencies and accumulate different amounts of phase. To the extent that they are out of phase at the time of the SE, signal is lost. The steeper the parabolic velocity profile (the greater the differences in velocity across the vessel) and the stronger the gradient, the greater the amount of dephasing.[61,64] Since the strength of the gradient is weaker when it is used for slice selection than for readout or phase encoding, less dephasing occurs for flow perpendicular to the plane than for flow within the plane. If laminar flow is steady and continues until a second echo is acquired, the dephasing seen on the first echo can be reconstituted on the second echo (see section on even-echo rephasing). When multiple echoes are acquired in a conventional or FSE train,[16] all the odd echoes will have decreased signal intensity (because of dephasing), whereas the even echoes will have increased intensity (because of even-echo rephasing). To understand the dephasing-rephasing phenomenon seen in laminar flow, a review of the mechanism of traditional SE formation is required.

Figure 11-16 is a schematic of the Carr-Purcell-Meiboom-Gill SE sequence.[16,33] Consider a hypothetical, microscopic group of protons that travel as a group and experience essentially the same magnetic field. Because they remain in phase, they are called *isochromats.*[33,34,59,63] After the 90-degree pulse, isochromats begin to get out of phase as a result of magnetic field nonuniformities. Isochromats in a slightly stronger part of the field precess at a higher frequency and tend to gain phase relative to those in weaker parts of the magnetic field. This results in flaring of the magnetization vectors in the rotating reference frame shown in Figure 11-16. The longer the time after the 90-degree pulse, the greater the relative phase accumulation by the more rapidly precessing protons.

After a 180-degree rotation about the *y* axis, dephased isochromats are flipped so that those which previously led now lag. Since they remain in a slightly stronger part of the magnetic field, however, they continue to precess at the higher frequency and eventually catch up to their more slowly precessing counterparts to generate an SE.[33]

The same phenomenon can be demonstrated by a spin-phase graph.[59] As shown in Figure 11-17, isochromats in a stronger part of the field gain phase until the 180-degree pulse. At this time, their phase is reversed, and they suddenly lose exactly the amount of phase they had just

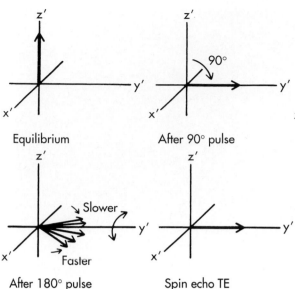

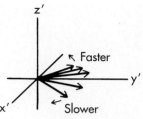

Equilibrium

After 90° pulse

After interpulse interval TE /2

After 180° pulse

Spin echo TE

FIGURE 11-16   Carr-Purcell-Meiboom-Gill SE sequence. In a rotating reference frame (indicated by primed axes), magnetization *(solid arrow)* is rotated into the x'-y' plane by a 90-degree RF pulse. Dephasing causes flaring of the magnetization because some protons precess faster and some slower than average because of relatively stronger and weaker local magnetic fields. After time TE/2, a 180-degree pulse is applied, causing rotation about the y' axis, and the flared magnetization vectors begin to rephase. At TE, rephasing is complete, and coherent SE is emitted.

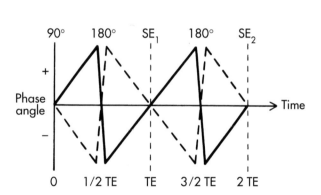

FIGURE 11-17   Spin-phase graph. Phase is either lost or gained relative to the average precessional frequency by protons in weaker and stronger parts of the magnetic field. The sign of the phase is reversed by each 180-degree pulse at 1/2 TE and 3/2 TE. Coherence is reestablished at the time of each SE.

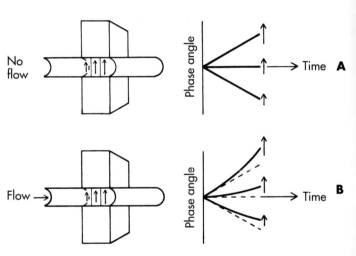

FIGURE 11-18   Accelerated phase gain caused by flow into an increasing magnetic field gradient. When a magnetic field gradient is present without flow **(A)**, phase accumulation occurs as it would in any other nonuniform magnetic field. When blood flows into this increasing magnetic field gradient **(B)**, phase is gained more rapidly (i.e., quadratically in time).

gained. They continue to gain or lose phase at the same rate and regain coherence with their more slowly precessing counterparts at the time of the SE. At this time, no difference exists in the phase angle among isochromats in different parts of the voxel. If the isochromats are allowed to again dephase after the first SE, they can again be rephased by a second 180-degree pulse, producing a second SE. Similarly repeated 180-degree pulses result in multiple SEs, producing an echo train.

The spin-phase graph can be used for the study of different types of flow.[59] Two types of gradients across the voxel determine the degree of dephasing that occurs with flow. These are the magnetic field gradient and the velocity gradient.[11,61-63] The strength of the magnetic field gradient encountered depends on the direction of flow. The component of flow into the weaker slice-selecting gradient experiences less dephasing than that into the stronger readout gradient. (The phase-encoding gradient varies from zero to the full strength of the readout gradient, so the dephasing-rephasing will be less than that resulting from flow along the readout gradient.) The velocity gradient across the vessel is zero both in the no-flow situation and in idealized plug flow. In laminar flow, the velocity gradient across the vessel and thus across each voxel spanning the vessel increases as the velocity increases.[5]

Figure 11-18 shows the change in phase angle (relative to that of protons in the main magnetic field) along the leading edge (stronger field) and lagging edge (weaker field) of the voxel.[63] When a magnetic field gradient exists but there is no flow, phase gain or loss relative to the main magnetic field changes linearly with time (Figure 11-18, *A*). Flow into an increasing gradient (Figure 11-18, *B*) increases rate of phase gain, which then becomes quadratic in time; that is, phase is gained in proportion to time squared. The more rapid the flow, the greater the phase gain.

Figure 11-19, *A*, is a spin-phase graph for plug flow during a double-echo sequence. Whereas protons on the leading edge of the voxel (in the stronger part of the field) gain phase more rapidly than those on the lagging edge, the incremental quadratic phase gain is the same at all positions within the voxel because the velocity is the same at all positions across the voxel in plug flow. Although the isochromats do not return to a zero phase angle at the time of the first echo, they do all acquire the same positive phase angle; thus coherence is reestablished. (With magnitude-reconstruction techniques,[46,63] the phase angle per se does not influence signal intensity, since real and imaginary components are combined as a root mean square.)

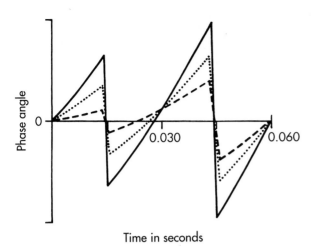

FIGURE 11-19 Computer simulation of plug flow. The phase angle of the isochromats in the stronger half of the field is plotted as a function of time, with SEs occurring at 0.030 and 0.060 sec. The positive phase angle at the time of the first SE is the result of a quadratic phase gain. Complete rephasing is seen to occur for both echoes.

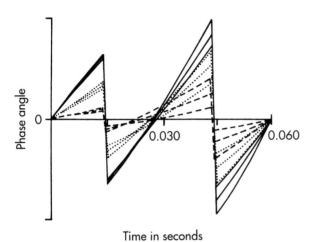

FIGURE 11-20 Computer simulation of laminar flow. The phase angles of the isochromats at different positions in the voxel are plotted as a function of time with SEs occurring at 0.030 and 0.060 sec. Three groups of three curves each are shown. Within each group the isochromats that gain phase most rapidly are in the center of the stream at the highest velocity. The group with solid lines is at the leading edge of the voxel, where the magnetic field is strongest; the dashed line corresponds to spins on the lagging edge of the voxel, where the field is weaker.

In laminar flow the situation is somewhat different (Figure 11-20). The spin-phase graph has three groupings of three curves each.[63] The major groupings reflect a front-to-back position along the slice-select gradient in the vessel. Those acquiring phase most rapidly are on the leading edge of the voxel in the strongest part of the gradient. The three curves within each major grouping reflect the different velocities across the lumen, with the center having the highest velocity and the periphery the lowest. At the time of the first echo, the phase curves do not converge at one point as they did in plug flow but rather spread out and criss-cross as a result of the different phases. This dephasing or loss of phase coherence at the time of the first echo results in signal loss (first-echo dephasing).

Even-Echo Rephasing

As shown in Figure 11-20, the phase curves that had previously spread out (as a result of loss of coherence at the time of the first echo) continue to cross at a point (reestablishing coherence) at the time of the second echo.[63] This rephasing phenomenon reconstitutes the signal that had been lost at the time of the first echo in a manner analogous to the

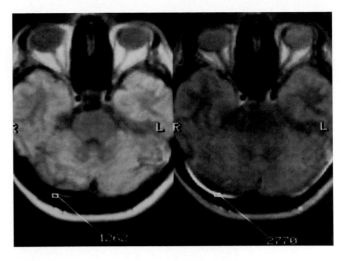

FIGURE 11-21 Even-echo rephasing. High signal is noted within the transverse sinuses *(boxes)* on the second echo image of this symmetrical double-echo acquisition (SE 2000/30 and 2000/60).

rephasing of a free-induction decay as an SE. As has been shown mathematically, the rephasing occurs only for flow of constant velocity into a linear gradient.[63] Thus when higher-order terms are present for either flow (i.e., acceleration, jerk) or the field gradient, complete even-echo rephasing does not occur.

Even-echo rephasing results in higher signal intensity for even echoes compared with the preceding odd echoes.[63] This can be demonstrated in veins,[35] dural sinuses, and large aneurysms[1] with slow (laminar) flow[42] on double-echo acquisitions (Figure 11-21). It is primarily seen on conventional SE images with symmetrical echoes (i.e., those in which the TE of the second echo is twice that of the first[16]) (Figure 11-21). Although it is much weaker, even-echo rephasing can also be seen to an extent in turbulent flow[12] and can be demonstrated mathematically if a gaussian distribution to the random component of motion is assumed.[22,23]

Stagnation

With stagnation the normal flow void is lost and high intraluminal signal can be seen, particularly on long-TR, proton density–weighted, and T2-weighted images (Figure 11-22). Such high signal can simulate an intraluminal mass or thrombus. Flow in the jugular vein can be slowed significantly merely by positioning the patient's head in the RF head coil. Figure 11-22 demonstrates high signal intensity on the first-echo image in an interior slice resulting from positional slowing of drainage through the left jugular vein. The accompanying CT scan and angiogram show no evidence of a pathological condition. Slow drainage through the left jugular vein was noted when the patient was placed in the Townes position for the cerebral angiogram. The patient was in a similar position in the RF head coil at the time of the MR study, resulting in slow flow and high signal in the jugular vein on that side. When confusing signal is found in the jugular vein, compression of the opposite jugular vein should force venous return through the side in question, creating a flow void (Figure 11-23).

Diastolic Pseudogating

The high signal resulting from stagnation can also be seen in arteries under certain conditions.[11] During a given cardiac cycle, flow is alternately rapid (during systole) and slow or absent (during diastole). When MR image acquisition is intentionally gated to the R wave of the electrocardiogram, higher intraluminal signal is observed in arteries during diastole then during systole (Figure 11-24).

It is possible for the cardiac and MR cycles to become synchronized without intentional cardiac gating.[11] For example, if the heart rate is 60 beats/min, a new cardiac cycle is initiated every second. If the TR of the MR imager also is set to 1.0 sec, the cardiac and MR cycles may remain

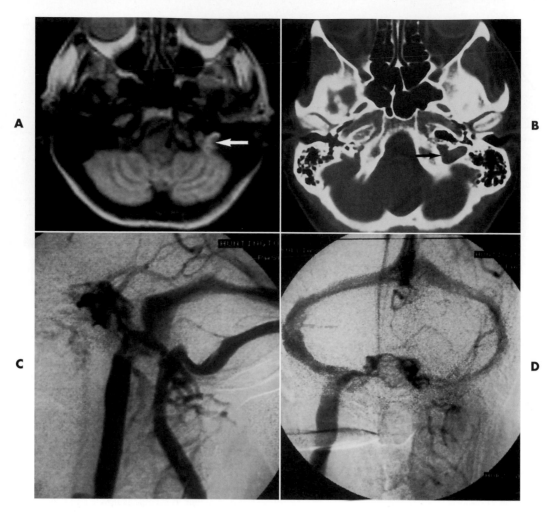

FIGURE 11-22   Positional flow through the left jugular vein. **A,** High signal intensity *(arrow)* is noted within the left jugular bulb in the first-echo image (SE 2000/28) on nonentry slice. In view of the clinical presentation (left-sided tinnitus), a glomus jugulare tumor was suspected. **B,** CT scan with bone windows demonstrates an enlarged jugular bulb with normal cortication *(arrow)* and no evidence of bone destruction to suggest a glomus tumor. **C,** Off-lateral digital subtraction angiography demonstrates a high-riding left jugular bulb. **D,** Slight flexing of the neck for a Townes projection results in marked slowing of flow through the left jugular system. The patient's head was in a similar position at the time of the MR scan. The high signal intensity noted in **A** thus represents positional slowing of venous flow on the left side.

in phase for a 2- to 4-minute acquisition. At a heart rate of 60 beats/min, approximately 30% of the cardiac cycle is spent in systole and 70% in diastole. If 10 slices were acquired during a 1.0-sec TR interval, it would be expected that three slices would show the flow void and seven slices would show higher signal because of the relatively slower flow. This is demonstrated in Figure 11-25. In this flow phantom experiment, the "heart rate" of the blood flow pump was set to 40 beats/min so that a new "cardiac cycle" began every 1.5 sec. The TR of the imager was also set to 1.5 sec, allowing 15 slices to be acquired sequentially. The resultant plot of signal intensity (relative to a stagnant standard) demonstrates high signal on the entry slices (see the section on FRE) and a central peak caused by diastolic pseudogating. The maximal signal resulting from diastolic pseudogating alone should not exceed that expected for stagnant, unclotted blood. Whenever signal higher than this is seen, it reflects the additional presence of a separate flow phenomenon such as FRE.

The position of the high-intensity slice in Figure 11-25 depends on the phase relationship between the cycles of the blood flow pump and the MR imager. Thus if the pump is started a few milliseconds later (relative to the initiation of the MR sequence), the peak would be shifted downstream (to the right). When the R-R interval is half the TR, it is possible to obtain *two* high-intensity peaks corresponding to diastolic acquisition at two regions within the imaging volume. This rep-

resents a beat frequency between the two cyclical processes. For example, if the heart rate had been 80 instead of 40 beats/min for the TR 1.5-sec acquisition in Figure 11-25, there would have been two peaks instead of one.

Whenever diastolic pseudogating is observed within an artery, the high signal may be mistaken for thrombus or tumor. In such cases, the study should be repeated with cardiac gating, and the patient should be positioned so that the slice in question is in the interior of the imaging volume rather than near an entry surface. If high signal is still seen on slices acquired with an R-delay corresponding to cardiac systole, then a lesion is truly present.[7]

Flow-Related Enhancement

When evaluating flow effects, it is important to remember that blood can become magnetized anywhere within the bore of the magnet, whereas imaging is performed only in the homogeneous region in the center of the magnet. This is where the RF coil is positioned both to selectively excite protons within a thin slice and to subsequently detect the SE signal emanating from that slice.

When slowly flowing blood enters the first slice of a multislice imaging volume, partially saturated (demagnetized) blood remaining from the previous sequence is replaced by totally unsaturated blood

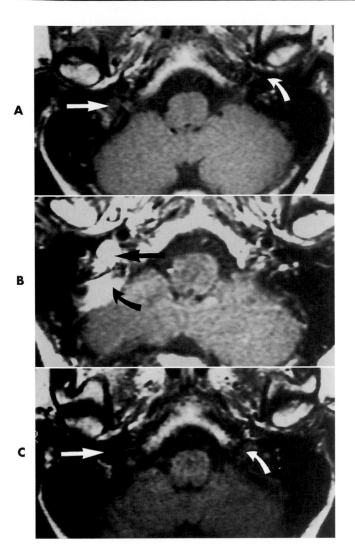

FIGURE 11-23   Contralateral jugular-compression maneuver. **A,** Intermediate signal intensity is noted in the expected position of the right jugular bulb (straight arrow) on this T1-weighted image as opposed to normal jugular flow void on the left (curved arrow) (SE 500/20). The patient had a known acoustic schwannoma (not shown) and this finding raised the question of an additional glossopharyngeal schwannoma. **B,** After the administration of gadolinium, high signal intensity is noted in the right sigmoid sinus *(curved arrow)* and jugular bulb *(straight arrow)*. It could not be determined whether this was slow flow enhancement caused by the gadolinium or an enhancing tumor. For this reason, the jugular-compression maneuver was implemented (SE 500/20). **C,** After mild compression of the left jugular vein, greater flow is diverted through the right jugular system, increasing the velocity and flow void *(arrow)*. Note increased signal *(curved arrow)* on compressed left side (SE 500/20). This was considerd evidence of slow blood flow; thus no other procedure was performed. (Courtesy R.B. Dietrich, Irvine, California).

(Figure 11-26). The strong signal elicited from unsaturated intraluminal blood reflects full magnetization, whereas the adjacent stationary tissue remains partially saturated to a degree depending on its own T1 and the selected TR. This is known as *flow-related enhancement (FRE)11* or *entry phenomenon*.

The signal elicited from the vessel in the entry slice comes from two populations of protons: a strong signal arising from the unsaturated, fully magnetized, upstream (inflowing) protons and a weaker signal arising from the protons in the downstream portion of the voxel that were within the slice at the time of the previous excitation (and are thus still partially saturated). The intraluminal signal is greatest at the velocity at which all the blood in the slice is just replaced in the interval (TR) between excitations.[11] This occurs at velocity V as follows:

(EQ. 7)

$$V = \Delta z / TR$$

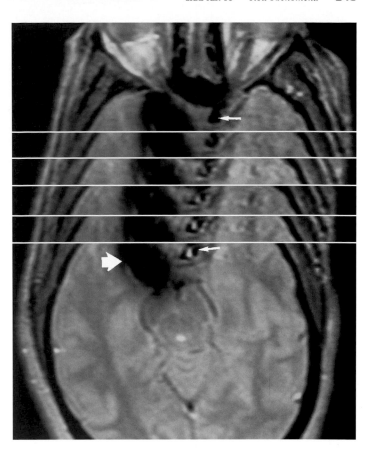

FIGURE 11-24   Diastolic pseudogating. Collage of multiple cardiac-gated images acquired throughout the cardiac cycle with R-delays of 300, 400, 500, 600, 700, and 750 ms. Note the metallic artifact from a previously clipped aneurysm *(large arrow)* in the right supraclinoid carotid as well as variable signal intensity in a newly diagnosed aneurysm *(small arrows)* in the left internal carotid artery resulting from variations in arterial velocity during the cardiac cycle. If the cardiac and MR cycles become unintentionally synchronized ("pseudogating") at one of these later R-delays during diastole, high intraluminal signal would result.

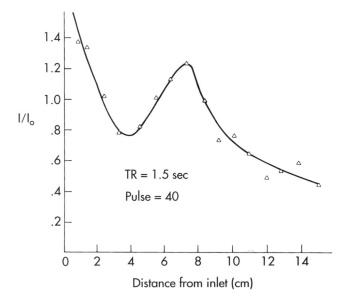

FIGURE 11-25   Diastolic pseudogating. Intensity profile in pulsatile flow phantom. The ratio of flowing to stationary water (I/I_0) is plotted as a function of the distance from the entry surface for a 15-slice acquisition. The increased intensity near the inlet is caused by FRE. The central peak is caused by acquisition during slower diastolic flow. Note that the intensity (I) of the peak is actually greater than that of the stagnant standard (I_o). This represents a breakthrough of flow-related enhancement.

Time =   t   t + TE

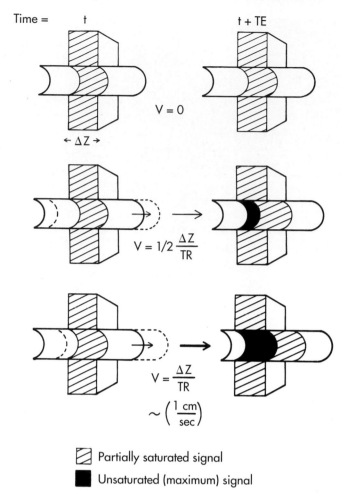

$V = 0$

$V = 1/2 \dfrac{\Delta Z}{TR}$

$V = \dfrac{\Delta Z}{TR}$

$\sim \left(\dfrac{1 \text{ cm}}{\text{sec}} \right)$

▨ Partially saturated signal

■ Unsaturated (maximum) signal

FIGURE 11-26   FRE. Under conditions of slow flow, unsaturated protons enter the section with full magnetization and emit a stronger signal than protons in the adjacent, partially saturated, stationary tissue. Maximal effect occurs when velocity *(v)* equals section thickness *(Δz)* divided by TR.

For example, if the slice thickness *(Δz)* is 1 cm and the TR is 1 sec, this corresponds to a velocity of 1 cm/sec (i.e., that typically seen in veins).

FRE is seen routinely during clinical MR imaging.[37] Figure 11-1 demonstrates FRE in the slowly flowing femoral veins, whereas signal from the adjacent rapidly flowing femoral arteries is absent. Figure 11-27 shows the lowest slices of a multislice imaging volume, which are the first sections encountered by the blood flowing cephalad in the inferior vena cava. When the inflowing protons are exposed to their first 90-degree RF pulse, they return the strongest signal (Figure 11-26). Exposure to subsequent 90-degree pulses deeper within the imaging volume elicits weaker signal (Figure 11-27), the maximal strength of which depends on the interval between excitations and the amount of recovery of longitudinal magnetization that has occurred (reflecting the T1 value of the unclotted blood).

When flow occurs at the velocity shown in Equation 7, maximal FRE is noted in the entry slice. The degree of relative enhancement of the inflowing blood also reflects the limited longitudinal recovery of the adjacent stationary tissue. FRE is thus more pronounced at shorter TRs on T1-weighted images. This is true for the entry slice of both two-dimensional (2D) (Figure 11-27) and 3D (Figure 11-28) acquisitions. The effect is also greater for stationary tissues with longer T1 relaxation times.[11] Equation 7 indicates that maximal FRE for short TRs occurs at higher velocities.

If the inflowing blood is able to avoid exposure to the 90-degree pulse in the first slice, it retains its full magnetization until it arrives at an inner slice, providing FRE deeper in the imaging volume (Figure 11-29). Thus for velocities above Δz/TR, the FRE can be seen in deeper slices.[12] As the velocity increases above the optimum in Equation 7, the FRE should be decreased somewhat in the entry slice as a result of the offsetting losses from increasing TOF effects and dephasing. Although this is certainly true for idealized plug flow in which all fluid elements move at the same velocity, it is less true for laminar flow in which the velocity varies across the vascular lumen. The continued increase in the cross-sectional area of the high-intensity center as the velocity increases reflects the fact that the more peripheral outer lamina reach the optimal velocity for the FRE in the entry slice.

Multislice FRE is illustrated in Figures 11-30 and 11-31. Unsaturated protons project several slices into the imaging volume with a parabolic, laminar flow profile. This appears as a cone as seen in three dimensions. Slicing across the cone produces a series of high-intensity dots in the center of the vessel, larger near the entry surface and smaller deeper in the imaging volume. This pattern of decreasing high-intensity

A   B

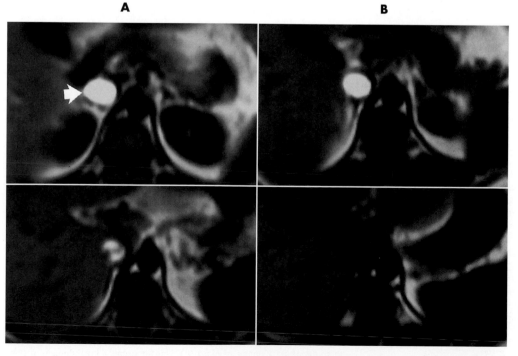

C   D

FIGURE 11-27   FRE. **A,** High signal intensity is noted in the inferior vena cava *(arrow)* in this lowest slice of a multislice imaging volume, which is particularly pronounced on this T1-weighted image (SE 300/10). **B to D,** Progressively lower signal intensity is noted in the inferior vena cava for higher slices, further removed from the entry surface (SE 300/10).

dots is demonstrated in Figure 11-31 in the right common carotid artery of an asymptomatic 30-year-old woman. If she were 80 years old with a right hemispheric infarct, the presence of intraluminal pathology might well be considered. Clearly, normal causes of high intraluminal signal must be excluded before a pathological condition is diagnosed or the patient is subjected to an unnecessary, invasive examination such as a catheter arteriogram.

Familiarity with a few details of the multislice imaging technique is required to understand the mechanism of FRE for slices deep to the entry slice. The 90-degree pulses for a given slice are separated in time by the interval TR. For the imaging volume as a whole, however, 90-degree pulses are applied more frequently, being separated by the interval TR/n between excitation of any number (n) of successive slices (Figure 11-32). For example, if 10 slices are acquired during a TR of 1.0 sec, the interval TR/n is 0.1 sec or 100 ms. In general, the minimum time TR/n required between excitations at successive levels depends on the TE of the last echo acquired, on the echo sampling time, and on the

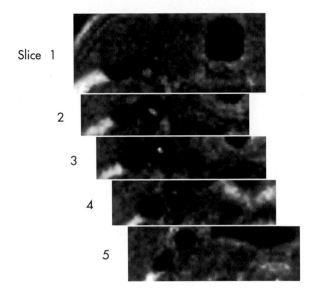

Slice 1
2
3
4
5

TR = 1.5 sec
TE = 28 ms

FIGURE 11-30 Multislice FRE in the right common carotid artery (SE 1500/28, nongated) of an asymptomatic 30-year-old woman. Decreasing intraluminal signal is noted for slices 1 to 5, deeper into the imaging volume and higher in the neck. If this were an 80-year-old patient with a right hemispheric infarct, an intraluminal thrombus or tumor might be considered.

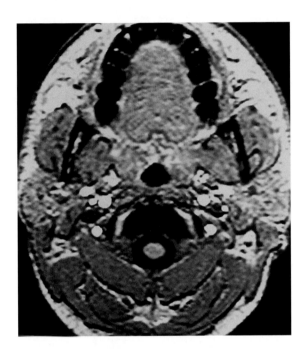

FIGURE 11-28 FRE in the entry slice of 3D acquisition. Enhancement is pronounced because of the marked T1-weighting on this RF-spoiled gradient-echo technique. It is also more pronounced because of the 1.5-mm partition thickness. High signal intensity is noted in all upflowing arteries (gradient-echo 24/9/30 degrees).

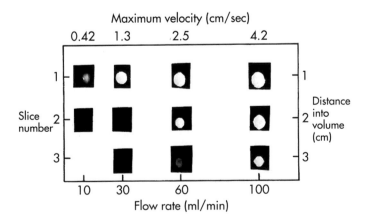

FIGURE 11-29 Multislice FRE. Signal intensities are demonstrated as a function of the volumetric flow rate, calculated maximum velocity, and distance into volume. The highest intensity is seen on the entry slice *(slice number 1)*, with decreasing signal and decreasing cross-sectional area noted on deeper slices (SE 500/28).

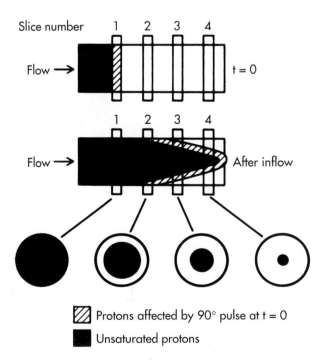

Protons affected by 90° pulse at t = 0
Unsaturated protons

FIGURE 11-31 Multislice FRE. Parabolic laminar flow profile projects several slices into the multislice imaging volume. Seen in three dimensions, the high signal inflowing protons form a cone. Cross sections of laminar profile result in central dots of high intensity caused by unsaturated protons. The dots are smaller deeper into the imaging volume and enlarge to fill the lumen on the entry slice.

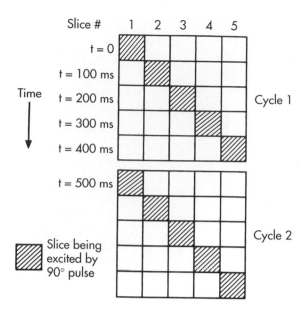

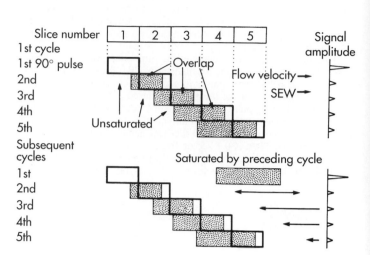

FIGURE 11-32 SEW. Cyclical excitation of consecutive slices is indicated by cross-hatching on two 500-ms TR cycles over two repetition periods. In this example, sequential slices are excited at 100-ms intervals (i.e., TR [500 ms]/5 slices).

FIGURE 11-34 Cocurrent FRE. When flow is in the same direction as the SEW, recently saturated protons (TR/n) flow into next slice to be excited and thus return a weak signal. The fraction of this overlap zone approaches 100% as the velocity of the blood approaches that of the SEW. (From reference 65.)

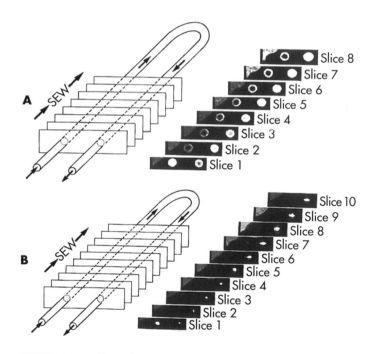

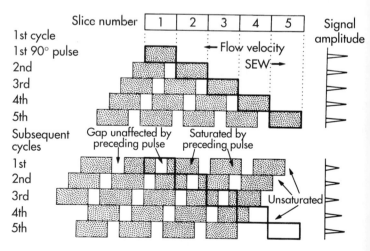

FIGURE 11-33 Comparison of cocurrent and countercurrent FRE. **A,** Low velocity (1 cm/sec). **B,** High velocity (10 cm/sec). Note the deeper penetration into the imaging volume of the unsaturated protons for flow countercurrent to SEW. At higher velocity, FRE is noted only in the center of the stream. Dephasing effects lead to loss of signal in the region of greatest shear (i.e., steepest velocity gradient) toward the periphery.

FIGURE 11-35 Countercurrent FRE. When flow is countercurrent to the SEW, gaps develop that contain protons that have had at least two TR intervals for the recovery of magnetization before flowing into the next slice to be excited. The size of this gap approaches that of the slice as the velocity approaches that of the SEW. The stronger signal from the protons flowing countercurrent (versus cocurrent) to the SEW is caused by the longer time available for longitudinal recovery. (From reference 65.)

dead time needed to allow the coils to "ring down." Excitation generally occurs for consecutive slices (i.e., 1, 2, 3 . . . n), although odd-even excitation (i.e., 1, 3, 5 . . . 2, 4, 6, . . . n) is also commonly used. (For purposes of discussion only consecutive-slice excitation is considered hereafter.)

As illustrated in Figure 11-32, the succession of 90-degree pulses appears as a slice excitation wave (SEW) moving through the imaging volume at a velocity (V_0) of one slice thickness (Δz) per interval TR/n, as follows:

(EQ. 8)

$$V_0 = \Delta z/(TR/n)$$

For example, if consecutive, contiguous 1-cm slices are excited at intervals of 0.1 sec, then the SEW velocity is 10 cm/sec.

Intraluminal signal intensity depends on whether flow is in the same direction as the SEW (i.e., cocurrent) or opposite to it (i.e., countercurrent).[65] As shown in the flow phantom experiments in Figure 11-33,

A   **B**

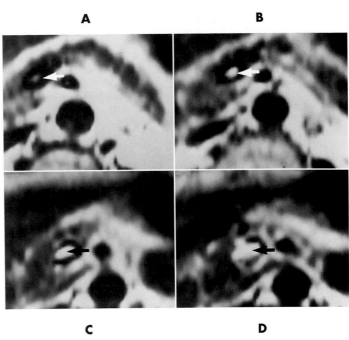

C   **D**

FIGURE 11-37   Countercurrent FRE in the superior mesenteric vein in a 72-year-old woman with abdominal pain referred for MRI to evaluate a "spot" on her pancreas seen on a CT scan. T1-weighted transverse axial sections (**A** to **D**) through the pancreas demonstrate variable signal intensity in the superior mesenteric vein *(arrow)*. On the most caudal section (**D**), upwardly flowing blood in the superior mesenteric vein manifests high signal intensity caused by FRE. On successively higher sections, the high-intensity dot decreases in size with a concomitant increase in the surrounding flow void. On the most cephalic sections (**A** and **B**), this pattern of countercurrent FRE simulates a pancreatic hematoma (SE 264/15).

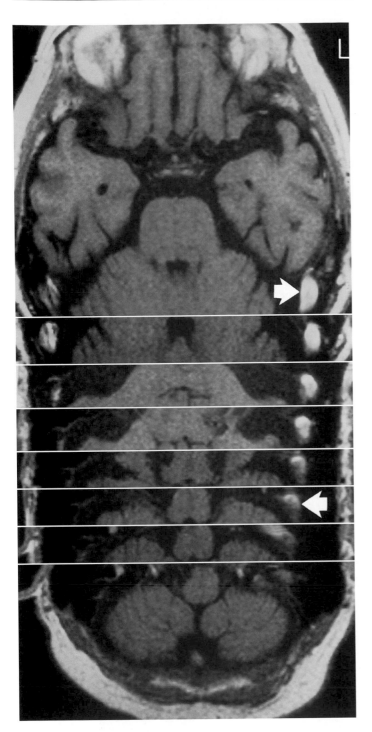

FIGURE 11-36   Countercurrent FRE in the sigmoid sinus. Nine sequential T1-weighted images acquired from bottom to top demonstrate countercurrent FRE in downflowing sigmoid sinuses (left > right) *(arrows)*.

FRE extends much deeper into the imaging volume for flow countercurrent to the SEW than for cocurrent flow. This is true at both low (Figure 11-33, A) and high (Figure 11-33, B) velocities, although the high-intensity dots are smaller with higher velocity as a result of competing dephasing effects.

The explanation for the differences in cocurrent and countercurrent FRE is shown in Figures 11-34 and 11-35.[65] These differences depend on the time available for the recovery of longitudinal relaxation during the time between excitations. When less time is available for recovery

of a significant fraction of the protons in the slice, the signal intensity is relatively decreased. As shown in Figure 11-34, cocurrent flow results in some of the protons in the slice just excited flowing immediately upstream into the next slice to be excited. These protons (indicated by the overlap zone in Figure 11-34) have only had time TR/n to recover magnetization and thus return a relatively weak signal. As the velocity approaches the SEW velocity, all the protons move in sync with the SEW. Thus when they are exposed to the next 90-degree pulse in the next slice time TR/n later, they are still saturated and return a weak signal. At velocities less than the SEW velocity, the percentage of protons remaining in the slice from the previous passage of the SEW increases. These protons have had a longer period of time (TR) to recover and thus return a stronger signal. As the velocity approaches zero, all the protons have had time TR to recover, which of course is the same as the time available for recovery by the stationary protons around the vessel. The actual signal intensity at a particular velocity depends on the relative proportions of these two populations and whether the velocity is closer to zero or to the SEW velocity.

For countercurrent flow, less saturated (or unsaturated) protons flow head-on into the next slice to be excited during the time interval TR/n. As shown in Figure 11-35, this motion produces gaps of less saturated protons that are exactly the same size as the overlap zones for cocurrent flow. These less saturated protons have had more time to recover magnetization since their last exposure to a 90-degree pulse, and thus they return a stronger signal. Therefore the intensity of protons flowing countercurrent to the SEW is always greater than those flowing in the same direction (except for the entry slices, which are the same).[65]

Countercurrent FRE is recognized on multislice acquisitions as high signal extending from the entry slice inward (Figure 11-36) in the direction of decreasing slice number (assuming the slice number reflects the order of slice excitation). Countercurrent FRE can simulate thrombus or hematoma (Figure 11-37).

COMBINED FLOW PHENOMENA

The flow phenomena already discussed often occur in combination and may have an additive or an offsetting effect. As the velocity increases from zero, the FRE initially increases in the slices near the entry surface. At V = Δz/TR, it is maximal in the first slice. As the velocity continues to increase, the FRE will be noted in deeper slices; however, the signal intensity will begin to decrease in the first slice because of offsetting TOF losses and dephasing.[11] Dephasing increases as the velocity increases because of a steepening parabolic velocity profile and a decreasing intravoxel coherence. This tendency toward signal loss partially decreases the signal gain that would have resulted from FRE. If a symmetrical second echo is acquired and laminar flow continues at the same velocity until the second TE, even-echo rephasing will reconstitute the signal loss that had occurred as a result of first-echo dephasing. However, signal loss caused by TOF effects will increase on the second echo image because a longer period is now available for the outflow of spins before exposure to the second 180-degree pulse. (This is because the spins must remain in the slice only for an interval TE/2 to acquire the 90- and 180-degree pulses for the first echo, but they must be in the slice for a period 3TE/2 to acquire the second 180-degree pulse for the second echo.) The signal of the second echo thus reflects offsetting influences: signal gain caused by even-echo rephasing and signal loss caused by increasing TOF losses. For comparable velocities and vascular diameters, decreasing the slice thickness increases the TOF losses, decreasing signal intensity. As the vascular diameter decreases for a given flow rate, the laminar parabolic profile steepens, increasing the dephasing-rephasing effects.

When high signal is seen in an artery, diastolic pseudogating may be present. The high signal noted in the carotid artery in Figure 11-30

probably reflects the influence of both FRE and diastolic pseudogating. Clinically it is important to distinguish flow-related causes of increased signal intensity in an artery from those caused by a tumor or thrombus. Since high signal should be seen in an artery only if diastolic pseudogating is present, the study should be repeated with cardiac gating. If high signal is noted in an interior slice during cardiac systole, flow-related causes of high signal have been excluded.

Flow Artifacts and Flow-Compensation Techniques

Motion artifacts may result from the movement of spins along any magnetic field gradient. Because this motion results in phase gain (or loss), motion artifacts appear only along the phase-encoding axis. (This is related to the fact that position along the readout axis is encoded as a specific frequency, whereas position along the phase axis is encoded as a specific phase.) Any phase shifts related to motion result in mismapping of signal along the phase-encoding axis. If the moving spins have high intensity (e.g., as a result of FRE), the intensity of the artifacts is also increased, producing ghost images of the vascular structure of origin.[49,58] As the flip angle is increased for gradient-echo images, the signal intensity of the ghosts increases (Figure 11-38). Ghosts can be positive or negative, depending on their phase relative to that of the background tissue. Positive ghosts are bright; negative ghosts are dark (Figure 11-39).

If flow is pulsatile, the spacing Δp between the ghosts can be predicted[49] (Figure 11-39):

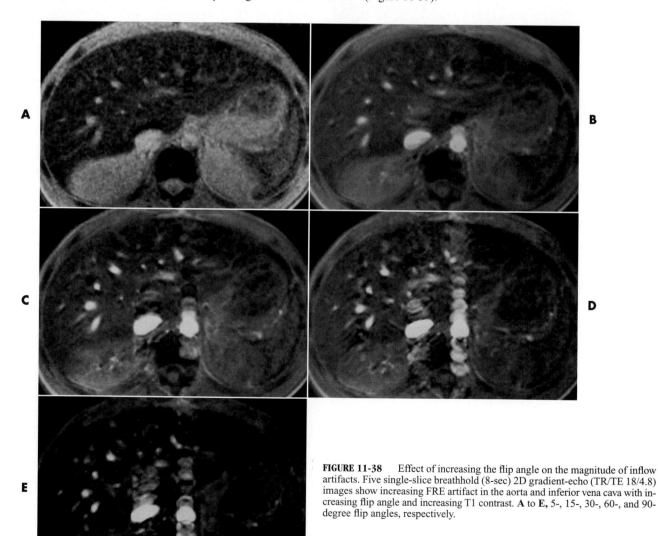

FIGURE 11-38   Effect of increasing the flip angle on the magnitude of inflow artifacts. Five single-slice breathhold (8-sec) 2D gradient-echo (TR/TE 18/4.8) images show increasing FRE artifact in the aorta and inferior vena cava with increasing flip angle and increasing T1 contrast. **A** to **E**, 5-, 15-, 30-, 60-, and 90-degree flip angles, respectively.

(EQ. 9)

$$\Delta p = \frac{TR \times N_p \times N_{ex}}{R \text{ - } R \text{ interval}}$$

where

Δp = Number of pixels separating the ghosts along the phase-encoding axis

N_p = Number of phase-encoding steps

N_{ex} = Number of excitations

R-R interval = Time between heartbeats

Ghosts can be eliminated if the entering spins are first demagnetized or saturated by exposure to a 90-degree pulse before they enter the imaging volume (Figure 11-40, *A*). Such spatial presaturation techniques[31] or *saturation pulses* are particularly effective for eliminating the signal arising from arteries because of their high velocity. They are less effective for eliminating FRE in veins as a result of the slower velocity and additional time available for the recovery of longitudinal magnetization before entry into the imaging volume. Spatial presatu-

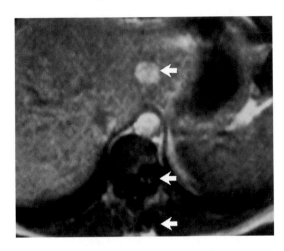

FIGURE 11-39   Ghost artifact caused by pulsatile flow. Ghost images of the aorta *(arrows)* are distributed along the phase-encoding axis, with spacing dependent on the TR, the number of excitations, the number of phase-encoding steps, and the R-R interval. These artifacts tend to be particularly prominent on gadolinium-enhanced images such as this. The lesion in the left lobe of the liver could simulate an enhancing metastasis. The lesion in the vertebral body and left pedicle could simulate a metastasis on an unenhanced image (GRE 100/4/80 degrees).

ration eliminates both FRE and the artifacts arising from it; therefore vessels appear dark (Figure 11-40, *B*).

A second method of eliminating motion artifacts is based on the principle of even-echo rephasing.[63] The signal lost from dephasing on the first echo is not really absent; it is merely mismapped along the phase-encoding axis. The phenomenon of even-echo rephasing replaces the signal arising from spins moving with constant velocity back in the vascular lumen, simultaneously increasing intraluminal signal intensity and decreasing flow artifacts. When extra gradient pulses are added, it is possible to produce the even-echo rephasing effect on the first echo (i.e., to achieve rephasing without the necessity of using a double-echo sequence). These techniques are known generically as *gradient-moment nulling,* although the terms *flow compensation, gradient-motion rephasing,* and *motion-artifact–suppression technique (MAST)* are synonymous[19,26-28,32] (Figures 11-41 and 11-42). The multiple 180-degree pulses in an FSE technique also accomplish natural flow compensation with even-echo rephasing after every pair of 180-degree pulses. This explains the high intravascular signal of FSE images as well as the excellent CSF motion compensation on FSE images acquired through the base of the brain (see Chapter 7).

As shown in Figure 11-41, gradient-moment nulling entails the use of additional gradient pulses so that moving spins have zero phase at the time of the echo. The magnitude, number, and duration of the gradient pulses are adjusted so that spins moving with constant velocity or constant acceleration have zero net-phase gain at the time of the SE. This is known as *first-* and *second-order flow compensation,* respectively. (NOTE: Zero-order motion is stationary, first-order [dx/dt] motion is velocity, second-order motion [d^2x/dt^2] is acceleration, and third-order motion [d^3x/dt^3] is jerk or pulsatility.)

As shown in Figure 11-41, the gradient pulses are balanced so that the area under the gradient versus time curves is equal at the center of the echo sampling time (TE). Thus the spins are not totally in phase during the full echo sampling interval, which is centered at time TE. In Figure 11-41, note that the additional gradient pulses have opposite signs for gradient-echo imaging and the same sign for SE imaging. As reflected in the phase diagrams, this reflects the phase reversal that occurs as a result of the 180-degree pulse in the SE.

Figure 11-42 shows the additional gradient pulses needed for second- and third-order flow compensation, leading to rephasing of spins traveling at constant acceleration and constant jerk (which is the time derivative of acceleration). Each additional order of flow compensation requires additional time for the additional gradient pulses and therefore increases the TE. As shown in Figure 11-42, the gradients can be placed to allow for variable or fixed TE. Balancing the gradient lobes on either side of the 180-degree pulse allows for variable TE. When the

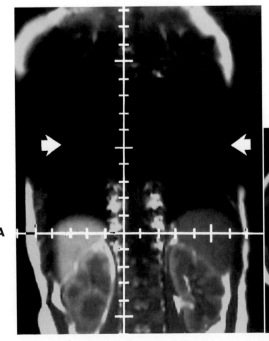

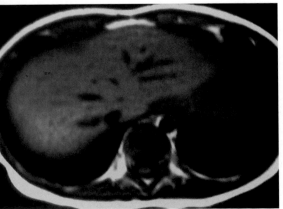

FIGURE 11-40   Presaturation pulse. **A,** Coronal scout view for subsequent axial acquisition demonstrates a saturation band *(arrows)* through the middle of the thorax. **B,** Axial section through the liver demonstrating the lack of flow artifact from the aorta; this image was taken after the saturation pulse indicated in **A** (SE 500/15).

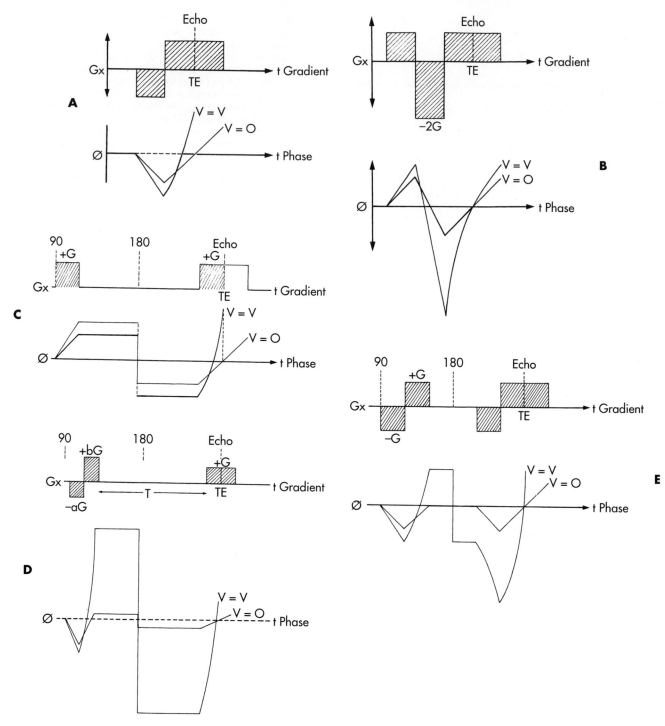

FIGURE 11-41 First-order flow compensation for gradient-echo and SE techniques. **A,** Timing diagram for the readout gradient *(G$_x$)* and associated phase change for stationary tissue and for fluid moving at velocity *V.* Note the positive phase angle at the time TE for the moving fluid on this in flow-compensated gradient-echo technique. **B,** First-order flow compensation for a gradient-echo technique. Note the additional lobes of the readout gradient, resulting in both stationary and flowing material rephasing at TE. **C,** Non–flow-compensated SE. Fluid flowing into an increasing gradient increases phase quadratically in time. At the time of the 180-degree pulse, all phase accumulated is reversed. At the time of the echo TE, fluid moving at velocity *V* has a positive phase angle on this non–flow-compensated SE technique. **D,** SE with first-order (velocity) compensation. The coefficients of the initial gradient pulses *(a* and *b)* are determined by the position of the 180-degree pulse and the time between the gradient pulses *(T).* Note the zero phase angle for moving spins at the midpoint of the echo sampling time (TE). **E,** Velocity-compensated SE with variable TE. Because the gradients are balanced on either side of the 180-degree pulse, time may be added equally on either side of the 180-degree pulse to increase the TE. (Courtesy N. Palmer, Cleveland.)

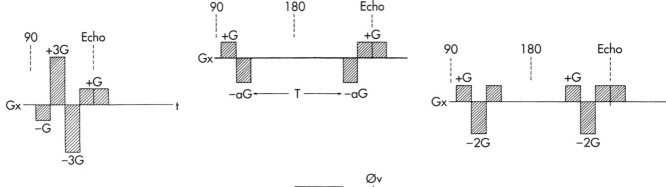

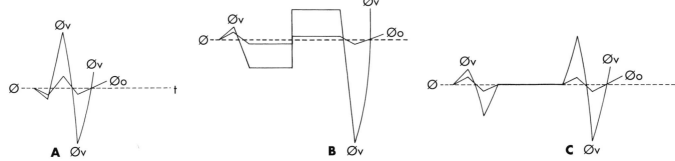

FIGURE 11-42 Second-order (acceleration) flow compensation. **A,** Acceleration-compensated gradient echo. Phase is gained as the third power of time but returns to zero at the time of the echo (TE). **B,** Acceleration-compensated SE. Note the cubic rise or fall in the phase angle with time in relation to acceleration and the complete phase reversal with the 180-degree pulse. At the time of the echo TE, the phase of accelerating spins is zero, indicating flow compensation. With this sequence, the coefficient *a* for the negative gradient lobes is the same for all "T." **C,** SE with third-order flow compensation (or second-order flow compensation with variable TE). Note the symmetry of the gradient lobes on either side of the 180-degree pulse, indicating the potential to vary TE. The phase plots are for constant acceleration, which results in zero phase angle at the time of the echo TE (for both constant acceleration and constant velocity). Whenever there is also zero phase at the time of the 180-degree pulse for the moving spins, the technique is also compensated for the next higher order of motion, in this case, the "jerk." (Courtesy N. Palmer, Cleveland.)

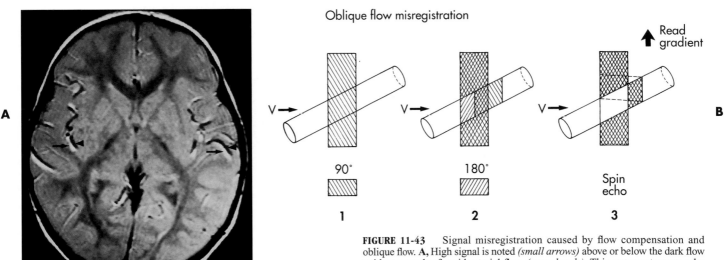

FIGURE 11-43 Signal misregistration caused by flow compensation and oblique flow. **A,** High signal is noted *(small arrows)* above or below the dark flow void as a result of rapid arterial flow *(arrowheads)*. This represents even-echo rephasing from gradient-moment nulling (i.e., flow compensation). The rephased high signal is not perfectly superimposed on the vascular flow void because flow is oblique to the imaging plane and is therefore displaced in the direction of the readout gradient (which is from top to bottom in this image) (SE 3000/22 with flow compensation). **B,** Oblique flow misregistration. Vessel contains blood flowing at velocoity v oblique to an imaging plane. *1,* Diagonal stripes indicate protons within the slice and within the blood vessel excited by the 90-degreee pulse initiating the spin echo. *2,* Protons exposed to the 180-degree pulse are indicated by the opposite diagonal striping. Note that stationary protons are now cross-hatched, indicating that they will give off a spin echo at time TE. At this velocity, approximately half the protons intitially exposed to the 90-degree pulse in *1* have moved out of the slice and therefore will not be exposed to a 180-degree pulse. Similarly, protons that have flowed into the slice during the interval TE/2 between the 90- and 180-degree pulses are only exposed to a 180-degree pulse and will not give off a spin echo. *3,* At the spin echo the protons within the vessel that were within the slice for both the 90- and 180-degree pulses have continued to flow obliquely relative to the imaging plane. These protons are now found in a stronger portion of the readout gradient near the top of the image. They will therefore be misregistered relative to the true lumen along the readout gradient.

phase of spins moving with a certain order of motion is zero at the initiation of the 180-degree pulse, the technique is also compensated for the next higher order of motion. For this reason, the pulsing sequence shown in Figure 11-42, *C,* is both flow compensated for constant acceleration with variable TE and jerk compensated.

Figure 11-43 is an MR image of the brain with first-order (i.e., constant velocity) flow compensation in the readout direction. Similar compensation is commonly performed in the slice-select direction as well. Because gradient-moment nulling recapitulates even-echo rephasing, intravascular signal is increased (Figure 11-43, *A*). To compensate for higher-order motion (e.g., acceleration, jerk), one needs additional gradient pulses. Since these would require additional time, the minimum

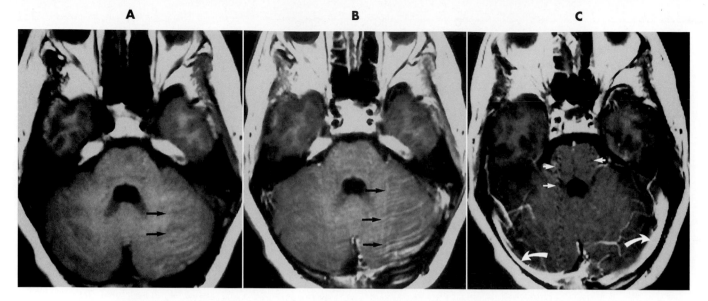

FIGURE 11-44 Use of flow compensation in gadolinium-enhanced imaging of the posterior fossa. **A,** Unenhanced T1-weighted image demonstrates mild artifacts arising from the left transverse sinus *(arrow)* up and down the phase-encoding axis (SE 600/15). **B,** After the administration of gadolinium, the intensity of the artifacts arising from the left transverse sinus increases *(arrows)* (SE 600/15). **C,** When first-order flow compensation is applied in the readout and slice-select directions, high signal remains in the transverse sinuses *(curved arrows),* and flow artifacts are minimized. Note the persistent artifact arising from the internal carotid arteries *(small arrows),* representing uncompensated higher orders of motion associated with pulsatile arterial flow (SE 600/22).

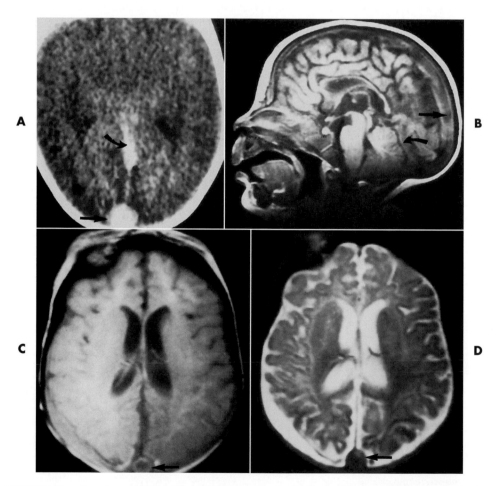

FIGURE 11-45 Superior sagittal sinus thrombosis in a 5-month-old girl. **A,** CT scan demonstrates hyperdensity in the superior sagittal sinus *(straight arrow)* and straight sinus *(curved arrow).* **B,** Midsagittal section demonstrates increased intensity in the superior sagittal sinus *(straight arrow)* and straight sinus *(curved arrow)* (SE 600/25). **C,** Proton density–weighted axial section demonstrates peripheral hyperintensity with central mixed intensity in the superior sagittal sinus *(arrow)* (SE 2600/30). **D,** T2-weighted axial section through the same level as **C** demonstrates markedly decreased signal intensity in the superior sagittal sinus *(arrow)* (SE 2600/30). **D,** T2-weighted axial section through the same level as **C** demonstrates markedly decreased signal intensity in the superior sagittal sinus *(arrow)* (SE 2600/120). These findings indicate that the thrombus is in the acute-early subacute state with intracellular deoxyhemoglobin and methemoglobin. (Courtesy R.B. Dietrich, Irvine, California.)

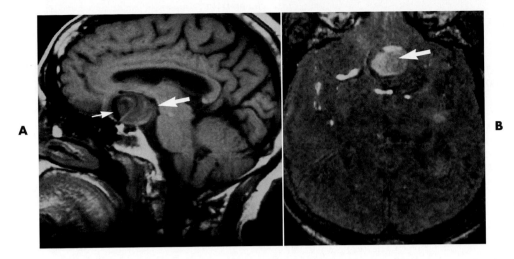

FIGURE 11-46   Slow flow versus thrombus in aneurysm. **A,** T1-weighted sagittal image demonstrates a giant intracranial aneurysm arising from the supraclinoid carotid artery. Note the black jet *(small arrow)* and intermediate signal filling the rest of the aneurysm *(large arrow),* which could represent slow flow or clot. **B,** An axial partition from the MR angiogram demonstrates the high signal in the bulk of the aneurysm *(arrow).* Because any increase in signal over the T1-weighted image in **A** can be related only to flow, this confirms the presence of slow flow rather than thrombosis as the cause of the intermediate signal in **A.**

TE would be increased, increasing the time available for dephasing to occur. Thus there is a tradeoff: Higher-order techniques compensate for additional motion but may lead to additional artifacts because of the longer TE. The author currently uses first-order flow compensation in the readout and slice-select directions on all long-TR conventional SE sequences. As new MR imaging systems with stronger gradients and faster rise times become available, greater flow compensation without undue prolongation of the TE will be possible.

Flow compensation is particularly useful in the posterior fossa when gadolinium is used.[51] Whereas flow artifacts normally arise from the transverse and sigmoid sinuses on unenhanced scans, these are particularly prominent on enhanced images (Figure 11-44). Thus flow compensation should always be used on gadolinium-enhanced T1-weighted images of the posterior fossa.

Cardiac gating is yet another technique for reducing motion artifacts.[29,30] Synchronizing the signal acquisition to a particular phase of the cardiac cycle reduces the view-to-view variation in the phase angle and thereby reduces motion artifacts. Cardiac gating can be performed by electrocardiographic triggering or by triggering from a finger plethysmograph. The primary disadvantage of cardiac gating is the restriction on the TR, which must be a multiple of the R-R interval.

A simple motion artifact is the spatial misregistration that results from flow oblique to the imaging plane.[2] As illustrated in Figure 11-43, *B,* any motion that occurs along the readout axis between the 180-degree pulse (at time TE/2) and the detection of the SE (at time TE) results in misregistration along the readout axis in the direction of flow (Figure 11-43). This effect is most pronounced in techniques that produce high intravascular signal: even-echo rephasing, gradient-moment nulling (flow compensation) (Figure 11-44), and FRE.

Distinguishing Thrombus from Slow Flow

Intermediate to high intraluminal signal on a particular pulse sequence may reflect the presence of thrombus, or it may be caused by slow flow. When high signal is found, normal flow-related causes of increased signal should first be excluded. These include FRE, diastolic pseudogating, and even-echo rephasing. FRE is most prominent for through-plane flow on the entry slice and is usually found in slowly flowing blood in veins. If FRE is found in an inner slice, high signal should be seen (Figure 11-36) in the same vessel on all slices back to the entry surface (countercurrent FRE). FRE is less marked for in-plane flow. Thus if thrombus is suspected, it should be documented on slices both parallel (Figure 11-45) and perpendicular to the vessel in question. If high signal is found in an artery, diastolic pseudogating might be suspected.

Even-echo rephasing is found only on the second-echo (Figure 11-21) or other even-echo images (or composites of even-echo images such as FSE) or if flow compensation has been implemented (Figure 11-43).

If determining the cause of the intraluminal signal—as caused by flow or thrombus from the routine acquisitions—is not possible, then additional MR maneuvers may be necessary. The acquisition of an MR angiographic sequence should provide high intraluminal signal if the vessel is patent because of its inherent tendency to maximize FRE (Figure 11-46). (The only thrombus that might appear as bright as FRE is late subacute hemorrhage, which is also bright on both T1- and T2-weighted images [see Chapter 58].) Comparison of luminal intensity for the same sequence applied in different imaging planes may provide a clue: If the signal changes, it suggests flow; if the signal does not change, it should be thrombus. If a saturation pulse can be applied upstream to the slice in question, the intensity of inflowing blood will decrease. If it is thrombus, it will not be affected. Rewindowing the image by reducing the background subtraction (i.e., the window center) to bring out motion artifacts may provide a clue as to the cause of the intravascular signal. If artifacts are seen along the phase-encoding axis, the signal is related to flow (Figure 11-47); if not, it is thrombus.

CEREBROSPINAL FLUID FLOW

The flow phenomena that influence the intensity of flowing blood also affect the appearance of flowing CSF.* CSF motion reflects the additive effects of slow flow caused by the production of CSF and more rapid flow related to superimposed cardiac pulsations.[4,9,25] The slow flow is caused by the production of CSF by the choroid plexus inside the ventricles at a volume of approximately 500 mm/day. CSF flows through the aqueduct, out the foramina of Luschka and Magendie, through the basal cisterns and spinal subarachnoid space, and eventually over the convexities, where it is absorbed by the arachnoid villi (see Chapter 66).

Superimposed on this slow, steady egress of CSF from the ventricle is a more rapid to-and-fro motion as a result of transmitted cardiac pulsations.[4,9,25] These pulsations arise from the general expansion of the cerebral hemispheres during systole,[8] as well as from the systolic expansion of the choroid plexus.[4] This to-and-fro motion of CSF occurs throughout the ventricles and basal cisterns, but it is most obvious through the narrowest portions of the ventricular system: the foramen of Monro (Figure 11-48) and the aqueduct (Figure 11-49). Pulsatile flow

---

*References 3, 9, 18, 29, 50, 57.

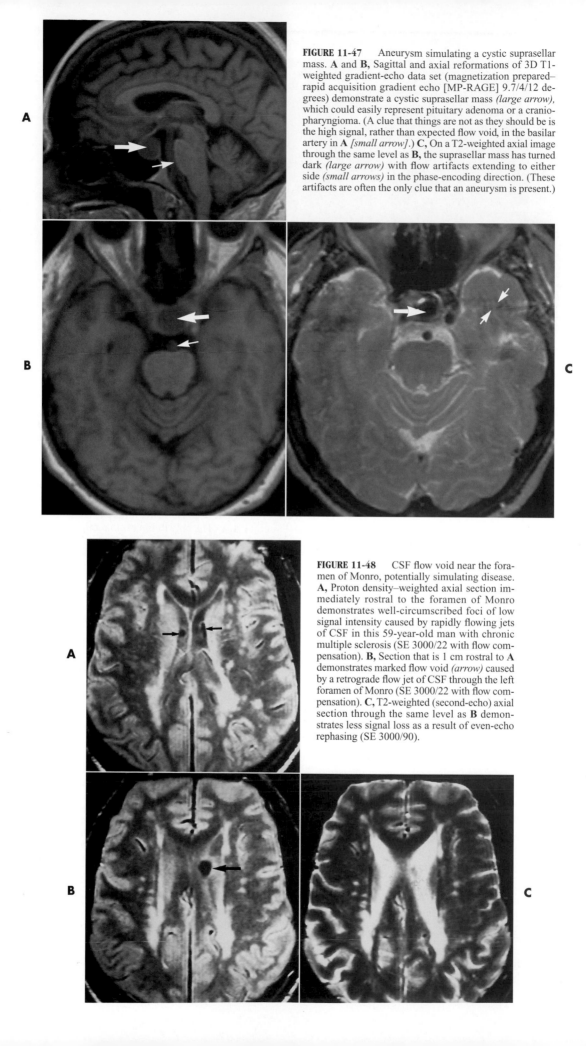

FIGURE 11-47 Aneurysm simulating a cystic suprasellar mass. **A** and **B,** Sagittal and axial reformations of 3D T1-weighted gradient-echo data set (magnetization prepared–rapid acquisition gradient echo [MP-RAGE] 9.7/4/12 degrees) demonstrate a cystic suprasellar mass *(large arrow),* which could easily represent pituitary adenoma or a craniopharyngioma. (A clue that things are not as they should be is the high signal, rather than expected flow void, in the basilar artery in **A** *[small arrow].*) **C,** On a T2-weighted axial image through the same level as **B,** the suprasellar mass has turned dark *(large arrow)* with flow artifacts extending to either side *(small arrows)* in the phase-encoding direction. (These artifacts are often the only clue that an aneurysm is present.)

FIGURE 11-48 CSF flow void near the foramen of Monro, potentially simulating disease. **A,** Proton density–weighted axial section immediately rostral to the foramen of Monro demonstrates well-circumscribed foci of low signal intensity caused by rapidly flowing jets of CSF in this 59-year-old man with chronic multiple sclerosis (SE 3000/22 with flow compensation). **B,** Section that is 1 cm rostral to **A** demonstrates marked flow void *(arrow)* caused by a retrograde flow jet of CSF through the left foramen of Monro (SE 3000/22 with flow compensation). **C,** T2-weighted (second-echo) axial section through the same level as **B** demonstrates less signal loss as a result of even-echo rephasing (SE 3000/90).

A   **B**   **C**

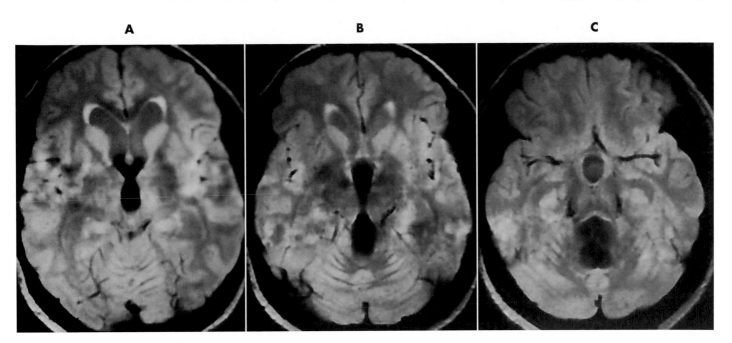

FIGURE 11-49   Marked CSF flow voids in a patient with chronic communicating hydrocephalus. **A,** Axial section through the foramen of Monro. **B,** Axial section through the aqueduct and upper fourth ventricle. **C,** Axial section through the fourth ventricle (SE 2500/25).

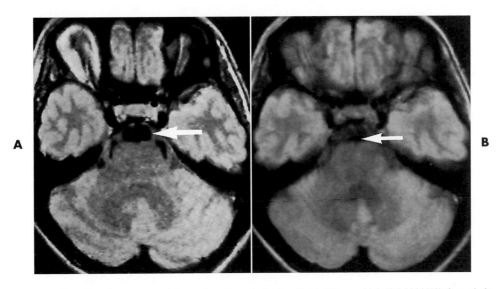

FIGURE 11-50   Pseudoaneurysm of the basilar artery. **A,** Section that is 2.5 mm thick (SE 2000/50) through the basilar artery demonstrates prominent flow void, suggesting aneurysm *(arrow)*. **B,** Section that is 1 cm thick (SE 2000/30) at the same level demonstrates a normal-diameter basilar artery *(arrow)*. The signal loss in **A** reflects dephasing from the radial motion of the CSF around the pulsating basilar artery.

can also be seen in the spinal subarachnoid space.[38,52,53] Because this flow originates at the foramen magnum, it is more prominent in the cervical and thoracic subarachnoid space and less prominent in the lumbar region.[53]

The pulsatile motion of the CSF in the brain and spine can generate the same flow phenomena as noted for blood; that is, it can lead to signal loss or gain. Signal loss is most often seen (Figure 11-49) in the aqueduct of Sylvius, where it produces a flow void.[9,18,54] Because the velocity increases as the cross-sectional area decreases (for a constant volumetric flow rate), TOF losses and dephasing are greatest in the aqueduct. This tends to be more pronounced on thinner slices and on more T2-weighted images, both of which increase the influence of TOF losses. Sections acquired through the upper fourth ventricle show signal loss, which may reflect turbulence as a result of the Venturi (nozzle) effect from the expanding jet of CSF[9] (Figure 11-5). Signal loss can

also be observed in the lateral and third ventricles, particularly near the foramen of Monro (Figures 11-48 and 11-49). Clinical conditions that decrease the velocity of CSF through the aqueduct reduce the degree of signal loss.[55] This is particularly obvious for cases of aqueductal stenosis or other causes of aqueductal obstruction.

Clinical conditions that increase the pulsatile velocity of CSF through the aqueduct increase the magnitude of the flow void.[9] As discussed in Chapter 66, the aqueductal flow void sign is particularly prominent in patients with chronic communicating hydrocephalus (Figure 11-49),[13,56] including any patient with a symptomatic normal-pressure hydrocephalus.[10,13]

Signal loss can also occur because of the radial to-and-fro motion of CSF around the basilar artery. On thin T2-weighted images, the signal loss can lead to the misdiagnosis of basilar artery aneurysm[15] (Figure 11-50).

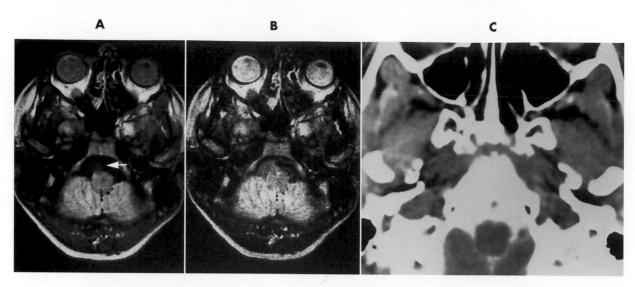

FIGURE 11-51 Pseudomass in the medullary cistern. **A,** First-echo image (SE 2000/40) demonstrates a well-marginated, intermediate-intensity "mass" in the right anterior medullary cistern that could be mistaken for an arachnoid cyst *(arrow)*. **B,** In the second-echo image (SE 2000/80), the mass has CSF intensity. The vertebral arteries are both to the left of midline. **C,** Metrizamide CT study shows no mass in the medullary cistern. The high signal intensity in the right anterior medullary cistern represents FRE caused by the to-and-fro motion of CSF. As upward-flowing, unsaturated protons enter this lowest slice of the imaging volume, they have increased signal intensity. The dephasing caused by the radial motion of CSF surrounding the vertebral arteries in the left medullary cistern leads to local signal loss.

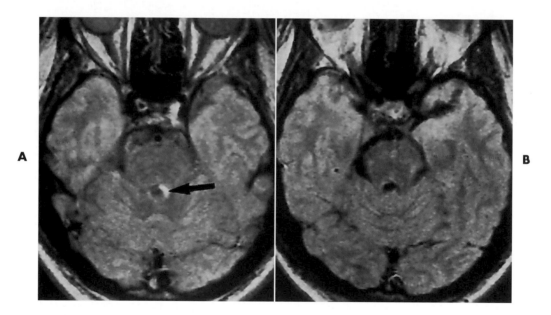

FIGURE 11-52 FRE of flowing CSF in the aqueduct, simulating subacute brainstem hemorrhage. **A,** High signal intensity is noted in the left periaqueductal region *(arrow)* on this lowest slice of a multislice acquisition. In this patient whose brainstem symptoms started 1 week earlier, this was originally interpreted as subacute hemorrhage. **B,** On a repeat section through the same level as **A** (now several slices in from entry surface), no evidence of high signal intensity is seen. The high signal noted in **A** (the lowest slice in the imaging volume) represents FRE as a result of the pulsatile motion of CSF back and forth through the aqueduct. The apparent location in the left periaqueductal tissues is related to oblique flow from slight head tilt.

High signal intensity caused by FRE from the pulsating CSF may be noted in the basal cisterns (Figure 11-51), particularly on slices near the entry surface of the imaging volume.[29] Such increased signal could be mistaken for an arachnoid cyst (Figure 11-51), a tumor, a lipoma, or even subacute hemorrhage, depending on the signal intensity.[7] When high signal intensity is observed in an entry slice, the study should be repeated, with the patient repositioned so that the slice in question is in the middle of the imaging volume (Figure 11-52).

REFERENCES

1. Alvarez O, and Hyman RA: Even echo MR rephasing in the diagnosis of giant intracranial aneurysm, J Comput Assist Tomogr 10:699, 1986.

2. Axel L: Blood flow effects in magnetic resonance imaging, Am J Roentgenol 143:1157, 1984.

3. Bergstrand G, Bergstrom J, Nordell B, et al: Cardiac gated MR imaging of cerebrospinal fluid flow, J Comput Assist Tomogr 9:1003, 1985.

4. Bering EA Jr: Choroid plexus and arterial pulsations of cerebrospinal fluid: demonstration of the choroid plexuses as a cerebrospinal fluid pump, Arch Neurol Psychiatry 73:165, 1955.

5. Bird RD, Stewart WE, and Lightfoot EN: Transport phenomena, New York, 1960, John Wiley & Sons.

6. Boros L, Thomas C, and Werner W: Larger cerebral vessel disease in sickle cell anemia, J Neurol Neurosurg Psychiatry 36:1236, 1976.

7. Bradley WG: Flow phenomena. In Bradley WG, and Bydder GM: MRI atlas of the brain, London, 1990, Martin Dunitz.

8. Bradley WG, Feinberg D, Openshaw KL, et al: Comparison of MR cardiac gated aqueductal flow velocity measurements in healthy individuals and in patients with hydrocephalus, Radiology 161(P):194, 1986.

9. Bradley WG, Kortman KE, and Burgone B: Flowing cerebrospinal fluid in normal and hydrocephalic states: appearance on MR images, Radiology 159:611, 1986.

10. Bradley WG, Scalzo D, Queralt J, et al: Normal-pressure hydrocephalus: evaluation with cerebrospinal fluid flow measurements at MR imaging, Radiology 198:523, 1996.

11. Bradley WG, and Waluch V: Blood flow: magnetic resonance imaging, Radiology 178:459, 1991.

12. Bradley WG, Waluch V, Lai KS, et al: The appearance of rapidly flowing blood on magnetic resonance images, Am J Roentgenol 143:1167, 1984.

13. Bradley WG, Whittemore AR, Kortman KE, et al: Marked cerebrospinal fluid void: indicator of successful shunt in patients with suspected normal-pressure hydrocephalus, Radiology 178:459, 1991.

14. Bryant DJ, Payne JA, Firmin DN, et al: Measurement of flow with NMR using a gradient pulse and phase difference technique, J Comput Assist Tomogr 8:588, 1984.

15. Burt TB: MR of CSF flow phenomenon mimicking basilar artery aneurysm, Am J Neuroradiol 162:527, 1987.

16. Carr HY, and Purcell EM: Effects of diffusion on free precession in nuclear magnetic resonance experiments, Phys Rev 94:630, 1954.

17. Chenevert TL, Brunberg JA, and Pipe JC: Anisotropic diffusion in human white matter: demonstration with MR techniques in vivo, Radiology 177:401, 1990.

18. Citrin CM, Sherman JL, Gangarosa RE, et al: Physiology of the CSF flow void sign: modification by cardiac gating, Am J Neuroradiol 7:1021, 1986.

19. Colletti PM, Raval JK, Benson RC, et al: Motion artifact suppression technique (MAST) in magnetic resonance imaging: clinical results, Magn Reson Imaging 6:293, 1988.

20. Crooks L, Sheldon P, Kaufman L, et al: Quantification of obstructions in vessels by nuclear magnetic resonance, IEEE Trans Nucl Sci NS-29:1181, 1982.

21. Crooks LE, Mills CM, Davis PL, et al: Visualization of cerebral and vascular abnormalities by NMR imaging: the effects of imaging parameters on contrast, Radiology 144:843, 1982.

22. DeGennes PG: Theory of spin echoes in a turbulent field, Phys Lett 29A:20, 1960.

23. Deville G, and Landesman A: Experiences d'echos de spins dan un liquide an ecoulement, J Physique 32:67, 1971.

24. Douglas R, Douglas R, Bradley WG, et al: Reliability of 3D time-of-flight MR angiography in sickle cell anemia, Am J Neuroradiol (in press).

25. DuBoulay GH: Pulsatile movements in the CSF pathways, Br J Radiol 39:255, 1966.

26. Duerk JL, and Pattany PM: Analysis of imaging axes significance in motion artifact suppression technique (MAST): MRI of turbulent flow and motion, Magn Reson Imaging 7:251, 1989.

27. Ehman RL, and Felmlee JP: Flow artifact reduction in MRI: a review of the roles of gradient moment nulling and spatial presaturation, Magn Reson Med 14:293, 1990.

28. Elster AD: Motion artifact suppression technique (MAST) for cranial MR imaging: superiority over cardiac gating for reducing phase-shift artifacts, Am J Neuroradiol 9:671, 1988.

29. Enzmann DR, and Augustyn GT: Improved MR images of the brain with use of a gated, flow-compensated, variable-bandwidth pulse sequence, Radiology 172:777, 1988.

30. Enzmann DR, Rubin JB, DeLaPaz R, et al: Cerebrospinal fluid pulsation benefits and pitfalls in MR imaging, Radiology 161:773, 1986.

31. Felmlee J, and Ehman RL: Spatial presaturation: a method for suppressing flow artifacts and improving depiction of vascular anatomy in MRI, Radiology 164:559, 1987.

32. Haacke EM, and Lenz GW: Improving MR image quality in the presence of motion by using rephasing gradients, Am J Roentgenol 148:1251, 1987.

33. Hahn EL: Spin echoes, Phys Rev 80:580, 1958.

34. Hahn EL: Detection of sea water by nuclear precession, J Geophys Res 65:776, 1960.

35. Hricak H, Amparo E, Fisher MR, et al: Abdominal venous system: assessment using MR, Radiology 156:415, 1985.

36. Kaufman L, Crooks L, Sheldon P, et al: The MR signal intensity patterns obtained from continuous and pulsatile flow models, Radiology 151:421, 1984.

37. Kucharczyk W, Kelly WM, Davis DO, et al: Intracranial lesions: flow related enhancement of MR images using time-of-flight effects, Radiology 161:767, 1986.

38. Lane B, and Kricheff II: Cerebrospinal fluid pulsations at myelography: a videodensitometric study, Radiology 110:579, 1974.

39. LeBihan D: Diffusion/perfusion MR imaging of the brain: from structure to function, Radiology 177:328, 1990.

40. LeBihan D: Magnetic resonance imaging of perfusion, Magn Reson Med 14:283, 1990.

41. LeBihan D, Breton E, Lallemand D, et al: Separation of diffusion and perfusion in intravoxel incoherent motion MR imaging, Radiology 168:497, 1988.

42. McMurdo SK Jr, Brant-Zawadzki M, Bradley WG, et al: Dural sinus thrombosis: study using intermediate field strength MR imaging, Radiology 161:83, 1986.

43. Merkel KH, Ginsberg PL, Parker JC, et al: Cerebrovascular disease in sickle cell anemia: a clinical pathological and radiological correlation, Stroke 9:45, 1978.

44. Mills CM, Brant-Zawadzki M, Crooks LE, et al: Nuclear magnetic resonance: principles of blood flow imaging, Am J Neuroradiol 4:1161, 1983.

45. Moran P: A flow velocity zeugmatographic interlace for NMR imaging in humans, Magn Reson Imaging 1:197, 1982.

46. Moseley ME, Cohen Y, Kucharczyk J, et al: Diffusion-weighted MR imaging of anisotropic water diffusion in cat central nervous system, Radiology 176:439, 1990.

47. Moseley ME, Kucharczyk J, Mintorovitch J, et al: Diffusion-weighted MR imaging of acute stroke: correlation with T2-weighted and magnetic susceptibility-enhanced MR imaging in cats, Am J Neuroradiol 11:43, 1990.

48. Motomiya M, and Karino T: Flow patterns in the human carotid artery bifurcation, Stroke 115:50, 1984.

49. Perman WH, Moran PR, Moran RA, et al: Artifacts from pulsatile flow in MRI, J Comput Assist Tomgr 10:473, 1986.

50. Quencer RM, Post MJD, and Hinks RS: Cine MR in the evaluation of normal and abnormal CSF flow: intracranial and intraspinal studies, Neuroradiology 32:371, 1990.

51. Richardson DN, Elster AD, and Williams DW III: Gd-DTPA-enhanced MR images accentuation of vascular pulsation artifacts and correction by using gradient-moment nulling (MAST), Am J Neuroradiol 11:209, 1990.

52. Rubin JB, and Enzmann DR: Harmonic modulation of proton MR precessional phase by pulsatile motion: origin of spinal CSF flow phenomenon, Am J Neuroradiol 8:307, 1987.

53. Rubin J, and Enzmann DR: Imaging of spinal CSF pulsation by 2DFT magnetic resonance: significance during clinical imaging, Am J Neuroradiol 8:297, 1987.

54. Sherman JL, and Citrin CM: Magnetic resonance demonstration of normal CSF flow, Am J Neuroradiol 7:3, 1986.

55. Sherman JL, Citrin CM, Bowen BJ, et al: MR demonstration of altered cerebrospinal fluid flow by obstructive lesions, Am J Neuroradiol 7:571, 1986.

56. Sherman JL, Citrin CM, Gangarosa RE, et al: The MR appearance of CSF flow in patients with ventriculomegaly, Am J Neuroradiol 7:1025, 1986.

57. Sherman JL, Citrin CM, Gangarosa RE, et al: The MR appearance of CSF pulsations in the spinal canal, Am J Neuroradiol 7:879, 1986.

58. Silverman PM, Patt RH, Baum PA, et al: Ghost artifact on gradient-echo imaging: a potential pitfall in hepatic imaging, Am J Roentgenol 154:633, 1990.

59. Singer JR: NMR diffusion and flow measurements and an introduction to spin phase graphing, Phys E Sci Instrum 11:821, 1978.

60. Singer JR, and Crooks LE: Nuclear magnetic resonance blood flow measurements in the human brain, Science 221:L664, 1983.

61. Valk PE, Hale JD, Crooks LE, et al: NMR of blood flow: correlation of image appearance with spin echo phase shift and signal intensity, Am J Roentgenol 146: 931, 1981.

62. Von Schulthess GK, and Higgins CB: Blood flow imaging with MR: spin phase phenomena, Radiology 157:687, 1985.

63. Waluch V, and Bradley WG: NMR even echo rephasing in slow laminar flow, J Comput Assist Tomogr 8:594, 1984.

64. Wedeen VJ, Rosen BR, Buxton R, et al: Projective MRI angiography and quantitative flow-volume densitometry, Magn Reson Med 3:226, 1986.

65. Whittemore AR, Bradley WG, and Jinkins JR: Comparison of cocurrent and countercurrent flow-related enhancement in MR imaging, Radiology 170:265, 1989.

12 Contrast Agents

Val M. Runge and Kevin L. Nelson

 KEY POINTS

- Paramagnetic contrast agents (e.g., the gadolinium chelates) function by shortening the T1 of nearby water protons, increasing signal intensity. At higher doses, the paramagnetic agents may also cause T2 shortening, decreasing signal intensity.
- As paramagnetic agents initially pass through the vascular bed of the brain, local T2 shortening can be used to monitor perfusion. For other organs lacking a blood-brain barrier, local T1 shortening provides a measure of perfusion.
- Superparamagnetic and ferromagnetic contrast agents induce spin dephasing, leading to T2 shortening and signal loss.

In just over a decade, magnetic resonance imaging (MRI) has become the imaging modality of choice for the study of central nervous system (CNS) disease, with additional broad applications in the abdomen, pelvis, and musculoskeletal system. Concurrent development of contrast media, now in widespread use, has aided the rapid expansion of this field and increased clinical efficacy. MRI offers high spatial res-

Parts of this chapter are from Nelson KL, and Runge VM: Basic principles of MR contrast, Top Magn Reson Imaging 7(3):124, 1995; and Runge VM, and Wells JW: Update: safety, new applications, new MR agents, Top Magn Reson Imaging 7(3):181, 1995.

olution and soft tissue contrast, with sensitivity to contrast-media greater than that of x-ray computed tomography (CT). First-pass brain studies now make possible the assessment of regional cerebral blood volume (rCBV), with high spatial and temporal resolution. New hardware developments, together with advances in contrast-media design, continue to drive expansion of contrast-media applications, building on the large base of current clinical use.

Because MRI provides excellent soft tissue contrast on unenhanced images, it was initially speculated that there would be no need for a contrast agent and that a noninvasive procedure would result. However, in the early 1980s it became apparent that contrast enhancement could substantially improve sensitivity and specificity in both the brain and the spine. For example, brain metastases that are unaccompanied by substantial vasogenic edema could easily be visualized after contrast enhancement because of disruption of the blood-brain barrier.[35] Small extraaxial tumors, such as meningiomas and acoustic neuromas, were also noted to be well visualized after gadolinium chelate administration, yet often unrecognized on precontrast scans. With the use of contrast enhancement, lesion conspicuity was dramatically increased.[34] As the benefits of the paramagnetic contrast agents became more obvious, their use increased exponentially. Today, contrast agents are commonly used in many indications for clinical MRI.

This chapter provides a brief review of the basic principles of contrast-media design, the mechanisms of MR image contrast, and relaxivity theory. Safety data concerning the gadolinium chelates in current clinical use, new agents and directions for future development, and new clinical applications are also discussed.

CONTRAST-AGENT DESIGN REQUIREMENTS

Certain criteria must be met in the design of an MR contrast agent.[45,64] The first and foremost of these criteria is the ability to alter the parameters responsible for image contrast in clinical MRI. MRI is unique in that there are multiple parameters responsible for signal intensity. The contrast agent must be efficient in its ability to influence these parameters at low concentration to minimize dose and potential toxicity.

Second, the contrast agent should possess some tissue specificity in vivo so that it is delivered to a tissue or organ in a higher concentration than to other areas in the body (Table 12-1). Additionally, once delivered to the desired tissue or organ, it must remain localized for a reasonable period of time so that imaging can be performed.

Third, the contrast agent must be substantially cleared from the targeted tissue or organ in a reasonable period of time, usually several hours after imaging, to minimize potential effects from chronic toxicity. The contrast agent must also be excreted from the body, usually by renal or hepatobiliary routes.

Fourth, the contrast agent must have low toxicity and be stable in vivo while being administered in doses that can affect the MR relaxation parameters sufficiently to result in visible contrast enhancement on the MR image. The dose levels of the contrast agent required to meet these criteria must be evaluated for potential mutagenicity, teratogenicity, carcinogenicity, and immunogenicity.

Finally, the contrast agent must possess a suitable shelf life for storage. It must remain stable in vitro for a reasonable period of time while being stored. A shelf life of months and preferably years is desirable.

MAGNETIC RESONANCE CONTRAST MECHANISMS

In conventional radiography and CT, image contrast is generated by differential attenuation of the x-ray beam by the tissues of the body. The degree of attenuation is directly related to the mass absorption coeffi-

Table 12-1 Targeting of MR Contrast Media

PROCESS/ LOCALIZATION	CHARACTERISTICS	EXAMPLE
Interstitial space	Excreted by glomerular filtration, excluded by intact blood-brain barrier	Gd-HP-DO3A, Gd-DTPA, Gd-DOTA, Gd-DTPA-BMA
Phagocytosis	Uptake of particles by macrophages	AMI-25
Metabolism	Internalization of contrast agent by cell surface receptors or transport mechanisms	Gd-BOPTA, Gd-EOB-DTPA
Cell surface	Antibodies targeted to tissue-specific antigens	
Vascular space	Molecular size larger than capillary pore size	AMI-227

cient of the tissue being imaged or, more specifically, the electron density and the effective atomic number of the tissue. Therefore in conventional radiography and CT the mechanism for contrast enhancement involves manipulation of the mass absorption coefficient alone. The use of a contrast agent with a high mass absorption coefficient, for example, any of the iodinated agents, results in attenuation of the x-ray beam to a greater degree, thereby producing contrast enhancement.

Compared with conventional radiography and CT, the mechanisms responsible for contrast enhancement in MRI are not singular but multiparametric. The large inherent differences of signal intensity between various tissues are what make MRI unique compared with other imaging modalities used in radiology today. In addition, the appropriate selection of operator-dependent imaging parameters is critical so that these signal intensity differences can be exploited to optimize MR image contrast.

The parameters that determine MR signal intensity and contrast are many.[122] The first of these, and easiest to understand, is spin density. Spin density refers to the fraction of protons that exists in the voxel of tissue being imaged and determines the maximum potential MR signal intensity that can be realized from that volume of tissue. Most protons in tissue are water protons. These far outweigh in number the protons that are associated with organic compounds in tissue. Because the in vivo water content of tissue cannot easily be altered by a contrast agent, compounds that affect spin density have received little attention.

Another common parameter exploited in generation of MR contrast is relaxivity. There are two relaxivity parameters that are unique to each tissue, T1 and T2. Longitudinal or spin-lattice relaxation time, known as *T1,* refers to the amount of time it takes for the tissue magnetization to return to its equilibrium state in the longitudinal direction of the main magnetic field after excitation with a radiofrequency (RF) pulse of energy. The excess energy that is absorbed by the magnetic spins from the RF pulse is transferred back to the environment or lattice during the relaxation process. The second relaxivity property of tissue is the transverse or spin-spin relaxation, referred to as *T2 relaxation.* In this relaxation process the excess energy deposited in the tissue by the RF pulse is transferred between the magnetic spins. This transferred energy results in loss of spin phase coherency in the transverse plane and spin dephasing.

Contrast-agent enhancement that is based on alteration of these two relaxivity parameters can be categorized according to the relative change it imparts on either T1 or T2.[19,29,54] A contrast agent that predominantly affects T1 relaxation is referred to as a *positive relaxation agent* because the enhanced shortening of T1 relaxation results in increased signal intensity on a T1-weighted image. By comparison, a contrast agent that predominantly affects T2 relaxation is referred to as a *negative relaxation agent* because reducing T2 results in decreased signal intensity on a T2-weighted image.

Another determinant of signal intensity in the MR image is magnetic susceptibility. Susceptibility describes the ability of a substance to become magnetized in an external magnetic field.[99] There are four categories of magnetic susceptibility. Most organic compounds are diamagnetic substances and have a small, negative magnetic susceptibility

when placed in an external magnetic field. Paramagnetic and ferromagnetic materials have very large net positive susceptibilities. Diamagnetic susceptibility has a negligible effect in clinical MRI, and therefore diamagnetic substances are of little interest as contrast agents.

Paramagnetic substances afford the greatest flexibility in contrast-agent design and have therefore received the greatest attention in contrast-media development. The presence of a paramagnetic ion can strongly influence the relaxation properties of nearby protons, leading to changes in tissue contrast. Paramagnetic contrast agents are predominantly used as positive T1 relaxation contrast agents, with little effect seen on T2 relaxation and then only at high concentrations. The positive net magnetic susceptibility on a paramagnetic ion has little influence as an actual enhancement mechanism in conventional MRI.

By comparison, the large net magnetic susceptibility of superparamagnetic and ferromagnetic compounds more directly influences tissue contrast, with little effect on relaxation per se. Superparamagnetic substances are individual particles that are large enough to be a domain. When these particles are exposed to an external magnetic field, they align with the field, resulting in a large net positive magnetization. When removed from the magnetic field, they return to random orientations and lose their net positive magnetization. By comparison, ferromagnetic compounds are large collections of interacting domains in a crystalline matrix. They exhibit an extremely large net positive magnetization in an external magnetic field and maintain this when removed from the field. Both superparamagnetic and ferromagnetic compounds have received substantial attention recently in regard to their application as clinically useful MR contrast agents. These agents function as negative contrast agents because their large net positive magnetic moments induce spin dephasing in tissue, with resultant signal loss.

The final two parameters that provide image contrast in MRI are diffusion and perfusion. The intensity of the MR signal is based on the magnitude of the bulk magnetization lying in the transverse plane. It is maximal when all the transverse spins are in phase coherence. Movement or diffusion of bulk water between tissues in a random motion leads to spin dephasing and loss of phase coherence in the transverse plane. Subsequently this results in the loss of MR signal intensity. Similarly, perfusion of blood in the microcirculation of the tissue being imaged also contributes to spin dephasing and a decrease in the intensity of the MR signal. In this manner, different degrees of diffusion and perfusion within tissue contribute to contrast in the MR image. The use of a relaxivity or susceptibility contrast agent to manipulate diffusion coefficients (and thus function as a contrast agent) has received limited attention to date. The presence of a susceptibility agent in the blood pool can cause large changes in signal intensity. This approach is being actively investigated as a means of contrast enhancement, specifically for the measurement of rCBV.

RELAXIVITY THEORY

Nearly all the attention in development of pharmaceutical MR contrast agents has focused on the use of paramagnetic compounds. The most commonly used paramagnetic ion is the gadolinium ion, which is complexed with various ligands (such as diethylene-triamine-pentaacetic acid [DTPA] and HP-DO3A) that act as chelating agents. Although an extensive review of relaxivity theory is beyond the scope of this chapter, a basic conceptual understanding is necessary to appreciate the intricate physics involved in paramagnetic contrast-agent enhancement.

The presence of unpaired electrons in the paramagnetic ion is a mandatory component to effect a change in the T1 and T2 relaxation rates of water protons.[37,53] The magnetic dipole moment created by the unpaired electrons can thereby enhance the relaxation rates of water protons, either by direct interaction with the water protons or by its local magnetic field influence. The relaxivity contributions of a paramagnetic ion are highly dependent on its spin state. If S denotes the spin quantum number of the total electron spin of the paramagnetic ion, then the relaxation rate is proportional to $S*(S + 1)$. Therefore a paramagnetic ion with the highest spin quantum number is desirable. The gadolinium ion (Gd^{+3}) of the lanthanide metal group has a high spin quantum number of 7/2, making it a desirable relaxivity contrast agent. Other ions that have received attention as potential MR contrast agents include Fe^{+3}, Dy^{+3}, and Mn^{+2} (all with $S = 5/2$). Although a high spin quantum number is theoretically desirable, it is not the only factor

Table 12-2   Properties of MR-Relevant Paramagnetic Metals

ION	CONFIGURATION	SPIN	ELECTRON SPIN (τ_s)	MAGNETIC MOMENT
Fe^{3+}	$3d^5$	5/2	10^{-9} to 10^{-10}	5.9
Mn^{2+}	$3d^5$	5/2	10^{-8} to 10^{-9}	5.9
Gd^{3+}	$4f^7$	7/2	10^{-8} to 10^{-9}	7.6
Dy^{3+}	$4f^9$	5/2	10^{-12} to 10^{-13}	10.6

τ_s, Electron spin relaxation time in seconds.

that determines whether an MR contrast agent will be efficacious (Table 12-2).

The interactions that occur between a paramagnetic contrast agent and protons of water molecules can be classified into two categories. *Inner-sphere relaxation* refers to the formation of a coordinate covalent molecular bond between a water molecule and the primary or intercoordination sphere of the paramagnetic ion. A chemical exchange occurs between the water molecule and the paramagnetic ion in this interaction, which leads to enhanced relaxation of the water protons on the basis of the magnetic influences and the efficiency of chemical exchange. It follows that the more water molecules that can bind with the paramagnetic ion, the greater its influence on relaxation enhancement. Therefore the shorter the residence time of the water molecule with the paramagnetic ion, the greater the relaxation enhancement effect because of the ability of the paramagnetic ion to interact with other water molecules. In contrast-agent design a rapid exchange ($\leq 10^6$ sec^{-1}) between water molecules and the paramagnetic ion is a desirable feature because it allows for greater relaxation enhancement. However, this factor is important only up to the point where the exchange contributes as a correlation time.

Outer-sphere relaxation is a more complex concept. It does not involve a direct bonding or chemical-exchange mechanism. It is the result of the relative rotational and translational diffusion of water molecules and the paramagnetic ion. Basically stated, the more water molecules that can approach the paramagnetic ion and interact with its dipole, the greater the relaxivity influence of the paramagnetic ion. The more the paramagnetic ion can move through space, the greater its ability to interact with other water protons. Additionally, the closer the water protons can approach the paramagnetic ion, the more efficient the relaxation enhancement. This interaction of the dipole moments of the paramagnetic ion and the water molecules in the environment has been termed a *dipole-dipole relaxation process*. Inner-sphere relaxation for Gd^{3+} is also a dipolar process ("through space"), since Gd^{3+} has no scalar relaxation ("through bond").

These factors are critical in contrast-agent design. For example, if the paramagnetic ion is complexed with a ligand such as DTPA, the molecular complex rotates more slowly and translates more slowly in space. This does not allow for as many water proton–paramagnetic ion interactions to occur, thereby limiting the relaxation effect of the molecular complex. Also, by complexing the paramagnetic ion, there is increased distance between the water-proton dipole and the paramagnetic ion dipole, decreasing the paramagnetic ion's relaxation enhancement effect.

The Solomon-Bloembergen-Morgan equation is a mathematical expression that describes the relaxation of water protons with a paramagnetic ion species.[3] This equation is used as a predictor of relaxation efficiency of a paramagnetic ion species in contrast-agent design. The Solomon-Bloembergen-Morgan equation can be thought of as essentially two terms. The first component of the equation, the dipole-dipole term, expresses a distance factor between the interacting species. In one dimension this is a statement of the inverse square law, in that the magnitude of the paramagnetic effect is related to the reciprocal of the square of the distance (d^{-2}). In three dimensions this becomes d^{-6} expressed as r^{-6} (r = radius). The dipole-dipole component is critically affected by the distance of the interacting species. Simply stated, the more closely a water molecule can approach the paramagnetic ion species, the more efficient the relaxation enhancement effect on the paramagnetic ion. Because the dipole-dipole component is critically affected by the distance, it is important in contrast-agent design to use

carrier ligands that minimize this distance effect. Some of the carrier ligands, however, may be quite large. These ligands cause an undesirable effect from the standpoint of relaxation enhancement by the paramagnetic ion. Use of such chelates is required because of the high toxicity of paramagnetic ions, such as gadolinium, when free in the body. Large carrier ligands and their surrounding water molecules of hydration tend to displace free or bulk water molecules from the surrounding inner sphere of influence of the paramagentic ion, decreasing proton-relaxation enhancement effects. Of all factors, this has the largest negative impact.

The total correlation time (τ_c) between the two interacting species can be expressed mathematically for both dipole-dipole and scalar interactions as follows:

$$1/\tau_c = 1/\tau_r + 1/\tau_s + 1/\tau_M$$

where
τ_c = Correlation time of interaction
τ_r = Correlation time of rotation
τ_s = Correlation time of electron relaxation
τ_m = Correlation time of chemical exchange

The critical feature of this mathematical expression is that, of the three components (τ_r, τ_s, and τ_m) comprising the total correlation time of any specific interaction, the component that is the smallest magnitude is the most important in determining the total correlation time of interaction.

Correlation times are important in paramagnetic contrast-agent design. As an example, the larger the carrier ligand to which the paramagnetic ion is bound, the more slowly it rotates and translates in space, thereby increasing the magnitude of τ_r. The total correlation time of interaction is thus increased in most instances of a large carrier-ligand molecule, somewhat offsetting the distance factor for these large carrier-ligands. Correlation times always reflect the interaction possessing the shortest time characteristic or the fastest dynamic behavior of the paramagnetic contrast agent, providing that chemical exchange is fast enough ($\leq 10^6$ sec^{-1}).

IMAGING TECHNIQUE

This section deals with the application of MR pulse sequences for visualization of contrast media, building on the knowledge of MR physics presented in the preceding paragraphs. As is now evident, the mechanisms responsible for MR contrast are multiparametric, including relaxivity effects of T1 and T2, spin density, susceptibility, perfusion, and diffusion. Similar to the multiple intrinsic MR properties of the tissues themselves, the methods of measurement of these parameters in clinical MR imaging are multiple. The type of MR pulse sequence used to generate a clinical MR image and its associated parameters also profoundly affects the contrast that is visualized from the tissues.

The ultimate goal in optimizing MR scanning technique for contrast-agent visualization is to suppress the contrast from unchanged tissue parameters and accentuate the contrast on the basis of the parameter that is altered by the contrast agent.[15] This requires knowledge of the mechanism of contrast-agent enhancement, the MR pulse technique being used to measure that parameter, and how the operator-dependent parameters can be altered to optimize the enhancement of the contrast agent being used. What follows is a discussion of the MR pulse sequences that are commonly used in conjunction with clinical MR contrast agents and the issues that are related to the optimization of these protocols. Although the scope of this discussion is limited, there are many extensive discussions in the literature.[37,64,122]

Conventional spin-echo imaging has remained the mainstay of MR pulse sequences used with MR contrast agents. This approach can provide images with T1, T2, and spin-density information. In spin-echo imaging a 90-degree RF pulse is followed by a 180-degree RF pulse, which generates an MR signal or echo at an operator-specified echo time (TE). This measurement is repeated at a repetition time (TR), which is also specified by the operator. In spin-echo imaging, short TRs and TEs produce an image with T1-weighted contrast. Long TRs and TEs produce images with T2-weighted contrast. During the same long-TR interval used to produce a T2-weighted image, a second image can be obtained with a short or intermediate TE (resulting in a second image with spin-density or intermediate T2 weighting). One of the major disadvantages of conventional spin-echo imaging when used to produce T2-weighted scans is the long imaging time. Imaging time is directly proportional to TR, which is long for a typical T2-weighted pulse sequence, usually 2 to 3 sec.

A recent innovation is fast, or turbo, spin-echo imaging, which permits T2-weighted scans to be acquired in a much reduced scan time. In this approach, multiple echoes are acquired with different phase encoding during each TR interval. Images with both proton density– and T2-weighted information can be obtained in times from one-fourth to one-sixteenth those required for conventional spin-echo techniques. Because the images generated from this approach are for multiple TE data measurements that are then averaged together for an effective TE image, the image contrast is somewhat different from that of a conventional spin-echo sequence. For example, the MR signal from fat remains more intense on a T2-weighted image obtained with this pulse technique, reflecting the brighter signal that fat produces on short-TE images. Despite these and other minimal shortcomings of fast spin-echo sequences, they have gained widespread popularity in clinical MR imaging of the central nervous system (CNS) and body.

Another pulse technique that has gained popularity in CNS and body applications is gradient-echo imaging. This offers an alternative imaging approach with substantially reduced imaging time and RF power deposition. A gradient-echo sequence differs from a spin-echo sequence in that a 180-degree RF pulse is not used. The initial RF pulse typically uses a flip angle of less than 90 degrees. Signal is then generated by manipulation of the gradient magnetic fields. By a change of the operator-dependent parameters of flip angle, TR, and TE, image contrast with T1, T2*, and spin-density information can be generated. One of the major disadvantages of this technique is that susceptibility effects become prominent. This enhanced susceptibility effect can be exploited to advantage, however, in certain clinical situations. For example, the high magnetic susceptibility of blood degradation products, such as deoxyhemoglobin, results in increased conspicuity of hemorrhage on gradient-echo scans.

Most of the contrast agents studied to date have been designed to affect relaxivity enhancement because most of the intrinsic contrast in MRI is dependent on T1 and T2 relaxation. Although these contrast agents can be imaged with a variety of different MR techniques, including spin-echo and gradient-echo pulse sequences, choosing appropriate imaging parameters to maximize visualization of the relaxation enhancement effect is paramount.

The gadolinium chelates, the major class of agents in use in clinical practice today, enhance T1 relaxivity and thereby result in visible contrast enhancement on T1-weighted pulse sequences with short TRs and TEs. Although these agents primarily affect T1 relaxation rates, producing positive contrast enhancement, their effect is biphasic in that at very high concentrations they can have T2 effects or negative contrast enhancement, even on T1-weighted pulse sequences (Figure 12-1). In most clinical situations the T2 effects have little contribution and the T1 effects are exploited to result in visible positive contrast enhancement. Their effects on proton density– and T2-weighted images are generally not clinically relevant. The signal intensity decrease seen with increasing concentrations of a paramagnetic ion species, on the basis of T2 effects, is usually not seen at current doses (other than with hyperconcentration of these agents in the urine).

As discussed, the positive T1 enhancement effects of the gadolinium contrast agents are well visualized on T1-weighted spin-echo images. T1-weighted gradient-echo imaging can also allow visualization of the contrast enhancement effect of the gadolinium chelates. These techniques can be particularly useful when obtained in a volumetric fashion. A volumetric or three-dimensional (3D) acquisition permits image manipulation on a work station, with reconstruction of high-resolution images in multiple planes without the need for additional scans.

Currently the US Food and Drug Administration (FDA) has approved three MR contrast agents for general use, all of which use the gadolinium ion as the paramagnetic metal species. These agents are Gd-HP-DO3A (gadoteridol or ProHance), Gd-DTPA (gadopentetate dimeglumine or Magnevist), and Gd-DTPA-BMA (gadodiamide or Omniscan), the first and last being nonionic. These three parenteral paramagnetic compounds function as extracellular contrast agents. After injection, they are distributed into the blood pool and extracellular fluid compartments of the body. All are rapidly excreted by glomerular filtration with half-lives between 1 and 2 hours. They act as positive

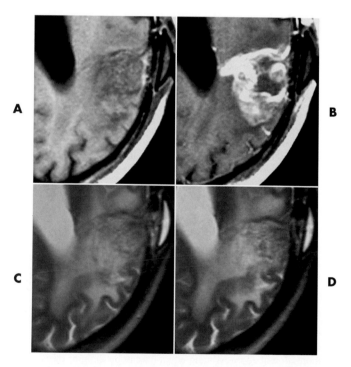

FIGURE 12-2   Gadolinium chelate (Gd-HP-DO3A, ProHance) enhances spin-echo scans with both T1 and T2 weighting in glioblastoma. Precontrast **(A)** and postcontrast **(B)** T1-weighted scans are compared with precontrast **(C)** and postcontrast **(D)** T2-weighted scans. On **B**, positive lesion enhancement is noted in the region of the blood-brain barrier disruption. Little change is seen in this region on **D**.

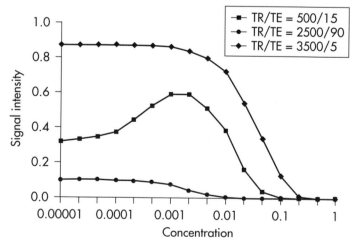

FIGURE 12-1   Image enhancement: Effect of gadolinium concentration and pulse technique. Effect of gadolinium chelate on signal intensity is nonlinear. With T1-weighted spin-echo techniques (TR/TE = 500/15) the initial increase in signal intensity with concentration is observed. This results in positive lesion enhancement, forming the basis for most clinical applications in neuroimaging. With both proton density– (TR/TE = 3500/5) and T2-weighted (TR/TE = 2500/90) spin-echo techniques, little change is seen except at high concentrations, where signal intensity drops. Presence of gadolinium ion enhances both T1 and T2 relaxation of nearby water protons. This effect on both T1 and T2, combined with dependency of signal intensity on both parameters, leads to this complex relationship between the concentration of contrast agent and signal enhancement.

T1 relaxation agents. In the CNS these agents are not distributed within normal brain and spinal cord tissue because of the presence of an intact blood-brain barrier. Slowly flowing venous structures, such as cortical veins and dural sinuses, however, demonstrate intense enhancement. When a pathological process, such as a high-grade tumor, results in disruption of the blood-brain barrier, administration of a gadolinium chelate produces positive contrast enhancement. This is best visualized on T1-weighted images, with little or no enhancement seen on proton density– and T2-weighted images (Figure 12-2). As has been extensively documented in the literature, contrast administration often proves very useful, increasing the conspicuity of diseases and providing physiological information regarding the status of the blood-brain barrier. For diseases outside the CNS, lesion enhancement depends on differential accumulation of the contrast agent between normal and abnormal tissue.

In the last few years, techniques using magnetization transfer (MT) have been introduced in clinical MRI.[127] The application of MT with spin-echo imaging can improve the enhancement effect produced by a gadolinium chelate in the brain. Water protons in tissue exist in three distinct pools. The protons in the free water pool exist in a narrow range of resonant frequencies and possess a long T2. These protons account for most of the MR signal recorded in clinical MRI. The fat pool is isolated from the water pool and normally absent in the brain and spinal cord. The third pool of protons is the restricted pool. These protons represent structural or bound water protons that are associated with large molecules, such as phospholipids in the brain and spinal cord. These protons have a large range of resonant frequencies and an extremely short T2. Because the restricted pool of water protons decays so quickly during MRI as a result of their short T2, it contributes little signal to the image. With the application of MT, magnetization is transferred from the restricted hydrogen pool to the freely mobile hydrogen pool. The result is a shortening of T1, with lower overall available magnetization and signal intensity. In theory, enhancement with gadolinium chelates is not mediated by macromolecular interactions and thus is not suppressed by the application of MT.[18] Accordingly, MT pulses preferentially suppress the signal from background tissue, improving the conspicuity of gadolinium-enhanced regions.[4] This can lead to improved visualization of abnormal contrast enhancement at a standard dose.

Contrast agents that principally affect T2 have received much less attention for application in clinical practice. In part this has been related to the fact that T2-weighted spin-echo images, as required to visualize such contrast-enhancement effects, require long TRs, resulting in long imaging times. Gradient-echo pulse sequences can be used, but their sensitivity to bulk susceptibility artifacts limits usefulness. One of the more promising groups of parenteral T2 contrast agents is the superparamagnetic contrast agents that incorporate ferrite particles. Ferrites are crystalline oxides, of which magnetite (Fe_3O_4) in a particle size of 0.5 to 1 μm has been used most commonly. Ferrite particles in this size range are phagocytosed by macrophages of the reticuloendothelial system, with prominent uptake in normal liver and spleen parenchyma. In such tissue there is selective T2 shortening with profound signal loss. Because MR signal intensity is decreased in normal liver and spleen, focal areas of replacement, such as metastatic disease, are seen as areas of higher signal intensity.[112] Ferrite particles exhibit a monophasic effect on signal intensity because progressively larger doses can only further reduce signal intensity until the level of background noise is reached.

One of the few compounds that has been investigated for use as a potential spin-density contrast agent is perfluoroctylbromide (PFOB). Perfluorobromides act as negative contrast-enhancement agents with possible clinical utility for gastrointestinal tract imaging (after oral administration). A negative contrast agent is likely preferable as a bowel contrast agent because signal intensity loss does not cause motion artifacts. Artifacts resulting from peristalsis of bowel contents can be seen with positive contrast agents, such as the gadolinium chelates, when administered orally. Perfluorobromides did not fare well clinically when introduced in 1994 because of substantial side effects. Suspensions of iron particles, which also serve as negative contrast agents, may find greater acceptance.

Echo-planar imaging (EPI), which is currently in use at a limited number of MRI centers worldwide, promises to provide another revolutionary change in clinical MRI. This ultrafast MR technique can provide high-quality images that are free of motion artifact and provide almost unlimited proton density–, T1-, and T2-weighted contrast in less than a second.[101] One of the primary advantages of EPI, when used in conjunction with contrast injection, is that it can provide information regarding physiological parameters previously inaccessible to MRI. Tissue perfusion and function can be assessed with high spatial resolution.[55] It is expected that EPI will soon become commonly available, further expanding MRI's clinical utility.

With the advent of ultrafast imaging techniques, such as EPI, the use of contrast agents in dynamic imaging has been investigated. With this approach, both quantitative and qualitative physiological information can be obtained. During controlled bolus injection of a susceptibility contrast agent, such as gadolinium or dysprosium HP-DO3A, ultrafast imaging techniques are applied with rapid sequential image acquisition. Decreases in brain signal intensity on these MR images are related to the presence of the susceptibility agent, which functions as a negative contrast-enhancement agent. The change in intensity of the MR signal is directly related to the concentration of the contrast agent, thus yielding data on tissue perfusion. Dynamic ultrafast imaging with susceptibility agents promises to be an exciting new area of investigation, particularly in brain imaging for the evaluation of rCBV.

EXTRACELLULAR GADOLINIUM CHELATES

Before 1982 the relaxation effects of the paramagnetic metals, which include gadolinium, were well known. However, the toxicity of these metals in their ionic form appeared to prevent use in humans. To design a safe agent, it was proposed that the metal ion be tightly bound by a chelate, permitting the metal to exhibit its paramagnetic effect yet limiting toxicity by achieving rapid and total renal excretion.[91] The gadolinium ion emerged as the most favorable choice with regard to paramagnetic effect and specifically enhancement of T1 relaxation.[123] Thus the clinical safety of a gadolinium chelate is to a large extent dependent on its stability in vivo. Key factors include thermodynamics, solubility, selectivity, and kinetics (see subsequent discussion). Gadolinium administered as the free metal ion is not suitable as a contrast agent because of its toxicity and biodistribution.[69]

Indications for contrast-media use in the head and spine have been well established through experience in clinical trials worldwide.[78,80,97] Administration of a gadolinium chelate can substantially improve lesion identification and characterization. With conventional spin-echo techniques, contrast enhancement occurs on the basis of either blood-brain (or blood-cord) barrier disruption or lesion vascularity, the latter with extraaxial lesions. In this setting the T1 effect of the agent on surrounding water protons, producing "positive" enhancement, is observed. At the dose most commonly used in clinical practice today, 0.1 mmol/kg, lesion enhancement on MRI with a gadolinium chelate is equivalent to or slightly superior to that observed on CT with iodinated agents. However, unlike CT, abnormal contrast enhancement is not obscured by adjacent bone or calcification. On MRI, small intraaxial and extraaxial lesions (e.g., metastases and meningiomas) can appear isointense on precontrast images, with only the administration of a gadolinium chelate providing lesion recognition. After therapeutic measures, recurrent disease can also be difficult to diagnose without contrast administration given the background of associated treatment-related tissue change. With perfusion studies, the contrast-agent bolus itself is tracked during the first pass through the brain. In this instance the T2 and susceptibility effects of the agent, producing "negative" enhancement, are observed.

In neoplastic disease of the CNS, MR contrast administration improves visualization of both intraaxial and extraaxial lesions. Only in the case of metastases confined to the vertebral body is lesion visualization generally not improved, and in this instance it may actually decrease. Small metastatic lesions within the CNS may not elicit sufficient edema to be recognized on unenhanced scans, mandating contrast administration for detection. Contrast use commonly improves lesion definition, permitting better evaluation of lesion margins and invasion of adjacent structures. Before surgery, contrast-enhanced scans are valuable for planning lesion resection and defining areas for biopsy. After surgery, contrast-enhanced scans are useful for definition of recurrent tumor.

In CNS infection, MR contrast administration is useful primarily for lesion characterization and assessment of lesion activity. Acute disease can be differentiated from chronic change, such as gliosis, and dis-

Table 12-3 Physicochemical Properties of the Gadolinium Chelates in Clinical Use in the United States

LIGAND	RELAXIVITY	LOG K_{eq}	k(obs)s^{-1}	OSMOLALITY	VISCOSITY
HP-DO3A	3.7	23.8	6.3×10^{-5}	0.63	1.3
DTPA	3.8	22.1	1.2×10^{-3}	1.96	2.9
DTPA-BMA	3.8	16.9	$>2 \times 10^{-2}$	0.65	1.4

ease progression or regression followed. Enhanced MRI is particularly superior to enhanced CT in this instance because of the lack of beam-hardening artifacts, which obscure visualization of tissue adjacent to bone. Meningeal inflammatory disease is well visualized with prominent enhancement, differentiating these processes from the normal falx and meninges. These latter tissues do not demonstrate substantial enhancement in the normal state, unlike on CT.

In ischemic disease involving the brain, MR contrast administration provides for temporal dating and assists in lesion characterization. Intravascular enhancement is observed in the first week after infarction, with parenchymal enhancement seen thereafter for up to 8 weeks. These patterns of enhancement also assist in differential diagnosis. Not all infarcts can be diagnosed as such by their involvement of a characteristic arterial distribution, with intravascular or gyriform enhancement in this instance providing important information for differential diagnosis.

In the spine,[79] as in the head, the indications for contrast-material use are also quite broad. Contrast enhancement is used routinely in the back after surgery for the differentiation of scar from recurrent or residual disk material.[77] In the first 20 min after contrast injection, scar tissue demonstrates enhancement because of its vascular nature, although disk material does not. On unenhanced scans, this differentiation may not be possible. Contrast administration also markedly improves the detection of leptomeningeal metastases. Identification of tumor enhancement can aid in the differentiation of a tumor syrinx from a congenital or posttraumatic syrinx.[70] For cord lesions, contrast administration improves differential diagnosis.

In the head and neck, postcontrast images can also provide additional diagnostic information.[42] In a clinical trial in which 0.1 mmol/kg Gd-HP-DO3A was administered to 122 patients, the additional information provided by contrast administration was judged by two blinded readers to be likely to have contributed to a change in the diagnosis of 16% of the patients.[132] The additional information available postcontrast consisted principally of improved lesion visualization and definition of lesion margins.

In body imaging the high intrinsic tissue contrast of MRI is notable, lessening to some degree the utility of contrast media. Administration of a gadolinium chelate is often reserved for specific problems, such as the differentiation of necrotic from viable tissue, the identification of active infection, the differentiation of benign from malignant disease, and the identification of recurrent neoplasia. Specific applications exist for disease involving the breast,[3 8,39,44] liver and spleen,[62] kidney,[103] pelvis,[40,41,65] and musculoskeletal system.[20]

Gadolinium chelates were developed because of the high relaxivity of the gadolinium ion and relative low toxicity of the complex with chelation of the metal ion. For all agents in clinical use in the United States, excretion is by glomerular filtration. The clinical safety of these agents is thus to a large extent dependent on the stability of the chelate in vivo. Key factors determining safety include thermodynamics, solubility, selectivity, and kinetics.[7,115,121] There must be a high affinity of the chelate for the metal ion, which is reflected by the thermodynamic binding constant of the complex. If the agent is not sufficiently soluble, precipitation of the gadolinium ion can occur, with potential toxicity. The chelate by necessity must have high selectivity for the gadolinium ion itself so that metal exchange with endogenous ions, such as zinc and copper, does not occur. And, last but not least the compound must exhibit slow kinetics in regard to release of the gadolinium ion, making possible near complete excretion of the complex in the setting of normal renal function. One way to assess kinetics is by the rate of dissociation of the complex in acid solution. Table 12-3 presents a comparison of the three agents available in the United States on the basis of these and other chemical characteristics. High thermodynamic stability, slow kinetics of dissociation (small k [obs] s^{-1}), low osmolality, and low viscosity are favorable features.

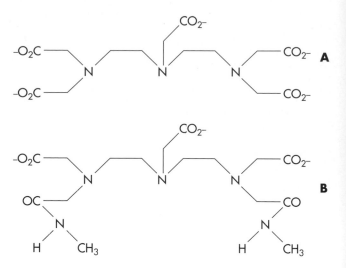

FIGURE 12-3 Chemical structures for DTPA **(A)**, the chelate in gadopentetate dimeglumine (Magnevist), and DTPA-BMA (diethylene-triamine-pentaacetic acid *bis*-methylamide) **(B)**, the chelate in gadodiamide (Omniscan). Both are linear chelates.

To date, two basic types of chelates—linear and macrocyclic—have been developed. Linear chelates (Figure 12-3) include Gd-DTPA and Gd-DTPA-BMA. In the United States, only one macrocyclic chelate, Gd-HP-DO3A, is available (Figure 12-4). In Europe a second macrocyclic compound, Gd-DOTA, is also in use. Both macrocycles exhibit higher thermodynamic and kinetic stability,[105,116] leading to lower long-term heavy-metal (Gd^{3+}) deposition (Figure 12-5). In any chelate preparation the addition of a small amount of excess ligand also diminishes (up to a point) the potential for metal-ion substitution.[25]

As a group the gadolinium chelates have a good overall safety profile with regard to acute toxicity. The majority of adverse events encountered are mild and transient. However, severe anaphylactoid reactions, although rare, have been documented. Radiologists should be aware of potential complications and adequately prepared for treatment of a major untoward event.[9]

Gd-DTPA

Gadopentetate dimeglumine (Gd-DTPA or Magnevist [Berlex Laboratories]) was the first extracellular gadolinium chelate to be developed for clinical use. It was approved for use in the United States by the FDA in 1988.[28] Currently this approval includes use in adult and pediatric patients (older than 2 years of age) at a single dose of 0.1 mmol/kg. The pharmaceutical preparation contains 0.2% of the excess ligand. There is extensive experience with this agent, as well as with Gd-DTPA-BMA and Gd-HP-DO3A in the head, neck, and spine.[6,71,81] As with any such agent, caution should be exercised in renally impaired patients. The safety of the agent depends to a large extent on its rapid excretion. Gd-DTPA, like Gd-DTPA-BMA and Gd-HP-DO3A, is cleared by dialysis. Debate continues, however, on the rate and degree to which the agents are cleared.

Concern has also been raised with regard to the use of Gd-DTPA in patients with hemolytic anemia because of early observations of a transient elevation in serum iron and bilirubin after injection. These laboratory abnormalities presumably result from the chelate's release of a small amount of gadolinium, which then causes blood hemolysis. In a large early clinical study, 11% (34 of 308) of men had abnormal serum iron levels and 2.9% (11 of 379) had abnormal bilirubin levels 24 hours after administration of Gd-DTPA. In healthy volunteers, when 0.25 mmol/kg Gd-DTPA was administered, an elevation in serum iron and total bilirubin could be observed by 3 hours, with a peak in levels

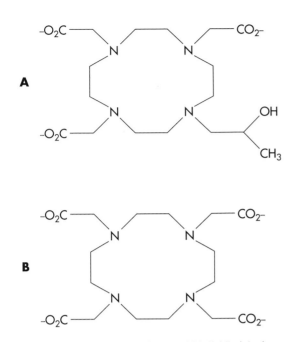

FIGURE 12-4 Chemical structures for HP-DO3A (1,4,7-tris(carboxymethyl)-10-2'-hydroxypropyl-1,4,7,10-tetraazacyclododecane) **(A)**, the chelate in gadoteridol (ProHance), and DOTA (1,4,7,10-tetraazacyclododecane tetraacetic acid) **(B)**, the chelate in gadoterate meglumine (Dotarem). Both are macrocyclic chelates.

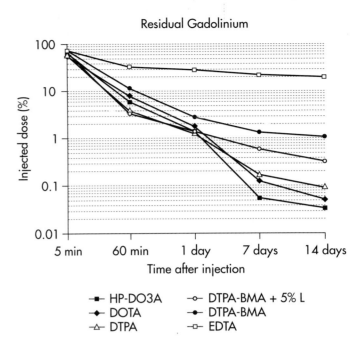

FIGURE 12-5 Whole-body residual gadolinium after IV administration of radiolabeled chelates. Gd-EDTA dissociates rapidly in vivo and is poorly tolerated. Stability of each chelate and the degree to which in vivo dissociation occurs are reflected by residual gadolinium at each time point. More stable chelates, with less release of gadolinium in vivo, leave less free metal ion. Of agents approved for clinical use, Gd-DTPA-BMA shows the greatest residual gadolinium. Addition of excess chelate (ligand L) improves excretion with this agent. Free gadolinium is deposited in liver and bone marrow, with potential for chronic heavy metal toxicity. (From reference 115.)

between 6 and 12 hours and return to baseline by 24 hours.[66] The implication of these findings in clinical application is unclear.

The effect of Gd-DTPA, as with all the gadolinium chelates, on the fetus is unknown. Injection during pregnancy is not recommended, except in extenuating clinical circumstances and with informed consent. The agent crosses the placenta[68] and is excreted in breast milk.[100] It is recommended that breast-feeding be discontinued for several days after the injection of contrast material in the mother.

As with the other gadolinium chelates with extracellular distribution and renal excretion, a 3% to 5% rate of adverse reactions is observed after intravenous administration. The majority of reactions are mild, including principally nausea and hives.[126] Caution should be exercised with bolus administration, particularly given the close confines of most MR units. In a large clinical trial of 4260 patients with bolus injection of Gd-DTPA, emesis was reported in 12.[43] Anaphylactoid-like reactions are rare but have been reported.[124] Administration of the agent in the presence of a physician is recommended, along with proper instruction and ready availability of equipment for treatment of possible untoward effects.

Gd-DTPA-BMA

Gadodiamide (Gd-DTPA-BMA or Omniscan [Nycomed]) is a neutral linear chelate that was approved for clinical use in the United States in 1993. The ligand, DTPA-BMA, is a derivative of DTPA. Neutrality is achieved by replacement of two anionic donors ($-CO_2^-$) with methylamide (*bis*-methylamide [BMA]). This leads to a substantial decrease in the thermodynamic stability constant for the complex: log K_{eq} for Gd-DTPA-BMA is 16.9 and for Gd-DTPA is 22.1 (Table 12-3). The pharmaceutical preparation contains 5% of the excess ligand as calcium DTPA-BMA. Questions have been raised concerning acute toxicological studies in animals and overall product tolerance.[110] A statistically significant change in serum iron has also been reported after administration of Gd-DTPA-BMA, as with Gd-DTPA.[117]

Transmetallation has been investigated in recent clinical studies.[26,27] Patients were randomized into three groups, comparing Gd-DTPA, Gd-DTPA-BMA, and Gd-HP-DO3A, all at a dose of 0.1 mmol/kg. Patients receiving Gd-DTPA-BMA experienced a significant drop in serum zinc after contrast injection. This result was not seen with either Gd-DTPA or Gd-HP-DO3A. Urine zinc was 26-fold higher in patients receiving Gd-DTPA-BMA, as compared with Gd-HP-DO3A. Urine zinc was also

increased after Gd-DTPA administration, although to a lesser degree than with Gd-DTPA-BMA. These results imply either substantial gadolinium release in vivo with Gd-DTPA-BMA or chelation of zinc by excess DTPA-BMA (in the drug formulation as administered). That Gd-DTPA can also minimally dechelate in vivo is supported by a case report of interference with a gallium-67 nuclear scan.[33]

No differences in lesion enhancement, at a dose of 0.1 mmol/kg, have been described as compared with Gd-DTPA or Gd-HP-DO3A. The conclusion from phase II and phase III trials in 439 patients was that Gd-DTPA-BMA is an effective MR contrast agent for imaging of the head and spine.[113] In a study of 73 patients at a dose of 0.1 mmol/kg, abnormalities in serum iron were described in 6 (8%). No abnormalities in total bilirubin were reported.[30] However, postcontrast blood samples were obtained only between 24 and 36 hours after injection. This avoided the early postcontrast time period, during which peak changes because of blood hemolysis would be anticipated. The most common adverse reactions reported are headache, dizziness, and nausea.

Gd-HP-DO3A

Gadoteridol (Gd-HP-DO3A or ProHance [Bracco Diagnostics]) is a neutral (nonionic) ring chelate that was approved for clinical use in the United States in 1992 for a dose range of 0.1 to 0.3 mmol/kg. The pharmaceutical preparation contains 0.1% of the excess ligand as calteridol calcium. Partly because of the ring (or macrocyclic) nature of the chelate, Gd-HP-DO3A is more stable in vitro and in vivo than either Gd-DTPA or Gd-DTPA-BMA (Figure 12-5). Gd-HP-DO3A is thus relatively inert to metal-ion substitution. With regard to potential long-term toxicity, on the basis of heavy metal deposition, this agent should be superior. A study of patients with end-stage renal disease has demonstrated that the agent is rapidly and safely dialysable.[51]

The effects of contrast-media extravasation in soft tissue have also been studied in animals.[13] Gd-HP-DO3A proved significantly less toxic than Gd-DTPA, which caused moderate necrosis, hemorrhage, and edema. The changes noted with Gd-DTPA were similar to those seen with a conventional radiographic contrast agent, meglumine diatrizoate.

Gd-HP-DO3A is approved for high-dose use (0.3 mmol/kg). Clinical trials with high doses have focused on the investigation of intracranial metastatic disease. Lesion enhancement is consistently improved at a high dose, with a mean increase of 107% at 0.3 versus 0.1 mmol/kg demonstrated in one study.[83] In a study of 27 patients with clinically suspected brain metastases, 46 new lesions were noted in 19 patients with a dose of 0.3 as compared with 0.1 mmol/kg.[129] A marked improvement in lesion conspicuity was also noted. In the phase III multicenter US trial, 49 patients were studied with evidence of at least one metastatic lesion on MRI.[130] On film review, both unblinded and blinded reviewers noted a marked improvement in diagnostic confidence and lesion detection at a high dose (Figure 12-6). The increase in number of lesions detected was 51% (unblinded) and 32% (blinded), respectively. Two patients with normal scans at 0.1 mmol/kg demonstrated a single metastatic lesion at 0.3 mmol/kg. A study of cost-effectiveness revealed lower overall cost of patient management, despite the higher cost of contrast administration.[61] Craniotomies and aggressive courses of radiation therapy were avoided in five patients because of detection of additional lesions at high dose.

Growing experience with gadolinium chelates has led to extensive discussion of the utility of a high dose (0.3 mmol/kg, as compared with 0.1 mmol/kg, the dose commonly used in most clinical practice). Whether given as a single dose or as a supplemental injection, a high dose has been shown to improve lesion enhancement over a broad range of pathological conditions. As noted in the previous paragraph, in studying patients with possible metastatic disease to the brain, high-dose contrast administration improves lesion detection and is strongly recommended. A high dose also improves reader confidence with regard to lesion identification and allows exclusion of abnormalities that might be questioned on the basis of the standard-dose postcontrast examination alone. First-pass perfusion studies are also improved, if injection time is kept short, with the use of a high dose.[17,86]

Cost concerns have limited high-dose trials and clinical acceptance. The use of a low dose, less than 0.1 mmol/kg, was advocated by numerous practitioners in the late 1980s and early 1990s, in part for financial reasons. This practice has fortunately been discontinued, with clinical experience demonstrating such scans to be nondiagnostic in many instances. Low contrast doses, such as 0.05 mmol/kg, have been shown to provide inferior tumor-brain contrast and inadequate lesion delineation.[102]

As requirements for a high dose have become more apparent, further research has been pursued to develop new agents with improved tolerance. Increased emphasis has been placed on physicochemical properties, including osmolality, viscosity, and stability of the metal chelate in vivo. Agents with lower osmolality and viscosity can be administered faster and generally at higher doses, important features for first-pass perfusion studies. Other avenues of research include development of compounds with higher relaxivity. Both approaches seek to lower the toxicity of the agent for a given effective dose. One step in development has paralleled the history of iodinated agents, with development of nonionic (neutral) compounds, such as gadoteridol, following the initial development of gadopentetate dimeglumine, an ionic (charged) compound.[114]

Other Chelates

Although not approved for clinical use in the United States, gadoterate meglumine (Gd-DOTA or Dotarem [Guerbet]) is currently used in many European and South American countries. Like Gd-HP-DO3A, Gd-DOTA is a ring chelate, with greater in vitro and in vivo stability than linear chelates. A randomized clinical trial comparing Gd-DOTA and Gd-DTPA in 300 patients found no difference in efficacy, with a similar frequency of adverse events.[5]

Gadobutrol (Gd-DO3A-butrol or Gadovist [Schering AG]) is a nonionic, cyclical, paramagnetic metal-ion chelate recently studied in phase II clinical trials in Germany.[24,118] Postcontrast MR examinations were obtained in 20 patients with metastatic disease, comparing doses of 0.1 and 0.3 mmol/kg Gd-DO3A-butrol with 0.1 mmol/kg Gd-DTPA. High-dose Gd-DO3A-butrol provided a statistically significant improvement in lesion enhancement, compared with the standard dose of either agent. Thirty-six additional metastatic lesions were noted in six patients at a high dose.

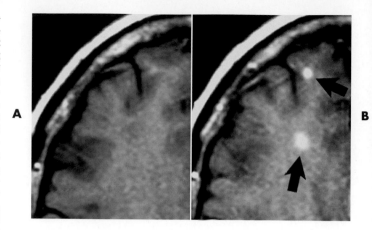

FIGURE 12-6 Brain metastases detected only after high-dose contrast administration (0.3 mmol/kg gadoteridol). **A,** The T1-weighted scan after administration of 0.1 mmol/kg, the current standard dose, is normal. **B,** Identification of two metastatic lesions *(arrows)* from primary lung carcinoma is possible only on the high-dose (0.3 mmol/kg) postcontrast T1-weighted scan. In a multiinstitutional study a 32% increase in the number of metastatic lesions detected was demonstrated with a dose of 0.3 mmol/kg in comparison with a dose of 0.1 mmol/kg.

Gadoversetamide (Gd-DTPA *bis*-methoxyethyl amide or Optimark [Mallinckrodt Medical]), a linear chelate, has recently been evaluated in normal volunteers at doses of 0.1 to 0.7 mmol/kg. Serum iron increased transiently after injection in a dose-dependent fashion.[14]

Although initially evaluated as a hepatobiliary contrast agent,[120] gadobenate dimeglumine (Gd-BOPTA [Bracco Diagnostics]) has recently received attention for CNS examinations (Figure 12-7). Published investigations have focused on the use of Gd-BOPTA in brain neoplasia and first-pass cerebral blood volume studies.[8] With a rat brain tumor model, lesion enhancement after a contrast dose of 0.1 mmol/kg has been shown to be substantially greater with Gd-BOPTA than with Gd-DTPA.[11]

Innovative research continues in the development of new extracellular paramagnetic metal-ion chelates and new formulations. Dimers have been investigated, with linkage flexibility demonstrated to play an important role in relaxivity per gadolinium unit.[107] Encapsulation of Gd-HP-DO3A into liposomes has been studied, with a marked decrease in liver signal intensity noted after contrast administration because of the susceptibility effect of Gd-HP-DO3A when compartmentalized within Kupffer's cells.[23]

NEW APPLICATIONS
High Dose

High-dose contrast administration with an agent such as Gd-HP-DO3A provides improved lesion detection, greater diagnostic confidence, and improved assessment of tissue perfusion, the last with first-pass studies. The original choice of contrast dose (0.1 mmol/kg for Gd-DTPA, first used in 1984) was determined by safety concerns and not on the basis of efficacy. Subsequent animal and clinical trials suggest efficacy for higher doses in a broad range of indications. The multicenter US trial comparing 0.1 and 0.3 mmol/kg Gd-HP-DO3A for the detection of brain metastases demonstrated an improvement of 32% in the number of lesions detected at a high dose (Figure 12-6). In this trial, patients received an initial injection of 0.1 mmol/kg, followed by a supplemental injection of 0.2 mmol/kg (for a total dose of 0.3 mmol/kg) 30 min later. A subsequent multicenter US trial compared doses of 0.1 and 0.3 given at different settings, separated by more than 1 day and less than 7 days. Results were similar, with the conclusion being that a high dose is efficacious regardless of whether given as a split injection or as a single dose.[95] Metastatic lesions show consistently greater enhancement at a high dose, leading to improved confidence in the diagnosis of lesions questioned on the basis of the standard-dose examination, as well as increased lesion detection. A high dose makes possible the detection of additional lesions by raising the level of enhancement above the threshold necessary for visualization.

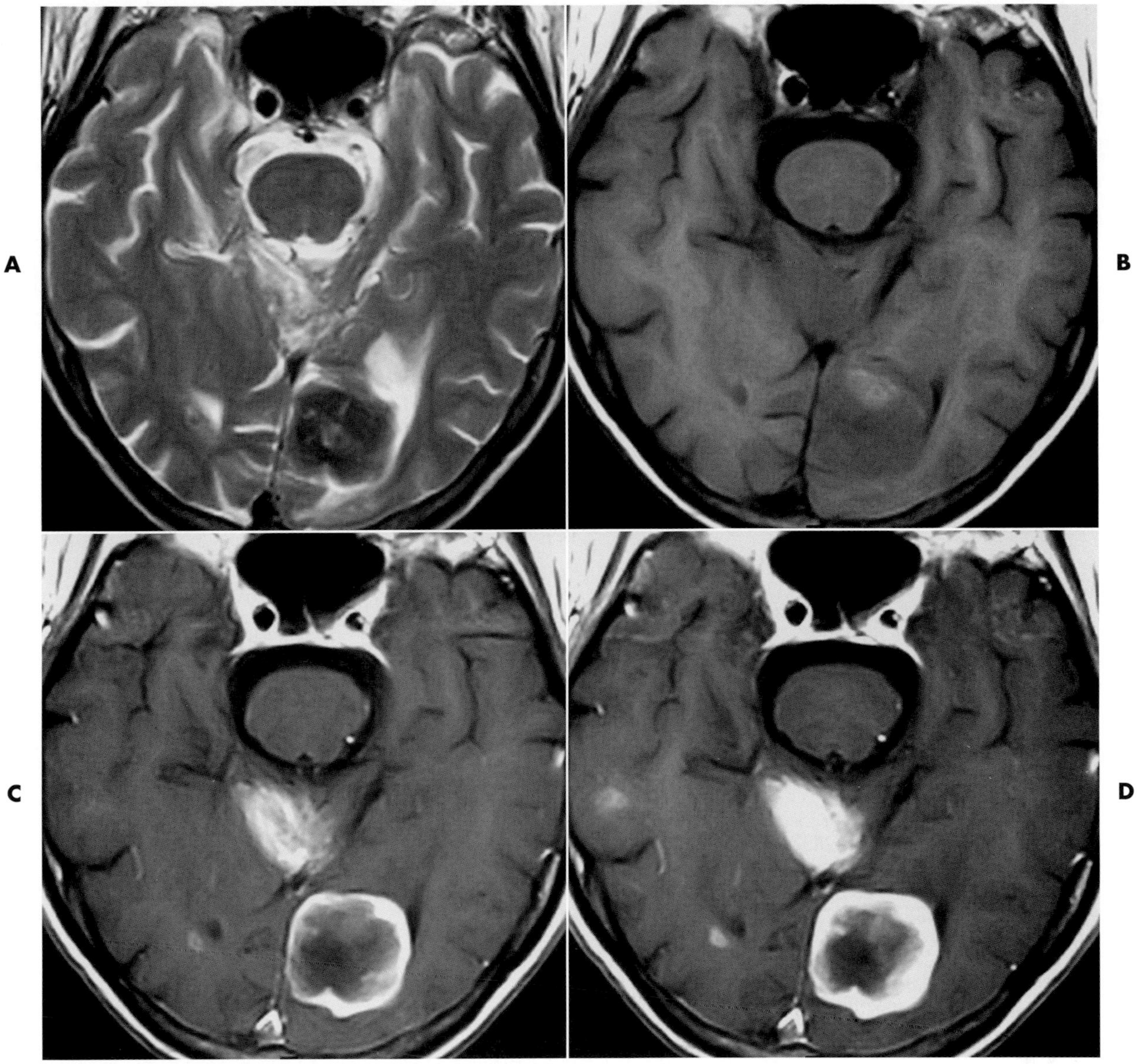

FIGURE 12-7 Brain metastases illustrating the use of Gd-BOPTA. Precontrast T2 **(A)** and T1-weighted **(B)** scans are compared with postcontrast T1-weighted scans using doses of 0.1 **(C)** and 0.2 **(D)** mmol/kg. Weak protein binding, which occurs with Gd-BOPTA, can substantially increase the enhancement effect of a gadolinium chelate. For example, in animal experiments, peak signal-intensity enhancement in brain tumors was 87% after administration of 0.1 mmol/kg Gd-BOPTA as compared with 64% after 0.1 mmol/kg Gd-DTPA (which has no protein binding). In this instance a higher dose improves enhancement of all lesions and makes more evident two small lesions, one near the right occipital horn and the other in the right temporal lobe.

There is limited experience with application of a high dose in brain neoplasia other than in metastatic disease. In a phase II clinical trial involving 14 patients with intracranial neoplastic disease, higher contrast doses (0.2 and 0.3 mmol/kg) consistently improved lesion enhancement.[82] A subsequent study, which combined phase II and III results in 40 patients with intracranial neoplastic disease, concluded that "improved enhancement, detection, and delineation" of CNS neoplasms resulted from injection of higher contrast doses. It was further suggested that findings at a high dose could be clinically significant and justify the higher cost.[128]

In gliomas of the brain the administration of a high contrast dose can lead to recognition of tumor outside the bounds defined by T2-weighted scans. In a study of 23 patients with pathologically proven gliomas, 12 "demonstrated enhancement on T1-weighted images extending beyond the zone of apparent signal abnormality demonstrated on T2-weighted images."[131] This was seen in none of the six patients receiving a contrast dose of 0.05 mmol/kg, in only one of five at 0.1

mmol/kg, in four of five at 0.2 mmol/kg, and in all of seven at 0.3 mmol/kg. Thus improved definition of neoplastic extent is possible at a high contrast dose in these infiltrative tumors by recognition of subtle blood-brain barrier disruption.

In early subacute cerebral infarction the degree of blood-brain barrier disruption may not be sufficient to produce abnormal contrast enhancement at a standard contrast dose.[86] In an experimental animal study, administration of 0.3 mmol/kg (as opposed to 0.1 mmol/kg) produced a statistically significant increase in enhancement—more than double. In six early subacute infarcts, abnormal contrast enhancement was noted in only three animals at 0.1 mmol/kg, yet in all at 0.3 mmol/kg. This phenomenon has also been observed in clinical studies (Figure 12-8).[92] Administration of a high dose enables recognition of characteristic parenchymal enhancement, providing information for lesion dating and differential diagnosis.

In brain infection, whether parenchymal[93] or meningeal[96] in nature, administration of high contrast doses also produces greater lesion en-

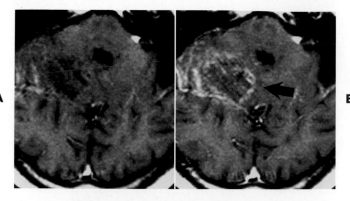

FIGURE 12-8 Blood-brain barrier disruption visualized in an acute cerebellar infarct at 0.3 mmol/kg, with absence of enhancement at 0.1 mmol/kg. **A,** Blood-brain barrier disruption in early infarction may be insufficient to manifest abnormal contrast enhancement at a standard dose. **B,** In such instances, administration of a high dose can reveal abnormal enhancement *(arrow)*. This confirms the acute nature of the lesion, with the patient in this instance being an elderly man studied 1 day after clinical presentation.

hancement (Figures 12-9 and 12-10). For early lesions or in the immunocompromised patient the use of a high dose permits identification of blood-brain barrier disruption, which might otherwise not be identified, confirming lesion activity. This finding can be critical clinically, changing the assessment of a lesion from chronic to active.

Triple-dose studies (0.3 mmol/kg) have recently been performed in patients with multiple sclerosis (MS). A high contrast dose permits detection of more enhanced MS plaques in the brain.[22] In addition, the size of enhanced lesions was larger and their conspicuity greater at a high dose.[21]

Initial studies comparing 0.1 and 0.3 mmol/kg in the head and neck and the spine suggest utility for high doses in both areas. In tumors of the head and neck, both the percent of lesion enhancement and the visual assessment rating were improved at 0.2 mmol/kg.[119] Better lesion detection and delineation, as well as greater diagnostic confidence, were reported at 0.3 mmol/kg in 14 patients with suspected spinal cord lesions. The final diagnosis was altered in 39% after the high-dose examination.[109]

Magnetic resonance angiography (MRA) has also been evaluated after contrast administration, with specific attention given to contrast dose (Figure 12-11).[84] Higher doses permit the concentration of the agent in the blood to be sustained for a longer time period at a higher level, with advantages in MRA specifically because of the long scan times.

Magnetization Transfer

MT techniques have recently been used in MRI to modulate tissue contrast. In this approach, off-resonance pulses are used to saturate protons in macromolecules. The addition of MT pulses to standard imaging sequences can improve the visualization of contrast enhancement in the brain, with this observation specifically demonstrated in cerebral infarction.[60] However, in a comparison of high and standard doses with and without MT, high doses with or without MT ranked superior to all other imaging approaches (Figure 12-12). The degree of lesion enhancement achieved with MT and a standard contrast dose does not approach that achieved with a high contrast dose, regardless of whether MT has been applied (Figures 12-9 and 12-10). Recent clinical studies have further investigated the use of a standard contrast dose (0.1 mmol/kg) combined with MT. This approach, however, is not recommended in place of imaging with a high contrast dose (0.3 mmol/kg).[46,72]

First-Pass Studies

First-pass studies can be acquired on either conventional 1.5 Tesla (T) MR systems or newer echo-planar units. By observing with rapid dynamic imaging the bolus of the contrast agent as it passes through the brain, one can make an assessment of rCBV and thus brain perfusion

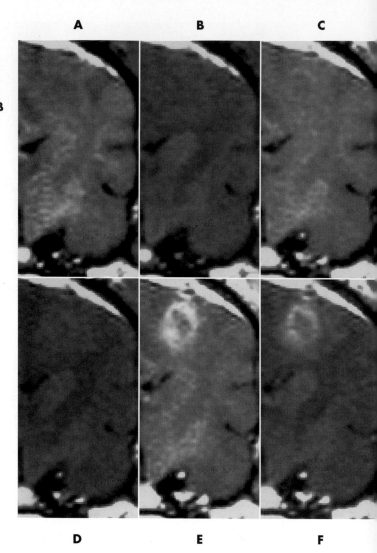

FIGURE 12-9 Early brain abscess. High-dose contrast and use of MT technique. Coronal T1-weighted scans are presented in a canine model 1 day after injection of bacterial suspension. Images are before **(A)** and after **(B)**, respectively, 0.1 mmol/kg **(C and D)**, and 0.3 mmol/kg **(E and F)** contrast injection (gadoteridol). Scans using the conventional spin-echo technique **(A, C,** and **E)** are compared with scans using MT **(B, D,** and **F)**. **A** and **B,** Precontrast, lesion is of low signal intensity. Normal brain parenchyma is of slightly lower signal intensity on **B** as compared with **A,** consistent with implementation of MT. **C** and **D,** At a standard dose there is minimal lesion enhancement. **E** and **F,** At a high dose there is prominent ring enhancement, which is well demonstrated on both scans. Enhancement on the high-dose scan without MT **(E)** is substantially greater than that on the standard dose scan with MT **(D)**. (From reference 93.)

(Figure 12-13). These studies typically depend on observation of the T2 or T2* effect of the contrast agent. Dose effects have been evaluated in three studies.[17,50,88] The conclusion of each investigation has been that there is a dose-dependent effect (Figure 12-14), with improved sensitivity and efficacy at higher doses (up to 0.5 mmol/kg). This type of MR study has found clinical application in the evaluation of brain ischemia (Figures 12-15 and 12-16) and neoplasia.

Recent publications have detailed additional applications for first-pass imaging. The hemodynamic impact of stenosis of the internal carotid artery can be assessed. Perfusion imaging can thus be used to determine appropriate clinical management, either surgical or medical.[67] In Alzheimer's disease, rCBV abnormalities can be quantified. This makes MRI a viable alternative to positron emission tomography (PET) and single photon emission computed tomography (SPECT) for the study of this disease.[58] Perfusion studies have also been used to determine the reduction of blood volume in astrocytomas and adjacent brain after radiotherapy. Thus tumor response and normal tissue effects can be monitored from a functional perspective.[125]

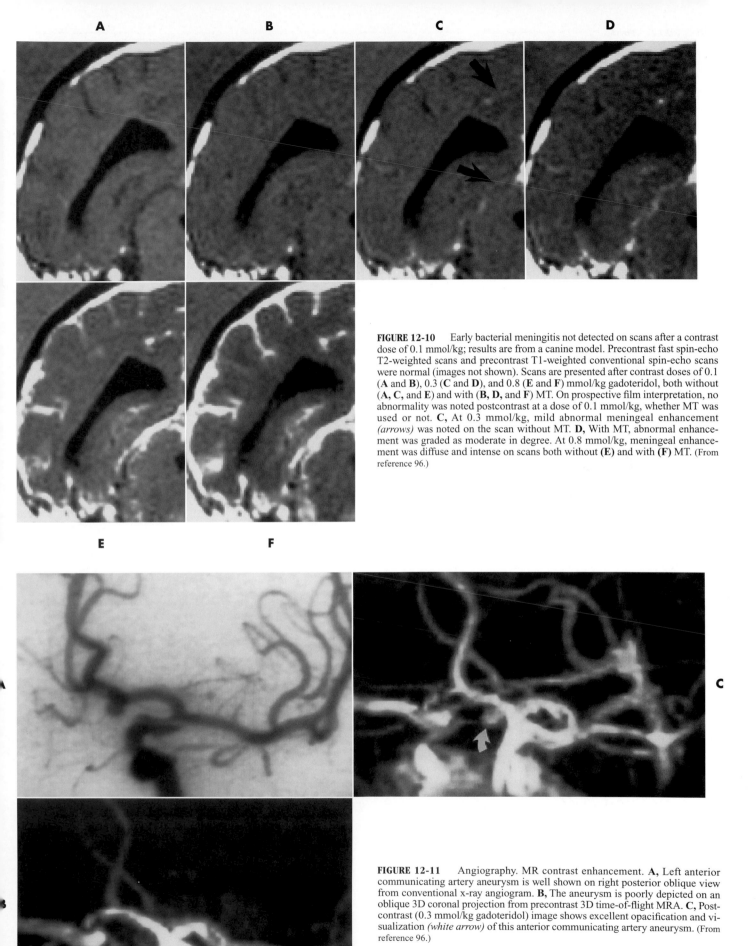

FIGURE 12-10 Early bacterial meningitis not detected on scans after a contrast dose of 0.1 mmol/kg; results are from a canine model. Precontrast fast spin-echo T2-weighted scans and precontrast T1-weighted conventional spin-echo scans were normal (images not shown). Scans are presented after contrast doses of 0.1 (**A** and **B**), 0.3 (**C** and **D**), and 0.8 (**E** and **F**) mmol/kg gadoteridol, both without (**A, C,** and **E**) and with (**B, D,** and **F**) MT. On prospective film interpretation, no abnormality was noted postcontrast at a dose of 0.1 mmol/kg, whether MT was used or not. **C,** At 0.3 mmol/kg, mild abnormal meningeal enhancement *(arrows)* was noted on the scan without MT. **D,** With MT, abnormal enhancement was graded as moderate in degree. At 0.8 mmol/kg, meningeal enhancement was diffuse and intense on scans both without (**E**) and with (**F**) MT. (From reference 96.)

FIGURE 12-11 Angiography. MR contrast enhancement. **A,** Left anterior communicating artery aneurysm is well shown on right posterior oblique view from conventional x-ray angiogram. **B,** The aneurysm is poorly depicted on an oblique 3D coronal projection from precontrast 3D time-of-flight MRA. **C,** Postcontrast (0.3 mmol/kg gadoteridol) image shows excellent opacification and visualization *(white arrow)* of this anterior communicating artery aneurysm. (From reference 96.)

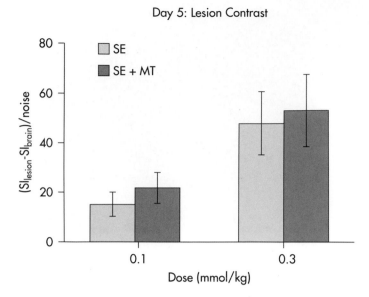

Day 5: Lesion Contrast

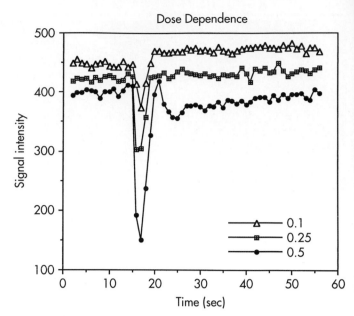

Dose Dependence

FIGURE 12-12   MT imaging of a brain abscess at the late cerebritis state (day 5 after implantation). The effects of the contrast dose dominate the effects of the scan technique (specifically application of MT). *SI,* Signal intensity; *SE,* spin-echo T1-weighted scan (without application of MT); *SE + MT,* spin-echo T1-weighted scan with MT. Results with MT are statistically superior to results without MT, when contrast dose is held constant. However, results at high dose (0.3 mmol/kg) are statistically superior to (and of substantially greater magnitude than) that at standard dose (0.1 mmol/kg), whether MT was applied or not. (From reference 93.)

FIGURE 12-14   First-pass effect in brain, as observed on MR images after bolus gadolinium chelate administration, is dose dependent. On steady state free precession and echo-planar imaging the presence of contrast within the capillaries during the first pass of the agent through brain reduces signal intensity because of T2 and susceptibility effects. A proportionally greater response, and thus more negative signal intensity change, is seen with higher contrast doses. Curves from normal brain are illustrated, comparing doses of 0.1, 0.25, and 0.5 mmol/kg. (From reference 88.)

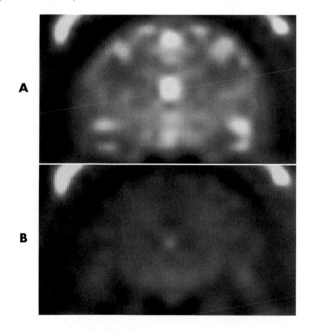

FIGURE 12-13   Cerebral perfusion assessed by first-pass, dynamic contrast-enhanced imaging using a gadolinium chelate (Gd-HP-DO3A, ProHance). Scans before contrast injection **(A)** and at peak of first pass **(B)**. After bolus IV contrast injection, a decrease in signal intensity is noted during the first pass of contrast agent through brain. Rather than observing the T1 effect of the agent, first-pass studies rely on observation of combined T2 and susceptibility effects.

Both Gd-HP-DO3A and Gd-DO3A-butrol can be formulated at a concentration of 1.0 M, twice that currently used clinically for all extracellular gadolinium chelates (0.5 M). Use of higher concentration formations in first-pass studies has been shown to improve the reliability of rCBV measurements (Figure 12-17). The smaller volume of contrast agent produces a sharper bolus.[36,94]

Magnetic Resonance Angiography

The latest major new application of MR contrast-media is for MRA. Clinically approved gadolinium chelates are used in combination with

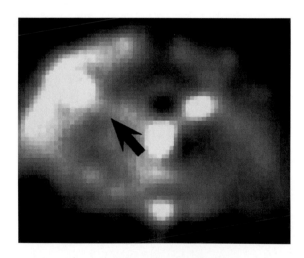

FIGURE 12-15   Acute left middle cerebral artery infarction *(arrow),* visualized on dynamic imaging immediately after bolus injection of a paramagnetic metal-ion chelate. Image displayed was that obtained at the peak of the first pass through brain. Information regarding rCBV is provided by first-pass studies, permitting detection of early ischemic injury. Normal left hemisphere demonstrates marked reduction in signal intensity because of the presence of the contrast agent. However, the right hemisphere remains hyperintense, demarcating the region of ischemic insult. This study was performed after occlusion of the middle cerebral artery in a cat. In acute infarction there may not be sufficient vasogenic edema to permit lesion detection on conventional T1- and T2-weighted scans, which were normal in this instance (images not shown).

breath-hold 3D time-of-flight scans. Improvements in imaging technique are ongoing; shorter imaging times (5 to 20 sec for a 3D slab) are generally superior. This approach represents a major advance in the study of the carotid arteries, aorta, renal arteries, and iliac arteries. The carotid arteries can be visualized from the aortic arch to the skull base.[12] The pulmonary vascular tree is exquisitely depicted. Imaging of aortic dissections and aneurysms is markedly improved.[48] The mesenteric arterial and venous circulation and the portal vein can also be directly visualized.[106] Major areas of clinical application include the study of renal arteries (for stenotic lesions)[108] and iliac arteries (for arteriosclerotic disease).

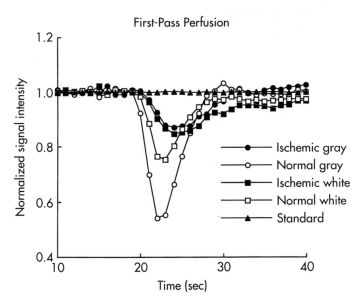

FIGURE 12-16   Perfusion changes tissue signal intensity during transit of contrast agent bolus through brain. Gadoteridol 0.5 mmol/kg was injected intravenously at a rate of 9 ml/sec. Normal and ischemic gray and white matter can be differentiated because of differences in perfusion, which are reflected by the magnitude of the signal-intensity change. (From reference 87.)

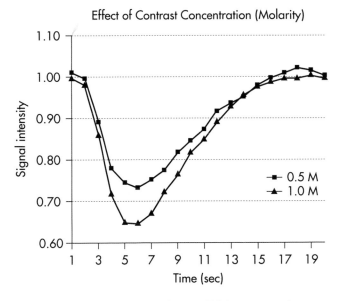

FIGURE 12-17   rCBV assessed by the use of higher-concentration contrast formulations. Results are compared for 0.5- and 1-M formulations of gadoteridol (Gd-HP-DO3A). The contrast dose was held constant. Nonionic agents, such as gadoteridol, can be formulated at higher concentrations than currently used clinically (0.5 M), with advantages in first-pass perfusion studies because of delivery of a more compact bolus. Region-of-interest measurements from normal white matter are illustrated, with higher concentration formulation resulting in greater magnitude of the signal-intensity reduction.

DYSPROSIUM CHELATES

For first-pass brain studies the T2 or T2* effect of the contrast medium is observed during bolus transit. Both gadolinium and dysprosium chelates have been used successfully in this application, at least in experimental investigation. In regard to dysprosium (Dy) chelates, to date reports exist only with formulations of Dy HP-DO3A (Figure 12-18) and Dy DTPA-BMA.[49,63] Improved results, specifically a greater magnitude of signal-intensity change during first pass, are seen with dysprosium chelates as compared with the corresponding gadolinium chelates at high magnetic fields, 1.5 to 2 T (Figure 12-19). This result is expected because of the higher T2 relaxivity and susceptibility effect of the dysprosium ion.

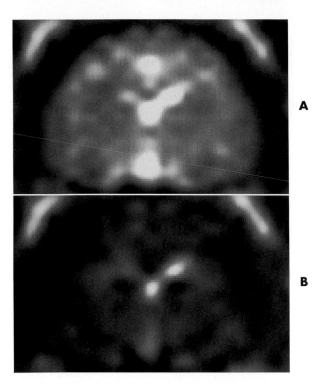

FIGURE 12-18   Cerebral perfusion assessed by first-pass, dynamic contrast-enhanced imaging using a dysprosium chelate (Dy HP-DO3A [Bracco Diagnostics]). Scans before contrast injection (**A**) and at peak of the first pass (**B**). Dysprosium has a negligible effect on T1 and yet the highest susceptibility effect of lanthanide metals, which include gadolinium. During the first pass of agent through brain, a decrease in tissue signal intensity is observed. This decrease is substantially greater in degree than that observed with equivalent gadolinium chelate injection (compare with Figure 12-13). Use of a dysprosium chelate could lead to greater accuracy and higher sensitivity in evaluation of cerebral perfusion. For example, differentiation of gray and white matter at the peak of bolus is greater with the dysprosium chelate, reflecting improved discrimination of tissues with higher (gray matter) as opposed to lower (white matter) blood volume.

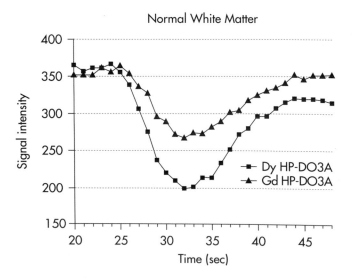

FIGURE 12-19   First-pass brain perfusion studies using a dysprosium chelate. In comparison of results with Gd-HP-DO3A and Dy HP-DO3A, with dose and imaging parameters held constant, effect of dysprosium agent is noted to be greater. Signal intensity curves during first pass are presented for normal white matter.

A

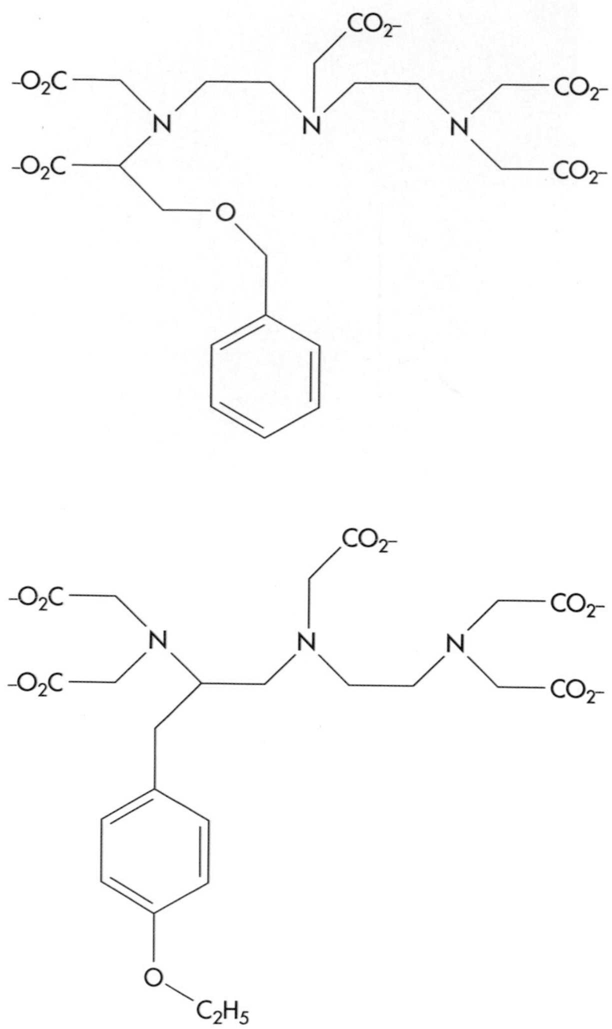

B

FIGURE 12-20 Chemical structures for benzyloxy-propionic-tetraacetic acid (BOPTA) **(A)**, the chelate in gadobenate dimeglumine, and ethoxybenzyl diethylene-triamine-pentaacetic acid (EOB-DTPA) **(B)**, the chelate in Eovist. The gadolinium compounds using these two chelates are in evaluation worldwide as potential hepatobiliary MR contrast media. Both are linear chelates.

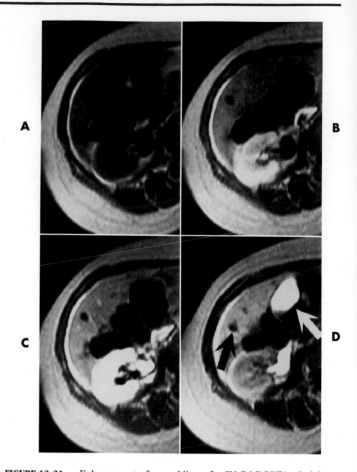

FIGURE 12-21 Enhancement of normal liver after IV Gd-BOPTA administration, permitting improved lesion characterization. T1-weighted scans are from before **(A)** and 1 **(B)**, 5 **(C)**, and 80 min **(D)** after contrast injection. Liver enhancement is noted immediately after contrast administration and persists with time. Excretion of contrast agent by both renal and hepatobiliary routes is demonstrated. The right kidney shows prominent early enhancement. The gallbladder *(white arrow)* is opacified on the delayed scan. On dynamic and delayed postcontrast scans a single lesion *(black arrow,* a simple cyst) that exhibits no change in appearance postcontrast and remains of low signal intensity is visible. On unenhanced MR images, simple cysts can be difficult to differentiate from hemangiomas. Both may be of uniform low signal intensity on T1-weighted scans and high signal intensity on heavily T2-weighted scans. Acquisition of dynamic postcontrast scans permits differentiation because cysts do not enhance.

HEPATOBILIARY CHELATES

Two gadolinium chelates with hepatobiliary excretion, Gd-BOPTA[111] and Gd-EOB-DTPA[73] (Figure 12-20), have recently been evaluated in clinical trials. Gd-BOPTA (gadobenate dimeglumine or MultiHance, Bracco Diagnostics) is in phase II and phase III trials worldwide, with more than 1000 patients studied to date.[120] Gd-EOB-DTPA is not as far along in clinical trials; phase II studies in 200 subjects are completed.[31,104] Both agents are taken up by hepatocytes and excreted in part in the bile. In this way they differ from the gadolinium chelates approved to date, which are excreted by glomerular filtration alone.

As previously noted, Gd-BOPTA is substantially further along in the approval process. It is also the only hepatobiliary gadolinium chelate evaluated to date in the United States. Approval of Gd-BOPTA for clinical use was granted in Great Britain in 1997. Doses up to 0.2 mmol/kg have been studied. A signal-intensity increase of more than 100% is seen postcontrast in normal liver on T1-weighted scans. Enhancement is maximum on delayed scans, with a broad temporal peak. Both dynamic and delayed postcontrast scans prove to be of value. Dynamic scans provide information principally concerning differential diagnosis (Figure 12-21). Lesion detectability can be markedly improved on delayed scans, in particular for small metastases (Figure 12-22).[10] The wide imaging window on delayed scans, made possible by the prolonged enhancement of normal liver parenchyma, provides flexibility in

scan acquisition and choice of imaging plane. Hepatobiliary gadolinium chelates may also find application in the assessment of liver function.[59] The safety profile for Gd-BOPTA appears identical to that of the other extracellular gadolinium chelates. Widespread approval is anticipated within a few years; agents in this class are expected to replace the current generation of gadolinium chelates for liver MRI.

It should be noted that gadolinium chelates with extracellular distribution, such as Gd-HP-DO3A, can also be used for improved detection of liver lesions.[85] In this application, scans are obtained in a dynamic fashion, with differential accumulation of the agent in normal as opposed to diseased tissue aiding lesion recognition (Figure 12-23). Valuable information regarding differential diagnosis is also provided in analogy with the use of extracellular iodinated contrast-media in x-ray CT. In this setting, improved results are obtained with higher contrast doses.[89]

Mn-DPDP (mangafodipir trisodium) was recently approved for use in the United States (Figure 12-24). The chelate carries a net charge of −3 and is formulated as the trisodium salt. In initial clinical trials, adverse events, including changes in heart rate and blood pressure and prominent flushing, were observed. Subsequent studies have used lower doses (5 μmol/kg), diluted for injection and given slowly (3 ml/min, 10- to 15-min infusion). Positive contrast enhancement of the liver is noted on T1-weighted scans.

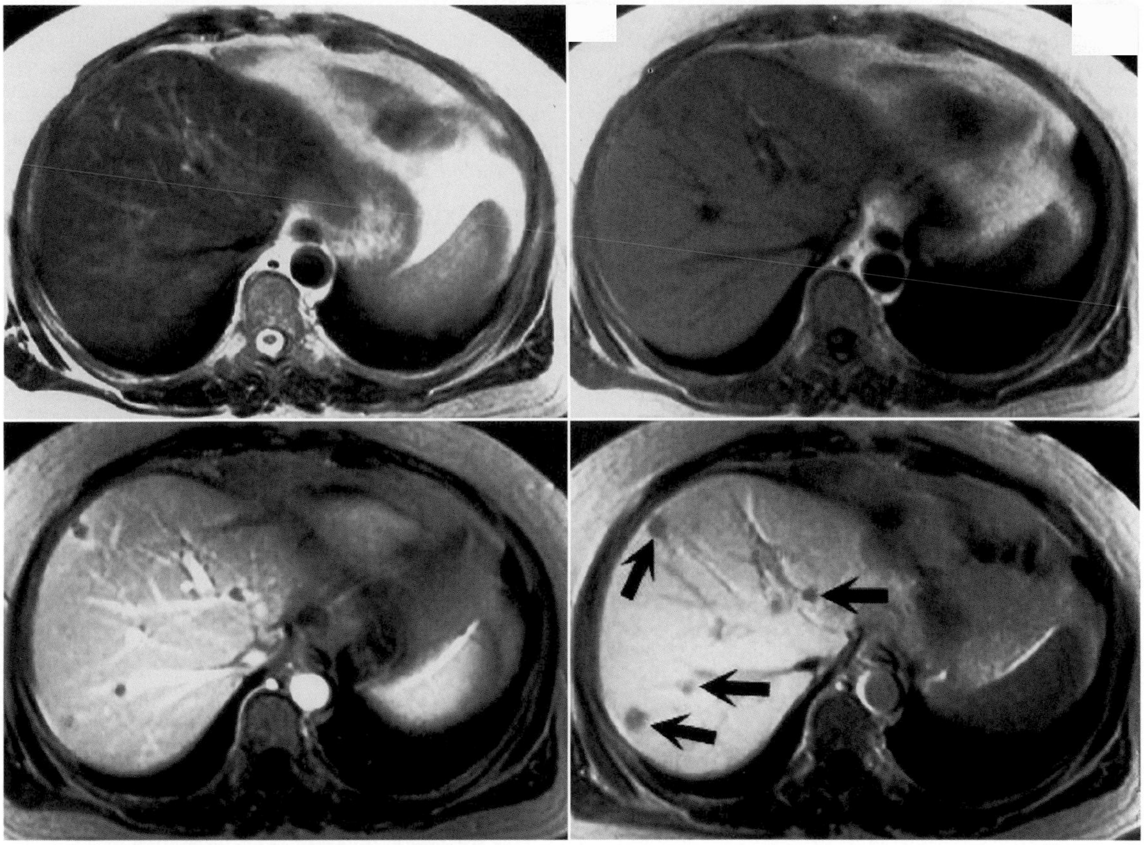

FIGURE 12-22   Improved detection of liver metastases after administration of a hepatobiliary gadolinium chelate, Gd-BOPTA (gadobenate dimeglumine or MultiHance [Bracco Diagnostics]). Precontrast T2- **(A)** and T1-weighted **(B)** scans are compared with postcontrast T1-weighted scans obtained at 1 **(C)** and 80 min **(D)** after injection. The T2-weighted scan is normal. On the precontrast T1-weighted scan, at most two lesions are visible and those only poorly. Postcontrast, there is intense enhancement of normal liver parenchyma, which improves detection of liver metastases. The latter remain of low signal intensity. On both dynamic **(C)** and delayed **(D)** postcontrast scans, four metastatic lesions *(arrows)* are well seen.

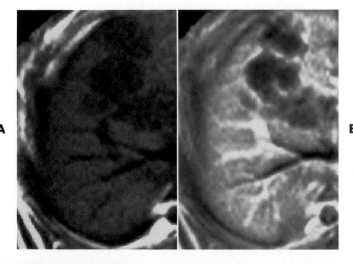

FIGURE 12-23   Dynamic enhancement of liver-lesion delineation with high-dose breath-hold immediate postcontrast scans. T1-weighted images obtained in first 1 to 2 min after gadoteridol (Gd-HP-DO3A) administration, using doses of 0.1 **(A)** and 0.3 **(B)** mmol/kg, are compared. A model of liver metastatic disease in a New Zealand white rabbit has been used for this comparison. Lesion conspicuity is highest on dynamic high-dose (0.3 mmol/kg) postcontrast scan. (From reference 90.)

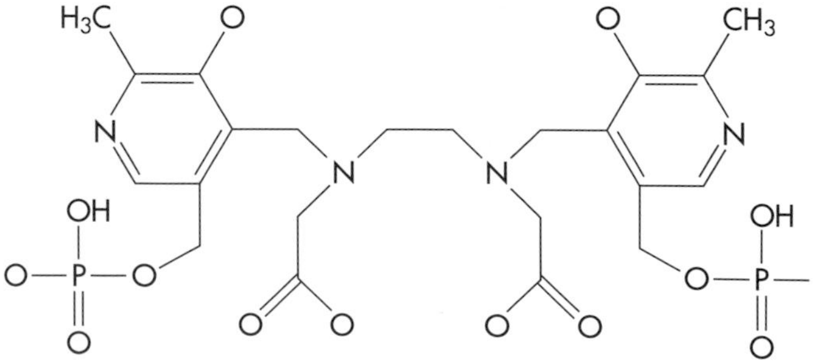

FIGURE 12-24   Chemical structure of dipyridoxyl diphosphate, Mn-DPDP.

BLOOD-POOL CHELATES

Gadolinium chelates that function as blood-pool agents are also being developed. This constitutes a third major class of MR contrast media; the extracellular gadolinium chelates are the first, and the hepatobiliary gadolinium chelates are the second.[75] Blood-pool agents should have a major impact; however, clinical approval is years away. These agents are designed to provide improved assessment of microscopic and macroscopic flow. MS-325 is the first to be evaluated in patients, with phase I trials completed. This agent reversibly binds to plasma albumin, achieving a substantial improvement in the magnitude and duration of blood-pool enhancement.[57]

PARTICULATE AGENTS

Iron particles of several sizes have been evaluated as potential MR contrast agents. In general, reaction rates have been higher than with gadolinium chelates.

Superparamagnetic Iron Oxide

Worldwide, 1535 patients have been studied with superparamagnetic iron oxide (AMI-25), which is now FDA approved and sold in the United States. US studies included 15 phase I and 213 phase II and phase III subjects. In phase II and III US trials the agent was diluted in 100 ml of 5% dextrose and given at a rate of 3 ml/min for an infusion time of 30 min.[76] Scans are obtained between ½ and 4 hours postcontrast. The agent is taken up by the reticuloendothelial system. A marked reduction in signal intensity of liver and spleen is seen postcontrast, with best results using intermediate T2-weighted scans. Increased lesion detectability was noted postcontrast in the initial clinical trial.[112] However, in subsequent work at high field, AMI-25 has failed to improve scan sensitivity.[16] Slow infusion is necessary to reduce the likelihood of hypotensive reactions. Other reported adverse events include low-back pain and flushing.

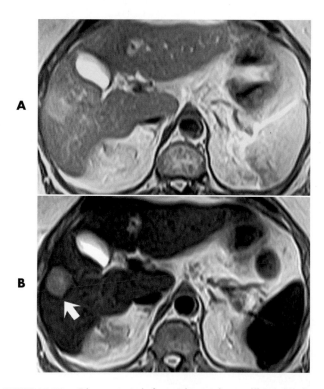

FIGURE 12-25   Liver metastasis from colon carcinoma, illustrating the use of an iron-particle nanocolloid. T2-weighted scans are illustrated before **(A)** and 30 min after **(B)** contrast administration. AMI-227 was administered as a slow IV infusion at a dose of 1.7 mg Fe/kg. On the postcontrast study the signal intensity of the normal liver parenchyma is markedly reduced. This improves recognition of the metastatic lesion (*arrow* in **B**), which remains hyperintense relative to normal liver.

Magnetite

Magnetite (Resovist or SHU 555 A) is in phase III clinical trials in Europe, with more than 100 patients studied to date. It represents a new formulation of superparamagnetic iron oxide (with slightly smaller particle size). Early clinical results appear favorable. In comparison with AMI-25, higher doses (up to 40 µmol/kg) and faster injection rates (including bolus injection) are possible.[32]

Iron Oxide Nanocolloids (Ultrasmall Superparamagnetic Iron Oxide)

Phase I and phase II US clinical trials with iron oxide nanocolloids (AMI-227) have been completed, with 55 normal volunteers and 220 patients studied. In phase II trials the agent was diluted in 100 ml of saline and given at a rate of 4 ml/min, for an infusion time of 25 min. T2 effects are dominant, with a decrease in signal intensity seen in well-perfused organs and the blood pool after injection. This agent can be used both for improved lesion detection, specifically in the liver (Figure 12-25),[98] and for lymph node studies (Figure 12-26). In a study of 12 patients with head and neck cancer, AMI-227 substantially improved

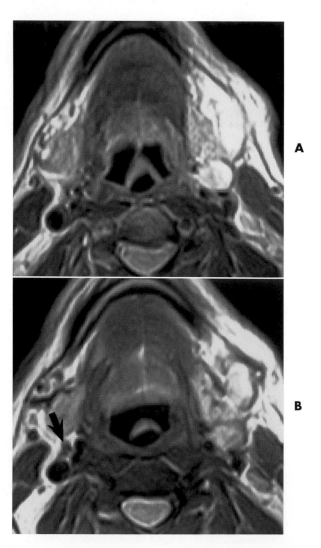

FIGURE 12-26   Lymph nodes. Differentiation of metastatic from normal tissue by use of iron oxide nanocolloid. The patient is a 53-year-old man with metastatic, poorly differentiated squamous cell carcinoma. Precontrast **(A)** and postcontrast **(B)** T2-weighted scans are presented. A dose of 1.7 mg Fe/kg was used. Before contrast administration, numerous enlarged lymph nodes are identified on the patient's left, with abnormal high signal intensity. After contrast administration, there is no substantial uptake of agent by these nodes, which through subsequent surgery were confirmed to be involved by metastatic disease. A small normal node in **B** (*arrow*), which demonstrates marked reduction in signal intensity postcontrast, is noted on the patient's right side.

the differentiation of metastatic and benign nodes, with a specificity of 84%.[2]

ORAL CONTRAST AGENTS

Opacification of the gastrointestinal tract is important on MR images, like CT, for differentiation of the gut from other normal structures and space-occupying lesions. Two basic classes of agents have been evaluated, those that cause an increase in signal intensity (positive contrast enhancement) and those that cause a decrease in signal intensity (negative contrast enhancement). LumenHance (Figure 12-27), Gd-DTPA,[52] and oil emulsions[56] have all been evaluated as possible positive oral contrast media. Unfortunately, positive enhancement can lead to image degradation on the basis of motion artifacts from bowel peristalsis. This can be minimized by careful selection of pulse technique and injection of a hypotonic agent, such as glucagon. Oral contrast media that reduce the signal intensity of the bowel contents offer a potential advantage because of the lack of motion-related image degradation (Figure 12-28). Superparamagnetic iron oxide particles have been evaluated in this role, with good bowel opacification demonstrated.[47,74] Susceptibility effects with this type of agent may diminish visualization of the bowel wall and pathological conditions therein.

SUMMARY

For Magnevist, Omniscan, and ProHance, which are the three gadolinium chelates in current clinical use in the United States, no difference in efficacy is observed when the agents are given at the same dose. However, macrocyclic chelates, such as ProHance, are more stable in vivo and offer a greater theoretical safety margin. For bolus injection, nonionic (neutral) chelates are favored, with these including ProHance and Omniscan. Growing areas of clinical application include the use of a high dose (0.3 mmol/kg), use in metastatic disease and other pathological conditions of the brain, and use in first-pass studies of the brain.

If future technological advances permit routine clinical application of breath-hold scans, then early dynamic postcontrast imaging will likely play a major role in liver MRI, as in CT. In particular, high-dose contrast administration with renally excreted gadolinium chelates, such as gadoteridol, can improve lesion detection and characterization. New contrast agents of innovative design will also likely play a major role in routine clinical MR studies in the future. Development is possible because of the lower required dose as compared with x-ray CT. In particular, the gadolinium chelates with hepatobiliary excretion appear promising as a new class of agents. As with the utility of MR itself, the impact of contrast media has far exceeded initial expectations, and its use continues to play a dominant role in this dynamic field.

ACKNOWLEDGMENT

With special thanks to Michael F. Tweedle, PhD, for his review of this material.

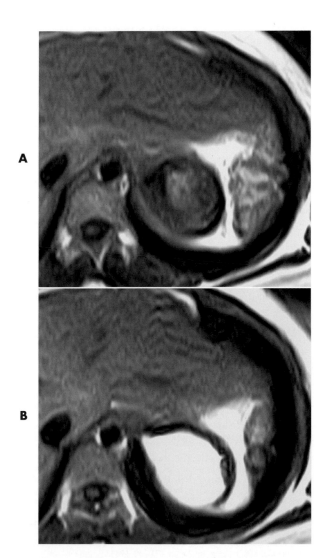

FIGURE 12-27   Bowel marking. Positive enhancement of the stomach contents after oral administration of an agent containing manganese chloride (LumenHance). Axial precontrast **(A)** and postcontrast **(B)** T1-weighted breath-hold scans are presented. Improved demarcation of bowel and bowel wall is provided postcontrast. The manganese in the preparation causes a reduction in the T1 of the bowel contents, and thus high signal intensity. FDA approval was recently granted.

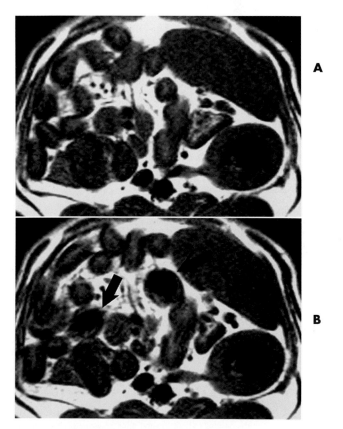

FIGURE 12-28   Bowel marking. Negative enhancement of the small bowel contents after oral contrast administration of PFOB, which affects proton density. Axial precontrast **(A)** and postcontrast **(B)** T1-weighted breath-hold scans are presented. Hydrogen atoms are replaced by halogen atoms in PFOB. The result is a material that appears black on all pulse sequences because of the lack of mobile protons. Before contrast administration **(A),** multiple small bowel loops are seen with intermediate signal intensity within the abdomen. The bowel wall is not well seen, and small intraluminal lesions cannot be excluded. On the axial postcontrast scan **(B),** two loops containing agent are identified *(arrows).*

REFERENCES

1. Aicher KP, Laniado M, Kopp AF, et al: Mn DPTP–enhanced MR imaging of malignant liver lesions: efficacy and safety in 20 patients, J Magn Reson Imaging 3:731, 1993.
2. Anzai Y, Blackwell KE, Hirschowitz SL, et al: Initial clinical experience with dextran-coated superparamagnetic iron oxide for detection of lymph node metastases in patients with head and neck cancer, Radiology 192:709, 1994.
3. Bloembergen N, and Morgan L: Proton relaxation time in paramagnetic solutions: effect of electron spin relaxation, J Chem Phys 34:842, 1961.
4. Boorstein JM, Wong KT, Grossman RI, et al: Metastatic lesions of the brain: imaging with magnetization transfer, Radiology 191:799, 1994.
5. Brugieres P, Gaston A, Degryse HR, et al: Randomized double blind trial of the safety and efficacy of two gadolinium complexes (Gd-DTPA and Gd-DOTA), Neuroradiology 36:27, 1994.
6. Bydder GM: Clinical use of contrast media in magnetic resonance imaging, Br J Hosp Med 43:149, 1990.
7. Cacheris WP, Quay SC, and Rocklage SM: The relationship between thermodynamics and the toxicity of gadolinium complexes, Magn Reson Imaging 8:467, 1990.
8. Caramia F, Huang Z, Hamberg LM, et al: Identification of peripheral areas of cerebral flow-volume mismatch in focal transient ischemia using susceptibility contrast dynamic MRI, Proceedings of the Society of Magnetic Resonance, Second meeting, Aug 1994.
9. Carr JJ: Magnetic resonance contrast agents for neuroimaging: safety issues, Neuroimaging Clin N Am 4:43, 1994.
10. Caudana R, Morana G, Pirovano GP, et al: Focal malignant hepatic lesions: MR imaging enhanced with gadolinium benzyloxypropionictetra-acetate (BOPTA)—preliminary results of phase II clinical application, Radiology 199(2):513, 1996.
11. Cavagna FM, Maggioni F, Castelli PM, et al: Contrast enhanced magnetization transfer MRI of rat brain tumors with Gd-BOPTA/dimeg and Gd-DTPA/dimeg, Proceedings of the Society of Magnetic Resonance, Third meeting, Aug 1995.
12. Cloft HJ, Murphy KJ, Prince MR, et al: 3D gadolinium-enhanced MR angiography of the carotid arteries, Magn Reson Imaging 14(6):593, 1996.
13. Cohan RH, Leder RA, Herbnerg AJ, et al: Extravascular toxicity of two magnetic resonance contrast agents: preliminary experience in the rat, Invest Radiol 26:224, 1991.
14. Coveney JR, Robison RO, and Leese PT: Phase 1 study of Optimark (Gadoversetamide injection) in healthy volunteers, Proceedings of the Society of Magnetic Resonance, Second meeting, Aug 1994.
15. Davis PL, Parker DL, Nelson JA, et al: Interactions of paramagnetic contrast agents and the spin echo pulse sequence, Invest Radiol 23:381, 1988.
16. Duda SH, Laniado M, Kopp AF, et al: Superparamagnetic iron oxide: detection of focal liver lesions at high field strength MR imaging, J Magn Reson Imaging 4:309, 1994.
17. Edelman RR, Mattle HP, Atkinson DJ, et al: Cerebral blood flow: assessment with dynamic contrast enhanced T2* weighted MR imaging at 1.5 T, Radiology 176:211, 1990.
18. Elster AD, Mathews VP, King JC, et al: Improved detection of gadolinium enhancement using magnetization transfer imaging, Neuroimaging Clin N Am 4:185, 1994.
19. Engelstad BL, and Wolf GL: Contrast agents. In Stark DD, and Bradley WB, eds: Magnetic resonance imaging, cd 1, St Louis, 1988, Mosby.
20. Erlemann R, Reiser M, Peters PE, et al: Musculoskeletal neoplasms: static and dynamic gadopentetate dimeglumine MR imaging, Radiology 171:767, 1989.
21. Filippi M, Campi A, Martinelli V, et al: Primary progressive multiple sclerosis: comparison of triple dose versus standard dose of gadolinium DTPA for detection of enhancing lesions, Proceedings of the Society of Magnetic Resonance, Third meeting, Aug 1995.
22. Filippi M, Yousry T, Campi A, et al: Comparison of triple dose versus standard dose of gadolinium DTPA for detection of multiple sclerosis enhancing lesions. Proceedings of the Society of Magnetic Resonance, Third meeting, Aug 1995.
23. Fossheim S, Fahlvik AK, and Klaveness J: Paramagnetic liposomes as liver contrast agents: evaluation of in vitro relaxivity and in vivo contrast efficiency, Proceedings of the Society of Magnetic Resonance, Third meeting, Aug 1995.
24. Geens V, Balzer T, and Niendorf HP: Results of 2 phase II studies with Gadovist, a new extracellular MRI contrast agent for CNS imaging, Proceedings of the Society of Magnetic Resonance, Third meeting, Aug 1995.
25. Gennaro MC, Aime S, Santucci E, et al: Complexes of diethylenetriaminepentaacetic acid as contrast agents in NMR image: computer simulation of equilibria in human blood plasma, Anal Chim Acta 233:85, 1990.
26. Gibby WA, Puttagunta NR, and Puttagunta VL: MRI contrast agents—does dechelation occur and does it matter? Proceedings of the Society of Magnetic Resonance, Third meeting, Aug 1995.
27. Gibby WA, Puttagunta NR, Smith GT, et al: Human comparative studies of zinc and copper transmetallation in serum and urine of MRI contrast agents, Proceedings of the Society of Magnetic Resonance, Second meeting, Aug 1994.
28. Goldstein HA, Kashanian FK, Blumetti RF, et al: Safety assessment of gadopentetate dimeglumine in US clinical trials, Radiology 174:17, 1990.
29. Gore JC: Contrast agents and relaxation effects. In Atlas SW, ed: Magnetic resonance imaging of the brain and spine, New York, 1991, Raven Press.
30. Greco A, McNamara MT, Lanthiez P, et al: Gadodiamide injection: nonionic gadolinium chelate for MR imaging of the brain and spine: phase II-III clinical trial, Radiology 176:451, 1990.
31. Hamm B, Staks T, Muhler A, et al: Phase I clinical evaluation of Gd-EOB-DTPA as a hepatobiliary MR contrast agent: safety, pharmacokinetics, and MR imaging, Radiology 195:785, 1995.
32. Hamm B, Staks T, Taupitz M, et al: Contrast-enhanced MR imaging of liver and spleen: first experience in humans with a new superparamagnetic iron oxide, J Magn Reson Imaging 4:659, 1994.
33. Hattner RS, and White DL: Gallium-67/stable gadolinium antagonism: MRI contrast agent markedly alters the normal biodistribution of gallium-67, J Nucl Med 31:1844, 1990.
34. Haughton VM, Rimm AA, Czervionke LF, et al: Sensitivity of Gd-DTPA enhanced MR imaging of benign extraaxial tumors, Radiology 166:829, 1988.
35. Healy ME, Hesselink JR, Press GA, et al: Increased detection of intracranial metastases with Gd-DTPA, Radiology 169:619, 1987.
36. Heiland S, Forsting M, Reith W, et al: Perfusion weighted magnetic resonance imaging of focal cerebral ischemia: use of the new paramagnetic contrast agent gadolinium-butriol, Proceedings of the Society of Magnetic Resonance, Second meeting, Aug 1994.
37. Hendrick RE, and Haacke EM: Basic physics of MR contrast agents and maximization of image contrast, J Magn Reson Imaging 3:137, 1993.
38. Heywang-Kobrunner SH: Contrast enhanced MRI of the breast, Munich, 1990, SH Karger.
39. Heywang-Kobrunner SH: Contrast enhanced magnetic resonance imaging of the breast, Invest Radiol 29:94, 1994.
40. Hricak H, Bush WH Jr, Cohan R, et al: Genitourinary radiology, Radiology 194:596, 1995.
41. Hricak H, and Kim B: Contrast enhanced MR imaging of the female pelvis, J Magn Reson Imaging 3:297, 1993.
42. Hudgins PA, Elster AD, Runge VM, et al: Efficacy and safety of gadopentetate dimeglumine in the evaluation of patients with a suspected tumor of the extracranial hcad and neck, J Magn Reson Imaging 3:345, 1993.
43. Kanal E, Applegate GR, and Gillen CP: Review of adverse reactions, including anaphylaxis, in 4260 intravenous bolus injections, Radiology 177(P):159, 1990 (abstract).
44. Kerslake RW, Fox JN, Carleton PJ, et al: Dynamic contrast enhanced and fat suppressed magnetic resonance imaging in suspected recurrent carcinoma of the breast: preliminary experience, Br J Radiol 67:1158, 1994.
45. Kirsch JE: Basic principles of magnetic resonance contrast agents, Top Magn Reson Imaging 3(2):1, 1991.
46. Knauth M, Forsting M, Hartmann M, et al: MR enhancement of brain lesions: increased contrast dose compared with magnetization transfer, Am J Neuroradiol 17(10):1853, 1996.
47. Kohl A, Allgayer B, Giovagnoni A, et al: Ferristene (USAN) as a contrast medium for rectal application in MRI of the pelvis: summary of clinical phase III trials, Proceedings of the Society of Magnetic Resonance, Third meeting, Aug 1995.
48. Krinsky GA, Rofsky NM, DeCorato DR, et al: Thoracic aorta: comparison of gadolinium-enhanced three-dimensional MR angiography with conventional MR imaging, Radiology 202(1):183, 1997.
49. Kucharczyk J, Asgari H, Mintorovitch J, et al: Magnetic resonance imaging of brain perfusion using the nonionic contrast agents Dy DTPA-BMA and Gd-DTPA-BMA, Invest Radiol 26:S250, 1991.
50. Kucharczyk J, Vexler ZS, Roberts TP, et al: Echo-planar perfusion-sensitive MR imaging of acute cerebral ischemia, Radiology 188:711, 1993.
51. LaFrance ND, Parker JR, Lucas TR, et al: Clinical investigation of the safety and pharmacokinetics of gadoteridol injection in renally-impaired patients or patients requiring hemodialysis, Proceedings of the Society of Magnetic Resonance, Third meeting, Aug 1995.
52. Laniado M, Kornmesser W, Hamm B, et al: MR imaging of the gastrointestinal tract: value of Gd-DTPA, Am J Roentgenol 150:817, 1988.
53. Lauffer RB: Paramagnetic metal complexes as water proton relaxation agents for NMR imaging: theory and design, Chem Rev 87:901, 1987.
54. Lauffer RB: Principles of MR imaging contrast agents. In Edelman RR, and Hesselink JR, eds: Clinical magnetic resonance imaging, Philadelphia, 1990, WB Saunders.
55. LeBihan D, Breton E, Lallemand D, et al: MR imaging of intravoxel incoherent motions: application to diffusion and perfusion in neurological disorders, Radiology 161:401, 1986.
56. Li KC, Ang PG, Tart RP, et al: Paramagnetic oil emulsions as oral magnetic resonance imaging contrast agents, Magn Reson Imaging 8:589, 1990.
57. Lin W, Abendschein DR, and Haacke EM: Contrast-enhanced magnetic resonance angiography of carotid arterial wall in pigs, J Magn Reson Imaging 7(1):183, 1997.
58. Maas LC, Harris GJ, Satlin A, et al: Regional cerebral blood volume measured by dynamic susceptibility contrast MR imaging in Alzheimer's disease: a principal components analysis, J Magn Reson Imaging 7(1):215, 1997.
59. Marzola P, Maggioni F, Vicinanza E, et al: Evaluation of the hepatocyte-specific contrast agent gadobenate dimeglumine for MR imaging of acute hepatitis in a rat model, J Magn Reson Imaging 7(1):147, 1997.
60. Mathews VP, King JC, Elster AD, et al: Cerebral infarction: effects of dose and magnetization transfer saturation at gadolinium-enhanced MR imaging, Radiology 190:547, 1994.
61. Mayr NA, Yug WTC, Muhonen MG, et al: Cost effectiveness of high dose MR contrast studies in the evaluation of brain metastases, Am J Neuroradiol 15:1053, 1994.
62. Mirowitz SA, Lee JKT, Gutierrez E, et al: Dynamic gadolinium enhanced rapid acquisition spin echo MR imaging of the liver, Radiology 179:371, 1991.
63. Moseley ME, Vexler Z, Asgari HS, et al: Comparison of Gd-and Dy chelates for T2 contrast enhanced imaging, Magn Reson Med 22:259, 1991.
64. Nelson KL, and Runge VM: Basic principles. In Runge VM, ed: Enhanced magnetic resonance imaging, St. Louis, 1989, Mosby.
65. Neuerburg JM, Bohndorf K, Sohn M, et al: Urinary bladder neoplasms: evaluation with contrast enhanced MR imaging, Radiology 173:739, 1989.
66. Niendorf HP, and Seifert W: Serum iron and serum bilirubin after administration of Gd-DTPA dimeglumine: a pharmacological study in healthy volunteers, Invest Radiol 23:S275, 1988.
67. Nighoghossian N, Berthezene Y, Meyer R, et al: Assessment of cerebrovascular reactivity by dynamic susceptibility contrast-enhanced MR imaging, J Neurol Sci 149(2):171, 1997.
68. Novak Z, Thurmond AS, Ross PL, et al: Gadolinium DTPA transplacental transfer and distribution in fetal tissue in rabbits, Invest Radiol 28:828, 1993.
69. Okesendal AN, and Hals PA: Biodistribution and toxicity of MR imaging contrast-media, J Magn Reson Imaging 3:157, 1993.

70. Parizel PM, Baleriaux D, Rodesh G, et al: Gd-DTPA enhanced MR imaging of spinal tumors, Am J Roentgenol 152:1087, 1989.
71. Powers TA, Partain CL, Kessler RM, et al: Central nervous system lesions in pediatric patients: Gd-DTPA enhanced MR imaging, Radiology 169:723, 1988.
72. Ramadan UA, Aronen HJ, Tanttu JI, et al: Improvement of brain lesion detection at 0.1 T by simultaneous use of Gd-DTPA and magnetization transfer imaging, Magn Reson Med 37(2):268, 1997.
73. Reimer P, Rummeny EJ, Daldrup HE, et al: Enhancement characteristics of liver metastases, hepatocellular carcinomas, and hemangiomas with Gd-EOB-DTPA: preliminary results with dynamic MR imaging, Eur Radiol 7(2):275, 1997.
74. Rinck PA, Smevik O, Nilsen G, et al: Oral magnetic particles in MR imaging of the abdomen and pelvis, Radiology 178:775, 1991.
75. Roberts HC, Saeed M, Roberts TP, et al: Comparison of albumin-(Gd-DTPA)30 and Gd-DTPA-24-cascade-polymer for measurements of normal and abnormal microvascular permeability, J Magn Reson Imaging 7(2):331, 1997.
76. Ros PR, Freeny PC, Harms SE, et al: Hepatic MR imaging with ferumoxides: a multicenter clinical trial of the safety and efficacy in the detection of focal hepatic lesions, Radiology 196:481, 1995.
77. Ross JS, Modic MT, Masaryk TJ, et al: Assessment of extradural degenerative disease with Gd-DTPA enhanced MR imaging: correlation with surgical and pathological findings, Am J Roentgenol 154:151, 1990.
78. Runge VM: Magnetic resonance imaging contrast agents, Curr Opin Radiol 4:3, 1992.
79. Runge VM, Awh MH, and Bittner DF: Neoplastic disease of the spine on MR, MRI Decisions International 2:11, 1995.
80. Runge VM, Carollo BR, Wolf CR, et al: Gd-DTPA: a review of clinical indications in central nervous system magnetic resonance imaging, Radiographics 9:929, 1989.
81. Runge VM, and Gelblum DY: The role of gadolinium diethylenetriaminepentaacetic acid in the evaluation of the central nervous system, Magn Reson Q 6:85, 1990.
82. Runge VM, Gelblum DY, Pacetti ML, et al: Gd-HP-DO3A in clinical MR of the brain, Radiology 177:393, 1990.
83. Runge VM, Kirsch JE, Burke VJ, et al: High-dose gadoteridol in MR imaging of intracranial neoplasms, J Magn Reson Imaging 2:9, 1992.
84. Runge VM, Kirsch JE, and Lee C: Contrast-enhanced MR angiography, J Magn Reson Imaging 3:233, 1993.
85. Runge VM, Kirsch JE, Wells JW, et al: Enhanced liver MR: contrast agents and imaging strategy, Crit Rev Diagn Imaging 34:1, 1993.
86. Runge VM, Kirsch JE, Wells JW, et al: Visualization of blood-brain barrier disruption on MR images of cats with acute cerebral infarction: value of administering a high dose of contrast material, Am J Roentgenol 162:431, 1994.
87. Runge VM, Kirsch JE, Wells JW, et al: Repeat cerebral blood volume assessment with first-pass MR imaging, J Magn Reson Imaging 4:457, 1994.
88. Runge VM, Kirsch JE, Wells JW, et al: Assessment of cerebral perfusion by first-pass, dynamic, contrast-enhanced, steady-state free-precession MR imaging: an animal study, Am J Roentgenol 160:593, 1993.
89. Runge VM, Kirsch JE, Woolfolk C, et al: Gadoteridol dose dependence in MR imaging of a liver abscess model, J Magn Reson Imaging 4:343, 1994.
90. Runge VM, Pels Rijcken TH, Davidoff A, et al: Contrast-enhanced MR imaging of the liver, J Magn Reson Imaging 4:281, 1994.
91. Runge VM, Stewart RG, Clanton JA, et al: Potential oral and intravenous paramagnetic NMR contrast agents, Radiology 147:789, 1983.
92. Runge VM, and Wells JW: Update: safety, new applications, new MR agents, Top Magn Reson Imaging 7(3):181, 1995.
93. Runge VM, Wells JW, and Kirsch JE: Magnetization transfer and high dose contrast in early brain infection on MR, Invest Radiol 30:135, 1995.
94. Runge VM, Wells JW, Kirsch JE, et al: Comparison of 0.5 molar and 1.0 molar gadoteridol for first pass brain perfusion studies, Proceedings of American Society of Neuroradiology, Thirty-second annual meeting, May 1994.
95. Runge VM, Wells JW, Nelson KL, et al: MR imaging detection of cerebral metastases with a single injection of high-dose gadoteridol, J Magn Reson Imaging 4:669, 1994.
96. Runge VM, Wells JW, Williams NM, et al: Detectability of early brain meningitis on MR, Invest Radiol 30:484, 1995.
97. Russel EJ, Schiable TF, Dillon W, et al: Multicenter double blind placebo controlled study of gadopentetate dimeglumine as an MR contrast agent: evaluation in patients with cerebral lesions, Am J Roentgenol 152:813, 1989.
98. Saini S, Edelman RR, Sharma P, et al: Blood-pool MR contrast material for detection and characterization of focal hepatic lesions: initial clinical experience with ultrasmall superparamagnetic iron oxide (AMI-227), Am J Roentgenol 164:1147, 1995.
99. Saini S, Frankel RB, Stark DD, et al: Magnetism: a primer and review, Am J Roentgenol 150:735, 1988.
100. Schmeidl U, Maravilla KR, Gerlach R, et al: Excretion of gadopentetate dimeglumine in human breast milk, Am J Roentgenol 154:1305, 1990.
101. Schmitt F, Stehling MK, Lodebeck R, et al: Echo-planar imaging of the central nervous system at 1.0 T, J Magn Reson Imaging 2:473, 1992.
102. Schubeus P, and Schoerner W: Dosing of Gd-DTPA in MR imaging of intracranial tumors, Workshop on contrast enhanced magnetic resonance imaging, Napa, California, 1991, Society of Magnetic Resonance in Medicine.

103. Semelka RC, Hricak H, Stevens SK, et al: Combined gadolinium enhanced and fat saturation MR imaging of renal masses, Radiology 178:803, 1991.
104. Shamsi K, Balzer T, Staks T, et al: Multicentric, double-blind phase II clinical trial of Gd-EOB-DTPA (Eovist): safety profile, Proceedings of the Society of Magnetic Resonance, Third meeting, Aug 1995.
105. Sherry AD: Lanthanide chelates as magnetic resonance imaging contrast agents, J Less Common Metals 149:133, 1989.
106. Shirkhoda A, Konez O, Shetty AN, et al: Mesenteric circulation: three-dimensional MR angiography with a gadolinium-enhanced multiecho gradient-echo technique, Radiology 202(1):257, 1997.
107. Shukla R, Fernandez M, Pillai RK, et al: Design of conformationally rigid dimeric MRI agents, Proceedings of the Society of Magnetic Resonance, Third meeting, Aug 1995.
108. Siegelman ES, Gilfeather M, Holland GA, et al: Breath-hold ultrafast three-dimensional gadolinium-enhanced MR angiography of the renovascular system, Am J Roentgenol 168(4):1035, 1997.
109. Simonson TM, Yuh WTC, Michalson LS, et al: Triple dose contrast studies in evaluation of spinal cord lesions, Proceedings of the Society of Magnetic Resonance, Second meeting, Aug 1994.
110. SMRM Workshop: Contrast enhanced magnetic resonance: discussion section, Magn Reson Med 22:229, 1991.
111. Spinazzi A, Pirovano G, Ratcliffe G, et al: Multicenter testing of gadobenate dimeglumine in magnetic resonance imaging of focal liver disease, Acad Radiol Suppl 2:S415, 1996.
112. Stark DD, Weissleder R, Elizondo G, et al: Superparamagnetic iron oxide: clinical application as a contrast agent for MR imaging of the liver, Radiology 168:247, 1988.
113. Sze G, Brant-Zawadzki M, Haughton VM, et al: Multicenter study of gadodiamide injection as a contrast agent in MR imaging of the brain and spine, Radiology 181:693, 1991.
114. Tweedle MF: Nonionic or neutral? Radiology 178:891, 1991.
115. Tweedle MF: Physicochemical properties of gadoteridol and other magnetic resonance contrast agents, Invest Radiol 27S:1, 1992.
116. Tweedle MF, Hagan JJ, Kumar K, et al: Reaction of gadolinium chelates with endogenously available ions, Magn Reson Imaging 9:409, 1991.
117. Valk J, Algra PR, Hazenberg CJ, et al: A double-blind, comparative study of gadodiamide injection and gadopentetate dimeglumine in MRI of the central nervous system, Neuroradiology 35:173, 1993.
118. Vogl TJ, Friebe CE, Mack MG, et al: MR evaluation of brain metastases: comparison of standard and high-dose gadobutrol versus standard-dose Gd-DTPA, Proceedings of the Society of Magnetic Resonance, Second meeting, Aug 1994.
119. Vogl TJ, Mack MG, Juergens M, et al: MR diagnosis of tumors of the head and neck: comparison of high dose gadodiamide injection and single dose Gd-DTPA in the same patient, Proceedings of the Society of Magnetic Resonance, Second meeting, Aug 1994.
120. Vogl TJ, Pegios W, McMahon C, et al: Gadobenate dimeglumine—a new contrast agent for MR imaging: preliminary evaluation in healthy volunteers, Am J Roentgenol 158:887, 1992.
121. Wedeking P, Kumar K, and Tweedle MF: Dissociation of gadolinium chelates in mice: relationship to chemical characteristics, Magn Reson Imaging 10:641, 1992.
122. Wehrli FW: The basis of MR contrast. In Atlas SW, ed: Magnetic resonance imaging of the brain and spine, New York, 1991, Raven Press.
123. Weinmann HJ, Brasch RC, Press WR, et al: Characteristics of gadolinium-DTPA complex: a potential NMR contrast agent, Am J Roentgenol 142:619, 1984.
124. Weiss KL: Severe anaphylactoid reaction after IV Gd-DTPA, Magn Reson Imaging 8:817, 1990.
125. Wenz F, Rempp K, Hess T, et al: Effect of radiation on blood volume in low-grade astrocytomas and normal brain tissue: quantification with dynamic susceptibility contrast MR imaging, Am J Roentgenol 166(1):187, 1996.
126. Wolf GL: Current status of MR imaging contrast agents: special report, Radiology 172:709, 1989.
127. Wolff SD, and Balaban RS: Magnetization transfer contrast (MTC) and tissue water proton relaxation in vivo, Magn Res Med 10:135, 1989.
128. Yuh WT, Fisher DJ, Engelken JD, et al: MR evaluation of CNS tumors: dose comparison study with gadopentetate dimeglumine and gadoteridol, Radiology 180:485, 1991.
129. Yuh WTC, Engelken JD, Muhonen MG, et al: Experience with high dose gadolinium MR imaging in the evaluation of brain metastases, Am J Neuroradiol 13:335, 1992.
130. Yuh WTC, Fisher DJ, Runge VM, et al: Phase III multicenter trial of high dose gadoteridol in MR evaluation of brain metastases, Am J Neuroradiol 15:1037, 1994.
131. Yuh WTC, Nguyen HD, Tali ET, et al: Delineation of gliomas with various doses of MR contrast material, Am J Neuroradiol 15:983, 1994.
132. Zoarski GH, Lufkin RB, Bradley WG, et al: Multicenter trial of gadoteridol, a nonionic gadolinium chelate, in patients with suspected head and neck pathology, Am J Neuroradiol 14:955, 1993.

13 Interventional Magnetic Resonance Imaging

Robert B. Lufkin, Dietrich H.W. Grönemeyer, and Rainer M.M. Seibel

---

 ## KEY POINTS

- The term *interventional MRI (IMRI)* implies using MRI to guide biopsy or treatment of a lesion.
- Current IMRI procedures include aspiration cytology, core biopsy, wire localization, depth electrode placement in the brain for EEG or pallidotomies, chemoablation, cryosurgery, and thermal ablation using laser, focused ultrasound, and radiofrequency energy.
- Open-architecture magnets and fast imaging sequences (MR fluoroscopy) allow probes to be placed and procedures to be performed with near–real time MR visualization.
- MR imaging data from a traditional "closed-architecture" superconducting system can be used to guide a procedure outside the magnet using an optical tracking system (also called *computer-assisted surgery* and *frameless stereotaxy*).
- IMRI can be used in the operating room to guide brain tumor resection after craniotomy.
- IMRI can be coupled with endoscopic procedures, providing both external and internal localization or visualization.

Despite its relatively short history, magnetic resonance imaging (MRI) has become a major diagnostic tool in almost all clinical specialties. The multiplanar capabilities, high spatial resolution, excellent soft tissue contrast, and absence of ionizing radiation and beam hardening from bony structure all have contributed to MRI's development as a powerful tool to guide interventional procedures.

New open designs of magnetic resonance (MR) scanners with in-room image monitors allow MR-guided interventional procedures. MR-compatible needles, catheters, and other instruments developed for interventional purposes (composed of high-nickel stainless steel and other MR-compatible materials) reduce the torque from the static magnetic field and minimize susceptibility artifacts.

Studies of MR interventional applications currently include aspiration cytology, stereotactic depth electrode placement for electroencephalography, chemoablation, cryosurgery, and thermal ablation using laser, focused ultrasound, and radiofrequency (RF) ablation. This chapter briefly discusses the various aspects of interventional MRI, including dedicated instrumentation, interventional techniques, and emerging clinical applications.

INSTRUMENTATION
Magnetic Resonance–Compatible Instruments

The first step toward practical interventional MRI is the development of instruments that can function satisfactorily and safely in the strong magnetic field of clinical MR scanners. There are several areas of concern.

Magnetism. A major concern is the properties of instruments constructed from materials with high magnetic susceptibility (such as standard surgical stainless steel). Such ferromagnetic objects may experience significant force when near the MR scanner (Figure 13-1, *A*). The potential for accidents caused by the magnetically induced force on surgical instruments or monitoring equipment cannot be ignored.

Image artifacts also may result from large magnetic susceptibility differences between introduced instruments and the diamagnetic patient (Figure 13-1, *B*). Susceptibility artifacts also depend on the pulse sequence applied. For instance, spin-echo sequences are less sensitive to time-independent local magnetic field variations, whereas gradient-echo sequences are sensitive to both time-dependent and time-independent local field changes. The degree of image distortion also depends on the strength of the main magnetic field and increases with higher field strengths.

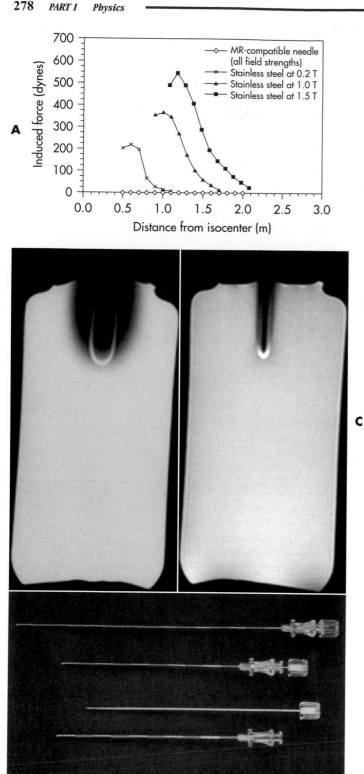

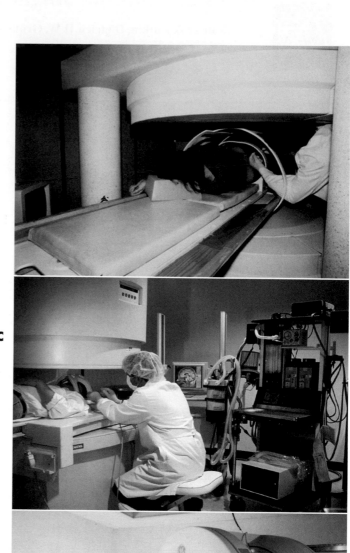

FIGURE 13-1 Noncompatible and MR-compatible instruments. **A,** Graph of torque versus distance from bore of the magnet for standard and MR-compatible needles at various field strengths. **B,** Standard (non-MR-compatible) needle produces a large image artifact. **C,** MR-compatible needle image obtained with the same imaging parameters as **B** shows considerably less artifact. **D,** Photograph of MR-compatible needles.

FIGURE 13-2 Representative interventional MR scanner with in-room monitors and associated equipment. **A,** Toshiba 0.064-T ACCESS, vertical field axis. **B,** Siemens 0.2-T OPEN vertical field axis. The instrument at right is an MR-compatible anesthesia machine. **C,** General Electric 0.5-T MRT, horizontal field axis.

Table 13-1   Comparison of Three Representative Open Interventional MR Scanners

	ACCESS (Toshiba)	OPEN (Siemens)	MRT (General Electric)
Field strength	0.064 T	0.2 T	0.5 T
Magnet	Permanent	Resis-	Superconducting
Design	Sandwich	tive	Open tube
Gantry opening	60 × 110 cm	C-arm	55/56 cm
Table centering	Manual	41 cm	Automatic
Projectile effect	0	Manual	+++
EMI	0 to +	++	+++
Gradient noise	+	++	+++
Image monitor in room	Yes	++	Yes
		Yes	
Fluoroscopy/ keyhole imaging	Yes	No	No
		No	
3D localizer	Yes		No
MR angiography	Yes	Yes	Yes
Weight	7 tons	Yes	5 tons
Cooling	None	12 tons	Cryogens
Electrical power	10 kVa	Water	60 kVa
	Yes	29 kVa	No
Diagnostic scans		Yes	

From reference 50.
0, Minimal; *+*, moderate; *++*, more; *+++*, much more.

Since the first MR-compatible needles were developed a decade ago by Mueller and Stark (Figure 13-1, *C*), various MR-compatible instruments have become available.[82,93] By optimizing pulse sequences, such as by using a shorter echo time, thinner slices, a smaller field of view (FOV), and higher readout gradients and by replacing standard medical-grade stainless steel with high-nickel-content stainless steel or other nonferrous alloys or ceramics, induced forces on interventional equipment and their associated artifacts can be minimized. MR-compatible needles, forceps, scissors, cannulas, and other instruments (Daum Inc., Germany; Cook Inc., Indianapolis; EFMT, Bochum, Germany; EZ-EM Westbury, New York; Micromed Inc., Bochum, Germany; and Radionics Inc., Burlington, Mass.) are manufactured at reasonable cost (Figure 13-1). Similar modifications have been made with other support instrumentation, such as anesthesia-monitoring equipment, lasers and RF generators, and tracking systems.

Electrical Conductivity. The fluctuating gradient field generated by the MR scanner to form images will induce voltage and current in a closed conducting loop according to Faraday's law of magnetic induction. The induced current may cause resistive heating of the metal device and pose a hazard to the patient and attending medical personnel. There is also the hazard of electrical arcing if two metal objects are placed near each other. In addition, the eddy currents induced in metal objects have long decay times and may distort the imaging field, causing artifacts. To ensure safety and reduce artifacts, the design of interventional devices must avoid closed or nearly closed metal loops and incorporate minimal-bulk metal.

Electromagnetic Effects. Electromagnetic interference (EMI) between the MR scanner and the interventional electronics may interfere with the MR scanner and physiological devices. For example, the RF generator used in RF thermal ablation may emit EM radiation, which interferes with the scanner's reception of MR signal from the patient's body, causing imaging artifacts. Conversely, the fluctuating magnetic field used in MRI may interfere with the operation of some monitoring equipment. Although MR-compatible monitoring devices are now commercially available from some manufacturers, all electronic equipment must first be tested for EMI in the MR scanning room before actual use in an interventional procedure.

Open Magnetic Resonance Systems

Current designs of interventional MR scanners emphasize maximum direct access to the patient so that therapy, monitoring, and anesthesia

can be achieved.[1,50,51] All systems have a similar design allowing improved access to the patient and are available from almost all major MR-scanner manufacturers. All interventional systems allow high-quality diagnostic studies and interventional procedures, with the exception of the GE therapy instrument, which is limited to interventional imaging. Certain other scanners also may be limited to imaging smaller body parts (extremities, breast, etc.).

Three representative systems are described here. The Toshiba ACCESS (Toshiba Medical Systems, San Francisco) 0.064-Tesla (T) scanner has an open four-sided permanent-magnet design allowing extensive horizontal access (Figure 13-2). The Magnetom OPEN scanner (Siemens Medical Systems, Iselin, New Jersey) consists of a vertically oriented 0.2-T iron-core resistive magnet that allows approximately 270 degrees horizontal access to the patient (Figure 13-2). The General Electric MRT magnet consists of two 0.5-T superconducting rings that allow the radiologist to slip in between the two rings and perform vertical and horizontal maneuvers (Figure 13-2). Features of these three scanners are summarized in Table 13-1.

Various other instruments are available from several manufacturers. In addition several new designs for machines are currently under development and testing (Figure 13-2).

Interventional Magnetic Resonance Imaging Pulse Sequences

Magnetic Resonance Imaging Temperature Monitoring and Related Sequences. MR-guided thermal ablation therapy would be greatly aided by the development of accurate MR thermal monitoring. Although tissue heating may be monitored by implanted transducers, such as thermocouples or thermistors, this procedure is invasive, is potentially hazardous, and can yield temperature measurements at only a few points limited by the number of the probes. Because several MR parameters, such as T1 relaxation time,[22,25,58,59,102] the diffusion coefficient (D),[75] and the chemical shift of the water peak,[63,125] are temperature dependent, MRI has long been proposed as a noninvasive technique to map in vivo temperature distribution.

Of the various parameters the temperature dependence of T1 relaxation was first studied in vitro, and there seemed to be a good correlation (Figure 13-3). T1 rose with heating, and signals decreased in T1-weighted images over a limited range (28° to 43° C). However, in vivo temperature measurement based on T1 showed profound influences of tissue perfusion and proton-density variations.[36,142] A significant hysteresis exists between signal intensity and temperature,[36] and with the high-energy depositions achieved during thermal ablation induced, T1 changes may be unpredictable and irreversible.[36,76] Currently, temperature monitoring remains unreliable.

Another parameter for MR temperature mapping is the diffusion coefficient of water (D). In the physiological temperature range the sensitivity of diffusion to temperature is about 2.4%, which is about double the sensitivity of T1.[75] However, because diffusion imaging is very sensitive to bulk motion and tissue anisotropy, it requires ultrafast acquisition schemes, such as echo-planar imaging (EPI), to avoid motion artifacts.

MR thermometry using water proton-chemical shift imaging[63,125] is of growing interest. The temperature dependency of water-proton chemical shift was measured comparing signal phase differences using a dynamic, multiplanar RF-spoiled fast field echo sequence.[125] The accuracy and efficacy of this method must be validated in further investigations.[21,74,89,101]

Fast Scanning and Magnetic Resonance Fluoroscopy. To approximate real-time imaging (fluoroscopic mode), image acquisition and image reconstruction have to be of very high speed. Spatial and temporal resolution are trade-offs for a given signal-to-noise ratio (SNR).

Currently, submillimeter spatial resolution can be achieved in a 0.2-T system with a standard spin-echo (SE) sequence within 5 min (8 slices, TR = 150 ms, 256 × 256 matrix) (Figure 13-4). A gradient-echo image (28-cm FOV, one slice, TR = 50 ms, 64 × 256 matrix) can be obtained in 3 sec, but these sequences suffer from a decrease in the SNR and a greater sensitivity to magnetic susceptibility artifacts.

Many recent studies focus on the development of high-speed sequences having a very short repetition time (TR). Several promising approaches have been made, including EPI, a hybrid of SE and echo-

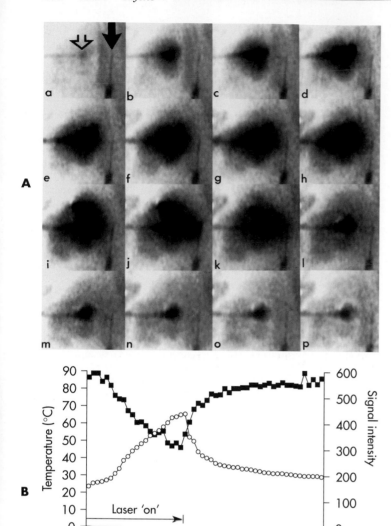

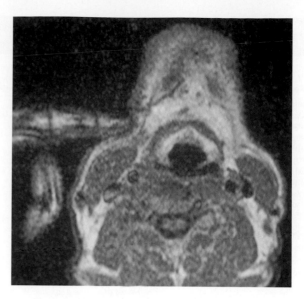

FIGURE 13-4 Gradient-echo acquisition during MR procedure. The rapid image acquisition combined with in-room monitors allows novel procedures. The physician's finger is used to localize a lesion before needle aspiration.

FIGURE 13-3 Temperature signal effects in MRI. **A,** Series of time-lapsed T1-weighted images acquired before *(a)*, every 25 sec during *(b to j)*, and after *(k to p)* laser irradiation of sheep brain in vitro. The tip of the laser probe *(open arrow)* and temperature probe 1.5 cm away *(bold arrow)* are shown. **B,** Graph of image signal intensity *(S)* and temperature *(T)* versus time during laser heating experiment, 1.5 cm away from probe top. (Courtesy Dr. K. Farahani.)

sion of the keyhole technique. By rotating each newly acquired raw data set, the entire κ space is updated after a few keyhole cycles.

The reconstruction method also can be modified to achieve faster imaging. Fourier-transform action covers an entire image plane (see Chapters 1 and 4). Wavelet transform is localized in space. With the wavelet technique, only the regions of an image affected by the movement of an interventional device are updated. A fluoroscopic mode with two images per second is achievable.

Localization Systems

Frame-based MR stereotaxis has been successfully employed in neurosurgery to guide biopsies, tumor resection, deep electroencephalography (EEG) electrode placement, functional target development and resection, and other interventional procedures* (Figure 13-5). Noninvasive visualization and localization provided by MRI greatly reduce the surgical invasion necessary to access the target and significantly lower patient morbidity. Several stereotactic systems with frames designed for MR localization are commercially available—the BRW and CRW (Radionics, Burlington, Mass.), Leksell (Elekta Instruments Inc., Atlanta, Ga.), Laitinen (Sandström Trade & Technology Inc., Welland, Ontario, Canada), and others.

Because MRI is more predisposed to geometric distortion than is computed tomography (CT), the accuracy of MR stereotaxis must be carefully calibrated. Localization error reported in the literature ranges from 1 to 5 mm. Variations in the reported error may be accounted for by the use of different stereotactic systems and different reference imaging modalities (CT, ventriculography, etc.) to which MRI is compared. The spatial accuracy of MRI depends on the linearity of magnetic field gradients and on magnetic susceptibility artifacts. Standardization and quality control should limit errors in magnetic field linearity and instrument calibration. MR sequences employing high bandwidth signal acquisition will reduce spatial distortion caused by susceptibility effects. Algorithms for mathematical correction may further improve the spatial accuracy of MRI.[8,26]

Conventional stereotactic systems require fixation of a frame to the patient's skull. Although generally accurate and reliable, these frames can be painful and are subject to migration. Frameless stereotactic systems will improve patient comfort, localization efficiency, and surgical access[70,87,127] (Figure 13-5).

planar methods (SE-EPI), keyhole imaging, Local-Look (LOLO) techniques, striped–κ space techniques, and wavelet-encoded data acquisition.[12,13,133,139]

EPI provides the shortest scan time. It requires substantial hardware modifications because a series of fast frequency and phase-encoding gradients are required to generate a train of gradient echoes after a single RF excitation. However, EPI suffers from a low SNR and is very sensitive to local field changes.

Other rapid imaging strategies involve a selective filling of the raw-data matrix (κ space). Restricted FOV strategies for fast imaging save time by updating only the low frequency domain of κ space and acquiring only a subset of the high frequency domain. Similar keyhole imaging or LOLO techniques use these subsampling methods to significantly shorten the imaging time.[133] LOLO uses a single-shot turbo SE and can acquire a 128 × 128 image matrix in 50 to 150 ms, nearly "real time." The striped–κ space data acquisition strategy is an exten-

---

*References 8, 10, 19, 26, 70, 72, 73, 84, 87, 127, 134.

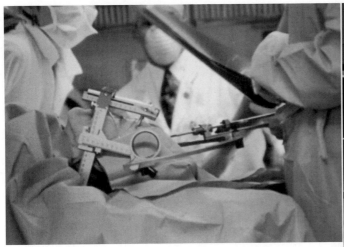
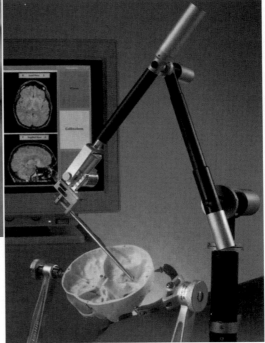

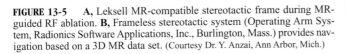

FIGURE 13-5 **A,** Leksell MR-compatible stereotactic frame during MR-guided RF ablation. **B,** Frameless stereotactic system (Operating Arm System, Radionics Software Applications, Inc., Burlington, Mass.) provides navigation based on a 3D MR data set. (Courtesy Dr. Y. Anzai, Ann Arbor, Mich.)

INTERVENTIONAL APPROACHES
Aspiration Cytology and Biopsy

Obviously lesions best visualized by MRI or not seen at all with x-ray methods will best be sampled under MR guidance. With fast MR scanners and in-room image display monitors, direct hand-guided biopsies are possible in more varied planes and without the radiation of x-ray fluoroscopy or CT.

Interstitial Laser Therapy

Treatment of neoplasms with lasers has been limited by the limited depth of tissue penetration achievable with surface illumination. Interstitial laser thermotherapy (ILT) is a new technique that transmits energy directly into deep tumors through a fiberoptic probe* (Figure 13-6). Nd-YAG lasers are commonly employed.

ILT causes thermal tissue injury through laser-energy deposition, resulting in coagulative necrosis. Unlike traditional hyperthermia, where the tissue is heated to 43° to 45° C for greater than 10 min (usually to augment some other therapy), in thermal ablation using laser or RF pulses the temperature is over 65° C, producing protein denaturation. ILT may create coagulative necrosis. Therefore accurate localization of the fiberoptic probe within a target tumor and careful monitoring with MRI are essential for successful treatment.

Advantages of ILT as a thermal-ablation technique are as follows:
1. The powerful heat source can destroy a large volume of tissue.
2. Few artifacts are caused by laser and fiber on MR images.
3. Small-caliber laser fibers do not require large-bore needles for insertion.
4. Thermal injury occurs independent of radiation sensitivity.
5. Adjacent normal structures incur minimal damage.

MRI facilitates tumor detection, instrument localization, and demonstration of thermal tissue injury. Fast MR images can show increased signal within brain tumors as temperature increases during ILT. MRI can show coagulative necrosis, with or without a central cavity, surrounded by high-signal edema on T2-weighted images. Histopathological correlation in chronic animal models shows that lesion size increases up to 1 week after laser treatment and gradually decreases in conjunction with infiltration of phagocytotic cells from adjacent vital tissue. Granulation will then form around the lesion, which eventually progresses to a fibrotic scar.

High-power ILT has a very steep thermal gradient, and the temperature around the fiber tip is extremely high such that tissue vaporization or charring may occur. High-power ILT is not ideal for treatment of lesions in closed spaces, such as the brain, because of the hazard of pressurized gas formation. Low power ILT (>4 Watt) requires longer treatment times, with the advantage of a more homogenous heating effect.

Radiofrequency Ablation

RF thermal ablation is a technique of tissue destruction by resistive heating using an RF (approximately 500 kHz)-alternating current.* A system consisting of active and dispersive electrodes is connected to the patient, completing an electrical circuit (Figure 13-6). The uninsulated tip of the active electrode (known as the *RF probe*) is placed at the center of target tissue, through which an alternating current is conducted. Because of the electrical impedance (resistance) of tissue surrounding the probe, ionic agitation causes frictional heating that results in tissue damage secondary to protein coagulation. The size of the RF lesion produced is a function of the length and diameter of the exposed electrode tip, as well as the energy delivered.

Before the development of MRI, RFs were used extensively in many neurosurgical applications, including thalamotomy, pallidotomy, and leucotomy for intractable pain and movement disorders. RF ablation for these functional disorders was guided by simply monitoring the patient's symptoms, such as tremor, dyskinesia, and pain. Imaging did not play a major role in the ablation procedure other than localization of the RF probe. Today, in interventional MR cases, MRI guides probe placement, RF energy delivery, and evaluation of the treatment effect.

The MR appearance of the RF-induced lesion is similar to that of laser-induced lesions, a well-defined ellipsoidal area of coagulative necrosis surrounded by edema. MR images can detect small degrees of thermal injury missed by CT and other imaging modalities. MRI sharply delineates lesions from surrounding normal tissue.

Focused Ultrasound Ablation

High-intensity focused ultrasound (HIFU) (frequency 0.5 to 10 MHz) can induce hyperthermia and destroy soft tissue lesions. This technique pro-

---

*References 2, 4, 5, 16, 30, 32, 62, 67, 68, 92, 105.

*References 6, 91, 99, 106, 120, 126.

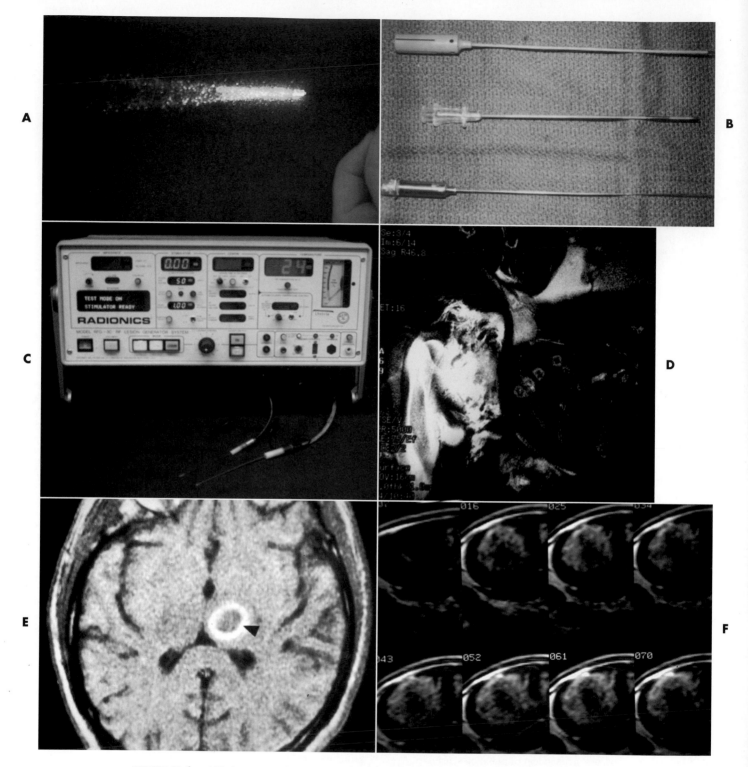

FIGURE 13-6 Ablation approaches. **A,** Laser energy delivered through a fiber. **B,** RF ablation electrodes. **C,** Typical RF generator system (Radionics Software Applications, Inc., Burlington, Mass.). **D,** High-intensity focused ultrasound ablation of rabbit thigh muscle. T2-weighted fast SE image shows the lesions circumscribed by hyperintense rings. The lesions were produced with the rabbit inside the MR scanner. **E,** T1-weighted image obtained several days after stereotactic cryothalamotomy shows the lesion well circumscribed by a hyperintense ring *(arrowhead)*. **F,** Sequential images of ablation of rabbit muscle after local ethanol infusion. (**D** Courtesy K. Hynynen et al, University of Arizona Health Sciences Center, Tucson.) (**F** Courtesy Dr. Y. Anzai, Ann Arbor, Mich.)

vides a nonincisional, transcutaneous ablation method using ultrasound energy to cause direct thermal coagulation necrosis and cavitation.*

HIFU beams are generated by piezoceramics. The beam is focused by lenses and reflecting surfaces to converge as a focal zone where the lesion is positioned. The relative ultrasound power deposition is highest in the focal zone and decreases significantly in the near and far fields. With sufficient intensity, very sharp temperature profiles can be produced so that an intense rise of temperature can be attained within a few seconds. Unlike other energy-delivery systems, such as RF and laser, HIFU can be moved easily throughout a solid lesion (Figure 13-6).

Destruction of tissues by HIFU is achieved by the following two mechanisms:

1. Rapid increase of temperature, causing protein denaturation
2. Generation of microbubbles (cavitation), which mechanically disrupts cellular structure

Phase I clinical trials, including treatment of breast, liver, and prostate tumors, have been performed. The sonic path must be clear of air and bone to avoid reflection or sonic distortion. Loss of acoustic coupling precludes application of HIFU in regions such as the lungs, skeleton, and bowel. HIFU does not cause tissue disruption as efficiently as RF or laser systems; hence multiple treatments may be required. Fifty minutes may be required to treat a 1-cm lesion volume. The profile of tissue destruction depends on the applied power, duration of sonication, tissue type, and vascularity. Most studies of HIFU to date have employed ultrasound for guidance and monitoring. It is expected that MRI also may be effective in guiding HIFU ablations. The dimensions of HIFU-induced lesions correlate well with findings on T2-weighted MR images.

Cryoablation

Cryosurgery is a therapeutic method that involves ablation of tissue by freezing, usually induced by direct contact with a cryoprobe. A cryogen, typically liquid nitrogen, is circulated through the probe, which is thermally insulated except at its tip. Thermal exchange occurs between the probe and the tissue, and a frozen region gradually extends outward from the probe's tip.† In experiments involving rabbit brain, 8 to 10 min of freezing were required to create a lesion 5 mm in depth; thawing the frozen tissue required approximately 8 min.

Intraoperative ultrasound is commonly used to guide cryosurgery in the prostate and the liver. Animal experiments demonstrate the ability of MRI to monitor the extent of cryoablation. Recently, MR-compatible cryoprobes were developed and tested on rabbit brain. Frozen regions are apparent on all MR pulse sequences as a well-defined signal void having a sharp interface with nonfrozen tissue. These changes can be tracked throughout the freeze-thaw process. The signal void of the frozen area is presumably the result of a significant increase in spin-spin (T2) relaxation rates as liquid water transitions to solid ice, rendering water protons invisible to MRI.

T1-weighted images display a bright band at the boundary of the freeze front, which represents cooled, nonfrozen tissue adjacent to the freeze front. On thawing, there is gadolinium enhancement at the margin of the frozen region, which correlates with vascular damage. Ischemic necrosis is seen at the center of the cryosurgical lesion (Figure 13-6).

Chemoablation

Percutaneous ethanol injection (PEI) is an example of chemoablation using high concentration ethanol to cause local dehydration necrosis. This technique has been used for treatment of liver tumors and parathyroid adenomas.‡ Spatially controlled chemoablation can be achieved in encapsulated lesions because the injected ethanol is constrained by organ capsules and tissue planes. In the absence of such anatomical barriers the hydrophilic nature of ethanol makes it difficult to produce a uniform or predictable lesion.

MRI can be useful to directly image ethanol within the tissue interstitium and assess proper delivery. Chemical-shift MRI can exploit the different resonance frequency of ethanol and water protons. Water signal can be selectively suppressed using a fast inversion recovery sequence.

After successful treatment, MR studies demonstrate that tumors treated with ethanol show decreased signal on T2-weighted images, presumably secondary to protein denaturation. Tumor recurrence may be manifested by an increasing signal on T2-weighted MR images (Figure 13-6).

CLINICAL APPLICATIONS
Brain

Brain Biopsy. MRI is widely recognized as the best imaging technique for the detection of most intracranial pathologies. With development of MR-compatible stereotactic frames, brain biopsy is now routinely performed at many institutions. Stereotactic coordinates and the optimum angle of probe insertion can be calculated with high accuracy. New interventional MR systems with open-magnet designs and in-room monitors enhance patient comfort and efficiency.

Electroencephalography. Intracerebral EEG is used in patients with medically intractable epilepsy to define the site and extent of the epileptogenic focus. Until recently, the most widely used method was stereoscopic x-ray angiography and a double-grid system to place intracranial electrodes for EEG. Stereoscopic x-ray angiography with digital subtraction identifies a safe trajectory for the electrode, avoiding intracranial vessels (such as the sylvian vessels and the vein of Labbé during temporal lobe electrode placement).

MRI can display tissue and vascular anatomy. Interventional MRI provides real-time feedback during insertion, noninvasive localization, assessment of positional accuracy, and the freedom to choose the target and the entry points (Figure 13-7).[71,79] After a seizure focus is localized, it may be possible to complete treatment in the same session, using RF or laser ablation. At present, patients are moved into the operating room for craniotomy and open resection (partial lobectomy) of the suspect tissue.

Brain Tumor Ablation. Trials are currently ongoing to assess the use of MR-guided thermal ablation of brain tumors. Groups in Dusseldorf, Paris, and Graz are evaluating the Nd-YAG laser. In the United States, RF ablation is under investigation.[3,7,69,107]

MR-guided brain tumor ablation (1) is less invasive than an open craniotomy for tumor resection (performed under local anesthesia with a 3-mm burr hole), (2) offers focal therapy with minimal adjacent vital tissue damage and may be repeated as often as necessary, (3) can be performed after a full dose of whole-brain radiation, and (4) is significantly less costly than open craniotomy.

The RF ablation technique currently employed at UCLA is as follows (Figure 13-8):

1. Pretreatment MR stereotaxis is preformed for localization of brain tumor.
2. Place biopsy needle (if necessary) or RF probe (Radionics, Burlington, Mass.) into the tumor through a 3-mm twist-drill hole.
3. RF power is applied to achieve an intratumoral temperature of 80° C for 1 min.
4. This 1-min treatment cycle is repeated until MRI demonstrates that the entire tumor volume and a small rim of normal tissue are destroyed.

The RF-induced ablation appears centrally as a focus of high signal on noncontrast T1-weighted images, presumably representing rapid, heat-induced degradation of hemoglobin to paramagnetic methemoglobin. The surrounding low–signal intensity ring is not yet explained but may represent coagulated, desiccated, nonhemorrhagic tissue. Peripheral to this low-signal ring, gadolinium-enhanced, T1-weighted images demonstrate a rim of enhancement, which represents the acute thermal lesion. As the lesion matures (3 to 7 days), a peripheral low-signal area appears on T2-weighted images, which is believed to represent hemosiderin. The RF lesion and adjacent edema increase in size for up to 1 week after RF therapy and then gradually decrease unless the tumor recurs (Figure 13-8).

---

*References 11, 17, 18, 27, 28, 31, 65, 88, 119, 121, 128, 132, 138, 141.
†References 29, 33-35, 90, 95-97, 108-110, 135.
‡References 45, 52, 77, 78, 117, 118, 122, 123, 130, 131.

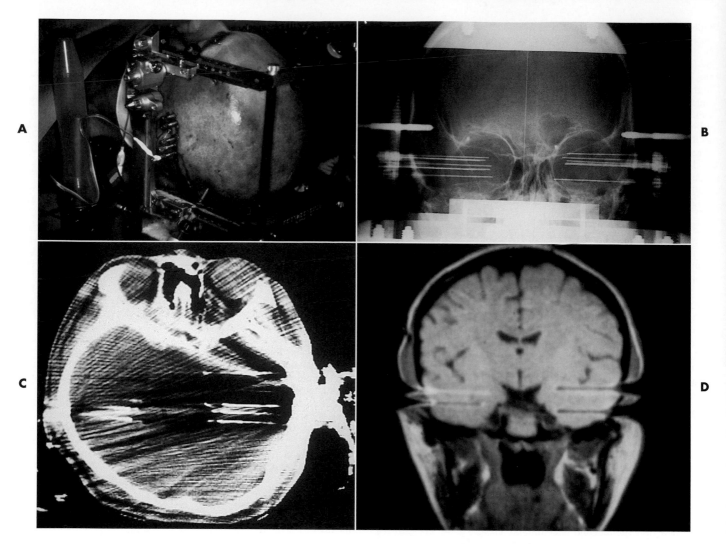

FIGURE 13-7 Stereotactic MR-compatible brain electrodes. **A,** Intraoperative implantation into the hippocampal region of a patient with refractory partial complex seizures. **B,** Plain radiograph shows the electrode position but fails to define possible soft tissue complications of the procedure. **C,** CT is nondiagnostic because of metallic artifacts. **D,** MR image shows MR-compatible deep EEG electrodes in place.

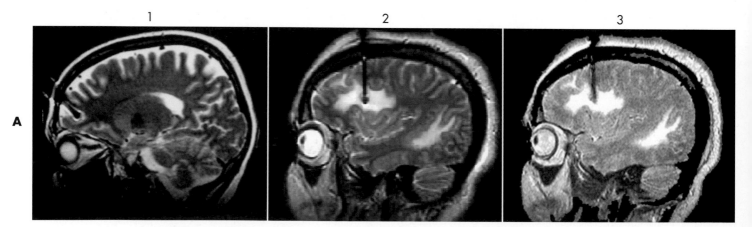

FIGURE 13-8 RF brain tumor ablation. **A,** RF electrodes and ablation. *1,* T2-weighted fast SE image of a patient with an anterior RF electrode in place. *2,* T2-weighted fast SE image of another patient with a more posterior RF electrode in place confirms the location of the electrode within the tumor. *3,* T2-weighted fast SE image obtained in same patient as 2 during RF ablation before the appearance of the RF lesion. Slight increased noise is seen as a result of RF energy delivery inside the MR unit; however, the image quality remains acceptable.

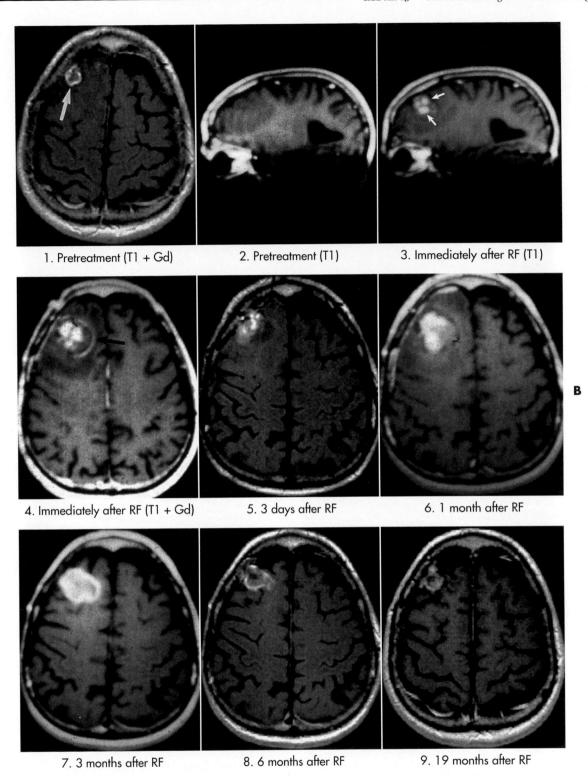

1. Pretreatment (T1 + Gd)   2. Pretreatment (T1)   3. Immediately after RF (T1)

4. Immediately after RF (T1 + Gd)   5. 3 days after RF   6. 1 month after RF

B

7. 3 months after RF   8. 6 months after RF   9. 19 months after RF

FIGURE 13-8, cont'd   B, A 44-year-old man with metastatic melanoma who had a previous open craniotomy and whole-brain radiation developed another brain metastasis in the right frontal lobe. The patient underwent MR-guided RF ablation with no additional treatment. *1,* Outside pretreatment axial T1-weighted MR image with enhancement shows a 1.2-cm mass in the right frontal lobe *(arrow). 2,* T1-weighted sagittal image before RF treatment shows the large area of edema without evidence of hemorrhage within the tumor. *3,* Non–contrast enhanced T1-weighted image immediately after RF ablation shows high signal foci in the central portion of the RF lesion *(arrows).* This finding is common in patients who had biopsy immediately before thermal ablation and is presumably related to heat-induced methemoglobin formation. *4,* Gadolinium-enhanced axial image immediately after thermal ablation shows well-defined ring enhancement of the RF lesion *(arrow).* Multiple high-signal foci seen outside the head represent fiducials in an MR-compatible stereotactic frame. *5,* Three days after the treatment the RF lesion covers the entire initial tumor volume. Contrast-enhanced MR images performed 1 month *(6),* 3 months *(7),* 6 months *(8),* and 19 months *(9)* after RF ablation show that the RF lesion gradually decreased in size. There has been no evidence of tumor progression observed over a 30-month follow-up period.

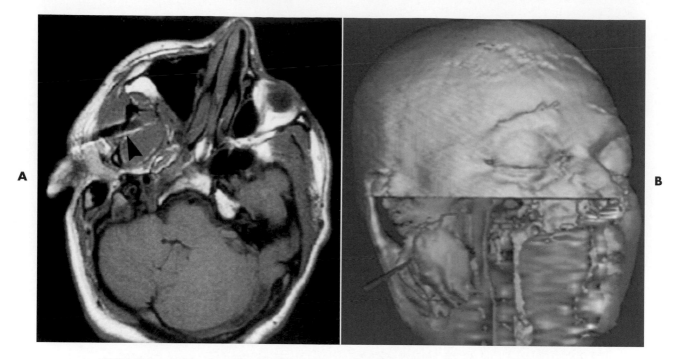

FIGURE 13-9 Head and neck approaches. **A,** Subzygomatic approach (arrowhead indicates needle position). Patient had a history of treated juvenile angiofibroma. Biopsy was performed to rule out recurrence. Cytology sample was negative. **B,** Three-dimensional rendered image of MR-guided laser treatment of a patient with metastatic cancer of the parotid.

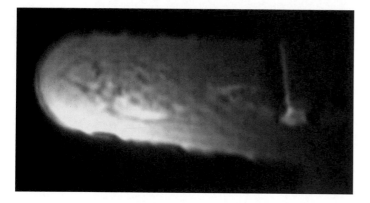

FIGURE 13-10 MR-guided breast biopsy. Needle is inserted into the breast under MR guidance. (Courtesy D. Gorcyzka.)

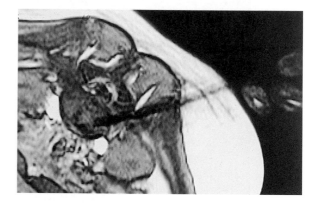

FIGURE 13-11 MR-guided approach to the spine. Percutaneous laser nucleotomy. The tip of the cannula is placed into the center of the disk.

MR-guided thermal ablation of brain tumors thus far appears to be a safe, minimally invasive treatment of brain tumors that deserves further study. Unlike radiation, it is not contraindicated by cumulative toxicity to adjacent normal brain tissue. Thermal ablation also may serve as palliation for end-stage patients who do not wish to undergo open craniotomy.

Head and Neck

Head and Neck Biopsy. MR-guided aspiration cytology for deep-seated head and neck lesions has been performed for more than 10 years and is now a standard procedure at many institutions.* Because of the complicated anatomy and close spacing of structures in this region, blind needle aspiration is technically difficult and dangerous. MRI permits visualization of vascular and neural structures near the skull base

where the effectiveness of CT is reduced by beam-hardening artifact. The multiplanar capability of MR also allows localization along the longitudinal course of the needle.

22-Gauge sheaths can be placed to guide multiple passes with a coaxial 26-gauge aspiration needle. MR-compatible coaxial needles of varying length and curvature are available.

The subzygomatic or infratemporal approach can be performed to access lesions in the parapharyngeal space, skull base, and infratemporal fossa. The patient's mouth is held open during the insertion. The triangle outlined by the zygoma, coronoid process, and mandibular condyle forms the landmark for needle insertion (Figure 13-9).

The retromandibular approach is useful in accessing the parapharyngeal, parotid, and lower masticator spaces. The needle is placed just posterior to the angle of the mandible and more than 1 cm below the tragus to avoid damaging the facial nerve (Figure 13-9).

The submastoid approach can be used to access lesions in the skull base. The needle is inserted 1 cm inferior to the mastoid tip along the anterior aspect of the sternocleidomastoid muscle.

*References 24, 25, 80, 81, 83, 129, 140.

Head and Neck Treatment. Lesions of the head, neck, and skull base often have close proximity to many cranial nerves and major vessels. Wide local resection of these lesions results in many functional and cosmetic deformities. Therefore most head and neck tumors are treated by limited surgery, radiation therapy, or both. MR-guided, minimally invasive thermal ablation offers an alternative, provided methods are developed to deliver thermal energy accurately and safely (Figure 13-9). Preliminary clinical trials of interstitial laser therapy have been reported.[11,96,99] Although the efficacy of this technique must be further proven in large series with long follow-up, the initial limited results are promising.

Breast

Breast Biopsy. Breast carcinoma is a leading cause of death for women in the United States. Because of high soft tissue contrast, MRI can detect breast carcinoma that is not visible with usual mammographic techniques. With a recent development of breast-biopsy surface coils, the breast can be compressed and stabilized while the patient is in a prone position. Although experience is limited to date, successful biopsy under MR guidance has been performed on lesions that are not detectable or easily localized by other modalities[98] (Figure 13-10).

Breast Treatment. A preliminary clinical trial of interstitial laser therapy for breast cancer followed by surgery was recently presented and showed excellent correlation of MR appearance and pathology. The study suggests that MR-guided ILT for breast cancer is potentially a useful tool.[60] Advanced study of MR-guided HIFU therapy for breast fibroadenomas is currently under way.[104]

Spine

Synovial Joints. MR-guided percutaneous injection of long-acting anesthesia (bupivacaine) and steroid (triamcinolone) to the facet joints and the sacroiliac joints has been performed to relieve pseudo-radicular pain. Preliminary results show a greater than 90% response rate.[39,53,54] Percutaneous laser diskectomy in the lumbar spine also is under investigation as an alternative to surgical disk resection.

Acute and chronic back pain with or without disk herniation is one of the major medical problems in health care worldwide. Low back pain has various causes. Radicular pain caused by herniations, pseudoradicular pain caused by facet joints, or local pain caused by the iliosacral joints may benefit from several surgical and less invasive ablative or resective treatments.

CT has been used to guide microinvasive periradicular therapy,[39,42,112] mechanical percutaneous nucleotomy,[114] and percutaneous laser nucleotomy,[55,113] as well as facet joint and iliosacral joint therapies.[51] Microinvasive interventional MRI is a new tool in spinal-guidance technology.[42,47,49,52] Most CT- or MR-guided treatments can be performed without general anesthesia and on an outpatient basis.

Facet joint anesthesia is used (1) to treat acute radicular pain caused by functional disorders and (2) to confirm the diagnosis before ethanol ablation. For pain treatment a combination of short- and long-acting anesthesia (mepivacaine 1% and bupivacaine 0.5%) is generally used. Steroids (10 to 40 mg of triamcinolone [Volon AR] and 1 ml 50% to 90% ethanol) are used to treat chronic facet joint pain. Care must be taken to avoid injection or leakage of ethanol into the spinal canal. Contraindications for cortisone injection include nonsterile inflammation, diabetes mellitus, and ulcers. Percutaneous ethanol instillation may be effective for treating chronic pain caused by spondyloarthrosis or chronic prolapse. Pain caused by postdiskectomy syndrome also can be treated with facet anesthesia, iliosacral joint therapy, or both.[41,50,52,111]

Sacroiliitis (sterile inflammation) may be treated with 10 to 40 mg of crystalline cortisone. This therapeutic method may be used in combination with facet joint therapy, periradicular and epidural treatments, and nucleotomy or diskectomy.[50,52]

Disk Spaces. Disk herniation is difficult to treat with open surgery. Less invasive periradicular therapy can be an effective alternative. Percutaneous laser nucleotomy is performed using a 1064-nm Nd-YAG or Hol-YAG laser (0.4-mm fiber, 10 W, 1-sec impulse, 1-sec gap, not to exceed 180 impulses). Periradicular treatments are performed three to

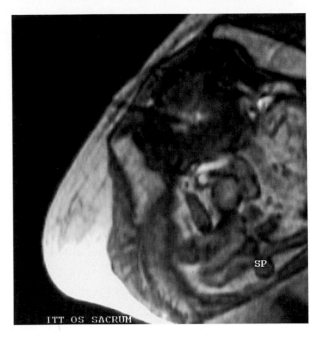

FIGURE 13-12   Axial T1-weighted image of MR-guided biopsy of a sacral mass.

six times, separated by time intervals of 21 days, using 18 to 21 Gauss (Micromed, Somatex, Daum, Cook, and EZM) nitinol, titanium, or stainless steel cannulas.

Percutaneous nucleotomy can be combined with flexible microendoscopy.[49,50] For these procedures an MR-compatible endoscopy system has to be installed near the gantry (a portable system is available from Micromed). Lower field strength MR systems are advantageous because they allow some conventional electronic equipment to be positioned inside the MRI suite.

Treatments in open magnets can be performed with the patient positioned prone or laterally. Under sterile conditions the entry point on the skin is marked by finger pressure and the instruments are inserted under local anesthesia. Mass herniation and sequestra are contraindications for percutaneous laser nucleotomy. For acute disk herniation (Figure 13-11),[54] Nd-YAG or Hol-YAG laser treatment may be performed after 6 weeks of unsuccessful conservative therapy.[41,49,50,52,111]

For chronic lumbar disk herniation or postoperative scar formation, instillation of 40 to 80 mg of crystalline cortisone may be effective.[41,50,52,111]

Treatment Planning. Conventional x-ray imaging and MRI of the affected region are important for diagnosis and, if necessary, for treatment planning functional studies. These imaging modalities may be used to rule out inflammation, degenerative disorders, tumors, osteoporosis, and spondylolisthesis. For more bony information CT may be useful. After 6 weeks of unsuccessful conservative treatment of back pain or in the presence of neurological deficits, an MR scan may be performed.

Abdomen and Pelvis

Percutaneous interventional procedures in the abdomen and pelvis are usually performed for biopsies, but they also are performed for drainages and sympathectomies. CT-, fluoro-, and ultrasound-guided punctures have been reported in the literature for nearly 30 years. In 1967, Nordenstrom reported the first series of percutaneous fluoro-guided lymph node biopsies.[93] Different approaches, such as transperitoneal, translumbar, and transvascular, using different image modalities are described.*

Fine-needle biopsies are most often performed for cytological and histological diagnosis in the abdomen, retroperitoneum, pelvis, lymph nodes, bones, and joints. In general the results with percutaneous aspiration techniques are very good (Figure 13-12). Success rates for ob-

---

*References 37, 41, 56, 57, 61, 64, 66, 85, 100, 111, 112, 116, 124.

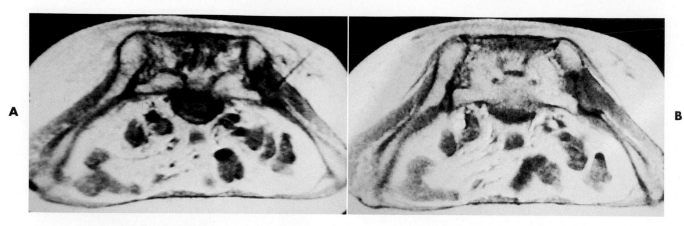

FIGURE 13-13   Percutaneous 96% ethanol instillation in breast carcinoma metastasis infiltrating the ilium. Guidance procedure before **(A)** and after **(B)** ethanol instillation.

taining cytologic diagnosis have been reported to be greater than 80%.[85,102,114]

Ultrasound-guided methods are increasingly supplanted by CT.[45] MRI diagnostic and therapeutic methods in the abdomen[43,46,48,92] have considerable potential. Premedication is not normally required. After diagnostic scanning, the puncture angle and depth are determined.

The puncture entry angle is calculated and transferred onto the patient by drawing the entry point and the slice level on the skin with a felt-tip pen localized using a positioning light. After the distance is measured on the skin using reference anatomical structures, such as ribs, spinous process, or muscles, the exact entry point is marked. Short-acting cutaneous anesthesia is injected immediately before the procedure is performed.[45]

For biopsies, special reduced-artifact instruments are available from Somatex, Daum, and EZM. Therapeutic sets for cancer therapy are available in addition from Micromed and Cook.

Tumor treatment may be performed directly after the biopsy through the same guidance cannula. Where tumor infiltrates bony structures, 1 to 4 ml of 96% ethanol instillation is reported to reduce pain in 75% of patients (Figure 13-13). If one treatment is not sufficient, a second or third ethanol instillation and an image-guided sympathectomy are often helpful. Contraindications to biopsy are anticoagulant therapy and blood clotting disorders.

FUTURE DEVELOPMENTS

In the near future more treatments in the abdomen and pelvis will be realized. RF, cryo, and laser techniques have great potential for treating of prostate tumors.[137] Drainage of large cysts and abscesses in the liver, pancreas, and retroperitoneum is another area of current development in MR-guidance procedures. Combined MRI and endoscopic therapy, especially for the uterus, gallbladder, urinary tract, and colon, may be used in routine techniques if endocoils or MR-compatible endoscopic systems are developed. The first experiences have been reported from DeSouza in London[20] and the Mulheim group.[54]

Technological advances in health care, such as MRI, are under great criticism because of their high cost. However, because it is minimally invasive compared with other open surgical approaches, interventional MRI may emerge as a means of actually lowering the overall cost of medical care.

Interventional MRI is clearly in its early stages of development. The future of MR-guided therapy remains to be proven by large clinical studies defining the ultimate effectiveness of this technique. With the new interventional MR units that are available, this work should be forthcoming.[40,51] As we look to the millennium it is possible to imagine dedicated interventional MR units for combined radiological and surgical approaches as the operating room of the twenty-first century.

REFERENCES

1. Anzai Y, Desalles A, Black K, et al: Interventional MR imaging, Radiographics 13(4):897, 1993.

2. Anzai Y, Lufkin R, Castro D, et al: MR imaging-guided interstitial Nd:YAG laser phototherapy: dosimetry study of acute tissue damage in an in vivo model, J Magn Reson Imag 1(5):553, 1991.

3. Anzai Y, Lufkin R, DeSalles A, et al: Preliminary experience with MR guided thermal ablation of brain tumors, Am J Neuroradiol 16:39, Jan 1995.

4. Anzai Y, Lufkin RB, Hirschowitz S, et al: MR imaging–histopathologic correlation of thermal injuries induced with interstitial Nd:YAG laser irradiation in the chronic model, J Magn Reson Imaging 2(6):671, 1992.

5. Anzai Y, Lufkin RB, Saxton RE, et al: Nd:YAG interstitial laser phototherapy guided by magnetic resonance imaging in an ex vivo model. I. Dosimetry of laser-MR-tissue interaction, Laryngoscope 101(7):755, 1991.

6. Aronow S: The use of radiofrequency power in making lesions in the brain, J Neurosurg 17:431, 1960.

7. Ascher P, Justich E, and Schrottner O: A new surgical but less invasive treatment of central brain tumours preliminary report, Acta Neurochir 52:78, 1991.

8. Bakker C, Moerland M, Bhagwandien R, et al: Analysis of machine-dependent and object-induced geometric distortion in 2DFT MR imaging, Magn Reson Imaging 10(4):597, 1992.

9. Blackwell KE, Castro DJ, and Lufkin R: MRI and ultrasound guided Nd:YAG laser phototherapy for palliative treatment of advanced head and neck tumors: clinical experience, J Clin Laser Med Surg, 11 (1):7, 1993.

10. Burchiel K: Image-based functional neurosurgery, Clin Neurosurg 39:314, 1992.

11. Burov A: High intensity ultrasonic oscillation for the treatment of malignant tumors in animals and man, Dokl Akad Nauk SSSR 106:239, 1956.

12. Busch M, Friebe MH, Hellwig, S et al: Keyhole sequence in two dimensions for high-speed fluoroscopic imaging on ultra-low-field MR systems, Magnetic SMR 8:38, 1994.

13. Busch M, Gronemeyer DHW, and Seibel RMM: Keyhole sequences for interventional procedures, Interventional MRI, 1994, Marina del Rey, California.

14. Castro D, Lufkin R, et al: Metastatic head and neck malignancy treated with MR guided laser therapy: an initial case report, Laryngoscope 102(1):26, 1992.

15. Castro D, Saxton RE, and Lufkin R: Interstitial photoablative laser therapy guided by magnetic resonance imaging for the treatment of deep tumors, Semin Surg Oncol 8:233, 1992.

16. Castro DJ, Saxton RE, Layfield LJ, et al: Interstitial laser phototherapy assisted by magnetic resonance imaging: a new technique for monitoring laser-tissue interaction, Laryngoscope 100(5):541, 1990.

17. Chen L, ter Haar G, Hill C, et al: Effect of blood perfusion on the ablation of liver parenchyma with high-intensity focused ultrasound, Phys Med Biol 38(11):1661, 1993.

18. Cline H, Hynynen K, Hardy C, et al: MR temperature mapping of focused ultrasound surgery, Magn Reson Med 31:628, 1994.

19. Derosier C, Delegue G, Munier T, et al: MRI geometric distortion of the image and stereotaxy, J Radiol 72:349, 1991.

20. deSouza NM, Flynn RJ, Coutts GA, et al: Endoscopic laser ablation of the prostate: MR appearances during and after treatment and their relation to clinical outcome, Am J Roentgenol 164(6):1429, 1995.

21. Dickinson R, Hall A, Hind A, et al: Measurement of changes in tissue temperature using MR imaging, J Comput Assist Tomogr 10(3):468, 1986.

22. Dickinson R, Hall A, Hind A, et al: Measurement of changes in tissue temperature using MR imaging, J Comput Assist Tomogr 10(3):468, 1986.

23. Duckwiler G, Lufkin R, and Hanafee W: MR-directed needle biopsies, Radiol Clin North Am 27(2):255, 1989.

24. Duckwiler G, Lufkin R, Teresi L, et al: Head and neck lesions: MR-guided aspiration biopsy, Radiology 170:519, 1989.

25. Ebner F, and Ebner RS: Temperature monitoring for tissue ablation by means of MRI, Interventional MRI Workshop, 1994, Marina Del Rey, California.

26. Fitzpatrick J, Chang H, Willcott M, et al: A technique for improving accuracy in position and intensity within images acquired in the presence of field inhomogeneity. In Book of abstracts: ninth annual meeting of the Society of Magnetic Resonance in Medicine, New York, 1990.

27. Foster R, Bihrle R, Sanghvi N, et al: High-intensity focused ultrasound in the treatment of prostatic disease, Eur Urol 23(Suppl 1):29, 1993.

28. Fry F, and Johnson L: Tumor irradiation with intense ultrasound, Ultrasound Med Biol 4(4):337, 1978.
29. Gage A: Current progress in cryosurgery, Cryobiology 25:483, 1988.
30. Gatenby RA, Hartz WH, Engstrom PF, et al: CT-guided laser therapy in resistant human tumors: phase I clinical trials, Radiology 163:172, 1987.
31. Gelet A, Chapelon J, Margonari J, et al: Prostatic tissue destruction by high-intensity focused ultrasound: experimentation on canine prostate, J Endourol 7(3):249, 1993.
32. Gewiese B, Beuthan J, Fobbe F, et al: Magnetic resonance imaging-controlled laser-induced interstitial thermotherapy, Invest Radiol 29(3):345, 1994.
33. Gilbert J, Onik G, Hoddick W, et al: Real time ultrasonic monitoring of hepatic cryosurgery, Cryobiology 22:319, 1985.
34. Gilbert J, Roos M, Wong, S et al: NMR monitored cryosurgery in the rabbit brain, Proceedings of The Society for Magnetic Resonance in Medicine, Berlin, 1992.
35. Gilbert J, Rubinsky B, Roos M, et al: MRI-monitored cryosurgery in the rabbit brain, Magn Reson Imaging 11:1155, 1993.
36. Goldhaber DM, Deli M, Gronemeyer DHW, et al: Measurement of tissue temperature by MRI, IEEE Nuclear Science & Medical Imaging 3: 1702, 1993.
37. Gothlin JH: Post-lymphographic percutaneous fine needle biopsy of lymph nodes, guided by fluoroscopy, Radiology 120:205, 1976.
38. Gronemeyer D, Seibel R, Erbel R, et al: Equipment configuration and procedures: preferences for interventional microtherapy, J Dig Imaging 9(2):81, 1996.
39. Gronemeyer D, Seibel R, Schindler O, et al: Microinvasive CT guided periradicular therapy for treatment of chronic functional disorders of the spine, Wiener Medizinische Wochenschrift 12:129, 1993.
40. Gronemeyer DHW, and Seibel RMM: Interventional CT and MRI, a challenge for safety and cost reduction in health care system, Health Care Technology Policy II, SPIE 2499:132.
41. Gronemeyer DHW, and Seibel RMM: Interventionelle Computertomographie, Wien, 1989, Ueberreuter Wissenschaft.
42. Gronemeyer DHW, and Seibel RMM: Interventionelle Computertomographie, Wien 1990, Ueberreuther Wissenscraft.
43. Gronemeyer DHW, and Seibel RMM: Intererventionelle Kernspintomographie. In Gronemeyer DHW, and Seibel RMM: Interventionelle Computertomographie, Wien, 1990, Ueberreuther Wissenschaft.
44. Gronemeyer DHW, and Seibel RMM: New forms of interventional tumor therapy in radiology. In Seibel RMM, and Gronemeyer DHW, eds: Interventional computed tomography, Oxford, 1990, Blackwell Science.
45. Gronemeyer DHW, and Seibel RMM: Microinvasive CT-guided cancer therapy of soft tissue and bone metastases, Wiener Medizinische Wochenschrift 12:312, 1993.
46. Gronemeyer DHW, Seibel RMM, Arnold WH, et al: Atlas of CT-guided biopsies. In Seibel RMM, and Gronemeyer DHW, eds: Interventional computed tomography, Oxford, 1990, Blackwell Sciencee.
47. Gronemeyer DHW, Seibel RMM, Busch M, et al: Interventional magnetic resonance imaging. In Seibel RMM, and Gronemeyer DHW, eds: Interventional computed tomography, Oxford, 1990, Blackwell Science.
48. Gronemeyer DHW, Seibel RMM, Kaufman L, et al: Interventional magnetic resonance imaging. In Seibel R, and Gronemeyer D, eds: Interventional computed tomography, Oxford, 1990, Blackwell Science.
49. Gronemeyer DHW, Seibel RMM, Kaufman L, et al: Interventional procedures in low field magnetic resonance imaging, Diagnostic Imaging International 11/12:32, 1990.
50. Gronemeyer DHW, Seibel RMM, Melzer A, et al: Image guided access technique, Endosc Surg Allied Technol 1:69, 1995.
51. Gronemeyer DHW, Seibel RMM, Melzer A, et al: Future of advanced guidance techniques by interventional CT and MRI, Minim Invasive Ther 2:251, 1993.
52. Gronemeyer DHW, Seibel RMM, Plasmann J, et al: Percutaneous drug instillation for local cancer and tumor pain therapy by CT and MRI guidance, Minim Invasive Ther, 1996 (in print).
53. Gronemeyer DHW, Seibel RMM, Schmid G, et al: Low back pain treatment with interventional MRI guidance, Soc of Magn Reson 011:39, 1994 (abstract).
54. Gronemeyer DHW, Seibel RMM, and Schmidt A: MRI- and CT-scopic microsurgery and drug instillation for outpatient treatments. In Lemke HU, Inamura K, Jaffe C, et al: Computer assisted radiology, Berlin, 1995, Springer-Verlag.
55. Gronemeyer DHW, Seibel RMM, Schmidt A, et al: Atraumatic CT-controlled percutaneous laser nucleotomy, Minim Invasive Ther 2:247, 1993.
56. Haaga JR, and Alfidi RJ: Precise biopsy localization by computed tomography, Radiology 118:603, 1976.
57. Haaga JR, Alfidi RJ, Havrilla TR et al: CT detection and aspiration of abdominal abscess, Am J Roentgenol 128:465, 1977.
58. Hall A, Prior M, Hand J, et al: Observation by MR imaging of in vivo temperature changes induced by radiofrequency hyperthermia, J Comput Assist Tomogr 14(3):430, 1990.
59. Hall L, and Talagala S: Mapping of pH and temperature distribution using chemical-shift-resolved tomography, J Magn Reson Imaging 65:501, 1985.
60. Hall-Craggs MA, Paley WM, Mumtaz H, et al: Laser therapy of breast carcinomas: MR/histopathological correlation, Interventional MRI Workshop, Boston, 1994.
61. Hancke S, Holm HH, and Koch F: Ultrasonically guided percutaneous fine needle biopsy of the pancreas, Surg Gynecol Obstet 140:361, 1975.
62. Higuchi N, Bleier A, Jolesz F, et al: Magnetic resonance imaging of the acute effects of interstitial neodymium:YAG laser irradiation on tissues, Invest Radiol 27:814, 1992.
63. Hindeman JC: J Chem Phys 44:4582, 1966.
64. Holm HH, Perderson JF, Kristensen JK, et al: Ultrasonically guided percutaneous puncture, Radiol Clin North Am 13:493, 1975.
65. Hynynen K, Darkazanli A, Unger E, et al: MRI-guided noninvasive ultrasound surgery, Med Phys 20(1):107, 1993.
66. Jaques PF, Staab E, Richey W, et al: CT-assisted pelvic and abdominal aspiration biopsy in gynecological malignancy, Radiology 128:651, 1978.
67. Jolesz F, Bleier A, Jokab P, et al: MR imaging of laser tissue interactions, Radiology 168:249, 1988.
68. Jolesz F, Moore G, Mulkern R, et al: Response to and control of destructive energy by magnetic resonance, Invest Radiol 24:1024, 1989.
69. Kahn T, Bettag M, Ulrich F, et al: MRI-guided laser induced interstitial thermotherapy of cerebral neoplasms, J Comput Assist Tomogr 18(4):519, 1994.
70. Kato A, Yoshimine T, Hayakawa T, et al: A frameless armless navigation system for computer-assisted neurosurgery, J Neurosurg 74:845, 1991.
71. Kelly P, Sharbrough F, Kall B, et al: Magnetic resonance imaging-based computer-assisted stereotactic resection of the hippocampus and amygdala in patients with temporal lobe epilepsy, Mayo Clin Proc 62:103, 1987.
72. Kondziolka D, Dempsey P, Lunsford L, et al: A comparison between magnetic resonance imaging and computed tomography for stereotactic coordinate determination, Neurosurgery 30(3):402, 1992.
73. Leksell L, Leksell D, and Schwebel J: Stereotaxis and nuclear magnetic resonance, J Neurol Neurosurg Psychiatry 48:14, 1985.
74. LeBihan D, Delannoy J, and Levin RL: Temperature mapping with MR imaging of molecular diffusion: application to hyperthermia, Radiology 161:401, 1989.
75. LeBihan D, Delannoy J, and Levin R: Temperature mapping with MR imaging of molecular diffusion: application to hyperthermia, Radiology 171:853, 1989.
76. Lewa C, and Majewska Z: Temperature relationships of proton spin-lattice relaxation time T1 in biological tissues, Bull Cancer (Paris) 67(5):525, 1980.
77. Livraghi T, Festi D, Monti F, et al: US-guided percutaneous alcohol injection of small hepatic and abdominal tumors, Radiology 16:309, 1986.
78. Livraghi T, Vettore C, and Lazzaroni S: Liver metastases: results of percutaneous ethanol injection in 14 patients, Radiology 179:709, 1991.
79. Lufkin R, Jordan S, Lylyck P, et al: MR imaging with topographic EEG electrodes in place, Am J Neuroradiol 9(5):953, 1988.
80. Lufkin R, and Layfield L: Coaxial needle system for MR and CT guided aspiration cytology, J Comput Assist Tomogr 13(6):1105, 1989.
81. Lufkin R, Teresi L, Chiu L et al: A technique for MR guided needle placement in the head and neck, Am J Roentgenol 151:193, 1988.
82. Lufkin R, Teresi L, and Hanafee W: New needle for MR-guided aspiration cytology of the head and neck, Am J Roentgenol 149(2):380, 1987.
83. Lufkin RB: MR-guided needle biopsy with a high-field-strength MR system, Am J Neuroradiol 12(6):1268, 1991.
84. Lunsford L, Martinez A, and Latchaw R: Stereotaxic surgery with a magnetic resonance-and computerized tomography-compatible system, J Neurosurg 64:872, 1986.
85. MacErlean DP, Bryan PJ, and Murphy JJ: Pancreatic pseudocyst: management by ultrasonically guided aspiration, Gastrointest Radiol 5:255, 1980.
86. Macintosh PK, Thomson KR, and Barbaric ZL: Percutaneous transperitoneal lymph-node biopsy as a means of improving lymphographic diagnosis, Radiology 131:647, 1979.
87. Maciunas R, Galloway RJ, Fitzpatrick J, et al: A universal system for interactive image-directed neurosurgery, Stereotact Funct Neurosurg 58(1-4):108, 1992.
88. Madersbacher S, Kratzik C, Szabo N, et al: Tissue ablation in benign prostatic hyperplasia with high-intensity focused ultrasound, Eur Urol 23(Suppl 1):39, 1993.
89. Matsumoto R, Mulkern R, Hushek S, et al: Tissue temperature monitoring for thermal interventional therapy: comparison of T1-weighted MR sequences, J Magn Reson Imaging 4(1):65, 1994.
90. Matsumoto R, Oshio K, and Jolesz F: Monitoring of laser and freezing-induced ablation in the liver with T1-weighted MR imaging, J Magn Reson Imaging 2:555, 1992.
91. Matsumoto S, Shima F, Hasuo K, et al: MR imaging of stereotactic thalamotomy using radiofrequency methods, Nippon Igaku Hoshasen Gakkai Zasshi 52:1559, 1992.
92. Matthewson K, Coleridge-Smith P, O'Sullivan JP, et al: Biological effects of intrahepatic neodymium:yttrium-aluminum-garnet laser photocoagulation in rats, Gastroenterology 93:550, 1987.
93. Mueller P, Stark D, Simeone J, et al: MR-guided aspiration biopsy: needle design and clinical trials, Radiology 161:605, 1986.
94. Nordenstrom B: Paraxiphoid approach to the mediastinum for mediastinography and mediastinal needle biopsy: a preliminary report, Invest Radiol 2:141, 1967.
95. Onik G, Cobb C, Cohen J, et al: US characteristics of frozen prostate, Radiology 168:629, 1988.
96. Onik G, Gilbert J, Hoddick W, et al: Ultrasonic monitoring of hepatic cryosurgery: preliminary report on an animal model, Cryobiology 21:715, 1984 (abstract).
97. Onik G, Porterfield B, Rubinsky B, et al: Percutaneous transperineal prostate cryosurgery using transrectal ultrasound guidance animal model, Urology 37:277, 1991.
98. Orel SG, Schnall MD, Newman RW, et al: MR imaging-guided localization and biopsy of breast lesions: initial experience, Radiology 193(1):97, Oct 1994.
99. Organ L: Electrophysiologic principles of radiofrequency lesion making, Appl Neurophysiol 39:69, 1976.
100. Pagani J: Biopsy of focal hepatic lesions: comparison of 18 and 22 gauge needles, Radiology 147:673, 1983.
101. Parker D: Applications of NMR imaging in hyperthermia: an evaluation of the potential for localized tissue heating and noninvasive temperature monitoring, IEEE Trans Biomed Eng 31(1):161, 1984.
102. Parker D, Smith P, Sheldon P, et al: Temperature distribution measurements in two-dimensional NMR imaging, Med Phys 10(3):321, 1983.
103. Pereiras PV, Meiers W, Kunhardt B, et al: Fluoroscopically guided thin needle aspiration biopsy of the abdomen and retroperitoneum, Am J Roentgenol 131:197, 1978.
104. Pomeroy O, Hynynen K, Singer S, et al: MR guided treatment of breast fibroadenomas by high intensity focused ultrasound, Interventional MRI workshop, Boston, 1994, p 62.
105. Robinson J, Lufkin R, Castro D, et al: Magnetic resonance imaging of laser phototherapy: initial experience, Eur J Radiol 2:24, 1992.

106. Rosomoff H, Brown C, and Sheptak P: Percutaneous radiofrequency cervical cordotomy: technique, J Neurosurg 23(5):639, 1965.

107. Roux FX, Merienne L, Leriche B, et al: Laser interstitial thermotherapy in stereotactical neurosurgery, Lasers Med Science 7:121, 1992.

108. Rubinsky B, Gilbert J, Onik G, et al: Monitoring cryosurgery in the brain and prostate with proton NMR, Cryobiology 30:191, 1993.

109. Rubinsky B, and Onik G: Cryosurgery: advances in the application of low temperatures to medicine, International Journal of Refrigeration 14:1, 1991.

110. Rubinsky B, and Shitzer A: Analysis of a Stefan-like problem in a biological tissue around a cryosurgical probe, Transactions of ASME Journal of Heat Transfer 98:514, 1976.

111. Ruttimann A: Iliac lymph node aspiration biopsy through paravascular approach: preliminary report, Radiology 90:150, 1968.

112. Seibel RMM, and Gronemeyer DHW: Interventional computed tomography, Oxford, 1990, Blackwell Science.

113. Seibel RMM, and Gronemeyer DHW: Microinvasive CT-guided dissection technique in the spinal canal, Endosc Surg Allied Technol 12:313, 1994.

114. Seibel RMM, Gronemeyer DHW, and Sorensen R: Percutaneous nucleotomy with CT and fluoroscopic guidance, J Vasc Interv Radiol 3:571, 1992.

115. Seibel RMM, Gronemeyer DHW, and Weigand H: Thorax-biopsy: lunge-pleura-mediastinum. In Seibel RMM, and Gronemeyer DHW: Interventional computed tomography, Oxford, 1990, Blackwell Science.

116. Seibel RMM, Gronemeyer DHW, Werner WR, et al: Die thorakale und abdominelle perkutane CT-gesteuerte Abszesdrainage. In Gronemeyer DHW, and Seibel RMM: Interventionelle Computertomographie, Berlin, 1989, Ueberreuter Wissenschaft.

117. Seki T, Nonaka T, Kubota Y, et al: Ultrasonically guided percutaneous ethanol injection therapy for hepatocellular carcinoma, Am J Gastroenterol 84:1400, 1989.

118. Sheu J Ch, Huang GT, Chen DS et al: Small hepatocellular carcinoma: intratumor ethanol treatment using new needle and guidance systems, Radiology 163:43, 1987.

119. Sibille A, Prat F, Chapelon J, et al: Characterization of extracorporeal ablation of normal and tumor-bearing liver tissue by high intensity focused ultrasound, Ultrasound Med Biol 19(9):803, 1993.

120. Siegfried J: 500 Percutaneous thermocoagulations of the gasserian ganglion for trigeminal pain, Surg Neurol 8(2):126, 1977.

121. Silverman R, Vogelsang B, Rondeau M, et al: Therapeutic ultrasound for the treatment of glaucoma, Am J Ophthalmol 111(3):327, 1991.

122. Sironi S, Livraghi T, Angeli E, et al: Small hepatocellular carcinoma: MR follow-up of treatment with percutaneous ethanol injection, Radiology 187:119, 1993.

123. Sironi S, Livraghi T, and DelMaschio A: Small hepatocellular carcinoma treated with percutaneous ethanol injection: MR imaging findings, Radiology 180:333, 1991.

124. Smith EM, Bartrum RJ Jr, Chang YC, et al: Percutaneous aspiration biopsy of the pancreas under ultrasonic guidance, N Engl J Med 292:825, 1975.

125. Stollberger R: Thermal monitoring using the water proton chemical shift, Interventional MRI workshop, Boston, 1994, p 12.

126. Sweet W, Mark V, and Hamlin H: Radiofrequency lesions in the central nervous system of man and cat, J Neurosurg 17:213, 1960.

127. Takizawa T: Isocentric stereotactic three-dimensional digitizer for neurosurgery, Stereotact Funct Neurosurg 60(4):175, 1993.

128. ter Haar G, and Robertson D: Tissue destruction with focused ultrasound in vivo, Eur Urol 23(Suppl 1):8, 1993.

129. Trapp T, Lufkin R, Abemayor E, et al: MR guided aspiration cytology of the head and neck, Laryngoscope 99:105, 1989.

130. Unger E: MR-guided alcohol ablation of the body. In Interventional MRI, Marina Del Rey, Calif, 1994, Medical Education Collaborative.

131. Unger E, Kartchner Z, and Karmann S: Measurement of intratumoral ethanol concentrations with CT in patients undergoing percutaneous ethanol injection (abstract 78). In Scientific Program of the 79th scientific assembly and annual meeting of RSNA, Chicago, 1993.

132. Vallancien G, Harouni M, Veillon B, et al: Focused extracorporeal pyrotherapy: feasibility study in man, J Endourol 6:173, 1992.

133. van Vaals J, Brummer M, Dixon W, et al: "Keyhole" method for accelerating imaging of contrast agent uptake, JMRI 3(4):671, 1993.

134. Villemure J, Marchand E, Peters T, et al: Magnetic resonance imaging stereotaxy: recognition and utilization of the commissures, Appl Neurophysiol 50:57, 1987.

135. Vining E, Duckwiler G, Udkoff R, et al: MRI of the thalamus following cryothalamotomy for Parkinson's disease and dystonia, J Neuroimaging 1(3):146, 1991.

136. Vogl TJ, Mack MG, Muller P, et al: Recurrent nasopharyngeal tumors: preliminary clinical results with interventional MR imaging–controlled laser-induced thermotherapy, Radiology 196(3):725, Sept 1995.

137. Vogl TJ, Muller PK, Hammerstingl R, et al: Malignant liver tumors treated with MR imaging–guided laser-induced thermotherapy: technique and prospective results, Radiology 196(1):257, July 1995.

138. Warwick R, and Pond J: Trackless lesions in nervous tissues produced by high intensity focused ultrasound, J Anat 102:387, 1968.

139. Wendt M, Lenz G, Batz L, et al: Dynamic tracking algorithm for interventional MRI using wavelet-encoding, In Proceedings of the annual meeting of the Society for Magnetic Resonance Imaging 2:1162, 1995.

140. Wenokur R, Andrews J, Abemayor E, et al: Magnetic resonance imaging–guided fine needle aspiration for the diagnosis of skull base lesions, Skull Base Surgery 2(3):167, 1992.

141. Yang R, Sanghvi NT, Rescorla FJ, et al: Liver cancer ablation with extracorporeal high-intensity focused ultrasound, Eur Urol 23(Suppl 1):17, 1993.

142. Young I, Hand J, Oatridge A, et al: Further observations on the measurement of tissue

14 Bioeffects and Safety

Frank G. Shellock and Emanuel Kanal

 KEY POINTS

- It is generally contraindicated to scan in an MR system patients with cardiac pacemakers or implanted cardiac defibrillators.
- Patients with ferromagnetic aneurysm clips should not undergo scanning; the risk of scanning other ferromagnetic objects depends on the location in the body (e.g., metal fragments in the eye).
- The FDA has set limits on the maximum field strength, the maximum rate at which the gradients can be changed, and the maximum amount of RF power deposition allowed.
- Scanning at fields higher than 2 T has been associated with vertigo resulting from induced currents in the semicircular canals.
- When strong gradients are changed too rapidly, peripheral nerve stimulation can occur.
- Excessive RF power deposition can lead to tissue heating.

During the performance of magnetic resonance imaging (MRI), the patient is exposed to three different forms of electromagnetic radiation: a static magnetic field, gradient magnetic fields, and radiofrequency (RF) electromagnetic fields. Each of these may cause significant bioeffects if applied at sufficiently high exposure levels.

Numerous investigations have been conducted to identify potentially adverse bioeffects of MRI.* Although none of these have determined the presence of any significant or unexpected hazards, the data are not comprehensive enough to assume absolute safety. In addition to bioeffects related to exposure to the electromagnetic fields used for MRI, there are several areas of health concern for both the patient and health practitioner with respect to the use of clinical MRI.

This chapter (1) discusses the bioeffects of static, gradient, and RF electromagnetic fields with an emphasis on the data that pertain to MRI; (2) describes and summarizes the investigations that specifically apply to MRI; and (3) provides an overview of other safety considerations and patient management aspects of this imaging technique.

Modified in part from Shellock FG, and Kanal E: Magnetic resonance: bioeffects, safety, and patient management, ed 2, New York, 1996, Lippincott-Raven.

*References 3, 9, 12, 19, 20, 23, 25, 26, 28, 31, 33, 38, 39, 44, 54, 59-61, 68, 72, 73, 75, 82, 86, 90, 92, 99, 101, 116-118, 121, 123, 126, 127, 137-141, 145-152, 157, 160, 165, 171, 180, 182, 185, 187, 192-196, 200, 201, 203-205, 207, 215-217, 221-226, 235, 240-243.

BIOEFFECTS OF STATIC MAGNETIC FIELDS
General Bioeffects of Static Magnetic Fields

There is a paucity of data concerning the effects of high-intensity static magnetic fields on humans. Some of the original investigations on human subjects exposed to static magnetic fields were performed by Vyalov,[227,228] who studied workers involved in the permanent-magnet industry. These subjects were exposed to static magnetic fields ranging from 0.0015 to 0.35 Tesla (T) and reported feelings of headache, chest pain, fatigue, vertigo, loss of appetite, insomnia, itching, and other, more nonspecific ailments.[227,228] However, exposure to other potentially hazardous environmental working conditions (elevated room temperature, airborne metallic dust, chemicals) may have been partially responsible for the reported symptoms in these study subjects. And because this investigation lacked an appropriate control group, it is difficult to ascertain whether there was a definite correlation between the exposure to the static magnetic field and the reported abnormalities. Subsequent studies performed with more scientific rigor have not substantiated many of the aforementioned findings.[11,119,142,212]

Temperature Effects

There are conflicting statements in the literature regarding the effect of static magnetic fields on the body and the skin temperatures of mammals. Reports have variously indicated that static magnetic fields either increase or both increase and decrease tissue temperature, depending on the orientation of the organism in the static magnetic field.[72,203] Other articles state that static magnetic fields have no effect on the skin and the body temperatures of mammals.[193,195,212,213]

None of the investigators who identified a static magnetic field effect on temperatures proposed a plausible mechanism for this response, nor has this work been substantiated. In addition, studies that reported static magnetic field–induced skin and/or body temperature changes used either laboratory animals known to have labile temperatures or instrumentation that may have been affected by the static magnetic fields.[72,203]

A recent investigation indicated that exposure to a 1.5 T static magnetic field does not alter the skin and the body temperatures in human beings.[213] This study was performed by using a special fluoroptic thermometry system demonstrated to be unperturbed by high-intensity static magnetic fields; therefore the skin and the body temperatures of human subjects are believed to be unaffected by exposure to static magnetic fields of up to 1.5 T.[193,195]

Electrical Induction and Cardiac Effects

Induced biopotentials may be observed during exposure to static magnetic fields and are caused by blood—a conductive fluid—flowing through a magnetic field. Induced biopotentials are exhibited by an augmentation of T-wave amplitude and by other, nonspecific waveform changes on the electrocardiogram (ECG). They have been observed at static magnetic field strengths as low as 0.1 T.[11,15,214]

The increase in T-wave amplitude is directly related to the intensity of the static magnetic field, such that at low static magnetic field strengths the effects are not as predominant as those at higher field strengths. The most marked effect on the T wave is thought to be caused when the blood flows through the thoracic aortic arch. This T-wave amplitude change can be significant enough to falsely trigger the RF excitation during a cardiac-gated MR examination.

Other portions of the ECG also may be altered by the static magnetic field, and this varies with the placement of the recording electrodes. Alternate lead positions can be used to attenuate the static magnetic field–induced ECG changes to facilitate cardiac-gating studies.[43] Once the patient is no longer exposed to the static magnetic field, these ECG voltage abnormalities revert to normal.

Because no circulatory alterations appear to coincide with these ECG changes, no biological risks are believed to be associated with the magnetohydrodynamic effect that occurs in conjunction with static magnetic field strengths of up to 2 T.[11,15,214]

Neurological Effects

Theoretically, electrical impulse conduction in nerve tissue may be affected by exposure to static magnetic fields; however, this is an area in the bioeffects literature that contains contradictory information. Some studies have reported remarkable effects on both the function and the structure of those portions of the central nervous system associated with exposure to static magnetic fields, whereas others have failed to show any significant changes.* Further investigations of potential unwanted bioeffects are needed because of the relative lack of clinical studies in this field that are directly applicable to MRI. At present, exposure to static magnetic fields of up to 2 T does not appear to significantly influence bioelectrical properties of neurons in humans.[96,177,184]

In summary, there is no conclusive evidence of irreversible or hazardous biological effects related to acute, short-term exposure of humans to static magnetic fields of strengths up to 2 T. However, as of 1998, there were several 3 and 4 T whole-body MR systems in operation at various research sites around the world. One study indicated that workers and volunteer subjects exposed to a 4 T MR system experienced vertigo, nausea, headaches, a metallic taste in their mouths, and magnetophosphenes (visual flashes).[157] As a result, considerable research is under way worldwide to study the mechanisms responsible for these bioeffects and to determine possible means, if any, to counterbalance them.

Cryogen Considerations

All superconductive MR systems in clinical use today use liquid helium. Liquid helium, which maintains the magnet coils in their superconductive state, will achieve the gaseous state ("boil off") at approximately −268.93° C (4.22° K).[96] If the temperature within the cryostat precipitously rises, the helium will enter the gaseous state. In such a situation the marked increase in volume of the gaseous versus the liquid cryogen (with gas-liquid volume ratios of 760:1 for helium and 695:1 for nitrogen) will dramatically increase the pressure within the cryostat.[96] A pressure-sensitive carbon "pop-off" valve will give way, sometimes with a rather loud popping noise, followed by the rapid (and loud) egress of gaseous helium as it escapes from the cryostat. In normal situations this gas should be vented out of the imaging room and into the external atmosphere. It is possible, however, that during such venting some helium gas might accidentally be released into the ambient atmosphere of the imaging room.

Gaseous helium is considerably lighter than air. If any helium gas is inadvertently released into the imaging room, the dimensions of the room, its ventilation capacity, and the total amount of gas released will determine whether the helium gas will reach the patient or the health practitioner, who is in the lower part of the room near the floor.[96] Helium vapor looks like steam and is odorless and tasteless, but it may be extremely cold. Asphyxiation and frostbite are possible if a person is exposed to helium vapor for a prolonged time. In a system quench a considerable quantity of helium gas may be released into the imaging room. This might make it difficult to open the door of the room because of the pressure differential. In such a circumstance the first response should be to evacuate the area until the offending helium vapor is adequately removed from the imaging room environment and safely redirected to an outside environment away from patients, pedestrians, or any temperature-sensitive material.[96]

Better cryostat design and insulation materials have allowed the use of liquid helium alone in many of the newer superconducting magnets. Nevertheless, a great number of magnets in clinical use still use liquid nitrogen as well. Liquid nitrogen within the cryostat acts as a buffer between the liquid helium and the outside atmosphere, boiling off at 77.3° K. In the event of an accidental release of liquid nitrogen into the ambient atmosphere of the imaging room, there is a potential for frostbite, similar to that encountered with gaseous helium release. Gaseous nitrogen is roughly the same density as air and is certainly much less buoyant than gaseous helium.

In the event of an inadvertent venting of nitrogen gas into the imaging room, the gas could easily settle near floor level; the amount of nitrogen gas within the room would continue to increase until venting ceased. The total concentration of nitrogen gas contained within the room would be determined on the basis of the total amount of the gas released into the room, the dimensions of the room, and its ventilation capacity (i.e., the existence and size of other routes of egress—doors,

---

*References 1, 30, 44, 73, 85, 96, 123, 177, 184, 205, 207, 224-226, 235.

windows, ventilation ducts, and fans). A pure nitrogen environment is exceptionally hazardous, and unconsciousness generally results as soon as 5 to 10 sec after exposure.[96] It is imperative that all patients and health practitioners evacuate the area as soon as it is recognized that nitrogen gas is being released into the imaging room. They should not return until appropriate measures have been taken to clear the gas from the room.[96]

Dewar (cryogen storage containers) storage should also be within a well-ventilated area, lest normal boil-off rates increase the concentration of inert gas within the storage room to a dangerous level.[71] At least one reported death has occurred in an industrial setting during the shipment of cryogens,[70] although to our knowledge no such fatality has occurred in the medical community. There is one report of a sudden loss of consciousness of unexplained cause by an otherwise healthy technologist (with no prior or subsequent similar episodes) passing through a cryogen storage area where multiple dewars were located.[4] Although there is no verification of ambient atmospheric oxygen concentration to confirm any relationship to the cryogens per se, the history is strongly suggestive of such a relationship.

Cryogens present a potential concern in clinical MRI despite an overwhelmingly safe record over the past 7 or more years of clinical service.[96] Proper handling and storage of cryogens, as well as the appropriate behavior in the presence of possible leaks, should be emphasized at each site. An oxygen monitor with an audible alarm, situated at an appropriate height within each imaging room, should be a mandatory minimum safety measure for all sites; automatic linking to and activation of an imaging room ventilation fan system when the oxygen monitor registers below 18% or 19% should be considered at each magnet installation.[96]

Electrical Considerations of a Quench

In addition to the potential for cryogen release, there is also a concern about the currents that may be induced in conductors (such as biological tissues) near the rapidly changing magnetic field associated with a quench.[96] In one study, physiological monitoring of a pig and monitoring of the environment were performed during an intentional quench from 1.76 T; there seemed to be no significant effect on the blood pressure, pulse, temperature, and electroencephalographic and ECG measurements of the pig during or immediately after the quench.[41] Although a single observation does not prove safety for humans undergoing exposure to a quench, the data do suggest that the experience would indeed be similar, and that there would be no deleterious electrical effects on humans undergoing a similar experience and exposure.

BIOEFFECTS OF GRADIENT MAGNETIC FIELDS

MRI exposes the human body to rapid variations of magnetic fields as a result of the transient application of magnetic field gradients during the imaging sequence. Gradient magnetic fields can induce electrical fields and currents in conductive media (including biological tissue) according to Faraday's law of induction. The potential for interaction between gradient magnetic fields and biological tissue is inherently dependent on the fundamental field frequency, the maximum flux density, the average flux density, the presence of harmonic frequencies, the waveform characteristics of the signal, the polarity of the signal, the current distribution in the body, and the electrical properties and sensitivity of the particular cell membrane.[96,177,184]

For animal and human subjects, the induced current is proportional to the conductivity of the biological tissue and the rate of change of the magnetic flux density.[18,96,161,177] In theory the largest current densities will be produced in peripheral tissues (i.e., at the greatest radius) and will linearly diminish toward the body's center.[18,96,161,177] The current density will be enhanced at higher frequencies and magnetic flux densities and will be further accentuated by a larger tissue radius with a greater tissue conductivity. Current paths are affected by differences in tissue types, such that tissues with low conductivity (e.g., adipose and bone) will change the pattern of the induced current.

Bioeffects of induced currents can result from either the power deposited by the induced currents (thermal effects) or direct effects of the current (nonthermal effects). Thermal effects caused by switched gra-

dients used in MRI are negligible and are not believed to be clinically significant.[30,96,177]

Possible nonthermal effects of induced currents are stimulation of nerve or muscle cells, induction of ventricular fibrillation, increased brain mannitol space, epileptogenic potential, stimulation of visual flash sensations, and bone healing.* The threshold currents required for nerve stimulation and ventricular fibrillation are known to be much higher than the estimated current densities that will be induced under routine clinical MR conditions.[30,96,161,177,184]

The production of magnetophosphenes is considered to be one of the most sensitive physiological responses to gradient magnetic fields.[30,96,177,184] Magnetophosphenes are supposedly caused by electrical stimulation of the retina and are completely reversible with no associated health effects.[30,96,177,184] These have been elicited by current densities of roughly 17 $\mu A/cm^2$. In contrast to this level, the currents required for the induction of nerve action potentials is roughly 3000 $\mu A/cm^2$, and those required for ventricular fibrillation induction of healthy cardiac tissue are calculated to be 100 to 1000 $\mu A/cm^2$.[30] Although to our knowledge there have been no reported cases of magnetophosphenes for fields of 1.95 T or less, magnetophosphenes have been reported in volunteers working in and around a 4 T research system.[157] In addition, a metallic taste and symptoms of vertigo also seem to be reproducible and associated with rapid motion within the static magnetic field of these 4 T systems.[157]

Time-varying, extremely low-frequency magnetic fields have been demonstrated to be associated with multiple effects, including clustering and altered orientation of fibroblasts, as well as increased mitotic activity of fibroblast growth, altered DNA synthesis, and reduced fentanyl-induced anesthesia.[96,152,200] Possible effects in multiple other organisms, including humans, have also been mentioned.[96] Although no study has conclusively demonstrated carcinogenic effects from exposure to time-varying magnetic fields of various intensities and durations, several reports suggest that an association between the two is plausible.[27,120,144]

BIOEFFECTS OF RADIOFREQUENCY ELECTROMAGNETIC FIELDS
General Bioeffects of Radiofrequency Electromagnetic Fields

RF radiation is capable of generating heat in tissues as a result of resistive losses. Therefore the main bioeffects associated with exposure to RF radiation are related to the thermogenic qualities of this electromagnetic field.† Exposure to RF radiation also may cause athermic, field-specific alterations in biological systems that are produced without a significant increase in temperature.‡ This topic is somewhat controversial because of assertions concerning the role of electromagnetic fields in producing cancer and developmental abnormalities, along with the concomitant ramifications of such effects.‡ A report from the U.S. Environmental Protection Agency (EPA) claimed that the existing evidence on this issue is sufficient to demonstrate a relationship between low-level electromagnetic field exposures and the development of cancer.[144] To date, there have been no specific studies performed to study potential athermal bioeffects of MRI. Those interested in a thorough review of this topic, particularly as it pertains to MRI, are referred to the extensive article written by Beers.[14]

Regarding RF-power deposition concerns, investigators have typically quantified exposure to RF radiation by means of determining the specific absorption rate (SAR).§ The SAR is the mass normalized rate at which RF power is coupled to biological tissue and is indicated in units of watts per kilogram. Measurements or estimates of SAR are not trivial, particularly in human subjects, and there are several methods of determining this parameter for RF-energy dosimetry.[50,65-67,119,124]

The SAR produced during MRI is a complex function of numerous variables: the frequency (which, in turn, is determined by the strength of the static magnetic field), type of RF pulse (i.e., 90 or 180 degrees), repetition time, pulse width, type of RF coil used, volume of tissue

---

*References 2, 18, 96, 161, 177, 230.
†References 14, 21, 22, 30, 40, 50, 65-67, 96, 124, 177, 184.
‡References 14. 40, 50, 65-67, 124.
§References 17, 22, 50, 65-67, 119, 124, 238.

within the coil, resistivity of the tissue, configuration of the anatomical region imaged, and other factors.[30,96,177,184] The actual increase in tissue temperature caused by exposure to RF radiation is dependent on the subject's thermoregulatory system (e.g., skin blood flow, skin surface area, and sweat rate).[96,177,184]

The efficiency and absorption pattern of RF energy are determined mainly by the physical dimensions of the tissue in relation to the incident wavelength.[50,65-67,124] Therefore if the tissue size is large relative to the wavelength, energy is predominantly absorbed on the surface; if it is small relative to the wavelength, there is little absorption of RF power.[50,65-67,124] Because of the relationship between RF energy and physical dimensions, studies designed to investigate the effects of exposure to RF radiation during MRI that are intended to be applicable to the clinical setting require tissue volumes and anatomical shapes comparable to those of human subjects. No laboratory animal sufficiently mimics or simulates the thermoregulatory system or responses of man. Thus results obtained in laboratory animal experiments cannot simply be "scaled" or extrapolated to human subjects.[65-67]

Magnetic Resonance Imaging and Exposure to Radiofrequency Radiation

Little quantitative data have been previously available on thermoregulatory responses of humans exposed to RF radiation before the studies performed with MRI. The few studies that existed did not directly apply to MRI because these investigations examined either thermal sensations or therapeutic applications of diathermy, usually involving only localized regions of the body.[40,50,65,124]

Several studies of RF-power absorption during MRI have been performed recently and have yielded useful information about tissue heating in humans.* During MRI, tissue heating results primarily from magnetic induction, with a negligible contribution from the electric fields, so that ohmic heating is greatest at the surface of the body and approaches zero at the center of the body. Predictive calculations and measurements obtained in phantoms and human subjects exposed to MRI support this pattern of temperature distribution.[21,22,180,185,187]

Although one paper reported significant temperature rises produced by MRI in internal organs,[201] this study was conducted on anesthetized dogs and is unlikely to be applicable to conscious adult human subjects because of factors related to the physical dimensions and dissimilar thermoregulatory systems of these two species. However, these data may have important implications for the use of MRI in pediatric patients because this patient population is typically sedated or anesthetized for MR examinations.

An investigation using fluoroptic thermometry probes that are unperturbed by electromagnetic fields demonstrated that human subjects exposed to MRI at SAR levels up to 4 W/kg (i.e., 10 times higher than the level currently recommended by the U.S. Food and Drug Administration [FDA]) have no statistically significant increases in body temperatures and elevations in skin temperatures and are not believed to be clinically hazardous.[194,238] These results imply that the suggested exposure level of 0.4 W/kg for RF radiation during MRI is too conservative for individuals with normal thermoregulatory function.[194] Additional studies are needed, however, to assess physiological responses of patients with conditions that may impair thermoregulatory function (e.g., elderly patients; patients with underlying health conditions, such as fever, diabetes, obesity, or cardiovascular disease; and patients taking medications that affect thermoregulation, such as calcium blockers, beta blockers, diuretics, and vasodilators) before subjecting them to MRI procedures that require high SARs.

Temperature-Sensitive Organs

Certain human organs that have reduced capabilities for heat dissipation, such as the testis and the eye, are particularly sensitive to elevated temperatures. Therefore these are primary sites of potential harmful effects if RF-radiation exposures during MRI are excessive. Laboratory investigations have demonstrated detrimental effects on testicular function (i.e., a reduction or cessation of spermatogenesis, impaired sperm motility, degeneration of seminiferous tubules) caused by RF radia-

tion–induced heating from exposures sufficient to raise scrotal or testicular tissue temperatures to 38° to 42° C.[17]

Scrotal skin temperatures (i.e., an index of intratesticular temperature) were measured in volunteer subjects undergoing MRI at a whole-body–averaged SAR of 1.1 W/kg.[192] The largest change in scrotal skin temperature was 2.1° C, and the highest scrotal skin temperature recorded was 34.2° C.[192] These temperature changes were below the threshold known to impair testicular function. However, excessively heating the scrotum during MRI could exacerbate certain preexisting disorders associated with increased scrotal or testicular temperatures (e.g., acute febrile illnesses and varicocele) in patients who are already oligospermic and lead to possible temporary or permanent sterility.[192] Therefore additional studies designed to investigate these issues are needed, particularly if patients are scanned at whole-body–averaged SARs higher than those previously evaluated.

Dissipation of heat from the eye is a slow and inefficient process because of the eye's relative lack of vascularization. Acute near-field exposures of RF radiation to the eyes or heads of laboratory animals have been demonstrated to be cataractogenic as a result of the thermal disruption of ocular tissues if the exposure is of a sufficient intensity and duration.[108,124] An investigation conducted by Sacks et al[171] revealed that there were no discernible effects on the eyes of rats by MRI at exposures that far exceeded typical clinical imaging levels. However, it may not be acceptable to extrapolate these data to humans, considering the coupling of RF radiation to the anatomy and tissue volume of the laboratory rat eyes compared with those of man.

Corneal temperatures have been measured in patients undergoing MRI of the brain by using a send-receive head coil at local SARs up to 3.1 W/kg.[180] The largest corneal temperature change was 1.8° C, and the highest temperature measured was 34.4° C. Because the temperature threshold for RF radiation–induced cataractogenesis in animal models has been demonstrated to be between 41° to 55° C for acute, near-field exposures, it does not appear that clinical MRI using a head coil has the potential to cause thermal damage in ocular tissue.[180] The effect of MRI at higher SARs and the long-term effects of MRI on ocular tissues remain to be determined.

Radiofrequency Radiation and "Hot Spots"

Theoretically, RF radiation "hot spots" caused by an uneven distribution of RF power may arise whenever current concentrations are produced in association with restrictive conductive patterns. It has been suggested that RF radiation hot spots may generate thermal hot spots under certain conditions during MRI. Because RF radiation is mainly absorbed by peripheral tissues, thermography has been used to study the heating pattern associated with MRI at high whole-body SARs.[196] This study demonstrated no evidence of surface thermal hot spots related to MRI of human subjects. The thermoregulatory system apparently responds to the heat challenge by distributing the thermal load, producing a "smearing" effect of the surface temperatures. However, there is a possibility that internal thermal hot spots may develop as a result of MRI.[180]

FOOD AND DRUG ADMINISTRATION GUIDELINES FOR MAGNETIC RESONANCE DEVICES

In 1988, MR diagnostic devices were reclassified from class III, in which premarket approval is required, to class II, which is regulated by performance standards, as long as the device (or devices) are within the "umbrella" of certain defined limits, addressed later.[52] Subsequent to this reclassification, new devices had to demonstrate only that they were "substantially equivalent" to any class II device that was brought to market using the premarket notification process (510[k]) or, alternatively, to any of the devices described by the 13 MR-system manufacturers that had petitioned the FDA for such a reclassification.

Four areas relating to the use of MR systems have been identified for which safety guidelines have been issued by the FDA. These include the static magnetic field, the gradient magnetic fields, the RF power of the examination, and the acoustical considerations.

On September 29, 1997, the office of Device Evaluation of the FDA issued a new guidance document for MR devices.[52] The new wording for those criteria that are considered significant risk investigations follow.

---

*References 102, 180, 185, 187, 192, 194, 201.

Magnetic Resonance Diagnostic Devices: Criteria for Significant Risk Investigations

Patient studies utilizing magnetic resonance diagnostic devices which are conducted under any one of the following operating conditions are considered significant risk investigations, and require approval of an investigational device exemption (IDE) by the Food and Drug Administration (FDA) Center for Devices and Radiological Health (CDRH):

1. Main static magnetic field greater than 4 Tesla;
2. Specific absorption rate (SAR) greater than
   a. 4 W/kg averaged over the whole body for any period of 15 minutes;
   b. 3 W/kg averaged over the head for any period of 10 minutes; or
   c. 8 W/kg in any gram of tissue in the head or torso, or 12 W/kg in any gram of tissue in the extremities, for any period of 5 minutes;
3. Time rate of change of gradient fields (dB/dt) sufficient to produce severe discomfort or painful nerve stimulation; or
4. Peak unweighted sound pressure level greater than 140 dB or A-weighted r.m.s. sound pressure level greater than 99 dBA with hearing protection in place.

These criteria apply only to device operating conditions. Other aspects of the study may involve significant risks and the study may therefore require IDE approval.

MAGNETIC RESONANCE IMAGING AND ACOUSTIC NOISE

The acoustic noise produced during MRI represents a potential risk to patients. Acoustic noise is associated with the activation and deactivation of electrical current that induces vibrations of the gradient coils. This repetitive sound is enhanced by higher-gradient duty cycles and sharper pulse transitions. Thus acoustic noise is likely to increase with decreases in section thicknesses and decreased fields of view, repetition times, and echo times.

Gradient magnetic field–related noise levels measured on several commercial MR scanners were in the range of 65 to 95 dB, considered to be within the recommended safety guidelines set forth by the FDA.[52] However, there have been reports that acoustic noise generated during MRI has caused patient annoyance, interference with oral communication, and reversible hearing loss in patients who did not wear ear protection.[28,189] A study of patients undergoing MRI without earplugs reported temporary hearing loss in 43% of the subjects.[28] Furthermore, the possibility exists that significant gradient coil–induced noise may produce permanent hearing impairment in certain patients who are particularly susceptible to the damaging effects of relatively loud noises.[28,189]

The safest and least expensive means of preventing problems associated with acoustic noise during clinical MRI is to encourage the routine use of disposable earplugs.[28,189] The use of hearing protection has been demonstrated to successfully avoid the potential temporary hearing loss that can be associated with clinical MR examinations.[28,189] MR-compatible headphones that significantly muffle acoustic noise are also commercially available.

An acceptable alternative strategy for reducing sound levels during MRI is to use an antinoise or destructive interference technique that effectively reduces noise and permits better patient communication.[63] This technique calls for a real-time Fourier analysis of the noise emitted from the MR system.[63] Next, a signal is produced that possesses the same physical characteristics of the sound generated by the MR system but of the opposite phase. The two opposite-phase signals are then combined, resulting in a cancellation of the repetitive noise, while allowing other sounds, such as music and voice, to be transmitted to the patient.[63] A recent investigation demonstrated no significant degradation of image quality when MRI is performed with MR systems that use this antinoise method.[63] Although this technique has not yet found widespread clinical application, it nevertheless has considerable potential for minimizing acoustic noise and its associated problems.

INVESTIGATIONS OF MAGNETIC RESONANCE IMAGING BIOLOGICAL EFFECTS

Many investigations have been performed to specifically study the potential biological effects of MRI. The results of these studies have been predominantly negative, supporting the widely held view that there are no significant health risks associated with use of this imaging modality. Experiments that yielded positive results either identified possible, non-specific biological responses, determined short-term biological changes that were not considered to be deleterious, or found biological effects that require further substantiation.*

While perusing these studies, the reader should note that the dosimetric aspects of the exposure to static, gradient, and/or RF electromagnetic fields are quite variable and include those that exceeded clinical exposures, simulated clinical exposures, or involved low-level, chronic exposures. In certain cases the effects of only one of the electromagnetic fields used for MRI were evaluated. Theoretically there is a possibility that the combination of static, gradient, and RF electromagnetic fields may produce some unusual or unpredictable biological effects that are unique to MRI.

"Window" effects are often present with respect to biological changes that occur in response to electromagnetic radiation. Window effects are those biological changes associated with a specific spectrum of electromagnetic radiation that are not observed at levels below or above this range.[119,124] Both field strength and frequency windows have been reported in the literature.[119,124] Virtually all the experiments conducted to date on MRI biological effects have been performed at specific windows, and the results cannot be assumed to apply to all of the various field strengths or frequencies used for clinical MRI.

A variety of different biological systems were used for these experiments. As previously mentioned, because the coupling of electromagnetic radiation to biological tissues is highly dependent on organism or subject size, anatomical factors, duration of exposure, the sensitivity of the involved tissues, and a myriad of other variables, studies performed on laboratory preparations may not be extrapolated or directly applicable to human subjects or to the clinical use of MRI. Therefore a cautionary approach to the interpretation of the results of these studies is advisable.

ELECTRICALLY, MAGNETICALLY, OR MECHANICALLY ACTIVATED IMPLANTS AND DEVICES

The FDA requires labeling of MR systems to indicate that the device is contraindicated for patients who have electrically, magnetically, or mechanically activated implants because electromagnetic fields produced by the MR system may interfere with the operation of these devices.[52] Therefore patients with internal cardiac pacemakers, implantable cardiac defibrillators, cochlear implants, neurostimulators, bone-growth stimulators, implantable electronic drug-infusion pumps, and other similar devices that could be adversely affected by the electromagnetic fields used for MRI should not be examined by means of this imaging technique.[5,49,58,81,189] Prior ex vivo testing of certain of these implants and devices may indicate that they are, in fact, MR compatible.

The associated risks of scanning patients with cardiac pacemakers are related to the possibility of movement, reed switch closures or damage, programming changes, inhibition or reversion to an asynchronous mode of operation, electromagnetic interference, and induced currents in lead wires.[49,58,81,189] At least one patient with a pacemaker has been scanned by MRI without incident.[5] One letter to a journal editor indicated that a patient who was not pacemaker dependent underwent MRI by having his pacemaker "disabled" during the procedure.[5] Although this patient sustained no apparent discomfort and the pacemaker was not damaged, it is inadvisable to routinely perform this type of maneuver on patients with pacemakers because of the potential to encounter the aforementioned hazards. There has been at least one MRI-related death of a patient with a pacemaker.[96]

Of particular concern is the possibility that the pacemaker lead wire (or wires) or other similar intracardiac wire configuration could act as an antenna in which the gradient or RF electromagnetic fields may induce sufficient current to cause fibrillation, a burn, or other potentially dangerous events.[49,58,81,96,189] Because of these theoretically deleterious and unpredicted effects, patients referred to MRI with residual external pacing wires, temporary pacing wires, Swan-Ganz thermodilution catheters, or any other type of internally or externally positioned con-

---

*References 3, 9, 12, 19, 20, 23, 25, 26, 28, 31, 33, 38, 39, 44, 54, 59-61, 68, 72, 73, 75, 82, 86, 90, 92, 99, 101, 116-118, 121, 123, 126, 127, 137-141, 145-152, 157, 160, 165, 171, 180, 182, 185, 187, 192-196, 200, 201, 203-205, 207, 215-217, 221-226, 235, 240-243.

ductive wire or similar device should not undergo MRI because of the possible associated risks.[48,96,189]

Some types of cochlear implants employ a relatively high–field strength cobalt samarium magnet used in conjunction with an external magnet to align and retain an RF transmitter coil on the patient's head; other implants are electronically activated.[45] Consequently, MRI is strictly contraindicated in patients with these implants because of the possibility of injuring the patient or damaging or altering the operation of the cochlear implant.

Because there is a potential for demagnetizing certain implants that involve magnets (e.g., dental implants, magnetic sphincters, magnetic stoma plugs, magnetic ocular implants, and other similar devices), which may necessitate surgery to replace the damaged implant, these implants should be removed from the patient before MRI, if possible.[45,109,178] Otherwise, MRI should not be performed on a patient with a magnetically activated implant or device. A patient with any other similar electrically, magnetically, or mechanically activated implant or device should be excluded from examination by MRI unless the particular implant or device has been previously demonstrated to be unaffected by the magnetic and electromagnetic fields used for MRI.[189]

PATIENTS WITH METALLIC IMPLANTS, MATERIALS, AND FOREIGN BODIES

MRI is contraindicated for patients with certain ferromagnetic implants, materials, or foreign bodies, primarily because of the possibility of movement or dislodgement of these objects.[96,177,184] Other problems may occur in patients with ferromagnetic implants, materials, or foreign bodies, including the induction of electrical current in the object, excessive heating of the object, and the misinterpretation of an artifact produced by the presence of the object as an abnormality.* These latter potentially hazardous situations, however, are encountered infrequently or are insignificant in comparison with movement or dislodgment of a ferromagnetic implant or foreign body by the magnetic fields of the MR system.

Many investigators have evaluated the ferromagnetic qualities of a variety of metallic implants, materials, or foreign bodies by measuring deflection forces or movements associated with the static magnetic fields used by MRI.† These studies were conducted to determine the relative risk of performing MRI on a patient with a metallic object with respect to whether the magnetic attraction was strong enough to produce movement or dislodgment (Table 14-1).

A variety of factors require evaluation when establishing the relative risk of performing an MR procedure on a patient with a ferromagnetic implant, material, device, or foreign body, such as the strength of the static and gradient magnetic fields, the relative degree of ferromagnetism of the object, the mass of the object, the geometry of the object, the location and orientation of the object in situ, and the length of time the object has been in place.[96,177] Each of these should be considered before allowing a patient with a ferromagnetic object to enter the electromagnetic environment of the MR system.

Aneurysm and Hemostatic Clips

Of the different aneurysm and vascular clips studied and reported in the literature, many of the aneurysm clips and none of the vascular clips were found to be ferromagnetic. Therefore only those patients who definitely have nonferromagnetic aneurysm clips should be exposed to the magnetic fields used for MRI; any patient with one of the previously tested hemostatic clips may safely undergo MRI.

Carotid Artery Vascular Clamps

Each of the carotid artery vascular clamps evaluated for ferromagnetism exhibited deflection forces. However, only the Poppen-Blaylock clamp was considered to be contraindicated for patients undergoing MRI because of the significant ferromagnetism shown by this object. The other carotid artery vascular clamps are believed to be safe for MRI

because of the minimal deflection forces relative to their use in an in vivo application (i.e., the deflection forces are insignificant, and therefore there is little possibility of significant movement or dislodgment of the implant).

Dental Devices and Materials

Various dental devices and materials have been tested for ferromagnetism. Although many of them demonstrated deflection forces, only a few are magnetically activated and pose a possible risk to patients undergoing MRI.

Heart Valves

Many of the commercially available heart valve prostheses have been tested for ferromagnetism. The majority of these displayed measurable deflection forces; however, the deflection forces were relatively insignificant compared with the force exerted by the beating heart. Therefore patients with these heart valve prostheses may safely undergo MRI.

Intravascular Coils, Filters, and Stents

Less than half of the intravascular coils, filters, and stents tested were ferromagnetic.[186,210] These devices are usually attached firmly into the vessel wall approximately 4 to 6 weeks after introduction.[210] Therefore it is unlikely that any ferromagnetic devices would become dislodged by magnetic forces presently used for MRI. Patients in whom there is a possibility that the intravascular coils, filters, or stents are not properly positioned or held firmly in place should not undergo MRI.

Ocular Implants

Various ocular implants have been evaluated for ferromagnetism. Of these, the Fatio eyelid spring and retinal tack made from martensitic stainless steel displayed measurable deflection forces. Although it is unlikely that the associated deflection forces would cause movement or dislodgement of these implants, it is possible that a patient with one of these implants would be uncomfortable or sustain a minor injury during MRI.

Orthopedic Implants, Materials, and Devices

Most orthopedic implants, materials, and devices tested for ferromagnetism are made from nonferromagnetic materials. Therefore patients with these particular orthopedic implants, materials, and devices may be safely imaged by MRI. The Perfix interference screw used for reconstruction of the anterior cruciate ligament, although composed of ferromagnetic material, does not pose a hazard to the patient undergoing MRI because of the significant force that holds it in place in vivo. However, the resulting imaging artifact precludes diagnostic assessment of the knee by means of MRI.

Otologic Implants

The cochlear implants evaluated for ferromagnetism are contraindicated for MRI. In addition to being attracted by static magnetic fields, these implants are electronically or magnetically activated. Only one of the remaining tested otologic implants has associated deflection forces. This implant, the McGee stapedectomy piston prosthesis composed of platinum and 17 Cr-4 Ni stainless steel, was made on a limited basis during mid-1987 and was recalled by the manufacturer. Patients with this otologic implant were issued warning cards instructing them to not be examined by means of MRI.

Pellets, Bullets, and Shrapnel

Most of the pellets and bullets previously tested for ferromagnetism are composed of nonferromagnetic materials.[186,211] Ammunition found to be ferromagnetic typically came from foreign countries or was used by the military. Shrapnel usually contains various amounts of steel and therefore presents a potential hazard for MRI. Furthermore, because pellets, bullets, and shrapnel may be contaminated with ferromagnetic materials, these objects represent relative contraindications for MRI.

---

*References 91, 96, 110, 153, 170, 184.
†References 7, 13, 29, 41, 46, 84, 89, 153, 156, 164, 176, 181, 183, 186, 190, 197, 198, 210, 211, 244.

Table 14-1   Metallic Implants, Materials, and Foreign Bodies that Are Potential Risks for Patients Undergoing MRI

Aneurysm clips
Drake (DR 14, DR 24), Edward Weck, Triangle Park, New Jersey
Drake (DR 16), Edward Weck
Drake (301 SS), Edward Weck
Downs multipositional (17-7 PH)
Heifetz (17-7 PH), Edward Weck
Housepian
Kapp (405 SS), V. Mueller
Kapp curved (404 SS), V. Mueller
Kapp straight (404 SS), V. Mueller
Mayfield (301 SS), Codman, Randolph, Massachusetts
Mayfield (304 SS), Codman
McFadden (301 SS), Codman
Pivot (17-7PH), V. Mueller
Scoville (EN58J), Downs Surgical, Decatur, Georgia
Sundt-Kees (301-SS), Downs Surgical
Sundt-Kees Multiangle (17-7 PH), Downs Surgical
Vari-angle (17-7 PH), Codman
Vari-angle micro (17-7 PM SS), Codman
Vari-angle spring (17-7 PM SS), Codman

Cartoid artery vascular clamp
Poppen-Blaylock (SS), Codman

Dental devices and materials
Palladium clad magnet, Parkell Products, Farmingdale, New York*
Titanium clad magnet, Parkell Products*
Stainless steel clad magnet, Parkell Products*

Intravascular coils, stents, and filters
Gianturco embolization coil, Cook, Bloomington, Idaho†
Gianturco bird nest IVC filter, Cook†
Gianturco zigzag stent, Cook†
Gunther IVC filter, Cook†

Intravascular coils, stents, and filters—cont'd
New retrievable IVC filter, Thomas Jefferson University, Philadelphia, Pennsylvania†
Palmaz endovascular stent, Ethicon, Sommerville, New Jersey†

Ocular implants
Fatio eyelid spring/wire*
Retinal tack (SS-martensitic), Western European

Otologic implants
Cochlear implant (3M/House)
Cochlear implant (3M/Vienna)
Cochlear implant, Nucleus Mini 22-channel, Cochlear, Englewood, Colorado
McGee piston stapes prothesis (platinum/17Cr-4Ni SS), Richards Medical, Memphis, Tennessee

Pellets, bullets, shrapnel§
BBs, Daisy
BBs, Crosman
Bullet, 7.62 × 39 mm (copper, steel), Norinco
Bullet, 0.380 inch (copper, nickel, lead), Geco
Bullet 0.45 inch (steel, lead), North America Ordinance
Bullet, 9 mm (copper, lead), Norma

Penile implants
Penile implant, OmniPhase, Dacomed Corp., Minneapolis, Minnesota*

Miscellaneous
Cerebral ventricular shunt tube, connector (type unknown)
Swan-Ganz catheter, Thermodilution, American Edwards, Irvine, California‡
Tissue expander with magnetic port, McGhan Medical, Santa Barbara, California*

NOTE: Manufacturer information is provided if indicated in previously published reference or if otherwise known.
SS, Stainless steel.
*The potential for these metallic implants or devices to produce significant injury to the patient is minimal. However, performing MRI in a patient with one of these devices may be uncomfortable for the individual or may result in damage to the implant.
†Ferromagnetic coils, filters, and stents typically become firmly incorporated into the vessel wall several weeks after placement; therefore it is unlikely that they will become dislodged by magnetic forces after a suitable period of approximately 6 to 8 weeks has passed.
‡Although there is no magnetic deflection associated with the Swan-Ganz thermodilution catheter, there has been a report of a catheter "melting" in a patient undergoing MRI. Therefore this catheter is considered contraindicated for MRI.
§The relative risks of performing MRI in patients with pellets, bullets, or shrapnel are related to whether these items are positioned near a vital structure.

Patients with these foreign bodies should be regarded on an individual basis with respect to whether the object is positioned near a vital neural, vascular, or soft tissue structure. This may be assessed by taking a careful history and using plain-film radiography to determine the location of the foreign body.

Penile Implants and Artificial Sphincters

One of the penile implants tested for ferromagnetism displayed significant deflection forces. Although it is unlikely that this implant, the Dacomed Omniphase, would cause serious injury to a patient undergoing MRI, it would undoubtedly be uncomfortable for the patient. Therefore this implant is regarded as a relative contraindication for MRI. Artificial sphincters that have been tested are made from nonferromagnetic materials. However, at least one artificial sphincter currently undergoing clinical trials has a magnetic component; patients with this device should not undergo MRI.

Vascular Access Ports

Of the various vascular access ports tested for ferromagnetism, two showed measurable deflection forces, but the forces were believed to be insignificant relative to the in vivo application of these implants.[190] Therefore it is considered safe to perform MRI for a patient that may have one of these previously tested vascular access ports. The exception to this is any vascular access port that is "programmable" or electronically activated. Patients with this type of vascular access port should not undergo MRI.

Miscellaneous

Various types of other metallic implants, materials, and foreign bodies also have been tested for ferromagnetism. Of these, the cerebral ventricular shunt tube connector (type unknown) and tissue expander that is magnetically activated exhibited deflection forces that may pose a risk to patients during MRI. An "O-ring" washer used as a vascular marker also showed ferromagnetism, but the deflection force was determined to be minimal relative to the in vivo use of this device.

Each of the contraceptive diaphragms tested for ferromagnetism displayed significant deflection forces. However, we have performed MRI on patients with these devices who did not complain of any sensation related to movement of these objects. Therefore scanning patients with diaphragms is not believed to be physically hazardous.

According to the *Policies, Guidelines, and Recommendations for MR Imaging Safety and Patient Management* information issued by the Society for Magnetic Resonance Imaging Safety Committee,[189] patients with electrically, magnetically, or mechanically activated devices, or electrically conductive devices should be excluded from MRI unless the particular device has been previously shown (i.e., usually by ex vivo testing procedures) to be unaffected by the electromagnetic fields used for clinical MRI and there is no possibility of injuring the patient. During the screening process for MRI, patients with these objects should be identified before their examination and before being exposed to the electromagnetic fields used for this imaging technique. There are implants, materials, devices, or other foreign bodies that have yet to be evaluated for MRI compatibility that may be encountered in the clinical setting. Patients with untested objects should not be allowed to undergo MRI.

SCREENING PATIENTS FOR METALLIC FOREIGN BODIES

Patients undergoing MRI may have a history of metallic foreign bodies, such as slivers, bullets, shrapnel, or other types of metallic fragments. The relative risk of scanning these patients depends on the ferromagnetic properties of the object, the geometry and dimensions of the object, and the strength of the static and gradient magnetic fields of the MR system. Also important is the strength with which the object is fixed within the tissue and whether it is positioned in or adjacent to a potentially hazardous site of the body, such as a vital neural, vascular, or soft tissue structure.

A patient who encounters the static magnetic field of an MR system with an intraocular metallic foreign body is at a particular risk for significant eye injury. The single reported case of a vitreous hemorrhage resulting in blindness occurred in a patient who underwent MRI on a 0.35 T scanner and who had an occult intraocular metal fragment that was 2 × 3.5 mm dislodge during the procedure.[100] This incident emphasizes the importance of adequately screening patients with suspected intraocular metallic foreign bodies before MRI.

Research has demonstrated that intraocular metallic fragments as small as 0.1 × 0.1 × 0.1 mm are detectable on standard plain-film radiographs.[239] Although thin-slice (i.e., ≤ 3 mm) computed tomography (CT) has been demonstrated to show metallic foreign bodies down to approximately 0.15 mm, it is unlikely that a metallic fragment of this size would be dislodged during MRI, even with a static magnetic field of up to 2 T.[239] Metallic fragments of various sizes and dimensions—ranging from 0.1 × 0.1 × 0.1 mm to 3 × 1 × 1 mm—have been examined to determine whether they were moved or dislodged from the eyes of laboratory animals during exposure to a 2 T MRI system.[239] Only the largest fragment (3 × 1 × 1 mm) rotated, but it did not cause any discernible damage to the ocular tissue.[239] Therefore the use of plain-film radiography may be an acceptable technique for identifying or excluding an intraocular metallic foreign body that represents a potential hazard to the patient undergoing MRI.[189] Patients for whom there is a high suspicion of an intraocular metallic foreign body (e.g., a metal worker exposed to metallic slivers and who has a history of an eye injury) should have plain-film radiographs of the orbits to rule out the presence of a metallic fragment before exposure to the static magnetic field. If a patient with a suspected ferromagnetic intraocular foreign body has no symptoms and a plain-film series of the orbits does not demonstrate a radiopaque foreign body, the risk in performing MRI is minimal.[189]

Using plain-film radiography to search for metallic foreign bodies is a sensitive and relatively inexpensive means of identifying patients who are unsuitable for MRI; it also may be used to screen patients who may have metal fragments in other potentially hazardous sites of the body.

Each MRI site should establish a standard policy for screening patients with suspected foreign bodies. This policy should include guidelines as to which patients require workup by plain-film radiographic procedures and the specific procedure to be performed (i.e., number and type of views, the position of the anatomy); each case should be considered individually. These precautions should be taken with regard to patients referred for MRI in any type of MR system, regardless of the field strength, magnet type, and the presence or absence of magnetic shielding.[189]

PERFORMING MAGNETIC RESONANCE IMAGING ON PREGNANT PATIENTS

MRI is not believed to be hazardous to the fetus, even though few investigations have examined its teratogenic potential (see Chapter 31). By comparison, thousands of studies have examined the possible hazards of ultrasound during pregnancy, and controversy still exists concerning the safe use of this nonionizing-radiation imaging technique.

Most of the earliest studies conducted to determine possible unwanted biological effects of MRI during pregnancy showed negative results.* More recently, one study examined the effects of MRI on mice exposed during midgestation. No gross embryotoxic effects were observed; however, there was a reduction in crown-rump length.[82] In another study, performed by Tyndall and Sulik,[222] exposure to the electromagnetic fields used for a simulated clinical MRI examination caused eye malformations in a genetically prone mouse strain. Therefore it appears that the electromagnetic fields used for MRI have the potential to produce developmental abnormalities.

A variety of mechanisms could produce deleterious biological effects with respect to the developing fetus and the use of electromagnetic fields during MRI.* In addition, it is well known that cells undergoing division, as in the case of the developing fetus during the first trimester, are highly susceptible to damage from different types of physical agents. Therefore, because of the limited data available at present, a cautionary approach is recommended for the use of MRI on pregnant patients.

In the United States the FDA requires the labeling of MRI devices to indicate that the safety of MRI when used to image the fetus and the infant "has not been established."[113] In Great Britain the acceptable limits of exposure for clinical MRI recommended by the National Radiological Protection Board in 1983 specify that "it might be prudent to exclude pregnant women during the first three months of pregnancy."[113]

According to the Safety Committee of the Society for Magnetic Resonance Imaging (this information also has been adopted recently by the American College of Radiology), MRI is indicated for use in pregnant women if other nonionizing forms of diagnostic imaging are inadequate or if the examination provides important information that would otherwise require exposure to ionizing radiation (i.e., x-ray, CT).[189] For pregnant patients, it is recommended to inform them that, to date, there has been no indication that the use of clinical MRI during pregnancy has produced deleterious effects. However, as noted by the FDA, the safety of MRI during pregnancy has not been proved.[52]

Patients who are pregnant or suspect they are pregnant must be identified to assess the risks versus the benefits of the MR examination. Because there is a high spontaneous abortion rate in the general population during the first trimester of pregnancy (>30%), particular care should be exercised with the use of MRI during the first trimester because of associated potential medicolegal implications.

MAGNETIC RESONANCE IMAGING AND CLAUSTROPHOBIA, ANXIETY, AND PANIC DISORDERS

Claustrophobia and a variety of other psychological reactions, including anxiety and panic disorders, may be encountered by as many as 5% to 10% of patients undergoing MRI. These sensations originate from several factors, including the restrictive dimensions of the interior of the scanner, the duration of the examination, the gradient-induced noises, and the ambient conditions within the bore of the scanner.†

Adverse psychological responses to MRI are usually transient. However, there was a report of two patients with no history of claustrophobia who tolerated MRI with great difficulty and had persistent claustrophobia that required long-term psychiatric treatment.[55] Because adverse psychological responses to MRI typically delay or even cause cancellation of the examination, several techniques have been developed to avert these problems.‡ These techniques include the following:

1. Brief the patient on the specific aspects of the MR examination, including the level of gradient-induced noise to expect, the internal dimensions of the scanner, and the length of the examination.
2. Allow an appropriately screened relative or friend to remain with the patient during the procedure.
3. Give the patient headphones with calming music to decrease the repetitive noise created by the gradient coils.
4. Maintain physical or verbal contact with the patient throughout the examination.
5. Place the patient in a prone position with the chin supported by a pillow. In this position the patient is able to visualize the opening of the bore and thus alleviate the "closed-in" feeling. An alternative method to reduce claustrophobia is to place the subject feet-first instead of head-first into the scanner.

---

6. Use scanner-mounted mirrors or prism glasses within the scanner to allow the patient to see out of the scanner.
7. Use a large light at either end of the scanner to decrease the patient's anxiety about being in a long, dark enclosure.
8. Use a blindfold on the patient so that he or she is unaware of the close surroundings.
9. Use relaxation techniques, such as controlled breathing and mental imagery.[113] Several case reports have shown hypnotherapy to be successful in reducing MRI-related claustrophobia and anxiety.
10. Use psychological "desensitization" techniques before the MR examination.

Recently, several investigators have attempted to compare the effectiveness of some of the aforementioned techniques in reducing MRI-induced anxiety or claustrophobia.[103,154,155] One study demonstrated that providing detailed information about the MRI procedure, in addition to "relaxation exercises," successfully reduced the anxiety level of a group of patients both before and during MRI. A similar anxiety reduction could not be shown in patients provided with only information or "stress reduction" counseling. Relaxation methods have also been shown to significantly decrease anxiety during other medical procedures. Certain MR-system architectures employing a vertical magnetic field offer a more open design that might reduce the frequency of psychological problems associated with MRI procedures.

MONITORING PHYSIOLOGICAL PARAMETERS DURING MAGNETIC RESONANCE IMAGING

Because the typical MR system is constructed such that the patient is placed inside a cylindrical structure, routine observation and vital signs monitoring is not a trivial task. Conventional monitoring equipment was not designed to operate in the MRI environment, where static, gradient, and RF electromagnetic fields can adversely affect the operation of these devices. Fortunately, MR-compatible monitors have been developed and are commonly used in MRI centers.*

Physiological monitoring is required for the safe use of MRI in patients who are sedated, anesthetized, comatose, critically ill, or otherwise unable to communicate with the MR-system operator. All such patients should be routinely monitored during MRI, and considering the current availability of MR-compatible monitors, there is no reason to exclude these types of patients from MRI. Every physiological parameter that can be obtained under normal circumstances in the intensive care unit or operating room can be monitored during MRI, including heart rate, skin blood flow, temperature, respiratory rate, systemic blood pressure, intracardiac pressure, oxygen saturation, and end-tidal carbon dioxide.† Table 14-2 lists examples of MR-compatible monitors that have been successfully tested and operated at field strengths of up to 1.5 T. In addition, there are now MR-compatible ventilators for patients who require ventilatory support.

Monitors that contain ferromagnetic components (i.e., transformers, outer casings) can be strongly attracted by mid- and high-field MR systems, posing a serious hazard to patients and possible damage to the MR system. Because the intensity of the standard static magnetic field falls off as the third power of the distance from the magnet, simply placing the monitor a suitable distance from the MR system is sufficient to protect the operation of the device and to help prevent it from becoming a potential projectile.[83,175] If monitoring equipment is not placed in a permanently fixed position, instructions should be given to all appropriate personnel regarding the hazards of moving this equipment too close to the MR system.[83,175]

In addition to being influenced by the static magnetic field, monitors may be adversely affected by electromagnetic interference from the gradient and RF pulses from the MR system.[83,175] In these instances, increasing the length of the patient-monitor interface and positioning the equipment outside the RF-shielded room (e.g., the control room) will enable the monitor to operate properly. It is usually necessary to position all monitors with cathode ray tubes at a location in the magnetic fringe field so that the display is not "bent" or distorted.

Certain monitors emit spurious electromagnetic noise that can result in moderate to severe imaging artifacts.[83,175] These monitors can be

*References 10, 47, 83, 97, 112, 175, 179, 237.
†References 47, 83, 97, 112, 175, 179, 237.

Table 14-2   Examples of MRI-Compatible Monitors and Ventilators*

DEVICE AND MANUFACTURER	FUNCTION
MRI Fiberoptic Pulse Oximeter Nonin Medical Inc. Plymouth, Minnesota	Oxygen saturation, heart rate
MR-Compatible Pulse Oximeter Patient Monitoring System Magnetic Resonance Equipment Corp. Bay Shore, New York	Oxygen saturation, heart rate
MR-Compatible Pulse Oximeter In Vivo Research, Inc. Orlando, Florida	Oxygen saturation, heart rate
Omega 1400 In Vivo Research, Inc. Orlando, Florida	Blood pressure, heart rate
Omni-Trak 3100 MRI Vital Signs Monitor In Vivo Research, Inc. Orlando, Florida	Heart rate, ECG, oxygen saturation, respiratory rate, blood pressure
Laserflow Blood Perfusion Monitor Vasomed, Inc. St. Paul, Minnesota	Cutaneous blood flow
Medpacific LD 500 Laser-Doppler Perfusion Monitor Medpacific Corporation Seattle, Washington	Cutaneous blood flow
Respiratory Rate Monitor, Models 515 and 525 Biochem International Waukesha, Wisconsin	Respiratory rate, apnea
MicroSpan Capnometer 8800 Biochem International Waukesha, Wisconsin	Respiratory rate, end-tidal carbon dioxide, apnea
Aneuroid Chest Bellows Coulborun Instruments Allentown, Pennsylvania	Respiratory rate
Datex CO_2 Monitor Puritan-Bennett Corporation Los Angeles, California	% Carbon dioxide
Wenger Precordial Stethoscope Anesthesia Medical Supplies Santa Fe Springs, California	Heart sounds
Fluoroptic Thermometry System, Model 3000 Luxtron Santa Clara, California	Temperature
Omni-Vent, Series D Columbia Medical Marketing Topeka, Kansas	Ventilator
Ventilator, Models 225 and 2500 Monaghan Medical Corporation Plattsburgh, Pennsylvania	Ventilator
Anesthesia Ventilator Ohio Medical Madison, Wisconsin	Ventilator
Infant Ventilator MVP-10 Bio-Med Devices, Inc. Madison, Connecticut	Ventilator
Siemens-Elema Model 900C Iselin, New Jersey	Ventilator

Modified in part from Shellock FG, and Kanal E: Magnetic resonance: bioeffects, safety, and patient management, ed 2 New York, 1996, Lippincott-Raven.
*Devices may require modifications to make them MR compatible. None should be positioned closer than 8 feet from the entrance of the bore of a 1.5 T MR system. Also, monitors with metallic cables, leads, or probes may cause mild to moderate imaging artifacts if placed near the imaging area of interest. Consult manufacturers to determine compatibility with specific MR systems.

modified to work during MRI by adding RF-shielded cables, using fiberoptic transmission of the signals (increasingly the method of choice in the MRI environment), or using special outer casing. In addition, special filters may be added to the monitor to inhibit electromagnetic noise.

Some monitoring equipment can be potentially harmful to patients if special precautions are not followed.[83,93,95,175,199] A primary source of adverse interactions between MR systems and physiological monitors has been the interface used between the patient and the equipment because this usually requires a conductive cable or other device. The presence of a conductive material in the immediate MR-system area is a safety concern because of the potential for monitor-related burns. For example, there was a report of an accident involving an anesthetized patient who sustained a third-degree burn of the finger associated with the use of a pulse oximeter during MRI.[199] Investigation of this incident revealed that the cable leading from the pulse oximeter to the finger probe may have been looped during MRI and the gradient or RF magnetic fields induced sufficient current to exorbitantly heat the finger probe, resulting in the finger burn.[199] This problem also may occur with the use of ECG lead wires or any other cable that may be looped or may form a conductive loop that contacts the patient.

Therefore the following precautions are recommended to prevent potential monitor-related accidents:

1. Monitoring equipment should be used only by trained personnel.
2. All cables and lead wires from monitoring devices that come into contact with the patient (e.g., the monitor-patient interface) should be positioned so that no conductive loops are formed.
3. Monitoring devices that do not appear to operate properly during MRI should be immediately removed from the patient and the magnetic environment.

The following is a brief description of some of the techniques of monitoring various physiological parameters.

Monitoring Blood Pressure

Noninvasive blood-pressure monitors typically use the oscillometric technique for measuring blood pressure, using a pressure transducer connected to a pressure cuff via a pneumatically filled hose. Certain monitors (e.g., Omega 1400, In-vivo Research Laboratories Inc., Broken Arrow, Oklahoma) have adjustable audible and visual alarms as well as a strip-chart recorder.

Occasionally the cuff inflation tends to disturb lightly sedated patients, especially pediatric patients, which may cause them to move and distort the MR image. For this reason the noninvasive blood-pressure monitor may not represent the optimal instrument for obtaining vital signs in all patient groups. Direct pressure monitoring of systemic or intracardiac pressures, if necessary, can be accomplished using a fiberoptic pressure transducer made entirely of plastic.

Monitoring Respiratory Rate, Oxygenation, and Gas Exchange

The monitoring of respiratory parameters during MRI of sedated or anesthetized patients is particularly important because the medications used for these procedures may produce complications of respiratory depression. Therefore as a standard of care, a pulse oximeter, capnograph, or capnometer should always be used to monitor patients who are sedated or anesthetized during MRI.

The respiratory monitors used successfully on sedated pediatric or adult patients (e.g., the model 515 Respiration Monitor and model 8800 Capnometer, Biochem International, Waukesha, Wisconsin) are relatively inexpensive and can be modified for use during MRI by simply lengthening the plastic tubing interface to the patient so that the monitors can be placed at least 8 feet from the unshielded MR imager.

Pulse oximeters are used to record oxygen saturation and heart rate. Commercially available, modified pulse oximeters that use hard wire cables have been used previously with moderate success to monitor sedated and anesthetized patients during the MRI study and the recovery period. These pulse oximeters tend to work intermittently during MRI as a result of interference from the gradient or RF electromagnetic fields. In certain instances, patients have been burned, presumably as a result of excessive current being induced in inappropriately looped conductive cables attached to the patient probes of the pulse oximeters.[93,95,199]

Portable fiberoptic pulse oximeters are now available for use during MR procedures.[191] The use of fiberoptic technology to obtain and transmit physiological signals from patients undergoing MRI has been demonstrated to have no associated MRI-related electromagnetic interference. It is physically impossible for a patient to be burned if a fiberoptic monitor is used during MRI because there are no conductive pathways formed by any metallic materials.

Monitoring Cutaneous Blood Flow

Cutaneous blood flow can be monitored during MRI by means of the laser-Doppler velocimetry technique. This noninvasive measurement technique uses laser light that is delivered to and detected from the region of interest by flexible, graded-index fiberoptic light wires. The Doppler-broadening of laser light scattered by the red blood cells moving within the tissue is analyzed in real time by an analogue processor that is indicative of instantaneous blood velocity and the effective blood volume and flow. A small circular probe can be attached to any available skin surface of the patient. Areas with a relatively high cutaneous blood flow (such as the toe, ear, foot, hand, or finger) yield the best results.

Hard-copy tracings obtained by laser-Doppler velocimetry can be used to determine the patient's heart rate, respiratory rate, and cutaneous blood flow. An audible signal may be activated to permit the operator to hear blood flow changes during monitoring. Because it is easily tolerated, this technique of continuous physiological monitoring is particularly useful when there is concern about disturbing a sedated patient.

Monitoring Heart Rate

The monitoring of the ECG during MRI is typically required for cardiac imaging, gating to reduce imaging artifacts from the physiological motion of cerebrospinal fluid in the brain and spine, and determining the patient's heart rate. Artifacts caused by the static, gradient, and RF electromagnetic fields may severely distort the morphology of the ECG, making determination of cardiac rhythm during MRI extremely difficult and unreliable. Although sophisticated filtering techniques can be used to attenuate the artifacts from the gradient and RF fields, the static magnetic field produces an augmentation of the T wave, as previously mentioned, and other nonspecific waveform changes that are in direct proportion to the strength of the field, which cannot be easily counterbalanced.

In some instances, static magnetic field–induced augmented T waves have a higher amplitude than the R waves, resulting in false triggering and an inaccurate determination of the beats per minute. ECG artifacts can be minimized during MRI by using special filters, using ECG electrodes with minimal metal, selecting lead wires with minimal metal, twisting or braiding the lead wires, and using special lead placements.[237]

The previously mentioned pulse oximeters also may be used to accurately record heart rate during MR examinations. These devices have probes that may be attached to the finger, toe, or earlobe of the patient.

CONTRAST MEDIA: SAFETY CONSIDERATIONS

Throughout the United States, roughly one third of all MR studies use contrast agents. Therefore familiarity with the safety aspects of using these medications that are so ubiquitous in the clinical MR environment is important.[77,134,167]

The three MRI contrast agents approved for intravenous administration by the FDA are gadopentetate dimeglumine injection (Magnevist, Berlex Laboratories, Wayne, New Jersey), gadodiamide injection (Omniscan, Sanofi-Winthrop Pharmaceuticals, New York; Nycomed Salutar, Oslo, Norway), and gadoteridol injection (ProHance, Squibb Diagnostics, Princeton, New Jersey). There is another agent approved internationally, gadoterate meglumine, Gd-DOTA (Dotarem, Guebet Laboratories, Aulnay-sous-Bois, France).

All these contrast agents are based on the element gadolinium and have similar mechanisms of action, biodistribution, and half-lives.[77,134,219,220] Drug equilibration and physiological biodistribution for each of the MRI contrast agents is in the extracellular fluid space, with biological elimination half-lives of roughly 1½ hours.[134]

Gadolinium-based MRI contrast agents are paramagnetic substances and therefore develop a magnetic moment when placed in a magnetic field. The relatively large magnetic moment produced by a paramagnetic agent results in a relatively large local magnetic field that can enhance the relaxation rates of water protons in the vicinity of the MRI contrast agent. When placed in a magnetic field, gadolinium-based MRI contrast agents decrease the T1 and T2 relaxation times in tissues where it accumulates (although the T1 relaxation time is mainly affected at the dosages used in the clinical setting) with the purpose of improving image contrast between two adjacent tissue compartments, thus producing a more conspicuous abnormality, if one exists.[134]

Free gadolinium ion is rather toxic, with a markedly prolonged biological half-life of several weeks. The predominant uptake and excretion of gadolinium are by the kidneys and liver. However, gadolinium ion is chelated to another structure that restricts the ion, which markedly decreases its toxicity and alters its pharmacokinetics.[134] This chelation also decreases the ability of the gadolinium ion to accomplish its task of T1 shortening. The science of MRI contrast agent design and development is often a tricky act of walking the tightrope between decreasing toxicity while not overly decreasing the T1 relaxivity.

As noted, the chelating process also alters the pharmacokinetics of the agent. For example, chelating the gadolinium ions allows for approximately a 500-fold increase in the rate of renal excretion of the substance.[32,36] In each case the chelating substance is what makes these various MRI contrast agents differ from one another.

In the case of Magnevist the chelating agent is the diethylene-tri-amine-pentaacetic acid (DTPA) molecule. For Omniscan, it is DTPA-BMA, and in ProHance it is the HP-DO3A molecule. Magnevist has a linear structure and is an ionic compound; Omniscan has a linear structure and is nonionic; ProHance is also nonionic and possesses a macrocyclical ring structure. Despite the marked differences in these chelating molecules, their ionic versus nonionic nature, and their linear versus ringlike molecular structure, these agents appear to have remarkably similar effectiveness and safety profiles. Some differences exist—both theoretically and on paper—and it is these differences that we will elaborate.

Multiple studies have documented the high safety index of MRI contrast agents, especially when compared with the iodinated contrast media used for CT.* However, from a safety profile standpoint, it is inappropriate to compare ionic and nonionic MRI contrast agents to ionic and nonionic CT contrast agents because of the drastically different osmotic loads associated with each of these drugs.

The median lethal dose (LD_{50})—the term used to denote the dose of an agent that, when administered, results in death of half of the population of recipients—of these agents, as studied in rodents, is quite high, being the highest for Omniscan (>30 mmol/kg), next highest for ProHance (12 mmol/kg), and the lowest for Magnevist (6 to 7 mmol/kg). In all cases the LD_{50} is generally in excess of roughly 300, 120, and 60 times the typical diagnostic dose of 0.1 mmol/kg, respectively.[134,233] There are also data to suggest that fewer acute cardiodepressive effects result from the nonionic drugs (specifically, ProHance was used in one study) than the ionic agent Magnevist when injected rapidly and into a central vein.[122] This finding may have limited clinical applicability, however, because MRI contrast agents are typically injected into peripheral veins, with only small total volumes being administered.[134]

Adverse Events Related to the Use of Magnetic Resonance Imaging Contrast Agents

The total incidence of adverse reactions of all types for each of the MRI contrast agents ranges from approximately 2% to 4%.[77,106,115] The most common reactions are hives, headaches, nausea, emesis, and local injection site symptoms, such as irritation, focal burning, or a cool sensation. With the use of Magnevist, transient elevations have also been reported in serum bilirubin levels (3% to 4% of patients), and with both Magnevist and Omniscan a transient elevation in iron (15% to 30% of patients) that seems to spontaneously reverse within 24 to 48 hours has been noted.[77,128] No such alterations in blood chemistry have been reported with the use of ProHance. There are no known contraindications for Magnevist, Omniscan, and ProHance.

The MRI contrast agent that has had FDA approval the longest, and thus the one for which there is the most clinical experience and infor-

mation, is Magnevist. There have been approximately 5.7 million doses administered worldwide since its approval in June 1988. This compares with the approximately 150,000 total administered doses for ProHance since its FDA approval in November 1992 and the approximately 100,000 doses for Omniscan since its FDA approval in January 1993. There have been rare reported incidents of laryngospasm or anaphylactoid reactions (necessitating interventional therapy with, for example, epinephrine) associated with the administration of each of these agents.*

In consideration of the above, it may be advisable to continue a prolonged observation period of all patients with a history of allergy or drug reaction. As stated in the package insert for Magnevist, for example:

> The possibility of a reaction, including serious, fatal, anaphylactoid, or cardiovascular reactions or other idiosyncratic reactions should always be considered especially in those with a known clinical history of asthma or other allergic respiratory disorders.

Delayed reactions of hypertension, vasovagal responses, and syncope also have been reported with the use of MRI contrast agents. Accordingly the product inserts for these drugs advise that all patients should be observed for several hours after drug administration.

Specific Adverse Events

The specific adverse events associated with the use of MRI contrast agents vary to a minor degree.† The majority of these adverse events occur at an incidence of less than 1%. Before proceeding, it might be helpful to clarify some commonly used and misused terminology pertaining to adverse events that occur with medications. An anaphylactoid reaction involves respiratory, cardiovascular, cutaneous, and possibly gastrointestinal or genitourinary manifestations.[6] This is not to say that all events in which such symptoms are involved are by definition anaphylactoid. However, it does become more difficult to make the diagnosis of anaphylaxis in the absence of such symptoms, especially the classic triad of upper airway obstructive symptomatology, decreased blood pressure (or other similar severe cardiovascular symptoms), and cutaneous manifestations, such as urticaria.

As defined by the FDA, a "serious reaction" is one in which an adverse experience from a drug proves fatal or life-threatening, is permanently disabling, necessitates in-patient hospitalization, or is an overdose.[51] A "life-threatening reaction" in FDA terminology is one wherein the initial reporter (i.e., the individual initially reporting the incident) believes that the patient was at immediate risk of death from the event. In consideration of these definitions, one may now understand how the interpretation of an adverse event may differ from that designated by the FDA.

Magnevist. As of June 1993, there have been 13 anaphylactoid reactions with Magnevist, for an estimated anaphylactoid reaction rate of 1:450,000.[61] One of the patients who had an anaphylactoid reaction died, and another patient suffered brain damage (at the time of this writing the patient is still in a coma) subsequent to administration of Magnevist. In each case there was a history of respiratory difficulty or allergic respiratory problem, such as asthma. As mentioned, the current package insert for Magnevist warns that caution should be exercised when administering this contrast agent to patients with known allergic respiratory disease.

The total reported incidence of adverse reactions of any kind to Magnevist is 2.4%, based on a retrospective review of 15,496 patients.[62] Of these cases only two reactions were labeled "serious" by FDA standards. In one of these cases a patient being evaluated for metastatic disease died of herniation from an intracranial tumor within 24 hours of the contrast-enhanced MR study. Because of the design of the present review process, this temporal association is sufficient to have the case reported as being "associated" with Magnevist administration, irrespective of any perceived or real causal relationship. The second serious reaction in this series of patients occurred in an individual who was undergoing evaluation for vertigo and had an acute progression of vertigo after administration of Magnevist. Seizures after administration of this drug have been reported.[76] In at least one case Magnevist injection was

---

*References 8, 16, 24, 34, 42, 53, 64, 74, 77, 98, 114, 115, 129, 130, 133, 168, 202, 206.

*References 35, 106, 128, 136, 158, 172, 188, 208, 209, 218, 236.
†References 6, 35, 37, 76, 94, 106, 111, 128, 136, 172, 188, 208, 209, 218, 236.

believed to induce a seizure in a patient with a history of grand mal seizures (see product insert information for Magnevist).

There are mild elevations in serum chemistries associated with the use of Magnevist that suggest that there may be a component of mild hemolysis associated in some unknown manner with the use of this drug. However, this association is not definite and there is no evidence demonstrating increased hemolysis as a result of Magnevist being administered to patients with hemolytic anemias.

The FDA has expressed concern via the package insert regarding the use of Magnevist, as well as the other gadolinium-based agents, in patients with sickle cell anemia. According to the package-insert information for MRI contrast agents, the enhancement of magnetic moment by Magnevist, Omniscan, or ProHance may possibly potentiate sickle erythrocyte alignment. This information was based on in vitro studies that showed that deoxygenated sickle erythrocytes align perpendicular to a magnetic field, and therefore vasoocclusive complications may result in vivo. However, no studies have assessed the effect of the use of these MRI contrast agents in patients with sickle cell anemia and other forms of hemoglobinopathies. In addition, there has been no report of sickle crisis precipitated by the administration of any of these drugs.

Of the three MRI contrast agents, Magnevist has the highest of the osmolaties, measuring 1960 mmol/kg of water, or roughly 6 to 7 times that of plasma (approximately 285 mmol/kg of water).[229] Doses greater than or equal to double that used in the United States (i.e., doses of up to 0.3 mmol/kg) have already been investigated in the clinical setting[78,128,131,132] and have been used for quite some time in Europe, with no apparent significant deleterious effects.[108]

In that the osmolality of Magnevist is 6 to 7 times the osmolality of plasma, one might expect local irritative reactions as a possible adverse response with the use of this relatively hyperosmolar substance. Indeed, there has been at least one incident of possible phlebitis necessitating hospitalization that was related temporally to the administration of an intravenous dose of Magnevist.[105] The mechanism(s) behind this are still unclear, although objective studies have demonstrated that tissue sloughing can occur as a result of extravasation of gadolinium-dimeglumine.[37,111]

There also have been several cases of erythema, swelling, and pain localized to the site of administration and proximally that were of delayed onset, typically appearing between 1 to 4 days after the intravenous administration of the gadolinium-DTPA. This typically progressed for several days, plateaued, and then resolved over several more days.[94] Nevertheless, severe adverse local reactions to even considerable quantities (>10 ml) of Magnevist extravasation seem to be quite rare, at best.

Magnevist is the only one of the three MRI contrast agents approved for use in the United States that has a package insert that recommends a slow, intravenous administration, at a rate not to exceed 10 ml/min. The FDA has approved rapid bolus intravenous administration of Omniscan and ProHance. Nevertheless, studies performed with rapid intravenous administration of Magnevist have indicated that there is no significant difference in the incidence of adverse effects compared with the slow, intravenous administration of this drug.[94,98,128]

Omniscan. Because Omniscan is the most recently FDA-approved MRI contrast agent, there are relatively little data available related to the safety aspects of this drug. Of the estimated 100,000 doses that have been distributed, there have been 28 reports of adverse reactions of any type, of which 20 were nausea and emesis. There was a single case of laryngospasm that was successfully treated with epinephrine, and a single case of a patient who had a seizure after receiving Omniscan. This patient had a history of seizure disorder. There have been no reports of patient hospitalizations or permanent disabilities related to the use of Omniscan.[159]

Omniscan has an osmolality value of 789 mmol/kg of water.[229] The manufacturer of Omniscan is in the process of applying for approval of higher total-dose administration for specified entities where this might be of clinical significance and benefit.[158]

ProHance. ProHance was approved for use 2 months before the release of Omniscan; therefore there is also a relative lack of postmarket safety data concerning this MRI contrast agent. Of the estimated 150,000 doses administered, there have been no deaths associated with the use of ProHance. Ten anaphylactoid reactions have occurred in association with the use of this MRI contrast agent, of which five caused hospitalization or ended in permanent disabilities.[163]

At this time, ProHance is the only MRI contrast agent with FDA approval to be administered for specific clinical indications up to a total dose of 0.3 mmol/kg, or a total of 3 times the standard dose for each of the other two FDA-approved MRI contrast agents. The relatively low 630 mmol/kg of water osmolality of ProHance may be one of the major factors that permits use of higher doses of this MRI contrast agent to be used without significant deleterious effects on the patient.[145] However, this is speculation. Here, too, total adverse effects of any type seem to total less than 4%, with nausea and taste disturbance each having an incidence of roughly 1.4% and all other adverse reactions being less than 1% each.[135]

The lower osmolality of ProHance compared with Magnevist was the subject of an investigation into the effect of extravasation of this agent versus that of Magnevist in the rat model.[138] The findings indicated that extravasation of Magnevist was associated with more necrosis, hemorrhage, and edema compared with ProHance, although the authors of this report cautioned about extrapolating the results of their study to contrast agent extravasation in human subjects.

Administration of Magnetic Resonance Imaging Contrast Agents to Patients with Renal Failure

As noted, toxicity may result from the dissociation of the gadolinium ion from its chelate. After intravenous administration of gadolinium-based contrast agents, intravascular copper and zinc (normally found in small amounts within the bloodstream), which have a competing affinity for the DTPA chelate, will displace some of the gadolinium from the chelating molecule, such as DTPA, which will be released as free gadolinium ion (Gd^{+3}). Although gadolinium is a highly toxic substance, the total concentration of the released free gadolinium is very low and is cleared rapidly, allowing for a low concentration of free ion to be maintained. In patients with normal renal function, the rate of dissociation is slower than that of clearance, thus preventing any accumulation phenomenon from occurring.[32] It is also believed that the macrocyclical molecules tend to bind the gadolinium more tightly than do the linear ones.[219,231]

As new physiological sources of copper and zinc ions are "leaked" into the intravascular space in an attempt to reestablish their concentration equilibrium, they also displace more gadolinium from its chelate. This cycle continues until all the gadolinium chelate is cleared from the body via the kidney by glomerular filtration. For this reason there is a potential concern for the level of free gadolinium ion in cases of renal failure, as there is in patients with a decreased rate of renal clearance of all such substances from the body.

The safety of administering MRI contrast agents to patients with impaired renal function or even overt renal failure has not been clearly established, although several studies suggest that it should be well tolerated.* Although there is a theoretical concern that decreasing the rate of clearance of the gadolinium chelate from the body might serve to increase the concentration of free gadolinium within the body, data suggest that, for a given level of renal function, administration of lower-volume doses may be safer than administering standard doses of iodine-based contrast agents to that same patient.[80] Similarly the safety of administering one of the MRI contrast agents to patients with elevated levels of copper (such as patients with Wilson's disease) or zinc has not been firmly established and will likely depend on factors such as the glomerular filtration rate and renal clearance rates, as well as the blood copper levels, of those patients.[32] It has also been shown that Magnevist is dialyzable, with more than 95% of the administered dose being removed by the third dialysis treatment.[102,165]

Chronic and Repeated Administration of Magnetic Resonance Imaging Contrast Agents

There is concern related to the total storage or accumulation of the MRI contrast agents, or even free gadolinium ion, after multiple doses are administered throughout a patient's lifetime. The amount of detectable

---

*References 57, 79, 80, 128, 130, 169.

drug still in the liver, kidneys, and bone days after administration seems to be higher in the case of Omniscan than for Magnevist,[77] and these both seem to be higher than the level for ProHance.[219,231] Currently there are no data available regarding the safety of long-term cumulative exposure to low doses of free gadolinium ion. Therefore there may be a clinical limitation regarding the number of times a patient is scanned safely with gadolinium-based contrast drugs. As of now, however, this question remains unanswered and warrants investigation.

Use of Magnetic Resonance Imaging Contrast Agents During Pregnancy and Lactation

Magnevist has been shown to cross the placenta and appear within the fetal bladder only moments after intravenous administration. It is assumed that the other MRI contrast agents behave in a similar fashion and cross the blood-placental barrier easily. From the fetal bladder, these contrast agents would then be excreted into the amniotic fluid and subsequently swallowed by the fetus. This fluid will then be filtered and excreted in the urine of the fetus, with the entire cycle being repeated innumerable times.

There are no data available to assess the rate of clearance of MRI contrast agents from the amniotic fluid cycle. Therefore it is our opinion that there is no information to support the safety of using MRI contrast agents in pregnant women. Our conservative approach is to recommend against the administration of any of the MRI contrast agents to a pregnant patient until more data become available. Pregnant patients should receive these drugs only if the potential benefit justifies the potential risk to the fetus. In any case, should it be decided to administer MRI contrast agents to pregnant patients to facilitate MRI, the patient should be provided written informed consent that stipulates specifically that the risk associated with the use of these drugs during pregnancy is presently unknown.

Magnevist has been shown to be excreted in very low concentrations (i.e., 0.011% of the total dose) in human breast milk over approximately 33 hours.[162,173] The concentration of this contrast agent in breast milk peaks at approximately 4.75 hours and decreases to less than a fifth of this level (down to <1 μmol/L) 22 hours after the injection.[162,173] For this reason and as an extra precaution, we recommend that nursing mothers express their breast milk and not breast-feed for 36 to 48 hours after the administration of an MRI contrast agent to ensure that the child does not receive the drug in any notable quantity by mouth. However, it should be noted that the LD_{50} of gadolinium chloride or gadolinium acetate (which easily release free gadolinium ions) when given intravenously is approximately 1000 times lower if taken orally because of the very low absorption of gadolinium from the gastrointestinal tract.[125] This finding supports other data that have demonstrated that 99.2% of orally administered Magnevist was fecally excreted and not absorbed.[232]

SAFETY UPDATE

For further up-to-date information regarding the continually changing issues involved in MR safety considerations, the reader is referrred to the MR Safety Central Web Site that can be found at http://kanal.arad.upmc.edu/mrsafety.html.

REFERENCES

1. Abdullakhozhaeva MS, and Razykov SR: Structural changes in central nervous system under the influence of a permanent magnetic field, Bull Exper Biol Med 102:1585, 1986.
2. Adey WR: Tissue interactions with nonionizing electromagnetic fields, Physiol Rev 61:435, 1981.
3. Adzamli IK, Jolesz FA, and Blau M: An assessment of blood-brain barrier integrity under MRI conditions: brain uptake of radiolabeled Gd-DTPA and In-DTPA-IgG, Nucl Med 30:839, 1989.
4. Aisen A: Personal communication, May 1989.
5. Alagona P, Toole JC, Maniscalco BS, et al: Nuclear magnetic resonance imaging in a patient with a DDD pacemaker, Pacing Clin Electrophysiol 12:619, 1989.
6. American College of Radiology: Manual on iodinated contrast media, 1991.
7. Augustiny N, von Schulthess GK, Meier D, et al: MR imaging of large nonferromagnetic metallic implants at 1.5 T, J Comput Assist Tomogr 11:678, 1987.
8. Ball WJ, Nadel S, Zimmerman R, et al: Phase III multicenter clinical investigation to determine the safety and efficacy of gadoteridol in children suspected of having neurologic disease, Radiology 168:769, 1993.
9. Barber BJ, Schaefer DJ, Gordon CJ, et al: Thermal effects of MR imaging: worst-case studies on sheep, Am J Roentgenol 155:1105, 1990.
10. Barnett GH, Ropper AH, and Johnson KA: Physiological support and monitoring of critically ill patients during magnetic resonance imaging, J Neurosurg 68:244, 1988.
11. Barnothy MF: Biological effects of magnetic fields, vols 1 and 2, New York, 1964 and 1969, Plenum Press.
12. Bartels MV, Mann K, Matejcek M, et al: Magnetresonanztomographie und Sicherheit: Elektroenzephalographische und Neuropsychologische Befunde vor und nach MR—Untersuchungen des Gehirns, Fortschr Rontgenstr 145(4):383, 1986.
13. Becker R, Norfray JF, Teitelbaum GP, et al: MR imaging in patients with intracranial aneurysm clips, Am J Neuroradiol 9:885, 1988.
14. Beers J: Biological effects of weak electromagnetic fields from 0 Hz to 200 MHz: a survey of the literature with special emphasis on possible magnetic resonance effects, Magn Reson Imaging 7:309, 1989.
15. Beischer DE, and Knepton J: Influence of strong magnetic fields on the electrocardiogram of squirrel monkey *(Saimiri sciures)*, Aerospace Med 35:939, 1964.
16. Berlex Laboratories: A two year report on the safety and efficacy of Magnevist (gadopentetate dimeglumine) injection, Wayne, NJ, 1990, Berlex Laboratories.
17. Berman E: Reproductive effects. In Biological effects of radiofrequency radiation, Environmental Protection Agency 600/8-83-026A, 1984.
18. Bernhardt J: The direct influence of electromagnetic fields on nerve and muscle and muscle cells of man within the frequency range of 1 Hz to 30 MHz, Radiat Environ Phys 16:309, 1979.
19. Besson J, Foreman EI, Eastwood LM, et al: Cognitive evaluation following NMR imaging of the brain, J Neurol Neurosurg Psychiatry 47:314, 1984.
20. Bore PJ, Galloway GJ, Styles P, et al: Are quenches dangerous? Magn Reson Imaging 3:112, 1986.
21. Bottomley PA, and Edelstein WA: Power disposition in whole body NMR imaging, Med Phys 8:510, 1981.
22. Bottomley PA, Redington RW, Edelstein WA, et al: Estimating radiofrequency power disposition in body NMR imaging, Magn Reson Med 2:336, 1985.
23. Bourland JD, Nyenhuis JA, Mouchawar GA, et al: Physiologic indicators of high MRI gradient-induced fields. In Book of abstracts, 1990, Society of Magnetic Resonance in Medicine.
24. Brasch R Safety profile of gadopentetate dimeglumine, MRI Decisions 3:13, 1989.
25. Brody AS, Sorette MP, Gooding CA, et al: Induced alignment of flowing sickle erythrocytes in a magnetic field: a preliminary report, Invest Radiol 20:560, 1985.
26. Brody AS, Embury SH, Mentzer WC, et al: Preservation of sickle cell blood flow patterns during MR imaging: an in vivo study, Am J Roentgenol 151:139, 1988.
27. Brown HD, and Chattopadhyay SK: Electromagnetic-field exposure and cancer, Cancer Biochem Biophys 9:295, 1988.
28. Brummett RE, Talbot JM, and Charuhas P: Potential hearing loss resulting from MR imaging, Radiology 169:539, 1988.
29. Buchli R, Boesiger P, and Meier D: Heating effects of metallic implants by MRI examinations, Magn Reson Med 7:255, 1988.
30. Budinger TF: Nuclear magnetic resonance (NMR) in vivo studies: known thresholds for health effects, J Comput Assist Tomogr 5:800, 1981.
31. Budinger TF, Fischer H, Hentschel D, et al: Physiological effects of fast oscillating magnetic field gradients, J Comput Assist Tomogr 15:909, 1991.
32. Cacheris W, Quay S, and Rocklage S: The relationship between thermodynamics and the toxicity of gadolinium complexes, Magn Reson Imaging 8:467, 1990.
33. Carson JJL, Prato FS, Drost DJ, et al: Time-varying fields increase cytosolic free Ca2+ in HL-60 cells, Am J Physiol 259:C687, 1990.
34. Carvlin M, DeSimone D, and Meeks M: Phase II clinical trial of gadoteridol injection, a low osmolal magnetic resonance imaging contrast agent, Invest Radiol 27:S16, 1992.
35. Chan C, Bosanko C, and Wang A: Pruritus and paresthesia after IV administration of Gd-DTPA, Am J Neuroradiol 10:S53, 1989.
36. Chang C: Magnetic resonance imaging contrast agents: design and physiochemical properties of gadodiamide, Invest Radiol 28(Suppl 1):S21, 1993.
37. Cohan RH, Leder RA, Herzberg AJ, et al: Extravascular toxicity of two magnetic resonance contrast agents: preliminary experience in the rat, Invest Radiol 26:224, 1991.
38. Cohen MS, Weisskoff R, Rzedzian R, et al: Sensory stimulation by time-varying magnetic fields, Magn Reson Med 14:409, 1990.
39. Cooke P, and Morris PG: The effects of NMR exposure on living organisms. II. A genetic study of human lymphocytes, Br J Radiol 54:622, 1981.
40. Coulter JS, and Osbourne SL: Short wave diathermy in heating of human tissues, Arch Phys Ther 17:679, 1936.
41. Davis PL, Crooks L, Arakawa M, et al: Potential hazards in NMR imaging: heating effects of changing magnetic fields and RF fields on small metallic implants, Am J Roentgenol 137:857, 1981.
42. DeSimone D, Morris M, Rhoda C, et al: Evaluation of the safety and efficacy of gadoteridol injection (a low osmolal MR contrast agent): clinical trials report, Invest Radiol 26(Suppl 1):S212, 1991.
43. Dimick RM, Hedlund LW, Herfkens RJ, et al: Optimizing electrocardiographic electrode placement for cardiac-gated magnetic resonance imaging, Invest Radiol 22:17, 1987.
44. Doherty JU, Whitman GJR, Robinson MD, et al: Changes in cardiac excitability and vulnerability in NMR fields, Invest Radiol 20:129, 1985.
45. Dormer KJ, Richard GJ, Hough JVD, et al: The use of rare-earth magnet couplers in cochlear implants, Laryngoscope 91: 1812, 1981.
46. Dujovny M, Kossovsky N, Kossowsky R, et al: Aneurysm clip motion during magnetic resonance imaging: in vivo experimental study with metallurgical factor analysis, Neurosurgery 17:543, 1985.
47. Dunn V, Coffman CE, McGowan JE, et al: Mechanical ventilation during magnetic resonance imaging, Magn Reson Imaging 3:169, 1985.
48. ECRI: Health devices alert: a new MRI complication? May 27, p 1, 1988.
49. Edelman RR, Shellock FG, and Ahladis J: Practical MRI for the technologist and imaging specialist. In Edelman RR, and Hesselink J, eds: Clinical magnetic resonance imaging, Philadelphia, 1990, WB Saunders.
50. Erwin DN: Mechanisms of biological effects of radiofrequency electromagnetic fields: an overview, Aviat Space Environ Med 59(Suppl 11):A21, 1988.

51. FDA Docket #85D-0249.

52. FDA (USDHHS), Center for Devices and Radiological Health, Office of Device Evaluation, Division of Reproductive, Abdominal, Ear, Nose, Throat and Radiological Devices, Computed Imaging Devices Branch, 1997 (http://www.fda.gov/cdrh/ode/magdev.html).

53. Felix R, and Schorner W: Intravenous contrast media in MRI: clinical experience with gadolinium-DTPA over four years. In Proceedings of the Second European Congress of NMR in Medicine in Biology, Berlin, 1988.

54. Fischer H: Physiological effects of fast oscillating magnetic field gradients, Radiology 173:(P)382, 1989.

55. Fishbain DA, Goldberg M, Labbe E, et al: Long-term claustrophobia following magnetic resonance imaging, Am J Psychiatry 145:1038, 1988.

56. Flaherty JA, and Hoskinson K: Emotional distress during magnetic resonance imaging, N Engl J Med 320:467, 1989.

57. Frank J, Choyke P, Girton M, et al: Gadopentetate dimeglumine clearance in renal insufficiency in rabbits, Invest Radiol 25:1212, 1990.

58. Gangarosa RE, Minnis JE, Nobbe J, et al: Operational safety issues in MRI, Magn Reson Imaging 5:287, 1987.

59. Garber HJ, Oldendorf WH, Braun LD, et al: MRI gradient fields increase brain mannitol space, Magn Reson Imaging 7:605, 1989.

60. Geard CR, Osmak RS, Hall EJ, et al: Magnetic resonance and ionizing radiation: a comparative evaluation in vitro of oncogenic and genotoxic potential, Radiology 152:199, 1984.

61. Gifford L, Director, Medical Affairs, Berlex Laboratories: Personal communication, June 1993.

62. Gifford L, Director, Medical Affairs, Berlex Laboratories: Personal communication, June 1993.

63. Goldman AM, Grossman WE, and Friedlander PC: Reduction of sound levels with antinoise in MR imaging, Radiology 173:549, 1989.

64. Goldstein H, Kashanian F, Blumetti R, et al: Safety assessment of gadopentetate dimeglumine in US clinical trials, Radiology 174:17, 1990.

65. Gordon CJ: Effect of radiofrequency radiation exposure on thermoregulation, ISI Atlas of Science, Plants and Animals 1:245, 1988.

66. Gordon CJ: Normalizing the thermal effects of radiofrequency radiation: body mass versus total body surface area, Bioelectromagnetics 8:111, 1987.

67. Gordon CJ: Thermal physiology. In Biological effects of radiofrequency radiation, Washington, 1984, EPA-600/8-830-026A, p. 4-1.

68. Gore JC, McDonnell MJ, Pennock JM, et al: An assessment of the safety of rapidly changing magnetic fields in the rabbit: implications for NMR imaging, Magn Reson Imaging 1:191, 1982.

69. Granet RB, and Gelber LJ: Claustrophobia during MR imaging, New Jersey Medicine 87:479, 1990.

70. Gray JE: Personal communication, August 1989.

71. Gray JE: Personal communication, September 1989.

72. Gremmel H, Wendhausen H, and Wunsch F: Biologische Effekte statischef Magnetfelder bei NMR-Tomographie am Menschen, Wiss, Radiologische, Klinik, Christian-Albrechts-Universitat zu Kiel, 1983.

73. Gulch RW, and Lutz O: Influence of strong static magnetic fields on heart muscle contraction, Phys Med Biol 31:763, 1986.

74. Hajek P, Sartoris D, Gylys-Morin V, et al: The effect of intra-articular gadolinium-DTPA on synovial membrane and cartilage, Invest Radiol 25:179, 1990.

75. Hammer BE, Wadon S, Mirer SD, et al: In vivo measurement of RF heating in Capuchin monkey brain. In Book of abstracts, 1991, Society of Magnetic Resonance in Medicine, p. 1278.

76. Harbury O: Generalized seizure after IV gadopentetate dimeglumine, Am J Neuroradiol 12:666, 1991.

77. Harpur E, Worah D, Hals P, et al: Preclinical safety assessment and pharmacokinetics of gadodiamide injection, a new magnetic resonance imaging contrast agent, Invest Radiol 28:S280, 1993.

78. Haustein J, Bauer W, Hibertz T, et al: Double dosing of Gd-DTPA in MRI of intracranial tumors. In Book of Abstracts, 1990, Society of Magnetic Resonance in Medicine, p. 258.

79. Haustein J, Niendorf H, Krestin G, et al: Renal tolerance of gadolinium-DTPA/dimeglumine in patients with chronic renal failure, Invest Radiol 27:153, 1992.

80. Haustein J, Niendorf H, and Louton T: Renal tolerance of Gd-DTPA—a retrospective evaluation of 1,171 patients, Magn Reson Imaging 8(S1):43, 1990.

81. Hayes DL, Holmes DR, and Gray JE: Effect of a 1.5 Tesla nuclear magnetic resonance imaging scanner on implanted permanent pacemakers, J Am Coll Cardiol 10:782, 1987.

82. Heinrichs WL, Fong P, Flannery M, et al: Midgestational exposure of pregnant Balb/c mice to magnetic resonance imaging, Magn Reson Imaging 6:305, 1988.

83. Holshouser BA, Hinshaw DB, and Shellock FG: Sedation, anesthesia, and physiologic monitoring during MRI. In Hasso AN, and Stark DD, eds: American Roentgen Ray Society, Categorical Course Syllabus, Spine and Body Magnetic Resonance Imaging, May 1991.

84. Holtas S, Olsson M, Romner B, et al: Comparison of MR imaging and CT in patients with intracranial aneurysm clips, Am J Neuroradiol 9:891, 1988.

85. Hong CZ: Static magnetic field influence on human nerve function, Arch Phys Med Rehabil 68:162, 1987.

86. Hong CZ, and Shellock FG: Short-term exposure to a 1.5 Tesla static magnetic field does not affect somato-sensory evoked potentials in man, Magn Reson Imaging 8:65, 1989.

87. Hricak H, and Amparo EG: Body MRI: alleviation of claustrophobia by prone positioning, Radiology 152:819, 1984.

88. Hurwitz R, Lane SR, Bell RA, et al: Acoustic analysis of gradient-coil noise in MR imaging, Radiology 173:545, 1989.

89. Huttenbrink KB, and Grobe-Nobis W: Experimentelle Untersuchungen und theoretische Betrachtungen uber das Verhalten von Stapes-Metall-Prothesen im Magnetfeld eines Kernspintomographen (Experiments and theoretical considerations on behaviour of metallic stapedectomy-prostheses in nuclear magnetic resonance imaging), Laryngologicie, Rhinologie, Otologie 66:127, 1987.

90. Innis NK, Ossenkopp KP, Prato FS, et al: Behavioral effects of exposure to nuclear magnetic resonance imaging. II. Spatial memory tests, Magn Reson Imaging 4:281, 1986.

91. Jackson JG, and Acker JD: Permanent eyeliner and MR imaging, Am J Roentgenol 149:1080, 1987.

92. Jehenson P, Duboc D, Lavergne T, et al: Change in human cardiac rhythm by a 2 Tesla static magnetic field, Radiology 166:227, 1988.

93. Kanal E, and Applegate GR: Thermal injuries/incidents associated with MR imaging devices in the US: a compilation and review of the presently available data. In Book of abstracts, 1990, Society for Magnetic Resonance Imaging, p. 274.

94. Kanal E, Applegate G, and Gillen C: Review of adverse reactions, including anaphylaxis, in 5260 cases receiving gadolinium-DTPA by bolus injection, Radiology 177(P):159, 1990.

95. Kanal E, and Shellock FG: Burns associated with clinical MR examinations, Radiology 175:585, 1990.

96. Kanal E, Talagala L, and Shellock FG: Safety considerations in MR imaging, Radiology 176:593, 1990.

97. Karlik SJ, Heatherley T, Pavan F, et al: Patient anesthesia and monitoring at a 1.5 T MRI installation, Magn Reson Med 7:210, 1988.

98. Kashanian F, Goldstein H, Blumetti R, et al: Rapid bolus injection of gadopentetate dimeglumine: absence of side effects in normal volunteers, Am J Neuroradiol 11:853, 1990.

99. Kay HH, Herfkens RJ, and Kay BK: Effect of magnetic resonance imaging on _Xenopus laevis_ embryogenesis, Magn Reson Imaging 6:501, 1988.

100. Kelly WM, Pagle PG, Pearson A, et al: Ferromagnetism of intraocular foreign body causes unilateral blindness after MR study, Am J Neuroradiol 7:243, 1986.

101. Keltner JR, Roos MS, Brakeman PR, et al: Magnetohydrodynamics of blood flow, Magn Reson Med 16:139, 1990.

102. Kido DK, Morris TW, Erickson JL, et al: Physiologic changes during high field strength MR imaging, Am J Neuroradiol 8:263, 1987.

103. Klonoff EA, Janata JW, and Kaufman B: The use of systematic desensitization to overcome resistance to magnetic resonance imaging (MRI) scanning, J Behav Ther Exp Psychiatry 17:189, 1986.

104. Lackner K, Krahe T, Gotz R, et al: The dialyzability of Gd-DTPA. In Bydder G, Felix R, and Bucheler E, eds: Contrast media in MRI, Bussum, 1990, Medicom Europe.

105. LaFlore, Medical Affairs, Berlex Laboratories: Personal communication, 1990.

106. LaFlore J, Goldstein H, Rogan R, et al: A prospective evaluation of adverse experiences following the administration of Magnevist (gadopentetate dimeglumine) injection. In Book of abstracts, 1989, Society of Magnetic Resonance in Medicine, p. 1067.

107. LaPorte R, Kus L, Wisniewski RA, et al: Magnetic resonance imaging (MRI) effects on rat pineal neuroendocrine function, Brain Res 506:294, 1990.

108. Leander P, Allard M, Caille J, et al: Early effect of gadopentetate and iodinated contrast media on rabbit kidneys, Invest Radiol 27:922, 1992.

109. Liang MD, Narayanan K, and Kanal E: Magnetic ports in tissue expanders: a caution for MRI, Magn Reson Imaging 7:541, 1989.

110. Lund G, Nelson JD, Wirtschafter JD, et al: Tattooing of eyelids: magnetic imaging artifacts, Ophthalmalic Surg 17:550, 1986.

111. McAlister W, McAlister V, and Kissane J: The effect of Gd-dimeglumine on subcutaneous tissues: a study with rats, Am J Neuroradiol 11:325, 1990.

112. McArdle CB, Nicholas DA, Richardson CJ, et al: Monitoring of the neonate undergoing MR imaging: technical considerations, Radiology 159:223, 1986.

113. McGuinness TP: Hypnosis in the treatment of phobias: a review of the literature, Am J Clin Hypn 26:261, 1984.

114. McLachlan S, Eaton S, and DeSimone D: Pharmacokinetic behavior of gadoteridol injection, Invest Radiol 27(Suppl 1):S12, 1992.

115. McLachlan S, Lucas M, DeSimone D, et al: Worldwide safety experience with gadoteridol injection (ProHance). In Book of abstracts, 1992, Society of Magnetic Resonance in Medicine, p. 1426.

116. McRobbie D, and Foster MA: Cardiac response to pulsed magnetic fields with regard to safety in NMR imaging, Phys Med Biol 30:695, 1985.

117. McRobbie D, and Foster MA: Pulsed magnetic field exposure during pregnancy and implications for NMR fetal imaging: a study with mice, Magn Reson Imaging 3:231, 1985.

118. Messmer JM, Porter JH, Fatouros P, et al: Exposure to magnetic resonance imaging does not produce taste aversion in rats, Physiol Behav 40:259, 1987.

119. Michaelson SM, and Lin JV: Biological effects and health implications of radiofrequency radiation, New York, 1987, Plenum Press.

120. Modan B: Exposure to electromagnetic fields and brain malignancy: a newly discovered menace? Am J Ind Med 13:625, 1988.

121. Montour JL, Fatouros PP, and Prasad UR: Effect of MR imaging on spleen colony formation following gamma radiation, Radiology 168:259, 1988.

122. Muhler A, Saeed M, Brasch R, et al: Hemodynamic effects of bolus injection of gadodiamide injection and gadopentetate dimeglumine as contrast media at MR imaging in rats, Radiology 183:523, 1992.

123. Muller S, and Hotz M: Human brainstem auditory evoked potentials (BAEP) before and after MR examinations, Magn Reson Med 16:476, 1990.

124. National Council on Radiation Protection and Measurements: Biological effects and exposure criteria for radiofrequency electromagnetic fields, Report No 86, Bethesda, 1986.

125. Nell G, and Rummel W: Pharmacology of intestinal permeation. In Csaky T, ed: Handbook of experimental pharmacology, Berlin, 1984, Springer-Verlag.

126. Ngo FQH, Blue JW, and Roberts WK: The effects of a static magnetic field on DNA synthesis and survival of mammalian cells irradiated with fast neutrons, Magn Reson Med 5:307, 1987.
127. Niemann G, Schroth G, Klose U, et al: Influence of magnetic resonance imaging on somatosensory potential in man, J Neurol 235:462, 1988.
128. Niendorf H, Dinger J, Haustein J, et al: Tolerance data of Gd-DTPA: a review, Eur J Radiol 13:15, 1991.
129. Niendorf H, and Ezumi K: Magnevist (Gd-DTPA): tolerance and safety after 4 years of clinical trials in more than 7000 patients. In Proceedings of Second European Congress of NMR in Medicine in Biology, Berlin, 1988.
130. Niendorf H, Haustein J, Cornelius I, et al: Safety of gadolinium-DTPA: extended clinical experience, Magn Reson Med 22:222, 1991.
131. Niendorf H, Haustein J, Louton T, et al: Safety and tolerance after intravenous administration of 0.3 mmol/kg Gd-DTPA, Invest Radiol 26:S221, 1991.
132. Niendorf H, Laniado M, Semmler W, et al: Dose administration of gadolinium-DTPA in MR imaging of intracranial tumors, Am J Neuroradiol 8:803, 1987.
133. Niendorf H, Valk J, and Reiser M: First use of Gd-DTPA in pediatric MRI. In Proceedings of Second European Congress of NRM in Medicine in Biology, Berlin, 1988.
134. Oksendal A, and Hals P: Biodistribution and toxicity of MR imaging contrast media, J Magn Reson Imaging 3:157, 1993.
135. Olukotun AY, and Rogan R, Squibb Diagnostics: Personal communication, June 1993.
136. Omohundro J, Elderbrook M, and Ringer T: Laryngospasm after administration of gadopentetate dimeglumine, J Magn Reson Imaging 1:729, 1992.
137. Osbakken M, Griffith J, and Taczanowsky P: A gross morphologic, histologic, hematologic, and blood chemistry study of adult and neonatal mice chronically exposed to high magnetic fields, Magn Reson Med 3:502, 1986.
138. Ossenkopp KP, Innis NK, Prato FS, et al: Behavioral effects of exposure to nuclear magnetic resonance imaging: I. Open-field behavior and passive avoidance learning in rats, Magn Reson Imaging 4:275, 1986.
139. Ossenkopp KP, Kavaliers M, Prato FS, et al: Exposure to nuclear magnetic imaging procedure attenuates morphine-induced analgesia in mice, Life Sci 37:1507, 1985.
140. Papatheofanis FJ, and Papthefanis BJ: Short-term effect of exposure to intense magnetic fields on hematologic indices of bone metabolism, Invest Radiol 24:221, 1989.
141. Peeling J, Lewis JS, Samoiloff MR, et al: Biological effects of magnetic fields on the nematode *Panagrellus redivivus*, Magn Reson Imaging 6:655, 1988.
142. Persson BR, and Stahlberg F: Health and safety of clinical NMR examinations, Boca Raton, Fla, 1989, CRC Press.
143. Phelps LA: MRI and claustrophobia, Am Fam Physician 42:930, 1990.
144. Pool R: Electromagnetic fields: the biological evidence, Science 249:1378, 1990.
145. Prasad N, Kosnik LT, Taber KH, et al: Delayed tumor onset following MR imaging exposure. In Book of abstracts, 1990, Society of Magnetic Resonance in Medicine, p. 275
146. Prasad N, Prasad R, Bushong SC, et al: Effects of 4.5 T MRI exposure on mouse testes and epididymis. In Book of abstracts, 1990, Society of Magnetic Resonance in Medicine, p. 606.
147. Prasad N, Bushong SC, Thornby JI, et al: Effect of nuclear resonance on chromosomes of mouse bone marrow cells, Magn Reson Imaging 2:37, 1984.
148. Prasad N, Lotzova E, Thornby JI, et al: Effects of MR imaging on murine natural killer cell cytotoxicity, Am J Roentgenol 148:415, 1987.
149. Prasad N, Lotzova E, Thornby JI, et al: The effect of 2.35-T MR imaging on natural killer cell cytotoxicity with and without interleukin-2, Radiology 175:251, 1990.
150. Prasad N, Wright DA, Ford JJ, et al: Safety of 4-T MR imaging: a study of effects of developing frog embryos, Radiology 174:251, 1990.
151. Prasad N, Wright DA, and Forster JD: Effect of nuclear magnetic resonance on early stages of amphibian development, Magn Reson Imaging 1:35, 1982.
152. Prato FS, Ossenkopp KP, Kavaliers M, et al: Attenuation of morphine-induced analgesia in mice by exposure to magnetic resonance imaging: separate effects of the static, radiofrequency and time-varying magnetic fields, Magn Reson Imaging 5:9, 1987.
153. Pusey E, Lufkin RB, Brown RKJ, et al: Magnetic resonance imaging artifacts: mechanism and clinical significance, Radiographics 6:891, 1986.
154. Quirk ME, Letendre AJ, Ciottone RA, et al: Anxiety in patients undergoing MR imaging, Radiology 170:463, 1989.
155. Quirk ME, Letendre AJ, Ciottone RA, et al: Evaluation of three psychological interventions to reduce anxiety during MR imaging, Radiology 173:759, 1989.
156. Randall PA, Kohman LJ, Scalzetti EM, et al: Magnetic resonance imaging of prosthetic cardiac valves in vitro and in vivo, Am J Cardiol 62:973, 1988.
157. Redington RW, Dumoulin CL, Schenck JL, et al: MR imaging and bio-effects in a whole body 4 Tesla imaging system. In Book of abstracts, 1988, Society of Magnetic Resonance Imaging, p. 20.
158. Reich L, Sanofi Winthrop: Personal communication, June 14, 1993.
159. Reich L, Sterling Winthrop: Personal communication, July 1, 1993.
160. Reid A, Smith FW, and Hutchison JMS: Nuclear magnetic resonance imaging and its safety implications: follow-up of 181 patients, Br J Radiol 55:784, 1982.
161. Reilly JP: Peripheral nerve stimulation by induced electric currents: exposure to time-varying magnetic fields, Med Biol Eng Comput 27:101, 1989.
162. Rofsky N, Weinreb J, and Litt A: Quantitative analysis of gadopentetate dimeglumine excreted in breast milk, J Magn Reson Imaging 3:131, 1993.
163. Rogan R, Squibb Diagnostics: Personal communication, June 15, 1993.
164. Romner B, Olsson M, Ljunggren B, et al: Magnetic resonance imaging and aneurysm clips, J Neurosurg 70:426, 1989.
165. Roschmann P: Human auditory system response to pulsed radiofrequency energy in RF coils for magnetic resonance at 2.4 to 170 MHz, Magn Reson Med 21:197, 1991.
166. Roth JL, Nugent M, Gray JE, et al: Patient monitoring during magnetic resonance imaging, Anesthesiology 62:80, 1985.
167. Runge V: Clinical application of magnetic resonance contrast media in the head. In Runge V, ed: Contrast media in magnetic resonance imaging: a clinical approach, Philadelphia, 1992, JB Lippincott.
168. Runge V, Bradley W, Brant-Zawadski M, et al: Clinical safety and efficacy of gadoteridol: a study in 411 patients with suspected intracranial and spinal disease, Radiology 181:701, 1991.
169. Runge V, Rocklage S, Niendorf H, et al: Discussion: gadolinium chelates. In Society of Magnetic Resonance in Medicine Workshop on Contrast Enhanced Magnetic Resonance, Berkeley, Calif, 1991.
170. Sacco DA, Steiger DA, Bellon EM, et al: Artifacts caused by cosmetics in MR imaging of the head, Am J Roentgenol 148:1001, 1987.
171. Sacks E, Worgul BV, Merriam GR, et al: The effects of nuclear magnetic resonance imaging on ocular tissues, Arch Ophthalmol 104:890, 1986.
172. Salonen O: Case of anaphylaxis and four cases of allergic reaction following Gd-DTPA administration, J Comput Assist Tomogr 14:912, 1990.
173. Schmiedl U, Maravilla K, Gerlach R, et al: Excretion of gadopentetate dimeglumine in human breast milk, Am J Roentgenol 154:1305, 1990.
174. Schwartz JL, and Crooks LE: NMR imaging produces no observable mutations or cytotoxicity in mammalian cells, Am J Roentgenol 139:583, 1982.
175. Shellock FG: Monitoring during MRI: An evaluation of the effect of high-field MRI on various patient monitors, Medical Electronics Sept:93, 1986.
176. Shellock FG: MR imaging of metallic implants and materials: a compilation of the literature, Am J Roentgenol 151: 811, 1988.
177. Shellock FG: Biological effects and safety aspects of magnetic resonance imaging, Magn Reson Q 5:243, 1989.
178. Shellock FG: Ex vivo assessment of deflection forces and artifacts associated with high-field MRI of "mini-magnet" dental prostheses, Magn Reson Imaging 7(Suppl 1):IT-03, 1989.
179. Shellock FG: Monitoring sedated patients during MRI, Radiology 177:586, 1990 (letter).
180. Shellock FG, and Crues JV: Corneal temperature changes associated with high-field MR imaging using a head coil, Radiology 167:809, 1986.
181. Shellock FG, and Crues JV: High-field MR imaging of metallic biomedical implants: an ex vivo evaluation of deflection forces, Am J Roentgenol 151:389, 1988.
182. Shellock FG, and Crues JV: Temperature, heart rate, and blood pressure changes associated with clinical MR imaging at 1.5 T, Radiology 163:259, 1987.
183. Shellock FG, and Crues JV: High-field MR imaging of metallic biomedical implants: an in vitro evaluation of deflection forces and temperature changes induced in large prostheses, Radiology 165:150, 1987.
184. Shellock FG, and Crues JV: MRI: safety considerations in magnetic resonance imaging, MRI Decisions 2:25, 1988.
185. Shellock FG, and Crues JV: Temperature changes caused by clinical MR imaging of the brain at 1.5 Tesla using a head coil, Am J Neuroradiol 9:287, 1988.
186. Shellock FG, and Curtis JS: MR imaging and biomedical implants, materials, and devices: an updated review, Radiology 180:541, 1991.
187. Shellock FG, Gordon CJ, and Schaefer DJ: Thermoregulatory responses to clinical magnetic resonance imaging of the head at 1.5 Tesla: lack of evidence for direct effects on the hypothalamus, Acta Radiol Suppl 369:512, 1986.
188. Shellock FG, Hahn P, Mink JH, et al: Adverse reaction to intravenous gadoteridol, Radiology 189:1, 1993.
189. Shellock FG, and Kanal E: Policies, guidelines, and recommendations for MR imaging safety and patient management, J Magn Reson Imaging 1:97, 1991.
190. Shellock FG, and Meeks T: Ex vivo evaluation of ferromagnetism and artifacts for implantable vascular access ports exposed to a 1.5 T MR scanner, J Magn Reson Imaging 1:243, 1991.
191. Shellock FG, Myers SM, and Kimble K: Monitoring heart rate and oxygen saturation during MRI with a fiber-optic pulse oximeter, Am J Roentgenol 158:663, 1992.
192. Shellock FG, Rothman B, and Sarti D: Heating of the scrotum by high-field-strength MR imaging, Am J Roentgenol 154:1229, 1990.
193. Shellock FG, Schaefer DJ, and Crues JV: Effect of a 1.5 Tesla static magnetic field on body and skin temperatures of man, Magn Reson Med 11:371, 1989.
194. Shellock FG, Schaefer DJ, and Crues JV: Alterations in body and skin temperatures caused by MR imaging: is the recommended exposure for radiofrequency radiation too conservative? Br J Radiol 62:904, 1989.
195. Shellock FG, Schaefer DJ, and Gordon CJ: Effect of a 1.5 T static magnetic field on body temperature of man, Magn Reson Med 3:644, 1986.
196. Shellock FG, Schaefer DJ, Grundfest W, et al: Thermal effects of high-field (1.5 Tesla) magnetic resonance imaging of the spine: clinical experience above a specific absorption rate of 0.4 W/kg, Acta Radiol Suppl 369:514, 1986.
197. Shellock FG, and Schatz CJ: High-field strength MRI and otologic implants, Am J Neuroradiol 12:279, 1991.
198. Shellock FG, Schatz CJ, Shelton C, et al: Ex vivo evaluation of 9 different ocular and middle-ear implants exposed to a 1.5 Tesla MR scanner, Radiology 177(P):271, 1990.
199. Shellock FG, and Slimp G: Severe burn of the finger caused by using a pulse oximeter during MRI, Am J Roentgenol 153:1105, 1989.
200. Shivers RR, Kavaliers M, Tesky CJ, et al: Magnetic resonance imaging temporarily alters blood-brain barrier permeability in the rat, Neurosci Lett 76:25, 1987.
201. Shuman WP, Haynor DR, Guy AW, et al: Superficial and deep-tissue increases in anesthetized dogs during exposure to high specific absorption rates in a 1.5-T MR imager, Radiology 167:551, 1988.
202. Soltys R: Summary of preclinical safety evaluation of gadoteridol injection, Invest Radiol 27(Suppl 1):S7, 1992.
203. Sperber D, Oldenbourg R, and Dransfeld K: Magnetic field induced temperature change in mice, Naturwissenschaften 71:100, 1984.
204. Stick VC, Hinkelmann ZK, Eggert P, et al: Beeinflussen starke statische magnetfelder in der NMR-Tomographie die gewebedurchblutung? (Strong static magnetic fields of NMR: do they affect tissue perfusion?), Fortschr Rontgenstr 154:326, 1991.
205. Stojan L, Sperber D, Dransfeld K: Magnetic-field-induced changes in the human auditory evoked potentials, Naturwissenschaften 75:622, 1988.

206. Sullivan M, Goldstein H, Sansone K, et al: Hemodynamic effects of Gd-DTPA administered via rapid bolus or slow infusion: a study in dogs, Am J Neuroradiol 11:537, 1990.
207. Sweetland J, Kertesz A, Prato FS, et al: The effect of magnetic resonance imaging on human cognition, Magn Reson Imaging 5:129, 1987.
208. Takebayashi S, Sugiyama M, Nagase M, et al: Severe adverse reaction to IV gadopentetate dimeglumine, Am J Roentgenol 14:912, 1990.
209. Tardy B, Guy C, Barral G, et al: Anaphylactic shock induced by intravenous gadopentetate dimeglumine, Lancet 339:494, 1992.
210. Teitelbaum GP, Bradley WG, and Klein BD: MR imaging artifacts, ferromagnetism, and magnetic torque of intravascular filters, stents, and coils, Radiology 166:657, 1988.
211. Teitelbaum GP, Yee CA, Van Horn DD, et al: Metallic ballistic fragments: MR imaging safety and artifacts, Radiology 175:855, 1990.
212. Tenforde TS: Magnetic field effects on biological systems, New York, 1979, Plenum Press.
213. Tenforde TS: Thermoregulation in rodents exposed to high-intensity stationary magnetic fields, Bioelectromagnetics 7:341, 1983.
214. Tenforde TS, Gaffey CT, Moyer BR, et al: Cardiovascular alterations in *Macaca* monkeys exposed to stationary magnetic fields: experimental observations and theoretical analysis, Bioelectromagnetics 4:1, 1983.
215. Teskey GC, Prato FS, Ossenkopp KP, et al: Exposure to time varying magnetic fields associated with magnetic resonance imaging reduces fentanyl-induced analgesia in mice, Bioelectromagnetics 9:167, 1988.
216. Tesky GC, Ossenkopp KP, Prato FS, et al: Survivability and long-term stress reactivity levels following repeated exposure to nuclear magnetic resonance imaging procedures in rats, Physiol Chem Phys Med NMR 19:43, 1987.
217. Thomas A, and Morris PG: The effects of NMR exposure on living organisms. I. A microbial assay, Br J Radiol 54:615, 1981.
218. Tishler S, and Hoffman JC: Anaphylactoid reactions to IV gadopentetate dimeglumine, Am J Neuroradiol 11:1167, 1990.
219. Tweedle M: Physiochemical properties of gadoteridol and other magnetic resonance contrast agents, Invest Radiol 27(Suppl 1):S2, 1992.
220. Tweedle M, Eaton S, Eckelman W, et al: Comparative chemical structure and pharmacokinetics of MRI contrast agents, Invest Radiol 23(Suppl 1):S236, 1988.
221. Tyndall DA: MRI effects on the teratogenicity of X-irradiation in the C57BL/6J mouse, Magn Reson Imaging 8:423, 1990.
222. Tyndall DA, and Sulik KK: Effects of magnetic resonance imaging on eye development in the C57BL/6J mouse, Teratology 43: 263, 1991.
223. Vogl T, Krimmel K, Fuchs A, et al: Influence of magnetic resonance imaging on human body core and intravascular temperature, Med Phys 15:562, 1988.
224. Von Klitzing L: A new encephalomagnetic effect in human brain generated by static magnetic fields, Brain Res 540:295, 1991.
225. Von Klitzing L: Do static magnetic fields of NMR influence biological signals, Clin Phys Physiol Meas (Bristol) 7:157, 1986.
226. Von Klitzing L: Static magnetic fields increase the power intensity of EEG of man, Brain Res 483:201, 1989.
227. Vyalov AM: Magnetic fields as a factor in the industrial environment, Vestn Akad Med Nauk SSSR 8:72, 1967.
228. Vyalov AM: Clinico-hygenic and experimental data on the effect of magnetic fields under industrial conditions. In Kholodov Y, ed: Influence of magnetic fields on biological objects, Moscow, 1971. Translated by the Joint Publications Research Service, JPRS 63-38:20, 1974.
229. Watson A, Rocklage S, and Carvlin M: Contrast media. In Stark D, and Bradley W, eds: Magnetic resonance imaging, ed 2, St Louis, 1991, Mosby.
230. Watson AB, Wright JS, and Loughman L: Electrical thresholds for ventricular fibrillation in man, Med J Aust 1:1179, 1973.
231. Wedeking P, Kumar K, and Tweedle M: Dissociation of gadolinium chelates in mice: relationship to chemical characteristics, Magn Reson Imaging 10:641, 1992.
232. Weinmann H, Brasch R, Press W, et al: Characteristics of gadolinium-DTPA complex: a potential NMR contrast agent, Am J Roentgenol 142:619, 1984.
233. Weinmann HJ, Gries H, and Speck U: Gd-DTPA and low osmolar Gd chelates. In Runge V, ed: Enhanced magnetic resonance imaging, St. Louis, 1989, Mosby.
234. Weinreb JC, Maravilla KR, Peshock R, et al: Magnetic resonance imaging: improving patient tolerance and safety, Am J Roentgenol 143:1285, 1984.
235. Weiss J, Herrick RC, Taber KH, et al: Bio-effects of high magnetic fields: a study using a simple animal model, Magn Reson Imaging 8(S1):166, 1990.
236. Weiss K: Severe anaphylactoid reaction after IV Gd-DTPA, Magn Reson Imaging 8:817, 1990.
237. Wendt RE, Rokey R, Vick GW, et al: Electrocardiographic gating and monitoring during NMR imaging, Magn Reson Imaging 6:89, 1988.
238. Wickersheim KA, and Sun MH: Fluoroptic thermometry, Medical Electronics Feb:84, 1987.
239. Williams S, Char DH, Dillon WP, et al: Ferrous intraocular foreign bodies and magnetic resonance imaging, Am J Ophthalmol 105:398, 1988.
240. Willis RJ, and Brooks WM: Potential hazards of NMR imaging: no evidence of the possible effects of static and changing magnetic fields on cardiac function of the rat and guinea pig, Magn Reson Imaging 2:89, 1984.
241. Withers HR, Mason KA, Davis CA, et al: MR effect on murine spermatogenesis, Radiology 156:741, 1985.
242. Wolff S, Crooks LE, Brown P, et al: Tests for DNA and chromosomal damage induced by nuclear magnetic resonance imaging, Radiology 136:707, 1980.
243. Yamagata H, Kuhara S, Eso Y, et al: Evaluation of dB/dt thresholds for nerve stimulation elicited by trapezoidal and sinusoidal gradient fields in echo-planar imaging. In Book of abstracts, 1991, Society of Magnetic Resonance in Medicine, p. 1277.
244. Yuh WTC, Hanigan MT, Nerad JA, et al: Extrusion of a magnetic eye implant after MR examination: a potential hazard to the enucleated eye. In Book of abstracts, 1991, American Society of Neuroradiology, p. 97.

CHAPTER

15 Breasts

Sylvia H. Heywang-Köbrunner and Petra Viehweg

Technique
   Pulse Sequences
   Contrast Enhancement
Tissue Characterization and Lesion Detection
   Unenhanced Magnetic Resonance Imaging
   Enhanced Magnetic Resonance Imaging
   Parenchymal Proliferation and Fibrocystic Disease
   Cysts
   Fibroadenomas
   Cancer
   Lymph Nodes
   Mammoplasty, Scarring, and Radiation Changes
Summary

 KEY POINTS

- Detection of breast cancer requires matched image sets; one obtained before and one or more sets obtained after bolus injection contrast material.
- Malignant lesions enhance more than many benign tissues; however, there is considerable overlap.
- Morphology and dynamics of contrast enhancement must be correlated with information from conventional imaging.
- MRI is most useful where sensitivity of conventional imaging is limited (e.g., dense tissue, scarring after tumorectomy, silicone implants) and where high-risk factors exist (e.g., cancer staging, treatment follow up).

Mortality can be reduced by as much as 50%, when high-quality mammographic screening is performed.[29,68,76] Although mammography is the best diagnostic method for early detection, problems still exist. Even with high-quality screening, about 40% of carcinomas are detected only when they are larger than 1.5 cm, and 20% to 40% of the carcinomas become apparent in the interval between the screening rounds.[6,7,40,52,83] A large number of these carcinomas were present at the time of earlier screening examination but were not detected. Besides the size and the histological condition of the tumor, the density of the surrounding tissue is the most important factor in determining when a lesion will be detected.[51,53,70]

The mammographic appearance of early carcinomas may mimic that of many benign conditions. Therefore further workup (ranging from additional imaging to needle biopsies and surgical excision) is necessary in 3 to 10 times as many patients as those who finally prove to have cancer.[18,58]

Detection and exclusion of malignancy in breasts with extensive scarring (after multiple or extensive surgeries, after irradiation, or around implants) may be difficult and sometimes unreliable. Sonogra-phy can help distinguish cysts from solid lesions, diminishing the number of unnecessary biopsies. Complementing mammography, sonography also shows palpable malignant tumors within dense breast tissue. However, in the case of small lesions sonography is not sensitive and specific enough to rule out early malignant disease.[3,4,13,71,74]

Image-guided core biopsy is an important tool used to reduce the number of biopsies of benign lesions.[17,21,63,72] Compared with aspiration cytology, core biopsy is specific, sensitive, and reliable. Damadian first suggested the use of nuclear magnetic resonance imaging (MRI) for the differentiation of cancer tissue from noncancer tissue.[11,14,33,64,66] Since MRI became possible in the early 1980s, its use for tissue characterization has been based on measured T1 and T2 values on the related "weighted" image signal intensities. Early hopes about a potential tissue differentiation[22,65,77] remain unfulfilled.[41,67,85] Signal intensities and (T1, T2) tissue parameters mainly depend on the content of water modified by structures, such as cells or fibrosis, which varies among different tissues. These parameters do not correlate with the biological nature of tumors. Carcinomas (e.g., scirrhous carcinomas) and dysplasias (e.g., fibrous dysplasia) may contain fibrosis and mimic the magnetic resonance (MR) appearance of simple scarring. Other carcinomas, such as most ductal invasive types, medullary carcinomas with a high content of cells or even water (e.g., mucinous carcinomas and fibrocystic disease), or dysplasias like fibrocystic changes with or without premalignant histology, show a long T2 characteristic of cancer. However, many benign fibroadenomas show similar MR characteristics. Therefore the fundamental MR tissue characteristics play no major role in the detection of breast cancer or in its differentiation from other lesions. MRI has proved important as the most sensitive imaging modality for the detection of rupture in breast implants (see Chapter 17).

A breakthrough in breast cancer detection was achieved by the demonstration that gadolinium diethylene-triamine-pentaacetic acid (Gd-DTPA) enhances virtually all cancers more than it enhances minimal glandular breast tissue.

The method of contrast-enhanced MRI of the breast was developed by the group of Heywang in 1985.[42] Since 1987, other groups have started to investigate the use of enhanced MRI for breast diagnosis as well,* and the present experience worldwide exceeds 10,000 MR examinations of the breast proved by histology or at least 1-year follow up.

On the basis of these experiences, contrast-enhanced MRI appears an interesting additional tool that can provide diagnostically valuable information in selected indications.

This chapter presents an overview of technique, interpretation guidelines, accuracy data, and indications for MRI of the breast.

TECHNIQUE

The necessary image quality can be achieved only when a dedicated breast coil is used. Most commercially available breast coils provide a sufficient signal-to-noise ratio (SNR).

---

*References 1, 2, 9, 10, 15, 23-28, 30-32, 34-39, 54-56, 59-62, 69-73, 79, 80, 84.

The signal intensity within 1 cm of the coil margin should vary by less than a factor of 2 from the center of the coil. Inhomogeneous reception may cause underestimation or overestimation of enhancement.

The latest equipment allows the imaging of both breasts with about the same image quality as with older single-breast coils. Because imaging of the contralateral breast may yield clinically important information (detection of multicentric carcinoma, simultaneous evaluation of bilateral problems, additional diagnostic information from comparison between both breasts), double-breast coils are favored. Figure 15-1 shows a typical double-breast coil.

High spatial resolution and high contrast are prerequisites to adequate visualization of small lesions. Slice thickness should be less than 4 mm—optimally 1 to 2 mm. In-plane resolution should be about 1 mm or less. Quantitative evaluations of small lesions are much more impaired by partial volume effect than are morphological assessments; therefore thin slices and motion reduction are important prerequisites for a reliable quantitative evaluation. Temporal resolution is necessary for evaluation of selective cancer enhancement, which deteriorates starting about 2 to 5 min after the intravenous injection of the contrast agent. The imaging time for thin-section visualization of the complete breast should not exceed 5 min after injection at maximum.

The reduction of breast motion is essential to maintain spatial resolution and SNR, and it is of utmost importance to allow reliable recognition of small enhancing areas by means of direct comparison of precontrast and postcontrast slices or by subtraction technique. The prone position helps reduce breast motion caused by respiration. The patient must be taught the importance of lying still. Vibration of the breast may be reduced by stuffing the breast coil with cotton or by having the patient wear a tight T-shirt. Compression devices are presently being investigated. Image postprocessing algorithms may permit retrospective correction of motion and help align precontrast and postcontrast data sets.

Cardiac artifact increases after the administration of Gd-DTPA. Cardiac motion artifacts are visualized bands that follow the phase-encoding gradient. Thus, depending on the direction of the phase-encoding gradient, cardiac artifacts may cross the left breast or both axillas. When imaging in the sagittal or coronal plane, the clinician can direct cardiac artifact away from the breasts and the axillae by orienting the phase encoding along the z axis. Thus, depending on the area of interest, the phase-encoding gradient direction must be carefully selected. Other methods, such as flow compensation or presaturation, cannot adequately reduce cardiac artifact without suppressing signals from other important structures.

Pulse Sequences

Fast three-dimensional (3D) gradient-echo sequences have proved most sensitive for visualization of paramagnetic contrast medium. Compared with two-dimensional (2D) techniques, they allow a high spatial and temporal resolution with high SNR. Moreover, 3D sequences may also be used with dosages exceeding 0.1 mmol/kg Gd chelate. Even though contrast with 2D sequences is lower, they may not be used with higher doses of paramagnetic contrast medium because they have a saturation effect.[44]

Fat usually exhibits high signal intensity and may interfere with the detection of small enhancing areas, unless each postcontrast image is diligently compared with the corresponding precontrast image. Therefore elimination of the fat signal appears desirable for facilitated reading of enhanced breast MRI. For this purpose, either selective fat saturation, selective water excitation,[16,38,39,81] or subtraction of the corresponding precontrast and postcontrast slices[30,32,44,49,55] has been recommended. Because of the narrow bandwidth of selective prepulses, signal inhomogeneities may result. Such inhomogeneities may result in overlooked or underestimated lesions.

Subtraction of precontrast and postcontrast slices may be the most robust method. Significant motion will compromise the diagnostic reliability of all methods.

Echo time (TE) must be adjusted in such a way that in-phase images result. At 1.5 Tesla (T), gradient-recalled echoes are in-phase at TEs of 3.6 and 6.0 ms or below 1.2 ms. At 1.0 T, in-phase gradient echoes occur at 4.8 and 7.2 ms or below 1.8 ms. At 0.5 T a gradient-echo TE of 10.8 or 18 ms or below 3.6 ms is preferred. Opposed-phase images must be avoided because fat-water signal cancellation may conceal enhancement, resulting in missed cancer diagnoses.[50]

Contrast Enhancement

A dosage of 0.1 to 0.2 mmol/L Gd chelate per kilogram of body weight is recommended.[67] Because the overall volume of paramagnetic contrast agent is low, injection of contrast agent must be followed by another injection of at least 20 ml of saline solution. This serves to flush the tube and the distal veins.

In addition to the precontrast T1-weighted image used as a subtraction mask, T2-weighted (long TR/TE) imaging may allow differentiation of cysts or fibrosed fibroadenomas from other well-circumscribed lesions. Thus the complete breast examination consists of a precontrast set of images and at least one postcontrast set of fast, high-resolution T1-weighted images (preferably fast 3D spoiled gradient echo) identical in geometry. The precontrast sets serve to assess the dynamics of enhancement. A single precontrast T2-weighted data set is optional.

On the T1-weighted gradient-echo images, which are commonly used for contrast-enhanced MRI, muscle, glandular tissue, and connective tissue display low signal intensity. Fat provides contrast for delineation of these tissues and as the reference standard for description of signal intensity. Fat shows intermediate to high signal intensity because of its short T1 relaxation time unless a frequency-selective or short tau inversion recovery (STIR) method is employed.

On T2-weighted images the signal intensity depends significantly on the water content of the tissue. Connective tissue always has very low signal intensity as a result of its short T2 relaxation time. The other benign and malignant tissues show a wide range in signal intensity on T2-weighted images. As known from mammography, the breast's composition of fatty versus nonfatty tissue depends on the patient's age and hormonal status. The water content of breast tissue is influenced by the menstrual cycle and by hormones.

On the postcontrast T1-weighted image, normal breast tissues usually exhibit no significant signal increase compared with the precontrast image. Exceptions with intermediate to strong enhancement, which may be diffuse or focal, do exist. They usually occur in post-

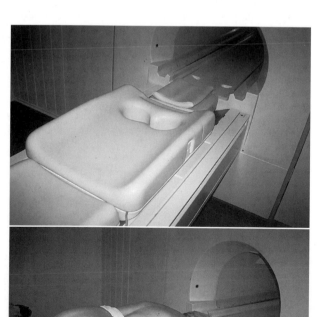

FIGURE 15-1   Double-breast coil.

menopausal patients who are receiving hormone-replacement therapy or in premenopausal patients predominantly during the first and fourth weeks of the menstrual cycle. Because focal or diffuse enhancement within normal tissue may obscure recognition of enhancing lesions and mimic malignant changes, enhanced MRI should not be preformed on very young patients (<35 years) unless strong indications exist. Enhanced-MR examinations should be performed between days 6 and 16 of the menstrual cycle (Figure 15-2).

TISSUE CHARACTERIZATION AND LESION DETECTION
Unenhanced Magnetic Resonance Imaging

Qualitative morphological information, such as central fibrosis or necrosis, visible on the T2-weighted images (Figure 15-3) can provide some useful biological information. Quantitative image analysis has not been reliable for tissue characterization (Figures 15-4 to 15-6).

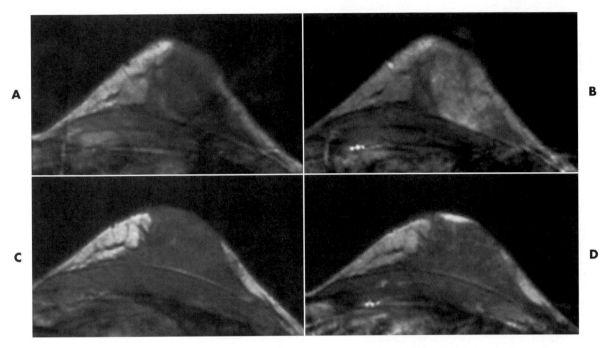

FIGURE 15-2   Influence of the menstrual cycle on Gd-DTPA enhancement in a premenopausal patient. **A,** Precontrast MR image, acquired during the fourth week of the menstrual cycle. **B,** Postcontrast MR image, acquired during the fourth week of the menstrual cycle. Strong enhancement is seen throughout large parts of the breast tissue. **C** and **D,** Precontrast and postcontrast images acquired in the same patient during the second week of the menstrual cycle. Except for some areolar enhancement—a normal finding in many patients—no significant enhancement is seen. Even though the differences are mostly not as striking as in this case of a 36-year-old woman, we generally recommend contrast-enhanced MR studies during the second or third week of the menstrual cycle.

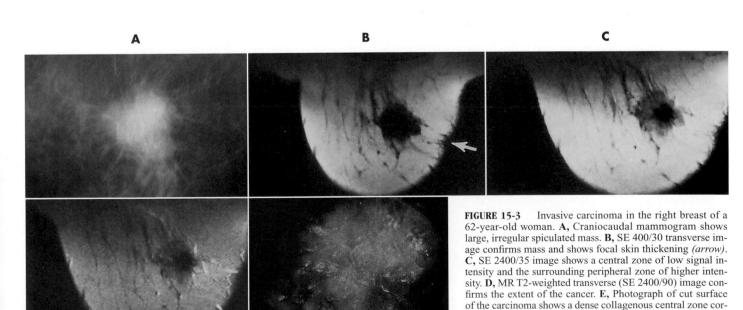

FIGURE 15-3   Invasive carcinoma in the right breast of a 62-year-old woman. **A,** Craniocaudal mammogram shows large, irregular spiculated mass. **B,** SE 400/30 transverse image confirms mass and shows focal skin thickening *(arrow).* **C,** SE 2400/35 image shows a central zone of low signal intensity and the surrounding peripheral zone of higher intensity. **D,** MR T2-weighted transverse (SE 2400/90) image confirms the extent of the cancer. **E,** Photograph of cut surface of the carcinoma shows a dense collagenous central zone corresponding to the low signal area in **C** and **D,** surrounded by a more loosely cellular zone corresponding to the higher signal–intensity area in **C** and **D.**

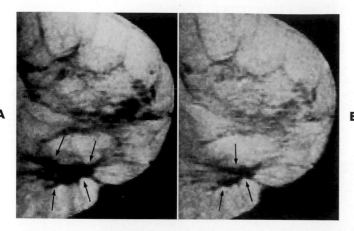

FIGURE 15-4   Scirrhous carcinoma in a 42-year-old woman. **A,** Sagittal SE 400/35 image shows a mass *(arrows)* of low signal intensity (similar to the breast tissue). **B,** SE 1600/70 image shows the carcinoma *(arrows)* as very low signal intensity (indicating dense collagen) relative to normal retroareolar breast tissue. (From reference 41.)

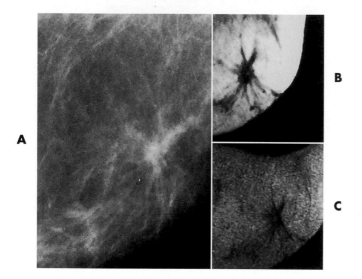

FIGURE 15-5   Suture granuloma mimicking carcinoma. **A,** Detail from craniocaudal mammogram shows a spiculated mass. **B,** SE 400/30 image. **C,** SE 2400/90 image shows that the lesion remains of low signal intensity; this appearance of the benign scan (nonspecific) is also consistent with scirrhous carcinoma.

Qualitative signal–intensity information has been useful for the diagnosis of cysts and fibrous fibroadenomas. However, most carcinomas show no characteristic signal behavior and can have the same appearance as the common benign lesions on unenhanced T1- and T2-weighted images.

Enhanced Magnetic Resonance Imaging

Although the majority of malignant tumors do enhance, overlap between enhancing benign and malignant tissues exists. Therefore, like all other imaging modalities, enhanced MRI often does not allow definitive tissue characterization. Indications where, however, contrast-enhanced MRI may provide valuable additional information and may thus improve diagnostic accuracy are summarized in Table 15-1. Table 15-2 summarizes the indications where because of too much overlap contrast enhanced MRI is not helpful or cost-effective.

Enhanced MRI includes evaluation of the amount (presence), the speed, and the morphology of the enhancement. Absence of enhancement excludes an invasive malignancy larger than the slice thickness, with a probability greater than 98%. This is based on the fact that the majority of the invasive carcinomas enhance significantly, that is, more than a "minimum threshold," which for a fast low-angle shot (FLASH) 3D technique is at about 50% enhancement[44] (2 to 3 min post injection of 0.16 mmol/L Gd chelate per kilogram of body weight).*

Because about 10% to 15% of in situ carcinomas may enhance only minimally, enhanced MRI must be combined with regular x-ray mammography.

When some type of enhancement above the minimum threshold exists, either benign or malignant disease may be present. Indicative of malignancy are irregular contours of an enhancing lesion, enhancement that follows the ducts or starts from the periphery, fast rise of enhancement, and, if present, wash-out. Indicative of benign disease are well-circumscribed contours of enhancement, diffuse milky or patchy enhancement, demonstration of typical septations within a well-circumscribed or lobulated mass, and slow rise of enhancement.

Lesions for which there is a high probability of malignancy must be biopsied even if conventional x-ray mammographic findings are negative because MRI may allow detection of otherwise occult malignancies. For lesions that are visible only by means of enhanced MRI, either an MR-guided core biopsy or surgical excision after MR- or CT-guided wire localization is performed.

Lesions for which there is a low probability of malignancy are managed as follows:

• If the suspicion is confirmed by x-ray mammographic or palpation findings, biopsy is performed.
• If there is no clinical or mammographic confirmation, routine clinical and mammographic follow-up is supplemented by a repeat MR examination within 1 year.

---

*The exact threshold depends on the chosen pulse sequence parameters and field strength.[50]

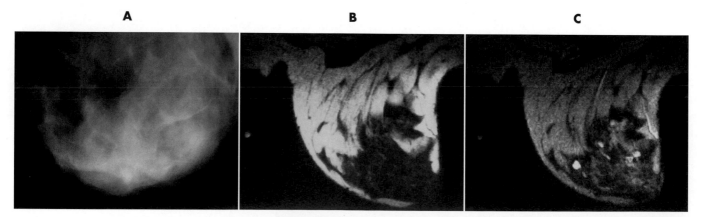

FIGURE 15-6   Proliferative glandular tissue with cysts. **A,** Craniocaudal mammogram shows dense retroareolar glandular tissue but fails to show any discrete masses. **B,** SE 400/35 image shows glandular tissue. Cysts are obscured by the surrounding low signal glandular tissue. **C,** SE 2400/90 image shows numerous small cysts.

Table 15-1   Indications for Contrast-Enhanced MRI

Indication

1. Scarring that is difficult to assess (1) after limited surgery (>6 months postoperatively); (2) after silicone implants (>6 months postoperatively); or (3) after limited surgery and irradiation (>12 months after irradiation)
2. Dense (difficult to assess) breast tissue and very high risk; (1) same or contralateral breast before limited surgery; (2) search for primary tumor, if other methods are negative; (3) high family risk*; (4) monitoring of neoadjuvant therapy

Reason

Accuracy of conventional imaging is limited, and detection of malignancy within fibrosed scarring is excellent by contrast-enhanced MRI (1, 2)
These indications combine high risk for breast cancer and difficult assessment by conventional imaging (1, 2)

*Further studies are necessary to exactly define the accuracy and thus establish this indication.

Table 15-2   Indications for which Contrast-Enhanced MRI Is Not Recommended

Indication

1. Differentiation of microcalcifications
2. Differentiation of inflammation and carcinoma
3. "Screening" in the dense or lumpy breast
4. Differentiation that is possible by percutaneous biopsy as well

Reason

High false-positive rate (1-4); false-negative by MRI alone possible (1)
Too much overlap (1-4)
Too high false-positive rate (1:10) compared with prevalence of malignancy (<1:100) (3)
Even though sensitivities of core biopsy and MRI are comparable, MRI is by far less specific and not cost-effective (4)

Parenchymal Proliferation and Fibrocystic Disease

The term fibrocystic disease, or dysplasia, describes an increased proliferation of fibrous mesenchymal or glandular tissue (frequently associated with cysts) as compared with the age-related normal breast.

Nonproliferative changes are characterized by increased fibrosis, with or without cyst formation; proliferative changes are characterized by epithelial hyperplasia, which may be intraductal (papillomatous, solid, or adenomatous) or extraductal (adenotic). Proliferative changes thus include lobular, ductal, and papillary hyperplastic changes and adenosis. When cellular atypias exist, the entity is named proliferative changes with atypias. Fibrocystic disease is most frequently seen in perimenopausal women. The real incidence is difficult to estimate because the criteria are subjective. Hormones play a role in its development, but the exact pathogenesis remains obscure. It is most often bilateral and diffusely distributed throughout the breasts, but its appearance may vary greatly within or between both breasts and may be focally and asymmetrically more pronounced.

Fibrocystic changes are important for several reasons.

- Sometimes they may simulate the clinical and radiographic appearance of focally or diffusely growing carcinomas and may thus pose diagnostic problems.
- Because of the frequently increased radiographic density of breasts involved with fibrocystic changes, mammographic detection of malignancy without microcalcifications is impaired.
- In about 5% of these cases, atypias are present. They are associated with a remarkably (about by a factor of 5) increased risk of malignancy, which is even greater (about by a factor of 10) when a family history of breast cancer exists. Only a slightly increased risk (up to a factor of 2) exists for patients with proliferative changes without atypias, and no relevant risk is associated with nonproliferative changes.[20,75]

Mammographically, fibrocystic changes are characterized by an increased density compared with the age-related "normal" breast tissue. This increase of density may be pronounced, but a definitive distinction from histologically normal breast tissue with reduced surrounding fat cannot be made radiologically. In addition, increased nodularity and microcalcifications may be present. As mentioned, diffuse changes may obscure malignancy, and focally pronounced changes may falsely mimic malignancy.

On unenhanced T1-weighted images, fibrocystic (like normal nonfatty) tissue shows low signal intensity because it is primarily composed of water (long T1) or fibrosis (short T2). On T2-weighted images the signal intensity of fibrocystic changes varies, presumably depending on the amount of water present in the tissue. The greater the water fraction, the greater the signal intensity on T2-weighted images (Figure 15-7). Because the tissue composition and the resulting signal intensity of carcinomas vary as much as those of changes, no reliable diagnostic criteria exist.

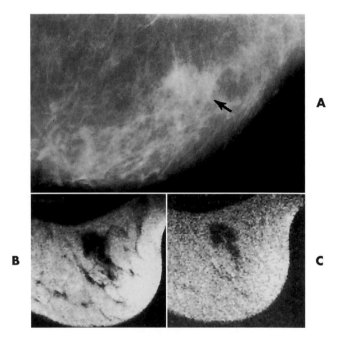

FIGURE 15-7   Focal fibrotic fibrocystic condition in the right breast of a 62-year-old woman. **A,** Craniocaudal mammogram shows focally increased density *(arrow)* in an otherwise normal fatty breast. **B,** SE 400/30 image shows low signal–intensity mass. **C,** SE 2400/90 image shows low signal intensity consistent with its collagenous composition.

Normal breast tissues and nonproliferative dysplasias in middle-aged (40 years) and older patients show little Gd chelate enhancement (Figure 15-8). Absence of enhancement has proved an important piece of information for improved exclusion of malignant disease.

Because both diffuse and focal enhancement may occur in the fourth and first weeks of the menstrual cycle[5,61] and are particularly frequent in the young patient, we do not recommend enhanced MRI as a routine method in the young patient (<35 years) with dense breast tissue. Enhanced MRI should be performed during the second or third week of the menstrual cycle (Figure 15-2). Because diffuse or focal enhancement also may be encountered during postmenopausal hormone-replacement therapy, we do not recommend enhanced MRI for patients who complain of breast tenderness during hormone-replacement therapy.[44] If hormone-replacement therapy is discontinued, enhancement subsides after a few months.

Proliferative dysplasia and adenosis may enhance to a variable degree. In most cases this enhancement is diffusely distributed, showing a milky or patchy signal increase throughout large parts or all of the

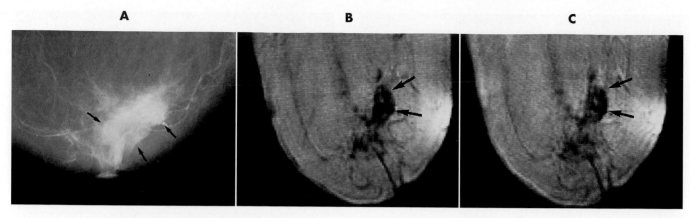

A   **B**   **C**

FIGURE 15-8   Nonproliferative fibrocystic changes (biopsy proven). MRI was performed to evaluate palpable asymmetry. **A,** Craniocaudal mammogram shows asymmetrical density *(arrows)* not present in the contralateral breast (not shown). **B,** 3D gradient-echo 40/14/50-degree image) shows the soft tissue density as a low signal–intensity mass *(arrows)*. **C,** Gd-DTPA does not enhance the mass, supporting the diagnosis of fibrocystic changes or scarring rather than malignant disease.

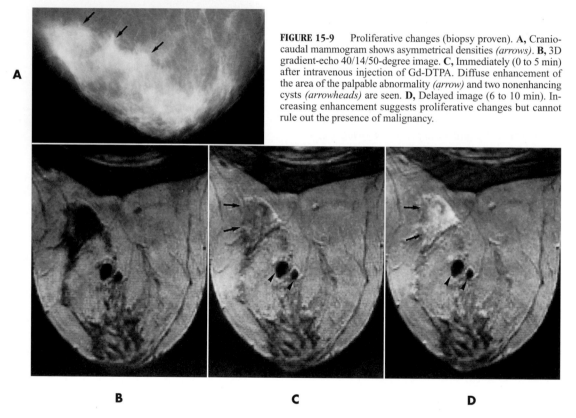

A

FIGURE 15-9   Proliferative changes (biopsy proven). **A,** Cranio-caudal mammogram shows asymmetrical densities *(arrows)*. **B,** 3D gradient-echo 40/14/50-degree image. **C,** Immediately (0 to 5 min) after intravenous injection of Gd-DTPA. Diffuse enhancement of the area of the palpable abnormality *(arrow)* and two nonenhancing cysts *(arrowheads)* are seen. **D,** Delayed image (6 to 10 min). Increasing enhancement suggests proliferative changes but cannot rule out the presence of malignancy.

B   **C**   **D**

breast tissue. The signal increase in proliferative dysplasias is usually delayed (Figure 15-9). Even though nonproliferative dysplasias in general do not enhance, there exists no reliable distinction from the premalignant atypias or proliferative dysplasias. In patients with proliferative dysplasia, only absence of enhancement allows exclusion of invasive malignancy with high probability.

When diffuse enhancement is present, early scanning after injection of Gd chelate will improve visualization of carcinomas. Because, however, a significant number of carcinomas (10% to 15%) enhance slowly or diffusely, diffuse or delayed enhancement can never exclude malignant disease. Focally enhancing proliferative dysplasia can mimic cancer (Figure 15-10).

Cysts

Simple cysts are retained fluid surrounded by a thin wall. Clinically harmless, they may become apparent as a mass on mammography or palpation. Occasionally they cause pain. MRI is (on T2-weighted im-

ages) highly sensitive and (using contrast enhancement) very specific for cyst detection and diagnosis. Sonography, by far more cost-effective, remains the principal method for diagnosis of cysts.

On T1-weighted unenhanced MR images, simple cysts exhibit very low to intermediate low signal intensity, depending on the protein contents of the cyst fluid. When surrounded by dense parenchyma of similar low signal intensity, they may vanish into the general low-signal background. Complicated cysts may contain blood products. Because of the shortening of T1 relaxation time, the fluid of these cysts shows high signal intensity. On T2-weighted images the cyst fluid is usually very intense, exceeding the intensity of fat (Figure 15-11). Blood products in breast cysts rarely are present in concentrations sufficient to reduce signal intensity on T2-weighted images.

Simple cysts do not enhance. A thin rim enhancement of the cyst wall may occur when an otherwise simple cyst becomes involved in inflammation (Figure 15-9). Irregular and nodular enhancement of the cyst wall morphologically may indicate cystic necrosis of a tumor, intracystic carcinoma, or papilloma.

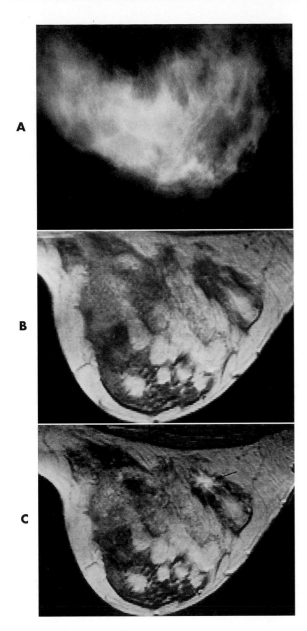

FIGURE 15-10 Focal proliferative changes. Dense asymmetrical tissue was palpated in the upper outer quadrant. **A,** Craniocaudal view. **B,** Precontrast T1 3D FLASH image is normal. **C,** Gd-DTPA–enhanced image shows stellate enhancing lesion *(arrow).* MR-guided biopsy after open needle localization yielded proliferative changes with atypia.

Fibroadenomas

Fibroadenomas are the most common breast tumor. They are usually oval or lobulated and well circumscribed. Their histological composition varies from myxoid to adenomatous to completely fibrosed (Figures 15-12 and 15-13).

On unenhanced T1-weighted images, fibroadenomas display low signal intensity. On T2-weighted images they display a spectrum of behavior, presumably resulting from the specific histological pattern and the fraction of water or fibrosis present in an individual fibroadenoma. Fibrous fibroadenomas that consist of densely packed collagen have a low signal intensity because of the short T2 of the water bound to collagen (Figure 15-14). The other fibroadenomas—adenomatous, myxoid, or mixed type—show increased signal intensity on T2-weighted images. This finding is explained by their higher cellularity and water content, which results in a longer T2. Because well-circumscribed malignancies (e.g., medullary, mucinous, or some papillary carcinomas, lymphomas, metastases, sarcomas, cystosarcomas, or involved lymph nodes) are also highly cellular or contain a high proportion of water, a

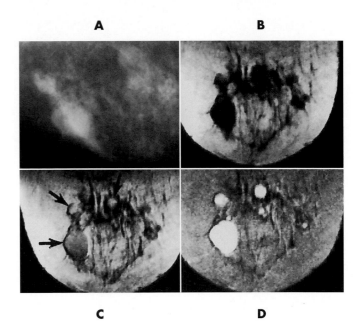

FIGURE 15-11 Multiple cysts. **A,** Craniocaudal mammogram. **B,** SE 400/30 image shows rounded lesions. **C,** SE 2400/35 image. **D,** SE 2400/90 image shows cyst signal intensity in excess of surrounding fat. Several very small cysts are now detectable.

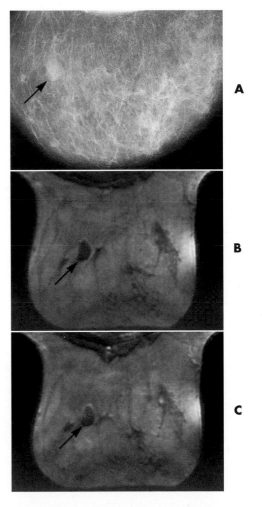

FIGURE 15-12 Fibroadenoma of the right breast. **A,** Craniocaudal mammogram. **B,** SE 400/30 image. **C,** On SE 2400/90 image the mass remains very low signal intensity consistent with its collagenous composition.

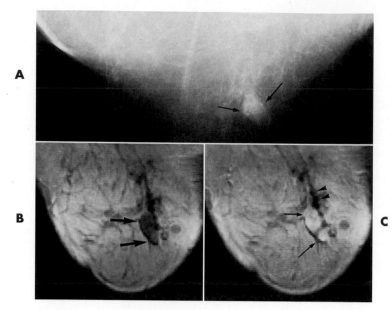

distinction between them and adenomatous or myxoid fibroadenomas is usually not possible. Both usually exhibit intermediate or high signal intensity on the T2-weighted images (Figure 15-15). However, fibrous fibroadenomas can be identified reliably because they exhibit low signal intensity on T2-weighted images.

Round or oval lobulation may be seen. The signal intensities of both the lobules and the surrounding connective tissue depend on their water content (Figure 15-16). If lobulation can be demonstrated on the T2-weighted image or postcontrast scan, a fibroadenoma is very probable. Rarely, lobulation may be seen in certain lymphomas or cystosarcomas.

Fibrous fibroadenomas enhance very little and can be distinguished from malignant disease. Unfortunately, adenomatous and myxoid fibroadenomas do enhance. Even though their enhancement is mostly delayed (whereas that of most carcinomas is fast), this distinction is not reliable. Caution is necessary because certain malignancies, including some of the well-circumscribed (medullary, papillary, and low-grade) carcinomas and lymphomas, also exhibit a delayed signal increase. Therefore core or excisional biopsy is recommended for all well-circumscribed lesions that enhance, and in the diagnostic workup of lesions that are visible by other imaging modalities or are palpable, core biopsy should be considered the method of choice.

Cancer

Breast carcinoma, the most common malignant tumor in women, is the leading cause of death in women ages 40 to 60. Integrity of the basal membrane distinguishes noninvasive (in situ) from invasive carcinoma. In situ carcinoma is a high-risk indicator; 20% to 50% of these patients may develop invasive carcinoma in the same or the contralateral breast. However, a high percentage of in situ carcinomas may

FIGURE 15-13 Cellular fibroadenoma (biopsy proven) and scar. **A,** Mammogram shows an indeterminate mass. **B,** 3D FLASH shows a low-intensity mass *(arrows)*. **C,** Gd-DTPA enhances a focal region *(arrows)* that can now be distinguished from nonenhancing scar tissue *(arrowheads)*. This appearance is consistent with the diagnosis of fibroadenoma; however, neither the lobular shape nor the amount of enhancement can exclude a well-circumscribed malignancy.

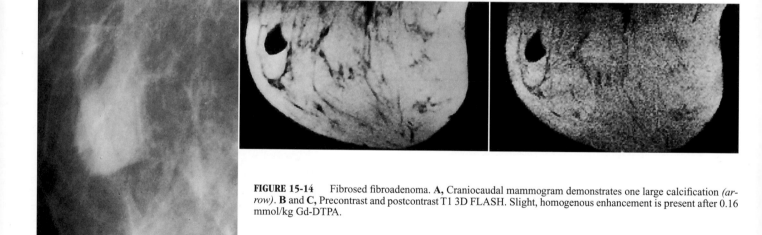

FIGURE 15-14 Fibrosed fibroadenoma. **A,** Craniocaudal mammogram demonstrates one large calcification *(arrow)*. **B** and **C,** Precontrast and postcontrast T1 3D FLASH. Slight, homogenous enhancement is present after 0.16 mmol/kg Gd-DTPA.

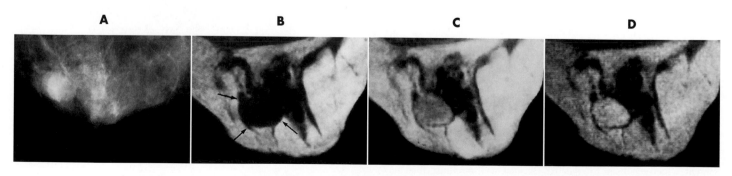

FIGURE 15-15 Mixed mucinous-medullary carcinoma. **A,** Craniocaudal mammogram. **B,** SE 400/35 image shows lesion *(arrows)* has low signal intensity similar to the adjacent dysplastic tissue. **C,** SE 1600/35 image shows inhomogeneity, excluding the diagnosis of a simple cyst. **D,** SE 1600/70 image. (From reference 41.)

never become invasive. Only invasive carcinomas have a risk of metastatic spread, a risk that increases with tumor size and histological grade.

Most invasive carcinomas are classified as ductal or lobular, according to their origin. Furthermore, numerous special types (e.g., medullary, mucinous, papillary, and tubular) exist. Within these groups great variation exists in differentiation, growth pattern, and tissue composition.

Breast cancer is detected by means of mammography and characterized primarily by morphological features or microcalcifications. About 30% of invasive carcinomas contain microcalcifications. Many invasive cancers tend to be irregular and have unsharp borders. Some grow along the ducts in diffuse or nodular patterns and cause uncharacteristic densities.

Because the majority of breast cancers have an x-ray density similar to that of nonfatty normal or dysplastic breast tissue, identification of carcinomas without microcalcifications is influenced by the appearance of surrounding fat or glandular tissue. Detection and diagnosis are impaired by dense breast tissue. Only a few of the in situ carcinomas cause (mostly uncharacteristic) palpable findings, an uncharacteristic x-ray density, or starlike configuration. The majority of the in situ carcinomas are identified by detection of microcalcifications. Microcalcifications cannot be visualized by means of MRI.

Unenhanced MRI shows carcinomas as low signal intensity on T1-weighted images and variably increased signal intensity on T2-weighted images (Figure 15-17). Because benign tissues display similar variations, no specific diagnostic features exist on unenhanced MRI. Even though morphology may sometimes be displayed very nicely, unenhanced MRI does not contribute significant information for the detection of breast cancer.

Enhanced MRI can contribute valuable additional information simply because the majority of invasive carcinomas enhance more than normal glandular tissue or fat.* This enhancement is generally fast, strong, focal, and irregularly circumscribed. Such type of enhancement is typical for malignancy (Figures 15-15 to 15-18). Early wash-out, which may be seen in part of the carcinomas, is another specific finding of malignancy. However, in about 10% of the invasive carcinomas, the enhancement may be delayed, well circumscribed, or diffuse (in diffusely growing carcinomas or in carcinomas, which are surrounded by diffusely enhancing benign tissue; Figure 15-19). Minimal† enhancement in invasive carcinomas is a rare finding. It may be the result of poor technique or a threshold too high for recognizing enhancement. Only few invasive carcinomas (lobular or mucinous) without significant enhancement have been reported (2%).

More than 80% of in situ carcinomas do enhance.‡ Because only 40% to 50% of in situ carcinomas exhibit an enhancement typical for malignancy, close correlation with mammography is even more important for the diagnosis of in situ carcinomas. Because the majority of in situ carcinomas contain microcalcifications, errors can be avoided when MRI is interpreted together with x-ray mammography. Only those in situ carcinomas that exhibit a so-called typical enhancement can be diagnosed by means of MRI alone, even in the absence of microcalcifications visible on x-ray films (Figures 15-19 to 15-21).

---

*References 1, 8, 9, 12, 23-28, 30, 32, 36, 38, 39, 41-50, 55, 79, 82.
†The exact threshold depends on the chosen pulse sequence parameters and field strength.[50]
‡References 10, 15, 31, 45, 47, 49.

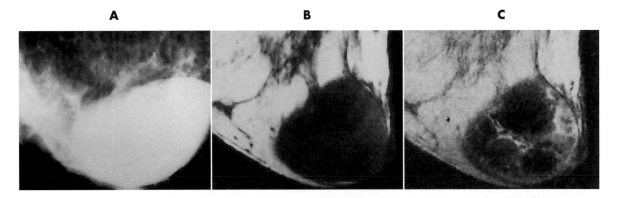

FIGURE 15-16   Large fibroadenomas. **A,** Craniocaudal mammogram. **B,** SE 400/30 image. **C,** SE 2400/90 image shows detailed internal architectural pattern of fibroadenoma, reflecting its inhomogeneous cellular composition.

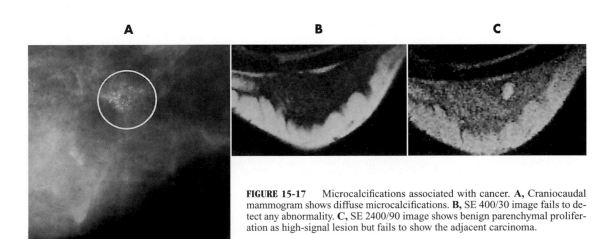

FIGURE 15-17   Microcalcifications associated with cancer. **A,** Craniocaudal mammogram shows diffuse microcalcifications. **B,** SE 400/30 image fails to detect any abnormality. **C,** SE 2400/90 image shows benign parenchymal proliferation as high-signal lesion but fails to show the adjacent carcinoma.

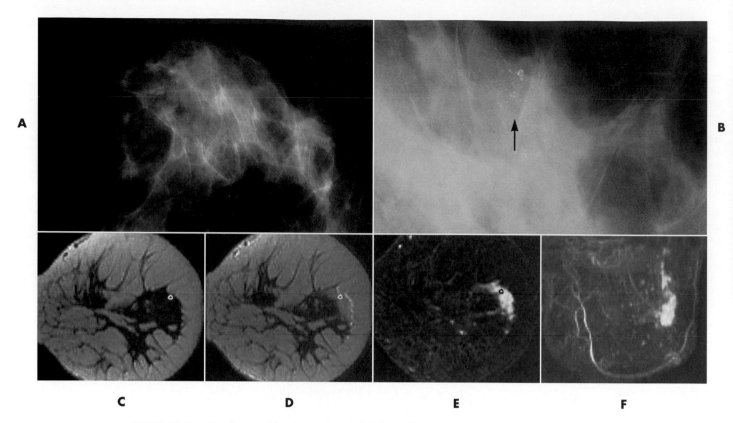

FIGURE 15-18 Carcinoma with enhancement typical for malignancy. **A,** Mammogram; craniocaudal view. **B,** Mammogram; magnified view. Suspicious microcalcifications *(arrow).* **C,** Precontrast image 3D gradient-echo 14/7/25-degree image. **D,** Post–0.2 mmol Gd-DTPA/kg. Enhancing carcinoma extends in a much larger area than suspected mammographically. **E,** Subtraction image (**D** minus **C**) demonstrates the strongly enhancing carcinoma and subcutaneous vessels (v). **F,** 3D reconstruction of the complete set of (individually) subtracted slices shows large extent of the invasive carcinoma *(arrow)* and intraductal extent of in situ tumor *(arrowheads)* toward the chest wall (histologically confirmed). Arrows show 5-mm enhancing intramammary lymph node, with biopsy-proven cancer.

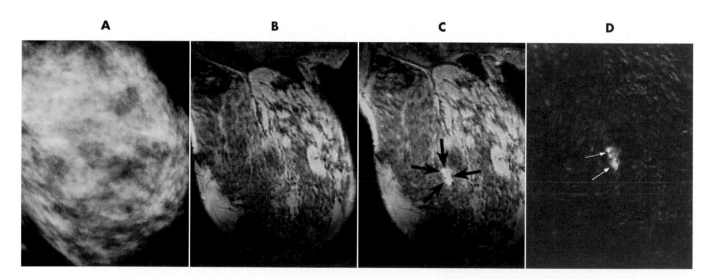

FIGURE 15-19 Ductal in situ carcinoma. Asymptomatic 38-year-old woman who had a small carcinoma removed previously during biopsy of a fibroadenoma. MRI was obtained to search for other malignancies. **A,** Mediolateral mammogram before biopsy. Dense breast shows no sign of malignant disease. **B** and **C,** Precontrast and postcontrast transverse 3D FLASH images show a suspicious enhancing lesion *(arrows)* far away from the initial biopsy site. **D,** Subtraction shows enhancement only within the carcinoma *(arrows)* and some vessels. This tiny lesion was nonpalpable and visible only on MRI; MR-guided needle localization was used to guide excision. (From Heywang SH, et al: J Comput Assist Tomogr 14[3], 1990.)

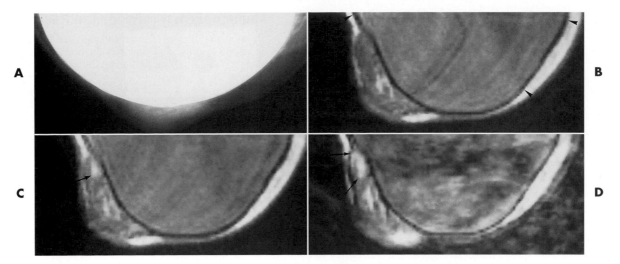

FIGURE 15-20   Recurrent lobular in situ carcinoma adjacent to a prosthetic implant. MRI was performed on this asymptomatic patient 1 year after subcutaneous mastectomy and silicone implant as a routine screening test for carcinoma. **A,** Craniocaudal mammogram shows remaining breast tissue behind the nipple, with evidence of scarring. There are no microcalcifications or other evidence of malignancy. **B,** Transverse 3D FLASH image shows the implant *(arrowheads)* and remaining retroareolar breast tissue. **C,** Gd-DTPA–enhanced images (0 to 5 min). **D,** Delayed images (7 to 10 min). Cardiac motion artifacts over breast. A slowly but strongly enhancing area is seen lateral to the implant *(arrows)*. Excision via MR-guided needle localization proved recurrent carcinoma in situ.

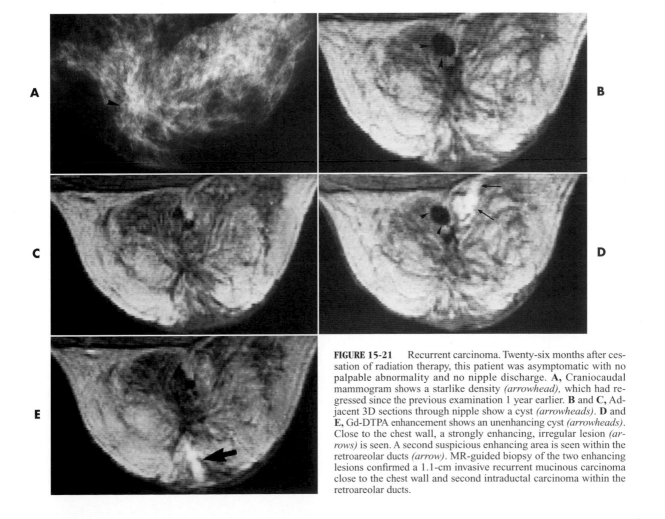

FIGURE 15-21   Recurrent carcinoma. Twenty-six months after cessation of radiation therapy, this patient was asymptomatic with no palpable abnormality and no nipple discharge. **A,** Craniocaudal mammogram shows a starlike density *(arrowhead)*, which had regressed since the previous examination 1 year earlier. **B** and **C,** Adjacent 3D sections through nipple show a cyst *(arrowheads)*. **D** and **E,** Gd-DTPA enhancement shows an unenhancing cyst *(arrowheads)*. Close to the chest wall, a strongly enhancing, irregular lesion *(arrows)* is seen. A second suspicious enhancing area is seen within the retroareolar ducts *(arrow)*. MR-guided biopsy of the two enhancing lesions confirmed a 1.1-cm invasive recurrent mucinous carcinoma close to the chest wall and second intraductal carcinoma within the retroareolar ducts.

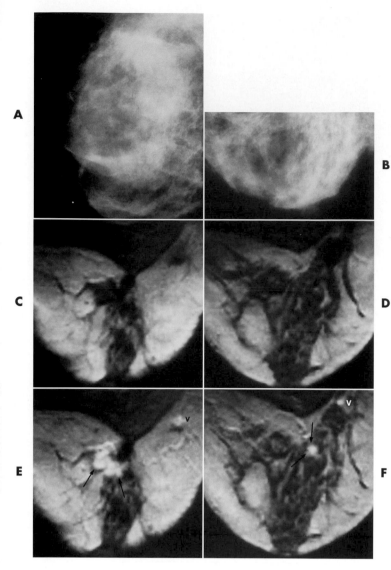

FIGURE 15-22   Recurrent malignancy within scar. MRI was performed in this patient because of persistent thickening within a surgical scar, which had not changed since excision of a stage T1 carcinoma 2 years previously. Oblique (**A**) and craniocaudal (**B**) mammograms. Suspicious irregular tissue in the upper outer quadrant had persisted since biopsy. **C**, T1-weighted 3D FLASH image at the level of the scar. **D**, 2 cm caudal to scar. **E**, Gd-DTPA–enhanced image shows significant focal enhancement *(arrows)*, indicating recurrent carcinoma within the unenhancing scar tissue. **F**, Image 2 cm caudal shows a second suspicious enhancing focus *(arrows)*. At surgery this proved to be a second 4-mm enhancing focus *(arrows)*. *V,* Enhancing vessel.

Lymph Nodes

MR examinations of the breast often fail to adequately image lymph nodes because of ghost artifacts overlying the retrosternal chain and the small field of view, which excludes the axillae.

Early claims that MRI can distinguish lymph nodes containing metastases on the basis of prolonged T2 have been widely discredited. Gd-DTPA enhancement may identify malignant involvement in lymph nodes because breast cancer will show enhancement in any of its locations. However, distinction between malignant and inflammatory changes often is not possible. Micrometastases to lymph nodes are not detectable by any imaging modality. Because micrometastases are common and clinically relevant, surgical sampling of axillary nodes continues to provide the most accurate diagnosis. It remains to be seen whether iron oxide particles or other functional contrast agents will be useful in a clinical setting.

Mammoplasty, Scarring, and Radiation Changes

Scarring after tumor resection and radiation therapy, cosmetic surgery, or wound healing may impair evaluation and diagnostic accuracy of palpation and imaging. Malignant disease may be either mimicked or obscured by scarring.

The tissue around silicone implants after reconstructive surgery is most difficult to evaluate because even with special mammographic views only part of the tissue is visualized.

Healing scars or granulation tissues enhance to a variable degree. Because most scars exhibit a delayed enhancement, whereas most carcinomas exhibit early enhancement, MRI may be quite helpful in the distinction between scarring and malignancy.*

More than 6 months after surgery, scar tissue (stable fibrosis) usually does not enhance. At this stage the distinction between malignancy and scarring is excellent (Figures 15-20 to 15-22).

During the first 12 months after irradiation, variable, early, and patchy enhancement is seen throughout the breast. At this stage, enhanced MRI is not useful. This enhancement usually abates 12 to 18 months after irradiation. More than 18 months after irradiation, little or no enhancement is present throughout the breast. At this stage, enhanced MRI can help exclude recurrent cancer.† Its major advantage, however, concerns very sensitive detection of early recurrence: Information that is most helpful within mammographically dense or distorted tissue (Figure 15-21).

In patients with silicone implants after reconstructive surgery, scar tissue behaves like that after surgery or like scarring after irradiation, depending on the preceding therapy. Breast tissue surrounding the implant can more easily be evaluated with MR than by means of x-ray mammography. In one study in which enhanced MRI was offered to 120 patients with silicone implants, 4 of 8 recurrences were detected with MRI alone. Some false-positive findings were proved to be inflammatory granulomas.[10,44,45] Inflammatory granulomas are nodular lesions with strong and mostly early enhancement. Because they cannot be distinguished from malignant disease by their enhancement, small enhancing nodules should be reexamined within 3 months.

SUMMARY

Unenhanced MRI is not useful in detecting or staging breast cancer. Contrast-enhanced MRI, however, may contribute valuable additional information to conventional x-ray mammography. Technical prerequisites for contrast-enhanced MRI are imaging with high spatial and fast temporal resolution (optimally every 1 to 3 min after intravenous injection of Gd chelate). Fat elimination (by subtraction or suppression) is necessary.

Clinical situations in which a high false-positive (or even false-negative) rate may be expected (Table 15-2) are to be avoided. MRI is most often indicated for detection or staging of cancers poorly seen with conventional x-ray mammography (e.g., scarring, dense tissue) and in patients with highly increased risk (e.g., exclusion of multicentricity in cases with proven small malignancy, follow-up studies after treatment of malignancy) (Table 15-1).

---

*References 8, 19, 28, 30, 32, 34, 44, 86.
†References 15, 44, 45, 47, 62, 78.

REFERENCES

1. Allgayer B, Hauck W, Jänicke F, et al: MRT-Diagnostik von Mammakarzinomen mit einem nicht-ionischen Kontrastmittel in 2D- und 3D-Gradientenecho-FFE-Technik, Radiologe 35/4(Suppl 1):S84, 1995.
2. Allgayer B, Imhof M, Kutschker C, et al: Dynamische MRT-Untersuchungen von Mammatumoren Vergleich: Kontrastenhancement vs. Vaskularisationsgrad, Radiologe 35/4(Suppl 1):S83, 1995.
3. Balu-Maestro C, Bruneton JN, Melia P, et al: High frequency ultrasound detection of breast calcifications, Eur J Ultrasound 3:247, 1994.
4. Bassett LW, and Kimme-Smith C: Breast sonography, Am J Roentgenol 156:449, 1991.
5. Beck R, Heywang-Köbrunner SH, and Untch M: Contrast-enhancement of proliferative dysplasia in MRI of the breast due to the menstrual cycle. In European Congress of Radiology 93, Book of abstracts. New York, 1993, Springer-Verlag
6. Bird RE, Wallace TW, and Yankaskas BC: Analysis of cancers missed at screening mammography, Radiology 184:613, 1992.
7. Bjurstam N: Early carcinoma, the great mimic, Vortrag beim Nicer Breast Imaging Course der Scandinavian Society of Mammography, Radiology 173:354, 1989.

8. Boetes C: Magnetic resonance imaging of breast cancer, a clinical study, Doktorarbeit an der Katholischen Universität Nimwegen, Nimwegen, 1995, Janssen Print.
9. Boetes C, Barentz JO, Mus RD, et al: MR characterization of suspicious breast lesions with a gadolinium-enhanced TurboFLASH subtraction technique, Radiology 193:777, 1994.
10. Bone B, Aspelin P, Isberg B, et al: Contrast-enhanced MRI of the breast in patients with breast implants after cancer surgery, Acta Radiologica 36:111, 1995.
11. Bovee WMMJ, Getreuer KW, Smidt J, et al: Nuclear magnetic resonance and detection of human breast tumors, J Natl Cancer Inst 61:53, 1978.
12. Buchberger W, Kapfer M, Stöger A, et al: Dignitätsbeurteilung fokaler Mammaläsionen: prospektiver Vergleich von Mammographie, Sonographie und dynamischer MRT, Radiologe 35/4(Suppl 1):S86, 1995.
13. Ciatto S, Roselli-del-Turco M, Catarzis, et al: The diagnostic role of breast echography, Radiol-Med (Torino) 88(3):221, 1994.
14. Damadian R: Tumor detection by nuclear magnetic resonance, Science 171:1151, 1971.
15. Dao TH, Rahmouni A, Campana F, et al: Tumor recurrence versus fibrosis in the irradiated breast: differentiation with dynamic gadolinium-enhanced MR imaging, Radiology 187:751, 1993.
16. Deimling M, and Loeffler W: Fast simultaneous acquisition of fat and water images, Society of Magnetic Resonance in Medicine 8th Annual Meeting, Amsterdam, In (Book of abstracts), Berkeley, 1989, The Society.
17. Dempsey P, and Rubin E: The roles of needle biopsy and periodic follow up in the evaluation and diagnosis of breast lesions, Semin Roentgenol 28:252, 1993.
18. D'Orsi CJ: To follow or not to follow, that is the question, Radiology 184:306, 1992.
19. Dresel V, Bühner M, Schulz-Wendtland R, et al: Intraduktale Karzinome der Mamma—ist eine Diagnose in der Kernspintomographie möglich? Radiologe 35/4(Suppl):S87, 1995.
20. Dupont WD, and Page DL: Risk factors for breast cancer in women with proliferative disease, N Engl J Med 312:146, 1985.
21. Elvecrog EL, Lechner MC, and Nelson MT: Nonpalpable breast lesions: correlation of stereotaxic large-core needle biopsy and surgical biopsy results, Radiology 188:453, 1993.
22. El Yousef SJ, Alfidi RJ, Duchesneau RH, et al: Initial experience with nuclear magnetic resonance (NMR) imaging of the human breast, J Comput Assist Tomogr 7:215, 1983.
23. Fischer U, Brinck U, Schauer S, et al: Korrelation von Anreicherungs verhalten in der MR-Mammographie mit immunhistochemischen Prognosefaktoren, Der Radiologe 35/4 (Suppl):S85, 1995.
24. Fischer U, Heyden D, Vosshenrich R, et al: Signal/time relation of malignant and nonmalignant lesions in contrast-enhanced MR imaging of the breast, Roe Fo 158:287, 1993.
25. Fischer U, Kopka L, Vosshenrich R, et al: Invasive mucinous carcinoma of the breast missed by contrast-enhanced MR mammography, Eur Radiol 6:929, 1995.
26. Fischer U, Vosshenrich R, Keating D, et al: MR-guided biopsy of suspect breast lesions with a simple stereotaxic add-on device for surface coils, Radiology 192:272, 1994.
27. Fischer U, Vosshenrich R, Probst A, et al: Preoperative MR mammography in patients with breast cancer—useful information or useless extravagance? Roe Fo 161/4:300, 1994.
28. Fischer U, Westerhoff JP, Brinck U, et al: Das Erscheinungsbild des duktalen Carcinoma in situ in der dynamischen MR-Mammographie, Roe Fo 164(4):290, 1995.
29. Fletcher SW, Black W, Harris R, et al: Report of the International Workshop on Screening for Breast Cancer, National Cancer Institute 85(28):1644, 1993.
30. Gilles R, Guinebretiere J, Lucidarme O, et al: Non-palpable breast tumors: diagnosis with contrast-enhanced subtraction dynamic MR imaging, Radiology 191:625, 1994.
31. Gilles R, Guinebretiere J, Shapeero LG, et al: Assessment of breast cancer recurrence with contrast-enhanced subtraction MR imaging: preliminary results in 26 patients, Radiology 188:473, 1993.
32. Gilles R, Guinebretiere J, Toussaint C, et al: Locally advanced breast cancer: contrast-enhanced subtraction MR imaging of response to preoperative chemotherapy, Radiology 191:633, 1994.
33. Goldsmith M, Koutcher JA, and Damadian R: NMR in cancer. XIII, Application of the NMR malignancy index to human mammary tumors, Br J Cancer 38:547, 1978.
34. Greenstein Orel SG, Schnall MD, Li Volsi VA, et al: Suspicious breast lesions: MR imaging with radiologic-pathologic correlation, Radiology 190:485, 1994.
35. Greenstein Orel SG, Schnall MD, Newman RW, et al: MR imaging-guided localization and biopsy of breast lesions: initial experience, Radiology 193:97, 1994.
36. Greenstein Orel SG, Schnall MD, Powell CM, et al: Staging of suspected breast cancer: effect of MR imaging and MR guided biopsy, Radiology 196:115, 1995.
37. Hachiya J, Seki T, and Okada M: MR imaging of the breast with Gd-DTPA enhancement: comparison with mammography and ultrasonography, Radiat Med 9:232, 1991.
38. Harms SE, Flaming DP, Hesley KL, et al: Fat suppressed three dimensional MR imaging of the breast, Radiographics 13:247, 1993.
39. Harms SE, Flaming DP, Hesley KL, et al: MR imaging of the breast with rotating delivery of excitation off resonance: clinical experience with pathologic correlation, Radiology 187:493, 1993.
40. Harvey JA, Fajardo LL, and Innis CA: Previous mammograms in patients with impalpable breast carcinoma: retrospective versus blinded interpretation, Am J Roentgenol 161:1167, 1993.
41. Heywang SH, Fenzl G, Hahn D, et al: MR of the breast: histopathologic correlation, Eur J Radiol 3/7:175-183, 1987.
42. Heywang SH, Hahn D, Schmid H, et al: MR imaging of the breast using gadolinium-DTPA, J Comput Assist Tomogr 10:199, 1986.
43. Heywang SH, Hilbertz T, Pruss E, et al: Dynamische Kontrastmitteluntersuchungen mit FLASH bei Kernspintomographie der Mamma, Digitale Bilddiagnostik 8:7, 1988.
44. Heywang-Köbrunner SH, and Beck R: Contrast-enhanced MRI of the breast, New York, 1996, Springer.
45. Heywang-Köbrunner SH, Beck R, Wendt T, et al: Stellenwert der Kontrastmittelkernspintomographie bei der Diagnostik des Lokalrezidivs. In Schmid L, and Wilmanns W, eds: Prakt Onkologie III, München, 1993, W. Zuckschwerdt.
46. Heywang-Köbrunner SH, Haustein J, Pohl C, et al: Contrast-enhanced MRI of the breast—comparison of two dosages of Gd-DTPA, Radiology 191:639, 1994.
47. Heywang-Köbrunner SH, Schlegel A, Beck R, et al: Contrast-enhanced MRI of the breast after limited surgery and radiation therapy, J Comput Assist Tomogr 17:891, 1993.
48. Heywang-Köbrunner SH, and Viehweg P: Sensitivity of contrast-enhanced MR imaging of the breast. In Davis PL, ed: Breast imaging, Magn Res Imag Clin North Am 2:527, 1994.
49. Heywang-Köbrunner SH, Viehweg P, Heinig A, et al: Contrast-enhanced MRI of the breast: accuracy, value, controversies, and solutions, Eur J Radiol 24:94, 1997.
50. Heywang-Köbrunner SH, Wolf HD, Deimling M, et al: Misleading changes of the signal intensity on opposed phase images after injection of contrast medium, J Comput Assist Tomogr 20:173, 1996.
51. Homer MJ: Breast imaging: pitfalls, controversies and some practical thoughts, Radiol Clin North Am 23:459, 1985.
52. Ikeda DM, Bondeson L, Helvie MA, et al: Evaluation of nonpalpable breast nodules: 4-month mammographic follow-up versus x-ray guided fine-needle aspiration, Breast Dis 4:205, 1991.
53. Jackson VP, Hendrick RE, and Feig FA: Imaging of the radiographically dense breast, Radiology 188:297, 1993.
54. Kaiser WA: MRM promises earlier breast cancer diagnosis, Diagn Imaging 88-93, 1992.
55. Kaiser WA: MR-mammographie, der Radiologe 33:292, 1993.
56. Kaiser WA, and Zeitler E: MR imaging of the breast: fast imaging sequences with and without Gd-DTPA, Radiology 170:681, 1989.
57. Knopp MV, Heβ T, Junkermann HJ, et al: Diagnostischer Stellenwert der MR-Mammographie bei nicht palpablen durch Vorsorgeuntersuchung detektierten Herden, Radiologe 35(4):81, 1995.
58. Kopans DB: Mammography screening for breast cancer, Cancer 72:1809, 1993.
59. Kuhl CK, Elevelt A, Gieseke J, et al: MR-mammographisch gesteuerte stereotaktische Markierung klinisch: mammographisch und sonographisch okkulter Läsionen durch eine Lokalisations- und Biopsiespule, Radiologe 35:S80, 1995.
60. Kuhl CK, Kreft BP, Hauswirth A, et al: MR-Mammographie bei 0.5 Tesla, Roe Fo 162:482, 1995.
61. Kuhl CK, Seibert C, Kneft BP, et al: Focal and diffuse contrast enhancement in dynamic MR mammography of healthy volunteers, Radiology 193:121, 1994.
62. Lewis Jones HG, Whitehouse GH, and Leinster SJ: The role of MRI in the assessment of local recurrent breast carcinoma, Clin Radiol 43:19, 1991.
63. Liberman L, Dershaw DD, Rosen PP, et al: Stereotaxic 14-gauge breast biopsy. How many core biopsy specimens are needed? Radiology 192:793, 1994.
64. Mansfield P, Morris PG, Ordidge R, et al: Carcinoma of the breast imaged by nuclear magnetic resonance (NMR), Br J Radiol 52:242, 1979.
65. McSweeney MB, Small WC, Cerny V, et al: Magnetic resonance imaging in the diagnosis of breast disease: use of transverse relaxation times, Radiology 153:741, 1984.
66. Medina D, Hazelwood CF, Cleveland GG, et al: Nuclear magnetic resonance studies on human breast dysplasias and neoplasma, J Natl Cancer Inst 54:813, 1975.
67. Murphy WA, and Gohagan JK: Breast. In Stark DD, and Bradley WG Jr, eds: Magnetic resonance imaging, ed 1, St. Louis, 1987, Mosby.
68. Nyström L, Rutqvist LE, Wall S, et al: Breast cancer screening with mammography: an overview of the Swedish randomized trials, Lancet 341:974, 1993.
69. Oellinger H, Heins S, Sander B, et al: Gd-DTPA enhanced MR breast imaging: the most sensitive method for multicentric carcinomas of the female breast, Eur Radiol 3(3):223, 1993.
70. Page DL, and Winfield AC: The dense mammogram, Am J Roentgenol 147:487, 1986.
71. Pamilo M, Soiva M, Anttinen I, et al: Ultrasonography of breast lesions detected in mammography screening, Acta Radiol 32:220, 1991.
72. Parker SH, Burbank F, Jackmann RJ, et al: Percutaneous large-core breast biopsy: a multiinstitutional study, Radiology 193:359, 1994.
73. Porter BA, and Smith JP: MRI enhances breast CA detection and staging, Diagn Imaging 18, 1993.
74. Potterton AJ, Peakman DJ, and Young IR: Ultrasound demonstration of small breast cancers detected by mammographic screening, Clin Radiol 49:808, 1994.
75. Prechtel K, Gehm O, Geiger G, et al: Die Histologie der Mastopathie und die kumulative ipsilaterale Mammakarzinomsequenz, Pathologe 15:158, 1994.
76. Roberts MM, Alexander FE, Anderson TJ, et al: Edinburgh trial of screening for breast cancer: mortality at seven years, Lancet 335:241, 1990.
77. Ross RJ, Thompson JS, Kim K, et al: Nuclear magnetic resonance imaging and evaluation of human breast tissue: preliminary clinical trials, Radiology 143:195, 1982.
78. Schutz-Wendtland R, Krämer S, Döinghaus K, et al: MR mammography in the diagnosis of local recurrences in breast cancer, Eur Radiol 7(Suppl):242, 1997.
79. Sittek H, Kessler M, Brendl T, et al: Dynamische FLASH-3D MR-Mammographie-Vergleich mit standardisierter Mammographie, Radiologe 35:S199, 1995.
80. Stack JP, Redmond V, Codd MB, et al: Breast disease: tissue characterization with Gd-DTPA-enhancement profiles, Radiology 174:491, 1990.
81. Szumowski J, Eisen JK, Vinitski S, et al: Hybrid methods of chemical shift imaging, J Magn Reson Med 9:379, 1989.
82. Tontsch P, Bauer M, Schulz-Wendtland R, et al: Dynamische MR-Mammographie bei 160 Hochrisikopatientinnen, Radiologe 35(4):83, 1995.
83. Van Dijck JAAM, Verbeek ALM, Hendriks JHCL, et al: The current detectability of breast cancer in a mammographic screening program, Cancer 72:1933, 1993.
84. Weinreb JC, and Newstead G: Controversies in breast MRI, Magn Reson Q 10(2):67, 1994.
85. Wiener JI, Chako AC, Merten CW, et al: Breast and axillary tissue MR imaging: correlations of signal intensities and relaxation times with pathologic findings, Radiology 160:299, 1986.
86. Zapf S, Halbsguth A, Brunier A, et al: Möglichkeiten der MRT in der Diagnostik nichtpalpabler Mammatumoren, Roe Fo 154:106, 1991.

16 Staging for Breast Cancer Treatment

Steven E. Harms

✓ KEY POINTS

- Breast MRI is cost-effective when used properly.
- Morphological criteria are helpful in predicting malignancy.
- Delineation of disease extent guides biopsy, excision, radiation, and other nonsurgical therapies.

Advances in breast cancer diagnosis have allowed earlier detection of the disease. The detection of small or early cancers has resulted from widespread screening programs. Conventional diagnostic methods, however, are limited in their ability to accurately determine disease extent. Decisions concerning breast cancer treatment are based on the extent of disease determined by clinical and imaging examinations and the estimated "subclinical" component that is projected from clinical trials information. This has led many treatment specialists to conclude that often more extensive therapy is being provided than is necessary to adequately treat the disease because treatment is based on the potential tumor extent rather than the actual demonstration of disease by diagnostic imaging in a particular patient.

High-contrast, high-resolution magnetic resonance imaging (MRI) methods have recently been developed for the accurate determination of disease extent within the breast. The use of high-quality MR staging can significantly alter treatment decisions, reducing morbidity and health care costs. In this chapter, the use of MRI for the clinical management of breast cancer is summarized, and the clinical integration of breast MRI is developed with several potential medical decision pathways.[12,30-37,65,66,71]

TECHNICAL CONSIDERATIONS

Effective breast MRI is based on high-contrast and high-spatial resolution with a rapid scan time.[12,30-37,65,66,71] Dynamic imaging studies demonstrate that tumor or background enhancement is adversely af-fected by scan times of longer than 5 min with a peak separation of around 2 to 3 min.[39,46,89] In contrast to many other cancers, breast cancer almost never forms a discrete margin with adjacent parenchyma. Instead, breast cancer is often intermixed with surrounding benign tissue. The cancer either extends as rays of infiltrating tumor cells into the surrounding area or is confined by the basement membrane of the ducts.[68] The demonstration of breast cancer by MRI is therefore significantly impaired by volume-averaging effects. Although the detrimental effects of volume averaging are best addressed with a combination of high-contrast and high-spatial resolution, there are tradeoffs. Lesion detectability at a lower spatial resolution could take place if a significantly higher contrast image is generated. The validation of diagnostic capability with a particular sequence cannot be readily extrapolated to methods with different contrast and spatial resolution.

Field Strength

The only MR methods validated for effective breast cancer staging at this time use 1.5 Tesla (T) scanners. The lower signal-to-noise ratio (SNR), reduced chemical shift, and different tissue contrast at mid and low fields could significantly impair the ability to produce the high-spatial and contrast resolution in a scan time of less than 5 minutes. Therefore the use of scanners of less than 1.5 T for breast cancer staging is not currently justified by scientific data.[12,30-37,65,66,71]

Staging Technique

Most commercially available breast MRI methods were inspired by the need for improved specificity of imaging diagnosis before biopsy is performed. The use of MRI before biopsy arose from centers where clinicians were concerned about surgical biopsies for false-positive results on mammograms. The success of core needle biopsies has reduced this problem in most centers. Needle biopsies can be performed for less cost than MRI and provide true histology.

The technical requirements for staging are significantly different from the MRI-before-biopsy application. The MRI-before-biopsy application is designed to improve the specificity of imaging diagnosis for a mammographically positive lesion. To achieve that goal, most users focus on dynamic imaging at the expense of lower spatial resolution. An example of the image quality typically obtained with low-resolution conventional MR sequences for MRI before biopsy is shown in Figure 16-1. The staging application has the goal of better demonstration of disease extending beyond the mammographically detected lesion. To better show this mammographically occult disease, the technology focuses on better spatial resolution and less temporal resolution while maintaining sufficient scan speed to preserve contrast resolution.

INTERPRETATION CRITERIA

There is consensus among almost all published series that the lack of MR contrast enhancement is a strong predictor for a benign lesion (> 95% negative predictive value). The sensitivity of high-resolution, high-contrast *r*otating *d*elivery of *e*xcitation *o*ff resonance (RODEO) MRI is very high, even when compared with serial pathological sectioning.[62] However, the presence of enhancement alone does not always indicate a malignant lesion because the specificity is only about 40%. The challenge for the development of diagnostic interpretation criteria for MR breast imaging is to maintain the high sensitivity for malignancy while improving specificity.*

---

*References 9, 13, 14, 21, 22, 27, 28, 38, 47, 60, 62, 64, 68, 80.

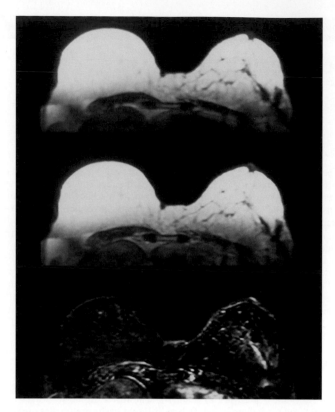

FIGURE 16-1 Conventional breast MRI. Two-dimensional, T1-weighted spin-echo images before *(top)* and after *(middle)* gadolinium contrast administration depict no obvious abnormality. The subtraction images *(bottom)* are used to detect differences in contrast enhancement. A subtle area of enhancement in the left breast was later found to be a false-positive result. The large field of view needed for both breasts reduces resolution. The subtraction method results in low SNR images. The thick slices are used to improve SNR and acquisition speed. Obviously, small lesions would be difficult to detect and characterize. Note the difficulty in obtaining suitable homogeneity over the large field of view needed to cover two breasts. The right breast is considerably more intense than the left. Motion artifacts are accentuated on the subtraction image, particularly along the chest wall, where false-positive hyperintense signal is seen as a result of image misregistration.

Morphological Criteria

As with mammography, the morphological appearance of a lesion with MRI greatly varies with the histology. Similar criteria developed for breast MRI have also closely correlated with the pathology.[1,2,74,87,88] The appearances used for morphological correlation are described in Table 16-1. Other characteristics visible on MRI include the following:

- Punctate or stippled areas of enhancement are almost always benign (98%), particularly if they are distributed widely throughout the breast or if they are located within the upper outer quadrant. This enhancement pattern most commonly is associated with fibrocystic change but can be seen with atypical hyperplasia, lobular carcinoma in situ (LCIS), and occasionally ductal carcinoma in situ (DCIS). This pattern is also seen in premenopausal women and can change during the menstrual cycle.
- Smoothly marginated enhancement is predictive of benign disease (95%). Smooth margination is often seen with sclerosing adenosis, fibroadenoma, atypical hyperplasia, and fibrocystic change.
- Lobulation and septation (Figure 16-2) are usually associated with fibroadenoma and are highly predictive of benign disease (95%). Mucinous carcinoma (2% of breast cancers) can have an appearance similar to that of fibroadenoma. The two mucinous carcinomas in our se-

Table 16-1 MR Morphological Findings and Usual Pathological Diagnosis

MR FINDING	USUAL PATHOLOGICAL FINDING
No enhancement	Benign
Diffuse, stippled enhancement	Benign, usually fibrocystic change
Smoothly marginated enhancement	Benign
Lobulated enhancement	Benign, usually fibroadenoma
Septated enhancement	Benign, usually fibroadenoma
Clumped globular enhancement	Malignant, usually DCIS
Clumped enhancement interspersed with tiny magnetic susceptibility effects	Malignant, usually comedo-type DCIS
Ductal pattern enhancement	Malignant, usually DCIS
Ring enhancement	Malignant, usually infiltrating cancer
Spiculated enhancement	Malignant, usually infiltrating cancer

DCIS, Ductal carcinoma in situ.

ries had lobulated margins with internal septations.[19] These lesions are also difficult to distinguish from fibroadenoma on physical examination, mammography, and ultrasonography. Recent reports indicate that these malignancies also have a dynamic enhancement pattern that is indistinguishable from that of fibroadenoma.

- Coalescent globules of abnormal enhancement (clumped) have been highly associated with DCIS (83%). Another sign of DCIS is the arrangement of clumped enhancement in a linear fashion along a duct extending like a ray toward the nipple. This duct pattern is highly predictive of DCIS involvement (100%) but was seen in only 15% of cases. Microcalcifications (Figure 16-3) seen as small foci of hypointensity amid the clumped enhancement are associated with comedo-type DCIS (90%).
- Spiculated enhancement is highly predictive of malignancy (85%), usually invasive cancer (Figure 16-4). Our invasive lobular carcinomas showed spiculated enhancement in 90% of cases. We had two cases of microabscesses that showed spiculated enhancement after surgical biopsy. Ring enhancement is even more predictive of malignancy (90%) but was much less common (18% of malignancies) and almost always seen with spiculation.

Extent Criteria

The goal for the development of extent criteria is to form methods of MR interpretation that would not only improve the specificity of diagnosis but also provide information that would be helpful in forming treatment decisions. Table 16-2 summarizes the extent criteria currently used for MR interpretation. Potentially, patients with S1, S2, and S3 disease would be eligible for breast-conservation surgery. Patients with S1 disease could be treated with lumpectomy alone, and patients with S2 or S3 disease would probably be treated with lumpectomy with radiation therapy (Figure 16-5). If the lesion/breast size ratio is large enough to preclude breast conservation, patients with S1, S2, S3, and M1 disease could undergo induction chemotherapy to downstage to less extensive disease before breast-conservation surgery (Figure 16-6). Patients who have a partial response to chemotherapy that results in postchemotherapy stages S1, S2, and S3 could be treated with breast conservation. Typically, stage M1, M2, and M3 disease would be treated with mastectomy. Complete response to chemotherapy would be classified as stage 0. Induction chemotherapy would be used in some of the patients with M2 and M3 disease in breasts that have locally advanced cancer at clinical presentation (Figure 16-7). Partial response to chemotherapy in these groups usually results in a reclassification to stage M1, M2, or M3 disease after therapy. The significance of these categories is further developed in the discussion of clinical decision making.[1,2,74,87,88]

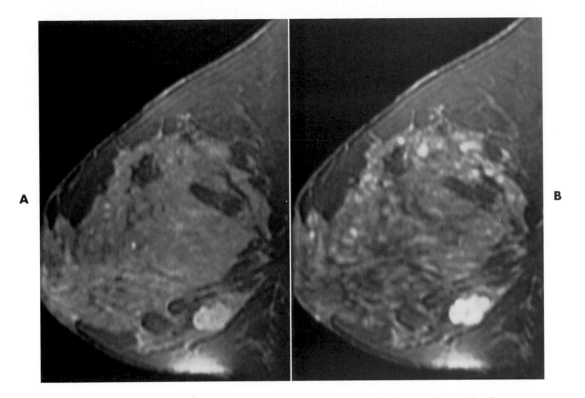

FIGURE 16-2   Lobulated margination. A well-marginated lobulated enhancing lesion with septations is seen on the precontrast **(A)** and postcontrast **(B)** sagittal RODEO images. This appearance is typical of a benign fibroadenoma but can be seen rarely in mucinous carcinoma.

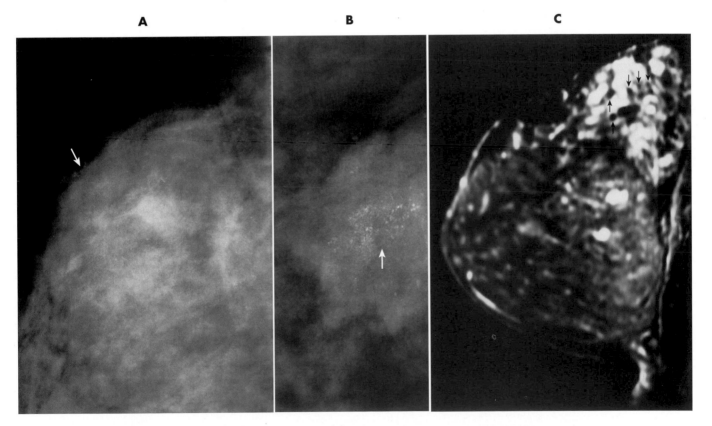

FIGURE 16-3   DCIS with microcalcifications. The mediolateral oblique **(A)** and craniocaudal **(B)** mammograms demonstrate several foci of suspicious microcalcifications *(arrow)* but do not depict the extent of disease as well as the coalescent clumped enhancement seen on the sagittal postcontrast RODEO image **(C).** Note the focal areas of magnetic susceptibility *(arrow)* within the abnormal enhancement on the RODEO image. RODEO detects microcalcifications in 85% of cases of DCIS when microcalcifications are seen on mammograms.

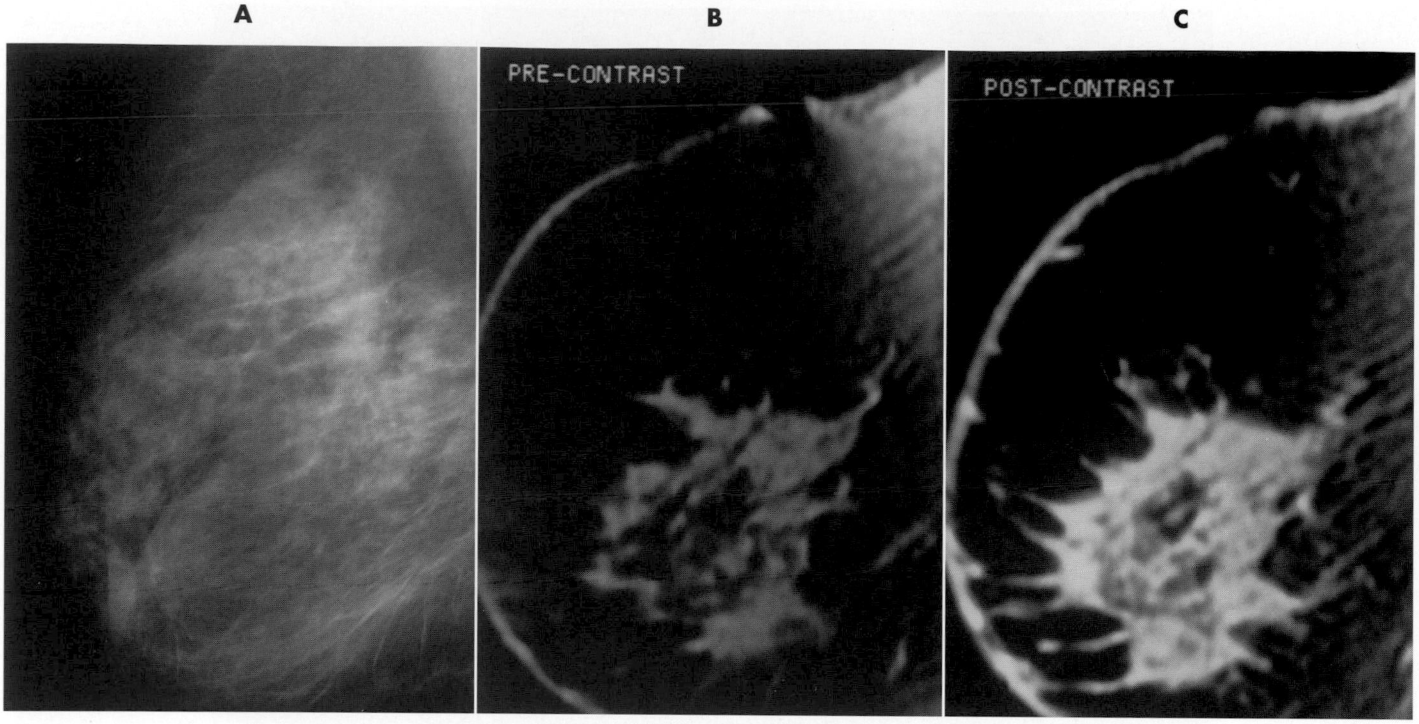

A
B
C

FIGURE 16-4   Spiculated enhancing invasive lobular carcinoma. The mediolateral oblique mammogram **(A)** fails to demonstrate a mass. The precontrast **(B)** and postcontrast **(C)** sagittal RODEO images depict a large spiculated enhancing mass typical of infiltrating carcinoma. Mammograms often poorly depict lobular carcinomas. RODEO MRI has been shown to accurately determine the extent of lobular carcinoma, which almost always is associated with spiculated margination.

Table 16-2   Extent of Disease Categories with Pathological and MR Findings

GRADE	DISEASE EXTENT	PATHOLOGICAL FINDINGS	BREAST MRI
0	No cancer	No gross or microscopic disease	No significant enhancement
S1	Solitary cancer in single quadrant	Solitary-focus malignancy in single quadrant	Solitary focus of abnormal enhancements in a single quadrant
S2	Multiple cancers but confined to a single quadrant	Multiple foci of cancer confirmed in a single quadrant only	Multiple foci of abnormal enhancement in a single quadrant
S3	Larger (>1 cm single-quadrant cancer with multiquadrant small foci (<1 cm) of disease	Solitary larger (>1 cm) malignancy with EIC-positive or other small (<1 cm), infiltrating lesions ≥ 2 quadrants	Solitary high-probability larger focus (>1 cm) with other foci of abnormal enhancement <1 cm in diameter ≥ 2 quadrants
M1	Single large cancer involving >1 quadrant	Solitary malignancy extending over >1 quadrant	Solitary focus of abnormal enhancement extending over >1 quadrant
M2	Multiple small cancers involving >1 quadrant	Multiple DCIS or infiltrating cancer (<1 cm) in >1 quadrant	Multiple foci of abnormal enhancement (<1 cm) in >1 quadrant
M3	Extensive disease in >1 quadrant	Multiple foci of gross disease (>1 cm) in >1 quadrant	Multiple foci of abnormal enhancement (>1 cm) in >1 quadrant

EIC, Extensive intraductal component.

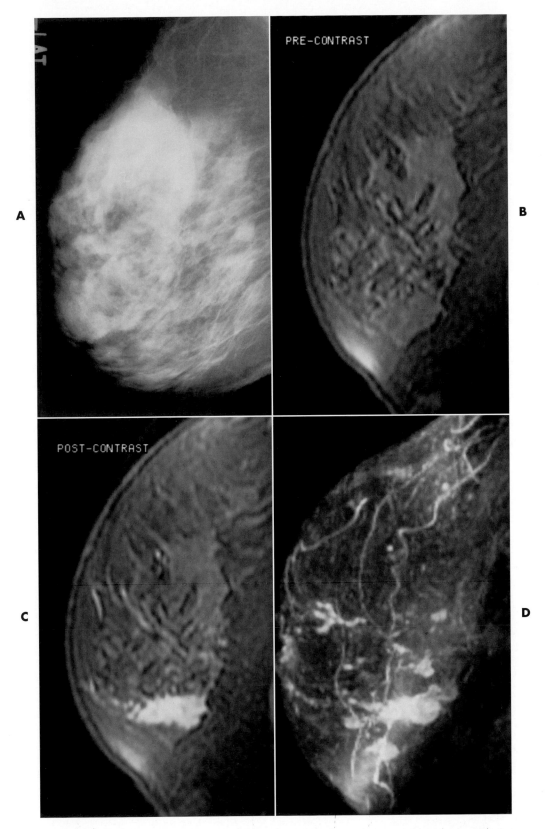

FIGURE 16-5   Multifocal infiltrating ductal carcinoma. The mediolateral oblique mammogram **(A)** and the physical examination failed to demonstrate a focal mass. The precontrast **(B)** and postcontrast **(C)** sagittal RODEO images demonstrate a spiculated enhancing mass typical of infiltrating carcinoma. The mediolateral projection **(D)** of the postcontrast RODEO images shows multiple smaller satellite lesions within the same quadrant. The extent would be classified as S2 and would remain eligible for breast-conservation surgery in some protocols.

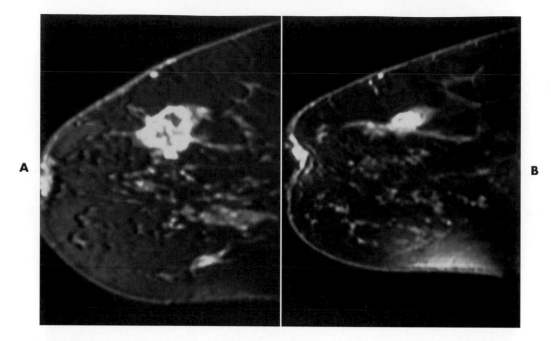

FIGURE 16-6 Induction chemotherapy before breast-conservation surgery. A spiculated, ring-enhancing mass typical of infiltrating carcinoma is seen on the postcontrast sagittal RODEO **(A)** image before treatment. The extent of disease (M1) was considered too great for adequate cosmesis with breast-conservation surgery. Induction chemotherapy was given to reduce the tumor size before lumpectomy. The postcontrast sagittal RODEO image **(B)** shows a response to chemotherapy, reducing the extent to S1. Successful breast-conservation surgery followed.

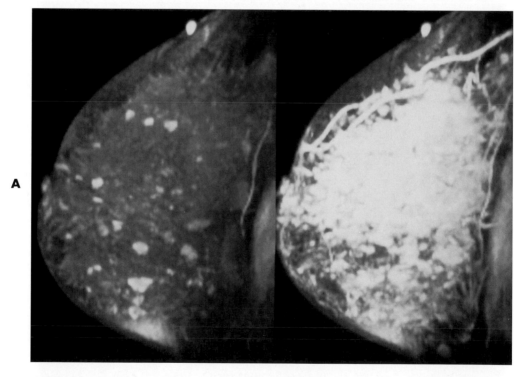

FIGURE 16-7 Induction chemotherapy for locally advanced breast cancer. The precontrast *(left)* and postcontrast *(right)* mediolateral projection RODEO images **(A)** demonstrate extensive multiquadrant disease classified as M3 in extent.

CLINICAL ROLES OF BREAST MAGNETIC RESONANCE STAGING
Breast-Conservation Surgery

With advances in early breast cancer detection comes the potential for breast-conservation surgery (i.e., lumpectomy, partial mastectomy, segmental mastectomy) with the goal of producing less deformity than radical mastectomy. Several prospective, randomized trials have compared mastectomy and breast-conservation treatment as defined by primary tumors of less than 4 or 5 cm with no distant metastases or fixed axillary nodes.[5-7,19,48,77,90] Whole-breast irradiation to doses of 4500 to 6000 cGy was used in all of these trials. Results after 8 to 10 years of follow-up have demonstrated that overall survival and relapse-free survival between mastectomy and breast conservation were not statistically different in any of the trials. Disease recurrence in the breast after breast-conservation treatment ranged from 3% to 19%, compared with

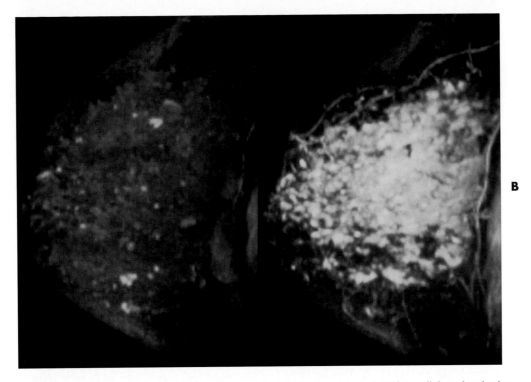

FIGURE 16-7, cont'd   After chemotherapy, the precontrast *(left)* and postcontrast *(right)* mediolateral projection RODEO images **(B)** show an overall reduction in the extent of abnormal enhancement, but the response is less than the 50% volume reduction needed to classify it as a partial response. The categorization of response to chemotherapy and the extent of residual disease is confounded clinically by the softening of the tumor and the association of postchemotherapy edema.

local recurrence after primary mastectomy of 2% to 9%. The clinical determination of which patients are candidates for breast-conservation treatment versus mastectomy is highly dependent on the imaging findings. Women with malignancies in more than one breast quadrant would not generally be candidates for breast conservation. Although tumor size is not an absolute contraindication to breast conservation, there is little evidence to support breast-conservation surgery in women with tumors larger than 4 to 5 cm. A large tumor in a small breast is also a relative contraindication because of the significant cosmetic alteration. Accurate definition of tumor size, number, and margins is absolutely critical in determining the staging for successful breast-conservation treatment.

Tumor Size and Multiple Tumors. Accurate determination of the disease extent is important in planning breast-conservation surgery. The size of the primary tumor in breast-conservation surgery does not appear to have any effect on recurrence rate. T1 (2-cm diameter) and T2 tumors (2- to 5-cm diameter) show equal recurrence rates.[48] There is no difference in local-regional recurrences for tumors up to 4.5 cm in diameter.[90]

The incidence of multicentric breast cancer ranges from 9% to 75%.* In patients with clinically occult, nonpalpable breast cancers detected on mammography, the incidence of multicentricity (greater than one quadrant) is 44%.[83] Of the tumors found to be microinvasive on pathological examination, 57% were multifocal (within the same quadrant). In another series, from Memorial Sloan-Kettering Cancer Center, 60% of patients in whom mastectomies were performed for in situ cancer had multicentric disease.[75] Mastectomy specimens show tumor foci outside a 5-cm radius of the reference tumor (the hypothetical border of a breast quadrant) in 20% of cases.[53] Residual tumor is found in 26% and 38% of patients with reference tumors smaller than 2 cm and larger than 2 cm in diameter, respectively.[76] The presence of multiple primary cancers has been associated with an increased risk of local recurrence after breast conservation. Patients with multiple lesions show a recurrence rate of 40%, compared with 11% when one lesion was present.[50,56] These findings indicate a fundamental difference in the efficacy of breast-conservation surgery when multiple primary tumors are present.

*References 42, 53, 55, 75, 76, 83.

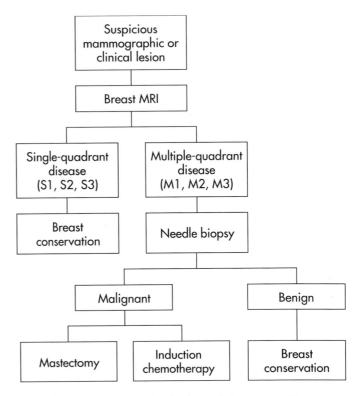

FIGURE 16-8   Potential algorithm for the surgical treatment of breast cancer based on MR extent classification.

Breast MR staging can be an effective method for determining the extent of disease before breast conservation. The decision process involved in the selection of patients for mastectomy versus breast conservation is shown in Figure 16-8. One important feature of clinical decision making is the determination of significant "subclinical" disease that would preclude breast-conservation treatment. As summarized in the following discussion, the size of lesion that is effectively treated with radiation therapy is not known. Many radiation oncologists agree that lesions larger than 1 cm in diameter are difficult to treat with radiation alone. Therefore we usually use core needle biopsy in cases involving lesions with diameters larger than 1 cm that are highly suspicious on MRI but are clinically and mammographically occult. Even though the lesions may be difficult to prospectively visualize by ultrasound, retrospectively ultrasound can usually identify MR-detected lesions that are larger than 1 cm in diameter. In such cases, we prefer ultrasound-directed biopsy over stereotaxic MR biopsy. We have achieved satisfactory results with ultrasound-directed biopsy of MR-detected disease in about 70% of cases.

Magnetic Resonance Imaging–Directed Stereotaxic Biopsy.

Mammographically directed core needle biopsies approach a failure rate of only about 1%.[45,69,70] The accuracy of stereotaxic core needle biopsies is comparable to that of surgery. A variety of prototype stereotaxic devices have been built for MRI-directed breast biopsy and needle localization.* These devices generally consist of the following components: breast immobilization, lesion localization from MR coordinates to spatial coordinates, and needle guidance. Localization methods are highly variable. All methods use some form of fiducial markers that reference the biopsy system to the MR coordinate system. Corrections for gradient nonlinearity are needed for accurate needle localization. MR-compatible localization wires and biopsy needles are currently under investigation and are not yet approved by the Food and Drug Administration.

We currently use a prototype C-arm stereotaxic unit (Fischer Imaging, Denver) (Figure 16-9). This device uses thermal-setting plastic to form a rigid exoskeleton for breast support rather than breast compression. A C-arm allows 360 degrees of freedom for the flexible selection of angle and positioning of the biopsy and localization needles. This approach is beneficial in the coordination of MR localization with surgical lumpectomy.

Ductal Carcinoma In Situ

The increased use of screening mammography over the past 2 decades has led to a marked increase in the number of patients in whom DCIS

*References 15, 16, 40, 44, 67, 79.

is diagnosed, and today in many centers, one DCIS lesion is diagnosed for every two to three mammographically detected invasive breast cancers. Multiple DCIS lesions are often present. However, these lesions are typically in a segmental pattern and are thus multifocal rather than multicentric. The distinction among DCIS, DCIS with microinvasion, and even frankly invasive cancer is problematic by conventional breast imaging. The histological distinction between DCIS and LCIS is sometimes difficult. Microinvasion can be mimicked by artifact, duct sclerosis, epithelial entrapment, microvessel proliferation, periductal fibroblasts, and mechanical implantation in needle tracts. Microinvasion is one of the most commonly revised diagnoses on pathological review. This difficulty in histological categorization has led to controversy over the interpretation of several treatment trials for DCIS.[52]

The presence of extensive intraductal component (EIC) is associated with an increased risk of recurrence.[39,46,65,66,89] In patients with EIC, 59% have residual carcinoma present farther than 2 cm from the index lesion, compared with 29% for specimens with no EIC. In addition, patients with EIC had residual carcinoma at the 4-cm distance from the index tumor in 32% of cases, compared with only 12% for those without EIC. At 6 cm or more from the index lesion, 21% of the group with EIC had residual carcinoma, compared with 8% for the group with no EIC.[41] Local recurrence rates for T1 and T2 lesions also depend on the size of the resection. For T1 tumors treated with small resections, the patients with EIC had a local recurrence rate of 29% compared with 10% for patients without EIC. For T2 lesions, patients with EIC treated with small resections had a local recurrence rate of 36%, but if a large resection was done, the local recurrence rate was 9%.[93] EIC status is an indicator of the potential for increased subclinical disease and a higher potential for positive margins. For these reasons, many surgeons prefer to perform a larger resection or mastectomy with histological findings of EIC. Unfortunately, the presence of EIC is often not known until after the initial lumpectomy. This problem might be

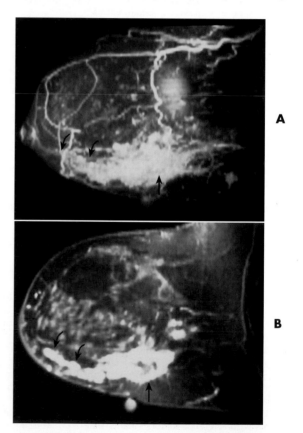

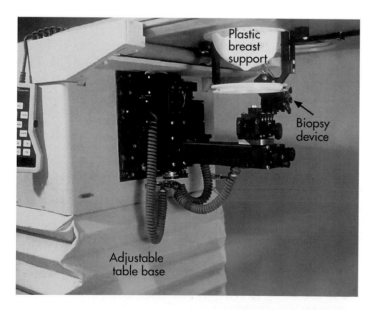

FIGURE 16-9   MR-directed stereotaxic table. The standard MRI docking table is replaced with a specially built stereotaxic table. The breast is placed through a hole in the table. Instead of compression plates as used in conventional mammographic stereotaxis, breast support is provided by thermal-setting plastic. A stereotaxic C-arm positioner allows flexibility in positioning of the needle. For needle localizations, it is important to place the wires in proximity to the operative field. The position of the needle in other stereotaxic systems is fixed.

FIGURE 16-10   Infiltrating carcinoma with EIC. The postcontrast oblique sagittal RODEO image **(A)** demonstrates a spiculated, ring-enhancing mass *(straight arrow)* in association with coalescent clumped enhancement extending along a ductal ray from the mass toward the nipple *(curved arrows)*. The spiculated mass represents an infiltrating ductal carcinoma. The coalescent clumped enhancement along a ductal ray is typical of DCIS. Mediolateral projection image **(B)** of the postcontrast RODEO series depicts the M1 extent.

addressed more appropriately by a more accurate imaging assessment of disease extent before surgery so that the size of the resection can be matched to the extent of disease.

Some clinicians have reported difficulty in demonstrating DCIS on breast MRI studies.[8,26,39] In a recent study using RODEO breast MRI, all of 22 DCIS lesions demonstrated abnormal enhancement in a characteristic clumped or linear pattern. In this series a 2.5-cm diameter DCIS with microinvasion was missed by mammography. RODEO breast MRI was more accurate than mammography in evaluating tumor extent. MRI accurately predicted single or multiquadrant disease in 21 of 22 patients (95%); mammography accurately predicted single or multiquadrant disease in only 14 of 19 patients (74%). In addition, high-resolution staging MR examinations were able to discriminate among DCIS, DCIS with microinvasion, and infiltrating carcinoma with EIC (Figure 16-10).[87]

Lumpectomy Localization

To improve breast conservation, many surgeons now prefer to match the lumpectomy size to the estimated size of the mass, including a margin of normal parenchyma. The inability to accurately determine the extent of disease by clinical and conventional breast imaging often results in inadequate tumor resection (Figure 16-11). Several large, retrospective reviews have demonstrated that involved margins lead to an increased risk of local or regional recurrence, whereas other studies indicate no effect from positive surgical margins.[24,52,92] These discrepancies probably reflect differences in the size of the initial tumor resection. Ghossein et al[24] report recurrence rates of 41% for tumorectomy, 15% for wide local excision, and 14% for quadrantectomy. Thus the larger resections provide greater certainty for negative margins, as reflected in decreased number of local recurrences. Many studies have not performed rigorous pathological analysis to guarantee adequate excision. The fact that most breast recurrences are located close to the original tumor site seems to confirm this impression. The incidence of positive margins in the lumpectomy specimen ranges from 30% to more than 95%.* This wide variation is attributed to the differences in the size of

---

*References 24, 29, 41, 48-50, 52, 53, 55, 56, 58, 72, 75, 76, 78, 83, 92.

the specimen (lumpectomy versus quadrantectomy) and the thoroughness of the pathological examination. A report from Japan indicated that when thorough pathological examination was performed, the positive margin rate was 95%.[29] The occurrence of positive margins could not be predicted by tumor size or distance from the nipple but did correlate with the presence of intraductal disease and tumor necrosis.[29] Schmidt-Ullrich et al[78] evaluated 108 women with AJC stage I and II invasive carcinoma for adequacy of the histopathological margins. Inadequate margins were found in the initial lumpectomy specimen in 32% of the T1 carcinomas and 49% of the T2 carcinomas. For patients with tumors more than 2 cm in diameter in whom excision was required, 71% had residual carcinoma. Incomplete tumor excision and residual microscopic carcinoma may be associated with higher recurrence rates, as suggested by the tendency of larger tumors to recur more frequently.[77] The problem of positive or close margins is addressed at many centers with the use of a radiation therapy boost to the primary site, but no randomized prospective studies have validated this concept. The ability of MRI to define and localize tumors could be used for the more accurate removal of primary tumors, thereby preventing positive lumpectomy margins.

The inability to effectively localize lesions by clinical and conventional imaging examinations often results in positive margins in the lumpectomy specimen. Positive margins frequently require either mastectomy or excision of the lumpectomy. The additional surgery is expensive and associated with increased morbidity rates. Our historical data indicate a positive margin rate of 70% when single-wire localizations are used. When two or more wires are used, the positive margin rate is reduced to 40%. These results are consistent with those of other investigators. Silverstein was able to reduce the positive margin rate to 30% by using four wires, compared with 7% with a single wire. It is expected that the improved capability of MRI to depict lesion margins can be used for improving lumpectomy localizations and excisions (Figure 16-12). Breast-conservation candidates (extent categories S1, S2, and S3) in whom conventional needle localization is needed (nonpalpable lesions) would be eligible for MR-guided stereotaxic localization. It is expected that MRI will experience a lower positive margin rate as a result of improved detection and localization of margins and the exclusion of patients with more extensive subclinical disease who are treated with mastectomy.

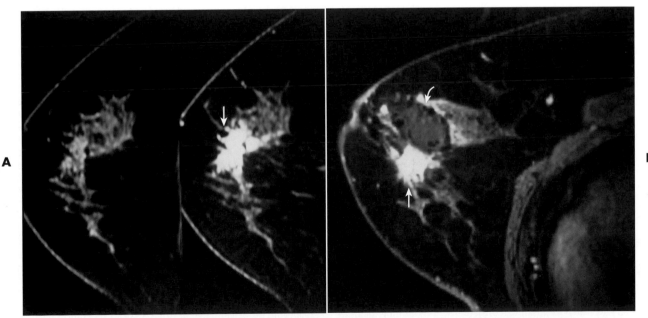

FIGURE 16-11   Residual tumor after lumpectomy. The rate of positive lumpectomy specimen margins ranges from 40% to 70%. This patient had positive pathological margins and still wanted breast conservation. The precontrast *(left)* and postcontrast *(right)* sagittal RODEO images **(A)** and an oblique axial reformatted axial postcontrast RODEO image **(B)** depict a spiculated enhancing mass *(straight arrow)* anteroinferior to the postoperative seroma *(curved arrow)*. Although many workers indicate that MRI is not effective in the postoperative period, a recent study demonstrates the effectiveness of RODEO staging for patients with positive pathological margins.

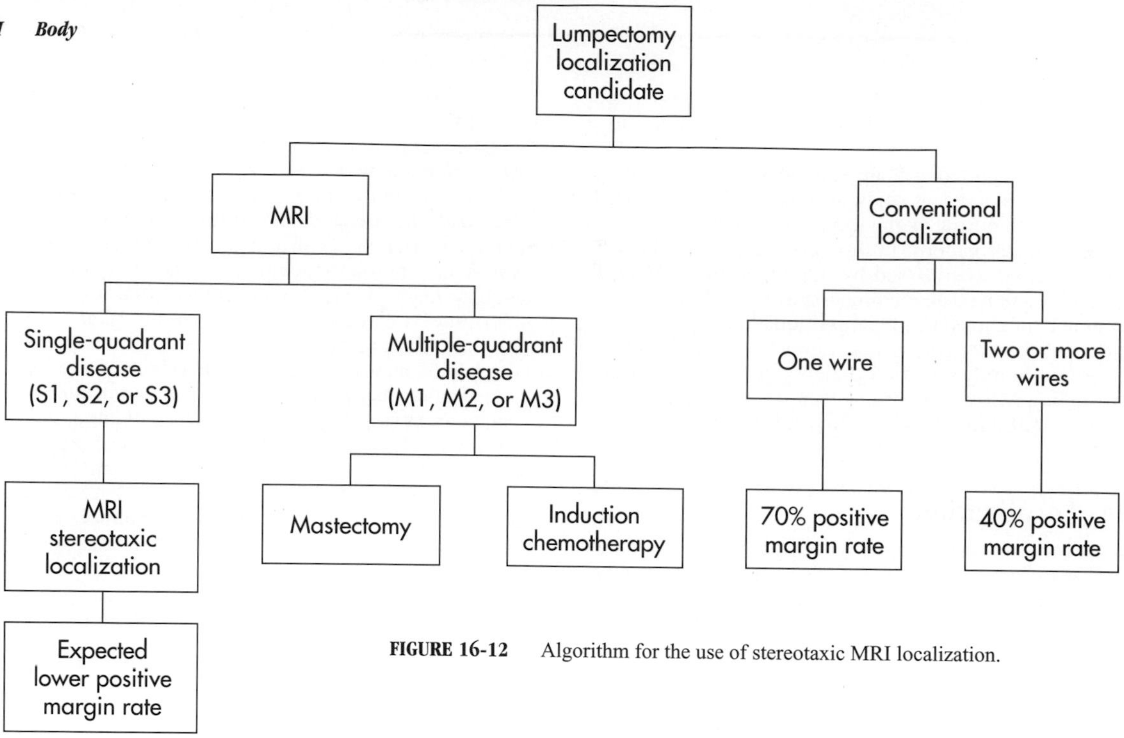

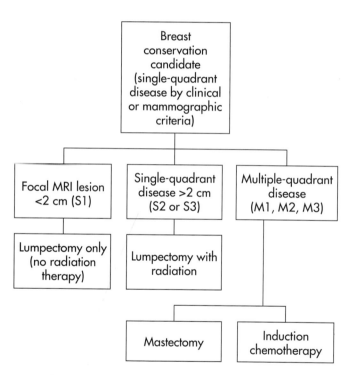

FIGURE 16-12 Algorithm for the use of stereotaxic MRI localization.

FIGURE 16-13 Algorithm for the selection of candidates for lumpectomy without radiation based on MR extent categories.

Radiation Therapy

The theoretical reason for radiation therapy in breast-conservation treatment is to supplement minimal surgery with a moderate radiation dose to eradicate residual microscopic foci of disease while preserving the cosmetic appearance of the breast. It is preferable to limit the extent of breast surgery as much as possible, consistent with obtaining local tumor control with radiation therapy. Microscopic disease is much less likely to contain hypoxic foci that are less susceptible to irradiation. It is estimated that a radiation dose of 500 cGy given over 5 weeks to the entire breast is sufficient to control 75% of subclinical disease.[20] It is a common practice to supplement the radiation treatment to the whole breast with a boost dose to the primary site so that the tumor area (region of lumpectomy) receives 6000 cGy. This strategy is based on the

assumption that the "subclinical" disease consists of microscopic foci that are effectively treated with radiation therapy.[41,42] However, as previously stated, more extensive "subclinical" disease may be present.

Lumpectomy without Radiation Therapy
Invasive carcinoma. Several treatment trials confirm the benefits of radiation therapy. The National Surgical Adjuvant Breast Project (NSABP)-B06 trial showed no difference in survival and recurrence rates for mastectomy versus lumpectomy with radiation therapy. However, the recurrence rate for lumpectomy with radiation therapy was 12% versus 43% local recurrence rate for lumpectomy alone, but the incidence of distant recurrences for both lumpectomy groups was the same. These findings confirm that radiation therapy can effectively treat residual subclinical disease.[19]

Although the randomized trials demonstrated a local control benefit of radiation therapy for some, the majority of patients treated with excision alone do not have disease recurrence. The NSABP-B06 trial demonstrated that radiation therapy benefited only about 30% of patients. (About 10% had recurrence even with radiation therapy, and 60% did not have recurrence with excision alone.) These analyses of the study results and the costs, inconvenience, morbidity, and potential late side effects of radiation therapy have prompted some groups to evaluate the selection of patients for which excision alone may be sufficient treatment. Previous trials indicate that even when the treatment fails, the recurrence will be local.[5-7,19,48,77,90] In the event of a recurrence, radiation therapy could be reserved for the recurrent disease. Randomized clinical trials using excision alone are under way for the evaluation of invasive tumors smaller than 2 cm.* MRI may have substantial benefit for the exclusion of significant subclinical disease and for patient follow-up.

Ductal carcinoma in situ. The NSABP-B17 trial, which randomized lumpectomy with and lumpectomy without radiation for DCIS, found the 5-year recurrence rate to be lower in the women treated with irradiation (7.5% versus 10.4%). Factors that could be used to predict recurrence include comedo-type and involved or uncertain margins.[17] Subsequent pathological review of the NSABP-B17 trial found the inclusion of atypical ductal hyperplasia and DCIS with microinvasion. Another criticism of the NSABP-B17 trial is the lack of systematic recording of size and extent of DCIS. The short-term benefit of radiation therapy in reducing the number of local recurrences after excisional biopsy for DCIS is well documented, but this benefit appears to decrease with longer follow-up. Lagios et al reported that a DCIS smaller than 25 mm is not associated with occult invasion or axillary metastasis at mastectomy, suggesting that excision alone may be sufficient

*References 10, 23, 57, 63, 73, 85, 91.

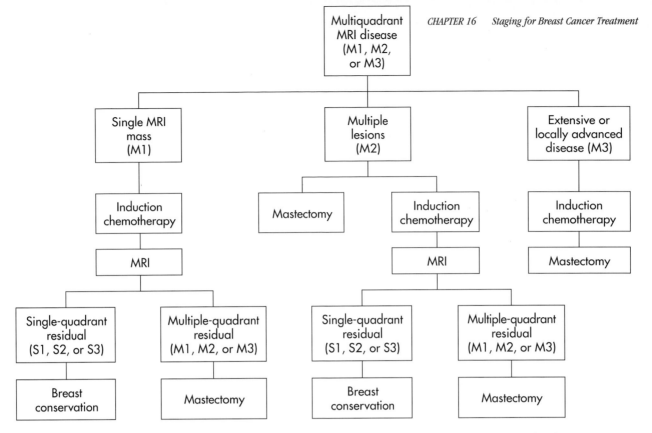

FIGURE 16-14   Algorithm for the selection of treatment of women with multiquadrant breast cancer based on the extent of disease seen on MRI.

treatment for some patients.[5,7] Investigators have examined the results of breast-conservation treatment of DCIS with surgical resection alone.* These studies indicate that with surgery with careful evaluation of margins and thorough specimen examination for evidence of microinvasion, treatment results comparable to those obtained with excision with radiation therapy can be achieved. Lagios et al[52] conclude, "Given the recurrence rates available from the published literature at 8 and 10 years, it may be more appropriate to reserve radiation therapy for invasive recurrences should they occur." A potential algorithm for using MR information to select patients for breast-conservation treatment without radiation is shown in Figure 16-13.

Induction Chemotherapy

Locally advanced cancer of the breast refers to breast carcinomas with significant primary or nodal disease but in which distant metastases cannot be documented (International Union against Cancer [UICC] and American Joint Commission on Cancer Staging and End Results Reporting [AJC] stage T3b to T4, N2 or N3, M0). These cancers have been shown to be poorly controlled by surgery alone. Patients with locally advanced disease may undergo combination chemotherapy before mastectomy (induction chemotherapy).[17,43,59,81] The NSABP recently performed a trial (B21) comparing induction chemotherapy before breast-conservation surgery with mastectomy.[86] One of the concepts of induction chemotherapy in this application is to reduce the tumor burden so that breast-conservation surgery is feasible. Unfortunately, chemotherapy often results in breast edema and softens the tumor, which confounds the estimation of response and extent of residual disease by clinical and mammographic methods.[61,86] An imaging examination that can accurately determine tumor bulk may have a role in determining the response to chemotherapy and extent of residual disease before breast-conservation surgery. This examination could be used to adjust chemotherapeutic regimens if a response is unsatisfactory.[1,2,25]

In some patients the disease is a solitary mass that can be palpated and shown on mammograms. On MRI these would be S1 or M1 lesions in extent. These masses often reduce in size concentrically when treated with induction chemotherapy. The patient with this clinical appearance would typically follow a protocol similar to that in the NSABP-B21

trial, wherein the therapy is designed to reduce tumor size to facilitate breast conservation. Most patients with locally advanced disease do not have solitary masses but instead have diffuse disease that cannot be readily palpated or assessed by mammograms. When this disease is treated with induction chemotherapy, it does not reduce in size in a concentric manner. Instead, the responding breast transforms into fibrosis and necrosis with islands of residual tumor. As a result, evaluation of the breast by clinical and conventional imaging methods after treatment can be very difficult.

MRI has considerable promise as a method for accurately evaluating chemotherapeutic response and residual disease. RODEO MRI was evaluated as a tool for determining tumor response and extent of residual disease after neoadjuvant chemotherapy. A total of 40 breasts in 39 patients with stage II, III, or IV breast carcinoma were prospectively evaluated before and after neoadjuvant chemotherapy by MRI, physical examination, and mammography. Assessment of response determined by the three methods was compared. In addition, detailed pathological correlation of residual disease was determined by serial sectioning of 31 mastectomy specimens from 30 patients. Nine patients had breast conservation and were included in the response evaluation only. Estimates of tumor response were made by both surgical and medical oncologists. Independent interpretations of MR studies without knowledge of clinical response were made by three radiologists. The surgical oncologists assessed complete response (CR), partial response (PR), and no response (NR) in 11, 22, and 7 cases, respectively. The medical oncologists assessed CR, PR, and NR in 12, 21, and 7 cases, respectively. The surgical and medical oncologists' clinical assessment of response agreed with the results of MRI in 52% and 55% of cases, respectively, and with each other in 75% (30 of 40) cases. Mammography correlated to MRI response in only 53% of cases. However, MRI accurately predicted the pathological determination of residual disease in 97% (30 of 31) of cases. There was no disagreement in the assessments of residual disease or response among the three radiologists. RODEO breast MRI accurately estimates residual disease after induction chemotherapy. It better assesses response to neoadjuvant chemotherapy than traditional methods of physical examination or mammography. The information obtained from this MR technique may be used as an objective tool during clinical trials and to better select patients for breast conservation after neoadjuvant chemotherapy for locally advanced disease[2] (Figure 16-14).

*References 3, 4, 11, 51, 54, 82, 84.

SUMMARY

The ability of breast MRI to better detect, characterize, and determine disease extent can be used in patients with inconclusive mammography (dense breasts), postoperative scar, silicone augmentation, or difficult histology (DCIS or invasive lobular carcinoma). This information may guide the surgical treatment of breast cancer (breast conservation versus mastectomy). Serial breast MR examinations can be used for the management of nonsurgical treatment (induction chemotherapy and interstitial hyperthermia). When used appropriately, breast MRI is a cost-effective tool for improved clinical care of patients with breast cancer.

REFERENCES

1. Abraham DC, Harms SE, Jones SE, et al: Evaluation by magnetic resonance imaging of neoadjuvant chemotherapeutic response in locally advanced breast cancer, Baylor Proceedings 8:29, 1995.
2. Abraham DC, Jones RC, Jones SE, et al: Evaluation of neoadjuvant chemotherapeutic response in locally advanced breast cancer by magnetic resonance imaging, Cancer 78:91, 1996.
3. Arnesson LG, Smeds S, and Fagerberg G: Follow-up of two treatment modalities for ductal cancer in situ of the breast, Br J Surg 76:672, 1989.
4. Arnesson LG, Smeds S, Fagerberg G, et al: Follow-up to two treatment modalities for ductal cancer in situ of the breast, Br J Surg 76:672, 1989.
5. Bader J, Lippman ME, and Swain SM: Preliminary report of the NCI early breast cancer (BC) study: a prospective randomized comparison of lumpectomy (L) and radiation (XRT) to mastectomy (M) for Stage I and II BC, Int J Radiat Oncol Biol Phys 13(Suppl 1):160, 1987 (abstract).
6. Blichert-Toft M, Brincker H, Andersen JA, et al: A Danish randomized trial comparing breast-preserving therapy with mastectomy in mammary carcinoma: preliminary results, Acta Oncol 27:671, 1988.
7. Blichert-Toft M: A Danish randomized trial comparing breast conservation with mastectomy in mammary carcinoma, Br J Cancer 62(Suppl 12):15, 1990.
8. Boetes C, Mus RDM, Holland R, et al: Breast tumors: comparative accuracy of MR imaging relative to mammography and US for demonstrating extent, Radiology 197:743, 1995.
9. Bydder GM, Steiner RE, Blumgart LH, et al: Imaging of the liver using short T1 inversion recovery sequences, J Comput Assist Tomogr 9:1084, 1985.
10. Cady B, Stone MD, and Wayne J: New therapeutic possibilities in primary invasive breast cancer, Ann Surg 218:338, 1993.
11. Carpenter R, Boulter PS, Cooke T, et al: Management of screen detected ductal carcinoma in situ of the female breast, Br J Surg 76:564, 1989.
12. Cross MJ, Harms SE, Cheek JH, et al: New horizons in the diagnosis and treatment of breast cancer using magnetic resonance imaging, Am J Surg 166:749, 1993.
13. Derby KA, Frankel SD, Kaufman L, et al: Differentiation of silicone gel from water and fat in MR phase imaging of protons at 0.064 T, Radiology 189:617, 1993.
14. Dixon WT: Simple proton spectroscopic imaging, Radiology 153:189, 1984.
15. Fischer U, Vosshenrich R, Bruhn H, et al: Breast biopsy guided with MR imaging: experience with two stereotaxic systems, Radiology 193:267, 1994.
16. Fischer U, Vosshenrich R, Keating D, et al: MR-guided biopsy of suspect breast lesions with a simple stereotaxic add-on-device for surface coils, Radiology 192:272, 1994.
17. Fisher B, and Anderson S: Conservative surgery for the management of invasive and noninvasive carcinoma of the breast: NSABP trials, World J Surg 18:63, 1994.
18. Fisher B, Contantino J, Redmond C, et al: Lumpectomy compared with lumpectomy and radiation therapy for the treatment of intraductal breast cancer, N Engl J Med 328:1581, 1993.
19. Fisher B, Redmond C, Poisson R, et al: Eight-year results of a randomized clinical trial comparing total mastectomy and lumpectomy with or without irradiation in the treatment of breast cancer, N Engl J Med 320:822, 1989.
20. Fletcher GH: Clinical dose-response curves of human malignant epithelial tumors, Br J Radiol 46:1, 1973.
21. Frahm J, Haase A, Hanicle W, et al: Chemical shift selective MR imaging using a whole-body magnet, Radiology 156:441, 1985.
22. Garrido L, Kwong KK, Pfleiderer B, et al: Echo-planar chemical shift imaging of silicone gel prostheses, Magn Reson Imaging 11:625, 1993.
23. Gelber RD, and Goldhirsch A: Radiotherapy to the conserved breast: is it avoidable if the cancer is small? J Natl Cancer Inst 86:652, 1994.
24. Ghossein NA, Alpert S, Barba J, et al: Importance of adequate surgical excision prior to radiotherapy in the local control of breast cancer in patients treated conservatively, Arch Surg 127:411, 1992.
25. Gilles R, Guinebretiere JM, Toussaint C, et al: Locally advanced breast cancer: contrast-enhanced subtraction MR imaging of response to preoperative chemotherapy, Radiology 191:633, 1994.
26. Gilles R, Zafrani B, Guinebretiere J-M, et al: Ductal carcinoma in situ: MR imaging-histopathologic correlation, Radiology 196:415, 1995.
27. Gorczyca DP, Litwer CA, Debruhl ND, et al: Silicone breast implant ruptures: comparison between fast multiplanar IR and fast SE MR imaging, Radiology 193:318, 1994.
28. Gorczyca DP, Schneider E, Debruhl ND, et al: Silicone breast implant rupture: comparison between three-point Dixon and fast spin-echo MR imaging, Am J Roentgenol 162:305, 1994.
29. Haga S, Makita M, Shimizu T, et al: Histopathological study of local residual carcinoma after simulated lumpectomy, Surg Today 25:329, 1995.
30. Harms SE, and Flamig DP: Present and future role of MR imaging. In Haus AG, and Yaffe MJ, eds: Syllabus: a categorical course in physics: technical aspects of breast imaging, Oak Brook, Ill, 1994, Radiological Society of North America.
31. Harms SE, and Flamig DP: MR imaging of the breast, J Magn Reson Imaging 3:277, 1993.
32. Harms SE, and Flamig DP: Staging of breast cancer with magnetic resonance, Magn Reson Imaging Clin N Am 2:4, 1994.
33. Harms SE, Flamig DP, Evans WP, et al: MR imaging of the breast: current status and future potential, Am J Roentgenol 163:1039, 1994.
34. Harms SE, Flamig DP, Evans WP, et al: Magnetic resonance imaging of the breast: present and future roles, Baylor Proceedings 7:21, 1994.
35. Harms SE, Flamig DP, Hesley KL, et al: Breast MRI: rotating delivery of excitation off-resonance: clinical experience with pathologic correlations, Radiology 187:493, 1993.
36. Harms SE, Flamig DP, Hesley KL, et al: Fat-suppressed three-dimensional MR imaging of the breast, Radiographics 13:247, 1993.
37. Harms SE, Jensen RA, Meiches MD, et al: Silicone-suppressed 3D MRI of the breast using rotating delivery of excitation off-resonance, J Comput Assist Tomogr 19:394, 1995.
38. Hasse A, and Frahm J: Multiple chemical shift selective NMR imaging using stimulated echoes, J Magn Reson 64:94, 1985.
39. Heywang SH, Wolf A, Pruss E, et al: MR imaging of the breast with GD-DTPA: use and limitations, Radiology 171:95, 1989.
40. Heywang-Koebrunner SH, Halle MD, Requardt H, et al: Optimal procedure and coil design for MR imaging-guided transcutaneous needle localization and biopsy, Radiology 193:267, 1994.
41. Holland R, Connolly JL, Gelman R, et al: The presence of an extensive intraductal component following a limited excision correlates with prominent residual disease in the remainder of the breast, J Clin Oncol 8:113, 1990.
42. Holland R, Veling SHJ, Mravunac M, et al: Histologic multifocality of TIs, T1-2 breast carcinomas: implication for clinical trials of breast-conserving surgery, Cancer 56:979, 1985.
43. Hortobagyi GN, Ames FC, Buzdar AU, et al: Management of state III primary breast cancer with primary chemotherapy, surgery, and radiation therapy, Cancer 51:2507, 1983.
44. Hussman K, Renslo R, Phillips JJ, et al: MR mammographic localization, Radiology 189:915, 1993.
45. Jackman RJ, Nowels KW, Shepard MJ, et al: Stereotaxic large-core needle biopsy of 450 nonpalpable breast lesions with surgical correlation I lesions with cancer or atypical hyperplasia, Radiology 193:91, 1994.
46. Kaiser WA, and Zeitler E: MR imaging of the breast: fast imaging sequences with and without GD-DTPA, Radiology 170:681, 1989.
47. Keller PJ, Hunter WW, and Schmalbrock P: Multisection fat-water imaging with chemical shift selective presaturation, Radiology 164:539, 1987.
48. Kurtz JM, Amalric R, Brandone H, et al: Local recurrence after breast-conserving surgery and radiotherapy, Helv Chir Acta 55:837, 1989.
49. Kurtz JM, Amalric R, Delouche G, et al: The second ten years: long term risk of breast conservation in early breast cancer, Int J Radiat Oncol Biol Phys 13:1327, 1987.
50. Kurtz JM, Jacquemier J, Amalric R, et al: Breast-conserving therapy for macroscopically multiple cancers, Ann Surg 212:38, 1990.
51. Lagios MD: Duct carcinoma in situ: pathology and treatment, Surg Clin North Am 70:853, 1990.
52. Lagios MD, Margolin FR, Westdahl PR, et al: Mammographically detected duct carcinoma in situ: frequency of local recurrence following tylectomy and prognostic effect of nuclear grade on local recurrence, Cancer 63:618, 1989.
53. Lagios MD, Richards VE, Rose MR, et al: Segmental mastectomy without radiotherapy: short-term follow-up, Cancer 52:2153, 1983.
54. Lagios MD, Westdahl PR, Margolin FR, et al: Duct carcinoma in situ: relationship of extent of noninvasive disease to the frequency of occult invasion, multicentricity, lymph node metastases, and short-term treatment failures, Cancer 63:619, 1982.
55. Lagios MD, Westdahl PR, and Rose MR: The concept and implications of multicentricity in breast carcinoma. In Sommers SG, and Rosen PP, eds: Pathology annual, New York, 1981, Appleton-Century-Crofts.
56. Leopold KA, Recht A, Schmitt SJ, et al: Results of conservative surgery and radiation therapy for multiple synchronous cancers of one breast, Int J Radiat Oncol Biol Phys 16:11, 1989.
57. Liljegren G, Holmberg L, Adami H-O, et al: Sector resection with or without postoperative radiotherapy for stage I breast cancer: five year results of a randomized trial, J Natl Cancer Inst 86:717, 1994.
58. Lindley R, Connolly J, and Geman R: Histologic features predictive of an increased risk of early local recurrence after treatment of breast cancer by local tumor excision and radical radiotherapy, Surgery 105:13, 1989.
59. Lopez MJ, Andriole DP, Kraybill WG, et al: Multimodal therapy in locally advanced breast carcinoma, Am J Surg 160:669, 1990.
60. Maudsley AA, Hilal SK, Perman WH, et al: Spatially revolved high resolution spectroscopy by "four dimensional" NMR, J Magn Reson 51:147, 1983.
61. Mauriac L, Durand M, Avril A, et al: Effects of primary chemotherapy in conservative treatment of breast cancer patients with operable tumors larger than 3 cm, Ann Oncol 2:347, 1991.
62. Meyer CH, Pauly IM, Macovski A, et al: Simultaneous spatial and spectral selective excitation, Magn Reson Med 15:287, 1990.
63. Moffat FL, Ketcham AS, Robinson DS, et al: Segmental mastectomy without radiotherapy for T1 and small T2 breast carcinomas, Arch Surg 125:364, 1990.
64. Monticciolo DL, Nelson RR, Dixon WT, et al: MR detection of leakage from silicone breast implants: value of a silicone-selective pulse sequence, Am J Roentgenol 163:51, 1994.
65. Nunes LW, Orel SG, Schnall MD: Diagnostic accuracy and lesion characteristic predictive values in the MR imaging evaluation of breast masses, Radiology 193:267, 1994.
66. Orel SG, Schnall MD, Livolsi VA, et al: Suspicious breast lesions: MR imaging with radiologic-pathologic correlation, Radiology 190:485, 1994.

67. Orel SG, Schnall MD, Newman RW, et al: MR imaging-guided localization and biopsy of breast lesions: initial experience, Radiology 193:97, 1994.
68. Page DL, and Anderson TJ: Diagnostic histopathology of the breast, New York, 1987, Churchill-Livingstone.
69. Parker SH, Jobe WE, Dennis MA, et al: US-guided automated large-core breast biopsy, Radiology 187:507, 1993.
70. Parker SH, Lovin JD, Jobe WE, et al: Nonpalpable breast lesions: stereotactic auto-mated large-core biopsies, Radiology 180:403, 1991.
71. Pierce WB, Harms SE, Flamig DP, et al: GD-DTPA enhanced MR imaging of the breast: a new fat suppressed three-dimensional imaging sequence, Radiology 181:757, 1991.
72. Rodenko GN, Harms SE, Pruneda JM, et al: MR imaging in the management before surgery of lobular carcinoma of the breast: correlation with pathology, Am J Roentgenol 167:1415, 1996.
73. Recht A, Pierce SM, and Abner A: Regional nodal failure after conservative surgery and radiotherapy for early-stage breast carcinoma, J Clin Oncol 9:1662, 1991.
74. Reed MW, and Morrison JM: Wide local excision as the sole primary treatment in el-derly patients with carcinoma of the breast, Br J Surg 76:898, 1989.
75. Rosen PP, and Kinne DE: The clinical significance of preinvasive breast carcinoma, Cancer 46:919, 1980.
76. Rosen PP, Fracchia AA, Urban JA, et al: "Residual" mammary carcinoma following simulated partial mastectomy, Cancer 35:739, 1975.
77. Sarrazin D, Le MG, Arriagada R, et al: Ten-year results of a randomized trial compar-ing a conservative treatment to mastectomy in early breast cancer, Radiother Oncol 14:177, 1989.
78. Schmidt-Ullrich R, Wazer DE, Tercilla O, et al: Tumor margin assessment as a guide to optimal conservation surgery and irradiation in early stage breast carcinoma, Int J Ra-diation Oncol Biol Phys 17:733, 1989.
79. Schnall MD, Orel SG, and Connick TJ: MR guided biopsy of the breast, Magn Reson Imaging Clin N Am 4:585, 1994.
80. Schneider E, and Chan TW: Selective MR imaging of silicone with the three-point Dixon technique, Radiology 187:89, 1993.
81. Schwartz GF, Cantor RI, and Biermann WA: Neoadjuvant chemotherapy before defin-itive treatment for state III carcinoma of the breast, Arch Surg 122:1430, 1987.
82. Schwartz GF, Finkel GC, Garcia JG, et al: Subclinical ductal carcinoma in situ of the breast: treatment by local excision and surveillance alone, Cancer 70:2468, 1992.
83. Schwartz GF, Patchesfsky AS, Feig SA, et al: Multicentricity of nonpalpable breast cancer, Cancer 45:2913, 1980.
84. Silverstein MJ, Cohlan BJ, Gierson ED, et al: Duct carcinoma in situ: 227 cases with-out microinvasion, Eur J Cancer 28:630, 1992.
85. Silverstein MJ, Furmanske MR, and Glerson ED: Cosmetic quadrantectomy: a new surgical approach for mid-sized breast cancer, Proc Surg Soc Oncl 46:159, 1993.
86. Singletary SE, McNeese MD, and Hortobagyi GN: Feasibility of breast conservation surgery after induction chemotherapy for locally advanced breast carcinoma, Cancer 69:2849, 1992.
87. Soderstrom CE, Harms SE, Copit DS, et al: Three-dimensional RODEO breast MRI of lesions containing ductal carcinoma in situ, Radiology 20:427, 1996.
88. Soderstrom CE, Harms SE, Farrell RS, et al: Detection with MR imaging of residual tu-mor in the breast soon after surgery, Am J Roentgenol 168:485, 1997.
89. Stack JP, Redmond OM, Codd MB, et al: Breast disease: tissue characterization with GD-DTPA enhancement profiles, Radiology 174:491, 1990.
90. Veronesi U, Banfi A, Del Vecchio M, et al: Comparison of Halsted mastectomy with quadrantectomy, axillary dissection, and radiotherapy in early breast cancer: long-term results, Eur J Cancer Clin Oncol 22:1085, 1986.
91. Veronesi U, Saccozzi R, and Del Vecchio M: Comparing radical mastectomy with quad-rantectomoy, axillary dissection, and radiotherapy in patients with small cancers of the breast, N Engl J Med 305:1097, 1981.
92. Veronesi U, Volterrani F, Luini A, et al: Quadrantectomy versus lumpectomy for small size breast cancer, Eur J Cancer 26:671, 1990.
93. Vicini FA, Eberlein TJ, Connolly JL, et al: The optimal extent of resection for patients with stages I or II breast cancer treated with conservative surgery and radiotherapy, Ann Surg 214:200, 1991.

17 Breast Implants and Soft Tissue Silicone

Michael S. Middleton

 KEY POINTS

- Diverse implant designs can be categorized and recognized with MRI.
- Silicone fluid "bleed" occurs for all intact silicone gel–filled implants but only rarely may be detected with MRI.
- Implant rupture, with escape of silicone from the implant and through the fibrous capsule, can be detected with MRI.
- Surgery is guided by MRI showing no evidence of rupture, intracapsular (contained) rupture, or extracapsular rupture with possible migration of silicone into surrounding tissues.

Silicone gel–filled implants were first placed in a patient in March 1962.[21,40]* Beyond the usual potential complications of any surgical procedure (pain, infection, hemorrhage), complications specifically related to breast implants (capsular contracture, rupture, silicone migration, granuloma formation, loss of nipple sensitivity, nipple areolar necrosis, and spontaneous extrusion) may occur with implant surgery.† In addition, possible links to immune and autoimmune disease, as well as to symptoms related to foreign body reaction, have been suggested.‡ Toluene diamine (TDA), a known rat liver and breast carcinogen, has been shown to be present in hydrolysis products of polyurethane coverings directly obtained from some breast implants.[12] Induction of plasmacytomas in mice with silicone gel implants has been reported,[111] on the basis of which further investigation in women with breast implants has been recommended.[118]

These and other concerns relating to cancer induction have been reviewed by Brinton and Brown.[25] If these concerns turn out to be valid and sufficiently common, silicone exposure may represent a health risk to women with breast implants and possibly even to those who have had implants removed. Estimates of the number of women with breast implants in the United States have ranged from fewer than 1 million to as many as 2 million. Analysis of a 1989 survey of 40,000 households yielded an estimate that there were 815,700 women with breast implants in the United States at that time.[39] Although the total number of implants per patient is not known, patients seen for problems or for suspected problems had 0.54 replacements per breast after the first implant was placed.[79]

Scientific evidence supporting an association between breast implants and autoimmune disease is being disputed.[123,140] Recent epidemiological studies have found no association between silicone gel–filled implants and classic autoimmune disease.[57,119] These negative results have been challenged on the basis that only a link to classic autoimmune disease was tested—that these studies did not test for a link to atypical immune or autoimmune disease.[127] In a more recent study an association of autoimmune disease with silicone breast implants was reported, but the incidence was low.[70] This study has been

Magnetic resonance (MR) evaluation of women with silicone gel–filled breast implants was first reported in 1991.[136] The main purpose of this examination is to determine whether implants are ruptured and whether silicone gel has escaped into the surrounding soft tissues. Magnetic resonance imaging (MRI) may also be helpful in determining the type and even the manufacturer of implants.[79]

---

*Letter from Dr. Thomas D. Cronin, of Baylor University, to Mr. Silas Braley, of the Dow Corning Center for Aid to Medical Research, dated April 11, 1962 (M-440043 and M-440048).
†References 17, 27, 32, 41, 42, 50, 55, 57, 62, 68, 71-73, 93, 94, 96, 97, 104, 110, 117, 125, 141.
‡References 9, 24, 35, 113, 126-128, 143.

criticized because the survey response rate was limited and the diseases were self-reported. Some of the difficulties encountered in proving that silicone has deleterious health effects include the variety of disease end points and the atypical nature of some of the suspected conditions.[135]

Information about the immunology of silicones and possible silicone toxicity may be found in two recently published collections.[22,112] A book on breast implant evaluation has been published,[64] and another is in press.[87]

The local complications of breast implants are not disputed. Gabriel et al[58] reported that 23.8% of implant patients required additional surgery as a result of a complication within 5 years of initial implant placement. The absolute rupture rate of implants in the general population of all implant patients has not yet been measured. Reported implant rupture rates for patients seen for known or suspected problems include 66.6%* by de Camara et al[43] (31 patients, 51 implants), 63.5%† by Robinson et al[114] (300 patients, 592 implants), 38.1%‡ by Rolland et al[115] (68 patients, 97 implants), 22.9%§ by Malata et al[74] (51 patients, 83 implants), 40%‖ by Peters et al[107] (57 patients, 102 implants), and 38%¶ by Middleton[79] (877 patients, 1626 implants). The rupture rates vary according to manufacturer, as well as implant type. Some polyurethane-coated implants (e.g., Aesthetech Même ME) have a rupture rate (for patients being seen for implant evaluation) of 92% for 10- to 14-year-old implants, compared with about a 34% rupture rate for non-polyurethane–coated implants of the same age.[79,90] Implant rupture rates were recently reviewed by Brown et al.[26]

Putting aside the question of whether there are systemic effects from silicone, there is still a clinical need to determine whether, on the basis of the known local complications of breast implants alone, implants have ruptured, and if so, whether silicone has extravasated into surrounding soft tissues. MRI can help answer these questions with sufficient confidence to be clinically useful on a routine basis.

TERMINOLOGY
Implant Materials

Silicon, Silica, Silanes, Silicates, and Silicones. Silicon (atomic number 14, chemical atomic weight 28.086) is below carbon in the Periodic Table, occurring naturally as a stable combination of ^{28}Si (92.2%), ^{29}Si (4.7%), and ^{30}Si (3.1%).[139] It can help form backbones of long chain molecules with room for side chains because of its tetravalent nature with four vacant p-electron subshell orbital locations.

Silica (SiO_2) can occur in amorphous or crystalline forms[103]; occurs naturally as quartz, tridymite, and cristobalite[139]; and comprises almost all of sandstone.[103] When inhaled as dust it causes silicosis, mostly for particles sized 0.5 to 5 μm in diameter.[103]

Silanes are reactive hydrides of silicon of the form SiH_4, Si_2H_6, or $SiH_3 — Si_xH_{2x} — SiH_3$.[139]

Silicates are compounds of silicon, oxygen, and various metals that make up most of meteorites, lunar rocks, and the earth's crust and include or are part of zircon, diopside, remolite, orthoclase, talc, and glass.[139]

Silicones are a class of long-chain molecules of variable length, which for medical purposes most often consist of polydimethylsiloxane (PDMS) subunits (— Si[CH$_3$]$_2$ — O —), typically 400 to 600 subunits in length, where various side chains may be substituted for the methyl groups. Silicone gel is composed of two components—a cross-linked matrix of long chains of silicone immersed effectively in a bath of non–cross-linked long chains of silicone. The cross-linking (vulcanization) is usually accomplished by allowing reactive side chains on adjacent molecules to form vinyl groups, connecting those molecules in

an exothermic reaction catalyzed by platinum. The non–cross-linked chains of silicone alone are called *silicone fluid.* Implant shells are usually made from silicone elastomer, a rubberlike substance consisting of a cross-linked silicone matrix usually of longer chains of silicone, to which fillers, such as amorphous silica, are sometimes added. Silicone fluid can permeate into and through silicone elastomer implant shells; this is called *bleed.* Starting in the early 1980s, the shells of some implants were designed to reduce silicone fluid bleed by adding a layer of fluorosilicone or some other such substance to the inner or outer surface of the implant shell or by sandwiching such a layer between two silicone elastomer layers.

Polyurethanes. In the 1950s various polyurethanes were used in the manufacture of sponge breast implants, including Etheron[6] and Surgifoam[54] implants. As with other early implants, some were enclosed in a polyethylene (plastic) bag. In the early 1970s some polyurethane sponges were inserted inside silicone elastomer shells, which were then inflated with saline, dextran,[101] or silicone gel. After a period of experimentation that began in about 1964,* the first silicone gel–filled polyurethane-coated single-lumen breast implant was introduced in 1968. It was called the *Ashley implant,* after Franklin Ashley, MD, who was involved in its design.[7,8,100] It was also called the *Natural-Y prosthesis* because it contained an internal Y-shaped baffle. In the early 1970s some implants, including some saline-filled and standard double-lumen types, were only partially covered with a layer of polyurethane foam; these were sometimes called *Capozzi* or *Pennisi implants,* after two of the physicians who advocated their use (Angelo Capozzi, MD, and Vincent R. Pennisi, MD).[30,31,33] Later American versions were the Même, Même Moderate Profile, Replicon, Vogue, and Optimam implants. Others have also become available from foreign manufacturers.

Polyurethane cannot be directly identified on routine clinical MR scans. The presence of polyurethane can instigate thin layers of intracapsular waterlike fluid surrounding implants, and this may be seen on MRI. Rarely, polyurethane may be appreciated on MRI as an apparent thickening or crinkling of the implant shell. Its presence in soft tissues after explantation is not detectable by using current MR methods.

Other Sponge Materials. Polyvinyl alcohol (Ivalon) solid and compound sponges,[102] polyethylene sponges,† SILASTIC silicone sponges,[44,51,69,133,138] and shredded polyethylene strips encased in a plastic bag[28,130] were among the types of early implants used before silicone gel–filled implants. Some may have been used as early as the late 1940s.[49,116] Sarcoma induction by Ivalon sponges and other substances in rodents was reported by Oppenheimer et al.[98,99] On that basis and on the basis of shrinkage, fistulization, and problems with sterilization, Ivalon implant material was largely replaced by polyurethane for sponge implants in the late 1950s and early 1960s. The literature is not clear on why the other materials were not widely used, but because citations to them are infrequent, we can probably conclude that they did not become or remain popular for purposes of breast augmentation. Sponges are identifiable on MRI on the basis of their shape and unique appearance. However, the various sponge materials, which may calcify[124] or be siliconized (sprayed or coated with silicone fluid),[20] may not be distinguishable from each other by means of MRI.

Dacron Mesh. Synthetic polyester textile fiber (Dacron) mesh was used in the first experimental silicone gel–filled breast implants from Dow Corning in 1962 to allow fixation by means of tissue ingrowth. Dacron mesh continued to be used by Dow Corning and other manufacturers until the 1980s to reinforce silicone elastomer and to provide fixation to surrounding tissues. Fine denier or coarse mesh Dacron suture tags were attached to some nonround implants from other manufacturers from about 1972 until the mid 1980s to allow fixation to surrounding tissues. Certain very early implants allowed fixation to surrounding tissues by attaching Dacron (and rarely polytetrafluoroethylene [Teflon]) felt to implants. Dacron material cannot be identified directly with MRI, but its presence in some implants may be in-

---

*Sum of their 52.9% "rupture" rate and their 13.7% "leakage" rate, as determined at surgery.

†Sum of their 36.1% "rupture" rate and their 27.4% "intact with severe bleed" rate, as determined at surgery.

‡Sum of their 11.3% "puncture" rate, 21.6% "torn" rate, and 5.2% "destroyed" rate, as determined at surgery.

§Implants with silicone gel on the outer surface of the implant were classified as ruptured, as determined at surgery.

‖As determined at surgery.

¶Includes all categories of rupture for single-lumen silicone gel–filled implants (only), as determined by MRI.

---

*"Augmentation mammaplasty," by Robert H. Pudenz, MD, Heyer-Schulte Corporation, dated July 1978 (MB 104861).

†References 18, 53, 61, 63, 75, 92, 95, 122.

ferred from the appearance of the implants known to include it in their manufacture.

Saline, Dextran, Polyvinylpyrrolidone, Antibiotics, and Steroids. In addition to saline-filled implants, which were used experimentally* and commercially[5] since the early 1960s, certain silicone gel–filled implants have compartments intended to contain (isotonic) saline. Some also are intended to have saline added directly to silicone gel–filled compartments. Despite manufacturers' warnings, it has been common practice since at least the early 1970s to add small amounts of saline solution directly into silicone gel–filled implants, usually by using a 30-gauge needle placed directly through the shell or the (thicker) implant back patch, as alluded to by Cronin et al.[41] Dextran was used to inflate some very early implants in the 1960s and early 1970s. Polyvinylpyrrolidone was used to inflate some implants from Bioplasty starting in about 1988. All these fluids show the typical MR signal of any waterlike fluid and cannot be distinguished from one another. Again, to our understanding, against the manufacturers' recommendations, small amounts of steroids or antibiotics were sometimes added directly to implants in hopes of reducing the incidence of infection, capsular contracture, or both. It is not possible with MRI to determine definitively whether this occurred.

Breast Implant Classification

On the basis of an evaluation of available evidence,† a breast implant classification scheme has been described, which now consists of the following 14 categories[78,85-87]: (1) single-lumen silicone gel–filled; (2) single-lumen adjustable (silicone gel and saline solution mixed in same lumen); (3) saline solution–, dextran–, or polyvinylpyrrolidone–filled; (4) standard double-lumen (silicone gel inner lumen, saline outer lumen); (5) reverse double-lumen (silicone gel outer lumen, saline inner lumen); (6) reverse-adjustable double-lumen (silicone gel inner and outer lumens, saline can be added to inner lumen); (7) gel-gel double-lumen (silicone gel inner and outer lumens); (8) triple-lumen (silicone gel inner and middle lumens, saline outer lumen); (9) Cavon "cast gel" (silicone gel, no shell); (10) custom; (11) pectus implants and early solid "spacers" (silicone elastomer); (12) sponge (solid or hollow, simple or compound); (13) sponge (adjustable, i.e., within an elastomer shell); and (14) "other" (e.g., soybean oil). Of the implants containing silicone gel in one or more compartments (for patients undergoing MRI because of suspected or known problems), about 81% are single-lumen; 15% standard double-lumen; 1.5% single-lumen adjustable; and the remainder account for less than 1% each.[79] Some of the major types are illustrated in Figure 17-1. That scheme is based on appearance on MR images. For example, saline-filled implants are grouped together with dextran-filled and polyvinylpyrrolidone-filled implants because on MRI all of those materials have essentially the same appearance.

Superimposed on this classification scheme are the following secondary groups of implant characteristics that can be thought of as crossing group boundaries: (1) polyurethane coating, (2) texturing of the implant surface, (3) valve type (diaphragm, retention, leaflet, plug, self-seal, internal tube, invertible tube, ligation), (4) fixation device (Dacron mesh patches, fenestration-style patches, Dacron felt patches, suture tags or loops), (5) orientation devices (bars, dots, disks), (6) shape (round, oval, teardrop, contoured, custom), (7) profile (very low, low, moderate, high), and (8) size.

Implant patients differ in the initial reason for obtaining implants, the number of current and prior implants in each breast, and the implant manufacturer. In one study‡ the reasons for implantation were given as follows: 79.2% for aesthetic reasons, 2.1% congenital deformities, 0.3% after trauma, 2.7% postoperative or after a major medical

procedure, 8.1% prophylactic mastectomy, and 7.6% known or suspected cancer.[79] Of the breasts studied, 64.6% had the first implant still in place, 21.6% the second, 5.8% the third, 2.7% the fourth, and less than 2.2% the fifth or greater implant.* Rarely, more than one implant at a time will be "stacked" in a single breast. (We have seen as many as three implants in a breast.)

American breast implant manufacturers and distributors have included Aesthetech, Bioplasty, Cox-Uphoff International (CUI), Dow Corning, Heyer-Schulte, McGhan, McGhan/3M, Mentor, Progress Mankind Technology (PMT), and Medical Engineering Corporation (MEC, Surgitek). Foreign manufacturers include Eurosilicone, Koken (distributed in the United States as Porex), Lab Sebbin (distributed in the United States as Unimed), Nagosil, Polytech, Prometel, Silicone Medicale Paris, Silimed, and Simaplast (distributed in the United States as Roger Klein). In some cases MRI can help determine the implant type and even the manufacturer.[79,86,87] A detailed catalogue of American implants and some foreign implants is currently being prepared by Middleton and McNamara.[87]

An understanding of implant styles and types is important for accurate evaluation of breast implant MR scans to help the clinician avoid false-positive diagnoses of implants that are rare or unusual, on the basis of not recognizing their normal appearances, and recognize signs of implant failure that may be particular to individual types of implants.[79,109] This point is well illustrated by the case of one patient with a triple-lumen implant that was determined to have ruptured on the basis of one computed tomography (CT) scan, one MR scan, and two mammograms. We repeated the MR scan and identified it as an intact triple-lumen implant. Our review of all four prior studies concluded that they all also showed the implant to be intact, with appearances characteristic of a triple-lumen implant. The patient canceled her emergency surgery but later changed her mind and had the implant removed anyway, at which time it was found to be intact.

Bleed

The slow escape from silicone gel–filled breast implants of very small amounts of silicone fluid, consisting of non-cross-linked silicone molecules, constitutes bleed.[10,16] All silicone gel–filled breast implants bleed. There is no such thing as a no-bleed implant; the best that have been attained are low-bleed implants. After the 1970s, when some implant shells were intentionally made thinner, there were efforts made to reduce the amount of silicone fluid escaping through the (intact semipermeable) shell that forms the outer surface of the implant device. Some implant shells were manufactured in layers by using techniques meant to reduce further the amount of bleed. Historically these efforts have been motivated by the desire to reduce capsular contracture thought by some to be caused in part by bleed.

Although the term *gel bleed* is used commonly, we recommend avoiding use of this term completely because of the ambiguity as to whether one is referring to the small amount of silicone fluid that normally escapes from intact breast implants or the silicone gel that escapes from ruptured implants. Instead of using the term *gel bleed,* we describe either silicone fluid (bleed) on the surface of an intact implant or silicone gel on the surface of a ruptured implant.

Rupture

We have observed that when silicone gel, as opposed to just silicone fluid (which would constitute only bleed), is found outside an implant shell, the implant is ruptured.[88] In those cases we investigated a hole was found in the shell or the back patch was separated from the shell, allowing silicone gel to escape.

On the basis of 1626 single-lumen silicone gel–filled implants studied, the MR appearance of rupture has been classified into six categories: (1) no evidence of rupture (64.9%), (2) indeterminate (7.9%), (3) uncollapsed rupture (13% intracapsular, 1.9% extracapsular), (4) minimally collapsed rupture (3% intracapsular, 0.5% extracapsular), (5) partially collapsed rupture (0.4% intracapsular, 0.7% extracapsu-

---

*Letter from Dr. Thomas D. Cronin to Mr. Silas Braley, dated June 27, 1962 (M-440020).

†Medical records from more than 3600 breast implant patients with histories of more than 8500 current or prior implants, more than 1400 silicone-related breast MR scans, direct visual examination of more than 4000 breast implants, and materials received directly from breast implant manufacturers and plaintiff attorneys.

‡For 1305 patients obtaining MR scans to evaluate current implants, residual silicone, or both.

---

*For 4328 current and prior implants for which an MR image was obtained or a second opinion offered, all breast implant types included–1455 patients, 2818 breasts.

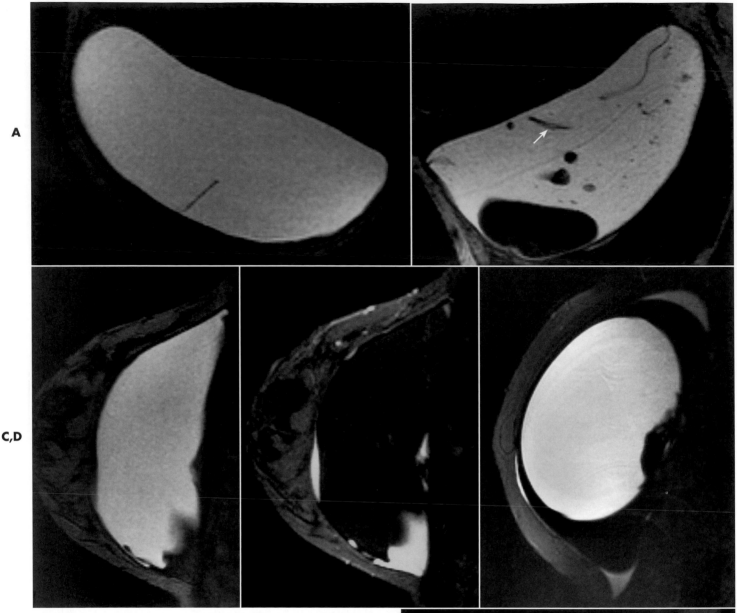

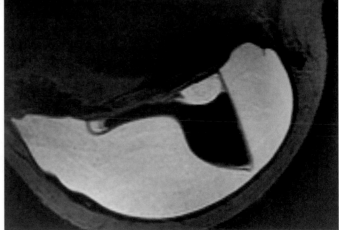

FIGURE 17-1   Common implant types. **A,** Single-lumen silicone gel–filled implant shown on an axial T2-weighted fast spin-echo (FSE) water-suppression image showing a normal fold as a dark line extending inward from the periphery. **B,** Single-lumen adjustable implant shown on an axial T2-weighted FSE water-suppression image showing silicone gel (bright) and saline (dark) mixed within the same lumen. A cross section of the leaflet valve is seen posteriorly *(arrow)*. **C,** Standard double-lumen (water-suppression) implant shown on a sagittal T2-weighted FSE image showing inner-lumen silicone gel (bright) and outer-lumen saline (dark). **D,** Standard double-lumen (silicone suppression) implant shown on a sagittal T2-weighted FSE image of the implant shown in **C,** showing inner-lumen silicone gel (dark) and outer-lumen saline (bright). **E,** Reverse double-lumen implant shown on a sagittal T2-weighted FSE silicone-suppression image showing inner-lumen saline (bright) and outer-lumen silicone gel (dark). Note the characteristic appearance posteriorly of the inner-lumen fill apparatus and the layer of intracapsular waterlike fluid surrounding the implant (bright). **F,** Reverse-adjustable double-lumen implant shown on an axial T2-weighted FSE water-suppression image showing outer-lumen silicone (bright) and inner-lumen silicone (bright) mixed with inner-lumen saline (dark). The inner lumen of this implant is not inflated to the maximum recommended capacity; if it were, the inner lumen would appear cylindrical.

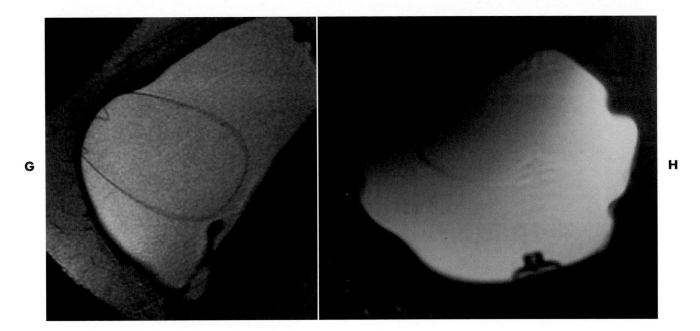

FIGURE 17-1, cont'd   G, Triple-lumen implant shown on a sagittal T2-weighted FSE water-suppression image showing the inner lumen typically overfilled with silicone gel (bright), the middle lumen less filled with silicone gel (bright), and the outer lumen filled with saline (dark). Note the characteristic anterior shell buckling (normal) between the inner and middle lumens. **H,** Saline-filled implant visible on an axial T2-weighted FSE silicone-suppression image showing the anterior diaphragm fill valve.

lar), and (6) fully collapsed rupture (3.6% intracapsular, 4.1% extracapsular).[79] For the 785 implants from that population that were removed, the sensitivity for rupture was 74%, specificity 98%, positive predictive value 98%, negative predictive value 79%, and accuracy 86%. For purposes of these statistics, "no evidence of rupture" and "indeterminate" implants were grouped together.

Fourteen percent of the single-lumen silicone gel–filled implants reported in that article that showed no evidence of rupture on MRI and were removed were found to be in a state of uncollapsed rupture at surgery. Some of those may have ruptured between the MR study and the surgery (mean delay time, 137 days), and others may have been unwittingly ruptured by the surgeon at time of removal. Of the cases considered indeterminate on MRI, 56% were found to be in a state of uncollapsed rupture at surgery.

There is little disagreement in the case of partially or fully collapsed rupture, where most or nearly all the gel has escaped. In a partially collapsed rupture the shell has "fallen into" the gel but not all the way. In a fully collapsed rupture the shell has fully fallen into the gel, resulting in the classic wavy line appearance of collapsed rupture,[79] also called the *linguini sign* by Gorczyca et al.[67] Controversy arises in cases of what we call *minimally collapsed rupture,* which is distinguished by finding silicone within folds outside the implant shell and away from the folds outside the shell, and *uncollapsed rupture,* which is distinguished by finding silicone only within folds outside the outer shell surface. Implants in these states can mistakenly be called *intact* if the significance of gel on the surface of the implant is not understood.

The reason some implants collapse and others do not is not entirely clear. Silicone from some older implants is often more cohesive, which probably makes the collapse of the implant after rupture less likely. The stiffness of some of the older implant shells, sometimes with associated fixation patches, probably also makes collapse less likely. It is possible that upper body exercise, other upper body activity, submuscular placement, trauma, closed capsulotomy, or mammography may facilitate collapse of an implant once rupture has occurred, but these issues have not yet been formally addressed.

In double- and triple-lumen implants the situation is more complex, in that any of the various shells can rupture and can be collapsed or uncollapsed. In addition to the silicone gel, the saline solution present in the various implant cavities can cross shell boundaries. Saline solution can escape the implant by leaking through the valve through which it was originally placed, or the saline compartment can overtly rupture,

with subsequent rapid resorption of most or all of the saline solution by the body, usually within a week. If all the saline solution is gone from a once saline-filled lumen, we refer to that lumen as *deflated.* We refer to a rupture of the shell separating a saline and a gel-filled lumen as *barrier disruption.* Rupture of the fibrous capsule (which is formed by all patients over time in response to the implant) surrounding an implant may occur with or without rupture of the implant itself; thus care should be taken not to confuse these separate processes.

Soft Tissue Silicone

A five-point confidence scale for evaluating soft tissue silicone by MRI has been described as follows: 1, no evidence of silicone; 2, possible silicone (confidence <50%); 3, suspicious for silicone (confidence >50%); 4, probable silicone present (confidence >90%); and 5, definite silicone present.[79] For the 496 breasts (without implants or with saline implants) described in that article, the percentages in these categories were 53.4%, 14.3%, 6.7%, 11.1%, and 14.5%, respectively.

Silicone Fluid Injection Migration Patterns

Migration patterns of silicone fluid injections into the breasts in 38 patients, the thighs in one patient, the lower legs in one patient, and a lip in one patient have been described.[79] In the breast patients, superior, medial, and lateral migration into adjacent soft tissues was the most common pattern observed. Spread into submuscular tissues, into the brachial plexus area, and inferior to the inframammary crease was also possible. The farthest migration reported was to the level of the hips and around the back. The thigh and leg injections spread into fatty tissues encircling the leg, as well as superiorly and inferiorly over about a 40-cm length of leg. The lip injection fully infiltrated all tissues of that lip.

Leakage

The term *leakage* has been used alternatively to refer to silicone (fluid) bleed and to implant rupture. Given this common ambiguity, we recommend avoiding the use of this term completely for the same reasons as given for the term *gel bleed.* Instead of using the term *leakage,* we describe whether we are referring to the normal and expected escape of small amounts of silicone fluid (i.e., bleed) from an intact implant or to the escape of silicone gel from a ruptured implant into surrounding tissues.

Other Terms

A variety of other terms are commonly used to describe the movement of silicone with respect to implants and soft tissues. Extrusion of silicone gel occurs through holes or other openings in an implant shell. Extrusion of contiguous collections of silicone gel also occurs through soft tissues, usually along tissue planes. We refer to infiltration of silicone into surrounding soft tissues to describe the gradual even spread that occurs, for example, when silicone fluid from direct injection infiltrates into breast fatty tissue or muscle. Extravasation and migration, more general terms, apply to those situations in which either extrusion or infiltration is occurring. We use the term *extension* for the special situation in which a contiguous collection of silicone gel extrudes in a defined direction, such as superiorly beyond the boundaries of the presumed location of the original fibrous capsule.

OTHER METHODS OF BREAST IMPLANT EVALUATION

The most important details to obtain before imaging evaluation are the age and type of implant, whether it is the first implant in that breast, whether prior implants were ruptured, the amount of saline solution added (and how it was added), and whether closed (or open) capsulotomy or capsulectomy has been performed. Useful documentation includes operative and pathology reports and notes, clinical notes, implant manufacturer's labels, and any prior MR, mammographic, CT, or ultrasound examination findings.

Physical examination alone, even if performed by a trained plastic surgeon, is not a substitute for further evaluation if an implant abnormality is suspected. Silent rupture, with or without systemic symptoms, is a known entity and cannot be excluded on the basis of physical examination alone. Commonly, neither the referring physician nor the patient suspects a rupture that is eventually discovered. Also, a physical examination may give the impression of implant rupture when the implant is intact. Whether or not the examining physician is able to determine or suspect a link to silicone, the role of the examining physician in excluding other diagnosable or treatable disease is important.

Implant history and clinical evaluation with physical examination, mammography, and ultrasound can be helpful in the evaluation of silicone gel–filled breast implants and of soft tissues suspected to contain silicone.* Mammoscopy has been investigated but is not generally used because it is an invasive procedure that can cause implant rupture.[48]

Mammography

Mammography usually does not allow for the detection of even fully collapsed rupture unless there is also extracapsular silicone present. It has been reported that, for patients being evaluated, extracapsular silicone is present in more than 25% of ruptures.[79] Xeroradiography and film-screen mammography can suggest an increased or decreased likelihood of implant rupture,[45] but most cases of uncollapsed rupture are missed. Mammography, if performed too vigorously, of ruptured implants may cause an increased risk of exacerbating the degree of implant collapse, the extrusion of gel into the extracapsular space, or the spread of silicone through soft tissues.[11,79]

Mammography often shows as intact those double-lumen (or triple-lumen) implants that still have saline solution in their outer lumen. However, if the saline is gone from its compartment, the mammographic and MR appearances may be indistinguishable from that of a single-lumen silicone gel–filled implant. Mammography can sometimes help in the definitive identification of implants as being saline filled, standard double-lumen, reverse double-lumen, triple-lumen, reverse double-lumen adjustable, or sponge and can sometimes be used to identify the implant manufacturer.

Ultrasound

Ultrasound can show rupture when the implant shell is collapsed and, in experienced hands, can also reveal uncollapsed rupture.[29,77,85] In cases of collapsed rupture, increased echogenicity within the gel is thought to represent microbubbles of body fluid that have permeated the silicone. In collapsed rupture a stepladder appearance represents segments of implant shell surrounded by gel. Uncollapsed rupture can be predicted when small amounts of intracapsular silicone are identified outside the visible implant shell.[85] Silicone gel within implants will be posteriorly displaced in relation to other tissues, such as the pectoralis muscles, whereas saline within or surrounding implants will not.[29,85]

Ultrasound may be more sensitive than MRI in the detection of soft tissue silicone and silicone in nodes, unless the silicone is deep to other silicone or calcification or is too deep within the patient's own tissue.[76,85] Soft tissue silicone granuloma and silicone in nodes show markedly increased echogenicity. Silicone fluid injected directly into patient's breasts (until the early 1970s in the United States) often extends all the way to the skin and nearly completely blocks penetration of the ultrasound signal to tissues deep to the skin. Calcification in the fibrous capsule can also block the ultrasound signal.

Computed Tomography

The role of CT in the evaluation of breast implant evaluation is limited, mainly because of the dose of ionizing radiation imparted but also because of the limited resolution available. A study of 23 cases of in vivo examination reported only a single case in which CT showed collapsed rupture.[1] It was concluded that MRI was preferable to CT for the detection of (collapsed) rupture, mainly because of the radiation dose imparted by CT. The issue of uncollapsed rupture—which in my experience is more common than collapsed rupture—was not directly addressed by that study.

Mammoscopy

In mammoscopy a flexible or rigid scope is placed through the skin and the fibrous capsule down to the level of the implant shell, and that surface is examined on a video screen.[48] Choosing to use this invasive procedure is in practice not much different from choosing to evaluate the patient surgically.

SILICONE IMAGING PRINCIPLES, EQUIPMENT, AND PROTOCOLS

The objectives in imaging silicone are twofold: to determine where the silicone is and to differentiate it from other materials or tissues (such as fat, water, or artifact). Of the many ways that silicone can be imaged, the method used most widely causes the silicone to be bright and all other materials and tissues to be dark.

The relaxation times (T1/T2) of relevant materials are (approximately, in milliseconds) as follows: silicone (1000/100), fat (250/40), and water (1000/350). Given these values, on T2-weighted images, with sufficient T2 weighting, fat tends to image with a darker signal, silicone a brighter signal, and water the brightest of all. In fast spin-echo (FSE) images the reason for the fat being dark is that for the long values of echo time (TE) used, the fat signal is much lower than the signal from silicone by virtue of its shorter T2 value. Fast multiplanar inversion recovery (FMPIR), with a value of T1 chosen to null fat, can be used instead of FSE, with potentially a greater reduction in the signal from fat.

One way to cause signal from water to be dark is to apply water suppression, in which case both fat and water are dark, theoretically leaving only silicone bright. The spectrum of water, fat, and silicone is schematically represented in Figure 17-2. The hydrogen protons on water molecules are less shielded from the main magnetic field than are the hydrogen protons on the methyl groups of fat molecules. This shielding is enough to cause the resonant frequency of the fat protons to be 3.5 parts per million (ppm) less than the water protons, which comes to about 220 Hz at 1.5 Tesla (T) (as shown in Figure 17-2), about 147 Hz at 1.0 T, and about 73 Hz at 0.5 T. We apply water suppression at 160% of the bandwidth usually applied for water suppression to increase its effectiveness. This results in some suppression of fat, which in this setting is acceptable, but very minimal (if any) suppression of silicone.

Because of additional shielding present around the methyl hydrogen protons on a silicone molecule, they resonate approximately 1.5 ppm downfield from the fat hydrogen protons. This is shown as an ap-

---

*References 2, 7, 34, 37, 59, 65, 108, 131, 137.

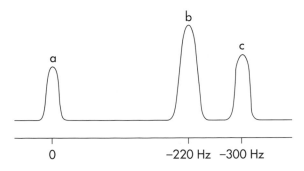

FIGURE 17-2   Schematic spectrum of water *(a)*, fat *(b)*, and silicone *(c)*. The separations of 220 Hz (water-fat) and 80 Hz (fat-silicone) assume a main magnetic field strength of 1.5 T.

proximately 80-Hz separation in Figure 17-2 between signal peaks from fat and silicone. In practice the shielding varies between about 80 and 100 Hz at 1.5 T, at least partly as a result of the viscosity and other microenvironmental characteristics of the silicone.

The trade-off between resolution and contrast is decided on the basis of the goal intended. A careful check of implant folds for uncollapsed rupture requires higher resolution, and the trade-off is lower contrast between soft tissues and silicone within those tissues. Alternatively, in a patient who has been explanted the highest priority is soft tissue contrast, and thus the resolution chosen for those scans is lower.

The equipment and methods used to image silicone can cause artifacts or fail to operate as expected, leading to potential pitfalls in image interpretation. These are discussed later in this chapter.

Imaging Protocols

A knowledge of the implant manufacturer and type, together with the date of placement, usually indicates which MR protocol should be used. On the basis of the initial MR images, we occasionally switch from one protocol to another in the middle of a scan. The monitoring of scans is perhaps more important when patients have come from far away because they cannot be easily called back for additional imaging.

Our protocols for breast implant imaging are directed toward optimizing the imaging of implants, soft tissues, or both. In practice, each scan is individually tailored to the needs of the patient.[79]

Scout Sequence. We start with a sagittal T2-weighted FSE scout sequence, which is intentionally unsuppressed (body coil in the prone position, head first with the arms above the head, TR >3000 ms, TE = 208 ms, echo train length [ETL] = 8, 36-cm field of view (FOV), 8-mm slice thickness skip 4 mm, number of excitations [NEX] = 2, 256 × 192 matrix, ~ 6 min). This sequence provides positional information and allows preliminary interpretation for the purpose of directing the remainder of the scan. Because this sequence is unsuppressed, we can determine when waterlike fluid collections are present either around implants or in soft tissues. Waterlike signal is much brighter on T2-weighted images than is the signal from silicone.

We then take one or both of two approaches for each breast independently. If we know from the scout sequence and other available information that an implant is ruptured or that no implant is present and the purpose of the scan is to evaluate for soft tissue silicone, we image that breast optimizing for high contrast. If on the basis of the scout sequence we see that rupture is not yet adequately determined, we image that breast optimizing for high resolution, and the soft tissues optimizing for high contrast as needed.

High Contrast. If there is a need to evaluate the soft tissues for silicone from current or prior implants or for prior silicone fluid or gel injections, we perform a T2-weighted FMPIR sequence with wideband water suppression to determine the location of possible silicone (breast coil in the unilateral position, TR >3000 ms, TE = 150 ms, TI = 180 ms, ETL = 16, 20-cm FOV, 4-mm slice thickness contiguous, NEX = 1, 256 × 192 matrix, ~ 4 min). If there are suspected foci of failure of water suppression or the anatomical relationships are not clear, we then obtain a T2-weighted FSE sequence with wideband silicone suppression over the same slices (breast coil in the unilateral position, TR

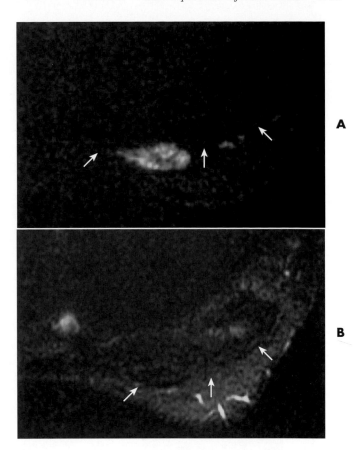

FIGURE 17-3   Soft tissue silicone granuloma anterior to pectoralis major 19 years after closed capsulotomy. Arrows indicate the anterior border of pectoralis major. **A,** Axial T2-weighted FMPIR fat-nulled water-suppression axial image showing silicone granuloma with bright inhomogeneous signal. **B,** Axial T2-weighted FSE silicone-suppression image at the same level showing anatomy and silicone granuloma with dark signal.

>3000 ms, TE = 130 ms, ETL = 16, 20-cm FOV, 4-mm slice thickness contiguous, NEX = 1, 256 × 192 matrix, ~ 3 min). If present in sufficient amount and concentration, silicone should appear bright on the first and dark on the second sequence (Figure 17-3). If the concentration of silicone in tissue drops too low, it can appear isointense to fat on the second sequence, and if it drops lower than that, it may not be distinguishable from surrounding tissues on the first sequence.

High Resolution. If an implant is old and the folds are thin (as is common with capsular contracture), we perform a sagittal and, if necessary, an axial high-resolution T2-weighted FSE wideband water-suppression sequence for that breast (breast coil in the unilateral position, TR >3000 ms, TE = 209 ms, ETL = 16, 15-cm FOV, 3-mm slice thickness contiguous, NEX = 2, 256 × 256 matrix, ~ 6 min). This sequence provides the best possible look at the folds themselves, which in our experience is the most sensitive way to detect uncollapsed rupture. If the implant shell is known to be textured or otherwise thick, we instead use moderate resolution (breast coil in the unilateral position, TR >3000 ms, TE = 208 ms, ETL = 8, 20-cm FOV, 4-mm slice thickness contiguous, NEX = 1, 256 × 256 matrix, ~ 4 min).

Upper Chest and Brachial Plexus Area. Finally, if the implant in a given breast is a second or greater implant and there is adequate suspicion of rupture of a prior implant extending into the upper chest, we take the patient off the table, remove the breast surface coil, put the patient back on the table on specially designed cushions, do a fast scout sequence using the body coil, and then do a high chest T2-weighted FSE water-suppression sequence (body coil in the prone position, head first with the arms above the head, TR >3000 ms, TE = 324 ms, ETL = 8, 36-cm FOV, 6-mm slice thickness contiguous, NEX = 2, 256 × 192 matrix, ~ 5 min). If that sequence is positive, we may also do a T2-weighted FSE silicone-suppression sequence over the same slices (~ 3 min).

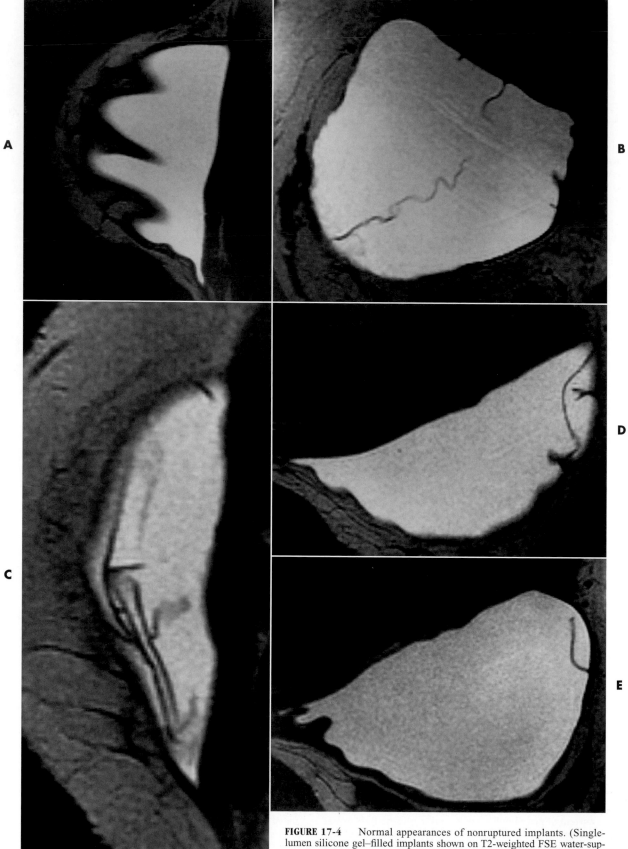

FIGURE 17-4   Normal appearances of nonruptured implants. (Single-lumen silicone gel–filled implants shown on T2-weighted FSE water-suppression images.) **A,** Undulating folds (sagittal, "soft" implant). **B,** Long, squiggly, thin folds extending inward from the periphery of the implant (axial). **C,** Complex folds (sagittal). **D,** Branching fold (axial). **E,** Floppy fold (axial).

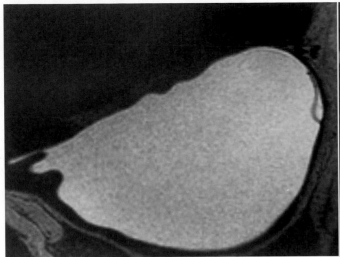
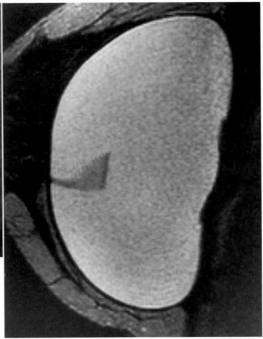

FIGURE 17-4, cont'd   F, Same floppy fold shown in **E** shown here on a nearby slice "touching" the internal surface of the implant shell, illustrating an appearance that could be incorrectly interpreted as rupture (axial). **G,** Traveling fold (sagittal).

Tailored Protocols. The aforementioned methods represent the most common pathways through our scans, but exceptions can occur. Our full protocols when monitored usually take about 45 to 60 min. Claustrophobic patients may require a shortened protocol. After an axial scout sequence, very good preliminary information can be obtained by using one graphically prescribed sagittal series, with a total examination time of about 15 min (breast coil in the bilateral prone position, head first with the arms above the head, TR >3000 ms, TE = 208 ms, ETL = 8, 20-cm FOV, 4-mm slice thickness contiguous through each breast graphically prescribed, NEX = 1, 256 × 256 matrix).

NORMAL AND ABNORMAL BREAST IMPLANTS

Findings associated with intact and herniated implants, as well as rupture with or without extracapsular migration of silicone, have been discussed by others* and by us.[79-90]

Intact

A tissue capsule develops around all implants soon after placement. It can be so thin as to be transparent, or it can be thick and constricted around the implant to the point of producing capsular contracture. Depending on the degree of capsular contracture and the amount of silicone gel fill (profile) of an implant, normal folds can take on a spectrum of appearances. For normal "soft" implants (i.e., without noticeable capsular contracture), the shell can be gently undulating (Figure 17-4, *A*). Folds can also appear as long squiggly lines extending from the edge inward, each representing two layers of implant shell (Figure 17-4, *B*). The fold pattern may be very complex, and the implant may still be intact (Figure 17-4, *C*). Normal folds can be branched (Figure 17-4, *D*) or floppy (Figure 17-4, *E*). In some cases in which they appear floppy, the innermost tip of the fold can be bent over so much that it is touching the inner surface of the implant shell, giving the false appearance of silicone outside the implant shell (Figure 17-4, *F*). A hint of this is when the fold "opens up" on other slices (Figure 17-4, *E*), it appears to be a double thickness of shell, and the angles the fold makes with the shell are near perpendicular on one side and obtuse on the other, as opposed to being almost equal to each other. If there is volume averaging and the fold is changing position from slice to slice, we call it a *traveling fold,* which can have a fanlike appearance (Figure 17-4, *G*). The posteromedial and posterolateral corners of the implant can be especially difficult to evaluate if silicone outside the shell is suspected

*References 4, 14, 23, 36, 47, 60, 67, 91, 109, 121, 129, 132, 134, 136.

there. Shells that are thicker (0.5 to 2 mm) are more easily visualized, whereas the thinnest shells (as thin as about 0.1 to 0.2 mm) can be very difficult to see even at the highest resolutions attainable.

Herniation

Contour abnormalities of the surface of an implant can represent implant rupture, herniation of an intact or ruptured implant through the fibrous capsule, or just variations in the shape of an intact fibrous capsule containing a nonruptured implant. These contour abnormalities are often seen on mammograms and are a common reason MR scans are requested. The presence of confirming signs of rupture should be searched for on MRI because these appearances on mammograms are often nonspecific. Herniation tends to have a classic appearance on MRI of "bunching of folds" at the point where the implant extrudes through the fibrous capsule (Figure 17-5).

Intracapsular Waterlike Fluid

Intracapsular waterlike fluid, often seen surrounding some breast implants (more often with textured and polyurethane-coated ones than with smooth ones), is of unknown significance. This phenomenon is known to plastic surgeons who can observe a small gush of fluid on entry into the fibrous capsule. The mechanism of production of this fluid is unknown. One possible explanation is that the fluid production is related to the textured surface or the polyurethane coating of the implants, but the mechanism of production may be different. Another possible explanation when there is audible sloshing is that third spacing of body fluids into the potential intracapsular space around the implants may be occurring because of decreased pressure at high altitudes, possibly exacerbated by cold weather—a scenario that has been reported.

The appearance of waterlike intracapsular fluid on nonsuppressed T2-weighted images is one of brightness greater than silicone within folds with an approximately 5-ppm chemical shift in the frequency-encoding direction (Figure 17-6, *A*). On water-suppressed T2-weighted images the waterlike fluid is darkened, sometimes giving rise to an apparent "thickening" of the folds (Figure 17-6, *B*). On silicone-suppressed images the waterlike fluid is seen within folds and sometimes as a layer of bright signal surrounding the implant (Figure 17-6, *C*).

Bubbles within Silicone Implants

Waterlike bubbles inside a single-lumen silicone gel–filled implant can be there because saline (and sometimes also a steroid or an antibiotic agent) was added to the implant at the time of placement or afterward. Fluid can be added through a valve provided by the manufacturer in a gel-saline single-lumen adjustable implant (Figure 17-1, *B*) or through a needle placed directly through the back patch or shell by the surgeon[41] (generally not according to manufacturers' recommendations). Although cases of rupture with waterlike bubbles seen adjacent to the ruptured shell are observed (Figure 17-7, *A* and *B*), it is not yet clear whether the rupture or the bubbles came first. One reason for the confusion is that often fluids added to single-lumen silicone gel–filled implants with a needle through the back patch or shell are not documented in the medical records. We know this because we observe gel–filled implants that are not ruptured and have internal waterlike bubbles, with no note of addition of fluid found in the medical records (Figure 17-7, *C*). We therefore consider waterlike bubbles within an implant to be a possible sign of rupture but require further evidence before predicting rupture with certainty. Evaluation of the medical records to determine implant type and whether saline solution or medication was added can be helpful. In determining whether the presence of the internal waterlike bubbles has any significance, it is useful to balance the amount of waterlike fluid inside the implant with the amount of gel observed outside the implant.

Waterlike bubbles can be seen in double- and triple-lumen implants that have had disruption of the internal shell separating the silicone gel and saline-filled cavities. This barrier disruption may appear like a mixed oil-water emulsion or may have a "salad oil" appearance, with waterlike bubbles in the gel compartment, globules of gel in the saline compartment, or both (Figure 17-8). Waterlike bubbles can be seen normally in some reverse double-lumen implants along the track of the inner-lumen filler tube that has been withdrawn. In addition, waterlike bubbles are normally present in the inner lumen of some reverse double-lumen adjustable implants (Figure 17-1, *F*).

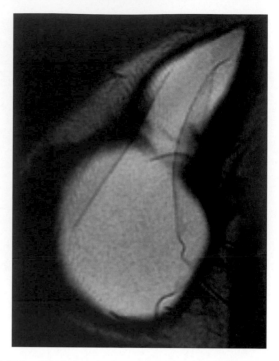

FIGURE 17-5 Herniation of an intact single-lumen silicone gel–filled implant through the fibrous capsule shown on a sagittal T2-weighted FSE water-suppression image.

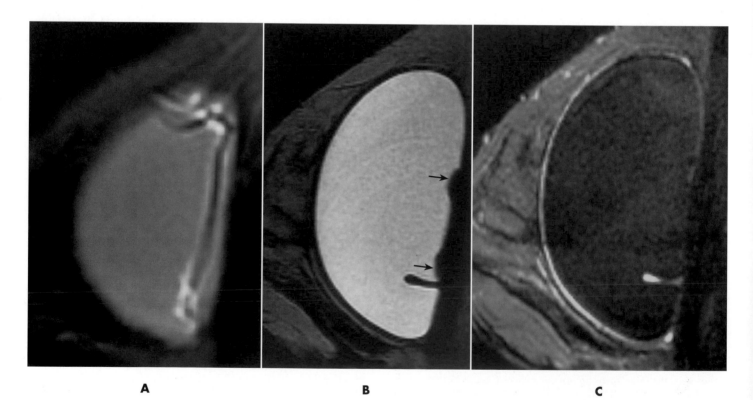

A **B** **C**

FIGURE 17-6 Intracapsular waterlike fluid surrounding implants. **A,** Waterlike fluid within folds. (Surgitek Replicon single-lumen, silicone gel–filled, polyurethane-coated implant shown on a sagittal T2-weighted FSE image without suppression.) Chemical-shift artifact is demonstrated between the water in the folds and the silicone gel in the implant. **B,** Thickened folds, partly on the basis of suppressed waterlike fluid in the folds. (McGhan Style 110 textured single-lumen silicone gel–filled implant shown on a sagittal T2-weighted FSE water-suppression image.) Silicone elastomer back patch seen posteriorly in the implant *(arrows)* is thicker than the implant shell because that is how it was made, not on the basis of water suppression. **C,** Same implant as in **B** showing intracapsular waterlike fluid around the implant with bright signal on a sagittal T2-weighted FSE silicone-suppression image.

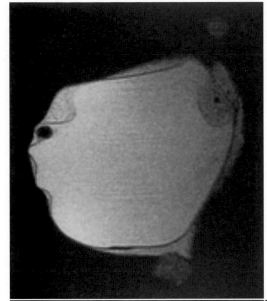

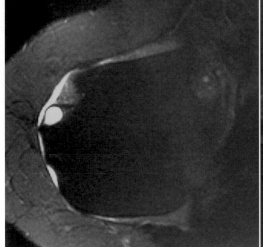

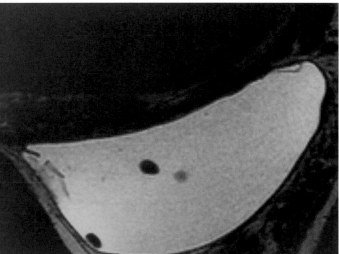

FIGURE 17-7   Waterlike fluid within single-lumen silicone gel–filled implants. **A,** Ruptured implant with silicone outside the implant and fibrous capsule (bright) and waterlike fluid inside and outside the implant in the form of large bubbles and microbubbles (dark) mixed with silicone gel shown on a sagittal T2-weighted FSE water-suppression image. **B,** Same implant as in **A** with applied silicone suppression, showing waterlike bubbles with bright signal on a sagittal T2-weighted FSE image. **C,** Waterlike bubbles (dark) within an intact implant on an axial T2-weighted FSE water-suppression image.

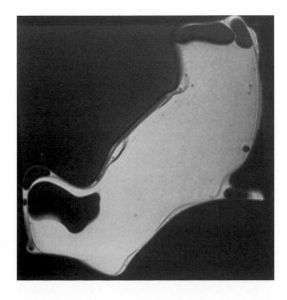

FIGURE 17-8   Standard double-lumen implant (shared back patch configuration) with waterlike bubbles in the inner gel compartment and gel globules in the outer saline compartment (in vitro image postexplantation after removal from the fibrous capsule) shown on a T2-weighted FSE water-suppression image.

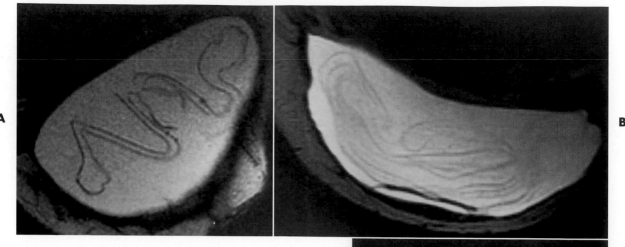

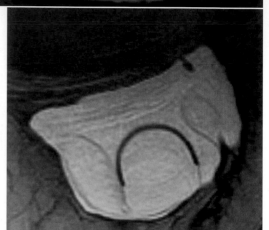

FIGURE 17-9   Signs of collapsed rupture as shown on T2-weighted FSE water-suppression images. **A,** Wavy line sign indicating collapsed rupture of a single-lumen silicone gel–filled implant (axial). This case is unusual in that actual breaks in the shell are seen. **B,** Double wavy line sign with twice as many lines seen, representing collapsed rupture of a standard double-lumen implant (shared back patch configuration, axial). **C,** C-sign indicating collapsed rupture of a single-lumen silicone gel–filled implant (axial).

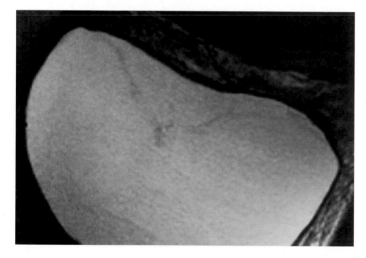

FIGURE 17-10   Cavon "cast gel" implant, formed silicone gel manufactured without a shell shown on an axial T2-weighted FSE water-suppression image. Dark waterlike signal internally represents fluid injected into the implant at the time of placement. Silicone fluid in the adjacent soft tissues as a result of direct injections this patient received in 1972 is incidentally noted.

Partially and Fully Collapsed Rupture

Signs of collapsed rupture include the wavy line sign (Figure 17-9, *A*; same as the linguini sign[67]), in which internal continuous wavy lines represent an implant shell totally enveloped and surrounded by silicone gel in a single-lumen implant[79]; the double wavy line sign[79] (Figure 17-9, *B*), which is the same as the wavy line sign but for a double-lumen implant, with twice as many lines; and the C-sign[79] (Figure 17-9, *C*), in which the back patch of an implant takes on the shape of the letter C and is fully surrounded by silicone gel. Implants are considered fully collapsed if the implant shell has a closely layered appearance and partially collapsed if the shell has not (yet) fully fallen in on itself.

In addition to the presence of internal wavy lines in cases of partially and fully collapsed rupture, peripheral folds generally are mostly or completely absent. Absence of peripheral folds with no evident internal wavy lines can occur where the internal wavy lines are not evident because of low MR scan resolution. This situation can occur because some implant shells, especially those used in the mid and late 1970s, were exceedingly thin (often visible only with high-resolution MRI). If intact implants are very soft, overfilled (high profile), or very large (700 to 800 cc or greater), there may be an absence of peripheral folds. Other unusual situations in which there are no peripheral folds include when implants were manufactured without a shell (the Cavon implant shown in Figure 17-10; manufactured by CUI and Aesthetech from about 1979 to 1985), when silicone gel was removed from the implant shell at the time of placement (with the shell being discarded) and the gel alone was placed directly into the patient,[56] or when "native" silicone gel was injected or implanted directly into soft tissues.[19,38,105]

False-positive findings may occur if complex implant folds are mistaken for the wavy line sign. Schmidt[120] described a special case in which a leaflet valve in a gel-saline implant was mistaken for a wavy line sign. Complex folds do not an abnormal implant make. A wavy line sign is not present unless (1) the shell is fully within the gel, (2) there are essentially no peripheral folds, and (3) the amount of waterlike bubbles within the implant, if they are present, is in some sense in proportion to the amount of silicone seen outside the implant shell. A knowledge of the kind of implant and its fill valve, where applicable, also helps the clinician recognize a normal appearance.

Uncollapsed and Minimally Collapsed Rupture

Uncollapsed rupture may be obvious but in some cases may be detectable only with high-resolution scanning. The best sign of uncollapsed rupture is the definitive presence of a small amount of intracapsular silicone gel within an implant fold or folds outside an implant,

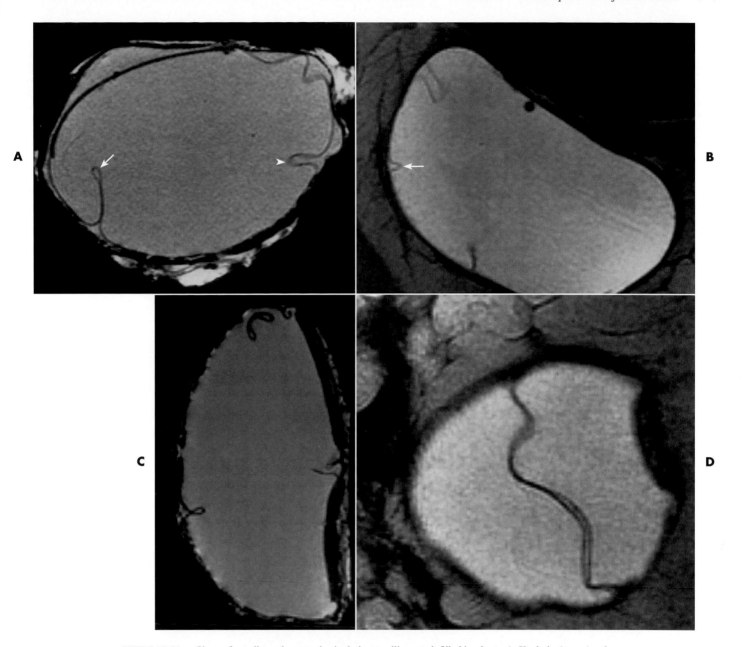

FIGURE 17-11   Signs of uncollapsed rupture in single-lumen silicone gel–filled implants. **A,** Keyhole *(arrow)* and pull-away *(arrowhead)* signs, where bright signal outside the implant shell represents silicone that has escaped the implant. If enough silicone is seen, as is the case here, these appearances can with confidence be taken to indicate rupture. This is an ex vivo image (3D spoiled GRASS [SPGR], 1.3-mm slice thickness) of an implant in a state of minimally collapsed rupture still in the fibrous capsule after explantation, shown here to illustrate the appearances of these signs in full detail. **B,** False-positive pull-away sign on an axial T2-weighted FSE water-suppression image. We examined this implant at the time of removal and found it to be intact. Thus the most likely explanation for this appearance is that the silicone seen on this image is actually silicone fluid (i.e., normal silicone fluid bleed) that has accumulated in a fold *(arrow)* in a quantity sufficient to be imaged. This is the only false-positive result we have had of this sign, representing less than 1% false-positive occurrences of this sign. Incidentally a waterlike bubble is also seen posteriorly within this intact implant. **C,** Pince-nez sign, where the bright signal outside the implant shell represents silicone that has escaped the implant (ex vivo image of implant still within fibrous capsule after explantation, 3D SPGR image, 1-mm slice thickness). This is a very rare appearance of uncollapsed rupture. This internal loop represents the tip of a complex fold with silicone outside it. Also seen in this Dow Corning 830 series ("four-quadrant") implant are two of the posterior fixation patches with a keyhole sign between them and another keyhole sign anteriorly. **D,** Parallel line sign, where the bright signal outside the implant shell represents silicone that has escaped the implant shown on a sagittal T2-weighted FSE water-suppression image. This is a very rare appearance of uncollapsed rupture representing silicone outside the shell, viewed lengthwise. Incidental note is made of a disk-shaped Dacron mesh fixation patch posteriorly on this Dow Corning 530 FP series implant.

the presumption being that if enough silicone is present to be seen in this setting, a thin layer of silicone gel must be surrounding the entire implant, and the only way it could have gotten there was through a hole or other defect in the shell. We call this appearance the *keyhole sign,* and if slightly more silicone is present outside the shell and the sides of

the keyhole do not touch each other, we call it the *pull-away sign* (Figure 17-11, *A*).[79] These are the same appearances that have been described as the *inverted teardrop,*[66,132] *open loop,*[52] and *noose signs.*[15]

Care must be taken if the amount of silicone seen is very small, that is, just barely detectable at high resolution (15-cm FOV, 256 × 256 matrix, 3-mm slice thickness), because it may represent just normal silicone fluid bleed from an intact implant (Figure 17-11, *B*). For this reason, our confidence that these are ruptured is only about 99%; about 1% of implants with this appearance may be intact.

In cases in which the keyhole or pull-away is quite small and is seen, for example, on only one slice, or we are not sure if it is real, we call the case *indeterminate*. The interpretation is that there is suspicion but not certainty of uncollapsed rupture. Just over half of the implants thus interpreted that have been removed were found to be in a state of uncollapsed rupture.[79]

Care also must be taken to avoid calling abnormal a pattern that represents just a complex fold mimicking one of those mentioned earlier, such as the pseudo–pull-away appearance (Figure 17-4, *F*). A real keyhole or pull-away will have a single thickness of implant shell; normal folds elsewhere in the same implant will have a double thickness of shell, and thus can be used as an internal reference for normal folds. The difference between a single and a double thickness of shell can often be appreciated on high-resolution imaging. Seeing this appearance remaining relatively constant over several slices helps to increase confidence that it is real. Variants of the keyhole and pull-away signs are the

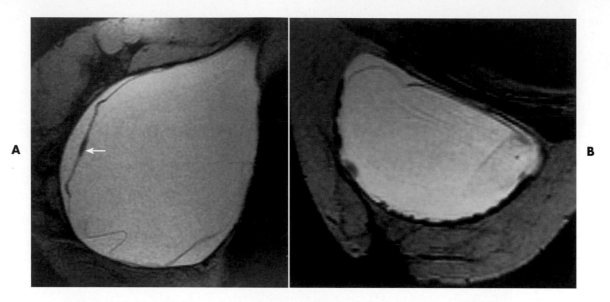

FIGURE 17-12   Signs of minimally collapsed rupture. (Single-lumen silicone gel–filled implants shown on T2-weighted FSE water-suppression images.) **A,** Back patch sign. Silicone is present behind the back patch in a quantity and with an appearance sufficient to predict rupture (sagittal). Slight central back patch thickening *(arrow)* represents the gel fill point (Heyer-Schulte Style 7000 implant). **B,** Anterior spiculation sign. Silicone present outside the implant shell with spiculated appearance represents penetration into interstices between broken plates of calcification lining the internal surface of the fibrous capsule (axial).

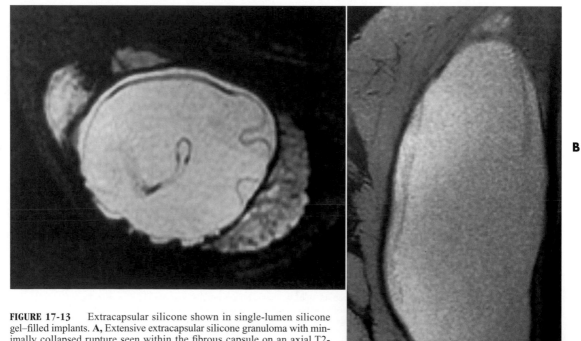

FIGURE 17-13   Extracapsular silicone shown in single-lumen silicone gel–filled implants. **A,** Extensive extracapsular silicone granuloma with minimally collapsed rupture seen within the fibrous capsule on an axial T2-weighted FMPIR fat-nulled water-suppression image. **B,** Extracapsular silicone granuloma superior to the intact current implant, all confirmed at surgery, shown on a sagittal T2-weighted FSE water-suppression image. The most likely explanation is that the extracapsular silicone is from a prior ruptured implant.

pince-nez (Figure 17-11, *C*) and parallel line (Figure 17-11, *D*) signs. These are just appearances of folds with silicone gel outside the shell viewed from different perspectives than in the keyhole and pull-away appearances.

If intracapsular silicone gel is present within folds and outside stretches of back patch or shell, we refer to the implant as being *minimally collapsed*—signs of which are the back patch sign (Figure 17-12, *A*) and the anterior spiculation sign (Figure 17-12, *B*).[79] Another pitfall is that silicone fluid bleed from an intact implant may collect between layers of a fixation patch, mimicking the back patch sign.

Small periimplant waterlike fluid collections surrounding implants, common in textured and polyurethane-coated implants, can make finding small amounts of silicone gel outside the shell of the implant more difficult. In these cases, small droplets of bright silicone may sometimes be seen within the dark (water-suppressed) waterlike fluid within the folds, which are often wider than usual.

Extracapsular Silicone

Silicone in the soft tissues outside an implant fibrous capsule is a very good sign of rupture of a present or a prior implant (Figure 17-13, *A*) unless there have been silicone fluid (or gel) direct injections into the breast; therefore taking an adequate history is important. The presence of silicone outside the fibrous capsule does not prove rupture of a current implant because the silicone may be remaining from a prior rupture or injection (Figure 17-13, *B*). It was the practice of some plastic surgeons to place small amounts of "native" silicone gel directly into soft tissue to "fix" small defects.[105] If appropriate high-resolution imaging is done, we expect one or more of the above-noted MR signs of rupture of a current implant to be present if the extracapsular silicone is arising from that implant. If no signs of silicone outside the shell of an implant are seen at all on high-resolution imaging, but silicone is clearly and definitively seen in the soft tissues outside the fibrous capsule, then the possibility of a prior implant having been ruptured or of soft tissue silicone otherwise having been placed should be considered, even if the history is to the contrary.

APPEARANCES OF SILICONE IN SOFT TISSUES

We have observed five appearances of soft tissue silicone (as noted in Table 17-1): two for silicone gel and fluid, and the other three mainly for silicone fluid.

Both silicone fluid and silicone gel are capable of persisting indefinitely in essentially their original state within soft tissue, especially if a surrounding scar or a fibrous capsule forms. In these states both appear homogeneous with their full expected T2 intensity on MR images, just as does silicone gel inside a normal implant (Figure 17-14), and currently we are not able to distinguish between them on the basis of their focal MR appearance.

Silicone fluid or gel in soft tissue may become infiltrated with scar tissue such that a firm white-yellow rubbery mass of tissue that feels greasy to the touch is formed, called a *silicone granuloma* or *siliconoma* (Figure 17-13, *A*).[13,142] The brightness of this tissue on T2-weighted sequences depends on the ratio of silicone to tissue within the granuloma or other tissue and in general appears inhomogeneous. The silicone granuloma appearance on MRI has been described by Persellin et al.[106] Ultralong TE sequences (TE = 300 to 350 ms) or fat-nulled FMPIR sequences are among the most sensitive to detect low concentrations of silicone. We expect silicone to be isointense to surrounding tissue at no less than about 5% to 15% concentration by volume. If sil-

icone is present in this range or lower, we expect that it will most likely escape detection by anyone using MRI. Again, on the basis of focal MR appearance alone, currently we are not able to distinguish silicone fluid from silicone gel if in the granulomatous state.

Silicone fluid usually is seen as a lacy, wispy infiltration extending over a wide area, often all the way to skin level. In our experience this appearance almost always occurs only with, and is pathognomonic for, silicone fluid. This usually means that there is a history of silicone-fluid breast injection. However, some rare implants manufactured in the early 1970s were reported to have been inflatable with silicone fluid, which could conceivably give the same appearance. Usually the intensity is moderately or very bright on T2-weighted sequences (Figure 17-15).

Silicone can infiltrate muscle. In our experience this usually occurs only with silicone fluid injections, which can form cysts and infiltrate extensively into the fatty tissue separating muscular groups and fibers

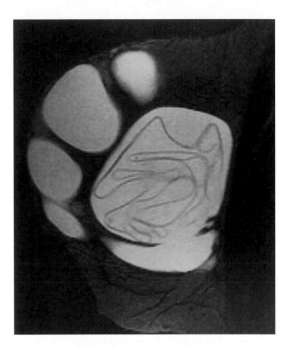

FIGURE 17-14   Cystic appearance of extensive soft tissue silicone shown on a sagittal T2-weighted FSE water-suppression image. Wavy line appearance of collapsed rupture is seen in the original implant pocket.

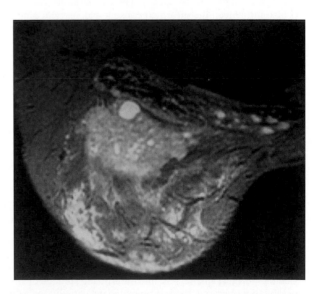

FIGURE 17-15   Direct silicone fluid injections shown on an axial T2-weighted FSE water-suppression image. Cystic and granulomatous silicone is present in the soft tissues. Wispy, lacy, infiltrative appearance of silicone fluid in the fatty breast tissues extends to the skin in places. Silicone fluid thoroughly infiltrates the pectoralis major muscle.

Table 17-1	Five Appearances of Silicone in Soft Tissue	
APPEARANCE	**SILICONE GEL**	**SILICONE FLUID**
Cyst	+++	++
Granuloma	+++	+++
Wispy, lacy infiltration of fatty breast tissues	++++	+
Infiltration of muscle	+++	+
Globules in muscle	++	+

Modified from reference 79.

++++, Universal; +++, very common; ++, common; +, rare.

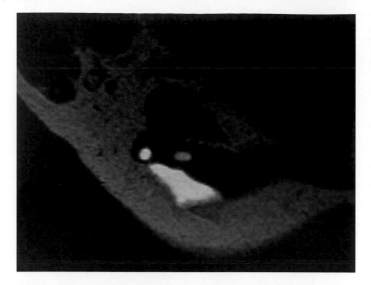

FIGURE 17-16   Penetration of silicone gel globules from a ruptured implant into the pectoralis major muscle shown on an axial T2-weighted FSE water suppression image. The upper portion of the implant is seen anterior to the muscle. There was a history of closed capsulotomy.

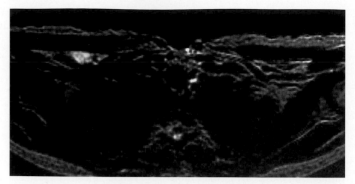

FIGURE 17-17   Silicone granuloma in the brachial plexus area causing thoracic outlet syndrome was relieved immediately on surgical removal. Part of the granuloma is shown here just posterior to the pectoralis major on an axial T2-weighted FSE water-suppression image.

(Figure 17-15). However, silicone gel also can rarely be found as globules or cysts within muscle (Figure 17-16).

SURGICAL EVALUATION AND OPERATIVE PLANNING

Of the first 204 patients with implants evaluated with MRI at our institution, we reported on the first 39 who also had their implants removed by one of our surgeons.[46] For nine of the 17 patients in whom MRI showed rupture, the MR finding was the decisive factor in the patient's request for explantation. In 10 of the 14 patients whose implants the surgeon did not consider ruptured on the basis of physical examination and history, but which were shown on MRI to be ruptured, the MR study was the decisive factor for the surgeon in recommending explantation. On the basis of history and physical examination, the surgeon felt certain that the implants were ruptured in four of the 39 patients. In one of those cases the implants were found to be intact, as predicted by MRI, when surgery was performed. Incidentally, in this limited series of 39 patients, MRI provided the correct interpretation for all but one implant, which was one of our six false-positives overall to date.

MRI also influenced the informed consent and surgical procedure. In one patient, silicone had encased the axillary artery, and its removal necessitated discussing the additional risk with the patient, as well as the departure from the usual surgical plan.

In another case, bilateral rupture was suspected clinically after a motor vehicle accident (both breasts suddenly became soft and formless), with emergency surgery planned for the following morning. An MR study obtained the night before showed no evidence of rupture, indicating that most likely only bilateral traumatic closed capsulotomy had occurred. The patient was informed, and she decided to have the implants removed anyway. Surgery was rescheduled electively, and the diagnosis of bilateral traumatic closed capsulotomy without implant rupture was confirmed.

MRI influences surgery in three principal ways:
1. If a patient and her physician have decided on surgery on the basis of an assumption that an implant has ruptured, a negative MR scan finding allows for a reconsideration of the decision to operate.
2. An implant may be ruptured but still be contained within the fibrous capsule. The surgeon may decide to remove the implant within the fibrous capsule as one unit, with the implant still inside the fibrous capsule, possibly minimizing spillage of silicone gel into the operative field. If no extracapsular silicone from the current or prior implants is seen or suspected on the basis of the MR scan or otherwise, the surgeon need not extensively explore adjacent soft tissues looking for silicone, and the patient can rest more easily knowing that none was detected with MRI and that any possible amount being missed is small.
3. Silicone can be seen in the soft tissues outside the fibrous capsule as a result of rupture of a current or prior implant, prior silicone fluid or gel injection or placement, or some combination of these factors. If the silicone is distant and removing it would entail greater risk, such as silicone in the brachial plexus area (Figure 17-17), then the patient can be properly informed and an appropriate decision made. If the silicone is deep and walled off under the pectoralis major muscle in a patient with subglandular implants or anywhere else not suspected by the surgeon, a plan can be made to attempt removal, thus avoiding a possible future operation. In these cases the MR scan serves as a kind of silicone road map to guide the surgeon in planning the operation.

INDICATIONS FOR BREAST IMPLANT IMAGING

Indications for obtaining an MR scan to evaluate breast implants or suspected soft tissue silicone are considered by some to be controversial in part because any possible deleterious effects of silicone or polyurethane have not yet been definitively proved or disproved to the satisfaction of all concerned (Table 17-2). In the previous section the possible medical benefits of a preoperative MR scan were outlined. The desire for this information on the part of the patient and physician has been the indication for MR evaluation of patients with implants. Market forces in balance with perceived benefits are currently dictating the terms on which MR scans are being requested.

Saline-filled implants are generally either inflated or deflated, and the difference is usually obvious to both the patient and the physician. Deflated saline implants have a characteristic appearance on mammograms. Medical records can be helpful, and prior mammograms can be reviewed if there is any question about whether a patient has saline- or silicone gel–filled implants.

When silicone gel–filled implants are removed and are reliably determined not to have ruptured and total capsulectomy with the implant still inside has been performed, it has been our experience that the chances of finding residual soft tissue silicone by using MRI are low.

For patients with double- or triple-lumen implants with outer-lumen saline still present as demonstrated with a mammogram or MR scan, we have found that the chance of finding detectable silicone outside that implant from that implant is low.

In those for whom the only question is whether breast cancer is present, an MR scan designed to detect rupture or soft tissue silicone will not answer the question and thus is not indicated. However, if an abnormality is suspected to be caused by silicone or an implant, then such an examination may be helpful, for example, by definitively finding a silicone granuloma.

For patients with a definite plan not to have their implants removed, even if an abnormality were to be discovered on the proposed MR scan, there is no clinical utility for obtaining that MR scan. In this case, both categories of clinical utility—to help decide whether surgery is indicated and to provide information for the surgeon to use during surgery—have been superseded by the patient's choice to avoid surgery.

Table 17-2 Main Relative Indications and Contraindications for Breast Implant MR Evaluation

Relative indications
1. To determine whether there is rupture of a silicone gel–filled implant
2. To determine whether there is detectable soft tissue silicone, and if so, the amounts and locations

Relative contraindications
1. Current saline-filled, dextran-filled, or PVP-filled implants in place, no history of silicone gel–filled implants or of silicone fluid or gel injections
2. Current saline-filled implants in place or no current implants in place, with a history of prior silicone gel–filled implants that definitely were not ruptured where total capsulectomies were performed
3. Current standard double- or triple-lumen implants in place with the outer-lumen saline still present as per MRI, mammography, or ultrasound; no history of prior silicone gel–filled implants or silicone fluid or gel injections
4. Current silicone gel–filled breast implants in place, or history of prior silicone gel–filled implants or silicone fluid or gel injections, but only question being asked clinically is whether breast cancer is present
5. Some saline-filled tissue expanders contain a metallic ring to allow in vivo localization for percutaneous filling (For example, the product literature for the McGhan MagnaSite series states that MRI is contraindicated. We did image one patient with this type of tissue expander without prior knowledge of its presence. She did not report discomfort during or after the scan. She did note a sense of movement entering and being removed from the scanner, reproducible when she turned around next to the scanner afterward. We have been informed that other tissue expanders [such as from PMT] are available with metallic inserts to aid in localization that are MR compatible. Confirmation of this from PMT has been requested but not yet received.)
6. Solid elastomer implants do not require "silicone-specific" imaging, MR or otherwise
7. Sponge implants do not require "silicone-specific" imaging, MR or otherwise
8. Breast MRI is relatively contraindicated if there has been a determination of a low pretest probability of a positive result, on the basis of:
   a) A prior adequate quality MR scan within 1 or 2 years that was reported to be negative for rupture, with no intervening history of any sudden change in breast shape or size, and no history of breast trauma
   b) Prior MR scan after explantation of comparable quality to the proposed scan, where the repeat scan is being requested to determine whether more silicone is detectable
   c) Adequate quality preexplantation MR scan was obtained that did not show evidence of extracapsular soft tissue silicone, where the explantation was performed by removing the implant still entirely within the fibrous capsule as a single unit, now seeking to determine whether residual silicone is present
9. No intention of undergoing surgery, no matter what results an MR scan may show

Modified from reference 79.

Some tissue expanders are manufactured with an embedded metallic piece to help localize the saline fill point with an external magnet for purposes of allowing percutaneous inflation. As per manufacturers' recommendations, MRI is contraindicated for some of these devices (Table 17-2).

EXPLANTATION

The importance to a patient and her surgeon of removing soft tissue silicone and avoiding a possible silicone spill during explantation may help determine whether an MR scan or ultrasound examination is performed preoperatively and, if so, how the operation is performed. As discussed by Ahn et al,[3] some think it necessary to remove the fibrous capsule along with the implant. One of three basic methods or a variant thereof is usually used to remove implants. The decision on which method to use often is made by the patient in consultation with her surgeon.

One method involves an initial incision and dissection down to the outer surface of the fibrous capsule, incision of the fibrous capsule, removal of the implant, and possible breakup of the fibrous capsule (capsulotomy), with no removal of the fibrous capsule.

A second method involves an initial incision and dissection down to the outer surface of the fibrous capsule, incision of the fibrous capsule, removal of the implant, and then partial or complete removal of the fibrous capsule (capsulectomy).

A third method involves incision and dissection down to the outer surface of the fibrous capsule, careful pericapsular dissection around the entire circumference of the fibrous capsule, removal of the fibrous capsule (unopened) with the implant still inside through an adequately sized skin incision, and then the opening of the fibrous capsule on a back table (or later) to remove and examine the implant.

SUMMARY

MRI allows us to accomplish the evaluation of silicone gel–filled implants with a high degree of confidence and the evaluation of soft tissue silicone to a lesser degree. Progress continues to be made in improving the equipment and the methods being used. However, because MRI is expensive, its use should be balanced against the capabilities of less expensive methods to evaluate implants, although often those methods may be less helpful. MRI and ultrasound can be considered complementary and overlapping in their capabilities to show these conditions, with MRI having the advantage with implants and ultrasound having the advantage with soft tissues.

Mammography generally is useful to evaluate only that small number of ruptures that result in observable extracapsular silicone. The notion that physical examination alone is sufficient to evaluate implants has lost credibility, given the large number of cases in which rupture or soft tissue silicone was detected with only MRI or ultrasound. In the future, blood tests may provide a reliable, inexpensive screen to determine whether further testing is required, but we are not there yet, and in any case blood tests cannot provide the surgeon a road map.

REFERENCES

1. Ahn CY, DeBruhl ND, Gorczyca DP, et al: Silicone implant rupture diagnosis using computed tomography: a case report and experience with 22 surgically removed implants, Ann Plast Surg 33:624, 1994.
2. Ahn CY, DeBruhl ND, Gorczyca DP, et al: Comparative silicone breast implant evaluation using mammography, sonography, and magnetic resonance imaging: experience with 59 implants, Plast Reconstr Surg 94:620, 1994.
3. Ahn CY, Shaw WW, Narayanan K, et al: Residual silicone detection using MRI following previous breast implant removal: case reports, Aesthetic Plast Surg 19:361, 1995.
4. Ahn CY, Shaw WW, Narayanan K, et al: Definitive diagnosis of breast implant rupture using magnetic resonance imaging, Plast Reconst Surg 92:681, 1993.
5. Arion HG: Presentation d'une prothese retromammaire, Comp Rend de la Soc Fran de Gyn 35:427, 1965.
6. Arons MS, Sabesin SM, and Smith RR: Experimental studies with Etheron sponge—effect of implantation in tumor-bearing animals, Plast Reconst Surg 28:72, 1961.
7. Ashley FL: Further studies on the Natural-Y breast prosthesis, Plast Reconst Surg 49:414, 1972.
8. Ashley FL: A new type of breast prosthesis: preliminary report, Plast Reconst Surg 45:421, 1970.
9. Bar-Meir E, Teuber SS, Lin HC, et al: Multiple autoantibodies in patients with silicone breast implants, J Autoimmun 8:267, 1995.
10. Barker DE, Retsky MI, and Schultz S: "Bleeding" of silicone from bag-gel breast implants, and its clinical relation to fibrous capsule formation, Plast Reconst Surg 61:836, 1978.
11. Bassett LW, and Brenner RJ: Considerations when imaging women with breast implants, Am J Roentgenol 159:979, 1992.
12. Batich C, Williams J, and King R: Toxic hydrolysis product from a biodegradable foam implant, Biomed Mater Res Appl Biomat 23:311, 1989.
13. Ben-Hur N, and Neuman Z: Siliconoma—another cutaneous response to dimethylpolysiloxane, Plast Reconst Surg 36:629, 1965.
14. Berg WA, Caskey CI, Hamper UM, et al: Diagnosing breast implant rupture with MR imaging, US, and mammography, Radiographics 13:1323, 1993.
15. Berg WA, Caskey CI, Hamper UM, et al: Single and double-lumen silicone breast implant integrity: prospective evaluation of MR and US criteria, Radiology 197:45, 1995.

16. Bergman RB, and van der Ende AE: Exudation of silicone through the envelope of breast prostheses: an in vitro study, Plast Reconst Surg 32:31, 1979.
17. Biggs TM, Cukier J, and Worthing LF: Augmentation mammaplasty: a review of 18 years, Plast Reconst Surg 69:445, 1982.
18. Bing JH: US Pat. #2,609,545, filed 11/24/50 in USA, 1/26/49 in Denmark, granted 9/9/52. Filling-body for surgical use, describing use of polyethylene as an implantable material. Assignor to Aktieselskabet Ferrosan, Copenhagen, Denmark.
19. Boo-Chai K: The complications of augmentation mammaplasty by silicone injection, Br J Plast Surg 22:281, 1969.
20. Braley SA: The medical silicones, Trans Am Soc Artif Intern Organs 10:240, 1964.
21. Braley SA: The use of silicones in plastic surgery, Plast Reconst Surg 50:280, 1973.
22. Brautbar N, ed: Special issue on silicone toxicity, Int J Occup Med Tox 4(1): 1995.
23. Brem RF, Tempany CMC, and Zerhouni EA: MR detection of breast implant rupture, J Comput Assist Tomogr 16:157, 1992.
24. Bridges AJ, Conley C, Wang G, et al: A clinical and immunological evaluation of women with silicone breast implants and symptoms of rheumatic disease, Ann Intern Med 118:929, 1993.
25. Brinton LA, and Brown SL: Breast implants and cancer, J Natl Cancer Inst 89:1341, 1997.
26. Brown SL, Silverman BG, and Berg WA: Rupture of silicone-gel breast implants: causes, sequelae, and diagnoses, Lancet 350:1531, 1997.
27. Burkhardt BR, Fried M, Schnur PL, et al: Capsules, infection, and intraluminal antibiotics, Plast Reconst Surg 68:43, 1981.
28. Calnan JS: Assessment of biological properties of implants before their clinical use, Proc R Soc Med 63:1115, 1970.
29. Campbell LA, Passodelis WE, Middleton MS, et al: Artifacts in breast implant imaging, 83nd Scientific Assembly and Annual Meeting of the RSNA, Chicago, Dec 1997 (poster).
30. Capozzi A: Long-term complications of polyurethane-covered breast implants, Plast Reconst Surg 88:458, 1991.
31. Capozzi A: Polyurethane-covered gel mammary implants, Plast Reconst Surg 69:904, 1982 (letter).
32. Capozzi A, Du Bou R, and Pennisi VR: Distant migration of silicone gel from a ruptured breast implant: case report, Plast Reconst Surg 62:302, 1978.
33. Capozzi A, and Pennisi VR: Clinical experience with polyurethane-covered gel-filled mammary prostheses, Plast Reconst Surg 68:512, 1981.
34. Caskey CI, Berg WA, Anderson ND, et al: Breast implant rupture: diagnosis with US, Radiology 190:819, 1994.
35. Coleman EA, Lemon SJ, Rudick J, et al: Rheumatic disease among 1167 women reporting local implant and systemic problems after breast implant surgery, J Women Health 3:165, 1994.
36. Collins JD, Shaver ML, Disher AC, et al: Compromising abnormalities of the brachial plexus as displayed by magnetic resonance imaging, Clin Anat 8:1, 1995.
37. Conant EF, Forsberg F, Moore JH, et al: Surgical removal of ruptured breast implants: the use of intraoperative sonography in localizing free silicone, Am J Roentgenol 165:1378, 1995 (technical note).
38. Conway H, and Goulian D Jr: Experience with an injectable Silastic RTV as a subcutaneous prosthetic material: a preliminary report, Plast Reconst Surg 32:294, 1963.
39. Cook RR, Delongchamp RR, Woodbury M, et al: The prevalence of women with breast implants in the United States, J Clin Epidemiol 48:519, 1996.
40. Cronin TD, and Gerow FJ: Augmentation mammaplasty: a new "natural feel" prosthesis. In Transactions of the Third International Congress of Plastic Surgery, Oct 13-18, 1963, Washington, DC, p. 41, 1964
41. Cronin TD, and Greenberg RL: Our experiences with the Silastic gel breast prosthesis, Plast Reconst Surg 46:1, 1970.
42. Davis PK, and Jones SM: The complications of Silastic implants: experience with 137 consecutive cases, Br J Plast Surg 24:405, 1971.
43. de Camara DL, Sheridan JM, and Kammer BA: Rupture and aging of silicone gel breast implants, Plast Reconst Surg 91:828, 1993.
44. Demergian P: Experiences with the newer subcutaneous implant materials, Surg Clin North Am 32:1313, 1963.
45. Destouet JM, Monsees BS, Oser RF, et al: Screening mammography in 350 women with breast implants: prevalence and findings of breast implant complications, Am J Roentgenol 159:973, 1992.
46. Dobke MK, and Middleton MS: Clinical impact of MRI on the surgical management of silicone gel–filled breast implant patients, Ann Plast Surg 33:241, 1994.
47. DeAngelis GA, de Lange EE, Miller LR, et al: MR imaging of breast implants, Radiographics 14:783, 1994.
48. Dowden RV, and Anain S: Endoscopic implant evaluation and capsulotomy, Plast Reconst Surg 91:283, 1993.
49. Edgerton MT: Augmentation mammaplasty—psychiatric implications and surgical indications, Plast Reconst Surg 21:279, 1958.
50. Edmond JA: Late complication of closed capsulotomy of the breast, Plast Reconst Surg 66:478, 1980 (letter).
51. Edwards BF: Teflon-silicone breast implants, Plast Reconst Surg 32:519, 1963.
52. Everson LI, Parantainen H, Detlie T, et al: Diagnosis of breast implant rupture: imaging findings and relative efficacies of imaging techniques, Am J Roentgenol 163:57, 1994.
53. Foged J: Hypoplasia mammae behandlet med polystanprotese, Ugeskrift for Læger 117:389, 1955.
54. Franklyn RA: Der neue kunststoff "Surgifoam" und seine chirurgische nutzbarkeit, Zentralblatt für Chirurgie 81:1192, 1956.
55. Freeman BS: Complications of subcutaneous mastectomy with prosthetic replacement, immediate or delayed, South Med J 60:1277, 1967.
56. Freeman BS: Reconstruction of the breast form by Silastic gel from breast prostheses, Br J Plast Surg 27:284, 1974.
57. Gabriel SE, O'Fallon WM, Kurland LT, et al: Risk of connective tissue diseases and other disorders after breast implantation, N Engl J Med 330:1697, 1994.
58. Gabriel SE, Woods JE, O'Fallon M, et al: Complications leading to surgery after breast implantation, N Engl J Med 336:677, 1997.
59. Ganott MA, Harris KM, Ilkhanipour ZS, et al: Augmentation mammaplasty: normal and abnormal findings with mammography and US, Radiographics 12:281, 1992.
60. Garrido L, Kwong KK, Pfleiderer B, et al: Echo-planar chemical shift imaging of silicone gel prostheses, Magn Reson Imaging 11:625, 1993.
61. Giacomelli V: Protesi sostitutiva con spugna di Polystan dopo mastectomia, Minerva Chir 8:584, 1953.
62. Goldwyn RM: An unusual complication of the use of the Cronin implant for augmentation mammaplasty, Br J Plast Surg 22:167, 1969.
63. Gonzalez-Ulloa M: Correction of hypotrophy of the breast by means of exogenous material, Plast Reconst Surg 25:15, 1960.
64. Gorczyca DP, and Brenner RJ, eds: The augmented breast-radiological and clinical perspectives, New York, 1997, Thieme.
65. Gorczyca DP, DeBruhl ND, Ahn CY, et al: Silicone breast implant ruptures in an animal model: comparison of mammography, MR imaging, US, and CT, Radiology 190:227, 1994.
66. Gorczyca DP, Schneider E, DeBruhl ND, et al: Silicone breast implant rupture: comparison between three-point Dixon and fast spin echo MR imaging, Am J Roentgenol 162:305, 1994.
67. Gorczyca DP, Sinha S, Ahn CY, et al: Silicone breast implants in vivo: MR imaging, Radiology 185:407, 1992.
68. Gurdin M, and Carlin GA: Complications of breast implantations, Plast Reconst Surg 40:530, 1967.
69. Hargiss JL: Silicone sponge implants, Arch Ophthalmol 74:527, 1965.
70. Hennekens CH, Lee IM, Cook NR, et al: Self reported breast implants and connective tissue diseases in female health professionals, JAMA 275:616, 1996.
71. Johnson HA: Silastic breast implants: coping with complications, Plast Reconst Surg 44:588, 1969.
72. Kelly AP Jr, Jacobson HS, Fox JI, et al: Complications of subcutaneous mastectomy and replacement by the Cronin Silastic mammary prosthesis, Plast Reconst Surg 37:438, 1966.
73. Little G, and Baker JL: Results of closed compression capsulotomy for treatment of contracted breast implants, Plast Reconst Surg 65:30, 1980.
74. Malata CM, Varma S, Scott M, et al: Silicone breast implant rupture: common/serious complication? Med Prog Technol 20:251, 1994.
75. Malbec EF. Mammary hypoplasia: corrective implants. In Transactions of the Third International Congress of Plastic Surgery, Oct 13-18. 1963, Washington, DC, p. 60, 1964.
76. McNamara MP, Lina M, Middleton MS, et al: Sonographic diagnosis of silicone adenopathy in breast implant and direct injection patients: radiologic/pathologic correlation. In 81st Scientific Assembly and Annual Meeting of the RSNA, Chicago, 1995 (abstract).
77. Mehta L, McNamara MP, Rzeszotarski MS, et al: Sonographic assessment of silicone gel breast implant integrity: radiologic-pathologic correlation with reported and new signs of rupture. In 82nd Scientific Assembly and Annual Meeting of the RSNA, Chicago, Dec 1996 (abstract).
78. Middleton MS: Breast implant classification. In Gorczyca DP, and Brenner RJ, eds: The augmented breast-radiological and clinical perspectives, New York, 1997, Thieme.
79. Middleton MS: MR evaluation of breast implants and soft tissue silicone, Top Magn Reson Imaging 9:92, 1998.
80. Middleton MS, Mattrey R, and Dobke MK: Accuracy of high resolution MRI breast implant imaging. In 80th Scientific Assembly and Annual Meeting of the RSNA, Chicago, 1994 (abstract).
81. Middleton MS, Mattrey R, and Dobke MK: Distinguishing breast implant silicone gel leakage from rupture using high resolution MR imaging. Presented at the 1993 SMRM 12th Annual Meeting, New York, 1993 (abstract).
82. Middleton MS, Mattrey R, Dobke MK, et al: Identification of rupture and/or residual silicone in breast implant patients. Presented at the 11th Annual Meeting of the Society of Magnetic Resonance Imaging, San Francisco, 1993 (abstract).
83. Middleton MS, Mattrey R, Dobke MK, et al: MR imaging of silicone gel-filled breast implants using conventional and silicone suppression techniques. Presented at the 11th Annual Meeting of the Society of Magnetic Resonance in Medicine, Berlin, 1992 (abstract).
84. Middleton MS, Mattrey R, Udkoff R, et al: MR evaluation of silicone gel–filled breast implants. Presented at the 25th National ACR Conference on Breast Cancer, Boston, 1992 (abstract).
85. Middleton MS, and McNamara MP: MR and ultrasound imaging of breast implants and soft-tissue silicone, Imaging 9:201, 1997.
86. Middleton MS, and McNamara MP: Breast implant classification and identification–a pictorial review. Presented at the 81st Scientific Assembly and Annual Meeting of the RSNA, Chicago, 1995 (abstract).
87. Middleton MS, and McNamara MP: Breast implant imaging, Philadelphia, 1998, Lippincott-Raven (in press).
88. Middleton MS, and McNamara MP: Does silicone *gel* really bleed? Presented at the 81st Scientific Assembly and Annual Meeting of the RSNA, Chicago, 1995 (abstract).
89. Middleton MS, and McNamara MP: Pitfalls in breast implant MR imaging. Presented at the 81st Scientific Assembly and Annual Meeting of the RSNA, Chicago, 1995 (abstract).
90. Middleton MS, McNamara MP, and Cross J: Increased rupture rate of polyurethane coated breast implants. Presented at the 81st Scientific Assembly and Annual Meeting of the RSNA, Chicago, 1995 (abstract).

91. Monticciolo DL, Nelson RC, Dixon WT, et al: MR detection of leakage from silicone breast implants: value of a silicone selective pulse sequence, Am J Roentgenol 163:51, 1994.
92. Naso A: Mastectomia e ricostruzione estetica della regione mammaria con spugna di polietilene, Riforma Medica 67:662, 1953.
93. Nelson GD: Complications of closed compression after augmentation mammoplasty, Plast Reconst Surg 66:71, 1980.
94. Nelson GD: Complications from the treatment of fibrous capsular contracture of the breast, Plast Reconst Surg 68:969, 1981.
95. Neuman Z: Use of the non-absorbable polyethylene sponge "Polystan Sponge" as a subcutaneous prosthesis in rats, Br J Plast Surg 9:195, 1957.
96. Nosanchuk JS: Silicone granuloma in breast, Arch Surg 97:583, 1968.
97. Oneal RM, and Argenta LC: Late side effects related to inflatable breast prostheses containing soluble steroids, Plast Reconst Surg 69:641, 1982.
98. Oppenheimer BS, Oppenheimer ET, Danishefsky I, et al: Further studies of polymers as carcinogenic agents in animals, Cancer Res 15:333, 1955.
99. Oppenheimer BS, Oppenheimer ET, and Stout AP: Sarcomas induced in rodents by imbedding various plastic films, Proc Soc Exp Biol Med 79:366, 1952.
100. Pangman WJ II: Compound prosthesis. U.S. Pat. # 3,559,214, filed 10/17/68, granted 2/2/71, describing what became known as the Natural-Y implant.
101. Pangman WJ II: Surgically implantable compound breast prosthesis. U.S. Pat. # 3,683,424, filed 1/30/70, granted 8/15/72, describing what became the Polyplastic Adjustable and the New Polyplastic Adjustable implants.
102. Pangman WJ II, and Wallace RM: The use of plastic prosthesis in breast plastic and other soft tissue surgery—clinical experience using Ivalon (polyvinyl) sponge in surgery, West J Surg Ob Gyn 63:503, 1955.
103. Pare JA, and Fraser RG: Synopsis of diseases of the chest, Philadelphia, 1983, WB Saunders.
104. Parsons CL, Stein PC, Dobke MK, et al: Diagnosis and therapy of subclinically infected prostheses, Surg Gynecol Obstet 177:504, 1993.
105. Perras C: The creation of a twin breast following radical mastectomy, Clin Plast Surg 3:265, 1976.
106. Persellin ST, Vogler JB, Brazis PW, et al: Detection of migratory silicone pseudotumor with use of magnetic resonance imaging, Mayo Clin Proc 67:891, 1992.
107. Peters W, Keystone E, and Smith D: Factors affecting the rupture of silicone gel breast implants, Ann Plast Surg 32:449, 1994.
108. Petro JA, Klein SA, Niazi Z, et al: Evaluation of ultrasound as a tool in the follow-up of patients with breast implants: a preliminary prospective study, Ann Plast Surg 32:580, 1994.
109. Piccoli CW, Greer JG, and Mitchell DG: Breast MR imaging for cancer detection and implant evaluation: potential pitfalls, Radiographics 16:16, 1996.
110. Planas J, Carbonell A, and Planas J: Salvaging the exposed mammary prosthesis. Aesthetic Plast Surg 19:535, 1995.
111. Potter M, Morrison S, Wiener F, et al: Induction of plasmacytomas with silicone gel in genetically susceptible strains of mice, J Natl Cancer Inst 86:1058, 1994.
112. Potter M, and Rose NR, eds: Immunology of silicones, Philadelphia, 1996, Springer-Verlag.
113. Press RI, Peebles CL, Kumagai Y, et al: Antinuclear autoantibodies in women with silicone breast implants, Lancet 340:1304, 1992.
114. Robinson OG, Bradley EL, and Wilson DS: Analysis of explanted silicone implants: a report of 300 patients, Ann Plast Surg 34:1, 1995.
115. Rolland C, Guidoin R, Marceau D, et al: Nondestructive investigations on ninety-seven surgically excised mammary prostheses, J Biomed Mater Res 23:285, 1989.
116. Rubin LR: Polyethylene—a three year study, Plast Reconst Surg 7:131, 1951.
117. Rudolph R, ed: Problems in aesthetic surgery: biological causes and clinical solutions, St Louis, 1986, Mosby.
118. Salmon SE, and Kyle RA: Silicone gels, induction of plasma cell tumors, and genetic susceptibility in mice: a call for epidemiologic investigation of women with silicone breast implants, J Natl Cancer Inst 86:1040, 1994.
119. Sanchez-Guerrero J, Colditz GA, Karlson EW, et al: Silicone breast implants and the risk of connective-tissue diseases and symptoms, N Engl J Med 332:1666, 1995.
120. Schmidt GH: False positive rupture on magnetic resonance imaging, Ann Plast Surg 33:683, 1994.
121. Schneider E, and Chan TW: Selective MR imaging of silicone with the three-point Dixon technique, Radiology 187:89, 1993.
122. Schnohr E: Anvendelse af polystan-mammaprotese ved progressiv lipodystrofi, Ugeskrift for Læger 116:1247, 1954.
123. Schusterman MA, Kroll SS, Reece GP, et al: Incidence of autoimmune disease in patients after breast reconstruction with silicone gel implants versus autogenous tissue: a preliminary report, Ann Plast Surg 31:1, 1993.
124. Schwartz AW, Dockerty MB, and Grindlay JH: Calcification of polyvinyl-formyl (Ivalon) sponge, Plast Reconst Surg 26:110, 1960.
125. Shah Z, Lehman JA, and Tan J: Does infection play a role in breast capsular contracture? Plast Reconstr Surg 68:34, 1981.
126. Silver RM, Sahn EE, Allen JA, et al: Demonstration of silicon in sites of connective tissue disease in patients with silicone-gel breast implants, Arch Dermatol 129:63, 1993.
127. Silverman BG, Brown SL, Bright RA, et al: Reported complications of silicone gel breast implants: an epidemiologic review, Ann Intern Med 124:744, 1996.
128. Silverman S, Gluck O, Silver D, et al: The prevalence of autoantibodies in symptomatic and asymptomatic patients with breast implants and patients with fibromyalgia. In Potter M, and Rose NR, eds: Immunology of silicones, Philadelphia, 1996, Springer-Verlag.
129. Sinha S, Gorczyca DP, DeBruhl ND, et al: MR imaging of silicone breast implants: comparison of different coil arrays, Radiology 187:284, 1993.
130. Smahél J, Schneider K, and Donski P: Bizarre implants for augmentation mammaplasty: long term reaction to polyethylene strips, Br J Plast Surg 30:287, 1977.
131. Soo MS, Kornguth PJ, Georgiade GS, et al: Seromas in residual fibrous capsules after explantation: mammographic and sonographic appearances, Radiology 194:863, 1995.
132. Soo MS, Kornguth PJ, Walsh R, et al: Complex radial folds versus subtle signs of intracapsular rupture of breast implants: MR findings with surgical correlation, Am J Roentgenol 166:1421, 1996.
133. Speirs AC, and Blocksma R: New implantable silicone rubbers: an experimental evaluation of tissue response, Plast Reconst Surg 31:166, 1963.
134. Steinbach BG, Hiskes SK II, Fitzsimmons JR, et al: Phantom evaluation of imaging modalities for silicone breast implants, Invest Radiol 27:841, 1992.
135. Swan SH: Epidemiology of silicone-related disease, Semin Arthritis Rheum 24(Suppl):38, 1994.
136. Udkoff R, Ahn C, Shaw W, et al: MR imaging in the evaluation of breast implants, Radiology 181(P):347, 1991 (abstract).
137. Venta LA, Salomon CG, Flisak ME, et al: Sonographic signs of breast implant rupture, Am J Roentgenol 166:1413, 1996.
138. Vinas JC: Surgical experience with silicone implants. Presented to 5th session of the Rio de la Plata Society for Plastic Surgery, Carmelo, UR, 1962.
139. Waser J, Trueblood KN, and Knobler CM: Chem one, New York, 1976, McGraw-Hill.
140. Weisman MH, Vecchione TR, Albert D, et al: Connective tissue disease following breast augmentation: a preliminary test of the human adjuvant disease hypothesis, Plast Reconst Surg 82:626, 1988.
141. Williams JE: Experiences with a large series of Silastic breast implants, Plast Reconst Surg 49:253, 1972.
142. Winer LH, Sternberg TH, Lehman R, et al: Tissue reactions to injected silicone liquids, Arch Dermatol 90:588, 1964.
143. Yoshida SH, Chang CC, Teuber SS, et al: Silicon and silicone: theoretical and clinical implications of breast implants, Reg Toxicol Pharmacol 17:3, 1993.

18 Mediastinum and Lung

Nadja M. Lesko and Kerry M. Link

KEY POINTS

- CT remains superior for evaluating the mediastinum, lung parenchyma, and pleura for most neoplasms and infections.
- MRI is used to resolve ambiguous CT findings, in particular the staging of apical or other peripheral lung–chest wall lesions and hilar adenopathy.
- MRI is useful for evaluation of suspected aneurysms, dissections, leaks, or thromboses of the thoracic aorta and other great vessels.

LUNG PARENCHYMA

The inability to adequately evaluate the lung parenchyma is perhaps the major reason why magnetic resonance imaging (MRI) is rarely used to image patients with known or suspected pulmonary disease. Current technology cannot overcome the poor signal-to-noise ratio (SNR) in lung magnetic resonance (MR) images. The poor SNR is the result of low proton density, magnetic-susceptibility artifact, and motion.

Essentially air, the lungs lack H[+], and appear black on MR images.[23,37,73] The middle and distal bronchial systems and the fissures of the lungs are not usually identifiable on MR images. Manipulations to increase spatial resolution (e.g., decreased field of view or decreased slice thickness) worsen SNR.

Lung structure consists of millions of air-tissue interfaces causing local magnetic gradients destructive to MRI.[14,16,23,37,67,73]

Respiration, cardiac motion, vascular perfusion, and molecular diffusion all degrade MR image quality.[17,23,67] Superimposed on these physiological causes of motion are voluntary and involuntary patient movement. Cardiac motion can be addressed with echocardiography (ECG)-gated spin-echo (SE) techniques; however, this adds to the overall length of the study and exacerbates problems with respiratory and patient motion. Respiratory-gating schemes have been used, but because of the irregularity and length of the respiratory cycle, this greatly increases the time of image acquisition. Respiratory-compensation schemes, such as respiratory-ordered phase encoding (ROPE),[10] reorder the phase-encoding line of κ space over the respiratory cycle. Although improving the quality of an image, this does not always eliminate motion artifact and MR images remain inferior to computed tomography (CT) scans.

MEDIASTINUM

MRI plays an important role in the evaluation of the mediastinum. Structures with markedly dissimilar tissue characteristics show substantial image contrast, allowing for identification and assessment of structural anomalies and pathological processes.

Anterior Mediastinum

Thyroid Lesions. Intrathoracic thyroid tissue almost always is the result of the inferior extension of a mass contiguous with the thyroid gland. Thyroid masses usually arise from the thyroid isthmus or anteriorly from a thyroid lobe. Because of their high fluid content, thyroid masses usually exhibit a low signal on T1-weighted images (Figure 18-1) and a bright signal on T2-weighted images. Multiplanar MRI provides an assessment of displacement or compression of surrounding anatomical structures. Intrathoracic thyroid tissue is not always homogeneous: calcification may result in a dark signal, and hemorrhage displays a variety of signal patterns depending on the age of the blood. Fat is uncommon in thyroid masses, and its presence would suggest the diagnosis of a teratoma.[40] MRI is not capable of differentiating between benign and malignant tumors.[32,102]

MRI has proved useful in the detection of parathyroid adenomas.[55] The majority are found in the neck near the esophagus. Ten percent are ectopic and most often found in the region of the thymus. Adenomas have a bright signal on T2-weighted images and a dark-to-gray signal on T1-weighted images.[61] They are typically enhanced with gadolinium–diethylene-triamine-pentaacetic acid (Gd-DTPA).[92] Fat-suppression techniques may be useful to separate adenomas from surrounding mediastinal fat. Surface-coil imaging is useful in establishing the location of 90% of these lesions.

Thymic Lesions. In childhood, the thymus has an asymmetrical bilobed appearance, with the left lobe slightly larger than the right.[43] The thymus usually is located anterior to the aorta but may on occasion be located in the posterior mediastinum.[89] Its signal intensity is less than that of fat on T1- and T2-weighted images. The thymus involutes after puberty and is eventually replaced by infiltrating fat. This makes it difficult to distinguish the normal thymus from mediastinal fat.

Lymphoma causes diffuse thymic enlargement, asymmetry of the lobes, focal contour abnormalities, and heterogeneous signal pattern (Figure 18-2). Thymic rebound can occur in patients who have undergone chemotherapy or radiation therapy.[25] It is important to differenti-

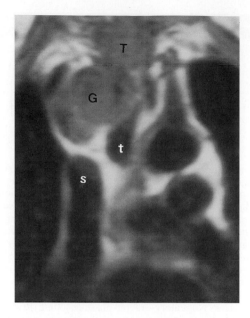

FIGURE 18-1   Intrathoracic goiter *(G)*. Coronal T1-weighted SE ECG-gated MR image shows intrathoracic extension of the thyroid gland *(T)*. *t,* Trachea; *s,* superior vena cava. (From reference 65.)

ate this phenomenon from recurrent lymphoma. The thymus is smooth, retains its bilobed appearance, and displays a homogeneous signal pattern in cases of thymic rebound.

Thymomas are the most common thymic tumors, accounting for approximately 20% of all mediastinal tumors. Myasthenia gravis is present or is subsequently diagnosed in about 50% of patients with a thymoma. On T2-weighted images, thymomas have a bright signal intensity that is similar to fat. However, the signal of thymomas is nonhomogeneous as opposed to the homogeneous pattern of fat.[12] On T1-weighted images, thymomas have a low signal intensity. Thymomas are usually difficult to differentiate from lymphomas or teratomas on the basis of signal characteristics. Malignant thymomas tend to be locally invasive and often extend along pleural reflections.[13,62,120] Once this occurs, they can spread to the posterior mediastinum or diaphragm or into the retroperitoneum. They can compress the trachea or major mediastinal vessels or invade the pericardium and heart (Figure 18-3).

Thymic cysts can be isolated or part of a complex pattern related to a thymoma. These cysts typically display a characteristically progressive bright signal on more heavily T2-weighted images. This behavior is thought to result from the proteinaceous fluid content of these cysts. Thymic cysts may be mistaken for solid tumors on CT because of their proteinaceous content.[69]

Thymolipomas are rare, benign tumors that are usually asymptomatic. They possess both fatty tissue and residual thymic tissue. They are therefore bright, even more so than normal fat, on T1- and T2-weighted images.[93]

A   **B**   **C**

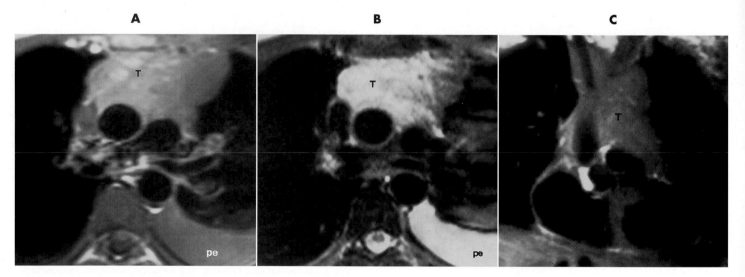

FIGURE 18-2   Thymic lymphoma *(T)*. T1- (**A** and **C**) and T2-weighted (**B**) SE ECG-gated MR images. *pe,* Pleural effusion. (From reference 65.)

A   **B**

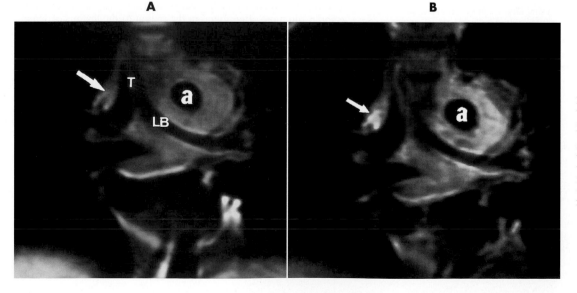

FIGURE 18-3   **A,** Malignant thymoma encases transverse aorta *(a)* and left main stem bronchus *(LB)*. The tumor *(T)* also extends into the right paratracheal space *(arrow)* on T-1-weighted axial image. **B,** Uniform tumor enhancement by Gd-DTPA on T1-weighted coronal image. (From reference 65.)

Teratoid Lesions. Teratomas are germ cell tumors that arise from primitive germ cells deposited within the mediastinum when their normal embryologic migration was prematurely stopped. They are part of the broad category of germ cell tumors, which includes choriocarcinomas, embryonal carcinomas, seminomas, and dermoid cysts. The tumor type determines the composition of the teratoma and can vary from almost exclusively a fluid to a composite of fluid, hemorrhage, fat, soft tissue, and calcification. MRI cannot differentiate a benign from a malignant tumor; however, it can determine the various elements of the tumor. A heterogeneous pattern is strong evidence of a teratoma (Figure 18-4) or other germ cell tumor as opposed to a thymoma.[91]

Lymphoma. MRI plays an important role in the evaluation and follow-up of patients with lymphoma. Multiplanar imaging graphically identifies the lymphomatous mass, as well as its relationship to, compression of, or invasion into adjacent mediastinal structures or the chest wall.[15] Multiplanar imaging may be especially useful in radiation treatment planning (Figure 18-2).[21]

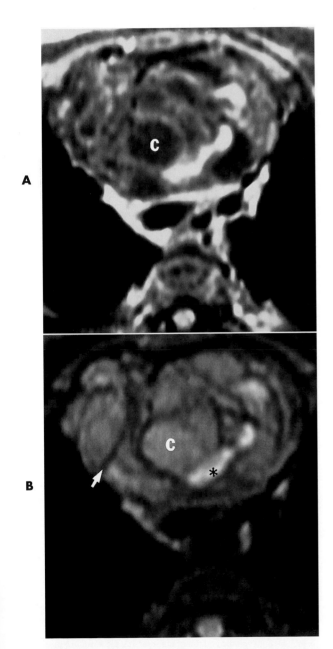

FIGURE 18-4   Benign teratoma is visible on proton density–weighted (**A**) and T2-weighted (**B**) SE ECG-gated transaxial images. The mass is cystic *(c)* with multiple septa *(arrow)* and contains foci of hemorrhage *(asterisk)*. (From reference 65.)

Although CT remains the initial modality for the identification and assessment of the lymphomatous mass, it is less useful in the assessment of tumor recurrence after therapeutic intervention. CT relies on measurements of tumor volume as the indication of recurrence or regression. Stable tumor size, however, does not guarantee a sterilized tumor.[64] Although there may be residual fibrous tissue, residual tumor may be present regardless of stable tumor size.[53,96] This situation can exist in up to 88% of patients with Hodgkin's disease and 40% of those with non-Hodgkin's lymphoma.[48,85]

MRI may be the better technique for evaluation of tumor recurrence or the presence of residual tumor after radiation therapy.* The MR signal is related to the concentration of water and protein within the tumor mass. Lymphoma cells, either residual or recurrent, have a larger water content, whereas fibrous tissue has a larger protein content, specifically polymerized protein. The differences in tissue composition result in different T2 relaxation times.[42] Fibrous tissue will have a low to intermediate signal on both T1- and T2-weighted images, and residual or recurrent lymphoma has a high signal on T2-weighted images (Figure 18-5). The ability of MRI to predict recurrent or residual tumor earlier than CT may affect follow-up planning and prognosis because 50% of patients with residual tumor will experience a relapse.[27]

There are a number of signal patterns associated with lymphoma. Homogeneous high signal on T2-weighted images is the hallmark of untreated lymphoma. A heterogeneous signal pattern on T2-weighted images, representing radiation inflammation, may be seen in the immediate posttherapeutic period and can last for as long as 6 months. After this time, heterogeneous T2-weighted signal is an indicator of recurrent or residual tumor. A heterogeneous T2-weighted signal pattern also can be seen in untreated nodular sclerosing Hodgkin's disease. A homogeneous low T2-weighted signal pattern represents fibrosis of the lymphoma after successful radiation therapy.[86]

Middle Mediastinum

Cystic Lesions. Cystic lesions of the mediastinum include pericardial cysts, thymic cysts, cystic hygromas, neurenteric cysts, and meningoceles. Some of these lesions may be suspected on the basis of their location, but all must be differentiated from solid masses. Many benign cysts are correctly diagnosed by CT, but MRI has a definite role in two areas: identification of meningoceles and evaluation of cysts with high protein content rather than serous fluid.[77] In the latter situation a cyst may be erroneously interpreted with CT as a solid tumor. With MRI these cysts will generally display an isointense to high signal on T1-weighted images and a high signal on T2-weighted images. The signal characteristics of meningoceles are similar to those of cerebrospinal

*References 80, 81, 86, 87, 105, 106, 118, 119.

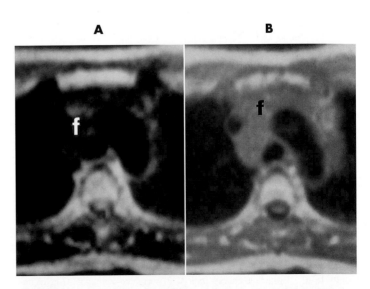

FIGURE 18-5   Posttherapy fibrosis *(f)* in a patient with superior mediastinal Hodgkin's disease. T1-weighted (**A**) and proton density–weighted (**B**) axial ECG-gated images. (From reference 65.)

fluid (CSF). It should be noted that ECG-gated T1-weighted images are not purely T1-weighted because of the long repetition time (TR) of the cardiac cycle (generally 800 to 1000 ms). As a result, purely serous cysts may appear intermediate in signal intensity. Proteinaceous cysts, mucinous cysts, or cysts with a hemorrhagic component have a higher signal than do simple cysts on T1-weighted images and may have a heterogeneous pattern (Figure 18-6). Rarely, a complex cyst will be difficult to differentiate from a solid tumor with MRI. On these occasions, Gd-DTPA will demonstrate lack of enhancement and possibly rim enhancement.

Lymphadenopathy. MRI and CT are equivalent in their usefulness in detecting mediastinal lymphadenopathy.[103,104] With multiplanar imaging capabilities and excellent contrast resolution, MRI can delineate many normal lymph nodes and most diseased nodes. Lymph nodes have an intermediate signal and are easily distinguished from the high signal of surrounding mediastinal fat. However, because of spatial resolution limitations, adjacent normal nodes may simulate a single large node and be erroneously interpreted as lymphadenopathy.[63] It remains to be seen what improvements if any will be gained with the use of dedicated chest coils. An additional limitation of MRI is its inability to detect minute amounts of calcium within a node,[38,51] which is important in differentiating between benign and malignant adenopathy (Figure 18-7). Furthermore, MRI, like CT, cannot differentiate benign lymph

node hyperplasia from lymphadenopathy caused by tumor involvement. Both in vitro and in vivo experiments demonstrate an overlap between benign and malignant nodes using T1 or T2 parameters.[39]

MRI has proved to be superior to CT in the detection of hilar, subcarinal, and aorticopulmonary adenopathy and in differentiating adenopathy from vascular structures (Figure 18-7).[11,33,107,109] MRI often helps solve the problems associated with ambiguous CT results when iodinated contrast material is contraindicated or when there is a specific interest in evaluating hilar, pericardial, aorticopulmonary, or lower left paratracheal nodes.[103,104,110]

Esophagus and Trachea. Peristaltic motion artifacts, spatial resolution limitations, and the fact that the esophagus is often collapsed or contains air or fluid complicate MRI. Esophageal tumors are difficult to distinguish from intraluminal fluid or the esophageal mucosa.[111]

MRI is most useful in the preoperative staging or radiation therapy planning of large esophageal and tracheal tumors (Figure 18-8). Multiplanar imaging in the coronal and sagittal planes coupled with the tissue conspicuity of the mediastinum on MRI are well suited to evaluat-

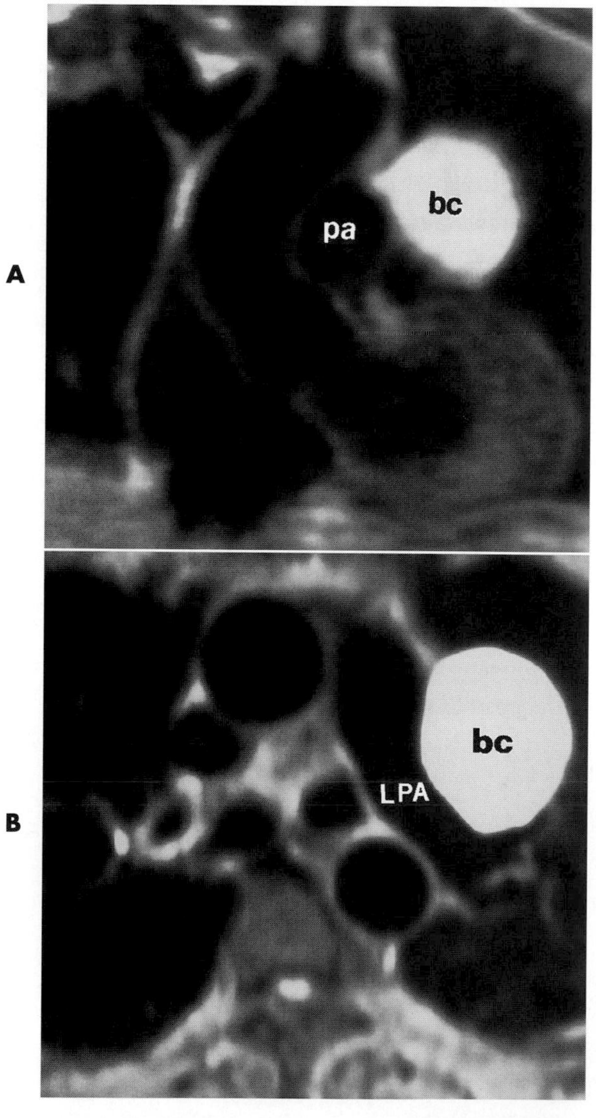

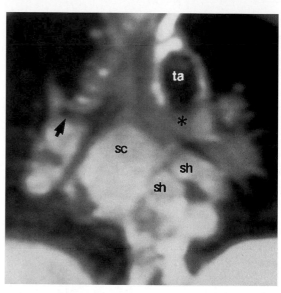

FIGURE 18-7 Diffuse adenopathy of subhilar *(sh)*, subcarinal *(sc)*, and aorticopulmonary window *(asterisk)* regions shown in T1-weighted coronal ECG-gated image. The right upper lobe bronchus is shown *(arrow)* above a large hilar node. *ta*, Transverse aorta. (From reference 65.)

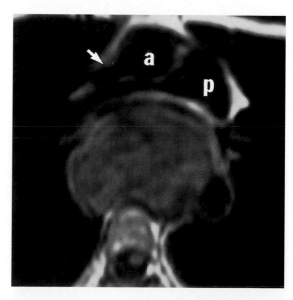

FIGURE 18-8 Benign spindle cell tumor compressing the aorta *(a)*, pulmonary artery *(p)*, and superior vena cava *(arrow)* on axial T1-weighted ECG-gated image. (From reference 65.)

FIGURE 18-6 Bronchogenic cyst *(bc)*. **A,** T1-weighted coronal ECG-gated image with high signal intensity indicating a high protein content. *pa,* Pulmonary artery. **B,** T2-weighted transaxial image through the compressed left pulmonary artery *(LPA)*. (From reference 65.)

ing tumor extension and its relationship to the surrounding structures (Figure 18-9).

Aorta. Arguably, thoracic aorta disease is best evaluated with MRI. The basic examination consists of SE ECG-gated multislice acquisitions; ECG-referenced single slice, multiphase cine; and velocity-mapping dynamic imaging. Transaxial scans are performed from the thoracic inlet to the level of the diaphragm, followed by a left anterior oblique (LAO) study through the thoracic aorta. On occasion it is necessary to perform transaxial and coronal scans through the abdominal aorta to evaluate the extension of a thoracoabdominal aneurysm or an aortic dissection. A long-axis study may be required to evaluate processes involving the aortic root. Because a large number of acquired anomalies are associated with atherosclerosis and hypertension, multiphase or dynamic imaging can be obtained using this view to determine the presence of left ventricular hypertrophy or dilatation and to calculate stroke volume and ejection fraction.

Aneurysms. In evaluating patients with aortic aneurysms, it is important to characterize the lesion in an attempt to delineate its cause and the patient's prognosis and need for surgery. In addition to measuring the true diameter of the vessel and the diameter of the patent lumen, it is extremely important to characterize the aneurysm in terms of location, shape, and extent and to determine its relationship to branch vessels and any effect it may have on adjacent structures. Evaluation

of the aortic wall for thickening, which can be seen with aortitis; for mural thrombosis, which may lead to thromboembolic disease; and for paraaortic hematomas should be a part of every examination.

Aneurysms are common anomalies involving the thoracic aorta and are found in up to 10% of autopsies. Atherosclerosis is the leading cause of aneurysms involving the thoracic aorta. The aneurysm itself results from a weakening of the media secondary to the atherosclerotic process. This leads to a progressive increase in the diameter of the aorta involving all layers of the vessel.[54] The atheroma and fibrous cap are not reliably depicted with MRI. Ectasia and tortuosity are easily identified on the LAO view. Because of the tortuosity, it is uncommon to see the entire aorta on a single section. Transaxial imaging can often lead to confusion because it can be difficult to differentiate tortuosity of the aorta from an aortic aneurysm.

Aneurysms can be classified on the basis of their configuration as being fusiform, saccular, or cylindroid. Atherosclerotic aneurysms usually involve long segments of the aorta circumferentially and generally assume a fusiform shape (Figure 18-10). The presence of a saccular aneurysm should always raise the question of an infectious cause or a false aneurysm. The number of saccular atherosclerotic aneurysms is small. When they do occur, saccular aneurysms are most commonly caused by atherosclerosis, as are the overwhelming number of thoracic aneurysms.

A clue to diagnosing the cause of an aneurysm hinges on its location in the thoracic aorta. It is rare for atherosclerosis to involve solely the ascending aorta. When an aneurysm of the ascending aorta is the result of atherosclerosis, it is usually associated with involvement of the aortic arch and descending aorta. Aneurysms localized to the ascending aorta are generally bulbous in configuration. Differential considerations include cystic medial necrosis, other degenerative processes of the media, and aneurysmal dilatation caused by aortic valvular disease. Effacement of the sinotubular segment of the aortic root is seen in patients with annuloaortic ectasia, cystic medial necrosis, and aortic regurgitation. This segment is normally preserved in cases of aortic valvular stenosis.

Marfan syndrome, or arachnodactyly, is an autosomal dominant disorder of the connective tissues. The syndrome includes abnormalities of the skeletal system, eye, and cardiovascular system. The most important abnormality in the cardiovascular system involves the aorta, an elastic artery. Large areas of the media are replaced by an accumulation of metachromatic mucopolysaccharide. A loss of elastic fibers occurs, and muscle cells enlarge and subsequently lose their normal circumferential orientation. This change results in an overall increase in the diameter of the aorta. Classically the process involves the aortic sinuses, the tubular portion of the aorta, and the proximal ascending aorta, resulting in a "pear-shaped" aortic root (Figure 18-11). The marked dilatation of

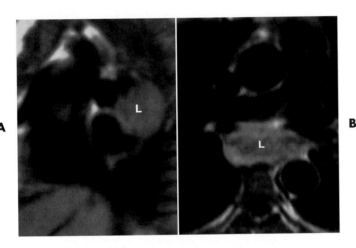

FIGURE 18-9 Leiomyoma *(L)* arising from the midesophagus. T1-weighted sagittal **(A)** and transverse **(B)** ECG-gated images. (From reference 65.)

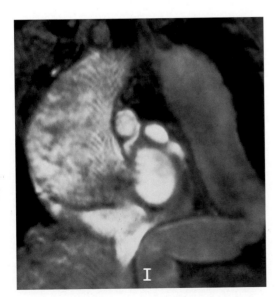

FIGURE 18-10 Atherosclerotic aneurysm involving the ascending and descending portions of the thoracic aorta is visible on this ECG-referenced LAO cine image. Kinking of the aorta above the level of the diaphragm *(I)* is common.

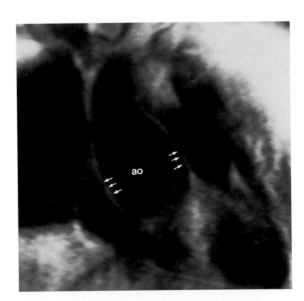

FIGURE 18-11 Marfan syndrome. Classic pear-shaped aortic root *(ao)*. This configuration, as shown on a T1-weighted ECG-gated coronal image, results from effacement of the sinotubular junction *(arrows)*. (From reference 65.)

the aortic root can, in turn, cause aortic insufficiency, aortic dissection, and hemopericardium.

Several reports have indicated the efficacy of MRI in studying the aortic findings in Marfan syndrome.[24,44,56,65,94] The classic pear-shaped aorta is nicely demonstrated with coronal (Figure 18-11) and LAO imaging. The effacement of aortic sinuses distinguishes Marfan syndrome from severe congenital bicuspid aortic valvular stenosis (Figure 18-12). When used in conjunction with cine MRI, these planes are helpful in detecting and quantifying any aortic insufficiency and in detecting aortic dissection or hemopericardium.

Marfan syndrome can involve the pulmonary arteries and result in isolated pulmonary artery aneurysms. The transaxial plane is used in the evaluation of the central pulmonary arterial tree. It is difficult to evaluate the more peripheral pulmonary arterial tree with standard SE techniques because of spatial-resolution limitations and the lack of contrast between the vessel and the surrounding lung. Theoretically, cine

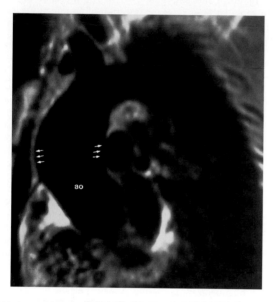

FIGURE 18-12   Bicuspid aortic valve shown in an LAO SE image through the thoracic aorta in an infant with critical stenosis. Although the aortic root has dilated markedly *(arrows)*, the sinotubular portion of the aortic root *(ao)* is not involved.

MRI and phase-velocity mapping techniques should be useful in searching for a more distal aneurysm.

Not all patients who have the skeletal and ocular manifestations of Marfan syndrome will exhibit aortic root changes. In addition, some patients exhibit a forme fruste of the classic pear-shaped aortic root. MRI provides an excellent noninvasive imaging modality for evaluating these patients on a regular basis for progression of aortic root involvement or associated complications. Knowledge of the normal transluminal diameters of the thoracic aorta is important for assessing these patients. At the level of the sinus of Valsalva the aorta measures 3.3 cm, the middle aspect of the ascending aorta measures 3 cm, the transverse portion of the aortic arch measures 2.7 cm, and the descending thoracic aorta measures 2.4 cm, with a range of ±0.4 cm.[56]

Patients can also be studied in the immediate postoperative period, as well as over the long term, for the presence of periaortic hematoma, aortic dissection, aortic rupture, false aneurysms at the distal anastomotic site, and hemopericardium.[45, 65]

The term *annuloaortic ectasia* refers to idiopathic dilatation of the aortic annulus and of the proximal aorta with pure aortic regurgitation. Annuloaortic ectasia accounts for 5% to 10% of patients receiving aortic valve replacement for pure aortic regurgitation.

Annuloaortic ectasia is the result of severe degenerative changes within the aortic wall. Cystic medial necrosis is usually the cause of the degenerative changes. Not surprisingly, 25% to 50% of patients with annuloaortic ectasia have some traits of Marfan syndrome. Recall that Marfan syndrome is a connective tissue disorder that, when involving the aorta, causes cystic medial necrosis. There is an overlap between these two entities. Patients with annuloaortic ectasia have cystic medial necrosis with no obvious cause.

With time, the aorta dilates as the degenerative process progresses. The process results in a bulbous-appearing aortic root, very similar in appearance to the aortic root in patients with Marfan syndrome (Figure 18-13). As the aortic root continues to dilate it involves the annulus, and regurgitation ensues. As with Marfan patients, these patients are predisposed to aortic dissection.

Aortic valve stenosis can be congenital or acquired. In congenital aortic valve stenosis, abnormal fusion of the tubercles of the conotruncus results in two asymmetrical aortic valves. Rheumatic disease is the most common cause of acquired aortic valve stenosis. These patients have three aortic valve leaflets, which fuse because of the inflammatory process. With time, both the bicuspid and tricuspid aortic valve stenoses can calcify. Both congenital and acquired aortic valve stenoses lead to progressive dilatation of the aortic root. Unlike acquired stenosis, the poststenotic dilatation associated with a congenital anomaly is usually localized to the aortic root (Figure 18-12).

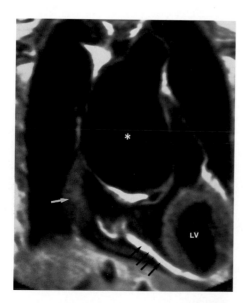

FIGURE 18-13   Annuloaortic ectasia *(asterisk)*. Aortic leakage resulted in hemopericardium with both acute *(white arrow)* and subacute *(black arrows)* hemorrhage. *LV,* Left ventricle. T1-weighted coronal ECG-gated image. (From reference 65.)

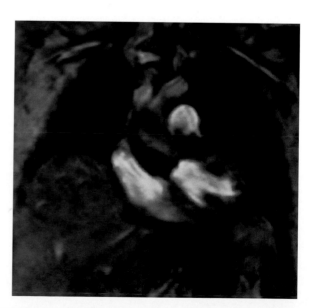

FIGURE 18-14   Aortic valve stenosis is shown on this coronal cine MR image through the middle aspect of the aortic root. The signal void that extends to the midportion of the ascending aorta represents turbulent flow.

It has long been recognized that turbulent flow generates a signal void on cine MR studies (Figure 18-14). Several studies have indicated that the severity of aortic valve stenosis can be graded by measuring the associated length of signal loss. In addition, associated aortic insufficiency is delineated by reversal of the signal void into the left ventricular chamber.[7,8,24,26,83] Comparison of biventricular stroke volumes can be used to calculate a regurgitant fraction. Cine MRI can also be used to evaluate stroke volume, ejection fraction, contraction dynamics, left ventricular hypertrophy, and left ventricular enlargement.[83,95,99] The availability of more reliable phase-velocity mapping techniques enables quantitative assessment of the velocity across the aortic valve in patients with stenosis. Because the precise angle of flow across the valve can be highly variable, depending on the severity and location of the stenosis, it is important to obtain velocity measurements in multiple planes (Figure 18-15).[19] The pressure gradient can be calculated using the modified Bernoulli equation.

Aneurysms greater than 6 cm in diameter have an increased incidence of aortic rupture and therefore require immediate surgery. Saccular aneurysms also have a greater tendency to rupture.[54]

MRI has proved useful for delineating the configuration, location, and extent of aneurysms and their involvement of branch vessels.[2,4,29,30] In addition, it is very accurate in determining the true diameter of the aneurysm. Mural thrombus has an intermediate to high signal intensity, depending on its age, and is easily differentiated from the aortic wall. Precise measurement of the patent lumen is therefore possible with MRI. It is important to specifically report the presence of exophytic mural thrombosis, which has a higher incidence of causing thromboembolic disease. Occasionally it can be difficult to differentiate slow-flowing blood from mural thrombus; both may display an intermediate to high signal. Patients with aneurysms commonly have an increased signal intensity because of slow or diastolic flow. This is because of the enlarged diameter of the aneurysm, which disturbs the normal flow pattern and results in a swirling of the blood, as well as

stasis, and therefore an increase in signal. In addition, because these patients commonly have associated atherosclerotic coronary arterial disease and decreased left ventricular function, it is not uncommon for them to have decreased cardiac output, slow flow, and associated increased signal. Double-echo techniques have been described for differentiating slow flow from mural thrombus; however, dynamic imaging techniques, especially phase-velocity mapping, can readily differentiate the two.[31,100]

MRI is effective in depicting paraaortic processes, including compression of adjacent structures by the aneurysm, paraaortic hematomas, and hemopericardium (Figure 18-13). It can sometimes be difficult to differentiate paraaortic blood from atelectasis. Atelectasis also mimics aortic dissection with thrombosis of the false lumen. In a study of seven patients we were able to differentiate atelectasis from paraaortic hematomas by the increased signal exhibited by atelectasis on T1-weighted images after injection of Gd-DTPA (Figure 18-16). After the diagnosis is established, MRI can be used to monitor patients for progression of disease before surgery. It also can be used to monitor patients for complications after surgical intervention or for progression of the underlying disease within the remainder of the thoracic aorta.

A false aneurysm is an encapsulated hematoma in communication with a ruptured aorta (Figure 18-17). The hematoma varies in signal intensity from intermediate to high, depending on its age. The site of rupture may not always be identified if the hematoma is well organized. Paraaortic hematomas tend to be more diffuse than hematomas associated with a false aneurysm.[72]

Dissections. Aortic dissection has been found in as many as one out of 400 autopsies.[5] It can occur at any age but is most commonly encountered in the sixth and seventh decades. Aortic dissection occurs in men three times as frequently as in women. The classic clinical picture consists of severe chest pain that radiates to the back. Often there will be differential pressures in the arms because of involvement of the branch vessel ostia. Aortic dissection results from degeneration of the

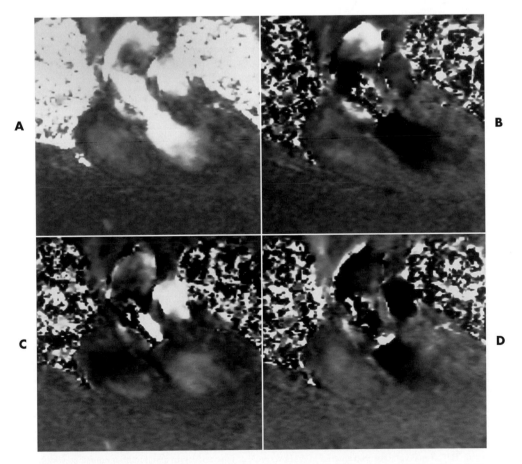

FIGURE 18-15   Phase-velocity mapping studies obtained through the middle aspect of the aortic root. Upper left-hand (coronal) image **(A)** represents a composite of phase velocities obtained in left-to-right **(B),** anteroposterior **(C),** and inferosuperior directions **(D).**

aortic media and was originally described as cystic medial necrosis. There is a loss of muscle and elastic fibers, which are replaced by metachromatic material. It is therefore not surprising that a high incidence of dissection is found in patients with Marfan syndrome and annuloaortic ectasia. Aortic dissection has a high association with hypertension, which occurs in more than 80% of patients. The degenerative process of the media eventually results in a hemorrhage or nondissecting dissection (Figure 18-18) and subsequent separation of the intima and media.[88] In most cases a disruption (tear) of the intima results in a false lumen. Blood leaving the heart with systemic pressure enters this channel and further undermines the intima and media, extending the dissection. Approximately 90% of cases have multiple flaps.[6] When this occurs, blood flows within both the true and false lumina of the aorta. As the dissection propagates, it may involve the ostia of the branch vessels or occlude their origins. About 10% of cases do not have an exit flap, and these cases are referred to as *incomplete dissections*.

More than 95% of aortic dissections start in the thoracic aorta. From 60% to 70% of dissections begin in the ascending aorta, with only 25% starting distal to the left subclavian artery in the region of the ligamentum arteriosum.[5] Dissections are classified by their location. The origin of dissections occurs where the aorta is relatively fixed. Type I dissections begin in the ascending aorta and extend into the descending thoracic aorta. Type II dissections are localized to the ascending aorta. Type III dissections begin just distal to the left subclavian artery. Types I and II constitute surgical emergencies because they often affect the coronary arteries and branch vessels; type III dissections are most often treated medically. Types I and III can involve the abdominal aorta and the iliac arteries. The branch vessels can be involved, with subsequent occlusion or extension of the dissection.

In the evaluation of the patient with suspected aortic dissection, it is important to document the presence of the lesion, its location and extent, and any involvement of the coronary arteries or branch vessels.

MRI is 98% sensitive and 98% specific for detecting aortic dissections.[79] It has been suggested that MRI is the best imaging modality for the evaluation of aortic dissection and should be the initial study performed in all hemodynamically stable patients.[79] Commonly the entrance site of the false lumen is identified with MRI.* The flap, which comprises the intima and part of the media, appears as a linear structure when contrasted by flowing blood in both the true and false lumens (Figure 18-19). The presence of a flap can sometimes be equivocal on SE studies even when blood flows in both the true and false lumens. Cine MRI usually clarifies or resolves the issue in these circumstances (Figure 18-20). Thrombosis within the false lumen or slowly flowing blood can give rise to an intermediate to high signal and may obscure the intimal flap. Differentiation between thrombosis and slowly flowing blood can be made through the use of cine MRI techniques or phase-velocity mapping techniques (Figure 18-21).[98,100,112]

MRI is highly effective in identifying occlusion or extension into the branch vessels by the dissection. Retrograde extension of the dissection to involve the aortic root and coronary arteries can be detected. When a coronary artery is involved, we perform T2-weighted studies in the long- and short-axis views to document the presence and extent of myocardial infarction. Cine MRI studies are performed in all type I and II dissections to access myocardial contraction and to assess the patient for associated aortic insufficiency (Figure 18-20).

A difficult task for any imaging modality is differentiating complete thrombosis of a false lumen from an aortic aneurysm with mural thrombus. Indirect signs of dissection include a longitudinal thrombus ex-

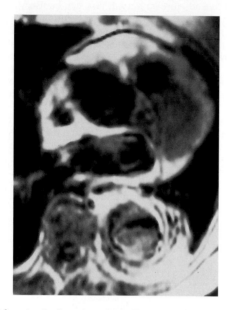

FIGURE 18-16 Aortic dissection. Gd-DTPA–enhanced transaxial SE image through the aortic root and descending aorta shows increased signal surrounding the descending aorta caused by atelectasis as opposed to periaortic hematoma or a thrombosed false lumen.

*References 3, 5, 29, 30, 41, 57.

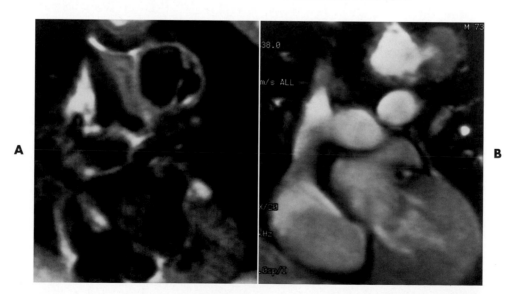

FIGURE 18-17 False aneurysm. **A,** Coronal SE image demonstrates narrow neck of dissection leading to a false aneurysm. **B,** Coronal velocity map anterior to **A** shows neck of false aneurysm and thrombus contained within adventitia.

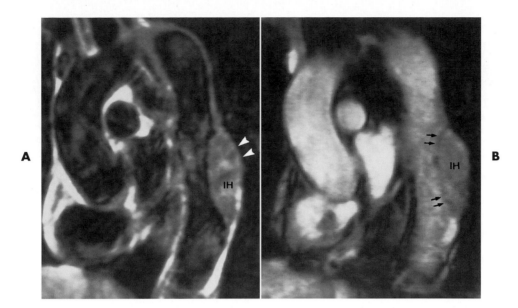

FIGURE 18-18   Intramural hematoma *(IH)* in the midportion of the descending aorta visible on LAO SE **(A)** and cine **(B)** images. Anterior bowing into the aortic lumen and a distinct posterior bowing or hump *(arrowheads)* are seen. On the cine study a raised intimal dissection flap is identified as a dark linear structure *(arrows)*.

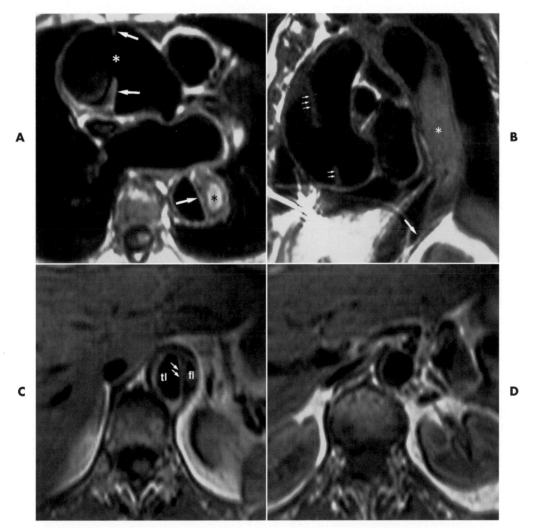

FIGURE 18-19   Incomplete type I aortic dissection. **A,** Transaxial image through the aortic root demonstrates the entrance site *(white asterisk)* and intimal flap *(arrows)*. Slow flow in both the ascending and descending aorta shows intermediate signal intensity. Subacute thrombus in the descending aorta *(black asterisk)* is bright. **B,** LAO view demonstrates intimal flap *(small arrows)* surrounding the entrance site. The asterisk marks slow flow in the descending aorta. The large arrow marks the closed (lower) end of dissection. **C,** Transverse section below the diaphragm demonstrates the intimal flap *(small arrows),* true lumen *(tl),* and false lumen *(fl).* **D,** At the level of the renal pedicle there is no evidence of dissection. (**B** and **C,** From reference 65.)

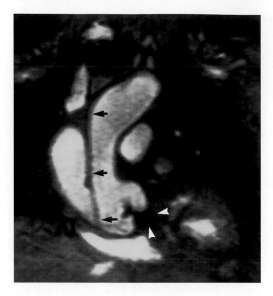

FIGURE 18-20 Type II aortic dissection. Coronal cine MR image through the ascending aorta demonstrates the intimal flap *(black arrows)*, as well as a small amount of aortic regurgitation *(white arrowheads)*.

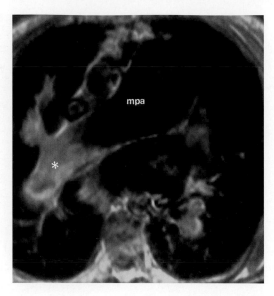

FIGURE 18-22 Dilated right main pulmonary artery *(mpa)* in a patient with severe pulmonary arterial hypertension. Axial T1-weighted ECG-gated image during systole shows signal from slow-flowing blood *(asterisk)*. (From reference 65.)

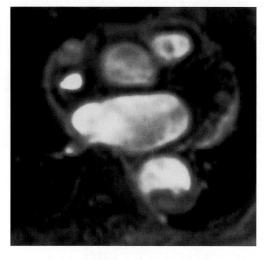

FIGURE 18-21 Thrombosed lumen, type III dissection. Phase-velocity mapped transaxial MR image through the midthoracic aorta demonstrates the patent true lumen *(white)* and thrombosed false lumen *(dark)*.

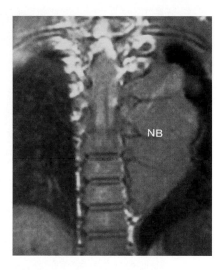

FIGURE 18-23 Paraspinous neuroblastoma *(NB)* spanning the length of eight vertebrae. (From reference 65.)

tension greater than 7 cm, which is not typically identified with aneurysms; a noncircular, compressed, patent lumen; and a change in the position of thrombus, that is, a spiral configuration corresponding to the path of the false lumen.[57,117]

In a small number of cases there is no evidence of an entrance or exit site. This situation has been variously termed *subintimal hematoma or aortic dissection without intimal rupture.*[115] Unlike a thrombosed false lumen or an aortic aneurysm with mural thrombus, the subintimal hematoma tends to have an elliptic configuration (Figure 18-18). The hematoma may exhibit an intermediate or high signal, depending on its age. We have found a characteristic anterior bowing toward the lumen and a posterior bowing or "hump." We believe that the uplifted intimal flap is represented by a dark, curvilinear structure on cine MR studies and is best demonstrated with the LAO plane.

MRI is extremely useful for studying patients after medical or surgical intervention.[6,113] Periaortic hematomas, infection, and progressive dilatation of the false lumen are easily identified. In patients who have undergone graft placement, it is possible to identify the graft and to identify anastomotic aneurysms or leakage. It is common, however, to see a residual false lumen in patients who have had a tacking procedure.

Pulmonary Artery. Standard MR techniques are limited in their ability to evaluate the pulmonary arterial tree, as are the other noninvasive modalities. The reason for this difficulty lies in the inability of these techniques to study the peripheral vasculature. Despite this limitation, MRI has proved useful for delineating both intrinsic and secondary processes involving the central pulmonary arterial tree.

Pulmonary artery hypertension. Diagnosing pulmonary artery hypertension can be difficult with angiography because of the increased risk associated with elevated pulmonary artery pressures and right-sided heart pressures. MRI nicely demonstrates pathophysiological consequences associated with pulmonary artery hypertension, including right ventricular hypertrophy, reversal of the normal curvature of the interventricular septum, dilatation of the central pulmonary arteries, and rapid tapering or "pruning" of the peripheral vasculature (Figure 18-22).[18]

In a normal pulmonary artery, a signal void appears within the artery during the systolic component of the cardiac cycle on standard SE pulse sequences. Signal activity normally increases during the diastolic phase of the cardiac cycle because of slow blood flow. On a multiphasic examination, patients with pulmonary arterial hyperten-

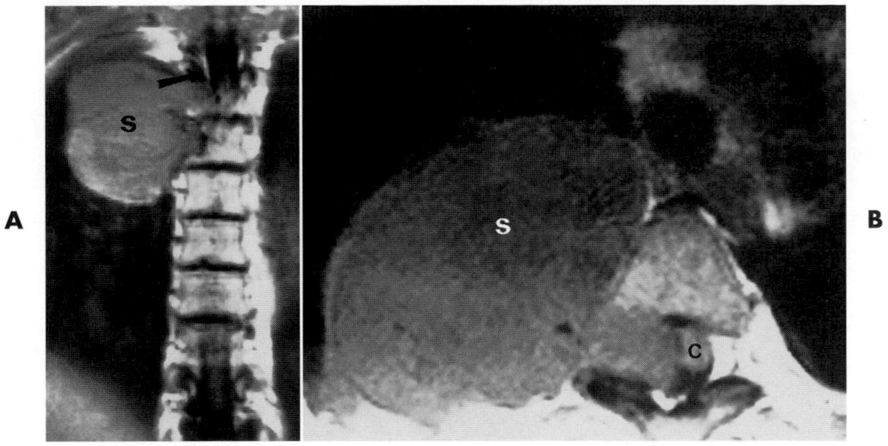

FIGURE 18-24   Schwannoma extending into the spinal canal *(S)*. (From reference 65.)

sion are noted to have an increased signal throughout the cardiac cycle. Therefore a high signal within the pulmonary artery during systole can be used as an indicator of pulmonary arterial hypertension (Figure 18-22).[28,101]

MRI has demonstrated this abnormal pattern in 92% of patients with pulmonary arterial hypertension. This increased signal in systole is noted in 100% of patients with pressures greater than 80 mm Hg and in 60% of patients with pressures less than 80 mm Hg.[114] Simple SE techniques therefore identify the presence of pulmonary artery hypertension, and they also grossly quantitate its severity. With phase-velocity techniques it should be possible to identify stagnation and reversal of flow.

Posterior Mediastinum

Neurogenic Tumors. The majority of tumors within the posterior mediastinum are of neural origin. Neurogenic tumors typically display intermediate signal on T1-weighted images and high signal on T2-weighted images.[20] MRI is not capable of distinguishing benign from malignant tumors. The fact that schwannomas and neurofibromas are enhanced uniformly with Gd-DTPA is useful in evaluating for intradural extension of these tumors. On T1-weighted images these tumors are isointense with the spinal cord, and tumor-tissue differentiation is difficult. Although the tumors display high signal on T2-weighted images, they are obscured by the high signal of the CSF.

Nerve sheath tumors can be extradural, intradural, or both. They may erode the pedicles and vertebral bodies or widen the neural foramen. Although MRI can display bone contour changes, CT provides better bone detail. MRI multiplanar acquisitions are very important in demonstrating the longitudinal extension of neurogenic tumors (Figure 18-23), the multiplicity of neurofibromas, and involvement of the adjacent soft tissues and bone marrow. MRI is also useful in evaluating for cord compression and extradural extension (Figure 18-24).

Neuroblastomas also may pass through the neural foramina and compress the spinal cord or invade bone. Lymphoma, inflammatory masses (Figure 18-25), bronchogenic cysts (Figure 18-26), and vertebral tumors (Figure 18-27) also may involve the posterior mediastinum and therefore must be distinguished from neurogenic tumors.

PERIPHERAL LUNG

Unlike the lung parenchyma, those structures at the periphery of the lung are well studied with MRI. As with the mediastinum, here there is significant tissue conspicuity between lung and the adjacent soft tissue structures to allow for assessment of pathological processes. This, coupled with a true multiplanar scanning ability, has resulted in an ability to evaluate those areas that are difficult for CT to study, even with reformatted image planes.

Superior Sulcus Tumors

Superior sulcus tumors are peripheral lung cancers that are located in the lung apex and that display a high incidence of chest wall involvement with extension to and involvement of the neurovascular structures of the brachial plexus and the spine. Because localized chest wall invasion is not a contraindication to surgical resection, it is imperative that the relationship of the tumor to adjacent structures be precisely outlined. Involvement of the brachial plexus, invasion into the spinal canal, gross vertebral body involvement, and encasement or invasion of arterial structures are contraindications for surgical resection. Here the multiplanar capacity of MRI, especially the use of the coronal and sagittal planes, is of obvious advantage over transaxial and reformatted CT.

Radiation therapy is almost always used in the treatment of these unique tumors, even when they are deemed surgically resectable. MRI can therefore be of tremendous value in radiation planning.

On T1-weighted images these tumors tend to be isointense with the musculature and brachial plexus. Their relationship to vascular structures is usually obvious because of the conspicuity with the low signal from within the vessels. These tumors tend to be bright on T2-weighted images and can generally be separated from adjacent tissues. On occasion, motion artifact can make interpretation equivocal, as can surface signal from shoulder coils. In these instances T1-weighted fat saturation sequences after Gd-DTPA administration may be very helpful. This technique is also helpful in evaluating for spinal cord involvement because the tumor-tissue demarcation is difficult to determine with T2-weighted images because of the bright signal of CSF.[48]

Pleura

Relatively little work has been done in the area of MR evaluation of the pleura. Undoubtedly this is related to the fact that most disease processes can be adequately evaluated using the chest radiograph and CT.[74] Where MRI is useful as an adjunct to these modalities is in depicting the entire extent of pleural neoplasms, with coronal or sagittal imaging, including their involvement of adjacent structures; in separating tumor from pleural effusions or atelectasis; and in evaluating pleural fluid collection (Figure 18-2, *A* and *B*).[68] With regard to the last, T1- and T2-weighted images are very good at identifying hemothoraces and chylothoraces, and Gd-DTPA may differentiate exudative fluid collections from a transudative one on the basis of their increased enhancement pattern.

Diaphragm

Axial imaging is inadequate in the evaluation of the complex anatomical configuration of the diaphragm. Coronal and especially sagittal imaging are far superior to axial imaging in the overall viewing of the diaphragm. This, coupled with the better contrast resolution of MRI, allows for assessment of the integrity of the diaphragm. Tumor in-

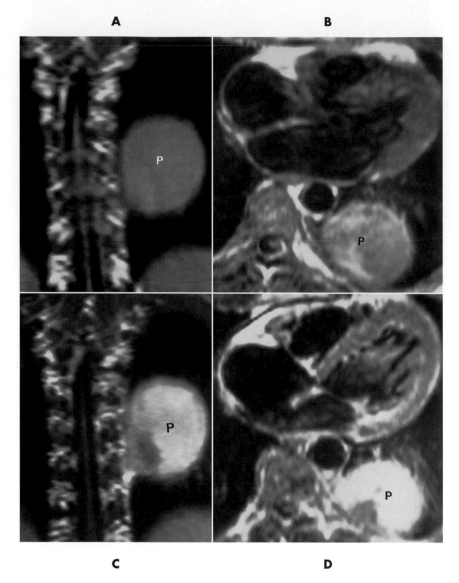

FIGURE 18-25 Paravertebral plasma cell granuloma *(P)* visible on T1-weighted (**A** and **B**) and Gd-DTPA enhanced (**C** and **D**) images. (From reference 65.)

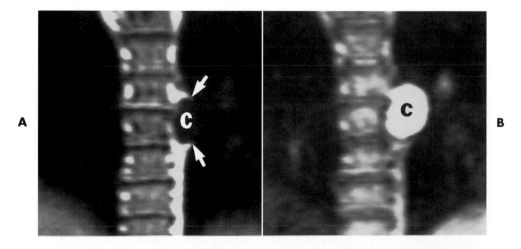

FIGURE 18-26 Bronchogenic cyst *(c)*. Visible on T1-weighted (**A**) and T2-weighted (**B**) images. (From reference 65.)

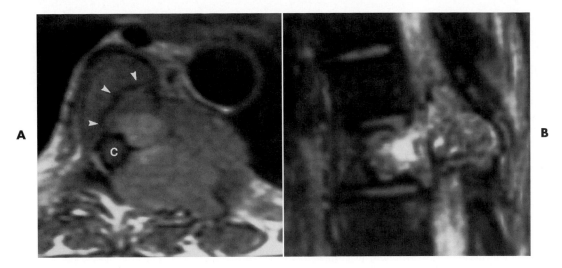

FIGURE 18-27   Giant cell tumor expanding the vertebral body, left pedicle, left transverse process, left lamina, and spinous process *(arrowheads)*. The spinal cord *(c)* is displaced as shown in T1-weighted axial **(A)** and T2-weighted sagittal **(B)** ECG-gated images. (From reference 65.)

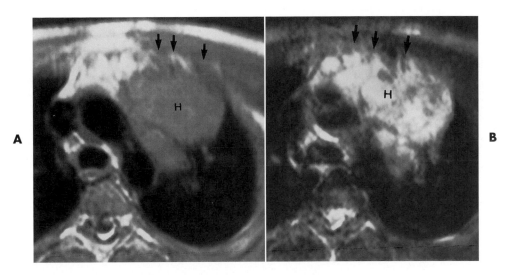

FIGURE 18-28   Hodgkin's disease *(H)*. Axial proton density–weighted **(A)** and T2-weighted **(B)** ECG-gated images show diffuse anterior chest wall invasion *(arrows)*. (From reference 65.)

volvement and penetration of the diaphragm from either pulmonary or abdominal tumors are best determined with MRI, as are diaphragmatic defects, whether they are caused by trauma or by hernias.[70]

On T1- and T2-weighted images the diaphragm appears as a discrete, curvilinear structure of bright signal intensity because of the presence of juxtaposed pleural fat. Tumors obliterating this fat plane indicate extension into the diaphragm. Tumors crossing the diaphragm are usually obvious on either T1- or T2-weighted images. The loss of continuity of this bright, curvilinear structure usually indicates a defect in the diaphragm. There may be abdominal contents bridging the defect.

Chest Wall

The chest wall is best studied with MRI,[47,105,106] especially when evaluating the area for primary tumors, metastatic lesions, and direct extension of pulmonary tumors. Tissue-tumor discrimination is usually evident with the use of T2-weighted images (Figure 18-28) and/or T1-weighted fat saturation Gd-DTPA–enhanced images. The sagittal plane is especially useful in both delineating the entire superior-inferior extent of chest wall pathology and simultaneously determining the anterior-posterior relationship of extrapulmonary tumors to the lungs and the extent of chest wall involvement by pulmonary tumors. Differentiating

benign from malignant tumors on the basis of signal characteristics alone is not possible with MRI. However, rib destruction and a diffuse invasive pattern with irregular borders are more typical of malignant neoplasms. Lipomas, the most common chest wall tumor, can herniate between the intercostal muscles and have a subpleural component. Lipomas, however, tend to be multilobulated and have a classic tissue characterization, mimicking subcutaneous fat on all imaging sequences.

Anterior and posterior mediastinal masses and peripheral lung masses may invade the chest wall. Resultant rib destruction is usually best determined by chest radiography. Early destruction of the vertebral bodies is best evaluated with CT. Because it is limited to the transaxial plane, CT is not well suited to evaluating the ribs, even on reformatted images. Likewise, its poor tumor-tissue discrimination has resulted in disappointing detection accuracy and early evaluation of invasion. MRI is well suited to study chest wall involvement and has proved to be more accurate than CT.[47,105,106] Superior contrast resolution allows for delineation of chest-wall fat, muscle, and bones and the processes that disturb them. Oblique scanning planes parallel and perpendicular to the ribs optimize the evaluation of chest wall invasion. Almost all malignant and inflammatory processes demonstrate increased signal intensity on T2-weighted images. The use of Gd-DTPA–enhanced, T1-weighted, fat-suppressed sequences will probably increase the sensitivity of MRI for evaluation of subtle chest wall invasion.[60] MRI is the preferred method for evaluating chest wall extension of mediastinal masses; its accuracy is 94% compared with 63% for CT.[76]

BRONCHOGENIC CARCINOMA

Despite the attributes of MRI previously discussed, CT remains the primary imaging modality for the evaluation of lung cancer, despite inherent limitations with CT itself.[46] The reason for this is the superior ability of CT to evaluate the pulmonary parenchyma, including the presence of minute amounts of calcium within pulmonary nodules.[34] Coupled with better spatial resolution and very short scan times with helical imaging—therefore decreasing noise—this makes CT a very powerful tool for staging bronchogenic carcinoma. Nevertheless, MRI is not without merit and does play an important role in working out problems encountered with CT imaging.[39,46]

After a suspected lung cancer has been detected, the role of an imaging modality is to stage the cancer for proper surgical or radiation treatment. The staging of lung cancer depends on the ability of an imaging technique to identify pathological conditions, including the primary tumor, nodal involvement, and metastatic disease. Perhaps the most important contribution of the imager is to distinguish between stage IIIb and stage IIIa carcinomas because all cancers up to and including stage IIIa are potentially resectable.[1] Therefore it becomes critically important to be able to determine the presence of mediastinal invasion, mediastinal adenopathy, hilar adenopathy, and distant metastases.

Detection of mediastinal invasion is one of the most important contributions of MRI in the staging of lung cancer.[108] Multiplanar imaging and excellent contrast resolution have firmly established MRI as a means of evaluating the heart and pericardium for tumor invasion by paracardiac masses.[4] MRI provides excellent delineation of the pericardium and distinguishes tumor involvement of the pericardium from involvement of the myocardium (Figure 18-29), the latter being a contraindication for surgical resection. Compression, encasement, and invasion of the mediastinum and its contents may be shown with combinations of standard SE techniques (Figure 18-30), cine MRI, phase-mapping imaging, and tagging techniques such as spatial modulation of magnetization (SPAMM) imaging.[9] Encasement or invasion of the vasculature, esophagus, and trachea, all contraindications for resection, are accurately detected with MRI (Figure 18-31). Erosion of the vertebral bodies and invasion into the spinal canal are also contraindications to resection. Marrow involvement with extension into the spinal canal is best visualized by use of a spine coil and is best displayed with fat suppression technique and Gd-DTPA administration.

In case of mediastinal invasion, MRI depicts vascular invasion, encasement, and tumor spread within the vasculature better than CT.[108] Cine and especially phase-mapping techniques are useful in differentiating slow blood flow within a vessel lumen from increased signal caused by tumor invasion. This is especially true regarding the superior vena cava.[35] Similarly, MRI is preferable for evaluation of myocardial and intracardiac involvement (Figure 18-29). Although neither MRI nor CT is capable of diagnosing microscopic invasion of medi-

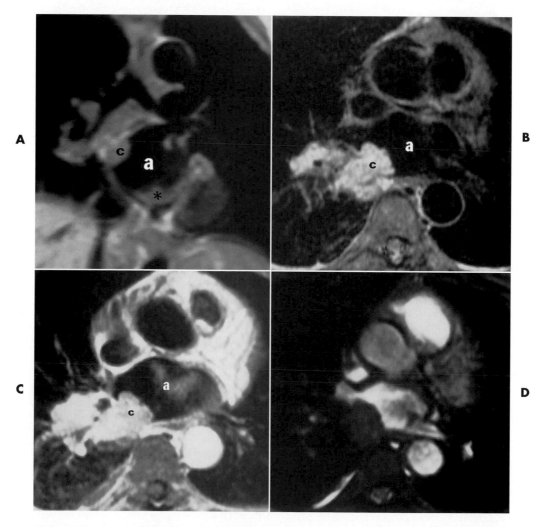

FIGURE 18-29   Large cell carcinoma *(c)* invading the left atrium *(a)*. **A,** T1-weighted ECG-gated coronal image. *Asterisk,* Slowly-flowing blood. **B,** T2-weighted axial ECG-gated image. **C,** T1-weighted ECG-gated axial image with Gd-DTPA enhancement. **D,** Transverse gradient-echo cine image enables detection of mobile intracardiac mass. (From reference 65.)

astinal fat, MRI may be better at showing subtle invasion because of its excellent contrast between tumor and fat (Figures 18-30 and 18-31).

MRI and CT are equally accurate in the detection of mediastinal lymphadenopathy, with sensitivities and specificities of approximately 65% and 75%, respectively.[46,84] Diagnosis of nodal involvement depends on size criteria, which in and of itself is far from an optimal way of assessment. As elsewhere, MRI is not capable of differentiating between benign and malignant nodes on the basis of T1 and T2 characteristics. There are preliminary data to suggest that dynamic contrast enhancement imaging may be useful in establishing nodal malignancy.[36] Although encouraging, this type of time-dependent contrast-enhancement analysis has been shown to have overlap between benign and malignant tissues elsewhere in the body. It remains to be seen if this will also occur in node evaluation.

MRI is superior to CT in detecting hilar node involvement.[11,33,107,109] This may be the result of coronal imaging coupled with excellent tumor-fat and tumor-vascular discrimination. As previously described, MRI is capable of differentiating a large central mass from a hilar mass with associated obstructive atelectasis.[50,60,97] In the latter cases the cholesterol pneumonitis associated with obstruction has a higher water content than the central mass.[22,59,75] Therefore the area of atelectasis has a higher signal on T2-weighted images than the central mass. Also areas of atelectasis tend to be enhanced to a greater degree than central

tumor masses after administration of Gd-DTPA.[60] Difficulties arise when the lung undergoes fibrosing pneumonitis.[52,58,90] When this occurs, both the lung and the central tumor can have overlapping signal characteristics on T2-weighted images.

CT remains the primary modality for assessing the abdomen for metastatic disease because lung scans typically include the liver and adrenal glands. Approximately one fifth of scans demonstrate an adrenal abnormality, of which two thirds are adenomas. In about 40% of these cases, CT cannot exclude malignant involvement.[78] Chemical-shift MRI or dynamic contrast-enhancement techniques may be helpful in such cases.[71] Similarly, MRI may aid in differentiating hemangiomas from liver metastases on the basis of increasing signal on increasingly more heavily T2-weighted imaging.

When bronchogenic tumors are unresectable, MRI can play a vital role in radiation therapy planning and in follow-up for residual tumor or recurrence. Coronal MRI may display the entire extent of tumor involvement. MRI may be performed along the actual plane along which radiation will be administered.

In bronchogenic carcinoma, as in lymphoma, postradiation fibrosis can be differentiated from tumor recurrence.[116] Both T1- and T2-weighted images show postradiation fibrosis as low-intensity signal. Recurrent or residual tumor has a high signal intensity on T2-weighted images. However, postradiation inflammation, which also has a high

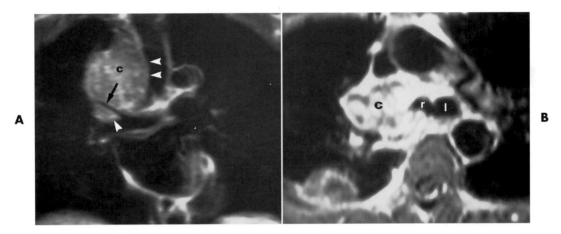

FIGURE 18-30   **A,** Large cell carcinoma *(c)* of the right upper lobe extending into the mediastinum and surrounding the right upper lobe pulmonary artery *(arrow). Arrowheads,* Tumor borders. **B,** Gd-DTPA produces heterogeneous enhancement of the tumor seen surrounding the right *(r)* and left *(l)* main stem bronchi. (From reference 65.)

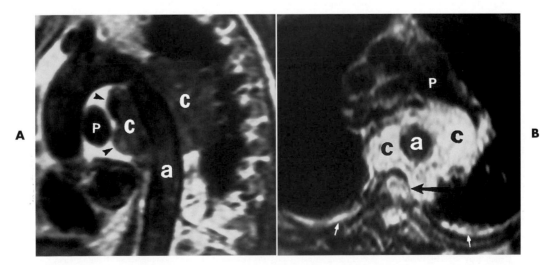

FIGURE 18-31   **A,** Large cell carcinoma *(c)* surrounding the descending aorta *(a)* and esophagus with extension into the mediastinal fat *(arrowheads).* **B,** T2-weighted axial image shows encasement of the descending thoracic aorta, displacement of the main and left pulmonary artery, and vertebral body invasion *(black arrow). Small white arrows,* Small bilateral pleural effusions. (From reference 65.)

signal intensity on T2-weighted images, can be mistaken for recurrent tumor. This phenomenon is seen up to 4 to 6 months after completion of radiation treatment. When in doubt, fat saturation T1-weighted Gd-DTPA–enhanced imaging may be of help. Typically, radiation inflammation is enhanced more than recurrent or residual tumor.[60]

Despite its attribute in studying the mediastinum and peripheral lung structures, the practical reality is that CT will serve as the primary imaging modality in the evaluation of all chest pathological conditions except for aortic diseases. Unless MRI can image the lung parenchyma, it will continue to serve a limited role as an adjunct to CT in studying the mediastinum and peripheral lung structures.

REFERENCES

1. American Joint Committee on Cancer: Manual for staging of cancer, Philadelphia, 1988, JB Lippincott.
2. Amparo EG: Magnetic resonance imaging of aortic disease: preliminary results, Am J Roentgenol 143:1203, 1984.
3. Amparo EG: Aortic dissection: magnetic resonance imaging, Radiology 155:399, 1985.
4. Amparo EG, Higgins CB, Farmer DW, et al: Gated MRI of cardiac and paracardiac masses: initial experience, Am J Roentgenol 143:1151, 1984.
5. Anagnostopoulos CE, Prabhakar MJ, Kittle CF, et al: Aortic dissections and dissecting aneurysms, Am J Cardiol 30:263, 1972.
6. Auffermann W: MR imaging of complications of aortic surgery, J Comput Assist Tomogr 11:982, 1987.
7. Aurigemma G: Cardiac cine magnetic resonance imaging: detection of mitral and aortic regurgitation, J Am Coll Cardiol 9:159A, 1987.
8. Aurigemma G: Evaluation of aortic regurgitation by cine magnetic resonance imaging, J Am Coll Cardiol 11:155A, 1988.
9. Axel L, and Dougherty L: Heart wall motion: improved method of spatial modulation of magnetization for MR imaging, Radiology 172:349, 1987.
10. Bailes DR: Respiratory ordered phase encoding (ROPE): a method for reducing respiratory motion artifacts in MR imaging, J Comput Assist Tomogr 9:835, 1985.
11. Batra P, Brown K, Steckel P, et al: MR imaging of the thorax: a comparison of axial, coronal, and sagittal imaging planes, J Comput Assist Tomogr 12:75, 1988
12. Batra P, Hermann C Jr, Mulder D, et al: Mediastinal imaging in myasthenia gravis: correlation of chest radiography, CT, MR and surgical findings, Am J Roentgenol 148:515, 1987.
13. Bergh NP, Gatzinski P, Larrson S, et al: Tumors of the thymus and thymic region: I. Clinicopathological studies on thymomas, Ann Thorac Surg 5:91, 1978.
14. Bergin CJ, Glover GH, Pauly JM, et al: Lung parenchyma: magnetic susceptibility in MR imaging, Radiology 180:845, 1991.
15. Bergin CJ, Healy MV, Zinone GE, et al: MR evaluation of chest wall involvement in malignant lymphoma, J Comput Assist Tomogr 14:928, 1990.
16. Bergin CJ, Noll DC, Pauly JM, et al: MR imaging of lung parenchyma: a solution to susceptibility, Radiology 183:673, 1992.
17. Bergin CJ, Pauly JM, Glover GH, et al: Lung parenchyma: projection reconstruction MR imaging, Radiology 179:777, 1991.
18. Bouchard A: Magnetic resonance imaging in pulmonary arterial hypertension, Am J Cardiol 56:938, 1985.
19. Bryant DJ: Measurement of flow with NMR imaging using a gradient pulse and phase difference technique, J Comput Assist Tomogr 8:588, 1984.
20. Burk DL Jr, Brunberg JA, Kanal E, et al: Spinal and paraspinal neurofibromatosis: surface coil MR imaging at 1.5 T, Radiology 162:797, 1987.
21. Carlsen SE, Bergin CJ, Hoppe RT, et al: MR imaging to detect chest wall and pleural involvement in patients with lymphoma: effect on radiation therapy planning, Am J Roentgenol 160:1191, 1993.
22. Carrillon Y, Tixier E, Revel D, et al: MR diagnosis of lipoid pneumonia, J Comput Assist Tomogr 12:876, 1988.
23. Case TA, Durney CH, Ailion DC, et al: A mathematical model of diamagnetic line broadening in lung tissue and similar heterogenous systems: calculations and measurements, J Magn Reson 73:304, 1987.
24. Cook SL: Effect of flow rate and orifice size on flow jets visualized by fast NMR imaging: a phantom study, J Am Coll Cardiol 11:56A, 1988.
25. Cory DA, Cohen MD, Smith JA, et al: Thymus in the superior mediastinum simulating adenopathy: appearance on CT, Radiology 162:457, 1987.
26. de Roos A: Cine MR imaging in aortic stenosis, J Comput Assist Tomogr 13:421, 1989.
27. DeVita VT Jr, Jaffe ES, and Hellman S: Hodgkin's disease and non-Hodgkin's lymphoma. In DeVita VT Jr, Hellman S, and Rosenberg SA, eds: Cancer: principles and practice of oncology, Philadelphia, 1985, JB Lippincott.
28. Didier D, and Higgins CB: Estimation of pulmonary vascular resistance by MRI in patients with congenital cardiovascular shunt lesions, Am J Roentgenol 146:919, 1986.
29. Dinsmore RE: Magnetic resonance imaging of thoracic aortic aneurysms: comparison with other imaging methods, Am J Roentgenol 146:309, 1986.
30. Dinsmore RE: MRI of dissection of the aorta: recognition of the intimal tear and differential flow velocities, Am J Roentgenol 146:1286, 1986.
31. Dinsmore RE: Phase-offset technique to distinguish slow blood flow and thrombus on MR images, Am J Roentgenol 148:634, 1987.
32. Dooms GC, Hricak H, Crooks LE, et al: Magnetic resonance imaging of the lymph nodes: comparison with CT, Radiology 153:719, 1984.
33. Epstein DM, Kressel H, Gefter W, et al: MR imaging of the mediastinum: a retrospective comparison with computed tomography, J Comput Assist Tomogr 8:670, 1984.
34. Feuerstein IM, Jicha DL, Pass HI, et al: Pulmonary metastases: MR imaging with surgical correlation—a prospective study, Radiology 182:123, 1992.
35. Finn JP, Zisk JHS, Edelman RR, et al: Central venous occlusion: MR angiography, Radiology 187:245, 1993.
36. Fujimoto K, et al: Gd-DTPA-enhanced dynamic MR imaging in pulmonary disease: evaluation of usefulness in differentiating benign from malignant disease, Radiology 189(P):438, 1993 (abstract).
37. Gamsu G, and Sostman D: Magnetic resonance imaging of the thorax, Am Rev Respir Dis 139:254, 1989.
38. Gamsu G, Stark DD, Webb WR, et al: Magnetic resonance imaging of benign mediastinal masses, Radiology 151:709, 1984.
39. Gefter WB: Magnetic resonance imaging in the evaluation of lung cancer, Semin Roentgenol 25:73, 1990.
40. Gefter WB, Spritzer CE, Eisenberg B, et al: Thyroid imaging with high-field-strength surface-coil MR, Radiology 164:483, 1987.
41. Geinsinger MA: Thoracic aortic dissections: magnetic resonance imaging, Radiology 155:407, 1985.
42. Glazer HS, Lee JKT, Levitt RG, et al: Radiation fibrosis: differentiation from recurrent tumor by MR imaging: work in progress, Radiology 156:721, 1985.
43. Goldstein G and Mackey IK: The human thymus, St Louis, 1969, Warren H. Green.
44. Gomes AS: Congenital abnormalities of the aortic arch: MR imaging, Radiology 165:91, 1987.
45. Gott VL: Surgical treatment of aneurysms of the ascending aorta in the Marfan syndrome, N Engl J Med 315:1070, 1986.
46. Grover FL: The role of CT and MRI in staging of the mediastinum, Chest 106:3915, 1994.
47. Haggar AM, and Froelich JW: MR imaging strategies in primary and metastatic malignancy, Radiol Clin North Am 26:689, 1988.
48. Heelan RT, Demas BE, Caravelli JF, et al: Superior sulcus tumors: CT and MR imaging, Radiology 170:637, 1989.
49. Henning J, Nauerth A, and Friedburg H: RARE imaging: fast imaging method for clinical MR, Magn Reson Med 3:823, 1986.
50. Herold CJ, Kuhlman JE, Zerhouni EA, et al: Pulmonary atelectasis: signal patterns with MR imaging, Radiology 178:715, 1991.
51. Higgins CB, Stark DD, McNamara M, et al: Multiplanar magnetic resonance imaging of the heart and major vessels: studies in normal volunteers, Am J Roentgenol 142:661, 1984.
52. Hsu BY, Edwards DK, Trambert MA, et al: Pulmonary hemorrhage complicating systemic lupus erythematosus: role of MR imaging in diagnosis, Am J Roentgenol 158:519, 1992.
53. Jochelson M, Mauch P, Balikian J, et al: The significance of the residual mediastinal mass in treated Hodgkin's disease, J Clin Oncol 3:637, 1985.
54. Joyce JW: Aneurysms of the thoracic aorta: a clinical study with special reference to prognosis, Circulation 29:176, 1964.
55. Kang YS, Rosen K, Clark OH, et al: Localization of abnormal parathyroid glands of the mediastinum with MR imaging, Radiology 189:1371993.
56. Kersting-Sommerhoff BA: MR imaging of the thoracic aorta in Marfan patients, J Comput Assist Tomogr 11:633, 1987.
57. Kersting-Sommerhoff BA: Aortic dissection: sensitivity and specificity of MR imaging, Radiology 166:651, 1988.
58. Kessler R, Fraisse P, Krause D, et al: Magnetic resonance imaging in the diagnosis of pulmonary infarction, Chest 99:298, 1991.
59. Kinsella D, Hamilton A, Goddard P, et al: The role of magnetic resonance imaging in cystic fibrosis, Clin Radiol 44:23, 1991.
60. Kono M, Adachi S, Kusomoto M, et al: Clinical utility of Gd-DTPA-enhanced magnetic resonance imaging in lung cancer, J Thorac Imaging 8:18, 1993.
61. Krubsack AJ, Wilson SD, Lawson TL, et al: Prospective comparison of radionuclide, computed tomographic, sonographic, and magnetic resonance localization of parathyroid tumors, Surgery 106:639, 1989.
62. LeGolvan DP: Thymomas, Cancer 39:2142, 1977.
63. Levitt RG, Glazer HS, Roper CL, et al: Magnetic resonance imaging of mediastinal and hilar masses: comparison with CT, Am J Roentgenol 145:9, 1985.
64. Libshitz HI, Jing BS, Wallace S, et al: Sterilized metastases: a diagnostic and therapeutic dilemma, Am J Roentgenol 140:15, 1983.
65. Link KM, Samuels LJ, Reed JC, et al: Magnetic resonance imaging of the mediastinum, J Thorac Imaging 8(1):34, 1993.
66. Mayo JR, McKay A, Muller NL, et al: MR imaging of the lungs: value of short TE spin-echo pulse sequences, Am J Roentgenol 159:951, 1992.
67. Mayo JR, McKay A, Muller NL, et al: T2 relaxation time in MR imaging of normal and abnormal lung parenchyma, Radiology 177(P):313, 1990 (abstract).
68. McLoud TC, and Flower CDR: Imaging the pleura: sonography, CT and MR imaging, Am J Roentgenol 156:1145, 1991.
69. Merine DS, Fishman EK, Zerhouni EA, et al: Computed tomography and magnetic resonance imaging diagnosis of thymic cyst, J Comput Assist Tomogr 12:220, 1988.
70. Mirvis SE, Keramati B, Buckman R, et al: MR imaging of traumatic diaphragmatic rupture, J Comput Assist Tomogr 12:147, 1988.
71. Mitchell DG, Crovello M, Matteucci T, et al: Benign adrenocortical masses: diagnosis with chemical shift MR imaging, Radiology 185:345, 1992.
72. Moore EH: MRI of chronic posttraumatic false aneurysms of the thoracic aorta. Am J Roentgenol 143:1195, 1984.
73. Morris AH, Blatter DD, Case TA, et al: A new nuclear magnetic resonance property of lung, J Appl Physiol 58:759, 1985.
74. Muller NL: Imaging of the pleura, Radiology 186:297, 1993.
75. Muller NL, Mayo JR, et al: Value of MR imaging in the evaluation of chronic infiltrative lung diseases: comparison with CT, Am J Roentgenol 158:1205, 1992.
76. Musset D, Grenier P, Carette MF, et al: Primary lung cancer staging: prospective comparative study of MR imaging with CT, Radiology 160:607, 1986.
77. Nakata H, Nakayama C, Kimoto T, et al: Computed tomography of mediastinal bronchogenic cysts, J Comput Assist Tomogr 6:733, 1982.
78. Nielson ME Jr, Heaston DK, Dunnick NR, et al: Preoperative CT evaluation of adrenal glands in non-small cell bronchogenic carcinoma, Am J Roentgenol 139:317, 1982.

79. Nienaber CA, von Kodolitsch Y, Nicolas V, et al: The diagnosis of thoracic aortic dissection by noninvasive imaging procedures, N Engl J Med 328:1, 1993.
80. Nyman R, Rehn S, Glimelius B, et al: Magnetic resonance imaging for assessment of treatment effects in mediastinal Hodgkin's disease, Acta Radiol 28:145, 1987.
81. Nyman RS, Rehn S, Glimelius BLG, et al: Residual mediastinal masses in Hodgkin disease: prediction of size with MR imaging, Radiology 170:435, 1989.
82. Olson EM, Bergin CJ, King MA, et al: Fast SE MRI of the chest: parameter optimization and comparison with conventional SE imaging, J Comput Assist Tomogr 19:167, 1995.
83. Pettigrew RI: Dynamic cardiac MR imaging: techniques and applications, Radiol Clin North Am 27:1183, 1989.
84. Pugatch RD: Radiologic evaluation in chest malignancies: a review of imaging modalities, Chest 107:2945, 1995.
85. Radford J A, Cowan RA, Flanagan MI, et al: The significance of residual mediastinal abnormality on the chest radiograph following treatment for Hodgkin's disease, J Clin Oncol 6:940, 1988.
86. Rahmouni AD, and Zerhouni EA: Role of MRI in the management of thoracic lymphoma: CT and MRI of the thorax. In Zerhouni EA, ed: Contemporary issues in computed tomography, New York, 1989, Churchill Livingstone.
87. Rehn SM, Nyman RS, Glomelius BLG, et al: Non-Hodgkin lymphoma: predicting prognostic grade with MR imaging, Radiology 176:249, 1990.
88. Roberts WC: Aortic dissection: anatomy, consequences, and causes, Am Heart J 101:195, 1981.
89. Rollins NK, and Currarino G: MR imaging of posterior mediastinal thymus, J Comput Assist Tomogr 12:518, 1988.
90. Rubin GD, Edwards DK III, Reicher MA, et al: Diagnosis of pulmonary hemosiderosis by MR imaging, Am J Roentgenol 152:573, 1989.
91. Ruzal-Shapiro C, Abrahamson SJ, Berdon WE, et al: Posterior mediastinal cystic teratoma surrounded by fat in a 13 month old boy: value of magnetic resonance imaging, Pediatr Radiol 20:107, 1989.
92. Seelos KC, DeMarco R, Clark OH, et al: Persistent and recurrent hyperparathyroidism: assessment with gadopentetate dimeglumine-enhanced MR imaging, Radiology 177:373, 1990.
93. Shirkhoda A, Chasen MH, Eftekhari F, et al: MR imaging of mediastinal thymolipoma, J Comput Assist Tomogr 11:364, 1987.
94. Soulen R: Marfan syndrome: evaluation with MR imaging versus CT, Radiology 165:697, 1987.
95. Stratemeier EJ: Ejection fraction determination by MR imaging: comparison with left ventricular angiography, Radiology 158:775, 1986.
96. Surbone A, Longo DL, DeVita VT JR, et al: Residual abdominal masses in aggressive non-Hodgkin's lymphoma after combination chemotherapy: significance and management, J Clin Oncol 6:1832, 1988.
97. Tobler J, Levitt RG, Glazer HS, et al: Differentiation of proximal bronchogenic carcinoma from postobstructive lobar collapse by magnetic resonance imaging: comparison with computed tomography, Invest Radiol 22:538, 1987.
98. Underwood SR: Magnetic resonance velocity mapping: clinical application of a new technique, Br Heart J 57:404, 1987.
99. Utz J A: Cine MR determination of left ventricular ejection fraction, Am J Roentgenol 148:839, 1987.
100. von Schulthess GK, and Augustiny N: Calculation of T2 values versus phase imaging for the distinction between flow and thrombus in MR imaging, Radiology 164:549, 1987.
101. von Schulthess GK, Fisher MR, Higgins CB, et al: Pathologic blood flow in pulmonary vascular disease as shown by gated magnetic resonance imaging, Ann Intern Med 103:317, 1985.
102. von Schulthess GK, McMurdo KK, Tscholakoff D, et al: Mediastinal masses: MR imaging, Radiology 158:289, 1986.
103. Webb WR: Magnetic resonance imaging of the hila and mediastinum, Cardiovasc Intervent Radiol 8:306, 1986.
104. Webb WR: The role of magnetic resonance imaging in the assessment of patients with ling cancer: a comparison with computed tomography, J Thorac Imaging 4(2):65, 1989.
105. Webb WR: Magnetic resonance imaging of the chest, Curr Opin Radiol 1:40, 1989.
106. Webb WR: MR imaging of treated mediastinal Hodgkin disease, Radiology 170:315, 1989.
107. Webb WR, Gamsu G, Stark DD, et al: Magnetic resonance imaging of the normal and abnormal pulmonary hila, Radiology 152:89, 1984.
108. Webb WR, Gastonis C, Zerhouni EA, et al: CT and MR imaging in staging non-small cell bronchogenic carcinoma: report of the Radiologic Diagnostic Oncology Group, Radiology 178:705, 1991.
109. Webb WR, Jenson BG, Gamsu G, et al: Coronal magnetic resonance imaging of the chest: normal and abnormal, Radiology 153:729, 1984.
110. Webb WR, and Moore EH: Differentiation of volume averaging and mass on magnetic resonance images of the mediastinum, Radiology 155:413, 1985.
111. Webb WR, and Sostman HD: MR imaging of thoracic disease: clinical uses, Radiology 182:621, 1992.
112. White EM: Intravascular signal in MR imaging: use of phase display for differentiation of blood-flow signal from intraluminal disease, Radiology 161:245, 1986.
113. White RD, Ullyot DJ, Higgins CB, et al: MR imaging of the aorta after surgery for aortic dissection, Am J Roentgenol 150:87, 1988.
114. White RD, Winkler NML, Higgins CB, et al: MR imaging of pulmonary arterial hypertension and pulmonary emboli, Am J Roentgenol 149:15, 1987.
115. Yamada T, Tada S, Harada J, et al: Aortic dissection without intimal rupture: diagnosis with MR imaging and CT, Radiology 168:352, 1988.
116. Yankelevitz DF, Henschke CI, Batata M, et al: Lung cancer: evaluation with MR imaging during and after radiation, J Thorac Imaging 9:41, 1994.
117. Zeitler E: Magnetic resonance imaging of aneurysms and thrombi, Cardiovasc Intervent Radiol 8:321, 1986.
118. Zerhouni EA: MRI in the management of lymphoma. In Margulis AR, et al, eds: Diagnostic radiology, St Louis, 1986, Mosby..
119. Zerhouni EA, Fishman EK, Jones R, et al: MR imaging of "sterilized" lymphoma, Radiology 161(P):207 Abstract, 1986.
120. Zerhouni EA, Scott WW Jr, Baker RR, et al: Invasive thymomas: diagnosis and evaluation by computed tomography, J Comput Assist Tomogr 6:92, 1982.

19 Magnetic Resonance Angiography: Great Vessels and Abdomen

Kerry M. Link and Nadja M. Lesko

KEY POINTS

- Gadolinium-enhanced breath-hold TOF is the most useful technique.
- Dynamic imaging techniques (cine and phase contrast) permit functional assessment of vascular disease.
- Thoracic and abdominal MRA is competitive with contrast-enhanced CT, ultrasound, and even angiography for selected applications.

Magnetic resonance angiography (MRA) has enjoyed clinical success in the assessment of the cranial, carotid, and vertebral vessels. Attempts to study the thoracic, abdominal, and peripheral vasculature have not been as successful and are used sparingly in the clinical arena. This chapter reviews the basic techniques, discusses the problems associated with their application to the body, and explores modifications addressing these problems.

MAGNETIC RESONANCE ANGIOGRAPHY TECHNIQUES
Time-of-Flight Magnetic Resonance Angiography

The two basic clinical MRA techniques are time-of-flight (TOF)[22,25,48,66] and phase-contrast (PC)[47,50,75] angiography. Although both techniques produce similar types of images of blood vessels, the way in which vascular images are produced is quite different. TOF angiography relies on flow-related enhancement, in which fully magnetized blood enters into the imaging plane. This enhancement is best accomplished by imaging perpendicular to the flow of blood. PC angiography produces an image by measuring the phase of the transverse magnetization as it moves along the magnetic field gradient. The contrast needed to produce an image is directly related to the change in the spin phase, or the phase angle, of the moving blood.

Perhaps the most commonly used MRA technique is two-dimensional (2D) TOF[23,35] imaging. This technique is based on standard 2D gradient-echo imaging. Blood flowing into the imaging slice is fully magnetized, whereas stationary tissue is partially saturated. Therefore blood will have a higher signal intensity than stationary tissue, from which signals are suppressed by selection of short repetition time (TR) pulse sequence parameters. To selectively visualize the arterial or venous structures, a saturation slab[15] is applied either above or below the slice. Saturated blood flowing into the slice yields no signal, whereas unsaturated blood flowing into the slice from the opposite side yields signal and is visualized. With the 2D technique, a volume of interest is created by stacking the individual, typically axial, slices and then subjecting them to some type of projection technique.[35] Commonly this is a ray-tracing technique known as a *maximum-intensity projection* (MIP) algorithm.[39] This technique allows for the display of multiple projection images oriented around the acquisition axis. For axial 2D TOF images, it allows for a set of coronal-to-sagittal images. Although MIP projection images are convenient for viewing all of the axial slices simultaneously and presenting the vasculature similar to standard angiography, the technique has its weaknesses. It decreases the apparent diameter of vessels, both normal and diseased. This effect may lead to overestimation of stenotic lesions. Similarly the technique does not always distinguish between overlapped vessels, and may present them as one. Therefore it is imperative that the individual axial slices ("source images") are reviewed in conjunction with the MIP projection images.[1]

Image contrast determines the overall quality of the TOF images. Poor manipulation of image-contrast parameters can lead to signal loss and therefore overestimation of stenoses. In addition, flow considerations must be taken into account when imaging any vascular bed to maximize flow-related enhancement and therefore image quality and accuracy.

MRA is well served by the increased signal-to-noise ratios (SNRs) of higher–field strength systems. T1-relaxation times increase with field strength. Therefore the signal intensity of stationary tissues decreases as field strength increases. The time to echo (TE) for fat-water phase cancellation on gradient-echo images is also field-strength dependent. Selection of such an opposed-phase gradient-echo sequence for MRA will help suppress signal from stationary (fatty) tissue. At 1.5 Tesla (T), fat and water protons are out of phase at TE = 2.2 ms and every 4.4 ms thereafter (i.e., 6.6, 11.0, 15.4, etc.). It is also important to use very short TEs in TOF MRA, and therefore TE = 2.2 ms is ideal. Care should be taken at longer TEs not to select a TE where fat and water are in phase (e.g., 8.8, 13.2, 17.6, etc.) because this will maximize the signal from stationary tissues, reducing their contrast with flowing blood.

The normal pulsatile flow situation results in acceleration, jerk, and higher-order motion that disperses the phase of transverse magnetization, resulting in signal loss. Dephasing caused by velocity (first-order motion) can be compensated for by gradient-moment nulling.[36,52] Although gradient-moment nulling can be applied to second- and higher-order motion, it takes time and adds complexity to the pulse sequence, which in turn causes other limitations. The best way to overcome dephasing caused by acceleration and higher-order motion is by using short TEs.[64] Very short TEs (e.g., 0 to 2.2 ms) can be obtained by use of asymmetrical echo sampling.

It is important to keep TR short to suppress signal from stationary tissues (background). However, at short TRs the blood also receives more radiofrequency (RF) excitations, lowering its SNR. When designing TOF angiography protocols, the clinician's knowledge of blood transit times, which vary among different areas of the body, can guide selection of optimal TRs.

Selection of a flip angle for gradient-echo sequences must take into account the relationship between stationary-tissue suppression and blood-signal enhancement. Larger flip angles more heavily suppress stationary-tissue signal but also saturate blood, resulting in signal loss.

Slow flow or conditions in which blood does not leave the imaging slice quickly will result in signal loss on TOF angiography because of saturation. This is a problem in imaging the venous system. Slow-flow problems also can occur in the arterial system. Within a vessel, there exists a velocity vector gradient, with fastest flow occurring in the center of the vessel and nearly stationary flow at the vessel wall.[8] Slowly flowing blood receives more excitations and becomes saturated, like stationary tissues. At bifurcations and vessel curves, slowly flowing (peripheral) blood moves away from the vessel wall (flow separation) and recirculates in the more central aspects of the vessel. Low-signal artifacts can mimic thrombus or dissection. Admixture of low-signal (saturated) blood to unsaturated blood reduces SNR, degrading image quality.

Vessel geometry is an important consideration in deciding how to image a particular vascular bed. Flow-related enhancement is maximized when blood flows perpendicular to the image slice. Whenever the vessel passes within or obliquely through the slice, it will be saturated to some degree, with resultant loss of intravascular signal. The vasculature to be studied should be aligned perpendicular to the imaging plane, and the thinnest possible slice thickness should be used to reduce in-plane flow.

Three-dimensional (3D) TOF angiography allows for small voxel sizes that decrease velocity vector gradients, thereby minimizing dephasing. As always, the shortest possible TE should be used. Another clear advantage of 3D TOF MRA is superior SNR.[24] However, the increased SNR inherent in 3D (over 2D) methods applies to both the blood vessel and the surrounding stationary tissue. This increases both SNR and contrast-to-noise ratio (CNR).

Three-dimensional techniques image a thick slab (a volume divided into thin slices selected by phase encoding in a second dimension), and the entire vasculature within the slab receives every excitation. The blood flow signal in the more downstream aspect of the volume imaged will start to fade out because of saturation accumulated once blood flows into the slab. This problem can be overcome with multiple thin-slab 3D acquisitions with a small amount of overlap between slabs, or multiple overlapping thin-slab angiography (MOTSA).[51]

Another TOF technique, not often thought of as an angiographic technique, is cine MRI.[20] This method involves 2D gradient-echo images acquired at a specific slice level at multiple time points within the cardiac cycle. Flowing blood pool appears bright, and when the images are displayed in a movie loop, blood pulsatility and the cardiac cycle are cinematically demonstrated. Cine MRI is best used in examining the heart and large-caliber vessels. Unlike plain, static MRA, the cine technique accommodates the cyclical velocity variations that occur during the cardiac cycle. As with static MRI, on cine images stagnant and retrograde flow result in signal loss. If the multiple time points, or "phases," of the cine study are evaluated, phases in which these phenomena are absent can be used to assess the true vessel lumen. As an alternative to cine MRA, cardiac gating can be used with TOF or PC MRA to prescribe imaging at a single phase or time point within the cardiac cycle.

Phase-Contrast Magnetic Resonance Angiography

TOF MRA uses movement of the longitudinal magnetization of blood to produce image contrast (CNR) through flow-related enhancement. PC MRA uses the movement of transverse magnetization to produce CNR. Changes in the phase (phase angle) of transverse magnetization in flowing blood are induced movement within one or more magnetic field gradients.[74]

These phase shifts, which are directly related to spin position, can be reversed by applying a second gradient pulse of equal duration but of opposite polarity. If nuclei have not moved during the interval between the first and the second gradient pulses, the reversal of the phase shift will be exact, canceling the effect of the original phase shift and resulting in no net phase shift (zero change in phase angle). However, nuclei such as flowing blood that have moved during the time interval between gradient pulses will not receive two equal, opposed gradient pulses, and the phase shift will not be corrected fully.[47,72] Therefore, after gradient-pulse reversal, the residual phase shift (or change in phase angle) is directly proportional to the change in location or the distance the nuclei moved between application of the first and second gradient pulses. These phase shifts are used by PC MRA to create angiographic images and measure flow velocities.[70]

Practical PC MRA methods consider only constant velocity to avoid prohibitively long scan times. This compromise is similar to the usual limitation in TOF MRI, wherein only first-order flow compensation (gradient-moment nulling) is performed because of timing considerations.

Depending on the vascular bed being studied, flow-encoded gradients can be applied in a single direction (e.g., superior-inferior for the extracranial carotids) or in three orthogonal planes (superior-inferior, anterior-posterior, and right-to-left).[16,53] These factors must be taken into account when setting up the pulse sequence.

To provide quantitative information, the velocity-encoding gradient (VENC, or V_{enc}) strength is set so that the highest velocity encountered will produce a phase shift near but not exceeding positive or negative 180 degrees. A positive 180 degrees corresponds to the maximum velocity measurable in one direction, and a negative 180 degrees corresponds to the maximum velocity measurable in the opposite direction. If the VENC is set at 50 cm/sec, the bipolar gradients are adjusted so that all velocities up to and including 50 cm/sec will be imaged. If the VENC is set too low, phase shifts exceeding 180 degrees become indistinguishable from the phase shift produced by flow in the opposite direction, an aliasing phenomenon. If the VENC is set too high, distinctions cannot be made between various intermediate flow velocities, and the procedure is no longer quantitative. Therefore some knowledge of normal arterial and venous velocity values is important when choosing the initial VENC value. After the first data are obtained and maximal velocities are correctly measured, repeat MRA can be performed with VENC selected optimally.

Time of Flight Versus Phase Contrast

Both TOF and PC MRA have advantages and disadvantages, and both suffer from artifactual signal losses. Selection of the proper technique depends on the available hardware and software, the vascular bed under investigation, the anatomical question that must be answered, whether quantitative information is needed, and whether cine or dynamic imaging is required. TOF MRA (both 2D and 3D) is less effective when blood flow is at low velocity (slow flow) because the progressive saturation occurs within the field of view (FOV). Slow flow does not limit PC MRA, provided only that the flow-encoding gradient strength is selected properly.

To properly image slowly flowing blood with PC MRA, the machine hardware must have minimal eddy currents. Eddy currents cause artifacts, wherein stationary tissue shows phase shifts that mimic blood flow. PC MRA requires longer scanning times than TOF MRA. This is a logistical problem and also potentiates image degradations resulting from patient movement and cardiac, respiratory, and abdominal content movements.

Both PC and TOF MRA have enjoyed success in studying the carotid vasculature.* However, the orientation of extracranial carotid vasculature parallel to the machine z axis is particularly well suited to axial TOF imaging. Blood flow is rapid, maximizing contrast, and the territory to be studied is short, permitting thin slices. Three-dimensional TOF can avoid in-plane flow and intravoxel phase dispersion, obtaining very small voxels with high SNR. On the other hand, PC angiography is advantageous for studying small, tortuous intracranial arteries and veins, especially where blood flow is slow and in plane.

Problems arise when MRA is applied to the rest of the body. First, vascular structures within the chest, abdomen, pelvis, and extremities cover a large territory, requiring very long acquisition times. Physiological motion of the heart, lungs, and abdominal contents is an additional challenge limiting the quality of MRA.

One way to overcome motion artifacts is to acquire data very quickly. Segmented κ-space data acquisition can be cardiac triggered, with data acquired during breath-holding.[3,9] Multiple phase-encoded lines (e.g., 4, 8, 16, of κ space) are acquired each cardiac cycle. If 16 phase-encoded lines are acquired per cardiac cycle, then 256 lines of κ space can be acquired over 16 cardiac cycles. However, as phase encoding is spread out over the cardiac cycle, blurring of the image may occur.

Recently, investigators have used gadolinium in an effort to reduce flow artifacts associated with TOF techniques.[55] This allows better visualization of larger caliber vessels when flow is slow (e.g., low car-

---

*References 11, 44, 45, 54, 62, 73.

diac output, aortic aneurysms, or dissections), as well as better visualization of smaller caliber vessels where flow is inherently slower.

Gadolinium gives blood a very bright signal on heavily T1-weighted images. This technique overcomes the limitations of the TOF techniques, since blood signal is now independent of the inflow of unsaturated spins. Therefore the image acquisition plane does not have to be perpendicular to the flow of blood. Large territories of vascular anatomy can therefore be imaged in a much shorter period of time. In addition, this method can be used in conjunction with breath-hold techniques, thereby decreasing respiratory motion artifacts.

To make the T1 of blood shorter than fat, a dose of at least 0.2 mmol/kg of gadolinium is required. Typically, double-dose gadolinium-enhanced MRA is used with a 3D-spoiled gradient-refocused echo (GRE) sequence. The SNR, which depends on the amount of T1 weighting, is influenced by a number of factors, including the speed of contrast injection, flip angle, and TR. The intricacies of the relationship between these parameters is beyond the scope of this chapter and the reader is referred to the excellent review by Prince.

CLINICAL APPLICATIONS
Thoracic Aorta

Electocardiographically gated spin-echo (SE) MRI of the thoracic aorta has accuracy equal to or better than computed tomography, transthoracic echocardiography (ECG), and transesophageal ECG for evaluating the entire spectrum of congenital anomalies and acquired diseases.[49] The technique does suffer from respiratory motion, in-plane flow, slow flow, and the inability to assess the aortic valve. Although the branch vessel ostia are often identified, comment usually cannot be made with regard to atherosclerotic disease. Cine MRI and cine 2D PC imaging are excellent for assessing the aortic valve, and they improve the ability to view the branch vessel ostia (Figure 19-1). Cine MRI may erroneously interpret thrombus within a false lumen as flow, depending on its stage of evolution. PC techniques, not being dependent on flow-tissue contrast differences, are not affected by this problem. Additionally, quantitative information regarding aortic stenosis, aortic regurgitation, and coarctation can be obtained if the VENC is correctly set.[20,26,70] The combination of SE and cine techniques is usually sufficient to study the thoracic aorta itself.

Improved MRA techniques are needed for evaluation of the branch vessels of the aorta (Figure 19-2), where SE and cine techniques are often nondiagnostic. To obliterate signal from the thoracic veins, multiple saturation slabs or a walking saturation pulse may be required. Because the flow of blood within these vessels is basically parallel to the longitudinal axis of the body, axial TOF MRA (Figure 19-3) may be used, preferably overlapping 3D MOTSA slabs.[51] Standard breath-hold turbo fast low-angle shot (turboFLASH) images do not image the aorta adequately.[26] However, ECG-gated breath-hold segmented TOF images in conjunction with double-dose gadolinium chelate have demonstrated good delineation of the arch and the branch vessels.[56]

By shortening the T1 of blood with a gadolinium chelate, it is possible to correct signal losses resulting from in-plane flow, slow flow, or swirling eddies within aneurysms. Gadolinium alleviates the reliance of TOF on the inflow of unsaturated spins for signal, and it becomes possible with TOF MRA to image in any plane, not just perpendicular to vessel direction. This allows coverage of large vascular territories in markedly less time than possible with unenhanced TOF MRA (Figure 19-4). Gadolinium enhancement gives TOF some of the flexibility of PC MRA. For evaluation of the thoracic and abdominal aorta, Prince[56] recommends a 3D Fourier-transform (FT) spoiled gradient-echo volume centered on the arteries of interest, 28 2-mm thick partitions within the slab, 36-cm FOV, 256 × 256 matrix, 6.9-ms TE (taking advantage of fat-water opposed phase), 24-ms TR, 40-degree flip angle, and first-order flow compensation. κ Space is sampled in the standard linear fashion, resulting in a scan time of 3 min 18 sec, during which 40 ml of gadopentetate dimeglumine (0.5 mol/L), gadoteridol (0.5 mol/L), or gadodiamide (0.5 mol/L) is infused continuously. Using this imaging protocol, a sensitivity of 1 and a specificity of 0.94 were achieved for the diagnosis of stenoses and occlusions of the aorta and branch vessels, with surgical results serving as the gold standard.

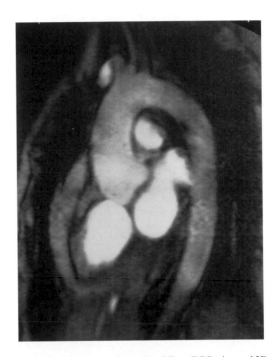

FIGURE 19-1   Thoracic aorta. Left anterior oblique ECG-triggered 2D cine MRI.

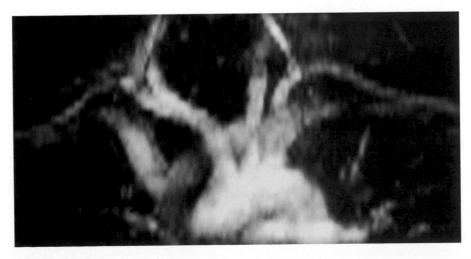

FIGURE 19-2   Branch vessels of the aortic arch better seen on 2D PC MRA than on 2D cine MRI (Figure 19-1).

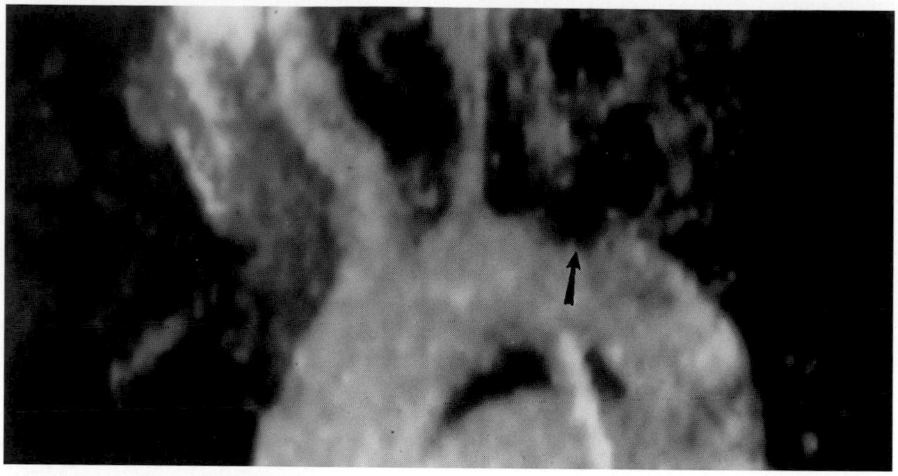

FIGURE 19-3   Atherosclerotic plaque *(arrow)* has encroached on the ostium of the left subclavian artery as seen on 3D TOF MRA.

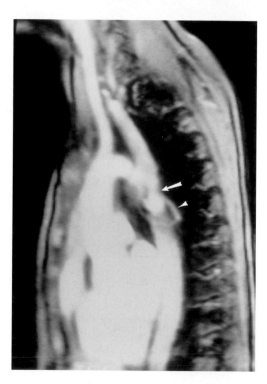

FIGURE 19-4   Coarctation *(arrow)* of the thoracic aorta showing a collateral vessel *(arrowhead)* and small intercostals. Left anterior oblique gadolinium-enhanced 3D MRA.

Abdominal Aorta and Its Branches

SE techniques have not been successful in evaluating the abdominal branch vasculature. ECG-gating with respiratory compensation schemes does not overcome motion-induced artifacts in the abdomen. Diaphragmatic excursion causes secondary movements of the abdominal organs, some traveling up to several centimeters per respiration. This movement greatly affects the ability to image the vessels feeding these organs, most notably the renal pedicle, the celiac axis, and the portal system. Breath-hold gadolinium chelate–enhanced TOF techniques have been most successful for studying these vessels. These techniques minimize organ motion and allow acquisition of the large FOVs needed in abdominal imaging. PC MRA also has a role in imaging the abdominal vasculature, especially in areas, such as the portal venous system, where flow direction is important in diagnosis and management.

SE MRI is a reliable method for detecting abdominal aortic aneurysms (AAAs)[32] and dissections, showing their location, extent, and relationship to the left renal vein (Figure 19-5). However, the technique is not reliable for detecting occlusive disease of the renal artery or other branch vessels. SE MRI cannot be used with confidence to detect accessory renal arteries. Similarly, cine techniques, although very accurate at detecting and localizing AAAs (Figure 19-6), are presently not sufficient for full presurgical workups of these patients.

Two-dimensional TOF MRA has demonstrated the ability to identify and localize AAAs. Unfortunately, evaluation of the visceral, renal, and pelvic arteries for related pathological conditions or anatomical demonstration of accessory renal arteries has been unreliable (Figure 19-7).[12,13] Even with addition of 3D TOF MOTSA only 64% of accessory renal arteries are detected.[34] Stenoses (>50%) of renal and visceral arteries are detectable with a sensitivity of only 67%; however, few false-positive diagnoses occur (specificity 98%).[34] These technical difficulties are the consequence of imaging slow flow, in-plane flow, and turbulence associated with the aneurysms.

Gadolinium-enhanced 3D TOF MRA was introduced to address the problem of signal loss.[57] This technique combines the high spatial resolution and SNR of 3D imaging with gadolinium, shortening T1 to obviate saturation problems. By dynamic imaging (i.e., within seconds of bolus injection), the arteries can be visualized separate from the veins. In one earlier study, MRA correctly diagnosed aneurysms of the aorta and iliac arteries, stenoses of the renal, mesenteric, and iliac arteries, and occlusion of the common iliac artery.[57]

AAAs imaged with enhanced 3D TOF MRA (Figure 19-8) yield sensitivities and specificities of 89% and 98%, respectively, for renal artery stenosis (>50%) and 100% and 91% for iliac artery stenosis; all (100%) main renal arteries are demonstrated, as are 78% of accessory renal arteries.[33] The proximal extent of the AAA can be shown in nearly 100% of patients, compared with 92% with conventional angiography.[33]

Breath-holding can further improve results obtained with a 3D gadolinium-enhanced spoiled gradient-echo MRA sequence.[58] With this method (2.6-ms TE, 14.1-ms TR, 45-degree flip angle, 2-mm slices, 256 × 128 matrix, and administration of 42 ml of gadolinium chelate over 25 sec), the abdominal aorta and the ostia of the pelvic, celiac, superior mesenteric, and renal arteries can be demonstrated in virtually all patients (Figure 19-9).[58] Of the 19 patients who underwent conventional

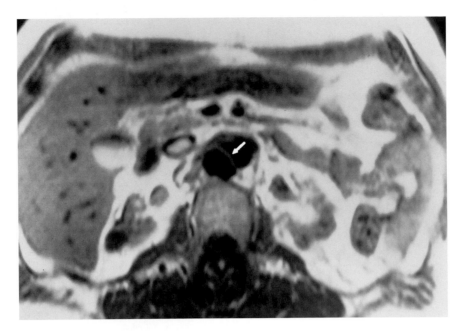

FIGURE 19-5   Dissection of the abdominal aorta demonstrating an intimal flap *(arrow)* on transaxial T1-weighted SE image.

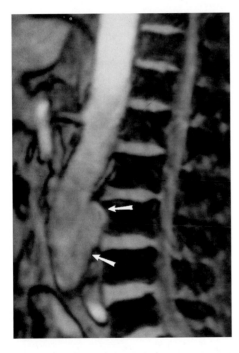

FIGURE 19-6   Eccentric distal abdominal aneurysm *(arrows)* of the abdominal aorta on sagittal ECG-triggered 2D cine MRI.

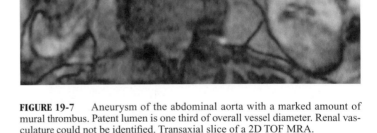

FIGURE 19-7   Aneurysm of the abdominal aorta with a marked amount of mural thrombus. Patent lumen is one third of overall vessel diameter. Renal vasculature could not be identified. Transaxial slice of a 2D TOF MRA.

angiography, Prince et al[58] identified 10 of 11 accessory renal arteries and 15 of 19 stenotic or occlusive lesions of the celiac, superior mesenteric, and renal arteries. In the last four discrepancies, MRA underestimated two stenoses and overestimated one stenosis. One normal renal artery was erroneously thought to have a moderate stenosis.

At this time, breath-hold gadolinium-enhanced 3D TOF MRA is perhaps the best technique for studying the entire abdominal aorta (Figure 19-10) in patients with known or suspected aneurysms.[10,38,71,78]

Renal Arteries

Renal artery stenosis is the most common cause of secondary hypertension, accounting for an increasing percentage of chronic renal in-

sufficiency and end-stage renal disease.[60] Two dimensional TOF MRA has been evaluated by several groups reporting sensitivities and specificities both in excess of 90% for detection of renal artery stenosis (>50% occlusion.)[10,37,67] Three-dimensional TOF MRA (Figure 19-11) has a reported sensitivity of 100% and specificity of 95%.[67] Unfortunately, these successes have not been repeatable in the hands of other authors using a variety of TOF techniques.[29,34,41]

In an effort to overcome the problems of in-plane flow and saturation, creative variations on the theme of TOF have been proposed. These variations include the use of signal targeting with alternating radiofrequency (STAR) in conjunction with a segmented ECG-gated turboFLASH sequence.[14] Blood in the suprarenal aorta is tagged with an inversion pulse, and imaging takes place at the renal arteries. By tag-

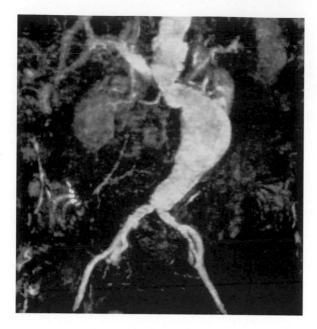

FIGURE 19-8   Diffuse atherosclerotic disease and fusiform infrarenal aneurysm. Contrast-enhanced 3D TOF MRA of the abdominal aorta acquired in the coronal plane.

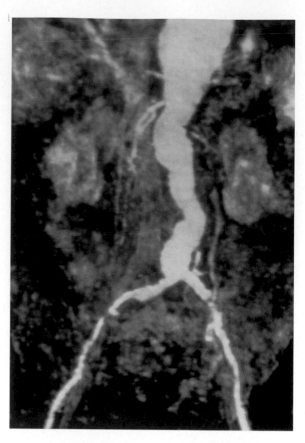

FIGURE 19-10   Diffuse atherosclerotic disease of the abdominal aorta and pelvic arteries showing a thoracoabdominal aneurysm. Dynamic breath-hold gadolinium-enhanced TOF MRA.

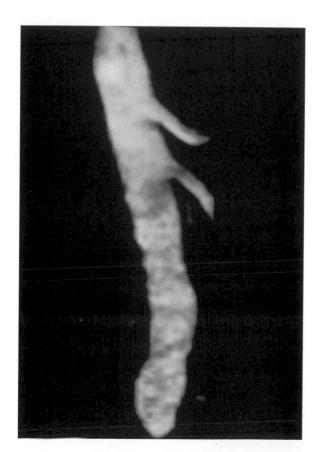

FIGURE 19-9   Inferior mesenteric artery occlusion. Dynamic, contrast-enhanced breath-hold 3D TOF MRA of the abdominal aorta demonstrating origins of celiac and superior mesenteric arteries.

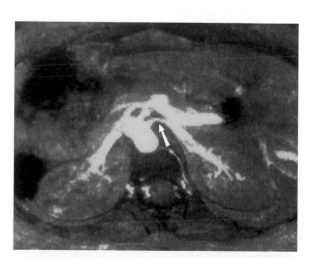

FIGURE 19-11   Renal artery stenosis. Individual partition of 3D TOF MRA of renal arteries demonstrates a smooth, focal, proximal left stenosis *(arrow)*.

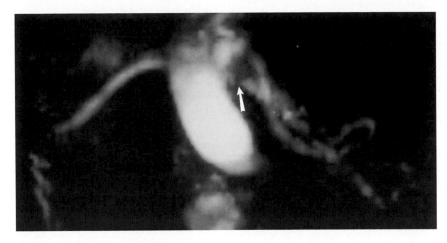

FIGURE 19-12   Renal artery stenosis. Contrast-enhanced breath-hold 3D TOF MRA of renal arteries demonstrates severe, focal, proximal stenosis *(arrow)* of one of the left renal arteries.

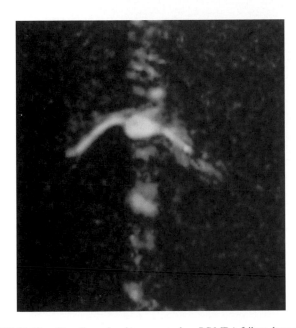

FIGURE 19-13   Two-dimensional transverse plane PC MRA fails to demonstrate distal renal branches. Note significant motion artifact on this non–breath-hold study.

ing. Non–breath-hold gadolinium-enhanced 3D TOF MRA reported sensitivity and specificity of 85% and 93% for significant proximal renal artery stenoses.[56]

PC MRA (Figure 19-13) potentially has the ability to quantitate flow within the renal arteries, providing a noninvasive measure of hemodynamic significance of stenoses. Cine MR phase (or velocity) mapping was used to measure blood flow throughout the aorta in 31 healthy human subjects.[4] Antegrade renal flow averaged 1037 ml/min, with retrograde diastolic flow measured at 54 ml/min. These measurements were indirect, based on differences in aortic flow above and below the renal arteries. Evaluation of the renal artery flow directly or determining peak velocity within the arteries is a much more difficult task. The latter can be addressed to a certain degree by using ECG triggering, although this does not guarantee that data acquisition can be coordinated with peak flow downstream at the level of the renal arteries. Movement of the renal arteries with diaphragmatic excursion may adversely affect such measurements.

One potential solution is to acquire data during a breath-hold, using a segmented κ-space technique. Conventional ECG-triggered velocity mapping has been compared with ECG-gated breath-hold segmented κ-space velocity mapping (Figure 19-14) for measurement of renal artery flow.[68] The breath-hold technique reduces vessel blurring and pulsatility artifacts. With this technique, in normal subjects the maximum renal artery velocity measured 230 ± 50 mm/sec, and the average left renal artery flow was 645 ± 80 ml/min. It remains to be seen how reliable this technique will be in patients with diseased vessels.

Abdominal Veins

The inferior vena cava and portal veins are large-caliber vessels, amenable to a variety of MR techniques, including SE, 2D cine gradient-echo, 2D cine PC, 2D or 3D TOF, and PC MRA. The combination of SE and cine gradient-echo techniques is highly accurate in establishing the diagnosis of inferior vena cava or portal vein thrombosis.[40,43,65] Thrombus appears as a filling defect that does not move during the course of the cine examination. Chronic thrombus appears dark on T1- and T2-weighted images. It is difficult to distinguish bland thrombus from tumor invasion unless a mass is seen within the liver or adjacent nonvascular structure (Figure 19-15).

Two-dimensional cine PC imaging has an added advantage in studying the portal system because of its ability to establish flow patency and flow direction and to calculate flow velocity, which is especially important in the study of patients with portal hypertension.

Breath-hold PC MRA of the portal system (Figure 19-16) is typically encoded for velocity in the superior-inferior or right-to-left planes with a VENC of 30 cm/sec.[2] MR measurements closely match Doppler ultrasound results with regard to patency and direction of flow.

ECG-triggered 2D cine PC with velocity encoding in three orthogonal directions also correlates well with Doppler ultrasound, angiography, and surgical findings.[6] MRA can detect varices in patients with portal venous hypertension (Figure 19-17). Dynamic contrast-

ging only on alternate acquisitions, one can subtract background tissue. The clinical utility of the sequence has not been proved.

Three-dimensional TOF, tilted optimized nonsaturating excitation (TONE) 3D TOF, and selective inversion recovery–rapid gradient echo (SIR-RAGE) 3D TOF MRA have been compared in one study.[5] For detection of stenosis, sensitivity and specificity were 94% and 94% for SIR-RAGE, 76% and 100% for TONE, and 73% and 100% for conventional 3D TOF MRA. For greater than 50% stenoses, sensitivity and specificity were 46% and 95% for SIR-RAGE, 23% and 90% for TONE, and 54% and 95% for conventional 3D TOF MRA. SIR-RAGE depicted greater lengths of the renal artery (34.8 ± 19.6 mm) than did TONE (21.8 ± 18.4 mm) or conventional 3D TOF (17.3 ± 15.4 mm).

Breath-hold 2D FLASH has been compared with non–breath-hold 3D TONE and 3D fast imaging with steady precession (FISP).[17] Forty-six patients were studied and had corresponding angiograms. Of the 92 vessels studied, there were 6 severe stenoses, 1 occlusion, 12 mild stenoses, and 73 normal arteries. Sensitivity and specificity for stenoses of greater than 60% were 100% and 89% for 3D TONE, 86% and 84% for 3D FISP, and 100% and 84% for 2D FLASH.

Breath-hold gadolinium-enhanced dynamic 3D TOF MRA (Figure 19-12) has been advocated for evaluation of the abdominal aorta and its branch vessels.[58] With gadolinium, 71% more renal and accessory renal arteries are visible, as compared with unenhanced breath-hold imag-

enhanced breath-hold 2D turboFLASH has also been successful in imaging the portal system.[61]

Burhart and Johnson[7] compared four 2D PC techniques (cine 2D PC with respiratory compensation, 2D cine PC without respiratory compensation, 2D PC with two signals acquired, and 2D PC with eight signals acquired) as they relate to image quality, vessel conspicuity, and SNR. The cine sequences produced 16 images (16 phases of the same slice), and the noncine studies produced one image. The 2D cine PC respiratory-compensated sequence produced the best image quality, vessel conspicuity, and SNR.

These studies and others have demonstrated the ability of MRA to evaluate the portal system. Considering the limitations of ultrasound and the dangers of angiography, MRA should be used more in the evaluation of patients with portal hypertension.

Pulmonary Arteries

Evaluation of the pulmonary arterial tree is difficult for any imaging modality, especially MRI. In addition to the problems of cardiac and respiratory motion and severe magnetic suspectibility artifacts, the oblique orientation of the pulmonary vessels, the different flow rates between the central and peripheral vessels, and the different flow directions make it difficult to study the vessels with either TOF or PC MRA techniques.

Although the central pulmonary vasculature can be visualized with SE cine or basic MRA techniques (Figure 19-18), for MRI to have a role in the workup of patients with pulmonary embolism, it must be able to reliably visualize the peripheral pulmonary vasculature. To this end, a multitude of MRA techniques have been used in studying the pulmonary arteries (Figure 19-19).[19,27,28,31,76] Most clinical work has

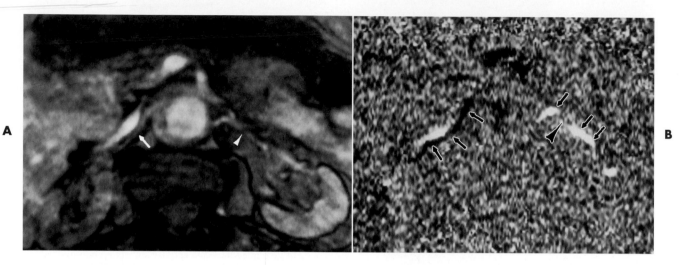

FIGURE 19-14   Velocity maps of the renal arteries. **A,** Magnitude image 2D breath hold demonstrates aneurysmal dilatation of the aorta with concentric mural thrombosis at the level of the renal artery. Right renal artery *(arrow)* is narrow but appears patent. Left renal artery is also diffusely narrowed, with suggestion of a proximal stenosis *(arrowhead)*. **B,** Velocity map demonstrates patent right renal artery (black signal indicating left-to-right flow *[arrows]*), flow in left renal artery (white signal indicating right-to-left flow *[arrows]*), and proximal stenosis *(arrowhead)*.

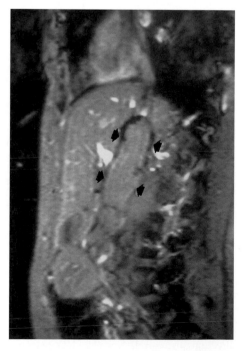

FIGURE 19-15   Renal cell carcinoma. Sagittal 2D cine MRI through the inferior vena cava (outlined by arrows) demonstrates invasion by tumor.

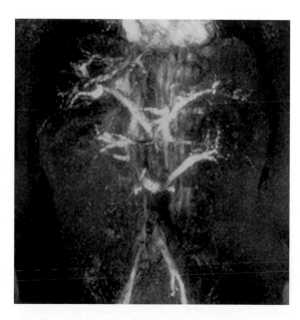

FIGURE 19-16   Normal veins on 2D breath-hold PC MRA, which demonstrates patency of splenic, portal, hepatic, and renal veins.

been done with 2D and 3D TOF techniques. Detection of pulmonary emboli by MRA yields sensitivities in the 85% to 90% range with modest (62%) specificity.[21,42] Initial results of MRA have been disappointing because of respiratory motion artifacts and poor embolus-blood contrast differences. The former problem can be overcome to a large degree by acquiring data in a simple breath-hold.[19] The latter problem is due to the inherent nature of TOF imaging and the peculiar aspects of the pulmonary vasculature, outlined earlier. With breath-hold techniques, phased-array coils have improved spatial resolution[19,27,28] but have not significantly solved the problem of CNR.

Despite its better spatial resolution, CT angiography (CTA) suffers from similar problems of respiratory motion and poor embolus-blood contrast. Review of the limited CTA and MRA data would suggest that CTA better identifies segmental pulmonary emboli than standard MRA techniques.[30,59,69,77] However, Meany et al[46] recently reported greater sensitivities and specificities (up to 100% and 95%, respectively) for detection of subsegmental pulmonary emboli using a gadolinium-enhanced 3D TOF MRA technique than has been previously reported with either MRI or CT. Although there is still debate over whether subsegmental pulmonary emboli are clinically significant and therefore whether they need to be treated, it would appear at this time that contrast-enhanced MRA has an edge on CTA as the technique of choice for non-invasive evaluation of patients for pulmonary emboli (Figure 19-19).

Mediastinal Veins

MRA has a definite role in the evaluation of the superior vena cava and its tributaries, for example, in the superior vena cava syndrome. In addition to demonstrating the site of obstruction and collateral vessels, MRI can help determine the origin, which in the majority of cases is a malignant process. Most MRA has been done with 2D breath-hold TOF (Figure 19-20) techniques.[18] We have found cine-PC studies to be just

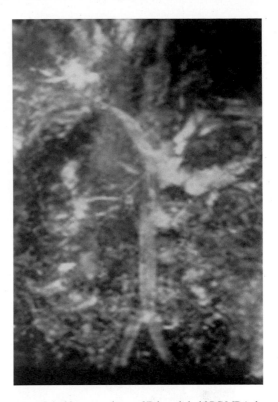

FIGURE 19-17   Portal hypertension on 2D breath-hold PC MRA demonstrates dilated splenic vein and collateral vessels consistent with hepatofugal flow.

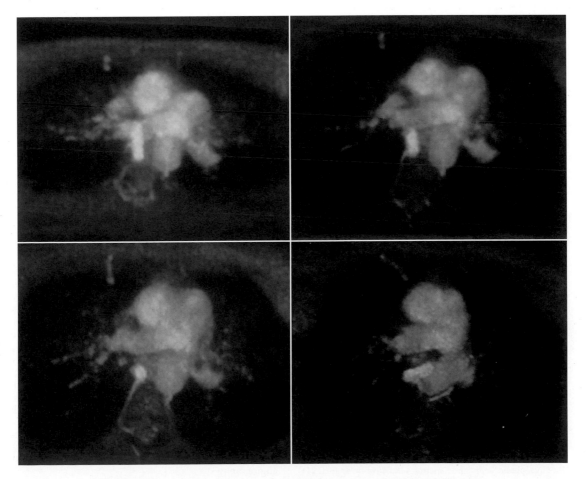

FIGURE 19-18   Central pulmonary arteries. Multiple rotations of a 3D TOF MRA MIP.

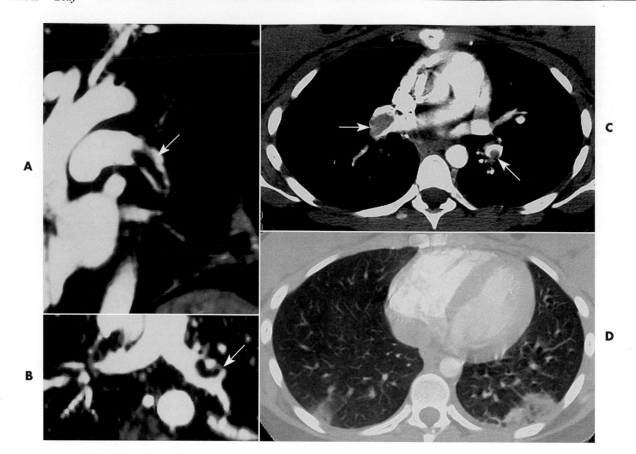

FIGURE 19-19   Pulmonary embolism. **A,** Coronal gadolinium-enhanced MRA shows filling defect *(arrow)* in descending left pulmonary artery. **B,** Transverse MRA (maximum-intensity projection) in the same patient as **A** also shows the left-sided pulmonary embolism *(arrow).* **C,** Transverse iodine-enhanced x-ray CTA (different patient than **A** and **B**) shows pulmonary emboli *(arrows)* in both left and right descending pulmonary arteries. **D,** CTA examination (photographed at lung windows) also shows bilateral peripheral posterior lung infarcts. (**B** Courtesy M. Prince, Ann Arbor, Michigan; **D** Courtesy D. Stark, Omaha, Nebraska.)

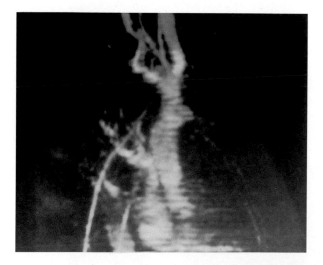

FIGURE 19-20   Brachycephalic veins and superior vena cava on sagittal 2D breath-hold TOF MRA.

as useful in determining the site of occlusion, invasion of the lumen, and the presence of collateral flow (Figure 19-21).

SUMMARY

The vasculature of the chest and abdomen presents unique obstacles to routine clinical application of MRA. Cardiac, respiratory, and abdominal motion, coupled with large vascular territories, complex vascular anatomy, and diverse flow patterns, challenges investigators and clinicians. Improved gradients and dedicated coils are having a major impact in improving SNR and spatial resolution and reducing scan times. At present, it would appear that the gadolinium-enhanced breath-hold techniques will be the cornerstone for studying the thoracic and abdominal vasculature. Breath-holding is a simple, reliable tool that can be applied to the wide variety of imaging circumstances. Its use directly follows the routine use of breath-holding in CT scanning.

In the future, we believe that velocity mapping techniques will assume a greater role. Such measurements would represent a fundamental and clinically important advance over traditional catheter angiography.

FIGURE 19-21   Velocity maps. Anterior **(A)** and posterior **(B)** coronal velocity maps of 2D PC MRA of the thoracic vasculature demonstrate occlusion of the distal superior vena cava *(arrow)* and reversal of flow in the azygous vein *(arrowhead)*, which serves as the major collateral vessel. Inferior flow is represented by bright signal, and superior flow is represented by dark signal. Stationary tissue is isointense.

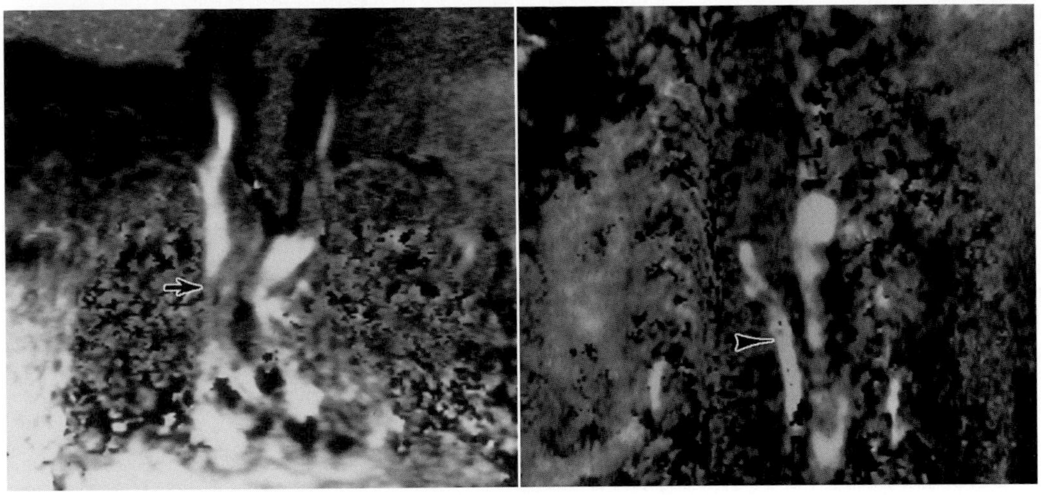

REFERENCES

1. Anderson CM, Saloner D, Tsuruda JS, et al: Artifacts in maximum-intensity-projection display of MR angiograms, Am J Roentgenol 154:623, 1990.
2. Applegate GR, Thaete Fl, Meyers SP, et al: Blood flow in the portal vein: velocity quantification with phase contrast MR angiography, Radiology 187:253, 1993.
3. Atkinson DJ, and Edelman RR: Cine-angiography of the heart in a single breath-hold with a segmented turboFLASH sequence, Radiology 178:357, 1991.
4. Bogren H, and Buonocore M: Blood flow measurements in the aorta and major arteries with MR velocity mapping, J Magn Reson Imaging 4:119, 1994.
5. Borrello JA, Li D, Vesely TM, et al: Renal arteries: clinical comparison of three-dimensional time-of-flight MR angiographic sequences and radiographic angiography, Radiology 197:793, 1995.
6. Burhart DJ, Johnson CD, Morton MJ, et al: Phase-contrast cine MR angiography in chronic liver disease, Radiology 187:407, 1993.
7. Burkart DJ, and Johnson CD: Upper abdominal phase-contrast MR angiography: comparison of cine and non-cine techniques, Radiology 195:101, 1995.
8. Caro CG, Pedley JG, Schroter RC, et al: The mechanics of circulation, Oxford, 1978, Oxford University Press.
9. Chien D, and Edelman RR: Ultra-fast imaging using gradient echoes, Magn Reson Q 7:31, 1991.
10. Debatin JF, Spritzer CE, Grist TM, et al: Imaging of the renal arteries: value of MR angiography, Am J Roentgenol 157:981, 1991.
11. Dumoulin CL, Cline HE, Souza SP, et al: Three dimensional time-of-flight magnetic resonance angiography using spin saturation, Magn Reson Med 11:35, 1989.
12. Durham JD, Hackworth CA, Tober JC, et al: Magnetic resonance angiography in the preoperative evaluation of abdominal aortic aneurysms, Am J Surg 166:173, 1993.
13. Ecklund K, Hartnell GG, Hughes LA, et al: MR angiography as the sole method in evaluating abdominal aortic aneurysms: correlation with conventional techniques and surgery, Radiology 192:345, 1994.
14. Edelman RR, Siewert B, Adamis M, et al: Signal targeting with alternating radio frequency (STAR) sequences: application to MR angiography, Magn Reson Med 31:233, 1994.
15. Edelman RR, Mattle HP, Kleefield J, et al: Quantification of blood flow with dynamic MR imaging and presaturation bolus tracking, Radiology 171:551, 1989.
16. Feinberg DA, Crooks LE, Sheldon P, et al: Magnetic resonance imaging of the velocity vector components of fluid flow, Magn Reson Med 2:555, 1985.
17. Fellner C, Strotzer M, Geissler A, et al: Renal arteries: evaluation with optimized 2D and 3D time-of-flight MR angiography, Radiology 196:681, 1995.
18. Finn JP, Zisk JH, Edelman RR, et al: Central venous occlusion: MR angiography, Radiology 187:245, 1993.
19. Foo TK, MacFall JR, Haues CE, et al: Pulmonary vasculature: single breath-hold MR imaging with phased-array coils, Radiology 183:473, 1992.
20. Glover GH, and Pelc NJ: A rapid-gated cine MR technique, Magn Reson Annu 299, 1988.
21. Grist TM, Sostman HD, MacFall JR, et al: Pulmonary angiography with MR imaging: preliminary clinical experience, Radiology 189:523, 1993.
22. Grover T, and Singer JR: NMR spin-echo flow measurements, J Appl Phys 42:938, 1971.
23. Gullberg GT, Wherli FW, Shimakawa A, et al: MR vascular imaging with a fast gradient refocusing pulse sequence and reformatted images from transaxial sections, Radiology 165:241, 1987.
24. Haacke EM, Masaryk TJ, Wielopolski PA, et al: Optimizing blood vessel contrast in fast three-dimensional MRI, Magn Reson Med 14:202, 1990.
25. Hahn EL: Detection of sea-water motion by nuclear precession, J Geophys Res 65:776, 1960.
26. Hartnell GG, Finn JP, Zenni M, et al: MR imaging of the thoracic aorta: comparison of spin-echo, angiographic and breath-hold techniques, Radiology 191:697, 1994.
27. Hatabu H, Gefter WB, Listerud J, et al: Pulmonary MR angiography utilizing phased-array surface coils: technique optimization and application, J Comput Assist Tomogr 16:410, 1992.
28. Hayes CE, and Roemer PB: Volume imaging with MR phased arrays, Magn Reson Med 16:181, 1990.
29. Hentz SM, Holland GA, Baum RA, et al: Evaluation of renal artery stenosis by magnetic resonance angiography, Am J Surg 168:140, 1994.
30. Holland GA, Gefter WB, Baum RA, et al: Prospective comparison of pulmonary MR angiography and ultrafast CT for diagnosis of pulmonary thromboembolic disease, Radiology 189(P):234, 1993 (abstract).
31. Isoda H, Masui T, Hasegawa S, et al: Pulmonary MR angiography: a comparison of 2D and 3D time-of-flight, J Comput Assist Tomogr 18:402, 1994.
32. Kandarpa K, Piwnica-Worums D, Chopra PS, et al: Prospective double-blinded comparison of MR imaging and aortography in the preoperative evaluation of abdominal aortic aneurysms, J Vasc Interv Radiol 3:83, 1992.
33. Kaufman JA, Geller SC, Peterson MJ, et al: MR imaging (including MR angiography) of abdominal aortic aneurysms: comparison with conventional angiography, Am J Roentgenol 163:203, 1994.
34. Kaufman JA, Yucel EK, Waltman AC, et al: Magnetic resonance angiography in the preoperative evaluation of abdominal aortic aneurysms: a preliminary study, J Vasc Interv Radiol 5:489, 1994.
35. Keller PJ, Drayer BP, Fram EK, et al: MR angiography with two-dimensional acquisition and three-dimensional display: work in progress, Radiology 173:527, 1989.
36. Keller PJ, and Wehrli FW: Gradient moment nulling through the Nth moment: application of binomial expansion coefficients to gradient amplitudes, J Magn Reson 78:145, 1988.
37. Kent KC, Edelman RR, Kim D, et al: Magnetic resonance imaging: a reliable test for the evaluation of proximal atherosclerotic renal arterial stenosis, J Vasc Surg 13:311, 1991.
38. Kim D, Edelman RR, Kent KC, et al: Abdominal aorta and renal artery stenosis: evaluation with MR angiography, Radiology 174:727, 1990.
39. Laub GA, and Kaiser WA: MR angiography with gradient motion refocusing, J Comput Assist Tomogr 12:377, 1988.
40. Levy HM, and Newhouse JH: MR imaging of portal vein thrombosis, Am J Roentgenol 151:283, 1988.
41. Loubeyre P, Revel D, Garcia P, et al: Screening patients for renal artery stenosis: value of three-dimensional time-of-flight MR angiography, Am J Roentgenol 162:847, 1994.

42. Loubeyre P, Revel D, Doek P, et al: Dynamic contrast-enhanced MR angiography of pulmonary embolism: comparison with pulmonary angiography, Am J Roentgenol 162:1035, 1994.
43. Martinoli C, Cittadini G, Pastrotino C, et al: Gradient echo MRI of portal vein thrombosis, J Comput Assist Tomogr 16:226, 1992.
44. Masaryk TJ, Modic MT, Ross JS, et al: Intracranial circulation: preliminary clinical results with three-dimensional (volume) MR angiography, Radiology 171:793, 1989.
45. Masaryk TJ, Modic MT, Ruggieri PM, et al: Three-dimensional (volume) gradient-echo imaging of the carotid bifurcation: preliminary clinical experience, Radiology 171:801, 1989.
46. Meaney JF, Weg JG, Chenevert TL, et al: Diagnosis of pulmonary embolism with magnetic resonance angiography, N Engl J Med 336:1422, 1997.
47. Moran PR: A flow velocity zeumatographic interlace for NMR imaging in humans, Magn Reson Imaging 1:197, 1982.
48. Morse O, and Singer JR: Blood velocity measurements in intact subjects, Science 170:440, 1970.
49. Nienaber CA, von Kokolitsch Y, Nicolas V, et al: The diagnosis of thoracic aortic dissection by noninvasive imaging procedures, N Engl J Med 328:1, 1993.
50. O'Donnell M: NMR blood flow imaging using multiecho, phase contrast sequences, Med Phys 12:59, 1985.
51. Parker DL, Yuan C, and Blatter DD: MR angiography by multiple thin slab 3D acquisition, Magn Reson Med 17:434, 1991.
52. Pattany M, Phillips J, Chiu L, et al: Motion artifact suppression technique (MAST) for MR imaging, J Comput Assist Tomogr 11:369, 1987.
53. Pelc NJ, Bernstein MA, Shimakawa A, et al: Encoding strategies for three-direction phase-contrast MR imaging of flow, J Magn Reson Imaging 1:405, 1991.
54. Pernicone JR, Siebert JE, Potchen EJ, et al: Three dimensional phase contrast MR angiography in the head and neck: preliminary report, Am J Radiol 155:167, 1990.
55. Prince MR: Contrast-enhanced MR angiography: theory and optimization, Magn Reson Imag 6(2):657, 1998.
56. Prince MR: Gadolinium-enhanced MR aortography, Radiology 191:155, 1994.
57. Prince MR, Yucel EK, Kaufman JA, et al: Dynamic Gd-DTPA enhanced 3D FT abdominal MR angiography, J Magn Reson Imaging 3:877, 1993.
58. Prince MR, Narasimham DL, Stanley JC, et al: Breath-hold gadolinium-enhanced MR angiography of the abdominal aorta and its major branches, Radiology 197:785, 1995.
59. Remy-Jardin M, Remy J, Wattinne L, et al: Central pulmonary thromboembolism: diagnosis with spiral volumetric CT with the single-breath-hold technique—comparison with pulmonary angiography, Radiology 185:381, 1992.
60. Rimmer JM, and Gennari FJ: Atherosclerotic renovascular disease and progressive renal failure, Ann Intern Med 118:712, 1993.
61. Rodgers DM, Ward J, Baudouin CJ, et al: Dynamic contrast-enhanced MR imaging of the portal venous system: comparison with x-ray angiography, Radiology 191:741, 1994.
62. Ruggiere PM, Laub GA, Masaryk TJ, et al: Intracranial circulation: pulse sequence considerations in three-dimensional (volume) MR angiography, Radiology 171:785, 1989.
63. Schiebler ML, Holland GA, Hatagu H, et al: Suspected pulmonary embolism: prospective evaluation with pulmonary MR angiography, Radiology 189:125, 1993.
64. Schmalbrock P, Yuan C, Chakeres DW, et al: Volume MR angiography: methods to achieve very short echo times, Radiology 175:861, 1990.
65. Silverman PM, Patt RH, Garra BS, et al: MR imaging of the portal venous system: value of gradient-echo imaging as an adjunct to spin-echo imaging, Am J Roentgenol 157:297, 1991.
66. Singer JR: Blood flow rates by nuclear magnetic resonance, Science 130:1652, 1959.
67. Smith HJ, and Bokke SJ: MR angiography of in situ and transplanted renal arteries: early experience using a three-dimensional time-of-flight technique. Acta Radiol 34:150, 1993.
68. Thomsen C, Cortsen M, Sondergaard L, et al: A segmented K-space velocity mapping protocol for quantification of renal artery blood flow during breath-holding, J Magn Reson Imaging 5:393, 1995.
69. Tiegen CL, Maus TP, Sheedy PF II, et al: Pulmonary embolism: diagnosis with electron-beam CT, Radiology 188:839, 1993.
70. Underwood SR: Cine magnetic resonance imaging and flow measurements in the cardiovascular system, Br Med Bull 45:948, 1989.
71. Vock P, Terrier F, Wegmuller H, et al: Magnetic resonance angiography of abdominal vessels: early experience using the three dimensional phase contrast technique, Br J Radiol 64:10, 1991.
72. von Schulthess G, and Higgins C: Blood flow imaging with MR: spin-phase phenomena, Radiology 157:687, 1985.
73. Wagle WA, Dumoulin CL, Souza SP, et al: 3D FT magnetic resonance angiography of carotid and basilar arteries, Am J Neuroradiol 10:911, 1989.
74. Wedeen V, Rosen B, Chesler D, et al: MR velocity imaging by phase display, J Comput Assist Tomogr 9:530, 1985.
75. Wehrli FW, Shimakawa A, MacFall JR, et al: MR imaging of venous and arterial flow by a selective saturation-recovery spin echo (SSRSE) method, J Comput Assist Tomogr 9:537, 1985.
76. Wielopolski PA, Haacke EM, and Adler LP: Three-dimensional MR imaging of the pulmonary vasculature: preliminary experience, Radiology 183:465, 1992.
77. Woodard PK, Sostman HD, MacFall JR, et al: Detection of pulmonary embolism: comparison of contrast-enhanced spiral CT and time-of-flight MR techniques, J Thorac Imaging 10:59, 1995.
78. Yucel EK, Kaufman JA, Prince MR, et al: Time of flight renal MR angiography in patients with renal insufficiency, Magn Reson Imaging 11:925, 1993.

20 Congenital Heart Disease

Daniel M. Chernoff and Charles B. Higgins

 KEY POINTS

- ECG is the procedure of choice for delineation of anatomy, but MRI can help visualize supracardiac and posterior mediastinal structures.
- Cardiac-gated spin-echo MRI effectively demonstrates preoperative and postoperative anatomy in the growing child or adult.
- Cine MRI offers functional information that lessens the need for repeated angiography.

This chapter describes a segmental anatomical approach to the diagnosis of congenital heart disease (CHD) using magnetic resonance imaging (MRI). This approach is effective for analyzing CHD and is particularly useful in complex cardiovascular malformations.[92] The description of the various congenital cardiovascular lesions is organized according to three segmental levels (atria, ventricles, and great arteries), their connections (atrioventricular and ventriculoarterial), and the visceroatrial situs. In addition to the anatomical depiction of CHD, MRI is capable of functional imaging, including measurement of intracardiac shunts,[15] differential pulmonary blood flow,[17] pressure gradients across valvular[32,53] and vascular[53] stenoses, and valvular regurgitant fraction.[18] These functional tools are useful in selected cases.

CURRENT CLINICAL ROLE

The effectiveness of MRI in the diagnosis of CHD is widely recognized,[24,36,42] but its appropriate role in an imaging armamentarium that includes echocardiography (ECHO) and angiocardiography is still evolving.

ECHO is currently used as the initial noninvasive imaging study for almost all patients with known or suspected CHD. MRI is unlikely to supplant ECHO as the first diagnostic procedure because of the portability, universal availability, and low cost of ECHO. ECHO is superior to MRI in depicting cardiac valves, real-time cardiac motion, and smaller intracardiac shunts. Conversely, MRI can demonstrate cardiovascular anatomy without the limitation of acoustic windows or ultrasound penetration of the body. Therefore the morphology of some regions, such as the supracardiac region and the posterior aspect of the heart, can be more clearly shown with MRI than with ECHO.[11,16,48] Furthermore, MRI can provide tomographic images in any imaging plane and with a wide field of view.[27] Clearly, in many cases the diagnostic capabilities of MRI and ECHO are complementary rather than competitive,[43,85] and patients may benefit from having both studies.

As surgical procedures and medical management of CHD improve, more patients are surviving into adulthood. These adult CHD patients may suffer from reduced cardiac function or complications related to their surgical procedure. MRI is particularly well suited to evaluation of adult CHD.[98] Sedation generally is not required, and the slower heart rates of adults compared with those of children allow more images to be obtained per cardiac cycle. Also, transthoracic ECHO in adult CHD patients often suffers from poor acoustic penetration through the thoracic cage and mediastinal scar tissue.

The capability of MRI in evaluating CHD includes both anatomical depiction and functional assessment. Cine MRI attains a temporal resolution almost equal to cine angiography, which is sufficient to calculate stroke volume, ejection fraction, regional ventricular wall motion, and wall-thickening dynamics.[66,82,83,90] Furthermore, MRI flow techniques (velocity-encoded cine MRI) can produce functional images depicting a map of blood velocity within the multiple cine MR images acquired throughout a cardiac cycle.[33,59,60,62,91] Cine MRI and velocity-encoded cine MRI can be used to assess cardiac chamber dimensions and function, as well as blood flow in the central circulation.

IMAGING TECHNIQUES

Electrocardiography (ECG)-gated, multislice, spin-echo sequences are used to evaluate the anatomy of CHD. Cine MRI (conventional or velocity encoded) is employed when functional information is required. Diagnostic image quality is obtained in more than 90% of appropriately selected patients.[49] Reduced image quality usually is due to patient motion; consequently, MRI is not effective in imaging uncooperative children.

Children older than 6 or 7 years usually can be studied without sedation if care is taken to explain the procedure in detail to the child and parent(s). For younger children, sedation is required. Effective sedation can be obtained with chloral hydrate (75 to 100 mg/kg body weight) administered orally approximately 45 min before the patient enters the magnet or pentobarbital (5 to 7 mg/kg) administered parenterally. The ECG signal is monitored and respiration is observed throughout the imaging procedure using an MR-compatible pulse oximeter to monitor oxygen saturation. In our experience the most effective and safest approach has been to have an anesthesiologist manage deep sedation and physiological monitoring during the MR study. In this setting an infusion of a short-acting drug, propofol, has been used.

Respiratory artifacts can be reduced by use of a prospective imaging algorithm called *respiratory-ordered phase encoding* (ROPE).[4] Phase-encoding steps are ordered in such a way as to reduce respiration-related motion artifacts by selecting a phase angle proportional to the current phase of the respiratory cycle. Although this method requires monitoring of respiration throughout the entire respiratory cycle, imaging time is not prolonged and image quality is greatly improved.

High-field strength (1.5-T) systems have some clear advantages over lower-strength systems, especially for the study of infants. The signal-to-noise ratio (SNR) from the high-field system is greater than that from lower-field systems, resulting in improved spatial resolution and shorter imaging times.[86] Importantly, a high-field system also provides an adequate SNR for the thin (3-mm) sections required to evaluate infants and small children effectively. Techniques for optimum placement of the ECG leads have been described for use with high-field systems.[26]

A standard transmit-and-receive head coil instead of a body coil is used for imaging infants with CHD, since it improves SNR, which in turn may be traded off for increased spatial resolution. Because the internal diameter of the head coil is relatively small (32 cm), older children are examined with the standard body coil or with a flexible surface coil wrapped around the torso.

Coronal images are first obtained to determine the location of subsequent transverse tomograms. Multislice transverse images are acquired from the top of the aorta to the diaphragm using spin-echo sequences. Echo time (TE) is set at 20 ms to reduce signal from slow-moving blood. Children are usually studied with contiguous 5-mm slices with two excitations. However, 5-mm slices are not always sufficient to depict small structures, such as diminutive pulmonary arteries in patients with pulmonary atresia. When anatomical details are required in a limited region, additional imaging with 3-mm slices and two to four excitations is performed. A field of view of 20 to 24 cm is used for infants; for older children the field of view is usually 32 cm. The typical scan time required for 7 to 12 transverse images is about 6 to 8 min. The transverse images are supplemented by sagittal, coronal, or oblique images, depending on the anatomy to be evaluated.

In general, anatomical structures oriented along a slice-select direction (e.g., right ventricular outflow tract on sagittal planes) are difficult to appreciate clearly because of partial volume averaging. In such a case imaging planes orthogonal to the axis of the anatomical structure (e.g., right ventricular outflow tract on transverse planes) may be preferable. Oblique imaging planes are accomplished by simultaneous application of two slice-select gradients. These oblique planes may help demonstrate anatomical structures with an oblique course through the body (e.g., the aortic arch and descending aorta).

For evaluation of ventricular function or blood flow in the central cardiovascular system, cine MRI or velocity-encoded cine MRI is performed.[1,5,62,81,84] These techniques may be used to evaluate the patency of systemic-pulmonary shunts and flow patterns associated with intracardiac shunts or valvular diseases. The slice thickness used for cine MRI is typically 5 to 10 mm.

SEGMENTAL ANATOMY

Multiple adjacent tomographic MR images provide three-dimensional evaluation of cardiovascular structures. A systematic approach to the identification of cardiac structures is required for comprehensive diagnosis of CHD. The efficacy of the segmental approach to analysis of the arrangement of cardiac structures in complex cardiovascular anomalies has been demonstrated and used in various diagnostic modalities.[79,93] The same approach can be applied to the diagnosis of CHD with MRI.

The human heart consists of three major cardiac segments (the atria, ventricles, and great arteries). CHD can be defined in terms of the abnormalities at each of the three segments or the connection between the segments (atrioventricular and ventriculoarterial connections). The first step of the segmental approach is to define the major cardiac segments.

Atria (Atrial Situs)

Identification of the atria is virtually determined by the connection to the inferior vena cava (IVC). In almost all cases the atrium to which the IVC is connected is the morphological right atrium (RA). On the other hand, the morphological left atrium (LA) is defined as not being connected to the IVC. The shape of the atrial appendage is also a specific indicator for differentiating the RA and LA. The right atrial appendage shows a triangular or bulbous shape with a wide connection to the atrial vestibule, whereas the left atrial appendage shows a finger-like shape with a *narrow* connection. These features can be identified on transverse or sagittal MR images (Figure 20-1).

The word *situs* (site) indicates the existing pattern of anatomical organization. Atrial site *solitus* indicates that the morphological RA is situated on the right side and the morphological LA is on the left side of the body. Atrial situs inversus indicates the opposite pattern of atrial location. Situs solitus of the abdominal or thoracic viscera indicates that the liver, IVC, and eparterial (on or over an artery) short main bronchus are right sided, whereas the hyparterial (below an artery) long main bronchus, the stomach, the spleen, and the abdominal aorta are left sided. In situs inversus of the abdominal or thoracic viscera, the locations of the viscera are the reverse of the situs solitus relationships.

The situs of abdominal or thoracic viscera is almost always concordant with the atrial situs (visceroatrial concordance). If the RA-IVC junction is observed on the right side of the spinal column, the visceroatrial situs is solitus; if on the left of the spinal column, the situs is inversus.

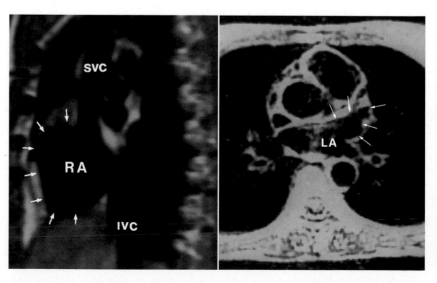

FIGURE 20-1   Identification of the right (**A**) and left (**B**) atria on MR images. The right atrium *(RA)* is identified by the continuation to the inferior vena cava *(IVC)*. The right atrial appendage (*arrows* in **A**) shows a bulbous shape with a wide connection to the atrial vestibule. The left atrial appendage (*arrows* in **B**) shows a fingerlike shape with a narrow connection. *SVC,* Superior vena cava; *LA,* left atrium.

A   B

In situs ambiguus, which is almost always associated with the asplenia or polysplenia syndromes, the situs of abdominal viscera is sometimes discordant with the atrial situs (visceroatrial discordance). Most patients with polysplenia syndrome show an interrupted IVC at the hepatic segment with continuation of venous connection to the superior vena cava (SVC) through the azygous or hemiazygous veins. In most patients with asplenia syndrome the IVC is located adjacent to the descending aorta on the same side of the spinal column (aortocaval juxtaposition). However, even in situs ambiguus, bronchial situs is almost always concordant with the atrial situs. Therefore bronchial morphology is helpful to estimate the atrial situs. The bronchial situs is best demonstrated on axial or coronal MR images. The morphological left bronchus is long and runs below the left pulmonary artery (hyparterial bronchus), whereas the morphological right bronchus is short and runs above the right pulmonary artery (eparterial bronchus). Asplenia syndrome is characterized by bilateral eparterial bronchi, bilateral anatomical RA (bilateral right-sidedness), and absence of the spleen. Polysplenia syndrome is characterized by bilateral hyparterial bronchi, bilateral anatomical LA (bilateral left-sidedness), and multiple spleens.

Transverse MR images of the upper abdomen may be used to identify the presence and morphology of the spleen. Distinguishing the posterior portion of one lobe of the liver from the spleen on a transverse image can occasionally be difficult. Both T1- and T2-weighted images can be useful for displaying the difference in signal intensity between the liver and spleen. The liver has higher signal intensity than the spleen on T1-weighted images, whereas the opposite relationship exists on T2-weighted images.

Ventricles (Ventricular Loop)

The next step in the segmental approach is to determine the ventricular loop, which indicates where the morphological right (RV) and left ventricles (LV) are located. The morphological RV and LV can be identified by structural features, which are usually well demonstrated on transverse MR images (Figure 20-2).

The major determining anatomical characteristic of the RV is the presence of an infundibulum, a myocardial tube separating the semilunar and the atrioventricular (AV) valves. The anatomical RV is also characterized by the presence of a tricuspid AV valve and a coarsely trabeculated septal and internal ventricular surface. Identification of the tricuspid valve is aided by identifying the attachment of its septal leaflet to the interventricular septum; this leaflet is positioned more closely to the apex than the septal leaflet of the mitral valve. The moderator band (anterior extension of the trabecula septomarginalis) is a prominent structure that passes from the interventricular septum to the anterior wall of the RV. The coarse trabeculation of the RV is most prominent at the septal surface near the apex.

The major determining anatomical characteristic of the LV is the absence of an infundibulum, one consequence of which is direct fibrous continuity between the semilunar and AV valves. The LV is also characterized by finer trabeculations than the RV, often most apparent at the apical septal surface, and the higher attachment of the AV valve. A moderator band is not present. Two large papillary muscles, representing attachments of the chordae tendineae of the mitral valve, are unique to the LV.

From these findings, each ventricle is defined as the morphological RV or LV. If the RV is situated to the right of the LV, the loop is defined as a D ventricular loop; if the RV is to the left, the loop is an L ventricular loop.

Great Arteries

The great arteries are identified by defining their branching or arch formation. The pulmonary artery is recognized on transverse images by its branching into right and left pulmonary arteries just above the base of the heart. The aorta is characterized by its continuation into the aortic arch. These findings can be recognized on adjacent multiple transverse MR images (Figure 20-3).

Transverse MR images of normally related great arteries show an anterior and leftward position of the pulmonary artery relative to the aorta at the base of the heart. In patients with discordant ventriculoarterial relationships (transposition), the aorta is usually located anterior to the pulmonary artery (Figure 20-4). Depending on whether the aortic valve is located to the right or left of the pulmonic valve, the transposition is designated as *D transposition* or *L transposition*, respectively.

Atrioventricular Connections

After the cardiac segments have been identified, the connections of these segments can be determined. Depending on the type of connections, they are divided into two major categories: concordant or discordant AV connections. When the anatomical RA connects to the anatomical RV and the LA connects to the LV, the AV connection is concordant. In contrast, a discordant AV connection implies an opposite pattern, characterized by the drainage of the RA to the LV and the LA to the RV. The AV connections are further subdivided into the following types:

1. *Usual alignment.* The interatrial septum and interventricular septum are aligned on almost the same plane. Consequently, each AV valve is appropriately located at the junction between each atrium and the ventricle.

2. *Crisscrossing.* Two AV routes rotate and cross each other in space. Each crossing route is usually difficult to demonstrate on the same imaging plane of MRI.[55,100] A series of adjacent images shows the crossing AV routes; the right-sided atrium connects to the left-sided ventricle, and vice versa.

3. *Overriding and straddling.* Overriding implies that the valve annulus overrides the interventricular septum. In this situation the interatrial septum and interventricular septum are extremely malaligned (Figure 20-5). Usually the AV valve belonging to the smaller ventricle overrides the interventricular septum, whereas the other AV valve is related entirely to the larger ventricle. With overriding the AV valve almost always straddles, which is defined as parts of the papillary muscle or tensor apparatus arising from both ventricles. If more than 1½ valves are committed to one of the ventricles, the connection is defined as double inlet.

4. *Double inlet.* Both AV valves insert into one large ventricle. The interatrial septum and interventricular septum are extremely malaligned. Depending on the structure of the predominant ventricle with a double inlet and the location of the other hypoplastic ventricle, a double-inlet RV or LV can be identified. This anomaly has

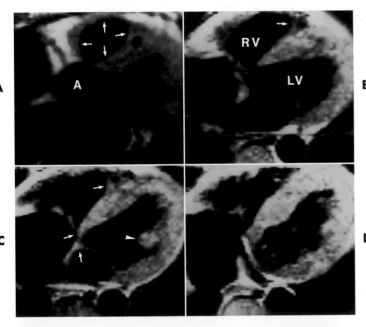

A   **B**   **C**   **D**

FIGURE 20-2   Identification of the right and left ventricles on MR images. Transverse images extend from cranial (**A**) to caudal (**D**). The right ventricle is characterized by the presence of an infundibulum (*arrows in* **A**), moderator band (*arrows in* **B** *and* **C**), and closer attachment of the atrioventricular valve to the apex (*arrows in* **C**). The left ventricle is characterized by the absence of infundibulum, the presence of papillary muscle (*arrowhead in* **C**), and higher attachment of the atrioventricular valve (*arrows in* **C**). (From Higgins CB, Hricak H, and Helms CA: Magnetic resonance imaging of the body, New York, 1992, Raven Press.)

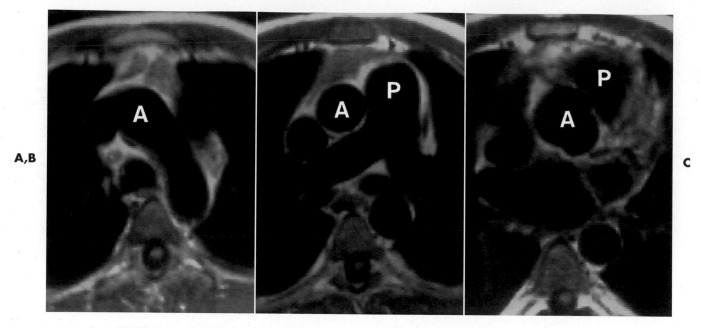

FIGURE 20-3   Identification of the normal great arteries on MR images. Transverse images extend from cranial **(A)** to caudal **(C)**. Two great arteries are recognized at the base of the heart **(A)**; one is located left anteriorly, the other right posteriorly. The left-sided, anterior artery branches first **(B)** and thus is identified as the pulmonary artery *(P)*. The right-sided, posterior artery continues to the arch at more cranial slices and is identified as the aorta *(A)*.

FIGURE 20-4   L transposition of great arteries. Transverse image **A** is cranial to image **B.** The right posteriorly located artery *(P)* branches first and therefore is the pulmonary artery. The other artery is located left and anterior to the pulmonary artery and is identified as the aorta *(A)* because it forms the arch (not shown). Note the presence of a subaortic infundibulum, which is a feature of transposition (*arrow* in **B**).

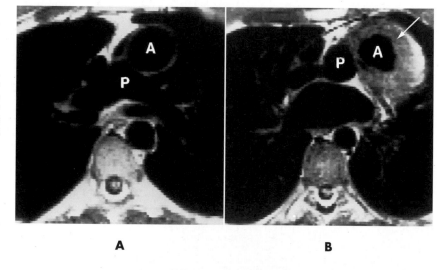

FIGURE 20-5   Overriding of the mitral valve. The interatrial septum and interventricular septum are malaligned. The left ventricle *(LV)* is hypoplastic. *RV,* Right ventricle; *LA,* left atrium; *RA,* right atrium.

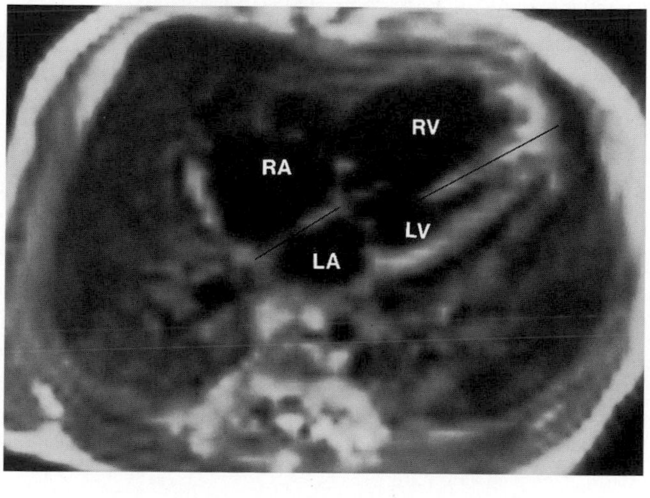

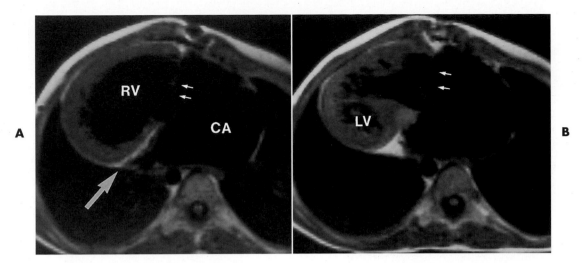

FIGURE 20-6   Absent unilateral atrioventricular connection. Image **A** is cranial to image **B**. Right AV connection is absent because of interposition of a muscular layer (*large arrow* in **A**). Rudimentary left ventricle *(LV)* is depicted at the right posterior aspect of the heart **(B)**. Therefore the absent right AV connection is considered to be mitral atresia. Note the delineation of the tricuspid valve *(small arrows)*. *RV,* Right ventricle; *CA,* common atrium. (From Higgins CB, Hricak H, and Helms CA: Magnetic resonance imaging of the body, New York, 1992, Raven Press.)

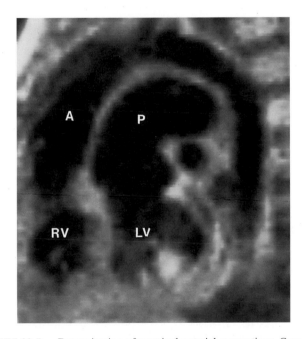

FIGURE 20-7   Determination of ventriculoarterial connections. Complete transposition is shown; the anteriorly located aorta *(A),* which is identified by the continuation to the aortic arch and branches to the head, is connected to the right ventricle *(RV).* The pulmonary artery *(P)* is located posteriorly and is connected to the left ventricle *(LV).* The coplanar relationship of the ascending aorta and main pulmonary artery is characteristic of complete transposition.

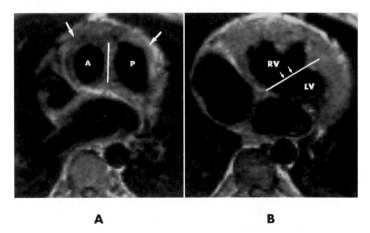

FIGURE 20-8   Double-outlet RV. Transverse images extend from cranial **(A)** to caudal **(B)**. More than 50% of the orifices of both the aorta *(A)* and the pulmonary artery *(P)* are committed to the right ventricle *(RV).* The plane of the infundibular interventricular septum is malaligned to the trabecular septum *(white lines* in **A** and **B**). Note the presence of bilateral infundibula *(arrows* in **A**) and subarterial, doubly committed ventricular septal defect *(arrows* in **B**). *LV,* Left ventricle; *RV,* right ventricle.

also been called *single ventricle* of the LV or RV types. When the predominant ventricle cannot be defined as the RV or LV, it may be defined as an indeterminate-type double-inlet ventricle.

5. *Absent unilateral AV connection.* This category includes two different types of AV atresia, depending on the nature of the atretic tissue. One type is *muscular atresia,* in which the interatrial septum and the interventricular septum are malaligned. The atrium is separated from the underlying ventricle by a layer of muscle and the AV sulcus (Figure 20-6). The other type is *membranous atresia,* in which the interatrial septum is correctly aligned to the interventricular septum. The tissue separating the atrium and ventricle is composed of the imperforate valve membrane.

Ventriculoarterial Connections

Concordant or discordant ventriculoarterial (VA) connections may exist. In *concordant* VA connections, the anatomical RV connects with the pulmonary artery and the anatomical LV with the aorta. In *discordant* VA connections, the RV connects with the aorta and the LV with the pulmonary artery. The term *transposition* implies these discordant VA relationships (Figure 20-7). If more than 1½ of the great arteries are committed to one of the ventricles, the connection is defined as a double-outlet VA connection (Figure 20-8). Double-outlet RV occurs more frequently than double-outlet LV, which is exceedingly rare.

The morphology of the infundibulum varies among the several forms of CHD. In normal hearts the infundibulum is present at the RV outflow. Although a general rule relating infundibular morphology and VA connections has been recognized, each VA anomaly has exceptions to the rule. The infundibulum can be divided into three parts: (1) the infundibular septum, which separates the two arterial valves; (2) the ventriculoinfundibular fold, which is a muscular bar separating the semilunar valves and AV valves; and (3) the parietal segment, which joins the infundibular septum and ventriculoinfundibular fold.

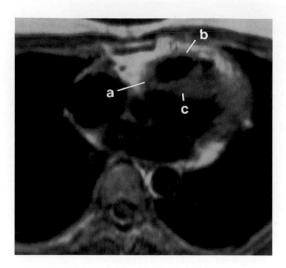

FIGURE 20-9   Infundibulum of the right ventricle. Three parts are recognized on transverse images: *a,* ventriculoinfundibular fold; *b,* parietal segment; and *c,* conus (or infundibular) septum.

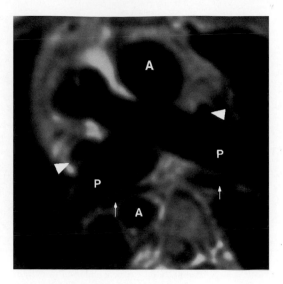

FIGURE 20-10   Right-sided isomerism. Transverse image shows a symmetrical ventral relationship of the right and left pulmonary arteries *(P)* to their respective bronchi *(arrows).* The main pulmonary artery is located to the right of the ascending aorta *(A).* Note the presence of bilateral superior venae cavae *(arrowheads).*

These three parts can be recognized on transverse or sagittal MR images (Figure 20-9).

ANOMALIES
Atria and Situs

This section describes abnormalities of atrial and abdominal visceral location, abnormal connections of the systemic or pulmonary veins to the atria, and atrial septal defects. Because MRI is not limited by the availability of acoustic windows or ultrasound penetration, venous structures behind the heart and their connections to the atria are more clearly demonstrated with MRI than with ECG.

Atrial isomerism is nearly always associated with complex CHD. Left-sided isomerism is usually associated with polysplenia and right-sided isomerism with asplenia. Isomerism is best demonstrated by symmetry of the bronchi and pulmonary arteries. This can be clearly shown by MRI on coronal sections as bilateral eparterial bronchi in right-sided isomerism (Figure 20-10) and bilateral hyparterial bronchi in left-sided isomerism. MRI is useful in demonstrating the complex congenital lesions associated with atrial isomerism[61,96] and has been shown to be equal to cardiac catheterization for this purpose.[39]

Persistent left superior vena cava (PLSVC) is recognized as a round structure with a flow void that is situated lateral to the main pulmonary artery on transverse images (Figure 20-11). PLSVC in most patients connects into an enlarged coronary sinus, which is shown on adjacent caudal slices. Rarely, drainage of the PLSVC connects directly to the roof of the left atrium (absence of the coronary sinus). This anomaly usually occurs in association with atrial septal defect and is known as *Raghib syndrome.*[68] PLSVC is easily diagnosed by MRI; a study of 34 patients with angiographically proven PLSVC showed that blinded MR interpretations correctly identified the PLSVC in every patient.[48]

Interruption of the IVC with azygous (or hemiazygous) continuation is recognized on transverse MRI as the absence of the hepatic portion of the IVC. This is associated with a greatly enlarged azygous or hemiazygous vein draining into the right or left SVC (Figure 20-12). These azygous or hemiazygous veins are located behind the diaphragm (retrocrural position) at the hepatic level. The enlarged azygous vein is seen in the thorax along the right anterior aspect of the spine, arching anteriorly to drain into the SVC. In hemiazygous continuation the dilated hemiazygous vein is recognized to the left of the spine and posterior to the aorta.[34,80] These anomalies are typically found in patients with polysplenia syndrome.

Total anomalous pulmonary venous connection is characterized by the following three major findings: (1) greatly enlarged RA and RV, (2) presence of an abnormal common pulmonary venous chamber (CPVC)

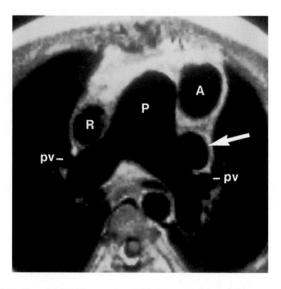

FIGURE 20-11   PLSVC in a patient with L transposition of the great arteries. PLSVC is recognized as a round structure *(arrow)* lateral to the main pulmonary artery *(P). A,* Aorta; *PV,* pulmonary vein; *R,* right SVC. (From Higgins CB, Hricak H, and Helms CA: Magnetic resonance imaging of the body, New York, 1992, Raven Press.)

behind the LA, and (3) continuation of the CPVC or pulmonary veins to the systemic vein or directly to the RA. This anomaly can be divided into supracardiac, cardiac, and infracardiac subtypes.[22]

Depending on the combination of drainage sites, the following can be recognized on transverse or coronal MR images: CPVC, dilated vertical or innominate vein, dilated coronary sinus, and the entry of the pulmonary veins into the abnormal sites (e.g., RA, SVC).[25,34]

Partial anomalous pulmonary venous connection occurs in almost all patients with sinus venosus defect. Possible sites for anomalous return of pulmonary vein(s) include the right SVC (Figure 20-13, *A*), RA (Figure 20-14), IVC, left innominate vein, and persistent left SVC. The normal (Figure 20-13, *B*) and abnormal connections of the pulmonary veins to the atrium can be depicted on transverse images.[25] The normal connection of the four pulmonary veins to the LA can be identified on transverse MR images in nearly all subjects. Occasionally on the transverse images the connection of the left upper vein

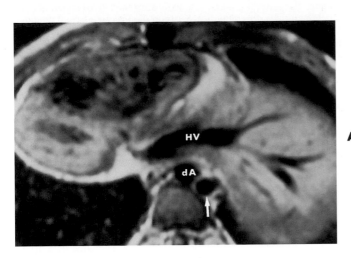

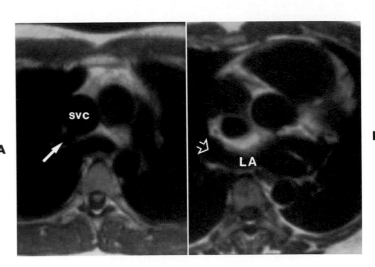

FIGURE 20-12 Interruption of the IVC with hemiazygous continuation in a patient with situs inversus totalis. Note the enlarged hemiazygous vein *(arrow)* to the left of the descending aorta *(dA)*, separate drainage of the hepatic veins *(HV)*, and inversion of the visceral and cardiac situs.

FIGURE 20-13 Partial anomalous pulmonary venous return. **A,** Right upper pulmonary vein *(arrow)* returns to the superior vena cava *(SVC)*. **B,** In normal subjects, return of the right upper pulmonary vein *(open arrow)* is identified at the most cephalic portion of the left atrium *(LA)*.

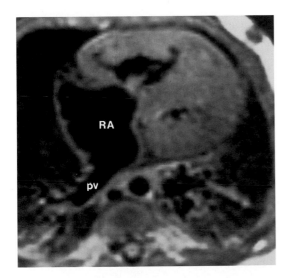

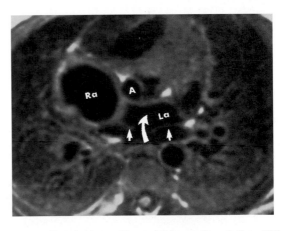

FIGURE 20-14 Partial anomalous pulmonary venous return. Drainage of the right inferior pulmonary vein *(pv)* into the right atrium *(RA)*. Note right ventricular hypertrophy (caused by right-to-right shunt) and left ventricular hypertrophy as a result of aortic arch hypoplasia (not shown).

FIGURE 20-15 Cor triatriatum. Transaxial image through the middle of the atrium shows pulmonary veins entering the posterior portion of the left atrial chamber. The posterior portion of the atrial chamber is separated from the anterior portion by a membrane *(arrows)*. There is a narrow ostium between the two portions of the atrium *(curved arrow)*. Note the increased signal of the lungs caused by pulmonary edema. *Ra,* Right atrium; *La,* left atrium; *A,* aortic valve.

cannot be distinguished from the LA appendage. In such a case coronal images are useful to define the entry of the upper vein. Because localization of anomalous pulmonary venous connection is sometimes difficult by ECG, MRI may be used as an alternative method of diagnosis.

Cor triatriatum is an anomaly in which one of the atrial chambers, usually the LA, is subdivided into two chambers. Basic anatomical features of cor triatriatum are as follows:

1. The LA is partitioned by an abnormal muscular shelf, which divides the pulmonary venous compartment (accessory chamber) from the true LA chamber, including the LA appendage and the AV vestibule.
2. Pulmonary venous blood returns normally to the accessory chamber, which usually drains to the true LA through a narrow ostium. Some pulmonary veins may separately return to the true LA chamber.

3. Patent foramen ovale or atrial septal defect, if present, is found between the RA and the true LA chamber.

Variations are found depending on whether the ostium between the accessory chamber and true LA is present and whether partial or total anomalous venous connection is an associated lesion.[56] The most common form is normal pulmonary venous connection to the accessory chamber, which drains to the LA chamber through a small ostium.

Transverse MR images show the accessory chamber partitioned from the true LA by a membranous or muscular shelf (Figure 20-15).[9,75] The accessory chamber is connected to dilated pulmonary veins (because of obstructed venous flow). High signal intensity in the accessory chamber on spin-echo sequences suggests slow blood flow. The accessory chamber of cor triatriatum should not be confused with a dilated coronary sinus caused by a total anomalous pulmonary venous connection. Similarly the shelf of cor triatriatum should not be confused with a supravalvular mitral ring. Cine MRI or phase-velocity mapping may facilitate identification of the ostium between the accessory chamber and LA.

In atrial septal defect (ASD) the normal interatrial septum extends from a posterocephalad to anterocaudal position. This is well depicted on transverse MR images. ASDs can be divided into subtypes according to their location within the interatrial septum. Ostium secundum ASD (most common) is centrally located. Sinus venosus ASD lies posterior to the fossa ovalis. Although the sinus venosus ASD is usually located high in the septum posteriorly adjacent to the SVC junction, rarely it may be positioned posteroinferior to the fossa ovalis near the IVC junction. Coronary sinus ASD is a rare anomaly that lies inferior and slightly anterior to the fossa ovalis at the anticipated site of the coronary sinus ostium.

The ostium secundum ASD is characterized by blunt ridges of thickened tissue along the margin of the defect on MR images (Figure 20-16). In some cases of intact interatrial septum the thinned region at the site of the fossa ovalis may produce little or no MR signal. In such an instance the septum gradually thins toward the site of signal absence, which facilitates differentiation between the fossa ovalis and secundum ASD. An alternative way to distinguish signal "dropout" at the fossa ovalis from an ASD is that signal dropout is confined to one imaging slice, with the adjacent slice showing the septum intact.

The sinus venosus ASD is displayed on MR images at the most posterior and cephalic portion of the interatrial septum[25] (Figure 20-17). This anomaly is frequently associated with partial anomalous connection of the right upper pulmonary vein.

Common atrium is a extreme form of ASD with virtual absence of the interatrial septum because of very large primum and secundum ASDs. In these patients a remnant of the interatrial septum is observed as a small ridge along the roof of the atrial wall at the junction of the SVC on MR images (Figure 20-18).

Atrioventricular Junction

This discussion includes abnormal AV connections and anomalies of valvular or subvalvular regions. Correct diagnosis of the AV connection is accomplished by a segmental approach. The wide field of view of MRI may be an advantage over ECG in defining atrial and ventricular structures from the apex to the base of the heart.

Atrioventricular septal defect is characterized by the malformation at the AV junction, including deficiency of the ostium primum septum, deficiency of the inlet interventricular septum, and malformed AV valves. The leaflets of the two AV orifices are attached to the interventricular septum at the same level, as opposed to the normal situation, in which the tricuspid annulus is positioned closer to the apex. Without a ventricular septal defect, this anomaly is called *ostium primum ASD*.

MR images of *ostium primum* ASDs show a defect in the lower portion of the interatrial septum adjacent to the AV valves. These AV valves are attached to a foreshortened interventricular septum because of a deficiency of the atrioventricular and inlet interventricular septum ("scooped out" interventricular septum). Both AV valves are found at the same level. On transverse MR images the origin of the ascending aorta is displaced anteriorly compared with the normal heart. The abnormal location of the aorta results in the elongation and narrowing of the LV outflow tract displayed on coronal images (goose-neck deformity). Attachment of chordal tissue from the AV valve to the crest of the interventricular septum is shown in patients with AV septal defect (Figure 20-19, *A*). A free-floating common AV valve can also be encountered (Figure 20-19, *B*). The MR features of AV septal defect have been reported.[45] Narrowing of the LV outflow tract caused by the abnormal

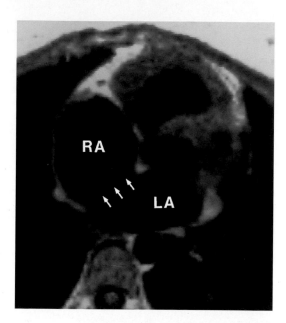

FIGURE 20-16   Ostium secundum ASD is recognized by the absence of the interatrial septum secundum *(arrows)*. *RA,* Right atrium; *LA,* left atrium.

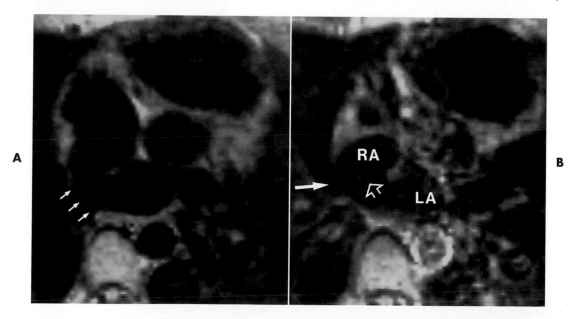

FIGURE 20-17   **A,** Sinus venosus ASD. Transverse image 1 cm cranial to image **B.** Sinus venosus ASD is depicted at the most posterior and cephalic portion of the interatrial septum *(open arrow* in **B**). Anomalous return of the right upper pulmonary vein *(arrow* in **B**) is associated with the ASD. Entrance of the right lower pulmonary vein *(arrows* in **A**) overrides the interatrial septum.

position of the aorta has been assessed quantitatively by using oblique MR images.[97]

Atrioventricular discordance is defined as a discordant AV connection, namely, the anatomical RA connects to the anatomical LV and the anatomical LA to the anatomical RV. This anomaly is most frequently accompanied by VA discordance. This anatomy is encountered in corrected transposition of the great arteries; the anatomical arrangement is hemodynamically "corrected." Typically a subaortic infundibulum is present and pulmonic-mitral valve fibrous continuity exists. Associated lesions in corrected transposition include subpulmonary perimembranous ventricular septal defect, valvular or subvalvular pulmonic stenosis, and Ebstein's malformation.

Several reports have demonstrated the capability of MRI to define AV discordance.[40,62] The anatomical RV can be identified by the presence of characteristic RV features shown on transverse MR images, as described earlier (Figure 20-20). Sagittal images may be useful to demonstrate subvalvular pulmonic stenosis. In AV discordance the interventricular septum frequently courses in an anteroposterior direction, causing ventricular septal defects (common in this disorder) to be depicted most effectively on coronal images.

The *double-inlet ventricle* set of anomalies has also been called *single ventricle*. Double-inlet left ventricle (DILV)[8] is characterized by both AV valves (or a common valve) entering the morphological LV, with a trabecular septum separating the rudimentary RV and main LV. The locations of the rudimentary RV are right-sided anterosuperior, left-sided anterosuperior, or occasionally directly anterior to the main chamber. When two valves exist, frequently either valve can show anomalies, including straddling, overriding, and atresia. A common valve also can show straddling and overriding. Most patients have a discordant VA connection (transposition). Other VA connections can be concordant (normal relation) or double outlet from the main LV or from the rudimentary RV. The pulmonic outflow tract is frequently stenotic. Aortic outflow tract stenosis can also be caused by a restricted bulboventricular foramen connecting the main chamber and the outlet chamber beneath the aortic valve in patients with VA discordance (transposition).

In double-inlet right ventricle (DIRV),[8] two AV valves (or a common valve) enter a morphological RV. The rudimentary LV is usually located posterior and to the left of the main RV but occasionally posterior and to the right. Similar anomalies of AV valves may occur as described for DILV. Pulmonic stenosis or atresia is frequently associated with DIRV.

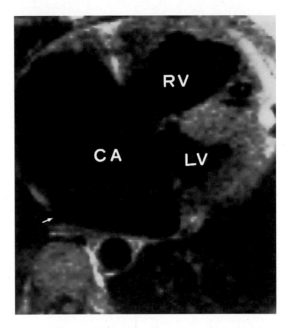

FIGURE 20-18   When both interatrial septum secundum and primum are deficient, the anomaly is called *common atrium (CA)*. *RV,* Right ventricle; *LV,* left ventricle; *arrow,* right lower pulmonary vein.

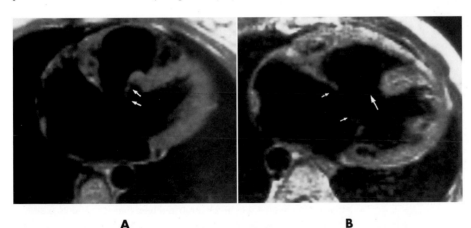

A   **B**

FIGURE 20-19   Atrioventricular septal defect. Deficiency of the interatrial septum primum and foreshortened (or "scooped out") interventricular septum are recognized on transverse images. Depending on the association with the ventricular septal defect and the form of the chordal attachment of the AV valves, subtypes can be defined. **A,** Chordal attachment to the crest of the interventricular septum *(arrows)* (Rastelli type A). **B,** Free-flowing AV valves *(small arrows)* (Rastelli type C). Note the absence of the interatrial septum and large VSD *(large arrow).*

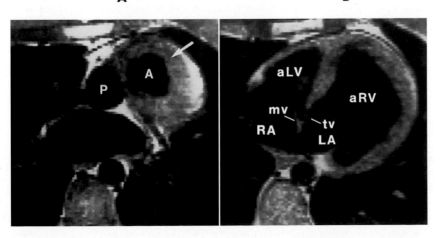

A   **B**

FIGURE 20-20   Atrioventricular discordance. Image **A** is cranial to image **B**. Anatomical RV *(aRV)* connects to the left atrium *(LA)*, and anatomical LV *(aLV)* connects to the right atrium *(RA)*. Identification of the ventricle is accomplished by the attachment of the tricuspid valve *(tv)* and mitral valve *(mv)*. The aRV possesses the infundibulum *(arrow in* **A***)*. *A,* Aorta; *P,* pulmonary artery.

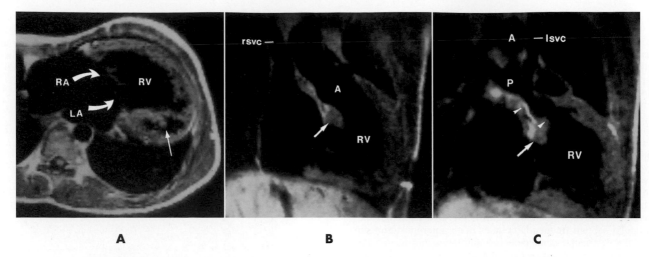

A **B** **C**

FIGURE 20-21 Double-inlet RV. **A,** Transverse image shows both sides of the AV connection committed to the right ventricle *(RV)*. Rudimentary LV *(arrow)* is posterior to the RV. **B** and **C,** Coronal images (**B** anterior to **C**) show both great arteries arising from the RV. The aorta *(A)* is located anterior to the pulmonary artery *(P)*. Subaortic and subpulmonic coni *(large arrows* in **B** and **C**). Subvalvular and supravalvular pulmonic stenosis *(arrowheads* in **C**). *lsvc,* Left superior vena cava; *rsvc,* right superior vena cava. (From Higgins CB, Silverman NH, Kerstein-Sommerhoff B, et al: Congenital heart disease, New York, 1990, Raven Press.)

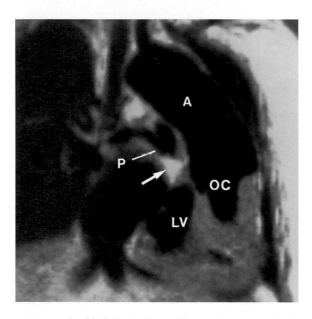

FIGURE 20-22 Double-inlet LV. Coronal image shows an outlet chamber *(OC),* which is a rudimentary RV lacking an inlet portion of the ventricle, located at a left-superior aspect of the heart. Because the aorta *(A)* is left sided and arising from the OC, the ventriculoarterial connection is an L transposition. Atresia of the main pulmonary artery *(P)* and confluent central pulmonary artery are depicted *(arrow)*. *LV,* Left ventricle. (From Higgins CB, Hricak H, and Helms CA: Magnetic resonance imaging of the body, New York, 1992, Raven Press.)

Double inlet to a sole ventricle without a rudimentary chamber may be classified as double inlet to an indeterminate ventricle.[8] In this type the trabecular pattern of the ventricle is coarser than that found for the normal RV.

MR images can be used to define the type of double-inlet ventricle. The initial step is to identify the morphology of the main chamber. The presence or absence of an infundibulum and the location of the rudimentary RV or LV to the main chamber on MR images can be used for ventricular identification (Figures 20-21 and 20-22). The trabecular pattern observed on transverse MR images is often misleading and should not be relied upon for ventricular identification.

Clinically important information obtained from MRI of double-inlet ventricle includes AV valve abnormalities. In DILV the presence or absence of narrowing at the bulboventricular foramen should be sought; a restrictive foramen has a cross-sectional area (diameter) less than the cross-sectional area of the aortic annulus. Coronal images frequently demonstrate the anatomy of the bulboventricular foramen. In patients with asplenia or polysplenia, total anomalous pulmonary venous return may be associated with a double-inlet ventricle. With recent advances in surgical repair for double-inlet ventricle, such as the modified Fontan and ventricular partition procedures, it is important that the AV valve size, the location of papillary muscles in the ventricle, and the presence of valvular regurgitation and stenosis be determined preoperatively. These diagnoses may be determined using cine MRI, as well as spin-echo sequences.

Tricuspid atresia can be divided into two types—muscular atresia and membranous atresia. In muscular atresia, the more frequently occurring form, the RA floor is muscular and has atretic tricuspid tissue, which is noted as a small dimple. Muscular atresia is usually associated with malalignment of the atrial and ventricular septa. Imperforate membranous atresia is a rare form in which the atrial and ventricular septa are normally aligned. Anomalies associated with tricuspid atresia include transposition of the great arteries, patent foramen ovale or ASD, ventricular septal defect, pulmonary stenosis or atresia, and patent ductus arteriosus. Juxtaposition of the atrial appendages is sometimes found in tricuspid atresia with discordant VA connections (transposition of great arteries).

Transverse MR images show that in muscular tricuspid atresia, a layer of muscle and fat is interposed between the RA and RV (Figure 20-23).[35,46] This finding is not present in patients with membranous atresia. Malalignment between atrial and interventricular septa is shown on transverse images.

In Ebstein's anomaly the essential pathological finding is displaced attachment of tricuspid valve leaflets from the AV junction into the RV cavity. The displaced valves are almost always limited to septal and inferior leaflets; rarely the anterosuperior leaflet is also involved. The extent of the displacement varies, depending on the severity of the disease. In the severe form the attachment of the septal or inferior valve leaflets to the ventricular wall may form a prominent muscular shelf.[2] As a consequence of the displaced tricuspid valve, the inlet part of the RV is physiologically "atrialized." In the severe form the atrialized ventricular wall is abnormally thin.

The anatomical features of Ebstein's anomaly are well demonstrated on axial and coronal MR images.[54] A greatly enlarged RA and atrialized RV are shown on axial images (Figure 20-24). The wall thickness of the atrialized ventricle may be diminished compared with the nonatrialized ventricle. The displaced attachment of the septal leaflet is found on axial images. In the severe form of this anomaly the attachment forms a muscular shelf, which is depicted as a strand a few millimeters thick, separating the atrialized portion of the RV from the nonatrialized portion.[54] Coronal images are sometimes more effective than axial images in displaying the displacement of the inferior leaflet.

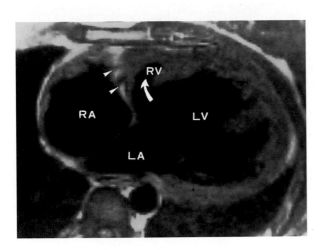

FIGURE 20-23   Tricuspid atresia. Continuation between the right atrium *(RA)* and right ventricle *(RV)* is interrupted by a layer of muscle and fat *(arrowheads),* which is characteristic of muscular tricuspid atresia. The RV is hypoplastic. Note the malalignment of the atrial and interventricular septi. Ventricular septal defect is also depicted *(curved arrow). LV,* Left ventricle; *LA,* left atrium.

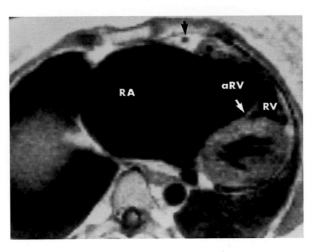

FIGURE 20-24   Ebstein's anomaly. Attachment of the septal leaflet of the tricuspid valve *(arrow)* is displaced toward the apex, resulting in a small right ventricular cavity *(RV).* In contrast, the right atrium *(RA)* is greatly enlarged. The inlet portion of the RV is physiologically "atrialized" *(aRV).* Note the location of the AV groove, indicated by the right coronary artery *(black arrow).*

Ventricular Septal Defects

The anatomical classification of ventricular septal defects (VSDs) can be based on two major components of the normal interventricular septum—membranous and muscular. The muscular component can be divided into inlet, trabecular, and outlet (infundibular) portions according to the location of the defect within the interventricular septum. The three muscular parts meet together at the membranous septum. Adjacent to the membranous septum, the AV septum is found between the LV and RA. The AV septum also consists of membranous and muscular components.

Three major types of VSDs can be distinguished: (1) perimembranous, (2) muscular, and (3) subarterial. Most VSDs are found around the membranous septum. The perimembranous defects almost always show extension from the membranous into the muscular septum. Depending on the direction of the extension, the defect can be classified as a perimembranous outlet, trabecular, or inlet defect. Perimembranous outlet defects are frequently associated with malalignment of the outlet septum with the trabecular septum. The malaligned outlet septum deviates into either the RV (e.g., tetralogy of Fallot) or the LV (e.g., coarctation of the aorta).

The muscular VSDs are characterized by being completely surrounded by the muscular component of the interventricular septum. The muscular defects therefore can be distinguished from the perimembranous defects because muscular tissue or a muscular bar exists between the defects and the central fibrous body and the mitral and tricuspid valvular attachments to the septum. The muscular defects can be classified into subtypes according to the location within the septum—outlet, inlet, or trabecular.

Subarterial VSDs are characterized by the defect's location at the outlet septum just beneath the aortic and pulmonic valves, without intervening muscular tissue (doubly committed subarterial defects). This classification of VSDs can be applied to the isolated defects and to the defects associated with various types of CIIDs, such as those with abnormal AV or VA connections.

Different components of the interventricular septum can be well depicted on transverse MR images extending from the base to apex of the heart (Figure 20-25).[23] The outlet (infundibular) muscular septum is depicted at the most cranial level. The next caudal section displays the anterior portion of the membranous septum just below the junction of the attachments of the right and noncoronary aortic cusps. More caudal sections show the membranous part of the AV septum, the inlet muscular septum, and the trabecular muscular septum (anterior to the muscular septum). Sagittal images through the base of the aorta may be used to display the outlet, membranous, and trabecular septum.

Each type of VSD is identified on transverse MR images (Figure 20-26). Detection of small VSDs may be aided by cine MR techniques (Figure 20-27). The perimembranous VSDs are frequently associated

with the formation of a membranous septal aneurysm, which is shown on transverse images (Figure 20-28). Extension of the perimembranous defects in any direction within the muscular septum can be shown by adjacent slices (Figure 20-29). Malalignment of the outlet septum to the trabecular septum can be seen on both transverse and sagittal images.

Inlet VSDs have been demonstrated in patients with AV septal defects. The location of the defect and the presence of the ostium primum ASD can be displayed at the correct level, including all four chambers of the heart.

Demonstration of VSDs by MRI can be improved in some patients by using an oblique imaging plane oriented parallel to the interventricular septum. Studies have examined the value of oblique planes in depicting inlet and trabecular components of the septum.[5,99] Such oblique section produced images comparable to seeing the inlet and trabecular septum directly. These oblique planes may have advantages over conventional orthogonal planes in detectection of multiple small muscular defects, since the oblique planes can employ in-plane resolution to display such small septal defects.

Ventricular Outflow Tract

This group of anomalies includes obstructive lesions at the ventricular outflow tract. Spin-echo MRI has limitations for depicting valvular structures because of problems with partial volume averaging caused by coarse slice thickness. However, cine MRI may be effective in showing valvular lesions by displaying abnormal flow patterns caused by valvular stenosis. When evaluating this group of anomalies, it is important to assess the exact location of the obstruction and the size of the narrowed outflow tract.

Tetralogy of Fallot consists of the classic anatomical features of (1) VSD, (2) overriding of the aorta, (3) infundibular pulmonic stenosis, and (4) RV hypertrophy. However, these anomalies can be understood as anatomical or hemodynamic consequences derived from one major feature, abnormal (anterior) alignment of the infundibular septum. Sequential transverse MR images display these anatomical features of tetralogy of Fallot (Figure 20-30). The anteriorly malaligned infundibular septum is seen on MR images through the RV outflow tract. The infundibular stenosis is shown as a space narrowed by the malaligned infundibular septum. At the same level the aortic valve is shown to be deviated both anteriorly and rightward compared with normal hearts and located at a position overriding the VSD. The adjacent caudal level displays the VSD. The location of the defect is usually perimembranous, with extension into the outlet septum. Occasionally the inferior rim of the VSD is muscular. A doubly committed subarterial defect can be encountered in this anomaly.

Sagittal images can be used to demonstrate the infundibular stenosis in tetralogy of Fallot. Although the stenosis is mainly caused by the

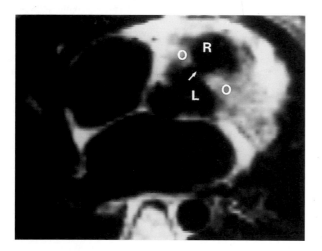

FIGURE 20-25   Components of the interventricular septum on axial MR images. Transverse images extend from cranial **(A)** to caudal **(D)**. **A,** The outlet muscular septum *(O)* is shown at the base of the heart. **B,** The next caudal section depicts the trabecular muscular septum *(T)* and membranous septum *(arrow)*. **C** and **D,** More caudally, the membranous part of the AV septum *(arrowhead* in **C)** and the inlet muscular septum *(I* in **D)** are shown. Note the correct alignment of the outlet septum and trabecular septum. *LV,* Left ventricle; *RV,* right ventricle; *RA,* right atrium. (From Higgins CB, Hricak H, and Helms CA: Magnetic resonance imaging of the body, New York, 1992, Raven Press.)

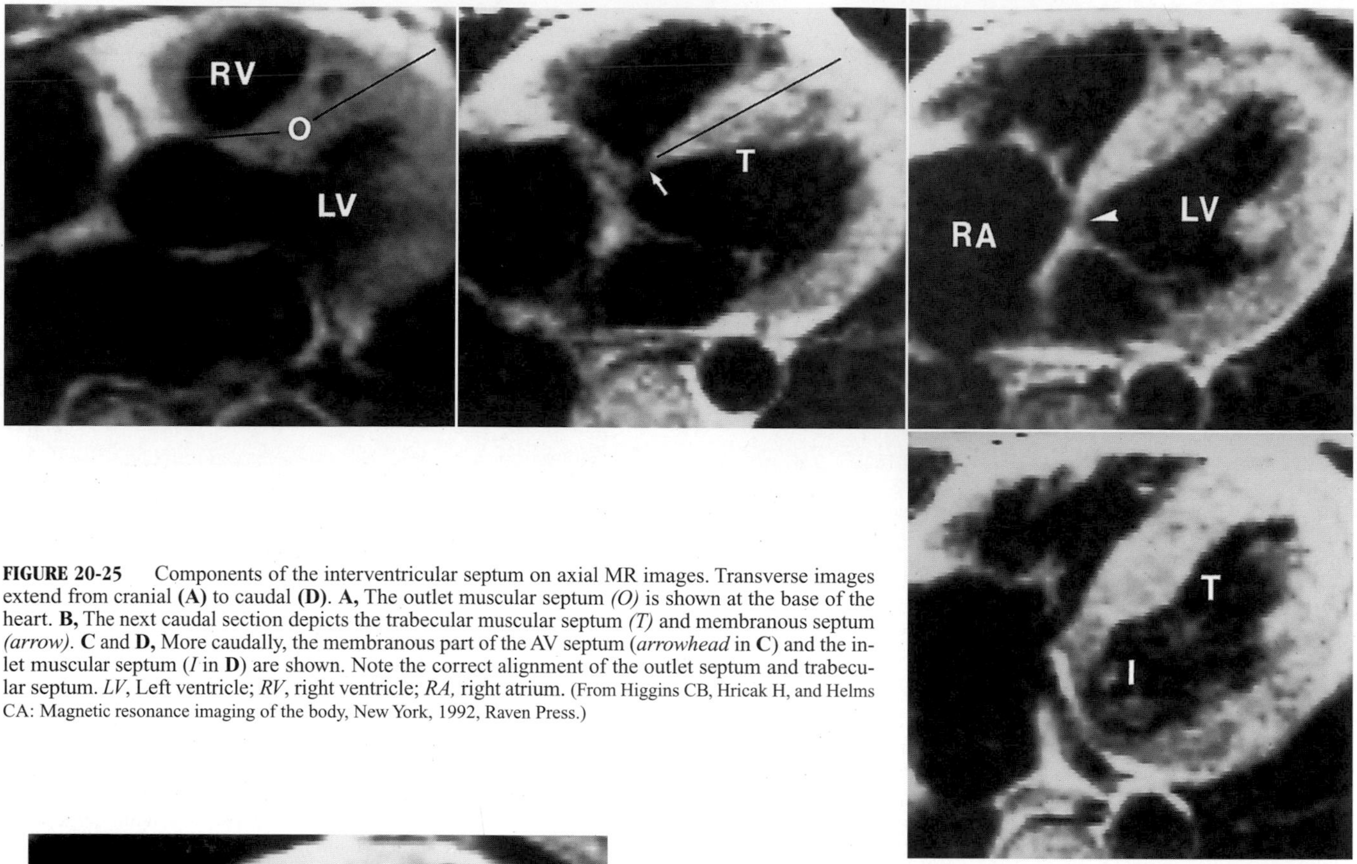

FIGURE 20-26   VSD at the muscular outlet septum *(O, arrow). R,* Right ventricle; *L,* left ventricle.

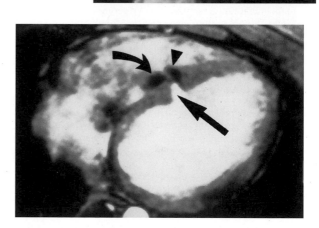

FIGURE 20-27   Cine MR images of a VSD at the muscular trabecular septum. Signal void *(curved arrow, arrowhead)*, caused by the turbulent jet of blood across the VSD *(arrow)*, is observed during systole.

FIGURE 20-28   Perimembranous VSD associated with a membranous septal aneurysm *(arrows)*, which is seen as a pouch protruding into the RV cavity below the septal attachment of the tricuspid valve.

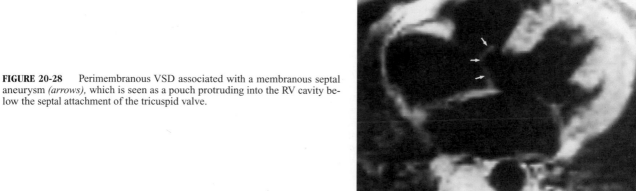

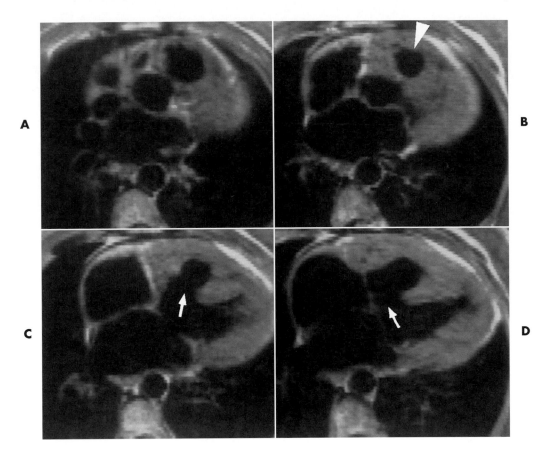

FIGURE 20-29   Perimembranous VSD with outlet extension. Transverse images (**A** to **D**) extend from cranial *(upper left)* to caudal *(lower right)*. VSD extends from the membranous septum *(arrow* in **D**) into the outlet muscular septum *(arrow* in **C**). Note the infundibular stenosis *(arrowhead* in **B**). (From Higgins CB, Silverman NH, Kerstein-Sommerhoff B, et al: Congenital heart disease, New York, 1990, Raven Press.)

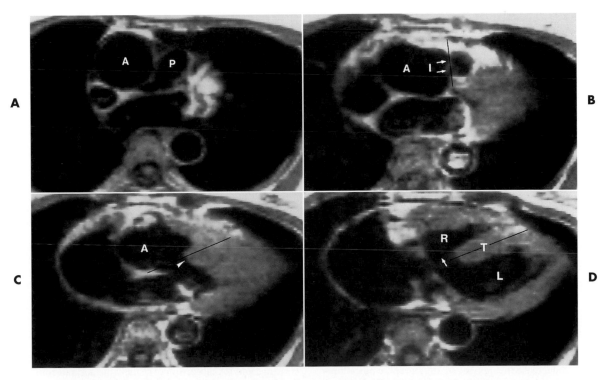

FIGURE 20-30   Tetralogy of Fallot, cranial (**A**) to caudal (**D**). Infundibular septum *(I)* is malaligned to the trabecular septum *(T)*. The aorta *(A)* is deviated anteriorly and rightward and overrides the interventricular septum. Ventricular septal defect *(arrow* in **D**) is perimembranous with outlet extension *(arrowhead* in **C**). *P,* Pulmonary artery; *R,* right ventricle; *L,* left ventricle.

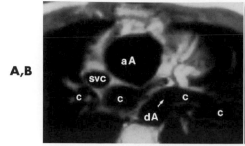
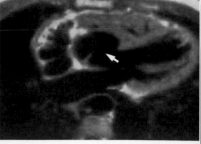

A,B

C

FIGURE 20-31 Pulmonary atresia with VSD. Transverse image **B** is caudal to image **A**. VSD (*arrow* in **B**) and atresia at the main pulmonary artery are shown. Many MAPCAs *(c)* are depicted. The origin of one of the MAPCAs from the descending aorta *(dA)* is shown *(arrow)*. Confluent central pulmonary artery is not found. **C,** Coronal image of another patient shows the origins of MAPCAs *(arrows)* from the descending aorta *(dA)*. *SVC,* Superior vena cava; *aA,* ascending aorta. (From Higgins CB, Silverman NH, Kerstein-Sommerhoff B, et al: Congenital heart disease, New York, 1990, Raven Press.)

anteriorly deviated infundibular septum, muscular hypertrophy of anterior trabeculations and septal trabeculations (trabecula septomarginalis) may exacerbate the degree of stenosis. A discrete infundibular chamber may be formed distal to these muscular stenotic structures.

Another clinically important finding depicted by MRI is the morphology of the pulmonary arteries. Pulmonary arterial caliber in patients with tetralogy of Fallot is usually smaller than in healthy individuals. Peripheral pulmonary stenosis can be found at the bifurcation of the main pulmonary artery, at the origin of the segmental branches, or both. This anatomy is depicted well on transverse and coronal MR images. The capability of MRI in localizing pulmonary stenosis and measuring pulmonary arterial size has been indicated in several reports.[16,37] Postoperative findings in tetralogy of Fallot are also well demonstrated by MRI.[38]

Pulmonary atresia with VSD is essentially an extreme form of tetralogy of Fallot in which the anteriorly deviated infundibular septum produces muscular atresia (Figure 20-31). The muscular infundibulum ends blindly and connects to a fibrous atretic pulmonary arterial trunk. Usually a considerable distance separates the blind end and the cavity of the proximal pulmonary artery, but the atresia can consist of merely a membrane at the valvular level. As seen in tetralogy of Fallot, the VSD is usually perimembranous with extension into the outlet septum.

Three types of pulmonary arterial supply can occur with this anomaly, depending on whether a *patent ductus arteriosus* (PDA) exists. The first type is associated with PDA. Blood to all portions of both lungs is supplied from central right and left pulmonary arteries. Major collateral arteries from the aorta are not present. Peripheral pulmonary stenosis or atresia is frequently found adjacent to the junction to a PDA. In the second type a PDA is not present. Blood supply to the lung comes from major aortopulmonary collateral arteries (MAPCAs) instead of a PDA. Confluent central pulmonary arteries coexist with the MAPCAs but frequently do not supply all the pulmonary circulation. The MAPCAs originate most frequently from the descending aorta and supply blood directly to the lung or via central pulmonary arteries. Occasionally the MAPCAs originate from subclavian arteries, the aortic arch, the abdominal aorta, or rarely coronary arteries. The third type of pulmonary arterial supply, in which PDA and the MAPCAs coexist, occurs infrequently.

Transverse MRI is effective in establishing the presence and size of central pulmonary arteries in patients who have pulmonary atresia with VSD (Figure 20-31).[16,51,72] MRI is at least as accurate as angiography for depicting right and left pulmonary arteries and the presence or absence of a central confluence.[72] Although MRI can depict MAPCAs, it is not as sensitive as angiography for this purpose.[51,72] However, if the origin of relatively large MAPCAs from the aorta can be displayed by MRI, it may serve to decrease the number of angiographic procedures needed in patients with pulmonary atresia (Figure 20-31). Furthermore, MRI may be useful in the serial assessment of pulmonary arterial growth and the postoperative status of these patients.

Ventriculoarterial Connections

Several cardiac anomalies, such as the double-outlet ventricle, transposition of the great arteries, and single-outlet ventricle (truncus arteriosus), are included in this group. The three-dimensional capability of MR tomographic imaging provides clear demonstration of VA connections. It is important to depict the dominant connection of each great artery to the ventricle, the location of VSDs, and their relation to the semilunar valves.

Double-outlet right ventricle is defined as the arrangement in which more than half of both arterial valves are committed to the RV. A bilateral infundibulum is associated with this anomaly but is not always present. Significant anatomical information for surgical correction includes the localization of the obligatory VSD and its relation to the great arteries. The locations of the great arteries can be divided into two groups: those with a right-sided aorta and those with a left-sided aorta. The location of the VSD can be divided into those with a (1) subaortic defect, (2) subpulmonic defect, (3) doubly committed subarterial defect, and (4) noncommitted defect.

In hearts with more or less normally related great arteries (i.e., the aorta is right sided and posterior to the pulmonary artery) the VSD is usually subaortic, although other locations can be encountered. The infundibular septum is malaligned and attaches to the interventricular septum anterior to the defect. The distance between the aortic valve and the VSD should be elucidated, because it may affect the procedures used for intracardiac repair. This distance is far or close, depending on the size of the ventriculoinfundibular fold. The distance becomes remote with an extensive ventriculoinfundibular fold or a noncommitted septal defect. When the ventriculoinfundibular fold is attenuated, the defect becomes perimembranous and close to the aortic valve. Subpulmonic stenosis is frequently associated with the subaortic VSD.

In hearts with a right-sided aorta that is side by side with or anterior to the pulmonary artery, the VSD is usually subpulmonic. These arrangements are more similar to complete transposition, and a spectrum between these two entities can be found. The proximity of the defect to the pulmonic valve varies, depending on the size of the ventriculoinfundibular fold. Aortic stenosis and coarctation of the aorta can frequently be found in patients with subpulmonic defects.

Transverse MR images can define the spatial relations of the great arteries in double-outlet RV. The location of the VSD is shown on transverse images (Figure 20-32). Sagittal images are useful for depicting the size of the ventriculoinfundibular fold and the origin of great arteries from the RV. Oblique imaging slices are useful for detecting the presence of subaortic or subpulmonic stenoses and for measuring the distance between the VSD and semilunar valves.[1,5]

Complete transposition is defined as the combination of AV concordance and VA discordance. Usually the aorta in complete transposition is located anterior and right in relation to the pulmonary artery. However, variations can be encountered with a directly anterior or left-sided and anterior aorta. The infundibular morphology of complete

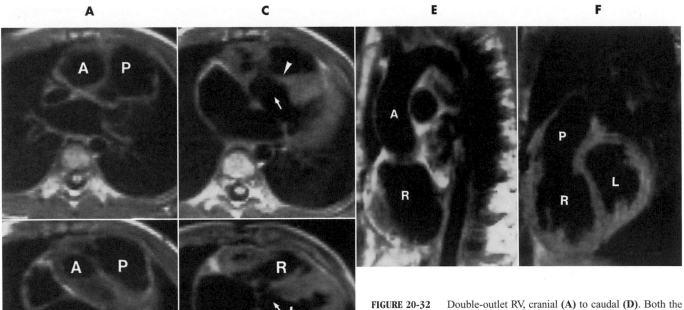

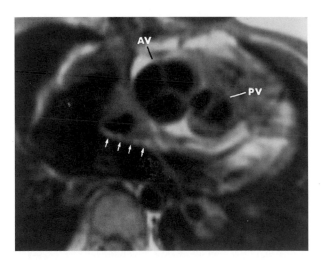

FIGURE 20-32 Double-outlet RV, cranial (**A**) to caudal (**D**). Both the aorta *(A)* and the pulmonary artery *(P)* are arising from the right ventricle *(R)*. The VSD *(arrow* in **C** and **D**) is perimembranous and subaortic. The infundibular septum is malaligned to the trabecular septum. Attachment of the infundibular septum *(arrowhead* in **C**) is anterior to the defect. **E** and **F,** Sagittal MR images of another patient show both great arteries *(A* and *P)* arising from the right ventricle *(R)*. *L,* Left ventricle.

transposition is usually opposite to that in normal hearts; that is, a subaortic infundibulum and pulmonic-mitral valve fibrous continuity are found. Sometimes, however, complete transposition with bilateral infundibula can be encountered. A VSD is frequently associated with complete transposition. Usually the VSD is an infundibular, malaligned type and located in the subpulmonic region. However, when the aorta is located left and anteriorly, the defect becomes subaortic. Pulmonic stenosis is caused by valvular or subvalvular stenosis. Subaortic stenosis does not occur often in complete transposition, but when present, it is frequently associated with aortic arch obstruction.

Spatial relations of great arteries in complete transposition are demonstrated on transverse MR images (Figure 20-33). MR images are effective for displaying the associated VSD, pulmonic stenosis, subaortic stenosis, and concurrent aortic arch anomalies. Ventricular wall thickness of both sides of the heart should be evaluated. Complete transposition with an intact interventricular septum typically shows a thin left and a thick right ventricular wall. In patients with pulmonary hypertension, both ventricles may show similarly thick walls. The wall thickness on MR images may be used to select candidates for arterial switch procedures to correct complete transposition and to assess the effectiveness of preswitch pulmonary artery banding in increasing left ventricular wall thickness (through increased afterload).

Truncus arteriosus is defined as a solitary arterial trunk exiting from the heart through a solitary arterial valve and supplying directly the coronary, at least one pulmonary, and systemic arteries.[20] In defining anatomical features, the following variables should be considered:

1. *Ventricular connection to the arterial trunk.* The truncal valve usually overrides the interventricular septum in approximately equal proportions to both ventricles. However, this valve may predominantly arise from one ventricle.
2. *Size and location of the VSD.* Determining whether the VSD is narrow and restrictive is significant for surgical correction. Usually the defect is a muscular infundibular type, but it can be perimembranous infundibular.
3. *Truncal valve.* This is most frequently tricuspid but may be quadricuspid, bicuspid, or hexacuspid.

FIGURE 20-33 D transposition of the great arteries. The aortic valve *(AV)* is located anterior and to the right of the pulmonic valve *(PV)*, the inverse of the usual anatomical arrangement. The valve leaflets are well demonstrated. A Senning baffle *(arrows)* has rerouted atrial blood flow.

4. *Variable patterns of origin of the pulmonary arteries from the trunk.* Usually, both pulmonary arteries arise separately from the left posterior aspect of the trunk (type II). A well-formed main pulmonary trunk may be found (type I). The pulmonary branches originating from the sides of the ascending trunk is relatively rare (type III). Another possibly associated anomaly is interruption of the aorta.

Transverse and sagittal MR images at the base of the heart can demonstrate a large arterial trunk arising above the VSD (Figures 20-34 and 20-35). MRI is valuable in defining the degree of overriding of the truncal valve in relation to the interventricular septum and the origin of the pulmonary arteries. Coronal or oblique images may be useful for

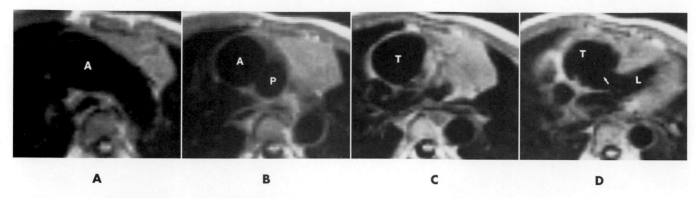

A   **B**   **C**   **D**

FIGURE 20-34   Truncus arteriosus, type I; cranial **(A)** to caudal **(D)**. Single arterial trunk *(T)* is arising predominantly from the right ventricle. VSD *(arrow* in **D)** is shown below the trunk. **B,** The trunk is divided into two arteries, the aorta *(A)* and pulmonary artery *(P)*.

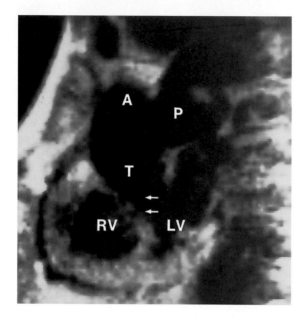

FIGURE 20-35   Single arterial trunk *(T)* overrides the interventricular septum. VSD *(arrows)* is shown below the trunk. Pulmonary artery *(P)* is originating from the trunk's posterior aspect. *A,* Aorta; *RV,* right ventricle; *LV,* left ventricle.

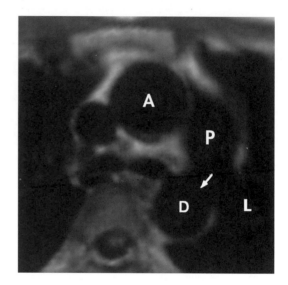

FIGURE 20-36   PDA. Communication *(arrow)* between the left pulmonary artery *(L),* just branching from the main pulmonary artery *(P),* and descending aorta *(D). A,* Ascending aorta.

determining the size and location of the VSD. Potential pulmonary artery stenoses should be sought after.

Great Arteries

MRI has been shown to be an effective imaging technique for defining abnormalities of the great arteries in the thorax.* Several different categories of congenital anomalies exist, including anomalous communication between the great arteries, obstructive lesions in the aortic arch, and abnormal branching patterns of the aorta or pulmonary artery.

Anomalous Communication Between Great Arteries. Aortopulmonary window is defined as a defect between the ascending portions of the aortic and pulmonary trunk. The presence of separate aortic and pulmonic valves distinguishes this anomaly from truncus arteriosus. The size of the defect varies from a small hole to a wide communication extending from the semilunar valvular rings to the pulmonary arterial bifurcation. The location of the defect also varies from the proximal ascending aorta to a more distal site adjacent to the right pulmonary artery.

PDA courses from the proximal descending aorta to the left pulmonary artery just beyond the pulmonary arterial bifurcation.

MR images can show the presence of a ductus arteriosus of relatively large size (Figure 20-36). A small ductus in infants, however, may not be diagnosed on MR images.[6] ECG is much more effective for this purpose.

Obstructive Aortic Arch Lesions. Coarctation of the aorta can be classified according to the shape and location of narrowing. The typical form of coarctation is a discrete shelflike lesion found within the proximal descending aorta (juxtaductal discrete coarctation). A less common form is tubular hypoplasia, which implies a uniform narrowing of a discrete segment of the aortic arch, usually involving the distal arch and isthmus region of the aorta. A discrete coarctation is usually found at the site of attachment of the ligamentum arteriosum and distal to the left subclavian artery but may occur proximal to the left subclavian, causing lower arterial pressure in the left arm and lower extremities. Coarctation may be associated with a wide variety of other congenital cardiac anomalies, notably PDA and VSD.

Interruption of the aorta can be considered an extreme form of tubular segmental hypoplasia of the aortic arch. As with tubular hypoplasia, the location of interrupted arch is found at the isthmus or between the left common carotid and subclavian arteries. Rarely the aortic interruption can be present between the right innominate artery and the left common carotid artery.

MRI has been found to be effective in the initial diagnosis of aortic coarctation and for patient evaluation after treatment (Figures 20-37

*References 6, 7, 10, 11, 13, 50, 74, 87, 94.

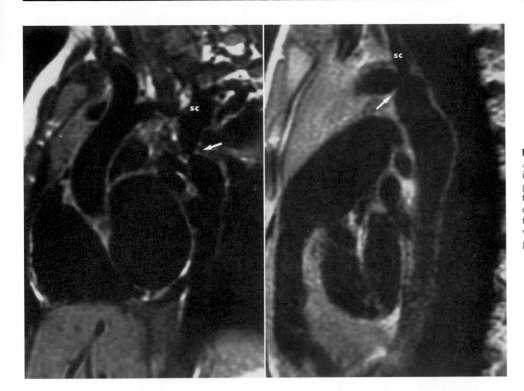

FIGURE 20-37 Coarctation of the aorta. **A,** Juxtaductal constriction of the aorta *(arrow)* is shown on an oblique sagittal image. The origin of a dilated left subclavian artery *(sc)* above the coarctation is also depicted. Note the presence of poststenotic dilatation. **B,** Oblique sagittal image in another patient with an anterior weblike coarctation *(arrow)* proximal to the origin of a nondilated left subclavian artery *(sc)*.

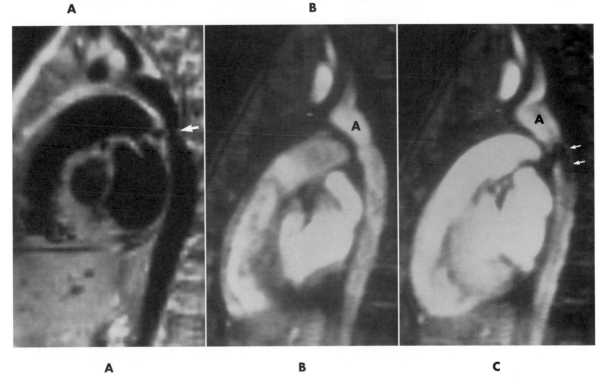

FIGURE 20-38 Flow patterns in aortic coarctation. **A,** Discrete juxtaductal coarctation is shown *(arrow)* in a spin-echo sagittal image. Cine MR frames obtained in diastole **(B)** and systole **(C)** depict flowing blood in white and the high-velocity poststenotic jet during systole as a signal void *(arrows in **C**)*. *A,* Aorta.

and 20-38).* To evaluate the coarctation, transverse and sagittal images are typically obtained. Additional oblique imaging planes, parallel to the aortic arch or perpendicular to the aorta at the site of coarctation, may improve anatomical depiction and sizing of the coarctation. By using this approach, MRI can depict all the anatomical information required for surgical repair, such as (1) the position of the coarctation, (2) its relation to the ductus arteriosus and the arteries arising from the aortic arch, (3) the length and diameter of the aortic isthmus, and (4) whether the coarctation is a discrete shelf or tubular lesion.[6] In addition, more recent studies have demonstrated the ability of velocity-encoded cine MRI to estimate the pressure gradient across the coarctation[58] and the proportion of collateral flow around the obstruction.[88] Therefore MRI can supplant angiography in the preoperative evaluation of patients with coarctation of the aorta.

After treatment of the coarctation with surgery or balloon angioplasty, serial evaluations may be required to detect complications, such as restenosis or pseudoaneurysm formation at the prior site of the coarctation. MRI has been shown to be the preferable method for this purpose.[7,15,74,87,94]

Aortic Arch Anomalies and Vascular Sling. Many different anomalies of the aortic arch are encountered in clinical practice. Most often these are incidental findings of no clinical significance, although many arch anomalies are encountered in association with other cardiovascular anomalies. In particular, right aortic arch is frequently associated with tetralogy of Fallot and truncus arteriosus. Aortic arch anomalies causing clinical symptoms are the rare types producing a vascular ring, encircling the trachea and esophagus, and compressing these structures.

Types of vascular rings include double aortic arch, the result of persistence of the embryonic double-arch system (left and right aortic arches); right aortic arch with aberrant left subclavian artery, producing a ring when the ductus arteriosus is located on the left; and vascular sling, a rare anomaly defined as the anomalous origin of one pulmonary artery from the other with bronchial compression. Anomalous origin of the left pulmonary artery from the right pulmonary artery occurs, and the vessel courses between the trachea and esophagus. Many other rarer variations of vascular rings have been reported.

Transverse spin-echo images are very effective in defining these aortic arch and pulmonary branch anomalies.[10,50] Because of the limitations of the acoustic window in this region available for ECG, the assessment of these anomalies is difficult with that modality. MRI is

currently the most effective noninvasive technique for evaluating vascular rings (Figure 20-39). Furthermore, compression of the esophagus and trachea by vascular rings can be directly documented by MRI.[10] Aberrant origin of the subclavian artery on transverse MR images is recognized as an "outpocketing" in the region of the proximal descending aorta (Figure 20-40). Adjacent cranial slices show the artery arising from the pocket.[50]

Coronary Arteries

Much progress has been made recently in MR angiography of acquired coronary artery disease,[30,31,63] although these techniques have yet to see widespread clinical application. In some types of congenital anomalies of coronary arteries, coronary artery caliber is sufficiently large that the origin and course of the coronary arteries in infants can be discerned with MRI; one example is coronary arteriovenous fistula. A dilated left anterior descending coronary artery connected to the RV has been demonstrated on transverse images and oblique sagittal images.[14] Another example is anomalous origin of the left coronary artery from the pulmonary artery (Bland-White-Garland syndrome). Sequential coronal images have demonstrated the normal origin of the dilated right coronary artery and differentiated the abnormal origin of the left coronary artery from the main pulmonary artery.[29] Other anomalous origins or courses of the coronary arteries have been demonstrated by MRI in case reports.[28,57] However, these cases were in adults, and the ability of MRI to demonstrate coronary artery anomalies in early infancy has not been established.

POSTOPERATIVE ASSESSMENT

The noninvasive nature of MRI makes it a useful method for sequential monitoring of children and adults after surgical intervention in CHD. Serial assessment is often required after both corrective and palliative procedures. Determination of the growth of the pulmonary arteries after systemic-pulmonary shunts is one of the critical factors in determining the prognosis and subsequent surgical management of patients with pulmonary stenosis or atresia. Because MRI is able to provide clear demonstration of supracardiac and intracardiac structures and to assess hemodynamics through cine and velocity-encoded cine imaging, it may be the ideal technique for following patients with CHD after surgery.

Many newer procedures for correction of complex heart disease involve surgical construction in the supracardiac area (Table 20-1). MRI

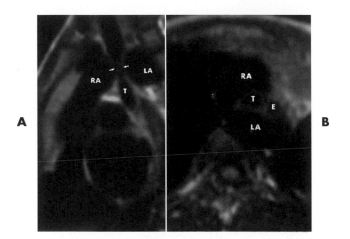

FIGURE 20-39 Double aortic arch. **A,** Sagittal image shows compression of the trachea *(arrows)* between the anterior right aortic arch *(RA)* and posterior left aortic arch *(LA)*. **B,** Transverse image shows the right and left arches surrounding the trachea *(T)* and esophagus *(E)*.

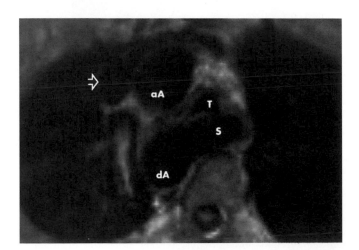

FIGURE 20-40 Right aortic arch with aberrant origin of the left subclavian artery. Left subclavian artery *(S)* arises from the descending aorta *(dA)* and courses behind the trachea *(T)*. *aA,* Ascending aorta; *open arrow,* superior vena cava.

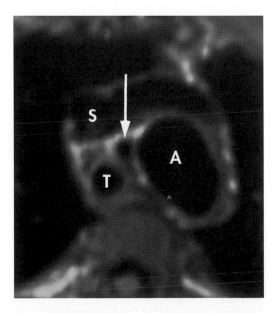

FIGURE 20-41 Blalock-Taussig shunt. A circular structure with central signal void *(arrow)* is shown adjacent to the aortic arch *(A)*. This signal void indicates that the systemic-pulmonary shunt is patent. *S,* Superior vena cava; *T,* trachea. (From Higgins CB, Silverman NH, Kerstein-Sommerhoff B, et al: Congenital heart disease, New York, 1990, Raven Press.)

has been shown to be as effective as angiography for evaluating the status and complications of these procedures.[52]

Many reports have shown the effectiveness of MRI after surgery for CHD. Patency of systemic-pulmonary shunts can be determined by spin-echo MRI. The patent shunt is shown as a circular structure with central signal void, arising from the subclavian artery or the ascending aorta and coursing to the pulmonary arterial branches (Figure 20-41).[47] Surgical baffles rerouting atrial blood from the systemic or pulmonary veins to the appropriate ventricles after the Mustard or Senning procedure for complete transposition can be shown by MRI (Figure 20-42).[15,77,89] Stenosis at the baffle can be shown correctly with MRI. Pres-

ence or absence of stenosis at the vascular anastomosis or external vascular conduit can be demonstrated in patients after various procedures, such as the Jatene for complete transposition of great arteries (Figure 20-43), Norwood for hypoplastic left heart syndrome (Figure 20-44), Fontan for tricuspid atresia (Figure 20-45),[21,71,78] and Rastelli for pulmonary atresia with ventricular septal defect (Figure 20-46).

One limitation of spin-echo MRI is that it is usually not adequate for evaluating valvular anomalies. Valvular regurgitation and the presence of a residual intracardiac shunt after surgery cannot be demonstrated well by spin-echo MRI, although cine MRI and velocity-encoded cine MRI are competitive with ECG for these types of flow measurements.

Table 20-1	Surgical Procedures in Congenital Heart Disease	
PROCEDURE	**STRUCTURAL ALTERATIONS**	**INDICATIONS**
Mustard or Senning	Atrial rerouting of venous blood flow	Transposition
Jatene	Switch in position of great arteries with reanastomosis of coronary arteries	Transposition
Glenn	Superior vena cava to right pulmonary artery anastomosis; bidirectional type provides flow to both pulmonary arteries	Tricuspid atresia; hypoplastic right ventricle; pulmonary atresia with intact ventricular septum; single ventricle
Fontan	Anastomosis of right atrium to pulmonary artery or conduit between the two	Tricuspid atresia; severe tricuspid stenosis; hypoplastic right ventricle, single ventricle
Rastelli	Conduit from right ventricle to pulmonary artery	Pulmonary atresia; severe infundibular stenosis; transposition with pulmonic stenosis
Waterston (Cooley)	Ascending aorta to right pulmonary artery anastomosis	Pulmonic stenosis; pulmonary atresia; tricuspid atresia
Blalock-Taussig	Subclavian to pulmonary artery anastomosis or conduit	Tricuspid atresia; pulmonary atresia; tetralogy of Fallot
Potts	Descending aorta to left pulmonary artery anastomosis	Tricuspid atresia; pulmonary atresia; tetralogy of Fallot
Central shunt	Conduit from aorta to pulmonary artery	Tricuspid atresia; pulmonary atresia; tetralogy of Fallot
Damus	End-to-side anastomosis of proximal main pulmonary artery to ascending aorta with shunt from aorta to disconnected distal pulmonary artery	Single left ventricle with transposition and subaortic stenosis; other complex CHD with subaortic stenosis
Norwood	*Palliative stage:* End-to-side anastomosis of main PA to ascending aorta, ligation of ductus arteriosus, systemic-to-PA shunt, creation of nonrestrictive ASD	Hypoplastic left heart
	Reparative stage: Modified Fontan and closure of systemic-pulmonary shunt	

ASD, Atrial septal defect; *CHD,* congestive heart disease; *PA,* pulmonary artery.

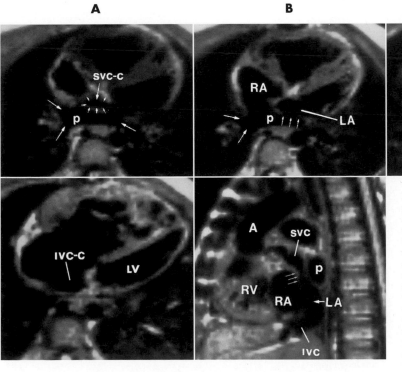

FIGURE 20-42 Complete transposition of great arteries after Senning procedure, cranial (**A**) to caudal (**D**). Pulmonary venous return (*long arrows* in **A** and **B**) is rerouted to the right atrium *(RA)* by way of a new venous channel *(p)*, which is formed by flaps (*small arrows* in **B**) of the interatrial septum and right atrial free wall. Consequently, systemic and pulmonary venous returns are switched at the atrial level (*curved arrows* in **C**). No obstruction is found at the pulmonary venous channel on the transverse images. However, obstructive systemic venous channel *(SVC-C)* from the superior vena cava *(SVC)* to the left atrium *(LA)* is shown on transverse (**A**) and sagittal (**E**) images (*small arrows* in **A** and **E**). *RV,* Right ventricle; *LV,* left ventricle; *A,* aorta; *IVC-C,* systemic venous channel from inferior vena cava to left atrium.

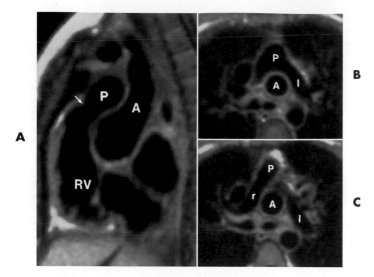

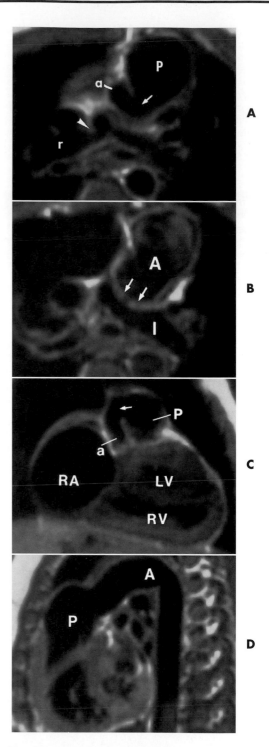

FIGURE 20-43 Complete transposition of great arteries after Jatene procedure. **A,** Sagittal image depicts the site of anastomosis *(arrow)* to the switched main pulmonary artery *(P)*, which does not have substantial stenosis. **B** and **C,** Transverse images show no stenoses between the main pulmonary artery *(P)* and the left *(l)* or right *(r)* pulmonary arteries. *RV,* Right ventricle; *A,* aorta.

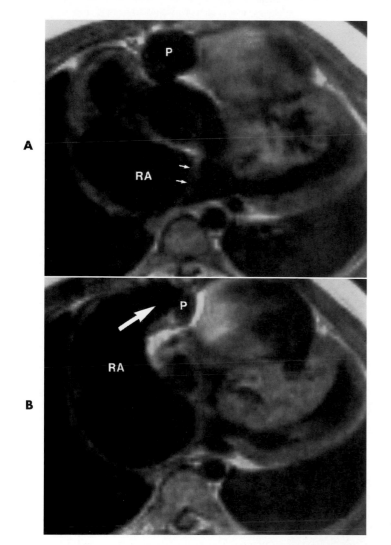

FIGURE 20-45 Tricuspid atresia after Fontan procedure. Transverse image **A** is cranial to **B.** Anastomosis *(arrow* in **B)** between the right atrium *(RA)* and the pulmonary artery *(P)* is shown. Bowing of the interatrial septum to the left *(short arrows* in **A)** indicates right atrial hypertension.

FIGURE 20-44 Hypoplastic left heart syndrome after Norwood procedure. Transverse (**A** and **B**) and coronal (**C**) images show a widely patent anastomosis *(arrow* in **A** and **C)** between the diminutive ascending aorta *(a)* and pulmonary artery *(P)*. Focal stenosis *(arrowhead* in **A)** is found at the origin of the right pulmonary artery *(r)*, and segmental stenosis *(arrows* in **B)** occurs at the left pulmonary artery *(l)*. **D,** Sagittal image shows the entire anatomy of the reconstructed aorta. No significant stenosis is found. *RA,* Right atrium; *RV,* right ventricle; *LV,* left ventricle.

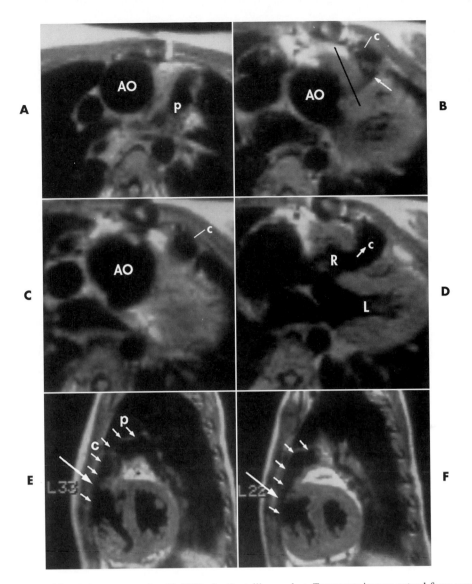

FIGURE 20-46   Pulmonary atresia with VSD after Rastelli procedure. Transverse images extend from cranial **(A)** to caudal **(D)**. Anastomosis between the right ventricle *(R)* and an external conduit *(c)* is shown in **D.** Stenosis of the conduit is found at the next cranial slice **(C).** Note the anteriorly malaligned infundibular septum *(black line* in **B)** and atretic right ventricular outflow tract *(small arrow).* **E** and **F,** Sagittal images show stenosis *(large arrow)* of the external conduit *(small arrows)* between the sternum and right ventricle wall. *P,* Pulmonary artery. (From Higgins CB, et al: Congenital heart disease, New York, 1990, Raven Press.)

FUNCTIONAL EVALUATION WITH CINE AND FLOW TECHNIQUES

Assessment of cardiac function is an important part of the complete evaluation of CHD. Advances in cine and velocity-encoded cine techniques have allowed MRI to become a comprehensive technique for evaluation of cardiovascular dimensions and function. Abnormal flow velocities and flow profiles can be recognized with cine sequences. Quantitative velocity and flow measurements in the heart and great vessels can be accomplished with velocity-encoded cine MRI.

Cine Techniques

Cine MRI produces multiple time-resolved images of the cardiac cycle at each level imaged, with flowing blood displayed as high signal intensity (bright) against a dark background of stationary tissue. By displaying images in a cinematic loop, blood flow and wall motion can be visualized, similar to cine angiography using contrast media.

Blood flow with abnormal flow patterns, such as jets or turbulent flow, is shown as a region of signal void within the bright blood pool on cine MRI (Figure 20-47). This signal difference caused by abnormal flow can be used to evaluate valvular regurgitation. Several reports have shown that the size of the signal void correlates with the degree of severity of valvular regurgitation in adults.[64,65,95] Signal void is also observed in the flow through VSDs, which is useful for identifying the atypical locations of these defects (Figure 20-28). Caval obstruction, which may be a complication after an intraatrial baffle procedure for complete transposition, can be detected by the presence of the signal void.[19] A study of coarctation of the aorta showed that the severity of the stenosis at the coarctation correlates well with the length of the signal void projected downstream from the coarctation.[84]

High temporal resolution attained by cine MRI enables the evaluation of RV and LV function by isolating images corresponding to end-systole and end-diastole. When such images are obtained in a volumetric fashion through both ventricles, left and right ventricular end-diastolic volumes, end-systolic volumes, and stroke volumes can be calculated without reliance on geometric assumptions. Because ventricular anatomy may be distorted in CHD, MRI may have an advantage over both ECG and angiocardiography, since the latter two rely on geometrical assumptions.

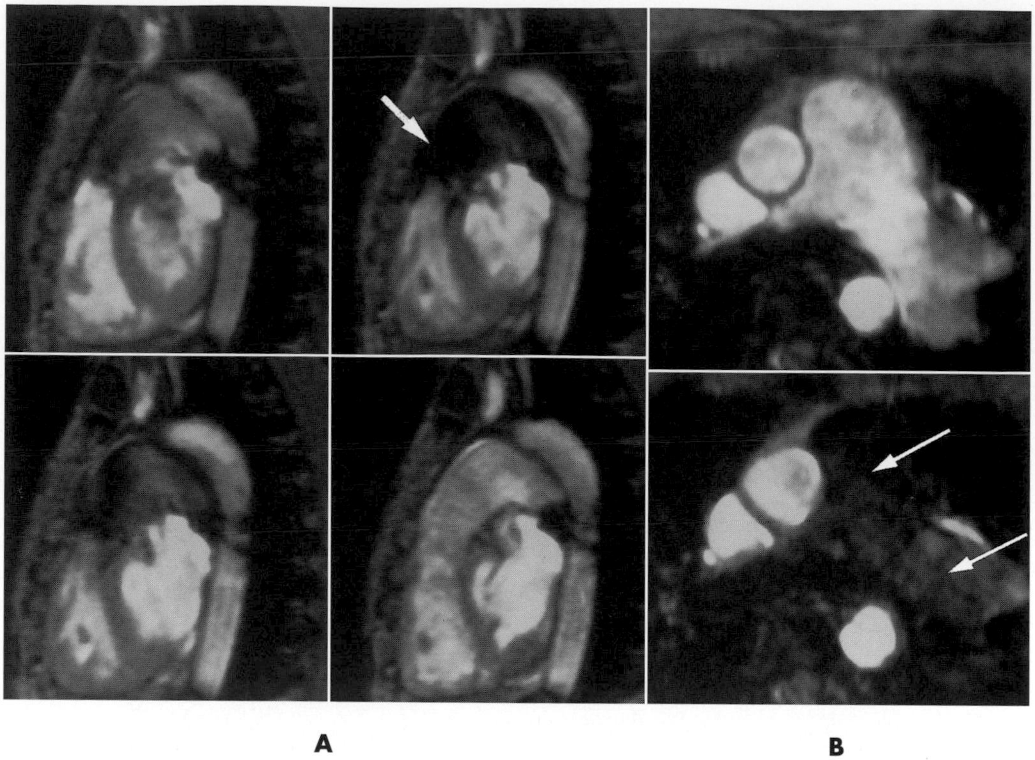

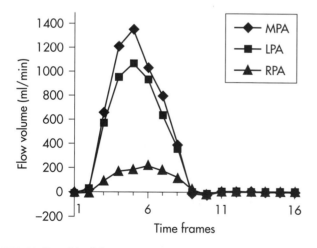

FIGURE 20-47   Cine MR images of valvular pulmonary stenosis. Sagittal **(A)** and transverse **(B)** images. Signal void caused by turbulent blood flow across the stenotic pulmonic valve during systole *(arrows)*. Increased signal intensity is seen in diastole.

FIGURE 20-48   Blood flow measurement in right pulmonary artery (RPA) stenosis. Instantaneous blood flow is calculated in the main pulmonary artery (MPA), left pulmonary artery (LPA), and RPA during each of 16 velocity-encoded cine MR frames, by multiplying the cross-sectional area of each vessel by the mean flow velocity within the vessel during the frame. Blood flow in the RPA is markedly diminished.

Velocity-Encoded Cine Techniques

MR velocity mapping, or velocity-encoded cine technique, is a more recently developed and powerful technique for the functional assessment of CHD.[12] Quantitative phase images provided by this technique contain two-dimensional velocity maps similar to duplex Doppler color flow mapping. Flow velocity in cardiac chambers along a desired direction can be displayed as gray-scale differences on MRI. Therefore shunt flow through ASDs[12,44] or VSDs[44] can be recognized on the velocity maps. Quantification of flow volume in the great arteries just above the RV or LV provides the blood volume ejected from each ven-

tricle, which correlates well with geometrical measurements obtained by the cine technique just described. Blood flow in the aorta, main pulmonary artery, and branch pulmonary arteries can be measured by the velocity-encoded cine technique. These data allow quantification of shunt fraction and differential pulmonary blood flow (Figure 20-48).[73] Velocity-encoded measurement of collateral blood flow in aortic coarctation has been described (Figure 20-49).[88] Velocity encoding has been used to assess valvular regurgitation after corrective surgery for tetralogy of Fallot,[69] tricuspid flow after Senning or Mustard surgeries,[70] and pulmonary blood flow after Fontan surgery.[71] Functional MRI can therefore assess both cardiac motion and cardiovascular flow dynamics. These may prove to be a useful adjunct to anatomical MRI techniques in many forms of CHD.

SUMMARY

MRI is an extremely powerful noninvasive tool for the anatomical depiction of CHD and evaluation of hemodynamics. At this time, several limitations of MRI still exist for the evaluation of CHD. Valvular lesions and abnormalities of the subvalvular tensor apparatus are difficult to demonstrate clearly on spin-echo MRI. This limitation is caused by partial volume averaging of cardiac structures within the slice thickness and by motion of structures during image acquisition. Although cine MRI reduces motion artifacts, spatial and temporal resolution still are not sufficient to depict such structures reliably. Structural evaluation of cardiac valves is clearly one area where ECG remains superior to MRI.

Another limitation of MRI is related to its relatively long time of examination. A full examination of a patient with CHD requires 30 to 60 min. This requires deep sedation for infants and small children. Ultrafast imaging sequences, such as echo-planar and turbo fast low-angle shot (FLASH),[3,41,76] may reduce or eliminate the need for sedation. By using these techniques, 8 or 16 images per cardiac cycle can be obtained within 20 sec. Fast versions of velocity-encoding sequences are also in development.[67] Although these techniques are currently limited by relatively low spatial resolution, future technical development may enable them to be applied effectively in evaluation of children with CHD.

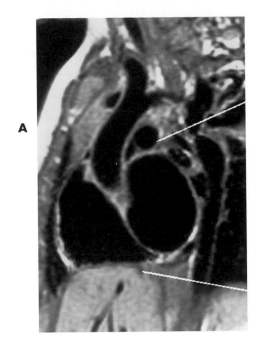

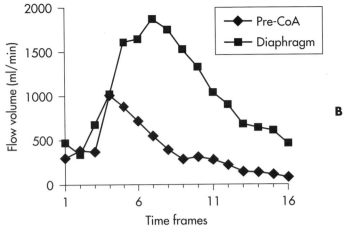

FIGURE 20-49 Collateral flow measurement in aortic coarctation. Velocity-encoded cine acquisitions just proximal to a severe aortic coarctation and at the diaphragm **(A)** produce flow-time curves **(B)** representing aortic flow at these two levels. The large increase in flow at the diaphragmatic level relative to the prestenotic level represents collateral contribution to abdominal aortic inflow.

REFERENCES

1. Akins EW, Martin TD, Alexander JA, et al: MR imaging of double-outlet right ventricle, Am J Roentgenol 152:128, 130, 1989.
2. Anderson KR, and Lie JT: Pathologic anatomy of Ebstein's anomaly of the heart revisited, Am J Cardiol 41:739, 1978.
3. Atkinson DJ, Burstein D, Edelman RR: First-pass cardiac perfusion: evaluation with ultrafast MR imaging, Radiology 174:757, 1990.
4. Bailes DR, Gilderdale DJ, Bydder GM, et al: Respiratory ordered phase encoding (ROPE), a method for reducing respiratory motion artifacts in magnetic resonance imaging, J Comput Assist Tomogr 9:835, 1985.
5. Baker EJ, Ayton V, Smith MA, et al: Magnetic resonance imaging at a high field strength of ventricular septal defects in infants, Br Heart J 62:305, 1989.
6. Baker EJ, Ayton V, Smith MA, et al: Magnetic resonance imaging of coarctation of the aorta in infants: use of a high field strength, Br Heart J 62:97, 1989.
7. Bank ER, Aisen AM, Rocchini AP, et al: Coarctation of the aorta in children undergoing angioplasty: pretreatment and posttreatment MR imaging, Radiology 162:235, 1987.
8. Becker AE, and Anderson RH: Pathology of congenital heart disease, London, 1981, Butterworth Publishers.
9. Bisset GS III, Kirks DR, Strife JL, et al: Cor triatriatum: diagnosis by MR imaging, Am J Roentgenol 149:567, 1987.
10. Bisset GS III, Strife JL, Kirks DR, et al: Vascular rings: MR imaging, Am J Roentgenol 149:251, 1987.
11. Blankenberg F, Rhee J, Hardy C, et al: MRI vs. echocardiography in the evaluation of the Jatene procedure, J Comput Assist Tomogr 18:749, 1994.
12. Brenner LD, Caputo GR, Mostbeck G, et al: Quantification of left to right atrial shunts with velocity-encoded cine nuclear magnetic resonance imaging, J Am Coll Cardiol 20:1246, 1992.
13. Boxer RA, LaCorte MA, Singh S, et al: Nuclear magnetic resonance imaging in evaluation and follow-up of children for coarctation of the aorta, J Am Coll Cardiol 7:1095, 1986.
14. Boxer RA, LaCorte MA, Singh S, et al: Noninvasive diagnosis of congenital left coronary artery to right ventricle fistula by nuclear magnetic resonance imaging, Pediatr Cardiol 10:45, 1989.
15. Campbell RM, Moreau GA, Johns JA, et al: Detection of caval obstruction by magnetic resonance imaging after intracardiac repair of transposition of the great arteries, Am J Cardiol 60:688, 1987.
16. Canter CE, Gutierrez FR, Mirowitz SA, et al: Evaluation of pulmonary arterial morphology in cyanotic congenital heart disease by magnetic resonance imaging, Am Heart J 118:347, 1989.
17. Caputo G, Kondo C, Masui T, et al: Right and left lung perfusion: in vitro and in vivo validation with oblique angle, velocity-encoded cine MR imaging, Radiology 180:693, 1991.
18. Caputo GR, Steiman D, Funari M, et al: Quantification of aortic regurgitation by velocity encoded cine MR imaging, Circulation 84(Suppl II):203, 1991.
19. Chung KJ, Simpson IA, Glass RF, et al: Cine magnetic resonance imaging after surgical repair in patients with transposition of the great arteries, Circulation 77:104, 1988.
20. Crupi G, Macarteney FJ, Anderson RH: Persistent truncus arteriosus: a study of 66 autopsy cases with special reference to definition and morphogenesis, Am J Cardiol 70:569, 1977.
21. Cynthia S, Martinez J, Rees S, et al: Evaluation of Fontan's operation by magnetic resonance imaging, Am J Cardiol 65:819, 1990.
22. Darling RC, Rathney MB, Cring JM: Total anomalous pulmonary venous drainage into the right side of the heart: report of 17 autopsied cases not associated with other major cardiovascular anomalies, Lab Invest 6:44, 1957.
23. Didier D, and Higgins CB: Identification and localization of ventricular septal defect by gated magnetic resonance imaging, Am J Cardiol 57:1363, 1986.
24. Didier D, Higgins CB, Fisher MR, et al: Congenital heart disease: gated MR imaging in 72 patients, Radiology 158:227, 1986.
25. Diethelm L, Déry R, Lipton MJ, et al: Atrial-level shunts: sensitivity and specificity of MR in diagnosis, Radiology 162:181, 1987.
26. Dimick RN, Hedlund LW, and Herfkens RJ: Optimizing electrocardiograph electrode placement for cardiac-gated magnetic resonance imaging, Invest Radiol 22:17, 1987.
27. Dinsmore RE, Wismer GL, Levine RA, et al: Magnetic resonance imaging of the heart: positioning and gradient angle selection for optimal imaging planes, Am J Roentgenol 143:1135, 1984.
28. Doorey AJ, Wills JS, Blasetto J, et al: Usefulness of magnetic resonance imaging for diagnosing an anomalous coronary artery coursing between aorta and pulmonary trunk, Am J Cardiol 74:198, 1994.
29. Duard H, Barat JL, Laurent F, et al: Magnetic resonance imaging of an anomalous origin of the left coronary artery from the pulmonary artery, Eur Heart J 9:1356, 1988.
30. Duerinckx AJ, Orman M: Two-dimensional coronary MR angiography: analysis of initial clinical results, Radiology 193:731, 1994.
31. Edelman RR, Manning WJ, Gervino E, et al: Flow velocity quantification in human coronary arteries with fast, breath-hold MR angiography, J Magn Reson Imag 3:699, 1993.
32. Eichenberger AC, Jenni R, von Schulthess GK: Aortic valve pressure gradients in patients with aortic valve stenosis: quantification with velocity-encoded cine MR imaging, Am J Roentgenol 160:971, 1993.
33. Firmin DN, Nayler GL, Klipstein RH, et al: In vivo validation of MR velocity imaging, J Comput Assist Tomogr 11:751, 1987.
34. Fisher MR, Hricak H, Higgins CB: Magnetic resonance imaging of developmental venous anomalies, Am J Roentgenol 145:705, 1985.
35. Fletcher BD, Jacobstein MD, Abramowsky CR, et al: Right atrioventricular valve atresia: anatomical evaluation with MR imaging, Am J Roentgenol 148:671, 1987.
36. Fletcher BD, Jacobstein MD, Nelson AD, et al: Gated magnetic resonance imaging of congenital cardiac malformations, Radiology 150:137, 1984.
37. Formanek AG, Witcofski RL, D'Souza VJ, et al: MR imaging of the central pulmonary arterial tree in conotruncal malformation, Am J Roentgenol 147:1127, 1986.
38. Greenberg SB, Faerber EN, Balsara RK: Tetralogy of Fallot: diagnostic imaging after palliative and corrective surgery, J Thorac Imaging 10:26, 1995.
39. Geva T, Vick GW, Wendt RE, et al: Role of spin echo and cine magnetic resonance imaging in presurgical planning of heterotaxy syndrome, Circulation 90:348, 1994.
40. Guit GL, Bluemm R, Rohmer J, et al: Levotransposition of the aorta: identification of segmental cardiac anatomy using MR imaging, Radiology 161:673, 1986.
41. Hasse A, Frahm J, Matthaei D, et al: FLASH imaging; rapid NMR imaging using low flip angle pulses, J Magn Reson 67:258, 1986.
42. Higgins CB, Byrd BF III, Farmer DW, et al: Magnetic resonance imaging in patients with congenital heart disease, Circulation 70:851, 1984.
43. Hirsch R, Kilner PJ, Connelly MS, et al: Diagnosis in adolescents and adults with congenital heart disease: prospective assessment of individual and combined roles of magnetic resonance imaging and transesophageal echocardiography, Circulation 90:2937, 1994.

44. Hundley WG, Li HF, Lange RA, et al: Assessment of left-to-right intracardiac shunting by velocity-encoded, phase-difference magnetic resonance imaging: a comparison with oximetric and indicator dilution techniques, Circulation 91:2955, 1995.

45. Jacobstein MD, Fletcher BD, Goldstein S, et al: Evaluation of atrioventricular septal defect by magnetic resonance imaging, Am J Cardiol 55:1158, 1985.

46. Jacobstein MD, Fletcher BD, Goldstein S, et al: Magnetic resonance imaging in patients with hypoplastic right heart syndrome, Am Heart J 110:154, 1985.

47. Jacobstein MD, Fletcher BD, Nelson AD, et al: Magnetic resonance imaging: evaluation of palliative systemic–pulmonary artery shunts, Circulation 70:650, 1984.

48. Julsrud PR, Ehman RL, Hagler DJ, et al: Extracardiac vasculature in candidates for Fontan surgery: MR imaging, Radiology 173:503, 1989.

49. Kersting-Sommerhoff BA, Diethelm L, Teitel DF, et al: Magnetic resonance imaging of congenital heart disease: sensitivity and specificity using receiver operating characteristic curve analysis, Am Heart J 118:155, 1989.

50. Kersting-Sommerhoff BA, Sechtem UP, Fisher MR, et al: MR imaging of congenital anomalies of the aortic arch, Am J Roentgenol 149:9, 1987.

51. Kersting-Sommerhoff BA, Sechtem UP, Higgins CB: Evaluation of pulmonary blood supply by nuclear magnetic resonance in patients with pulmonary atresia, J Am Coll Cardiol 11:166, 1988.

52. Kersting-Sommerhoff BA, Seelos KC, Hardy C, et al: Evaluation of surgical procedures for cyanotic congenital heart disease by using MR imaging, Am J Roentgenol 159:255, 1990.

53. Kilner PJ, Firmin DN, Rees RS, et al: Valve and great vessel stenosis: assessment with MR jet velocity mapping, Radiology 178:229, 1991.

54. Link KM, Herrera MA, D'Souza V, et al: MR imaging of Ebstein anomaly: results in four cases, Am J Roentgenol 150:363, 1988.

55. Link KM, Weesner KM, Formanek AG: MR imaging of the criss-cross heart, Am J Roentgenol 152:809, 1989.

56. Lucas RV: Anomalous venous connections, pulmonary and systemic. In Adams FH, and Emmanouilides GC, eds: Heart disease in infants, children and adolescents, ed 3, Baltimore, 1983, Williams & Wilkins.

57. Machado C, Bhasin S, Soulen RL: Confirmation of anomalous origin of the right coronary artery from the left sinus of Valsalva with magnetic resonance imaging, Chest 104:1284, 1993.

58. Mohaddin RH, Kilner PJ, Rees S, et al: Magnetic resonance volume flow and jet velocity mapping in aortic coarctation, J Am Coll Cardiol 22:1515, 1993.

59. Moran PR, Moran RA, Karstaedt NK: Verification and evaluation of internal flow and motion, Radiology 154:433, 1985.

60. Nayler GL, Firmin DN, Longmore DB: Blood flow imaging by cine magnetic resonance, J Comput Assist Tomogr 10:715, 1986.

61. Niwa K, Uchishiba M, Aotsuka H, et al: Magnetic resonance imaging of heterotaxia in infants, J Am Coll Cardiol 23:177 1994.

62. Park ET, Han MC, Kim C: MR imaging of congenitally corrected transposition of the great vessels in adults, Am J Roentgenol 153:491, 1989.

63. Paschal CB, Haacke EM, Adler LP, et al: Magnetic resonance coronary artery imaging, Cardiovasc Intervent Radiol 15:23, 1992.

64. Pflugfelder PW, Landzberg JS, Cassidy MM, et al: Comparison of cine MR imaging with Doppler echocardiography for the evaluation of aortic regurgitation, Am J Roentgenol 152:729, 1989.

65. Pflugfelder PW, Sechtem UP, White RD, et al: Noninvasive evaluation of mitral regurgitation by analysis of left atrial signal loss in cine magnetic resonance, Am Heart J 117:1113, 1989.

66. Pflugfelder PW, Sechtem UP, White RD, et al: Quantification of regional function by rapid cine MR imaging, Am J Roentgenol 150:523, 1988.

67. Pike GB, Meyer CH, Brosnan TJ, et al: Magnetic resonance velocity imaging using a fast spiral phase contrast sequence, Magn Reson Med 32:476, 1994.

68. Raghib G, Ruttenberg HD, Anderson RC, et al: Termination of left superior vena cava in left atrium, atrial septal defect, and absence of coronary sinus: a developmental complex, Circulation 31:906, 1965.

69. Rebergen SA, Chin JGJ, Ottenkamp J, et al: Pulmonary regurgitation in the late postoperative followup of tetralogy of Fallot: volumetric quantification by MR velocity mapping, Circulation 88:2257, 1993.

70. Rebergen SA, Helbing WA, van der Wall EE, et al: MR velocity mapping of tricuspid flow in normal children and patients who have undergone Mustard or Senning repair, Radiology 194:505, 1995.

71. Rebergen SA, Ottenkamp J, Doornbos J, et al: Postoperative pulmonary flow dynamics after Fontan surgery: assessment with MR velocity mapping, J Am Coll Cardiol 21:123, 1993.

72. Rees RSO, Somerville J, Underwood SR, et al: Magnetic resonance imaging of the pulmonary arteries and their systemic connections in pulmonary atresia: comparison with angiographic and surgical findings, Br Heart J 58:621, 1987.

73. Rees S, Firmin D, Mohiaddin R, et al: Application of flow measurements by magnetic resonance velocity mapping to congenital heart disease, Am J Cardiol 64:953, 1989.

74. Rees S, Somerville J, Ward C, et al: Coarctation of the aorta: MR imaging in late postoperative assessment, Radiology 173:499, 1989.

75. Rumancik WM, Hernanz-Schulman M, Rutkowski MM, et al: Magnetic resonance imaging of cor triatriatum, Pediatr Cardiol 9:149, 1988.

76. Rzedzian RR, and Pykett IL: Instant images of the human heart using a new, whole-body MR imaging system, Am J Roentgenol 149:245, 1987.

77. Sampson C, Kilner PJ, Hirsch R, et al: Venoatrial pathways after the Mustard operation for transposition of the great arteries: anatomical and functional MR imaging, Radiology 193:211, 1994.

78. Sampson C, Martinez J, Rees S, et al: Evaluation of Fontan's operation by magnetic resonance imaging, Am J Cardiol 65:819, 1990.

79. Satomi G, and Takao A: Systematic diagnosis method of two-dimensional echocardiography in congenital heart disease, Heart Vessels 1:101, 1985.

80. Schultz CL, Morrison S, Bryan PJ: Azygous continuation of the inferior vena cava: demonstration by NMR imaging, J Comput Assist Tomogr 8:774, 1984.

81. Sechtem U, Pflugfelder P, Cassidy MC, et al: Ventricular septal defect: visualization of shunt flow and determination of shunt size by cine MR imaging, Am J Roentgenol 149:689, 1987.

82. Sechtem U, Pflugfelder P, Gould R, et al: Measurement of right and left ventricular volumes in healthy individuals with cine MR imaging, Radiology 163.697, 1987.

83. Sechtem U, Pflugfelder PW, White RD, et al: Cine MRI: potential for the evaluation of cardiovascular function, Am J Roentgenol 148:239, 1987.

84. Simpson IA, Chung KJ, Glass RF, et al: Cine magnetic resonance imaging for evaluation of anatomy and flow relations in infants and children with coarctation of the aorta, Circulation 78:142, 1988.

85. Simpson IA, and Sahn DJ: Adult congenital heart disease: use of transthoracic echocardiography versus magnetic resonance imaging scanning, Am J Card Imaging 9:29, 1995.

86. Smith MA, Baker EJ, Ayton VT, et al: Magnetic resonance imaging of the infant heart at 1.5 T, Br J Radiol 62:367, 1989.

87. Soulen RL, Kan J, Mithell S, et al: Evaluation of balloon angioplasty of coarctation restenosis by magnetic resonance imaging, Am J Cardiol 60:343, 1987.

88. Steffens JC, Bourne MW, Sakuma H, et al: Quantification of collateral blood flow in coarctation of the aorta by velocity encoded cine magnetic resonance imaging, Circulation 90:937, 1994.

89. Theissen P, Kaemmerer H, Sechtem U, et al: Magnetic resonance imaging of cardiac function and morphology in patients with transposition of the great arteries following Mustard procedure, Thorac Cardiovasc Surg 39:221, 1991.

90. Utz JA, Herfkens RJ, Heinsimer JA, et al: Cine MR determination of left ventricular ejection fraction, Am J Roentgenol 148:839, 1987.

91. van Dijk P: Direct cardiac NMR imaging of heart wall and blood flow velocity, J Comput Assist Tomogr 8:429, 1984.

92. van Praagh R: The segmental approach to diagnosis in congenital heart disease, Birth Defects 8:4, 1972.

93. van Praagh R: The importance of segmental situs in the diagnosis of congenital heart disease, Semin Roentgenol 20:254, 1985.

94. von Schulthess GK, Higashino ST, Higgins SS, et al: Coarctation of the aorta: MR imaging, Radiology 158:469, 1986.

95. Wagner S, Auffermann W, Buser P, et al: Diagnostic accuracy and estimation of the severity of valvular regurgitation from the signal void on cine magnetic resonance images, Am Heart J 118:760, 1989.

96. Wang JK, Li YW, Chiu IS, et al: Usefulness of magnetic resonance imaging in the assessment of venoatrial connections, atrial morphology, bronchial situs, and other anomalies in right atrial isomerism, Am J Cardiol 74:701, 1994.

97. Wenink ACG, Ottenkamp J, Guit GL, et al: Correlation of morphology of the left ventricular outflow tract with two-dimensional Doppler echocardiography and magnetic resonance imaging with atrioventricular septal defect, Am J Cardiol 63:1137, 1989.

98. Wexler L, and Higgins CB: The use of magnetic resonance imaging in adult congenital heart disease, Am J Cardiac Imag 9:15, 1995.

99. Yoo SJ, Lim TH, Park IS, et al: Defects of the intraventricular septum of the heart: en face MR imaging in the oblique coronal plane, Am J Roentgenol 157:943, 1991.

100. Yoo SJ, Seo JW, Lim TH, et al: Hearts with twisted atrioventricular connections: findings at MR imaging, Radiology 188:109, 1993.

21 Acquired Heart Disease

David A. Bluemke and Jerrold L. Boxerman

 KEY POINTS

- MRI is the procedure of choice for evaluation of cardiac and paracardiac tumors.
- Breath-hold MR sequences for cardiac imaging are becoming the standard for imaging cardiac function.
- MRI with myocardial tagging is the only noninvasive method for quantitatively assessing myocardial mechanics in a three-dimensional manner, accounting for through-plane motion.
- Coronary MR angiography techniques remain preliminary because of the limited resolution available, but progress is being made using navigator echoes to compensate for respiratory motion for three-dimensional acquisitions.
- MRI has become the gold standard for analysis of cardiac structure and morphology.

Magnetic resonance imaging (MRI) is becoming the noninvasive gold standard for the assessment of cardiac structure and function. The high contrast between moving blood and the myocardium, high spatial resolution, and lack of ionizing radiation make MRI a superb technique for myocardial assessment. This chapter reviews technical considera-

tions in magnetic resonance (MR) evaluation of cardiovascular disease, with emphasis on newer rapid imaging techniques, describes established clinical MR applications, and demonstrates novel approaches to cardiovascular disease diagnosis.

TECHNICAL CONSIDERATIONS

Cardiac motion poses a fundamental problem that is unique when compared with other MR applications. The current generation of MR scanners has primarily been designed to image the central nervous system, which is relatively free from motion. Thus imaging times on the order of 1 to 10 min or more are acceptable. Cardiac motion, however, demands time resolution on the order of 25 to 50 ms. Furthermore, the ideal imaging planes for cross-sectional analysis of the heart are generally not the orthogonal axes of the body. Although a new generation of dedicated cardiovascular MR scanners is being designed to specifically accommodate these requirements, cardiovascular imaging using the majority of currently available MR hardware platforms requires meticulous attention to technique.

Cardiac Gating

MR images of the heart must be restricted to a constant portion of the cardiac cycle or "gated" to avoid blurring. Coordination of pulse-

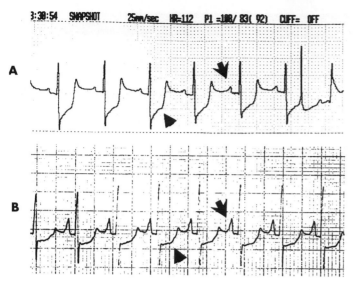

3:30:54 SNAPSHOT   25mm/sec   HR=112 P1 =108/ 83(92)   CUFF= OFF

A

B

FIGURE 21-1   MR scanner effect on ECG. **A,** ECG from a dog instrumented with a flow reducer in the left anterior descending artery. The ST segment is depressed *(arrowhead),* and a small P wave is present *(arrow).* **B,** ECG from the same experiment taken while the animal was adjacent to a 1.5 T MR scanner. Note that the amplitude of the P wave is enlarged and the T wave is diminished. The ST depression has virtually disappeared in the high field. The heart rate was slightly increased at MRI. Both ECGs were recorded with 1 mV/cm and 25 mm/sec. (Courtesy D. Kraitchman, Baltimore.)

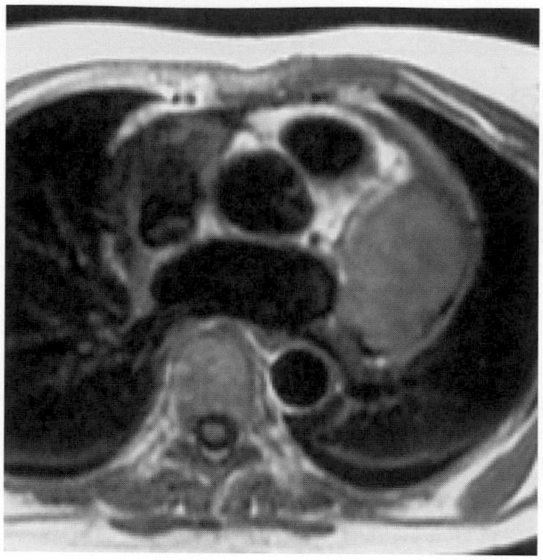

FIGURE 21-2   Mesothelioma of the pericardium. Axial T1-weighted image shows intermediate–signal intensity mass adjacent to the pericardium.

sequence timing relative to the cardiac contraction reduces flow and motion artifacts. The two methods that achieve gating are (1) triggering to the QRS complex of the electrocardiogram (ECG) and (2) triggering to a peripheral pulse. Because of the substantial delay time from the QRS complex to the onset of the peripheral pulse, ECG gating is strongly recommended. Only in the most difficult cases, such as extremely low–voltage ECG (e.g., patients with cardiac failure), is peripheral-pulse gating used as an alternative method.

Triggering to the ECG is complicated by distortion of the normal ECG pattern that is a result of the magnetic field. The so-called magnetohydrodynamic effect refers to the generation of an electric current when a conducting fluid (blood) moves in a magnetic field.[41] Although only a small current is generated by this effect, there are substantial alterations of the ECG. The magnetohydrodynamic effect is a function of the velocity of moving blood, the direction of blood flow, and the magnetic field strength. The effect is greater at higher field strengths and is greatest at high blood velocities (systole). No direct physiological effect of this induced current has been described.

The magnetohydrodynamic effect has a detrimental effect on ECG and causes an increase in the size of T waves. With dobutamine stimulation of the heart (dobutamine stress MRI), T waves increase further in amplitude as the velocity of ejected blood from the left ventricle (LV) increases. Under these circumstances, the gating subsystem of the MR scanner may have difficulty in distinguishing the R wave from the T wave. Ischemia that could occur during MR scanning may potentially be masked on the ECG because of elevation of the ST segment (Figure 21-1). Repositioning the ECG leads may aid in reducing the size of the T waves. The changing magnetic field gradients may also lead to an induced current in the ECG signal. This appears as noise on the ECG. Most modern gating subsystems either have built-in filters or ignore the ECG after successful detection of an R wave.

Patients with dysrhythmias impose an additional limitation. Using breath-hold imaging techniques (discussed later), the number of cardiac phases or slices may have to be reduced substantially to accommodate reasonable breath-hold times. Moreover, patients with very slow heart rates (often secondary to β-blocking cardiac medications) have relatively long imaging times because each R wave corresponds to one or more lines of κ-space. As the R-R interval increases, the imaging time increases proportionally.

Electrodes that are commonly used for ECG measurement outside of the MR environment frequently have metal components. For MRI,

electrodes with metal components should be avoided because they can result in substantial image artifacts and a signal void that may project over the anterior portion of the heart, particularly on gradient-echo images. Carbon fiber electrodes are commercially available, and these do not cause artifacts on MR images. ECG leads should be placed according to the MR manufacturer's recommendations; typically, four leads are placed anteriorly on the chest. The skin should be cleaned with alcohol, and electrode conducting gel is applied to the skin surface to improve the quality of the ECG signal. Posterior placement of ECG leads on the chest is occasionally used, particularly in female patients because breast tissue may prevent optimum lead placement.

Spin-Echo/Fast Spin-Echo Cardiac Imaging

Conventional Spin-Echo Imaging. The most common pulse sequence traditionally used for cardiac imaging is a conventional spin-echo (CSE) sequence gated to the cardiac cycle in a multislice mode. In this technique the repetition time (TR) is equal to the R-R interval and the minimum echo time (TE) of 10 to 20 ms is used. Because the T1 time of the myocardium is on the order of 800 ms, only moderate T1 weighting is achieved using this method. These images are commonly referred to as *black blood images* because saturation bands are placed above and below the imaging planes and blood in the ventricle is dark. Because the TR depends on the R-R interval, imaging times are typically long (e.g., 6 to 8 min with 192 phase-encoding steps and two signal averages). Image quality is only moderate and depends on consistent ECG gating and lack of patient motion during the relatively long acquisition times. However, the contrast difference between the heart, epicardial fat, and the ventricular cavities is relatively good (Figure 21-2).

T2 weighting for CSE images is achieved by gating at several multiples of the R-R interval, together with a TE of 80 to 100 ms. Imaging times are quite long. The quality of T2-weighted images is lower than the quality of T1-weighted images because of the lower signal-to-noise ratio (SNR) typically associated with long-TE images and the respiratory and cardiac motion, the effects of which may be pronounced as a result of long imaging times. T2-weighted images are usually not necessary for anatomical evaluation of the heart but are more helpful for characterization of cardiac or paracardiac masses (Figure 21-3). In these cases the mass frequently has somewhat restricted motion relative to the myocardium, so that image quality is often adequate.

For both T1- and T2-weighted images the axial plane is typically imaged. Images at multiple cardiac phases typically are not obtained using this method, because each cardiac phase would require a separate image acquisition (i.e., six cardiac phases would require 6 times the total imaging time). Images should be acquired so that the most inferior axial slices are obtained as soon as possible after the R wave of the ECG signal. Each subsequent image slice is obtained at a progressively increasing time delay after the R wave. Note that the duration of the R-R interval shows approximately 5% beat-to-beat variability[72]; the majority of this variability occurs during diastole, with systole relatively more constant in duration. In a multislice acquisition of 15 slices, the initial slices are thus obtained at a more consistent interval from the beginning of the R wave. Thus axial image prescription in an inferior to superior manner substantially improves image quality.

Fast Spin-Echo Imaging. Fast spin-echo (FSE) T2-weighted images should be used, if available, because they provide shorter imaging times and better image resolution than CSE images. Typical echo train lengths (ETLs) are 8 to 16. Because of the high signal intensity of fat on FSE images, chemical shift–fat suppression is frequently used with this method. This technique also has the benefit of decreased respiratory motion artifacts related to motion of otherwise high–signal intensity fat in the anterior chest wall.

FSE with multiple inversion-recovery pulses can be used to obtain black blood images.[143] Using a long ETL of 32, single-slice cardiac images can be obtained during a 20- to 30-sec breath-hold. Overall, the quality of these images is generally much better than that of CSE T1- or T2-weighted images, with substantially reduced imaging times.

Cine Gradient-Echo Imaging

Cine imaging for cardiac MRI consists of a motion picture loop of various phases of the cardiac cycle. Because of advantages with speed of acquisition, gradient-echo techniques are used for image acquisition. To generate cine images, images must be gated to the cardiac cycle. The two general schemes for obtaining the gated images are retrospective and prospective gating. Prospective gating, using segmented κ-space acquisition, is the predominant mode of cine imaging and has widespread applications.

Prospective Cine Acquisition. In prospective cine acquisitions, lines of κ space are acquired beginning immediately after the R wave. In this method, the phase-encoding gradient is incremented for each successive R wave. Thus, if 128 phase-encoding steps are acquired, the pulse sequence would take 128 heartbeats to fill κ space.

Segmented κ-space acquisition allows 12 to 18 phases of the cardiac cycle (referred to later as *movie frames* of a cine sequence) to be acquired in a single breath-hold using prospective cardiac gating.[6] The pulse sequence (Figure 21-4) consists of a fast gradient-recalled echo (GRE) acquisition with a relatively short TR (e.g., 5 to 10 ms), combined with a very short TE (approximately 2 ms) and a flip angle of 10 to 20 degrees. The TR and TE are usually the minimum values achievable by the MR gradient system, so these parameters may be automatically set by the system software. These acquisition parameters result in saturation of stationary tissues, and inflowing blood with unsaturated spins has higher signal (flow-related enhancement).

The unique aspect of the segmented κ-space pulse sequence is the manner in which individual lines of phase-encoded data are acquired (Figure 21-4, *A*). During each heartbeat, the R-R interval of the cardiac cycle is divided into multiple cine "frames" typically of 20- to 80-ms duration.[13] Only a portion, or "segment," of κ space is then collected over the duration of each cine frame. The number of lines of κ space acquired over the duration of a cine frame is referred to as the *number of views per segment* (NVS; also referred to as *number of views per phase [NVP]*). NVS multiplied by the TR equals the duration of the cine frame. By collecting multiple lines of κ space per R-R interval, the imaging time decreases by a factor of NVS. As an example, to complete 128 total phase-encoding steps of κ space with an NVS of 8 requires 128 (size of κ space) divided by 8 (NVS), which equals 16 R-R intervals (or heartbeats). The total acquisition time is thus determined by the patient's heart rate; for an R-R interval of 1 sec (60 beats per minute), the breath-hold time is 16 R-R intervals times 1 sec, which equals 16 sec. In this example, if TR is 10 ms, the duration of the cine

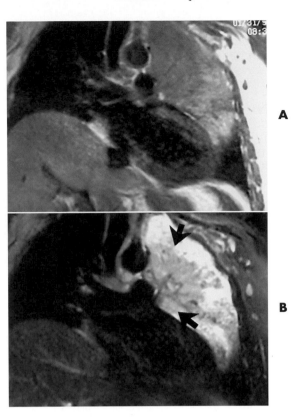

FIGURE 21-3   Lymphoma. **A** and **B**, Axial T1- and T2-weighted coronal images of a patient referred for evaluation of paracardiac mass and left upper lobe atelectasis. The T1-weighted image shows the extent of atelectasis, but on the T2-weighted image (with fat saturation), the central paracardiac masses are depicted as intermediate-intensity masses *(arrows)*, adjacent to the left hilum. Peripheral atelectatic lung shows a somewhat higher signal intensity.

frame is 8 (NVS) times 10 ms (the TR interval), which equals 80 ms. Because the R-R interval is 1 sec long (1000 ms), 1000 ms minus 80 ms equals 920 ms remaining that can be used to collect other lines of κ space for different phases of the cardiac cycle (single-slice, multiple cardiac phase mode). The NVS value is user defined and analogous to a "turbo factor" or ETL with FSE imaging; a higher value reduces the imaging time in direct proportion to the NVS. Similar to using a high ETL (but for different reasons), higher NVS values can result in image blurring. As NVS is increased, each cine frame captures a longer portion of the cardiac cycle (frame duration = NVS × TR); cardiovascular structures are moving rapidly. Also, as NVS is increased, the number of "movie frames" available for cine display correspondingly decreases. For example, for a movie frame duration of 80 ms (NVS × TR = 8 × 10 ms), the maximum number of cardiac cycles is the R-R (interval) divided by the segment duration, or 1000 ms divided by 80 ms, which equals approximately 12 frames. If NVS is 16, the number of separate cardiac frames available is reduced to 6, so the cine display appears less smooth.

"View sharing" is a technique used to interpolate between cine frames. For example, if cine frames are obtained beginning every 50 ms during the cardiac cycle, data from sequential cine frames are interpolated to generate an image at 25-ms intervals. Cine loops of cardiac contraction appear "smoother" with view sharing, and the display is more realistic.[128] Alternatively, if multiple frames of the cardiac cycle are not necessary, the R-R interval can be used to collect lines of κ space for other slice locations (multislice, single cardiac phase mode[128] (Figure 21-4, *B*). In a "multislice" acquisition, similar to a multislice SE image, additional slice locations are acquired, albeit each at a different point in time in the cardiac cycle. Thus instead of 12 cine movie frames in these examples where NVS equals 8, 12 different slice locations can be acquired in a breath-hold. Typically a 10- to 20-degree flip angle is used for these studies, with interslice spacing of up to 20% of the slice thickness. One application of a "multislice" acquisition is the rapid

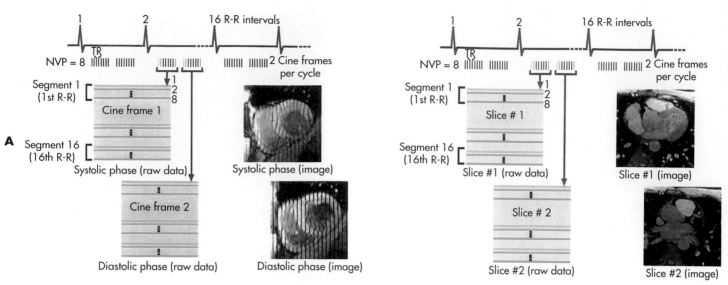

FIGURE 21-4   Segmented κ-space technique. **A,** Single-slice, multiphase mode. Each R-R interval is divided into multiple cardiac phases (cine frames) of relatively short duration, so only a portion or "segment" of κ space for each frame is acquired every heartbeat. Multiple RF pulses are applied during every segment, and each pulse corresponds to one line of κ space. NVS equals 8 in this diagram. For a TR of 5 ms, the temporal resolution of each cine frame is 5 ms × 8 = 40 ms; thus multiple cine frames can be acquired during a typical R-R interval. One of the two segments illustrated here was obtained during systole and the other during diastole. Note that "segments" of κ space are usually not contiguous (like the contiguous segments shown here) but are interleaved to minimize image artifacts. To complete 128 phase-encoding steps requires 128/8 = 16 R-R intervals. **B,** Multislice, single cardiac phase mode. Each R-R interval is again divided into short intervals, each yielding NVS lines of κ space, but each interval now corresponds to a different slice location obtained during different portions of the cardiac cycle. In this example, one slice location is obtained during systole, and the other during diastole. Because flow-related enhancement is greater during systole, using only the first portion of the cardiac cycle increases vascular signal at the expense of slightly increased image acquisition time. (From reference 17.)

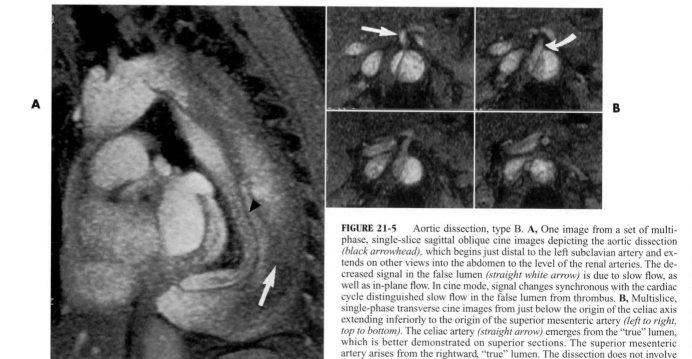

FIGURE 21-5   Aortic dissection, type B. **A,** One image from a set of multiphase, single-slice sagittal oblique cine images depicting the aortic dissection *(black arrowhead),* which begins just distal to the left subclavian artery and extends on other views into the abdomen to the level of the renal arteries. The decreased signal in the false lumen *(straight white arrow)* is due to slow flow, as well as in-plane flow. In cine mode, signal changes synchronous with the cardiac cycle distinguished slow flow in the false lumen from thrombus. **B,** Multislice, single-phase transverse cine images from just below the origin of the celiac axis extending inferiorly to the origin of the superior mesenteric artery *(left to right, top to bottom).* The celiac artery *(straight arrow)* emerges from the "true" lumen, which is better demonstrated on superior sections. The superior mesenteric artery arises from the rightward, "true" lumen. The dissection does not involve the superior mesenteric artery *(curved arrow).* (From reference 17.)

screening of the length of the aorta to determine whether there is involvement of branch vessels in cases of aortic dissection (Figure 21-5).

Rapid image acquisition with a segmented κ-space technique is also beneficial for evaluating ill and potentially unstable patients. Single-phase, multislice acquisitions with multiple signal averages (n = 4 to 8) may provide a rapid examination in sedated or uncooperative patients for whom breath-holding is not possible (Figure 21-6).

Retrospective Cine Acquisition.   In retrospective cine acquisition, rather than gating the acquisition to the cardiac cycle, images are acquired continuously while the ECG signal is recorded. At the end of the acquisition, the cardiac cycle is divided into 10 to 15 cine frames. For each cine frame, κ space is filled with phase-encoding data at the same delay time after the R-R interval. Using this method requires extra imaging time because the duration of the R-R interval varies slightly throughout the cardiac cycle. The images taken using this technique show flowing blood as bright signal intensity relative to the adjacent myocardium. The overall image acquisition time is on the order of 4 to 5 min (varying, depending on the heart rate), and during this time, between two and four separate cine locations can be acquired. The primary disadvantage of this technique is that more rapid methods for acquiring multiple phase-encoding steps of κ space (i.e., segmented κ-space acquisition) are difficult to implement using retrospective gating.

Segmented κ-Space and Echo-Planar Hybrid Techniques

The imaging speed of the standard segmented κ-space technique may be further improved by sampling additional echoes with extra readout-gradient lobes, as is done in echo-planar imaging (EPI). For instance, each additional readout lobe requires approximately an additional 2 ms per radiofrequency (RF) excitation but halves the total number of TR excitations required, thereby reducing the overall imaging time by 30% to 40%. Acquiring additional echoes per TR excitation further reduces the imaging time. Therefore for fixed (constant breath-hold) NVS the temporal resolution (NVS × TR) improves because the "effective TR" per κ-space line decreases. Alternatively, for a given temporal resolution the breath-hold can be reduced because NVS can increase to offset the decreased effective TR.

Hybrid spoiled gradient-recalled echo/echo-planar imaging (SPGR/EPI) reduces several problems associated with standard single-shot EPI yet maintains some of the speed advantage. Single-shot echo-planar images obtained in one heartbeat are susceptible to severe artifacts caused by field inhomogeneities, chemical shift, and motion. However, with a hybrid sequence, the shorter TE reduces image distortion that results from susceptibility differences, ECG gating with shorter temporal resolution helps minimize motion-induced blurring of the heart, and flow sensitivity is inversely proportional to the number of interleaves or echoes per excitation. A hybrid SPGR/EPI sequence[27,93,161] offers a compromise between the speed and high SNR of EPI and the robust image quality and reproducibility of SPGR imaging.

Blood Flow Mapping with Phase-Contrast Techniques

Contrast between the myocardium or aorta and flowing blood may be provided by one of two general techniques: time-of-flight (TOF) or phase-contrast (PC) methods. In TOF imaging, unlabeled spins from blood outside of the imaging plane or volume continually wash in and wash out of the image. Because stationary tissues are relatively saturated by multiple RF pulses, flowing blood has a much higher signal intensity. This phenomenon is referred to as *flow-related enhancement.* Alternatively, PC methods generate contrast between stationary and moving tissues as a result of velocity-induced phase shifts of moving spins in a magnetic field gradient.[155] Images are then reconstructed from the phase of the MR signal rather than the amplitude of that signal. Using this method, the induced phase shift is directly proportional to the velocity so that PC methods allow quantitative measurement of the velocity of flow.[75] Absolute flow (in milliliters per minute) can then be calculated by multiplying the linear blood velocity by the cross-sectional area of the blood vessel (Figure 21-7). This approach has been applied to the measurement of coronary artery blood flow; flow in the aorta, pulmonary arteries, or ventricular cavities of patients with congenital heart defects; and flow across cardiac valves. The primary limiting factor is that motion of any kind, such as respiration or patient movement, also induces a phase shift that cannot be distinguished from actual blood flow. In addition, moderately sophisticated analysis software is required and can necessitate significant amounts of postprocessing time.

Imaging Parameters

The field of view (FOV) is adjusted for patient size (e.g., 28 to 36 cm) to avoid wrap-around artifact. Antialiasing ("no phase wrap") is used only for SE imaging. For breath-hold sequences, antialiasing requires two signal averages and doubles the acquisition time. The matrix size is typically 256 in the frequency-encoding direction and 128 to 256 in the phase-encoding direction. Fractional echo sampling is routinely used for segmented κ-space sequences to reduce the TE. An additional pa-

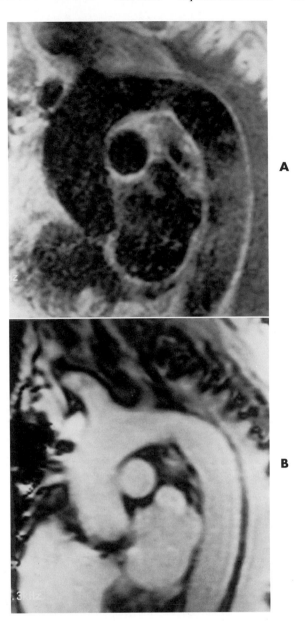

FIGURE 21-6   Aortic valve replacement evaluated for aortic dissection. Breath-holding was not possible for this sedated patient. **A,** CSE T1-weighted sagittal oblique image is contaminated by motion artifact that projects over the descending aorta. Two averages (n = 2) were obtained in 319 sec. **B,** One image from a 5-slice, single-phase set of cine images demonstrating the absence of a dissection. Eight averages (n = 8) were obtained in 71 sec. Because of averaging, the cardiac and respiratory motion artifact is minimal, and dissection was ruled out. (From reference 17.)

rameter, referred to as the *delay time,* indicates when imaging should start in relationship to the QRS complex. Normally the delay time is the minimum value accepted by the system (i.e., image during systole), although coronary arteries are more optimally visualized during diastole. View sharing[128] is used if available and results in a smoother cine animation loop. First-order flow compensation can be used to increase the vascular signal, but flow artifact can also be reduced by using a very short TE (<2.5 ms).

Coil Selection

The body coil can be used for cardiac imaging and has the primary advantage of a large FOV with uniform signal intensity. Pixel sizes, however, must be relatively large (2 mm) to achieve an adequate SNR within reasonable imaging times. Lower bandwidths (±16 kHz) must be used to increase the SNR. It is usually more desirable, however, to

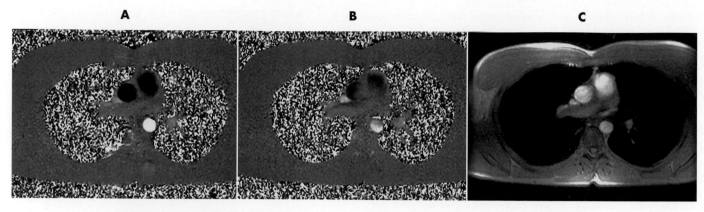

FIGURE 21-7   Aortic flow evaluated with segmented κ-space cine PC acquisition, using 19-ms resolution. Velocity maps obtained 105 ms **(A)** and 257 ms **(B)** after the R wave. Flow was encoded in the superior-to-inferior (black and white signal intensity, respectively) direction. Measured velocities were 20.9 and 14.1 cm/sec in the ascending aorta **(C).** The area of the ascending aorta in the corresponding magnitude image multiplied by the flow rate yields the absolute flow.

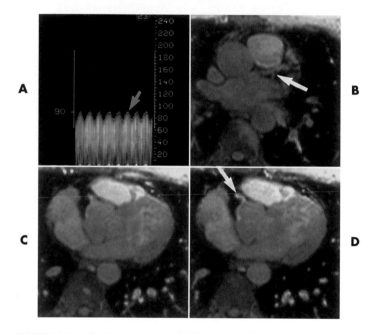

FIGURE 21-8   Navigator echo–based 3D coronary MRA using retrospective respiratory gating. **A,** Sample diaphragm tracking using navigator echoes. The white dotted line *(arrow)* demonstrates the scanner's ability to track the diaphragm at the interface of the lungs *(above)* and liver *(below).* Segments of κ space are acquired during successive heartbeats. If the segment is acquired during an acceptable diaphragm position, the segment is used to construct the appropriate slice; otherwise, it is rejected and not included in image construction. **B,** Sample slice from the 3D coronary MR image set at the level of the left main coronary artery, bifurcating into the left anterior descending and left circumflex *(arrow)* arteries. **C** and **D,** Sample slices from the 3D coronary MR image set at the level of the right coronary artery ostium *(arrow).*

use a phased-array surface coil, if available. The torso coil allows increased bandwidths (±32 kHz or greater) with an adequate SNR, which in turn reduces the minimum TR and TE values, allowing more lines of κ space to be collected per unit time. Dedicated cardiac coils are currently uncommon. The FOV is somewhat smaller than typical torso coils so that optimum placement is necessary for good coverage of the entire LV, as well as the atriums. Coil placement greatly affects the quality of the examination, and optimal results are obtained when the coil is centered around the heart.

Navigator Echoes

Inconsistencies in breath-holding result in lack of anatomical registration between imaging sections, as well as image blurring. Cardiac pa-

tients may be incapable of breath-holding because of sedation, poor respiratory status, or inability to cooperate. The so-called navigator echoes allow tracking of diaphragmatic motion (Figure 21-8), so that cardiac imaging may take place when the position of the heart is consistent.[34] Navigator echoes have been suggested in particular for imaging coronary arteries, in which a small degree of blurring otherwise obscures the fine detail necessary.[28] Using navigator echoes, the operator sets a limit on the superior-inferior position of the diaphragm; only when the diaphragm is at this position do phase-encoding steps contribute to the final image. A current difficulty with this approach is the poor time efficiency; the diaphragm may be in an optimal position for image acquisition for only 5% to 15% of the respiratory cycle. Nevertheless, the technique may be feasible for three-dimensional (3D) image acquisitions, for which complete image acquisition cannot be accomplished within a single breath-hold.

Cardiac Magnetic Resonance Scan Prescription

A limitation of cardiac imaging to date has been the lack of rapid, highly interactive prescription algorithms. With echocardiography, a transducer is easily positioned at well-defined but readily adjusted angles to the chest wall to optimize the long- and short-axis views of the heart. Although MRI is capable of multiangle oblique imaging, the scan prescription time needed to define the double-oblique orientation of the LV, for example, relative to the chest wall, is time consuming. As a result, many studies are performed with axial, coronal, and sagittal imaging planes. However, more rapid pulse sequences, such as segmented κ-space acquisitions, allow true long- and short-axis imaging planes to be prescribed more quickly. Furthermore, real-time MR fluoroscopy has been demonstrated.[48] Integration of fluoroscopic images with control over imaging gradients allows real-time prescription of imaging planes ideally suited to the cardiac anatomy.

Relative to the chest wall, the cardiac axis is oriented along the following two oblique planes:

1. The cardiac apex is pointed toward the left.
2. Relative to the base of the heart, the apex is pointed anteriorly.

Images that are perpendicular to the long axis of the heart (i.e., short-axis images) (Figure 21-9) can be prescribed through a series of steps (Figure 21-10). First, an orthogonal imaging plane to the body is acquired (Figure 21-10, *A*). The sagittal plane is usually convenient because it also allows the superior-to-inferior position of a surface coil to be checked and repositioned if necessary. From the sagittal image the anterior angulation of the cardiac apex, relative to the base, is determined. A series of oblique images is acquired parallel to this plane. These images are then inspected, and the leftward angulation of the cardiac apex can be determined (Figure 21-10, *B*). Images parallel to the short axis of the heart can then be prescribed graphically, perpendicular to a line that defines the leftward angulation of the heart. Horizontal and vertical long-axis images are then prescribed, relative to the short-axis images.

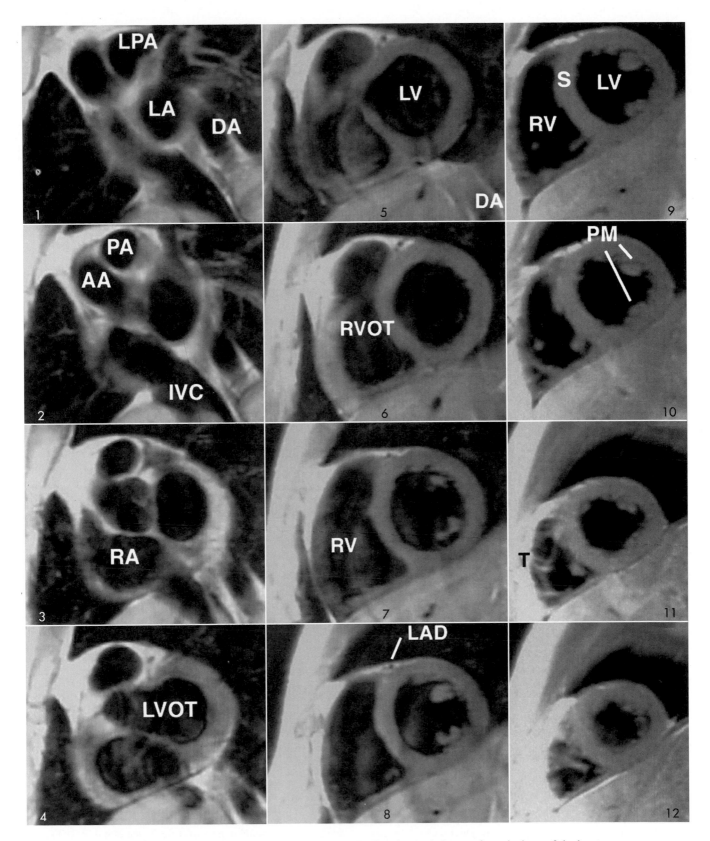

FIGURE 21-9   Normal short-axis cardiac anatomy. Twelve short axis images from the base of the heart *(1)* through the cardiac apex *(12)*. *AA,* Ascending aorta; *DA,* descending pulmonary artery; *IVC,* inferior vena cava; *LA,* left atrium; *LAD,* left anterior descending coronary artery; *LPA,* left pulmonary artery; *LV,* left ventricle; *LVOT,* left ventricular outflow tract; *PA,* pulmonary artery; *PM,* papillary muscles; *RA,* right atrium; *RVOT,* right ventricular outflow tract; *RV,* right ventricle; *S,* septum; *T,* trabeculations in RV.

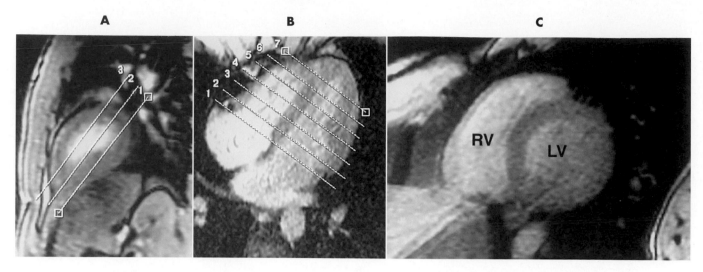

FIGURE 21-10   Short-axis cardiac prescription. **A,** Based on a sagittal localizing image, several pseudo–long axis slices of the LV are graphically prescribed. **B,** True short-axis images are then obtained by graphic prescription based on the pseudo–long axis, obtained from **A. C,** The resulting short-axis image is shown at the mid-ventricle level. *RV,* Right ventricle; *LV,* left ventricle.

MYOCARDIUM
Normal Anatomy

On SE sequences the ventricular and atrial cavities generally have low signal intensity when the images are acquired with superior and inferior saturation bands. "Ghosting" artifacts, caused by respiratory motion in the phase-encoding direction, are common. FSE sequences may show subendocardial blood as areas of increased signal intensity, which may be the result of slow-moving blood during diastole. The normal myocardial signal is similar to or slightly greater than that of skeletal muscle on T2-weighted images.

Left Ventricle. The normal LV wall thickness is 9 to 11 mm at end diastole. Focal areas of thinning of the myocardium are associated with remodeling after myocardial infarction (MI). In both the transverse and short-axis views, the LV anterolateral and inferoposterior papillary muscles are visualized, beginning at the midventricular level (Figure 21-9).

Right Ventricle. The right ventricle (RV) wall is approximately 3 mm in thickness. Near the apex, blurring caused by respiratory and cardiac motion may make the ventricular wall difficult to visualize on SE imaging. The trabeculations of the RV are readily visualized relative to the less trabeculated LV. The primary intraventricular structure visualized is the moderator band, extending from the distal portion of the intraventricular septum to the apical portion of the free wall of the RV (Figure 21-11). The moderator band is a segment of muscle through which the right bundle branch of the interventricular conduction system travels. The papillary muscles of the RV extend from the free wall toward the tricuspid valve.

Atriums. The walls of the atriums are thin and best identified on transaxial or long-axis images. On SE images the interatrial septum may not be identified in normal individuals; however, lack of identification on SE images does not indicate an atrial septal defect. The coronary sinus may be routinely identified on axial images at the inferior surface of the heart. The coronary sinus enters the right atrium at the level of the diaphragm. On axial images the inferior and superior venae cavae are identified entering the right atrium. The pulmonary veins are also best identified on transaxial images as they enter the left atrium.

Assessment of Cardiac Function

Morphological Indices of Cardiac Function. LV volume is an important diagnostic and prognostic factor after MI and in patients with valvular abnormalities[160]; essentially all indices of LV function derive from measurements of volume and pressure.[18] Current ap-

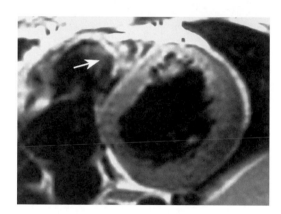

FIGURE 21-11   Axial image of the heart. Because of the geometry of the heart in this patient, the axial image demonstrates prominent trabeculae and moderator band in the apex of the RV *(arrow).*

proaches to patient therapy depend on knowledge of systolic performance of the LV.[24] Ejection fraction and cardiac output measures, although dependent on afterload, provide an overall index of global ventricular performance.[18] LV hypertrophy and mass are strong predictors for cardiovascular disease morbidity or mortality.[11,22,66,77] However, measures of global LV function using echocardiography or ventriculography depend on geometrical assumptions that are inaccurate in patients whose ventricles do not conform to ideal geometrical models. MR methods use Simpson's rule and therefore avoid introduction of geometrical assumptions that lead to inaccuracy. MR evaluation of cardiac chamber dimensions is facilitated by the ability to obtain images with good spatial resolution in any tomographic plane. Thus errors associated with geometrical assumptions, as is the case with echocardiography, are avoided.[142]

Accurate LV volume measurements may be obtained during normal respiration with SE and conventional cine MR techniques[117] or during a breath-hold, using a segmented κ-space cine technique.[133] Compared with cast volume displacement of the LV, a correlation of 99% can be achieved, with standard error of the estimate of 4.9 cm³.[125] Interstudy variability has been determined to be less than 4% to 6% for cine MR assessment of the LV mass.[117,140,141] Standard deviation of MRI-determined LV ejection fraction is 4%.[117] Cardiac index and end systolic wall stress interstudy variability is slightly greater at 8% to 10% and likely a result of physiological variation in afterload.[117]

RV functional assessment is complex because of the unusual shape of that cavity.[128] Echocardiography is of limited value in assessing the

RV because of difficulties with visualizing the endocardial borders and the complex geometry.[102] MR assessment of the RV is based on Simpson's rule and like LV assessment does not require geometrical assumptions.

MR validation data for the RV are less extensive than for the LV.[116] Excellent correlation, however, has been found between MRI and indicator dilution methods (r = 0.93) and ventriculography (r = 0.96).[65,102] In healthy individuals, RV stroke volume is equal to LV stroke volume.[102,136] Impairment of RV diastolic function may be a more sensitive marker of myocardial disease than is RV ejection fraction.[116] In patients with dilated cardiomyopathy, although ejection fraction was normal, the time to peak filling rate was prolonged and filling fraction of the RV was reduced.[150] RV mass allows detection of early RV hypertrophy.[118] Interobserver and intraobserver variation of RV ejection fraction by MRI in one study was approximately 6% using Simpson's rule for cavity size measurement.[111]

Atrial assessment is important in acquired valvular disease and systemic or pulmonary hypertension, although its role has largely been ignored in population-based studies. As a compliant reservoir for delivery of blood to the ventricle, atrial function augments ventricular function.[73,149] Because of the marked volume response of the atriums to pressure changes, atrial volume may be an early indicator of subclinical cardiovascular disease. Atrial volume assessment also has been limited previously by the lack of a method to noninvasively and accurately assess chamber dimensions.

Atrial assessment with MRI showed 7% underestimation of cavity dimension compared with atrial casts. Information regarding reproducibility of measurements and intraobserver and interobserver variability has not been specifically studied or described in the literature.[58]

Stroke volume and cardiac output may be assessed by cine PC imaging[36,109] in the aorta at the level of the pulmonary artery bifurcation using breath-hold techniques.[14] Signal intensity is mapped to velocity-induced phase shifts of moving spins in the presence of a magnetic field gradient. Thus phase shift is proportional to velocity. Stroke volume is derived from velocity and the cross-sectional area of the aorta, and cardiac output is obtained from stroke volume multiplied by the average heart rate. These aortic measurements improve accuracy compared with stroke volume/cardiac output by LV volumetric methods, if mitral regurgitation or intracardiac shunt is present. Aortic measurements, however, do not account for the fraction of cardiac output that goes to the coronary arteries.

Myocardial Tagging. Myocardial tagging involves labeling a region or strip of voxels via magnetic saturation. This labeled zone can be followed anatomically throughout the cardiac cycle (Figure 21-12). Measurement of local myocardial wall motion using myocardial tagging has become a simple and reproducible examination using single breath-hold cine methods. Direct visualization of the myocardium provides important insights into regional myocardial mechanics. In contrast to global measures of systolic function, such as ejection fraction, MRI myocardial tagging makes it possible to quantify the severity and extent of subtle regional heart wall motion abnormalities both at rest and during stress.[8,168]

The three stages of myocardial tagging are (1) placement of a saturation band pattern (either a grid or parallel tag lines) over the myocardium, with spatially selective RF pulses; (2) MR image acquisition, during which time tag motion is observed (Figure 21-12); and (3) detection of myocardial tag motion. The motion of the saturation pattern is then used to compute the regional myocardial function. Throughout these steps, image acquisition is gated to the ECG.

The fundamental improvements in regional function assessment using MR tagging techniques rather than echocardiography and nontagged MRI are (1) the same volume of myocardium can be tracked over the heart cycle to map the function in a specific region and (2) very precise quantitative estimates of myocardial shortening and wall thickening can be computed from the images. With myocardial tagging techniques, the normal contraction patterns of the human LV are consistent from heart to heart.[105] The regional mechanical behavior after infarction (Figure 21-13)[84] and during ischemia[106] has been characterized using myocardial tagging. On day 5 after a first anterior MI with single-vessel disease, patients demonstrate reduced intramyocardial circumferential shortening throughout the LV, including remote noninfarcted regions.[69] These observations are relatively subtle and require

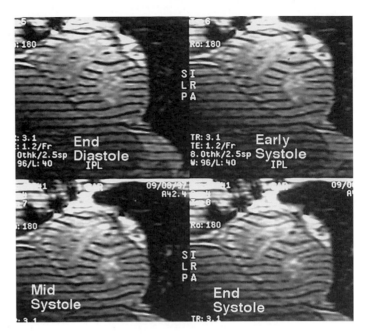

FIGURE 21-12 Myocardial tagging. MR images show normal change in position of parallel tag lines from end diastole to end systole.

the analysis of myocardial-tagged images to be detected. Reduced magnitude and reorientation of principal strains and reduction in segmental rigid-body motion characterize nonreperfused transmural MIs 1 week after coronary occlusion.[79] Quantitative functional analysis in patients treated with angiotensin-converting enzyme inhibition shows a reduction in LV remodeling and preserved function in the adjacent noninfarcted region.[68]

Tag detection is extremely precise and accurate.[4,95,108,166] Reproducibility is maintained by consistent adherence to acquisition methods and analysis techniques that use intrinsic cardiac landmarks. The position of a myocardial tag can be estimated to within 0.1 pixels, corresponding to tag localization to within approximately 150 μm. In healthy volunteers imaged once, imaged a second time later the same day, and imaged again 4 weeks later, the mean differences in end-diastolic wall thickness, end-systolic wall thickness, and percent wall thickening mean between the baseline and 4-week studies were −0.05 ± 0.7 mm, 0.0 ± 0.9 mm, and 0.98% ± 17%, respectively.[135] Correlation coefficients for wall thickness measures performed on the same day and repeated 4 weeks later were 0.94 and 0.95. Although tagging allows calculation of the full 3D displacement field over the entire LV,[84,105,107,112] currently two-dimensional (2D) analysis in the circumferential and radial directions is more practical because the analysis is much more rapid.

Displacement of tag points is determined from "material points" that intersect the imaging plane at the time of imaging. Computer software has been developed that allows tracking of the tag points over the cardiac cycle; this allows the deformation of a material point in the heart to be calculated. Cardiac motion may be sampled in three orthogonal directions. If this is done with sufficient resolution, the 3D displacement field over the entire LV may be reconstructed.[11,117,133,142,155]

Although 3D strain maps describe the complete motion of the heart (Figure 21-14), the clinical need for this thorough description has not been demonstrated. A more practical quantitative tool for characterizing myocardial function may instead be the use of LV strain maps. LV strain maps are 2D plots of strain versus time curves during the cardiac cycle (Figure 21-15); the spatial location on the LV for each box in this chart is given by the coordinates on the axes. In this plot, age- and gender-matched population normal curves at ±2 standard deviations are overlaid on the specific patient's data being examined. The normal population shows a tight distribution, implying that quantitative metrics can be used to compare each individual against the expected normal strain pattern.

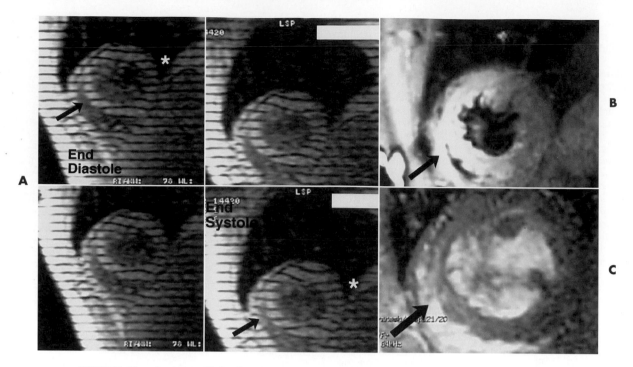

FIGURE 21-13   Anteroseptal infarction. **A,** Myocardial tagging images at a single level identify lack of wall motion in the anteroseptal distribution *(arrow)*. At the asterisk, normal wall motion is indicated for comparison. **B,** T2-weighted FSE sequence shows increased signal intensity in the septum and anterior wall *(arrow)*. **C,** Myocardial perfusion study shows increased signal intensity in the same distribution *(arrow)* as **A.**

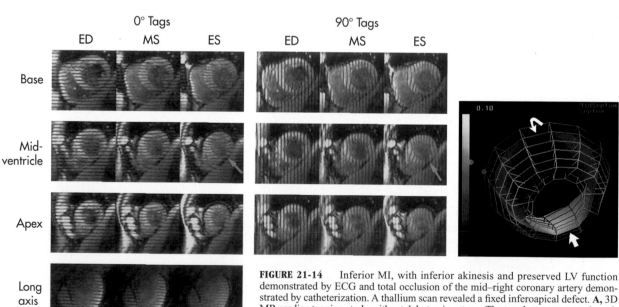

FIGURE 21-14   Inferior MI, with inferior akinesis and preserved LV function demonstrated by ECG and total occlusion of the mid–right coronary artery demonstrated by catheterization. A thallium scan revealed a fixed inferoapical defect. **A,** 3D MR cardiac tagging study without dobutamine stress. The top three rows contain end-diastolic *(ED)*, midsystolic *(MS)*, and end-systolic *(ES)* time frames from short-axis slices through the base, midventricle, and apex. The tag orientations of the left and right set of time frames are orthogonal. The fourth row contains three time frames from a long-axis slice intersecting the inferior and anterior walls with tags parallel to the short-axis imaging planes. Inferoseptal akinesis is demonstrated by a lack of tag contraction most notable at end systole in the midventricular and apical short-axis slices *(white arrows)*, as well as the long-axis slice. **B,** Tag displacement information in the three orthogonal tag directions was used to estimate 3D myocardial displacement and strain values over the entire LV. Shown here is a 3D color-coded display of the eigenvector of the strain tensor describing endocardial circumferential shortening. The blue vectors on the anterior wall describe normal contraction *(curved arrow)*, whereas the yellow vectors on the inferoseptal wall correspond to abnormal stretching *(straight arrow)*. (From reference 17.)

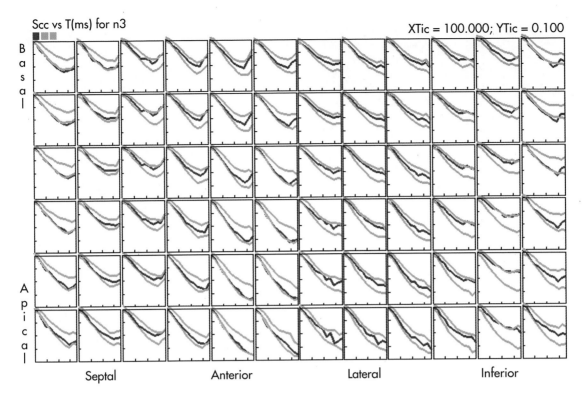

FIGURE 21-15   LV strain map showing the normal circumferential shortening versus time at 72 midwall locations around the LV. Each graph represents the behavior of approximately 1.5 g of myocardial tissue the position of the tissue is given on the labels of the array of graphs. Green lines indicate the normal range of circumferential shortening, and the yellow curves show the patient being examined. The patient's values are within the expected range of a normal LV. (Courtesy E. McVeigh, Baltimore.)

Assessment of Ischemic Heart Disease

Noncontrast Magnetic Resonance Imaging of Myocardial Infarction. Early studies using SE techniques required several minutes to acquire each image,[120] and the regional increase in signal intensity observed on SE T2-weighted images resulted from edema formation, which takes several hours to develop.[153] Acute MI results in local edema and changes in the T1 and T2 times of the damaged myocardium. Experimentally, T1 relaxation times are prolonged 30 min after coronary occlusion, and T2 prolongation has been reported within 3 to 6 hours.[51] These changes in T1 and T2 times may be detected on gated-SE images of the myocardium. Experimentally, however, changes in the T1 time of the myocardium have not correlated well with the extent of MI by comparison with histological examination until 3 weeks after the infarction in a dog model.[164] Quantification of infarct size using T2-weighted images, however, has been more successful. Good correlation between infarct size and T2 signal changes has been identified in animal models using a 6-hour model of coronary occlusion.[127] Moderate overestimation of infarct size has been reported by correlation of infarct size with radioactive microsphere–detected perfusion changes at 1 week after infarction in a closed-chest canine model of infarction.[15]

Human studies of MI using noncontrast T1- and T2-weighted images have shown mixed results. In autopsied hearts, T1 times of infarcted tissue are greater than those of normal regions (459 ms versus 272 ms, respectively.). Similarly, T2 prolongation occurred in the area of infarction (49 ms versus 35 ms, infarcted versus noninfarcted, respectively).[54] In comparison with pyrophosphate scanning 5 to 7 days after MI, good correlation is seen between T1 maps of the myocardium and single-photon emission tomography assessment of infarct size.[154] Although increased T2 signal corresponding to areas of infarction on thallium images has been demonstrated,[94] healthy patients and patients with unstable angina with similar signal-intensity changes have been reported.[1,35] These signal changes are probably the result of technical differences in the quality of the T2-weighted images. Also, after infarction, focal hypokinesia or akinesia results in slow-moving blood near the MI. Because the T2 relaxation time of oxyhemoglobin is long,

slow flow causes increased signal near the endocardial border, which makes identification of the endocardium difficult.[52]

Inversion-recovery pulses to null signal both from blood and fat combined with rapid, breath-hold FSE imaging[143] can produce high-resolution images of the myocardium that show increased signal in the area of the infarction, consistent with edema. This breath-hold approach to high-quality SE imaging can be very useful in myocardial evaluation.

Contrast Magnetic Resonance Imaging of Myocardial Infarction. Gadolinium diethylene-triamine-pentaacetic acid (Gd-DTPA)–enhanced MRI has a significant role in the evaluation of MI, as well as in assessing microvascular perfusion.[26,115,129,165] Animal[163] and human[83,86] studies assessed myocardial perfusion by rapidly imaging the first pass of extravascular paramagnetic contrast agents, such as Gd-DTPA, and characterizing the enhancement patterns that occurred during the first 1 to 2 min after administration of contrast agent (Figure 21-16).[80] Signal intensity of myocardial territory corresponding to microvascular occlusion was reduced (hypoenhanced) when compared with normal myocardium immediately after contrast administration (Figure 21-17).[163] In reperfused infarcts, myocardial image intensity was increased (hyperenhanced), as illustrated in Figure 21-18.[59,130] The ability to discern these changes with fidelity may play a role in the detection of MIs and the determination of their size.

Patterns of myocardial contrast enhancement have been studied in experimental models of MI. Regions of the myocardium that become hyperintense several minutes after contrast administration are primarily nonviable (Figure 21-19).[59] Furthermore, patients with reperfused infarction whose regions of hyperenhancement increase over time ultimately develop larger scars 6 months after infarction.[82] This delayed contrast enhancement (up to 10 min after contrast administration) is probably caused by increased concentration of the gadolinium molecule, and impaired wash-out of the molecule relative to more rapid wash-out from normal myocardium (Figure 21-20). Areas of myocardium characterized as hypoenhanced "no-reflow" regions centrally within the MI 1 to 2 min after contrast administration correlate with

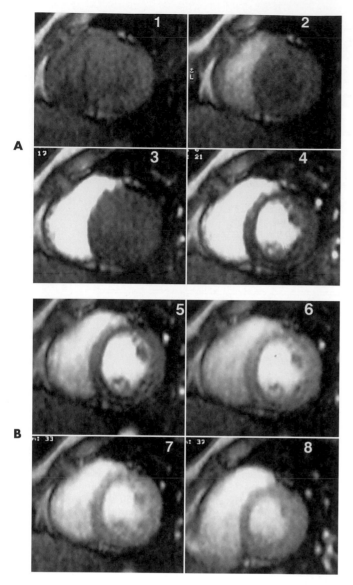

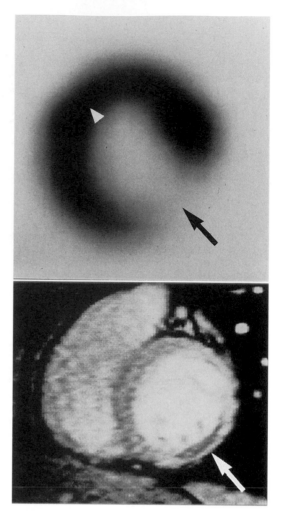

FIGURE 21-16   First-pass cardiac perfusion. Normal short-axis images, obtained at 1 slice per heartbeat. **A,** Normal enhancement of the RV, followed by the LV, is shown. Images obtained in sequence from the base to the apex are numbered 1 to 4, respectively. **B,** Subsequent enhancement of the myocardium and papillary muscles occurred over the next four heartbeats (5 to 8).

FIGURE 21-17   Occlusion of a circumflex artery, status after streptokinase therapy with partial resolution of symptoms. The bottom image is one frame from the first pass of a magnetization-driven SPGR perfusion study. Within the first minute after administration of contrast agent, a subendocardial hypoenhanced zone *(white arrow)* is observed, extends toward the epicardium, and corresponds pathologically to a region with microvascular obstruction and delayed delivery of contrast agent. The hypoenhanced region on the MR image matches anatomically a fixed defect on the corresponding thallium scan *(black arrow, top image).* The fixed defect on the thallium scan is mildly larger than the area of microvascular obstruction depicted on the MR perfusion image. The patient underwent rescue percutaneous transluminal coronary angioplasty. *White arrowhead,* Ventricular septum. (Courtesy J. Lima, Baltimore. From reference 17.)

FIGURE 21-18   Reperfusion study in a canine model. The left anterior descending coronary artery was occluded for 90 min with a balloon catheter, and the heart was then reperfused for 48 hours. On the left, the TTC-stained heart demonstrates an absence of stain (infarction) in the endocardial left anterior descending artery territory *(curved white arrow).* The right image was obtained approximately 10 min after a bolus injection of Gd-DTPA using an MD-SPGR technique. This "delayed-phase" image depicts endocardial hyperenhancement *(curved black arrow)* in a region that anatomically matches the infarct region on the TTC-stained heart. (Courtesy C. Rochitte, Baltimore.)

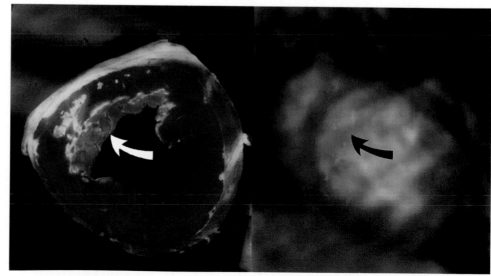

regions of extremely low blood flow (Figure 21-17). The primary feature thought to cause low blood flow is widespread microvascular damage, which is characteristic of no-reflow regions. Microvascular damage is the result of neutrophil plugging, microvascular thrombosis, endothelial cell swelling, extravascular compression by tissue edema, or a combination of these factors. Accordingly, large human infarcts, which are associated with prolonged obstruction of the infarct-related artery, frequently have central areas of hypoenhancement during the first several minutes after MI. Smaller, reperfused infarcts tend to demonstrate more uniform signal hyperenhancement.[81]

First-Pass Magnetic Resonance Perfusion Imaging. First-pass myocardial perfusion sequences must be capable of rapidly establishing T1 contrast for multiple slices with high temporal resolution (usually 1 to 2 heartbeats). Early segmented κ-space approaches typi-

cally used single-slice inversion-recovery–fast low-angle shot (IR-FLASH) techniques,[5,67,163] and multislice IR-prepped sequences were subsequently developed.[157] Because the relationship between image intensity and 1/T1 for IR-prepped sequences is largely nonlinear, particularly for the blood pool, a single-slice magnetization-driven SPGR (MD-SPGR) technique was developed that drives magnetization to steady state with a train of "dummy" RF pulses before imaging with a 45-degree flip angle.[61] This technique broadens the range over which image intensity is linearly related to 1/T1 and contrast-agent concentration. The magnetization sampled by IR-prepped and MD-SPGR sequences depends on the extent of T1 relaxation during the previous R-R interval and thus is dependent on heart rate. "Dysrhythmia-insensitive" perfusion sequences use saturation recovery with a 90-degree saturation pulse[60,74] to eliminate sensitivity of contrast to fluctuations of cardiac rhythm and rate.

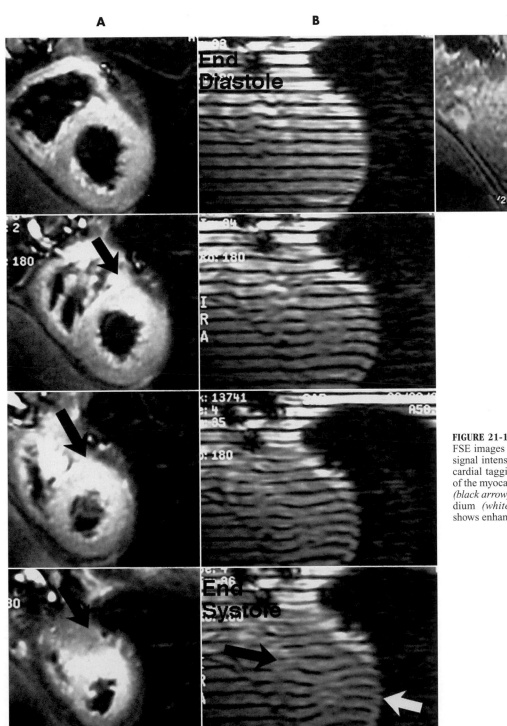

FIGURE 21-19   Acute MI. **A,** T2-weighted FSE images show a diffuse area of increased signal intensity anteriorly *(arrows).* **B,** Myocardial tagging demonstrates lack of motion of the myocardial tagging lines during systole *(black arrow)* compared with normal myocardium *(white arrow).* **C,** Perfusion image shows enhancement of the infarct *(arrow).*

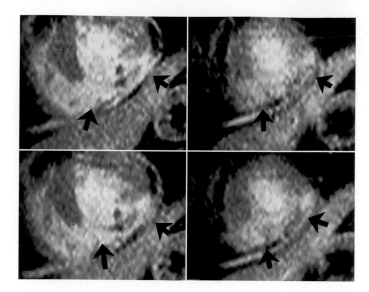

FIGURE 21-20   Acute inferoseptal MI. Short-axis perfusion images obtained 8 min after contrast administration demonstrate a large area of delayed enhancement *(arrows)* in a septal and inferior wall distribution.

First-pass myocardial perfusion methods may be applied to assess coronary flow reserve. Coronary flow reserve is defined as the ratio of blood flow at maximal vasodilatation divided by flow at rest. Maximal flow is measured under conditions of vasodilatation, as achieved with dipyridamole or adenosine. Typically, coronary flow reserve ranges from 3 to 5 in healthy individuals. In the presence of fixed coronary stenoses, coronary flow reserve is markedly reduced.[163] Coronary flow reserve may be measured with an intracoronary Doppler flow ultrasound probe, but first-pass contrast MRI is also useful for assessment of flow reserve. In both animal and human studies a linear relationship between coronary flow reserve and first-pass MRI has been found. This relationship indicates that patients with microvascular dysfunction, either from epicardial vascular disease or from diseases altering the microvasculature (e.g., hypertension or diabetes), may be assessed using these methods.[162]

Chronic Myocardial Infarction.   Chronic MI results in thinning of the LV wall (remodeling) that is distinct from the normal myocardial wall thickness. These changes are better seen during systole because of the increased thickness of the normal myocardium relative to the region of infarction. Focal myocardial wall thinning is specific for chronic MI on MRI.[49,94]

LV aneurysms may occur after MI and are depicted as areas of focally protruding myocardium (Figure 21-21) with transmural thinning and associated mural thrombus. Although distinguishing between a true aneurysm and false aneurysm (ruptured myocardium contained by pericardium) is usually straightforward by echocardiography, MRI is useful in cases in which an adequate acoustic window is not obtained. Pseudoaneurysms are characterized by a relatively small neck communicating with the LV cavity, whereas true aneurysms have a relatively wide neck.[46]

Cardiac Masses

Primary cardiac tumors are rare, with an incidence of 0.001% to 0.5% based on postmortem studies.[47,71] Approximately 80% are benign and can be effectively treated with surgical resection. Secondary tumors involving the heart are somewhat more common, resulting from metastatic disease to the myocardium or pericardium or from tumors of the adjacent lung or mediastinal structures with myocardial invasion.

Although echocardiography is frequently used for the diagnosis of heart tumors, MRI is able to fully represent the heart and also the thorax, mediastinum, pleura, and lungs. MRI is also very useful for presurgical evaluation and for assessment of response after chemotherapy or surgical treatment. Using conventionally gated T1- and T2-weighted images, cardiac and paracardiac myocardial tumors are usually readily distinguished from normal myocardial structures on the basis of their signal intensity (Figure 21-22, *A* and *B*).[96] Gated-cine images further assist in depicting the origin of tumors through improved contrast between blood and the adjacent tumor (Figure 21-22, *C*). Myocardial tagging by MRI may further help to define tissue planes and differentiate contractile from noncontractile tumor.[16]

In equivocal cases in which the signal intensity of the myocardium is similar to that of the myocardial tumor, Gd-DTPA contrast-enhanced images have been shown to be useful to provide differential signal enhancement from the myocardium.[40] On SE images, contrast-enhanced images help resolve myocardial signal from tumor, although both increased and decreased signal of the tumor compared with the myocardium has been reported. With first-pass cine gradient-echo images, all cardiac tumors showed increased signal enhancement in a small series of 15 patients.[139] Importantly, thrombus, which commonly occurs in the atriums but may occur in any cardiac chamber, showed no increase in signal intensity after contrast administration. Thus contrast enhancement may play a role in the differential diagnosis of cardiac masses.

The most common of the true cardiac tumors is the myxoma, which accounts for approximately 50% of cardiac masses within the heart. The majority of myxomas are found within the left atrium (70%), followed by the right atrium (25%) and ventricles. The clinical presentation of myxoma may mimic other systemic diseases or lymphoma. Symptoms may include night sweats, thoracic outlet syndrome (from distal embolization), stroke, mitral stenosis (a result of tumor prolapse across the mitral valve), weight loss, and finger clubbing. It is important to distinguish this tumor from mural thrombus, which may occur in similar locations. Thrombus invariably has a broad-based attachment to the endocardium, whereas myxoma is identified by a characteristic stalk, which in some cases allows the pedunculated tumor to prolapse across the mitral valve. The signal intensity of myxoma on SE images is similar to that of myocardium but shows decreased signal on cine images. After contrast enhancement, one series showed enhancement of six myxomas,[139] whereas a separate report identified enhancing tumor, but central areas of low signal intensity corresponded to necrosis.[91]

Other primary cardiac tumors include rhabdomyomas and rhabdomyosarcomas, angiosarcomas (Figure 21-23), lipomas, ectopic endocrine tissue, fibromas, and melanomas. Except for lipoma, which has signal intensity similar to that of subcutaneous fat on all sequences, the signal intensity of other cardiac tumors is not specific for tumor etiology. As opposed to myxoma, primary malignant tumors have been reported to have a wide point of attachment or involvement of the myocardium (Figure 21-24) and may demonstrate areas of heterogeneous signal as a result of necrosis,[144] as well as pericardial or extracardiac extension. Teratoma (Figure 21-25) and lymphoma are common mediastinal masses that may be paracardiac in location.

Pseudotumors of the atria have been reported on MRI as a result of prominent intraatrial structures, including the crista terminalis and Chiari network.[96] Prominent intraatrial structures were reported in 59% of subjects, including a single prominent nodule in 36%, an intraatrial strand in 13%, and both in 10%. Although these structures are seen more commonly with MRI than other modalities, familiarity with normal MR appearances prevents the inappropriate diagnosis of a pathological mass when none is present. Furthermore, occasional pseudomasses on echocardiography, such as hiatal hernia, tortuous descending aorta, fatty infiltration of the atrioventricular groove, pericardial effusion (Figure 21-26), and hematoma after surgery (Figure 21-27), are usually resolved with the use of MRI and are distinguished from true cardiac or paracardiac masses.[97]

Cardiomyopathy

The cardiomyopathies represent a diverse group of disorders that are generally defined as muscular disorders of the heart. Strictly speaking, these disorders are limited to idiopathic entities, although certain diseases, such as hemochromatosis, amyloid disease, scleroderma, and congestive vascular etiologies, are often referred to as *cardiomyopathy* during the initial stages of clinical evaluation. Given idiopathic forms, cardiomyopathy is subdivided into three categories, each with unique pathological and physiological characteristics: (1) hypertrophic cardiomyopathy, with symptoms of dyspnea, chest pain, and palpitations and clinical features of hypertrophy and heart failure; (2) dilated cardiomyopathy, with clinical features of cardiac enlargement, increased

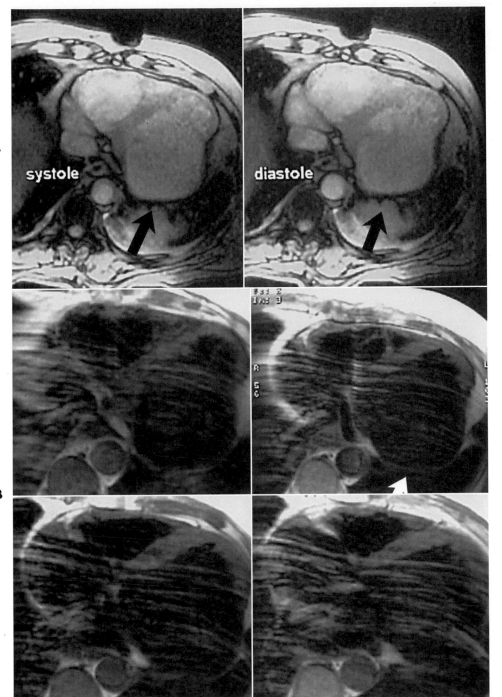

FIGURE 21-21 Myocardial infarction with LV aneurysm formation. **A,** Systolic and diastolic cine images demonstrate a wide-mouthed out-pouching from the posterior aspect of the LV, a result of a true aneurysm after MI. **B,** Corresponding T1-weighted axial images at several levels show the extent of the aneurysm.

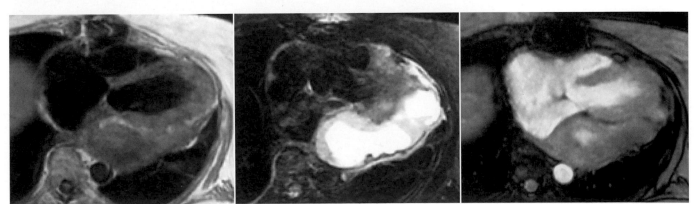

FIGURE 21-22 Hemangiopericytoma. Axial T1- and T2-weighted (**A** and **B**) and cine gradient-echo (**C**) images show a large mass posterolateral to the LV. On T2-weighted images, focal bright areas within the mass are present as a result of blood-filled spaces within the mass. The cine images (**C**) demonstrate the mass effect limiting filling of the left side of the heart.

cardiac volume, and congestive failure; and (3) restrictive cardiomyopathy, with reduced cardiac filling and emptying that result from infiltrative disorders of the myocardium.

Because of the diverse range of disease entities, the potential value of MR in these entities also demonstrates a wide range of contributions to disease management. In most cases, however, MRI has primarily been used as an investigative tool that aids in the understanding of the physiological and anatomical features of the disorder.

Hypertrophic Cardiomyopathy. The morphological changes of hypertrophic cardiomyopathy (HCM) may be demonstrated on conventional SE or FSE images. Although transaxial images may be obtained, more information regarding the site of muscular wall hypertrophy is typically gained when true short-axis images are obtained from the base of the heart to the apex. Additional four-chamber or vertical long-axis images complement short-axis views.

The major role of MRI has been to identify the site of localized hypertrophy and its extent. MRI is useful in identifying asymmetrical septal hypertrophy as well as apical hypertrophy.[114] Two-dimensional echocardiography is typically used to identify regions of hypertrophy, but MRI adds additional anatomical visualization, particularly at the apical portion of the LV.[43] Echocardiography and MRI correlate best in the assessment of thickness of the septum wall ($r = 0.93$) compared with the posterolateral wall ($r = 0.74$) in 23 patients.[134] In 5 of these patients (22%), the assessment of the distribution of hypertrophy as defined by echocardiography was changed after MRI. When standardized scoring schemes of hypertrophy are used, MRI allowed a complete evaluation of the Spirito-Maron and Wigle scores in 49 of 52 patients (94%), whereas echocardiography allowed complete assessment of anatomical features in 33 of 52 patients (63%). Thus MRI provides the more comprehensive diagnostic information for patients with HCM.[123] Additional findings in patients with asymmetrical septal HCM demonstrated by MRI include increased end-diastolic thickness of the septal wall, decreased systolic thickening of the septal wall, systolic anterior motion of the mitral valve, and a signal void area within the LV outflow tract during systole.[3] However, despite more complete assessment of patterns of hypertrophy with MRI, the only clinical measure found to correlate with this anatomical information was the presence of an abnormal depolarization pattern of the ECG in patients with HCM.[122] Thus the value of MRI relative to echocardiography in affecting clinical outcome in patients with HCM has yet to be demonstrated.

MR tagging has provided unique insight into myocardial mechanics in HCM. Circumferential and longitudinal myocardial shortening is depressed in subjects with hypertrophied segments compared with that in normal subjects.[10,70] Compared with healthy subjects, patients with HCM demonstrate reduced intramyocardial circumferential end-systolic shortening in the septum and inferior and anterior regions.

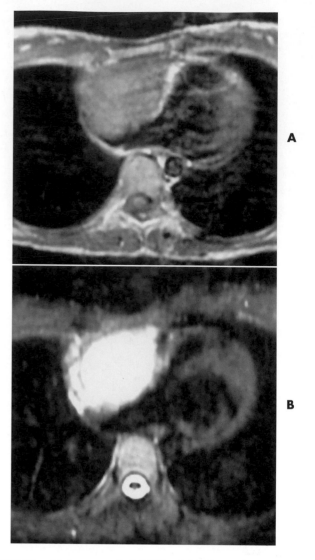

FIGURE 21-23 Angiosarcoma. **A,** Axial T1-weighted image shows a mass anterior to the right atrium and RV, deforming the cardiac border. **B,** Axial T2-weighted image shows a high–signal intensity mass. Biopsy demonstrated angiosarcoma of the heart.

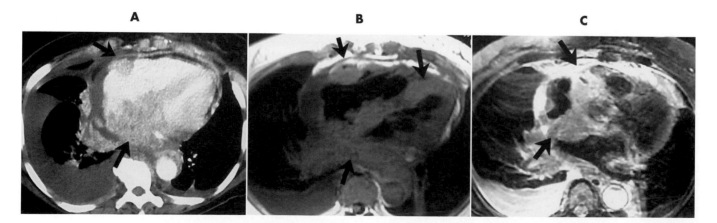

FIGURE 21-24 High-grade malignant neoplasm. **A,** Computed tomographic scan demonstrates right pleural effusion, pericardial effusion, and thickening of the septum and left atrium *(arrows)*. **B,** T1-weighted MR image shows marked thickening of all cardiac chambers *(arrows),* as well as pericardial effusion adjacent to the RV. **C,** T2-weighted MRI at a more superior level than **B** shows tumor encasing the right atrium and pulmonary veins *(arrows).* A right pleural effusion is again noted. The patient died 2 weeks after the MR scan.

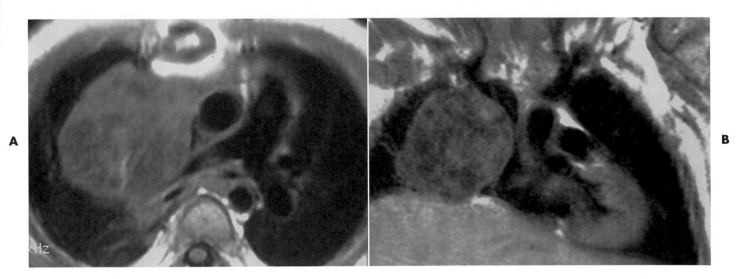

FIGURE 21-25   Teratoma. **A** and **B,** Axial and coronal T1-weighted images show a large paracardiac mass with compression of the right atrium and inferior vena cava.

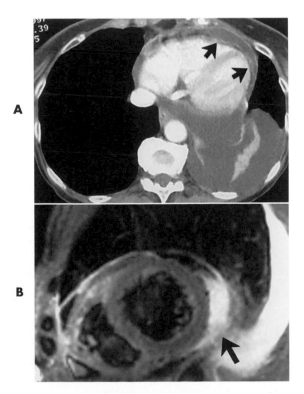

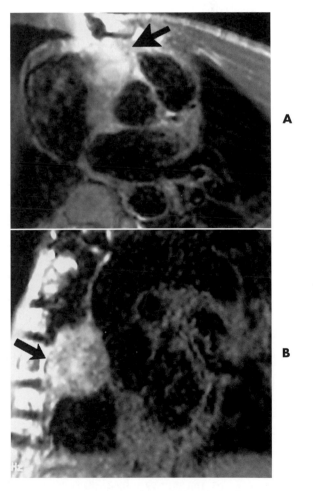

FIGURE 21-26   Suspected mass (false-positive echocardiogram). **A,** CT scan with contrast shows pericardial enhancement *(arrows),* with left pleural effusion and left lower lobe atelectasis. MRI was performed to evaluate the pericardial effusion for intrapericardial mass. **B,** T2-weighted short-axis view of the heart shows flowing, bright fluid in the pericardium posteriorly *(arrow),* similar to that of the posterior pleural effusion. No solid masses were present.

FIGURE 21-27   Aortic root hematoma in a patient after cardiac surgery with paraaortic mass on echocardiogram. **A** and **B,** Axial and sagittal oblique planes in MRI show a mass *(arrow)* extrinsic to the aortic root, adjacent to the surgical site, with increased signal. No flow was identified within the mass. Follow-up scan (not shown) showed a decrease in the size of the mass, which is compatible with hematoma.

End-systolic shortening is reduced compared with that in healthy subjects at all levels from the apex to the base. In patients with HCM, septal and inferior wall circumferential end-systolic shortening values were the most depressed.[70] Depressed myocardial shortening has been related primarily to myofibrillar disarray and associated myocardial fibrosis rather than to only increased wall thickness.

Although a consistent finding in HCM is abnormal LV function, RV function may also be affected. In one study, the mean thickness of the RV free wall was 2.9 mm in healthy subjects but 4.4 mm in patients with HCM.[151] The peak filling rate of the RV and the filling fraction are reduced relative to the LV according to MR findings.[150]

Dilated Cardiomyopathy. Dilated cardiomyopathy (DCM) is the common end point of a variety of factors and disorders. Alcohol, toxins, ischemia, viral disease, and hereditary factors may all lead to morphological changes of a grossly dilated heart. By definition, however, coronary atherosclerosis, valvular disease, and other specific cardiac abnormalities are absent in DCM. Pathologically, there are LV dilatation and thinning of the wall; RV and atrial dilatation may also be present. Despite the thinned wall, there typically is morphological enlargement of the myocardium. Pathologically, underlying myocardial fibrosis is present, accounting for the reduced contractility despite the increased muscle mass.

MRI may be helpful in distinguishing the etiologies of cardiac dilatation other than those of DCM. For example, isolated RV dilatation

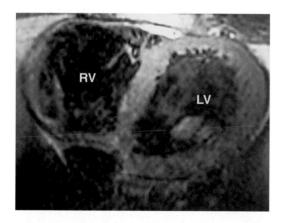

FIGURE 21-28 RV dysplasia. FSE image showing marked dilatation of the RV and thinning of the anterior wall. The main differential diagnosis for this appearance is RV infarct, which can be excluded by factors including the patient's age and symptoms.

identified on short-axis images is more likely to indicate right ventricular infarction or ischemia. Normal ejection fractions and volumes have been reported in DCM.[150] Segmental dilatation of the LV is also more likely to be a result of coronary occlusion rather than DCM.[39] Ejection fractions are reduced in DCM and correlate well with the findings from radionuclide ventriculography studies.[44]

Functional MR tagging has shown markedly reduced cross-fiber shortening at the endocardium compared to that in normal individuals. The normal pattern of cross-fiber shortening as the dominant direction of myocardial fiber shortening in the endocardium is preserved in DCM.[85] End-systolic wall stress is elevated throughout the LV in DCM patients compared to that in normal individuals.[38]

Restrictive Cardiomyopathy. Restrictive cardiomyopathy is uncommon, and no large series using MRI have been described. Restrictive cardiomyopathy results from infiltrative conditions leading to myocardial stiffness and restriction. Clinically, this disorder may have a presentation similar to that of constrictive pericarditis. Hemodynamic studies show increased and equalized diastolic pressures in atrial and ventricular chambers. An indirect finding of impaired RV diastolic filling (e.g., dilatation of the inferior vena cava and right atrium) is present in both constrictive pericarditis and restrictive cardiomyopathy. MRI can identify increased pericardial thickness, thus allowing the clinician to make the diagnosis of constrictive pericarditis[37,90] and to differentiate it from restrictive disease.[37]

Restrictive cardiomyopathy is characterized by enlarged atria and ventricles of relatively normal size.[62] Increased blood signal may be present in the atria secondary to slow-moving blood in these cavities. MR cine images show reduced diastolic filling and emptying of the ventricles.

Dysrhythmogenic Right Ventricular Dysplasia

Dysrhythmogenic RV dysplasia is a primary disorder of the RV characterized by partial or total thinning and replacement of muscle by adipose or fibrous tissue and enlargement of end-diastolic diameter[88] (Figure 21-28). Fat extends from the epicardial surface through the interstitium and displaces myocardial fibers. Reduced fractional shortening in the RV and LV, trabecular disarray and segmental wall-motion abnormalities, bulges, and aneurysms also occur in some patients.[103] Most individuals, however, have regional segmental RV thinning and akinesia or dyskinesia as well as ventricular fibrillation or tachycardia (Figure 21-29). Inheritance patterns suggest that RV dysplasia is autosomal dominant with variable expression and penetrance. RV dysplasia is found predominantly in male patients, and symptoms frequently occur with exercise.

RV dysplasia must be differentiated from RV outflow tract tachycardia, which presents a substantially lower risk of sudden death, and

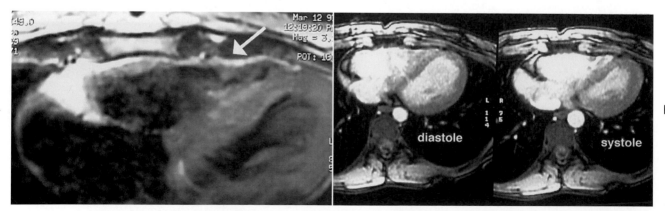

FIGURE 21-29 RV dysplasia. **A,** T1-weighted axial image shows bright signal compatible with fatty infiltration in the free wall of the RV *(arrow)*. **B,** Axial gradient-echo cine images during diastole and systole show poor function of the RV. This 36-year-old woman declined placement of an implanted defibrillator and died 1 month later as a result of ventricular fibrillation.

from nonpathological fatty infiltration, which usually does not cause clinical symptoms. The diagnosis is based on the identification of specific anatomical and functional abnormalities of the RV. RV angiography is considered a gold standard but cannot visualize pathological structural changes in the myocardium. MRI recently has shown promise in clarifying the diagnosis of RV dysplasia and can provide useful information about cardiac function, regional wall motion, and myocardial thinning and fatty infiltration of the RV free wall.[7,12,126] In a patient with RV dysplasia, the RV may appear normal in size or dilated, and the free wall may appear globally thinned or have focal areas of marked myocardial thinning. T1-weighted images demonstrate increased myocardial signal because of fatty infiltration. Breath-hold cine acquisitions are used to identify focal or global wall-motion abnormalities (Figure 21-30). Localization of dyskinesia to the RV outflow tract helps distinguish RV outflow tract tachycardia from RV dysplasia.[21]

CORONARY MAGNETIC RESONANCE ANGIOGRAPHY

Clinical applications of existing coronary MR angiography (MRA) techniques[29,156] include determining the patency and direction of flow in native coronary arteries[55,87]; evaluating the patency of coronary artery bypass grafts[42] and native vessels after coronary stent placement[30]; evaluating congenital[92] and acquired coronary variants; following the progress of known proximal lesions, such as after treatment with angioplasty; and identifying anomalous coronary arteries and their anatomical course.[31] Coronary MRA can also be used to screen and evaluate ischemic heart disease and coronary artery disease. Several clinical comparisons between coronary MRA and cardiac catheterization have been made.[32,87,119,124] No MRI technique has emerged that can provide the sensitivity and specificity for lesion detection equal to that of catheterization-based x-ray angiography, although preliminary clinical studies appear promising. Coronary MRA can routinely depict the proximal and middle portion of major coronary arteries and some coronary artery branches in most patients. The current limitations of coronary MRA include the inability to visualize the more distal portion of the coronary arteries and coronary artery branches. At its current stage of development, coronary MRA may be most helpful for excluding clinically important stenoses in patients referred for diagnostic contrast angiography. As techniques continue to improve, they may become an integral part of the evaluation with ischemic heart disease.

Respiratory and cardiac motion, plus the small caliber and tortuosity of the coronary arteries, make coronary MRA a technical challenge. ECG-gated segmented κ-space acquisitions with breath-holding to minimize cardiac and respiratory motion artifacts, respectively, have made coronary MRA possible. The low flip angle and short TR of segmented κ-space acquisitions, with the addition of fat suppression to eliminate epicardial fat, provide a good TOF effect that accentuates the coronary arteries. Both 2D and 3D techniques are used; 2D TOF single breath–hold cardiac-gated imaging has been implemented using segmented κ-space SPGR, an NVS of 8, and a κ space of 128 (16-heartbeat acquisition).[6,33] Oblique 4-mm slices were acquired in mid-diastole to minimize heart motion and maximize coronary flow. Later improvements included spectrally selective RF pulses to suppress epicardial fat and a surface coil to increase SNR; similar 2D techniques have been implemented using spiral scanning with interleaved spiral trajectories through κ space[98] that provide high temporal and spatial resolution with relative insensitivity to flow and motion artifacts.

Tortuous vessels make the selection of 2D imaging planes difficult. Anatomical approaches[132] comparable to those used with conventional angiography and echocardiography have been particularly useful. For imaging the right coronary artery (RCA), a transaxial slice through the LV and RV is used to select an oblique plane through the RV that transects the RCA in two points (Figure 21-31). This oblique image is used to select a plane through the anterior atrioventricular groove that contains the RCA. Scout scans for slice localization typically use a high NVS (short breath-hold) and multislice, single-phase acquisitions for obtaining gross landmarks. A low NVS with multiphase, single-slice acquisitions is then obtained within one breath-hold once the vessel plane is identified. Cine display of the images is used to provide better visualization of the coronary arteries, as illustrated in Figure 21-32.[132] Parallel overlapping slices are obtained to cover tortuous vessels. Oblique,[131] as well as fixed, transverse planes have been used to image the left main artery and left anterior descending artery. Infusion of Gd-DTPA during the acquisition improves the contrast-to-noise ratio of the vessel relative to adjacent tissue (Figure 21-33).

Non–breath-hold 3D MRA techniques use navigator echo–based retrospective respiratory gating and respiratory triggering[124,158] according to the superoinferior position of the diaphragm (Figure 21-8). Thin, contiguous slices are acquired with less partial-volume effects and a more accurate estimation of vessel size than in 2D techniques (Figure 21-34). These techniques offer several advantages over 2D techniques, including higher spatial resolution, increased SNR, continuous coverage of the coronaries, a capacity for multiplanar reconstruction after processing, and suitability for patients who cannot manage with breath-holding requirements. Also, 3D volume acquisitions are less operator dependent than iterative 2D approaches that require multiple oblique prescriptions. However, 3D acquisitions require approximately 30 minutes or more to scan the entire heart in three acquisition slabs, which may be substantially longer than that required by 2D techniques. Irregular breathing patterns may be problematic, and the accuracy with which the diaphragm is tracked greatly determines whether the coronaries are imaged at a constant position.

VALVULAR DISEASE

With SE MRI, evaluation of valvular disease was primarily limited to identification of large valvular masses or cardiac masses located adjacent to the cardiac valves. Because of long imaging times and low temporal resolution, SE imaging does not routinely allow the identification of primary valvular disorders. Although cine MRI and phase-mapping techniques offer substantial improvement in the depiction of valvular abnormalities, MRI is currently used as an adjunct to echocardiography. Quantitative signal-analysis packages for the MR evaluation of valvu-

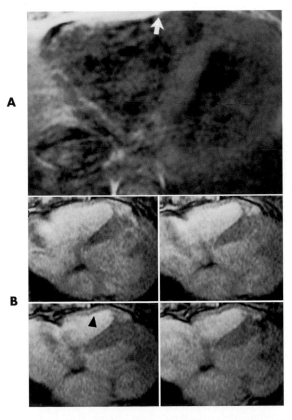

FIGURE 21-30 RV dysplasia in a 55-year-old man. **A,** SE T1-weighted image demonstrates thinning and fatty infiltration of the anterior and inferior wall of the RV *(arrow),* which is separated from pericardial fat by the dark pericardial line. **B,** Single-slice, multiphase transverse cine images through systole *(left to right, top to bottom)* show akinesis of the RV apex *(arrowhead)* and dyskinesis of the RV base. Mild right atrial and ventricular enlargement is also noted. (From reference 17.)

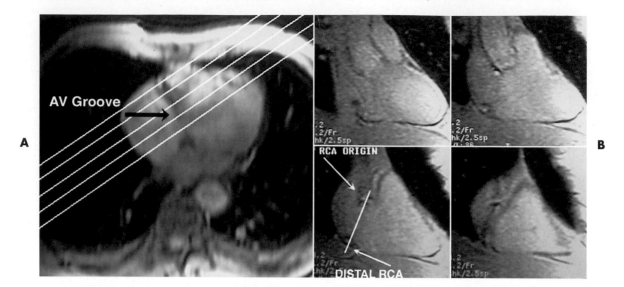

FIGURE 21-31   Coronary artery prescription. **A,** Long segment of the RCA can usually be obtained by first identifying the atrioventricular groove in the axial plane. Multiple slices perpendicular to this are then prescribed. **B,** The origin and distal portions of the RCA are next located. Prescription of several parallel slices along a line containing the origin and distal vessel yields images such as those shown here. (From reference 17.)

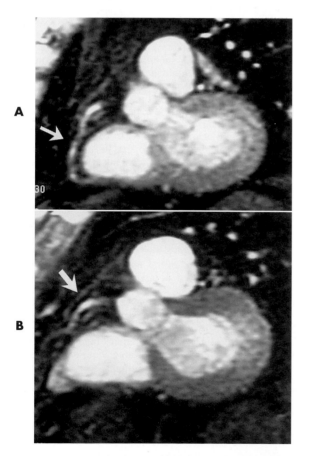

FIGURE 21-32   Coronary MRA of the RCA. **A,** Oblique 2D TOF single breath-hold cine acquisition with fat suppression reveals the middle and distal segments of the RCA *(arrow).* Using a segmented κ-space technique, 13 cardiac phases were then imaged within one breath-hold through the prescribed slice. Cine display of the images was used to better visualize the coronary arteries. The cardiac phase depicted here corresponds to middiastole. The proximal RCA is out of the imaging plane in **A** and is best seen on an adjacent view **(B),** parallel to the imaging plane.

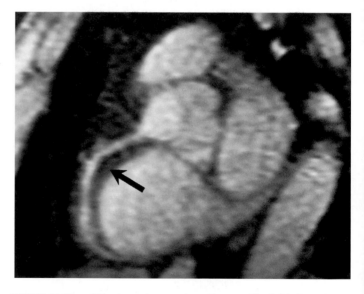

FIGURE 21-33   Gd-enhanced coronary angiogram. The RCA *(arrow)* was obtained using a 2D spoiled gradient-echo acquisition after administration of Gd-DTPA.

lar stenoses and regurgitation are not widely available; thus MRI is most commonly used to assess the secondary anatomical changes that occur from valvular disorders.

Technique

Using bright blood cine techniques, segmented κ-space acquisitions allow good temporal resolution when a small NVS is used,[4-6] so temporal resolution is on the order of 25 ms. Thin slices (5 mm) allow improved depiction of valvular motion. Typically, 12 to 15 images are acquired at a single level in relationship to the valve plane. These images are then played back in a movie loop to demonstrate the valvular

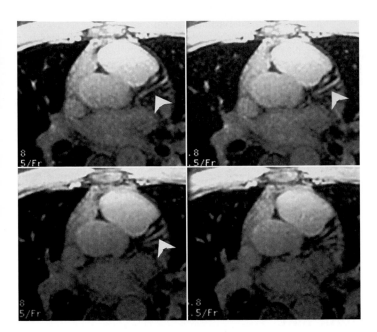

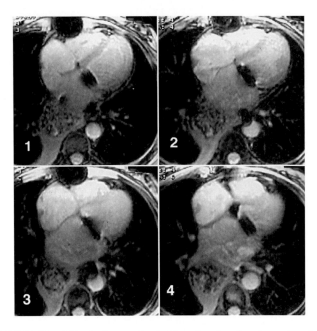

FIGURE 21-34   Navigator-based coronary artery acquisition. Overlapping 2-mm thick slices are shown at the level of the left anterior descending coronary artery *(arrow)*. (From reference 17.)

FIGURE 21-35   Mitral valve prosthesis. Four-chamber cine views of the heart demonstrate susceptibility artifact because of the metal components of a mitral valve prosthesis. Valve function is normal, without turbulence from regurgitation or stenosis.

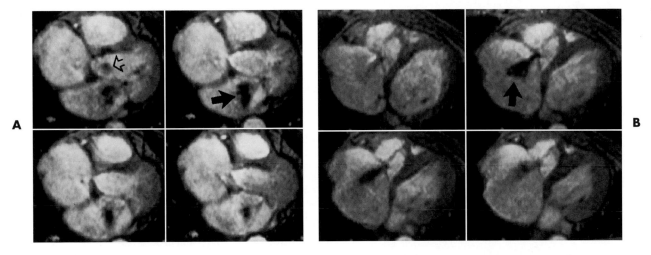

FIGURE 21-36   Mitral and tricuspid regurgitation diagnosed using cine MRI in a 76-year-old woman evaluated for constrictive pericarditis. **A,** Sequence of four transverse slices intersecting the mitral valve plane covering systole *(left to right, top to bottom)*. Mitral regurgitation appears as a signal void that results from a turbulent jet that worsens during systole *(arrow)*. Aortic insufficiency is also noted in the late diastole, early systole frame in the upper left *(open arrow)*. The left atrium is dilated. **B,** Sequence of four transverse slices intersecting the tricuspid valve plane covering systole *(left to right, top to bottom)*. Tricuspid regurgitation also appears as a jet of signal void that worsens during systole *(arrow)*. Marked right atrial enlargement is noted. The study was negative for constrictive pericarditis. Moderate mitral regurgitation, moderate aortic insufficiency, severe tricuspid regurgitation, and mild pulmonary hypertension were also demonstrated on the ECG. (From reference 17.)

motion and any evidence of blood flow disturbance. Disturbances in blood flow because of valvular turbulence are depicted as areas of signal loss and are described as a signal void. These signal voids indicate the location of the valvular abnormality, and the size of the void is related to the severity of disease. Metal components of valve prostheses yield susceptibility artifact (Figure 21-35).

In valvular stenosis, turbulent flow results in spin dephasing and signal loss downstream from the valve plane. In regurgitant lesions, signal voids propagate in a retrograde manner in the same direction of regurgitant flow. Signal voids appear during ventricular systole in mitral and tricuspid regurgitation (Figures 21-36 and 21-37). Pulmonic and aortic regurgitation has signal voids during ventricular diastole.

Unfortunately, the size and character of the signal void provide only qualitative information about the severity of the valvular lesion. The size of the signal void is greatly influenced by the TE and flip angle.[147] Furthermore, depending on these factors, signal void resulting from turbulence across normal valves may also be identified.[100] The signal void jets are complex 3D phenomena that are only partially seen on a single 2D imaging plane and vary considerably in size during the cardiac cycle. Therefore attempts to quantify the extent of a valvular regurgitant or stenotic lesion are only partially quantitative but correspond well to qualitative evaluation using echocardiography.[23,101]

Quantitative assessment of the extent of valvular lesion is possible using volumetric or phase-mapping techniques.[53] Although this is time

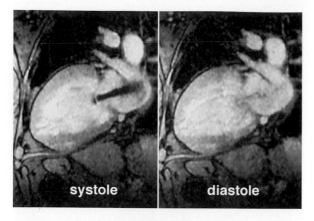

FIGURE 21-37 Mitral valve regurgitation. Signal void from the LV to the left atrium during systole is due to turbulence and signal dephasing. The overall size of the signal void is proportional to the extent of regurgitation but depends highly on the pulse sequence and imaging parameters used.

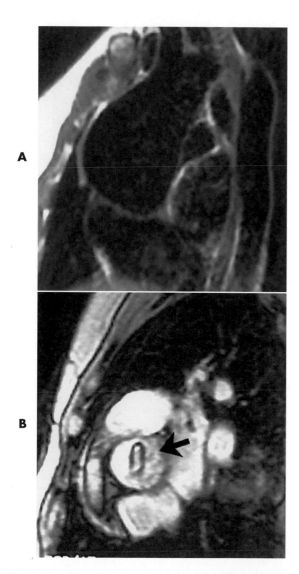

FIGURE 21-38 Bicuspid aortic valve. **A,** T1-weighted sagittal oblique image shows marked dilatation of the ascending aorta, secondary to long-standing aortic stenosis. **B,** Cine gradient-echo image of the aortic valve shows a bicuspid, stenotic conformation *(arrow).*

consuming and automated methods remain in a developmental stage, MRI is the gold standard for the assessment of cardiac chamber volumes using planimetry of each chamber and Simpson's rule to calculate total chamber volumes. In comparison, echocardiographic assessments of left and right atrial volumes, as well as RV structure and function, are particularly limited when compared with MRI.[76] The normal RV shape is difficult to model by geometrical assumptions,[25] and the atria are relatively inaccessible to multiplane echocardiographic imaging because of their intrathoracic location away from the anterolateral aspect of the chest wall. MRI has allowed for reduced variability of measurements in clinical[20,113,167] and experimental[69,79,142] studies of cardiac pathology. Since the stroke volumes for the LV and RV are normally equal, the difference in stroke volume between the regurgitant and normal ventricle is equal to the regurgitant volume. The regurgitant fraction is the regurgitant volume divided by the total stroke volume.

Phase-mapping techniques[145] may be used to measure regurgitant flow by obtaining images parallel to the annulus of the valve. Velocity profiles throughout the cardiac cycle are directly proportional to the strength of the phase-encoding gradient using this method. Total flow during the cardiac cycle is calculated as the product of the valve area and the velocity. Selected examples of common valvular abnormalities are discussed further.

Aortic Valve

Congenital aortic stenosis can occur as an isolated anomaly or may be associated with thoracic or cardiac anomalies. Subvalvular aortic stenosis is most commonly seen in pediatric patients and occurs in male more often than female patients, with a ratio of 2.5:1. A bicuspid aortic valve (Figure 21-38) is the most common cause of congenital aortic stenosis. Approximately 20 to 30 years pass before sufficient valvular degeneration has occurred and the condition becomes symptomatic and warrants valve replacement. Supravalvular aortic stenosis is the least common form of aortic stenosis and occurs in isolation or as part of Williams syndrome (Figure 21-39). In these patients, sagittal oblique views of the ascending aorta demonstrate the anatomical site of the stenosis.

Marfan syndrome is a connective tissue disorder characterized by skeletal, ocular, and cardiovascular involvement. Aortic disease is the most serious and lethal cardiovascular complication in patients with Marfan syndrome. Without surgical repair of the aorta, patients have decreased life expectancy resulting primarily from progressive aortic root dilatation (Figures 21-40 and 21-41) with a propensity for aortic dissection, rupture, or regurgitation. Repair of the ascending aortic aneurysm with aortic valve ectasia can be achieved using a composite graft technique with coronary artery ostial reattachment[9] (Figure 21-42). Despite repair of the ascending aorta and aortic valve, in approximately 30% of patients, there are progression of aortic dilatation and new onset or progression of aortic dissection, requiring subsequent surgery.[63] MRI is valuable for the complete monitoring of such patients for postoperative complications at the surgical site, as well as evaluation of the thoracoabdominal aorta.

Mitral Valve

The mitral valve is best visualized in the vertical and horizontal long-axis views. Associated LV hypertrophy and dysfunction are best evaluated in the short-axis plane. In-plane phase mapping may be performed through the center of a signal void jet in the presence of mitral stenosis. The resulting velocity-time plot is displayed, and the peak atrial systolic velocity is used in the modified Bernoulli equation to calculate peak atrial systolic pressure.[64]

Rheumatic fever is the most common cause of mitral valve stenosis and regurgitation; other common etiologies of stenoses include congenital deformity and bacterial endocarditis. Increased atrial pressures and volume result in left atrial enlargement, with subsequent pulmonary venous hypertension and eventual RV hypertrophy. Either cine or SE MRI readily demonstrates the size of the cardiac chamber. Mitral valve regurgitation is commonly associated with coronary artery disease. After MI, progressive LV dilatation causes enlargement of the valve orifice and distortion of the chordae tendineae. Infarction or trauma can also result in mitral regurgitation. Trauma can result in ruptured papillary muscles and valve dysfunction (Figure 21-43).

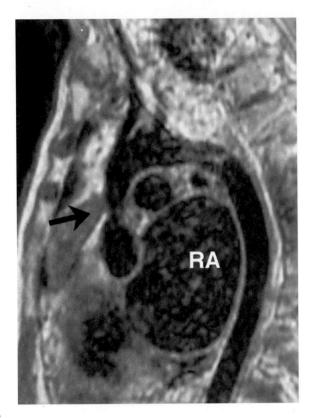

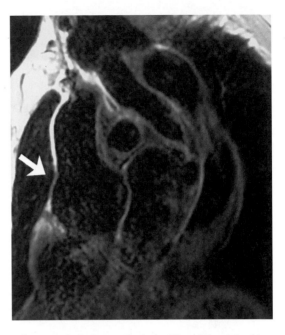

FIGURE 21-39 Supravalvular aortic stenosis in 48-year-old man with Williams syndrome. Sagittal oblique view shows marked narrowing of the supravalvular aorta *(arrow)*. There is also marked dilation of the left atrium *(LA)*.

FIGURE 21-40 Marfan's disease. Sagittal, oblique T1-weighted image shows a classic "tulip-bulb" enlargement of the aortic root that is characteristic of this disorder.

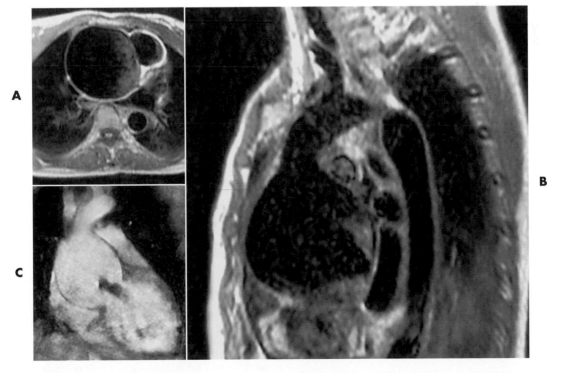

FIGURE 21-41 Marfan's disease. **A** and **B,** Axial and sagittal oblique T1-weighted images show marked dilation of the aortic root. The aortic annulus is also dilated. **C,** Cine gradient-echo image shows turbulence across the aortic valve because of aortic regurgitation.

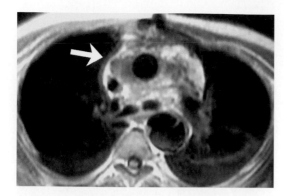

FIGURE 21-42   Normal postoperative aortic root after composite graft replacement in a 46-year-old man with Marfan's disease. The aortic graft is surrounded by intermediate signal intensity *(arrow)*, which is a result of postoperative fluid and hemorrhage. After graft placement, the native aorta is "wrapped" around the graft to contain potential leaks at the graft site. A residual dissection is present in the descending aorta.

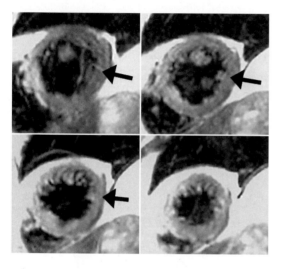

FIGURE 21-43   Papillary muscle rupture in a 36-year-old man with acute onset of mitral valve dysfunction after a motor vehicle accident. Short-axis views demonstrate that posterior leaflet papillary muscle is small and discontinuous *(arrow)*, a result of disruption. The patient underwent mitral valve replacement.

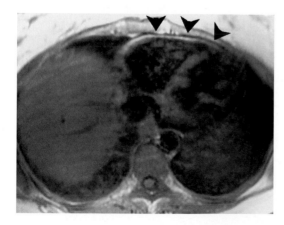

FIGURE 21-44   Normal pericardium. Axial T1-weighted image shows 2 to 3 mm of dark pericardial signal, best seen anterior to the RV *(arrowheads).*

PERICARDIUM

Although echocardiography is the primary modality by which pericardial disease is identified, MRI has an established role in the evaluation of the pericardium. MRI is commonly used (1) when clinical symptoms are inconsistent with the echocardiographic diagnosis, (2) when the echocardiographic examination is technically inadequate (e.g., patients with severe emphysema or large pleural effusions), and (3) when more precise characterization of lesions is necessary (e.g., evaluation of tumor relationship to the pericardium). In these circumstances, MRI is typically the examination of choice; the exception is the identification of calcific pericarditis, in which computed tomography (CT) should be used. MRI provides a complete anatomical view of the heart, pericardium, and myocardium and, unlike echocardiography, is not limited by the need for acoustic "windows."

Normal Pericardium

The pericardium is composed of an outer fibrocollagenous layer and an inner serous membrane. The inner serosal layer is closely applied to the epicardial surface of the heart and is termed the *visceral pericardium.* The serosal layer doubles back on itself to become the inner lining of the outer fibrous layer. These two layers thus form the parietal pericardium. A potential space between the serosal layers normally contains about 15 to 50 ml of fluid. Pericardial fluid is an ultrafiltrate of plasma, with protein content about one third that of plasma.[45]

The normal pericardial signal on MRI is derived from three potential sources: visceral pericardium, parietal pericardium, and pericardial fluid. The visceral pericardium consists of a single layer of mesothelial cells and therefore is not imaged by MRI in normal subjects.[104] The parietal pericardial signal is primarily from fibrous tissue, which shows low signal on both T1- and T2-weighted images. Pericardial fluid has low signal on T1-weighted images and high signal on T2-weighted images, as verified by cadaver studies.[56] In normal patients, the pericardial signal measures less than 2 mm in thickness, as defined on T1-weighted images[138] (Figure 21-44). Since the pericardium anatomically is only 0.8 to 1 mm thick, the wider pericardial signal observed on MRI likely results from flow-related loss of pericardial fluid signal on T1-weighted images.[56,138] Overall, pericardial signal is somewhat better seen during systole, probably because of an increased pericardial space during cardiac ejection. Similar observations have been made using M-mode echocardiography and angiography.[19] Pericardial signal is easily identified on T1-weighted or proton density–weighted images anterior to the RV, where its dark signal contrasts with that of the high fat signal of mediastinal or subepicardial fat. However, posterolateral to the LV the pericardial signal is often not seen against the low–signal intensity lung parenchyma.

Perhaps contrary to expectations of a "fluid-derived" signal, the normal pericardial signal on T2-weighted images is frequently lower than that expected of simple fluid.[138] This lower signal probably results from loss of phase coherence of the pericardial fluid from bulk motion or nonlaminar fluid flow, particularly during systole. In patients with large, simple effusions without loculations, pericardial signal is frequently nonuniform on T2-weighted images and sometimes has areas of both high and intermediate signal. Flow effects in the pericardium can also be demonstrated on cine gradient-echo imaging, in which flow-related enhancement of pericardial fluid is frequently detected (Figure 21-45).

Pericardial Effusions

Pericardial effusion is serous, bloody, or lymphatic in nature. Frequently, effusions have an increased protein content and a higher cellular content than normal pericardial fluid. Effusions as small as 30 to 50 ml may be detected with MRI. Since the upper limit of pericardial thickness on MRI is considered to be approximately 2 mm, pericardial dimensions exceeding 3 mm are abnormal. Effusions are regions of low signal on T1-weighted and proton density–weighted images that displace the parietal pericardium and associated fat away from the myocardial wall (Figure 21-46). Thickened pericardium is distinguished from effusion by the elliptical shape of the effusion posterolaterally to the LV. The T2-weighted signal of effusions is variable depending on the nature of the effusion. Moderate effusions, as judged by echocardiography, contain between 100 and 500 ml of fluid.[89] Comparison to

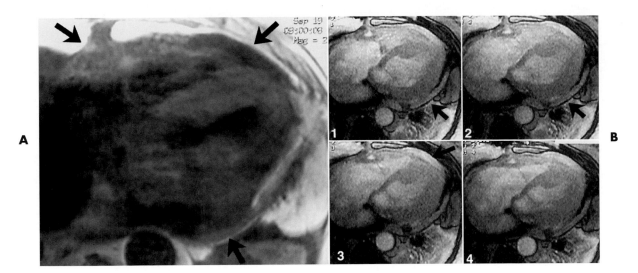

FIGURE 21-45   Pericardial effusion evaluated by cine images. **A,** Gated axial T1-weighted image in a 59-year-old woman after cardiac transplant shows complex signal intensity surrounding the heart. The effect of the fluid, some of which is expected after cardiac surgery, on cardiac mechanics cannot be shown using this method. **B,** Segmented κ-space cine acquisition shows normal sequence of contraction of the LV and RV. The pericardial fluid *(arrow)* changes in signal intensity during the cardiac cycle, suggesting flowing fluid rather than constriction.

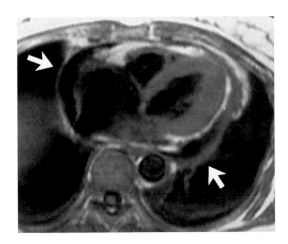

FIGURE 21-46   Pericardial effusion. Axial T1-weighted image shows increased width of the dark pericardial stripe anterior to the RV, as well as posterior to the LV *(arrows),* compatible with effusion.

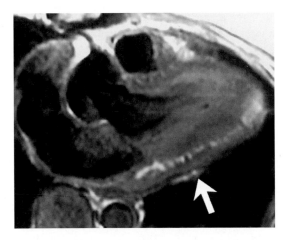

FIGURE 21-47   Pericardial thickening. A T1-weighted image shows 5-mm thickening of the pericardium posterior to the LV *(arrow).* Epicardial fat remains intact. Thickening was the result of a treated cardiac malignancy.

MR has shown that moderate effusions are associated with a pericardial space that is larger than 5 mm and is anterior to the RV.

Loculated pericardial effusions are diagnosed when adhesions are visualized between the visceral and parietal pericardium. An associated pericardial inflammation may be separately recognized as thickened pericardium with a higher signal intensity. For loculated effusions or inflammatory exudate adhering to the pericardium, fluid motion is diminished. Correspondingly, flow-related phase loss is also reduced, and loculated effusions show regions of higher signal intensity on T2-weighted images.[99,137,148]

Pericardial Thickening

Thickening of the pericardium on MRI appears as a widened pericardial line of low signal on T1-weighted images (Figure 21-47). This is also the case for pericardial effusion and calcific pericarditis, so an attempt should be made to distinguish between these entities. Several features help the clinician identify and differentiate thickening from other pericardial lesions. First, inflammatory thickening is accompanied by changes in the normal low pericardial signal to a medium or high signal.[137] Second, calcifications are often associated with fibrous pericarditis. Calcifications appear as focal areas of decreased signal with irregular borders. Gradient-echo images show calcifications that are apparently larger because of susceptibility effects. Third, the distribution of focal or diffuse thickening is not similar to the elliptical accumulation of pericardial fluid, which is typically seen posterolaterally to the LV.[137] Furthermore, an enlarged anterosuperior pericardial recess is associated with effusion but not thickening. On cine images, a thickened pericardium has a constant width throughout the cardiac cycle, whereas the pericardium in pericardial effusion has cyclical changes in width.

Constrictive Pericarditis

Constrictive pericarditis results from progressive pericardial fibrosis, leading to restriction of the cardiac ventricles during diastole. The disease progresses over a period of years, leading to increased systolic and pulmonary venous pressures. Symptoms include fatigue, dyspnea, and chest pain accompanied by ascites, hepatomegaly, and peripheral edema. Atrial fibrillation is present in one fourth of patients. Constriction may follow any pericardial injury that invokes an inflammatory response. Tuberculosis accounts for about 20% of cases, with other etiologies including infectious pericarditis, connective tissue disease,

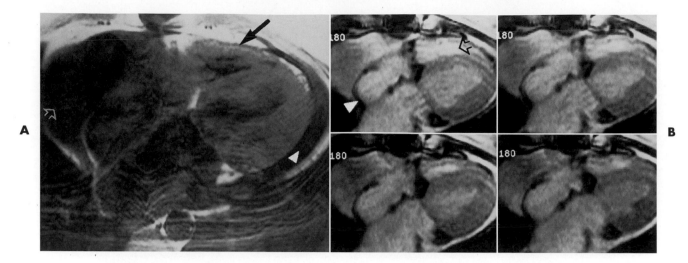

FIGURE 21-48   Constrictive pericarditis in a 40-year-old woman after cardiac transplant. **A,** SE T1-weighted image demonstrates moderate inhomogeneous effusion around the LV *(arrowhead)* leading to constrictive physiology. The left atrium is enlarged, and the right atrium is compressed by loculated pericardial fluid *(open arrow).* The RV is elongated, tubular, and diminished in volume *(black arrow).* The image artifact is due to respiratory motion during image acquisition. **B,** Single-slice, multiphase transverse cine images through systole *(left to right, top to bottom)* show mild dyskinesis and decreased contractility of the LV, decreased contractility of the RV *(open arrow),* compression of the right atrium *(arrowhead),* and decreased diastolic filling of the right atrium and RV. The patient subsequently underwent pericardial stripping and symptoms were relieved. (From reference 17.)

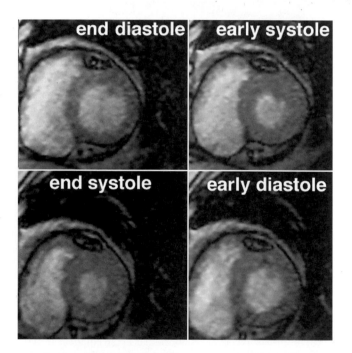

FIGURE 21-49   Normal cardiac function excluding constrictive pericarditis in a 59-year-old man after cardiac surgery with question of failed cardiac transplant versus constrictive pericarditis. Separate images of the pericardium (not shown) were equivocal because of pericardial changes after surgery. Short-axis cine images, however, demonstrate normal or slightly increased size of the RV, with normal filling and slightly reduced ejection fraction. Biopsy confirmed cardiac rejection.

neoplasm, and trauma. Constriction is also a recognized complication of long-term dialysis for renal failure, cardiac surgery (Figure 21-48), and radiation therapy (more than 4000 rads).

The major difficulty in diagnosing constrictive pericarditis is distinguishing it from restrictive cardiomyopathy (e.g., amyloid heart disease).[57,110] Echocardiography excludes conditions such as pericardial effusion, tamponade, valvular dysfunction, and dilated cardiomyopathy mimicking constrictive disease. However, echocardiographic findings, such as early pulmonic valve opening, abnormal septal wall motion, and diastolic posterior wall flattening, may also be seen with restrictive disease. Cardiac catheterization demonstrates equalization of LV and RV pressures in both conditions. Treatment of constrictive pericarditis, however, requires surgery (pericardiectomy) and has a success rate of 75%. If medical management is applied (appropriate for cardiomyopathy), the patient's condition progressively deteriorates.

On MRI, pericardial thickening greater than 4 mm supports the diagnosis of constriction.[146] In chronic constriction, the thickened pericardium has a lower signal intensity than other causes of pericarditis-associated thickening because of the low signal intensity of fibrous tissue. Thickening in subacute forms of constrictive pericarditis that result from uremia, radiation therapy, or cardiac surgery has moderate to high signal intensity.[50] Structural abnormalities are observed in association with constriction. A small, tubular RV is seen on MRI. The right atrium, inferior vena cava, and superior vena cava are dilated. Cine images show reduced diastolic filling and hypokinesis of the RV (Figures 21-48, *B,* and 21-49).

Pericardial and Paracardiac Masses

MR evaluation of masses related to the pericardium primarily involves the identification of abnormal structures and boundaries rather than characterization of relative tissue intensities. Notable exceptions include pericardial cyst, lipoma, and fibroma, each of which has a distinctive signal intensity. The value of MRI evaluation of tumors related to the pericardium lies in treatment planning and preoperative assessment.

Pericardial cysts are congenital in origin, arising from embryologically separated lacunae of pericardial tissue.[78] The majority are right-sided lesions (70%), and 90% are located in the right or left costophrenic sulcus. Both MRI and CT provide specific diagnoses of pericardial cysts. On CT, the cysts are smooth-walled, fluid-filled structures with densities of up to 20 Hounsfield units (HU). On MRI, the diagnosis is equally specific: a paracardiac mass with long T1 and T2 relaxation times (Figure 21-50). The cyst wall is smooth and of low signal intensity.[137] The true pericardial cyst does not communicate with the pericardium. Pericardial diverticula may be congenital in origin or acquired through a defect in the parietal pericardium. These contain all layers of the pericardium and communicate with the pericardiac space. Their signal intensity is the same as that of normal pericardial fluid on all pulse sequences.

Primary pericardial neoplasms are much less common than metastatic disease and include fibrosarcoma, angiosarcoma, and teratoma. Paracardiac tumors include pheochromocytoma and lipoma. Lipoma and teratoma have areas of high signal intensity on T1-weighted images because of fat content. Neoplastic involvement of the pericardium

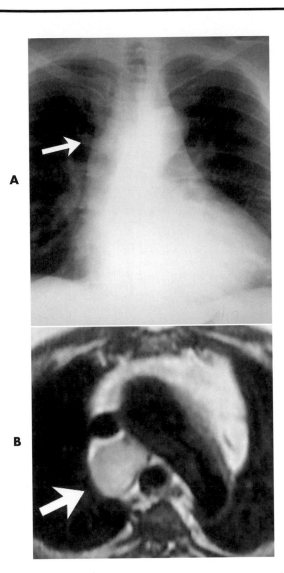

FIGURE 21-50   Pleuropericardial cyst. **A,** Chest x-ray film shows fullness in the right paratracheal region *(arrow)*. **B,** Axial T2-weighted image shows a right paratracheal mass *(arrow)* that is high in signal intensity. This mass is a congenital diverticulum, typically discovered incidentally in young adults.

results in focal or diffuse obliteration of the normal low-signal pericardium. For malignancy adjacent to the pericardium, preservation of the pericardial signal is evidence that pericardial invasion has not occurred.

Metastatic disease involving the pericardium has an incidence of 1.5% to 22%.[104] Some 80% of metastatic diseases to the pericardium also involve breast cancer, leukemia, and lymphoma.[2,152] Metastatic disease involving the pericardium is characterized by large effusions that are out of proportion to the amount of tumor present; this occurs to the extent that neoplasm is the most common cause of tamponade. Focal or diffuse thickening of the pericardium may occur, obliterating the pericardial space. MRI of metastatic disease to the pericardium demonstrates excellent anatomical detail, and tumor deposits are identified more distinctly from associated effusion than on CT.[121,159]

CONCLUSION

The role of MRI in the evaluation of acquired heart disease has expanded from the traditional role of anatomical characterization. Particularly with the advent of more rapid breath-hold pulse sequences, MRI is increasingly used outside of specialized centers for the evaluation of cardiac function and blood flow. Specialized cardiovascular MR scanners are under development; these scanners will incorporate software improvements to allow real-time fluoroscopic imaging, echoplanar techniques, and rapid cine image review, as well as software for spe-

cialized analysis. These developments can improve acceptance among radiologists and cardiologists, as well as decrease examination time for patients. Thus cardiac imaging appears to be a key area in which MR applications can continue to expand over the next several years.

REFERENCES

1. Ahmad M, Johnson R Jr, Fawcett HD, et al: Magnetic resonance imaging in patients with unstable angina: comparison with acute myocardial infarction and normals, Magn Reson Imaging 6:527, 1988.
2. Applefeld MM, and Pollock SH: Cardiac disease in patients who have malignancies, Curr Probl Cardiol 4:1, 1980.
3. Arrive L, Assayag P, Russ G, et al: MRI and cine MRI of asymmetric septal hypertrophic cardiomyopathy, J Comput Assist Tomogr 18:376, 1994.
4. Atalar E, and McVeigh ER: Optimum tag thickness for the measurement of position with MRI, IEEE Trans Med Imaging 13:152, 1994.
5. Atkinson D, Burstein D, and Edelman R: First-pass cardiac perfusion: evaluation with ultrafast MR imaging, Radiology 174:757, 1990.
6. Atkinson D, and Edelman R: Cineangiography of the heart in a single breathhold with a segmented turboFLASH sequence, Radiology 178:359, 1991.
7. Auffermann W, Wichter T, Breithardt G, et al: Arrhythmogenic right ventricular disease: MR imaging vs angiography, Am J Roentgenol 161:549, 1993.
8. Axel L, and Dougherty L: Heart wall motion: improved method of spatial modulation of magnetization for MR imaging, Radiology 172:349, 1989.
9. Bentall HH, and De Bono A: A technique for complete replacement of the ascending aorta, Thorax 23:338, 1968.
10. Beyar R: Hypertrophic cardiomyopathy: functional aspects by tagged magnetic resonance imaging, Adv Exp Med Biol 382:293, 1995.
11. Bikkina M, Levy D, Evans JC, et al: Left ventricular mass and risk of stroke in an elderly cohort, JAMA 272:33, 1994.
12. Blake L, Scheinman M, and Higgins C: MR features of arrhythmogenic right ventricular dysplasia, Am J Roentgenol 162:809, 1994.
13. Bluemke D, Boxerman J, Atalar E, et al: Segmented κ-space cine breath-hold cardiovascular MR imaging. I. Principles and technique, Am J Roentgenol 169:395, 1997.
14. Bluemke D, Boxerman J, Mosher T, et al: Segmented κ-space cine breath-hold cardiovascular MR imaging. II. Evaluation of aortic vasculopathy, Am J Roentgenol 169:401, 1997.
15. Bouchard A, Reeves RC, Cranney G, et al: Assessment of myocardial infarct size by means of T2-weighted 1H nuclear magnetic resonance imaging, Am Heart J 117:281, 1989.
16. Bouton S, Yang A, McCrindle BW, et al: Differentiation of tumor from viable myocardium using cardiac tagging with MR imaging, J Comput Assist Tomogr 15:676, 1991.
17. Boxerman JL, Mosher T, McVeigh ER, et al: Advanced MRI techniques for the evaluation of the heart and great vessels, Radiographics 18:543, 1998.
18. Braunwald E: Assessment of cardiac function. In Braunwald E, ed: Heart disease: a textbook of cardiovascular medicine, ed 4, Philadelphia, 1992, WB Saunders.
19. Bryk D, Kroop IG, and Budow J: The effect of heart size, cardiac tamponade, and phase of the cardiac cycle on the distribution of pericardial fluid, Radiology 93:273, 1969.
20. Buck T, Hunold P, Wentz KU, et al: Tomographic three-dimensional echocardiographic determination of chamber size and systolic function in patients with left ventricular aneurysm: comparison to magnetic resonance imaging, cineventriculography, and two-dimensional echocardiography, Circulation 96:4286, 1997.
21. Carlson M, White R, Trohman R, et al: Right ventricular outflow tract ventricular tachycardia: detection of previously unrecognized anatomic abnormalities using cine magnetic resonance imaging, J Am Coll Cardiol 24:720, 1994.
22. Casale PN, Devereux RB, Milner M, et al: Value of echocardiographic left ventricular mass in predicting cardiovascular morbid events in hypertensive men, Ann Intern Med 105:173, 1986.
23. Colletti PM, DeFrance A, Tak T, et al: Cardiac MRI cine and color Doppler in valvular disease: correlative imaging, Magn Reson Imaging 9:343, 1991.
24. Conway J: Clinical assessment of cardiac output, Eur Heart J 11:148, 1990.
25. Czegledy FP, and Katz J: A new geometric description of the right ventricle, J Biomed Eng 15:387, 1993.
26. De Roos A, van der Wall EE, Bruschke AV, et al: Magnetic resonance imaging in the diagnosis and evaluation of myocardial infarction, Magn Reson Q 7:191, 1991.
27. Deichmann R, Adolf H, Noth U, et al: Calculation of signal intensities in hybrid sequences for fast NMR imaging, Magn Reson Med 34:481, 1995.
28. Duerinckx AJ: Coronary MR angiography, Magn Reson Imag Clin North Am 4:361, 1996.
29. Duerinckx AJ: MR angiography of the coronary arteries, Top Magn Reson Imaging 7:267, 1996.
30. Duerinckx AJ, Atkinson D, Hurwitz R, et al: Coronary MR angiography after coronary stent placement, Am J Roentgenol 165:662, 1995.
31. Duerinckx AJ, Bogaert J, Jiang H, et al: Anomalous origin of the left coronary artery: diagnosis by coronary MR angiography, Am J Roentgenol 164:1095, 1995.
32. Duerinckx AJ, and Urman M: Two-dimensional coronary MR angiography: analysis of initial clinical results, Radiology 193:731, 1994.
33. Edelman R, Manning W, Burstein D, et al: Coronary arteries: breath-hold MR angiography, Radiology 181:641, 1991.
34. Felmlee JP, Ehman RL, Riederer SJ, et al: Adaptive motion compensation in MRI: accuracy of motion measurement, Magn Reson Med 18:207, 1991.
35. Filipchuk NG, Peshock RM, Malloy CR, et al: Detection and localization of recent myocardial infarction by magnetic resonance imaging, Am J Cardiol 58:214, 1986.
36. Firmin DN, Nayler GL, Klipstein RH, et al: In vivo validation of MR velocity imaging, J Comput Assist Tomogr 11:751, 1987.

37. Frustaci A, Chimenti C, and Pieroni M: Idiopathic myocardial vasculitis presenting as restrictive cardiomyopathy, Chest 111:1462, 1997.
38. Fujita N, Duerinckx AJ, and Higgins CB: Variation in left ventricular regional wall stress with cine magnetic resonance imaging: normal subjects versus dilated cardiomyopathy, Am Heart J 125:1337, 1993.
39. Fujita N, Hartiala J, O'Sullivan M, et al: Assessment of left ventricular diastolic function in dilated cardiomyopathy with cine magnetic resonance imaging: effect of an angiotensin converting enzyme inhibitor, benazepril, Am Heart J 125:171, 1993.
40. Funari M, Fujita N, Peck WW, et al: Cardiac tumors: assessment with Gd-DTPA enhanced MR imaging, J Comput Assist Tomogr 15:953, 1991.
41. Gaffey CT, and Tenforde TS: Alternations in the rat electrocardiogram induced by stationary magnetic fields, Bioelectromagnetics 2:357, 1981.
42. Galjee M, van Rossum A, Doesburg T, et al: Value of magnetic resonance imaging in assessing patency and function of coronary artery bypass grafts: an angiographically controlled study, Circulation 93:660, 1996.
43. Gaudio C, Pelliccia F, Tanzilli G, et al: Magnetic resonance imaging for assessment of apical hypertrophy in hypertrophic cardiomyopathy, Clin Cardiol 15:164, 1992.
44. Gaudio C, Tanzilli G, Mazzarotto P, et al: Comparison of left ventricular ejection fraction by magnetic resonance imaging and radionuclide ventriculography in idiopathic dilated cardiomyopathy, Am J Cardiol 67:411, 1991.
45. Gibson AT, and Segal MB: A study of the composition of pericardial fluid, with special reference to the probable mechanism of fluid formation, J Physiol 277:367, 1978.
46. Gomes AS, Lois JF, Child JS, et al: Cardiac tumors and thrombus: evaluation with MR imaging, Am J Roentgenol 149:895, 1987.
47. Grande AM, Ragni T, and Vigano M: Primary cardiac tumors: a clinical experience of 12 years, Tex Heart Inst J 20:223, 1993.
48. Hardy CJ, Darrow RD, Nieters EJ, et al: Real-time acquisition, display, and interactive gahic control of NMR cardiac profiles and images, Magn Reson Med 29:667, 1993.
49. Higgins CB: MRI in ischemic heart disease: acute infarction, chronic infarction and contrast media in ischemic myocardial disease, Radiol Med 79:680, 1990.
50. Higgins CB: Overview of MR of the heart—1986, Am J Roentgenol 146:907, 1986.
51. Higgins CB, Herfkens R, Lipton MJ, et al: Nuclear magnetic resonance imaging of acute myocardial infarction in dogs: alterations in magnetic relaxation times, Am J Cardiol 52:184, 1983.
52. Higgins CB, and McNamara MT: Magnetic resonance imaging of ischemic heart disease, Prog Cardiovas Dis 28:257, 1986.
53. Higgins CB, Wagner S, Kondo C, et al: Evaluation of valvular heart disease with cine gradient echo magnetic resonance imaging, Circulation 84:1198, 1991.
54. Hsu JC, Johnson GA, Smith WM, et al: Magnetic resonance imaging of chronic myocardial infarcts in formalin-fixed human autopsy hearts, Circulation 89:2133, 1994.
55. Hundley W, Clarke G, Landau C, et al: Noninvasive determination of infarct artery patency by cine magnetic resonance angiography, Circulation 91:1347, 1995.
56. Im JG, Rosen A, Webb WR, et al: MR imaging of the transverse sinus of the pericardium, Am J Roentgenol 150:79, 1988.
57. Isner JM, Carter BL, Bankoff MS, et al. Computed tomography in the diagnosis of pericardial heart disease, Ann Intern Med 97:473, 1982.
58. Järvinen VM, Kupari MM, Hekali PE, et al: Right atrial MR imaging studies of cadaveric atrial casts and comparison with right and left atrial volumes and function in healthy subjects, Radiology 191:137, 1994.
59. Judd RM, Lugo-Olivieri CH, Arai M, et al: Physiological basis of myocardial contrast enhancement in fast magnetic resonance images of 2-day-old reperfused canine infarcts, Circulation 92:1902, 1995.
60. Judd R, Parrish T, Ramani K, et al: Comparison of first-pass and delayed MRI contrast enhancement to rest-redistribution 201Tl SPECT in patients with chronic LV dysfunction, Presented at the fifth annual meeting of the International Society of Magnetic Resonance in Medicine, Vancouver, 1997.
61. Judd R, Reeder S, Atalar E, et al: A magnetization-driven gradient echo pulse sequence for the study of myocardial perfusion, Magn Reson Med 34:276, 1995.
62. Kastler B, Germain P, Dietemann JL, et al: Spin echo MRI in the evaluation of pericardial disease, Comput Med Imaging Graph 14:241, 1990.
63. Kawamoto S, Bluemke DA, Traill TA, et al: Thoracoabdominal aorta in Marfan syndrome: MR imaging findings of progression of vasculopathy after surgical repair, Radiology 203:727, 1997.
64. Kilner PJ, Firmin DN, Rees RS, et al: Valve and great vessel stenosis: assessment with MR jet velocity mapping, Radiology 178:229, 1991.
65. Kondo C, Caputo GR, Semelka R, et al: Right and left ventricular stoke volume measurements with velocity-encoded cine MR imaging: in vitro and in vivo validation, Am J Roentgenol 157:9, 1991.
66. Koren MJ, Devereux RB, Casale PN, et al: Relationship of left ventricular mass and geometry to morbidity and mortality in uncomplicated essential hypertension, Ann Intern Med 114:345, 1991.
67. Kraitchman D, Wilke N, Hexeberg E, et al: Myocardial perfusion and function in dogs with moderate coronary stenosis, Magn Reson Med 35:771, 1996.
68. Kramer CM, Ferrari VA, Rogers WJ, et al: Angiotensin-converting enzyme inhibition limits dysfunction in adjacent noninfarcted regions during left ventricular remodeling, J Am Coll Cardiol 27:211, 1996.
69. Kramer CM, Lima JA, Reichek N, et al: Regional differences in function within noninfarcted myocardium during left ventricular remodeling, Circulation 88:1279, 1993.
70. Kramer CM, Reichek N, Ferrari VA, et al: Regional heterogeneity of function in hypertrophic cardiomyopathy, Circulation 90:186, 1994.
71. Lam KY, Dickens P, and Chan AC: Tumors of the heart: a 20-year experience with a review of 12,485 consecutive autopsies, Arch Pathol Lab Med 117:1027, 1993.
72. Lanzer P, Botvinick EH, Schiller NB, et al: Cardiac imaging using gated magnetic resonance, Radiology 150:121, 1984.
73. Lau V-K, and Sagawa K: Model analysis of the contribution of atrial contraction to ventricular filling, Ann Biomed Eng 7:167, 1979.
74. Laub G, and Simonetti O: Assessment of myocardial perfusion with saturation-recovery turboFLASH sequences, Presented at the fourth annual meeting of the International Society of Magnetic Resonance in Medicine, New York, 1996.
75. Lee VS, Spritzer CE, Carroll BA, et al: Flow quantification using fast cine phase-contrast MR imaging, conventional cine phase-contrast MR imaging, and Doppler sonography: in vitro and in vivo validation, Am J Roentgenol 169:1125, 1997.
76. Levine RA, Gibson TC, Aretz T, et al: Echocardiographic measurement of right ventricular volume, Circulation 69:497, 1984.
77. Levy D, Garrison RJ, Savage DD, et al: Prognostic implications of echocardiographically determined left ventricular mass in the Framingham heart study, N Engl J Med 322:1561, 1990.
78. Lilley WI, McDonald JR, and Clagett OT: Pericardial celomic cysts and pericardial diverticula: a concept of etiology and reports of cases, J Thorac Surg 20:494, 1950.
79. Lima JA, Ferrari VA, Reichek N, et al: Segmental motion and deformation of transmurally infarcted myocardium in acute postinfarct period, Am J Physiol 268:H1304, 1995.
80. Lima J, Judd R, Bazille A, et al: Regional heterogeneity of human myocardial infarcts demonstrated by contrast-enhanced MRI: potential mechanisms, Circulation 92:1117, 1995.
81. Lima JA, Judd RM, Bazille A, et al: Regional heterogeneity of human myocardial infarcts demonstrated by contrast-enhanced MRI: potential mechanisms, Circulation 92:1117, 1995.
82. Lima JAC, Judd RM, Lugo-Olivieri CH, et al: Myocardial perfusion pattern by contrast enhanced MRI in the acute post-infarct period can predict myocardial necrosis and eventual extent of scar formation, Circulation 90:1, 1994.
83. Lima J, Judd R, Zerhouni E, et al: Contrast enhanced ultrafast MRI demonstrates perfusion in infarcted myocardium supplied by patent coronary artery despite thallium defect, Circulation 88(Suppl):I275, 1993.
84. Lugo-Olivieri CH, Moore CC, Poon EG-C, et al: Temporal evolution of three dimensional deformation in the ischemic human left ventricle: assessment by MR tagging, Soc Magn Reson Abstr 3:1482, 1994.
85. MacGowan GA, Shapiro EP, Azhari H, et al: Noninvasive measurement of shortening in the fiber and cross-fiber directions in the normal human left ventricle and in idiopathic dilated cardiomyopathy, Circulation 96:535, 1997.
86. Manning W, Atkinson D, Grossman W, et al: First-pass nuclear magnetic resonance imaging studies of patients with coronary artery disease, J Am Coll Cardiol 18:959, 1991.
87. Manning W, Li W, and Edelman R: A preliminary report comparing magnetic resonance coronary angiography with conventional angiography, N Engl J Med 328:828, 1993.
88. Marcus F, Fontaine G, Guiraudon G, et al: Right ventricular dysplasia: a report of 24 adult cases, Circulation 65:384, 1982.
89. Martin RP, Rakowski H, French J, et al: Localization of pericardial effusion with wide angle phased array echocardiography, Am J Cardiol 42:904, 1978.
90. Masui T, Finck S, and Higgins CB: Constrictive pericarditis and restrictive cardiomyopathy: evaluation with MR imaging, Radiology 182:369, 1992.
91. Matsuoka H, Hamada M, Honda T, et al: Morphological and histologic characterization of cardiac myxomas by magnetic resonance imaging, Angiology 47:693, 1996.
92. McConnell M, Ganz P, Selwyn A, et al: Identification of anomalous coronary arteries and their anatomic course by magnetic resonance coronary angiography, Circulation 92:3158, 1995.
93. McKinnon G: Ultrafast interleaved gradient-echo-planar imaging on a standard scanner, Magn Reson Med 30:609, 1993.
94. McNamara MT, and Higgins CB: Magnetic resonance imaging of chronic myocardial infarcts in man, Am J Roentgenol 146:315, 1986.
95. McVeigh ER, and Zerhouni EA: Noninvasive measurement of transmural gradients in myocardial strain with magnetic resonance imaging, Radiology 180:677, 1991.
96. Meier RA, and Hartnell GG: MRI of right atrial pseudomass: is it really a diagnostic problem? J Comput Assist Tomogr 18:398, 1994.
97. Menegus MA, Greenberg MA, Spindola-Franco H, et al: Magnetic resonance imaging of suspected atrial tumors, Am Heart J 123:1260, 1992.
98. Meyer C, Hu B, Nishimura D, et al: Fast spiral coronary artery imaging, Magn Reson Med 28:202, 1992.
99. Miller SW, Brady TJ, Dinsmore RE, et al: Cardiac magnetic resonance imaging: the Massachusetts General Hospital experience, Radiol Clin North Am 23:745, 1985.
100. Mirowitz SA, Lee JK, Gutierrez FR, et al: Normal signal-void patterns in cardiac cine MR images, Radiology 176:49, 1990.
101. Mitchell L, Jenkins JP, Watson Y, et al: Diagnosis and assessment of mitral and aortic valve disease by cine-flow magnetic resonance imaging, Magn Reson Med 12:181, 1989.
102. Møgelvang J, Stubgaard M, Thomsen C, et al: Evaluation of right ventricular volumes measured by magnetic resonance imaging, Eur Heart J 9:529, 1988.
103. Molinari G, Sardanelli F, Gaita F, et al: Right ventricular dysplasia as a generalized cardiomyopathy? Findings on magnetic resonance imaging, Eur Heart J 16:1619, 1995.
104. Moncada R, Kotler MN, Churchill RJ, et al: Multimodality approach to pericardial imaging, Cardiovasc Clin 17:409, 1986.
105. Moore CC, Lugo-Olivieri CH, Lee L, et al: 3D deformation of the normal human left ventricle: assessment by MR tissue tagging, Soc Magn Reson Abstr 4:1567, 1995.
106. Moore CC, McVeigh ER, Mebazaa A, et al: Use of striped tagging to measure three-dimensional endocardial and epicardial deformation throughout the canine left ventricle during ischemia, J Magn Reson Imaging 3P:124, 1993.
107. Moore CC, O'Dell WG, McVeigh ER, et al: Calculation of three-dimensional left ventricular strains from biplanar tagged MR images, J Magn Reson Imaging 2:165, 1992.

108. Moore CC, Reeder SB, and McVeigh ER: Tagged MR imaging in a deforming phantom: photographic validation, Radiology 190:765, 1994.
109. Nayler GL, Firmin DN, and Longmore DB: Blood flow imaging by cine magnetic resonance, J Comput Assist Tomogr 10:715, 1986.
110. Nishimura RA, Connolly DC, Parkin TW, et al: Constrictive pericarditis: assessment of current diagnostic procedures, Mayo Clin Proc 60:397, 1985.
111. Niwa K, Uchishiba M, Aotsuka H, et al: Measurement of ventricular volumes by cine magnetic resonance imaging in complex congenital heart disease with morphologically abnormal ventricles, Am Heart J 131:567, 1996.
112. O'Dell WG, Moore CC, Hunter WC, et al: Three-dimensional myocardial deformations: calculation with displacement field fitting to tagged MR images, Radiology 195:829, 1995.
113. Palmon LC, Reichek N, Yeon SB, et al: Intramural myocardial shortening in hypertensive left ventricular hypertrophy with normal pump function, Circulation 89:122, 1994.
114. Park JH, Kim YM, Chung JW, et al: MR imaging of hypertrophic cardiomyopathy, Radiology 185:441, 1992.
115. Pattynama PM, and de Roos A: MR evaluation of myocardial ischemia and infarction, Top Magn Reson Imaging 7:218, 1995.
116. Pattynama PM, de Roos A, van der Wall EE, et al: Evaluation of cardiac function with magnetic resonance imaging, Am Heart J 128:595, 1994.
117. Pattynama PM, Lamb HJ, van der Velde EA, et al: Left ventricular measurements with cine and spin-echo MR imaging: a study of reproducibility with variance component analysis, Radiology 187:261, 1993.
118. Pattynama PM, Willems LNA, Smit AH, et al: Early detection of cor pulmonale with MR imaging of the right ventricle, Radiology 182:375, 1992.
119. Pennell D, Bogren H, Keegan J, et al: Assessment of coronary artery stenosis by magnetic resonance imaging, Heart 72:127, 1996.
120. Peshock R, Malloy C, Buja L, et al: Magnetic resonance imaging of acute myocardial infarction: gadolinium diethylenetriamine pentaacetic acid as a marker of reperfusion, Circulation 74:1434, 1986.
121. Pizzarello RA, Goldberg SM, Goldman MA, et al: Tumor of the heart diagnosed by magnetic resonance imaging, J Am Coll Cardiol 5:989, 1985.
122. Pons-Llado G, Carreras F, Borras X, et al: Comparison of morphologic assessment of hypertrophic cardiomyopathy by magnetic resonance versus echocardiographic imaging, Am J Cardiol 79:1651, 1997.
123. Posma JL, Blanksma PK, van der Wall EE, et al: Assessment of quantitative hypertrophy scores in hypertrophic cardiomyopathy: magnetic resonance imaging versus echocardiography, Am Heart J 132:1020, 1996.
124. Post J, van Rossum A, Hofman M, et al: Three-dimensional respiratory-gated MR angiography of coronary arteries: comparison with conventional coronary angiography, Am J Roentgenol 166:1399, 1996.
125. Rehr RB, Malloy CR, Filipchuk NG, et al: Left ventricular volumes measured by MR imaging, Radiology 156:717, 1985.
126. Ricci R, Longo R, Pagnan L, et al: Magnetic resonance imaging in right ventricular dysplasia, Am J Cardiol 70:1589, 1992.
127. Rokey R, Verani MS, Bolli R, et al: Myocardial infarct size quantification by MR imaging early after coronary artery occlusion in dogs, Radiology 158:771, 1986.
128. Sacks MS, Chuong CJ, Templeton GH, et al: In vivo 3-D reconstruction and geometric characterization of the right ventricular free wall, Ann Biomed Eng 21:263, 1993.
129. Saeed M, Wendland MF, Lauerma K, et al: First-pass contrast-enhanced inversion recovery and driven equilibrium fast GRE imaging studies: detection of acute myocardial ischemia, J Magn Reson Imaging 5:515, 1995.
130. Saeed M, Wendland M, Masui T, et al: Reperfused myocardial infarctions on T1- and susceptibility-enhanced MRI: evidence for loss of compartmentalization of contrast media, Magn Reson Med 31:31, 1994.
131. Sakuma H, Caputo G, Steffens J, et al: Breath-hold MR cine angiography of coronary arteries in healthy volunteers: value of multiangle oblique imaging planes, Am J Roentgenol 163:533, 1994.
132. Sakuma H, Caputo G, Steffens J, et al: Breathhold MR angiography of coronary arteries with optimal double-oblique imaging planes and cine display, Presented at the seventy-ninth annual meeting of the Radiological Society of North America, Chicago, 1993.
133. Sakuma H, Fujita N, Foo TKF, et al: Evaluation of left ventricular volume and mass with breath-hold cine MR imaging, Radiology 188:377, 1993.
134. Sardanelli F, Molinari G, Petillo A, et al: MRI in hypertrophic cardiomyopathy: a morphofunctional study, J Comput Assist Tomogr 17:862, 1993.
135. Sayad D, Willet DW, Chwialkowski M, et al: Rapid, noninvasive quantitation of regional left ventricular function using gradient-echo MRI with myocardial tagging: interstudy reproducibility, Am J Cardiol 76:985, 1995.
136. Sechtem U, Pfulgfelder PW, Gould RG, et al: Measurement of right and left ventricular volumes in healthy individuals with cine MR imaging, Radiology 163:697, 1987.
137. Sechtem U, Tscholakoff D, and Higgins CB: MRI of the abnormal pericardium, Am J Roentgenol 147:245, 1986.
138. Sechtem U, Tscholakoff D, and Higgins CB: MRI of the normal pericardium, Am J Roentgenol 147:239, 1986.
139. Semelka RC, Shoenut JP, Wilson ME, et al: Cardiac masses: signal intensity features on spin-echo, gradient-echo, gadolinium-enhanced spin-echo, and turboFLASH images, J Magn Reson Imaging 2:415, 1992.
140. Semelka RC, Tomei E, Wanger S, et al: Interstudy reproducibility of dimensional and functional measurements between cine magnetic resonance studies in the morpholgically abnormal left ventricle, Am Heart J 119:1367, 1990.
141. Semelka RC, Tomei E, Wagner S, et al: Normal left ventricular dimensions and function: interstudy reproducibility of measurements with cine MR imaging, Radiology 174:763, 1990.
142. Shapiro EP, Rogers WJ, Beyar R, et al: Determination of left ventricular mass by magnetic resonance imaging in hearts deformed by acute infarction, Circulation 79:706, 1989.
143. Simonetti OP, Finn JP, White RD, et al: "Black blood" T2-weighted inversion-recovery MR imaging of the heart, Radiology 199:49, 1996.
144. Siripornpitak S, and Higgins CB: MRI of primary malignant cardiovascular tumors, J Comput Assist Tomogr 21:462, 1997.
145. Sondergaard L, Thomsen C, Stahlberg F, et al: Mitral and aortic valvular flow: quantification with MR phase mapping, J Magn Reson Imaging 2:295, 1992.
146. Soulen RL, Stark DD, and Higgins CB: Magnetic resonance imaging of constrictive pericardial disease, Am J Cardiol 55:480, 1985.
147. Spielmann RP, Schneider O, Thiele F, et al: Appearance of poststenotic jets in MRI: dependence on flow velocity and on imaging parameters, Magn Reson Imaging 9:67, 1991.
148. Stark DD, Higgins CB, Lanzer P, et al: Magnetic resonance imaging of the pericardium: normal and pathologic findings, Radiology 150:469, 1984.
149. Suga H: Importance of atrial compliance in cardiac performance, Circ Res 35:39, 1974.
150. Suzuki J, Caputo GR, Masui T, et al: Assessment of right ventricular diastolic and systolic function in patients with dilated cardiomyopathy using cine magnetic resonance imaging, Am Heart J 122:1035, 1991.
151. Suzuki J, Sakamoto T, Takenaka K, et al: Assessment of the thickness of the right ventricular free wall by magnetic resonance imaging in patients with hypertrophic cardiomyopathy, Br Heart J 60:440, 1988.
152. Theologides A: Neoplastic cardiac tamponade, Semin Oncol 5:181, 1978.
153. Tscholakoff D, Higgins C, Sechtem U, et al: Occlusive and reperfused myocardial infarcts: effect of Gd-DTPA on ECG-gated MR imaging, Radiology 160:515, 1986.
154. Turnbull LW, Ridgway JP, Nicoll JJ, et al: Estimating the size of myocardial infarction by magnetic resonance imaging, Br Heart J 66:359-63, 1991.
155. van der Geest RJ, de Roos A, van der Wall EE, et al: Quantitative analysis of cardiovascular MR images, Int J Card Imaging 13:247, 1997.
156. van Rossum A, Post J, and Visser C: Coronary imaging using MRI, Herz 21:97, 1996.
157. Walsh E, Doyle M, Lawson M, et al: Multislice first-pass myocardial perfusion imaging on a conventional clinical scanner, Magn Reson Med 34:39, 1995.
158. Wang Y, Rossman P, Grimm R, et al: Navigator-echo-based real-time respiratory gating and triggering for reduction of respiration effects in three-dimensional coronary MR angiography, Radiology 198:55, 1996.
159. Westcott JL, and Steiner RM: Clinical applications of magnetic resonance imaging (MRI) of the heart, Cardiovasc Clin 17:323, 1986.
160. White HD, Norris RM, Brown MA, et al: Left ventricular end-systolic volume as a major determinate of survival after recovery from myocardial infarction, Circulation 76:44, 1987.
161. Wielopolski P, Manning W, and Edelman R: Single breath-hold volumetric imaging of the heart using magnetization-prepared 3-dimensional segmented echo planar imaging, J Magn Reson Imaging 5:403, 1995.
162. Wilke N, Jerosch-Herold M, Wang Y, et al: Myocardial perfusion reserve: assessment with multisection, quantitative, first-pass MR imaging, Radiology 204:373, 1997.
163. Wilke N, Simm C, Zhang J, et al: Contrast-enhanced first pass myocardial perfusion imaging: correlation between myocardial blood flow in dogs at rest and during hyperemia, Magn Reson Med 29:485, 1993.
164. Wisenberg G, Prato FS, Carroll SE, et al: Serial nuclear magnetic resonance imaging of acute myocardial infarction with and without reperfusion, Am Heart J 115:510, 1988.
165. Yokota C, Nonogi H, Miyazaki S, et al: Gadolinium-enhanced magnetic resonance imaging in acute myocardial infarction, Am J Cardiol 75:577, 1995.
166. Young AA, Axel L, Dougherty L, et al: Validation of tagging with MR imaging to estimate material deformation, Radiology 188:101, 1993.
167. Young AA, Imai H, Chang C, et al: Two-dimensional left ventricular deformation during systole using magnetic resonance imaging with spatial modulation of magnetization, Circulation 89:740, 1994.
168. Zerhouni EA, Parish DM, Rogers WJ, et al: Human heart: tagging with MR imaging—a method for noninvasive assessment of myocardial motion, Radiology 169:59, 1988.

22 Liver

Donald G. Mitchell and Richard C. Semelka

 KEY POINTS

- A comprehensive MR examination of the liver, including T1-weighted, T2-weighted, chemical-shift, and contrast-enhanced images, can substitute for a battery of other imaging tests.
- MRI is the most accurate method for detection, differential diagnosis, and staging of benign and malignant liver tumors.
- Diffuse fatty liver and iron overload can be diagnosed accurately. These disorders do not interfere with detection of focal lesions by MRI.
- Cirrhosis and its complications can be imaged effectively, as can various vascular disorders of the liver.

TECHNIQUES FOR ABDOMINAL MAGNETIC RESONANCE IMAGING

The general subject of magnetic resonance imaging (MRI) has been covered in earlier chapters. However, we will briefly review the types of MR techniques that are particularly important for hepatic imaging.

T1-Weighted Images

There are a variety of reliable techniques for achieving high T1 contrast between normal abdominal viscera and focal lesions, and for depicting fat planes. These include motion-compensated spin-echo (SE), inversion recovery, multislice spoiled gradient-echo, and magnetization-prepared rapid gradient-echo techniques.[200,232] The optimum technique varies, depending on the details of implementation on specific instruments.

The three most important considerations for choosing techniques for imaging the liver are contrast, motion artifact, and coverage. Adequate T1 contrast is possible with a wide variety of T1-weighted pulse sequences, provided that repetition time (TR) is kept moderate to short (e.g., less than 500 ms for 1.5 Tesla [T] and even shorter for lower field strengths) and echo time (TE) is minimized (e.g., less than 15 ms for SE techniques and less than 7 ms for gradient-echo techniques at 1.5 T; higher TEs may be acceptable for lower field strengths). Motion artifact can be controlled for SE pulse sequences using a combination of respiratory monitoring techniques, averaging, and presaturation pulses. However, respiratory artifact is controlled best with breath-hold techniques, which are beginning to replace SE techniques for most users of up-to-date MR equipment (Figure 22-1). Breath-hold techniques are also essential for MR-guided biopsy (Figure 22-2). Even with adequate compensation for ghost artifacts, movement of structures into and out of an image section causes substantial partial volume averaging, which reduces contrast and lesion conspicuity.[19] Most users prefer multisection spoiled gradient-echo images with TR between 100 and 150 ms and TE 5 ms or less because of generally high signal-to-noise ratios (SNRs) and adequate contrast. Heavier T1 contrast and reduced pulsation artifact, at the expense of lower SNR and lower resolution, may be achieved using magnetization-prepared gradient-echo techniques.[14]

T2-Weighted Images

High T2 contrast between normal viscera, lesion, and fluid can be achieved using motion-compensated SE techniques. More recently, techniques using multiple SEs acquired at numerous TEs have been introduced, yielding effective T2-weighted images of the abdomen when motion artifact is corrected via averaging or suspended respiration[113,144] (Figure 22-3). These techniques are all based on a pulse sequence called *RARE* (rapid acquisition with relaxation enhancement). In this chapter we refer to these techniques as *multishot fast spin echo (FSE)*; other common terms include *hybrid RARE* and *turbo SE*. In some comparisons there is a slight loss of contrast between liver and lesion with multishot FSE, but the dramatic improvement in efficiency more than compensates for this, provided that the multishot FSE images are appropriately optimized.

A further advantage of multishot FSE techniques is that high-quality, heavily T2-weighted images with TEs approaching or exceeding 200 ms can be obtained in only a few minutes. These images depict ducts and other fluid clearly and may be used to obtain MR cholangiopancreatograms (MRCP).[7,171]

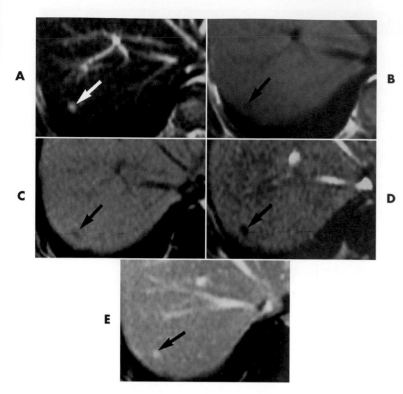

FIGURE 22-1 Small cavernous hemangioma *(arrow)*. **A,** SE 2500/100 image. **B,** SE 400/11 image. The lesion is barely visible as a result of motion-induced blurring. **C,** Gradient-echo 102/2.3/90 image. **D,** Snapshot inversion recovery 12/2.5/30 image, TI 500, centric-phase ordering. SNR is lower than in **C,** but contrast is higher because signal from the hemangioma is nulled. Vessels have high signal because of wash-in TOF effects (single-slice technique). **E,** Gradient-echo 102/2.3/90 image, after administration of Gd chelate. (From Mitchell DG, and Stark DD: Hepatobiliary MRI, St Louis, 1993, Mosby.)

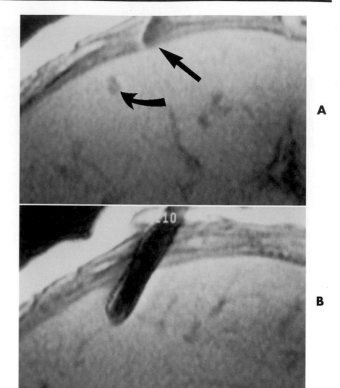

FIGURE 22-2 Biopsy of a 5-mm solitary liver lesion in a patient with breast carcinoma. T1-weighted gradient-echo 83/3.5/70 image obtained using a surface coil. **A,** The tip of the needle can be seen just superficial to the liver capsule *(straight arrow)*. *Curved arrow,* Lesion. **B,** Only blood and endothelial cells were obtained, and follow-up examination 1 year later showed no change. The diagnosis is cavernous hemangioma.

Chemical-Shift Images

Chemical-shift imaging (CSI) techniques are sensitive to differences in resonance frequency (i.e., chemical shift) between protons in water and triglyceride. Current CSI techniques include opposed-phase images, featuring signal cancellation within voxels that contain triglyceride and water, and suppression techniques, in which signal from either triglyceride or water is reduced by one or more different mechanisms.

At 1.5 T, TEs of approximately 2.1, 6.3, and 10.5 ms yield opposed-phase images, whereas TEs of approximately 4.2, 8.4, and 12.6 ms yield in-phase images.[141,254] At lower field strengths, the difference between in-phase and out-of-phase TEs is greater.

Lipid signal can be reduced or eliminated via the chemical shift between fat and water. The most commonly used chemical shift–fat suppression techniques involve transmitting a narrow-band excitation pulse designed to saturate triglyceride protons selectively without affecting water protons.[149,197] Fat-suppression techniques can improve image quality by reducing artifacts from fat and by improving dynamic range, but fat-suppressed images are less sensitive for detecting fatty liver than are opposed-phase images. Opposed-phase images are more sensitive to small quantities of lipid, whereas fat-suppressed images more reliably identify tissues with large quantities of lipid[142] (Figure 22-4).

Chemical-shift selective fat suppression must be distinguished from short tau inversion recovery (STIR). In STIR images, fat is suppressed because of its short T1 rather than its chemical shift relative to water. STIR techniques can be implemented with fast SE, in which a 180-degree inversion pulse and a 90-degree excitation pulse are followed by several 180-degree refocusing pulses. STIR techniques are relatively insensitive to fatty liver and do not reliably distinguish between fat and other tissues with short T1.

Magnetic Resonance Angiography

Gradient-echo images are valuable for depicting abdominal vascular anatomy as high signal intensity. Until recently, most techniques for de-

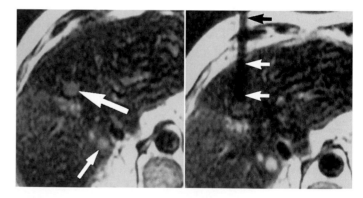

FIGURE 22-3 Aspiration of abscess not visible by CT. Multishot FSE 1500/120 echo-train length (ETL) 16, five 12-sec slices. (From reference 144.)

picting abdominal blood vessels as bright used time-of-flight (TOF) principles, where blood flowing into an image section has higher magnetization than the partially saturated stationary tissue within the section. MR angiographic images can be created by combining the data from multiple two-dimensional, TOF (2D-TOF) single sections.[51] Three-dimensional TOF techniques are usually suboptimal for imaging abdominal vessels because of their lower sensitivity to slow flow.

In the abdomen, 2D-TOF images provide reliable depiction of most vessels using the following parameters: thin sections (e.g., 2 to 7 mm), minimized TE (as short as possible, preferably ≥7 ms), gradient-moment nulling (unless TE is ≥3 ms), TR of approximately 25 to 50 ms, flip angle of 30 to 60 degrees, and no signal averaging (Figure 22-5). Thinner sections improve depiction of slow flow but require more time. Suspended respirations are beneficial, but they also increase examina-

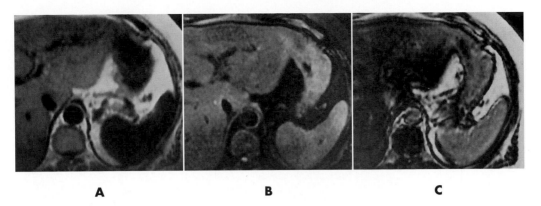

FIGURE 22-4   Fatty liver depicted by SE fat-suppression and gradient-echo opposed-phase techniques. **A,** SE 400/12 image. The liver is brighter than the spleen. **B,** SE 400/14 image with fat suppression (by combined-saturation and opposed-phase techniques). Relative signal of the liver is decreased. **C,** T1-weighted gradient-echo 103/2.3/90 image. At 1.5 T the fat and water phases are opposed with a TE of 2.3 ms, causing intravoxel signal cancellation. (From Mitchell DG, and Stark DD: Hepatobiliary MRI, St Louis, 1993, Mosby.)

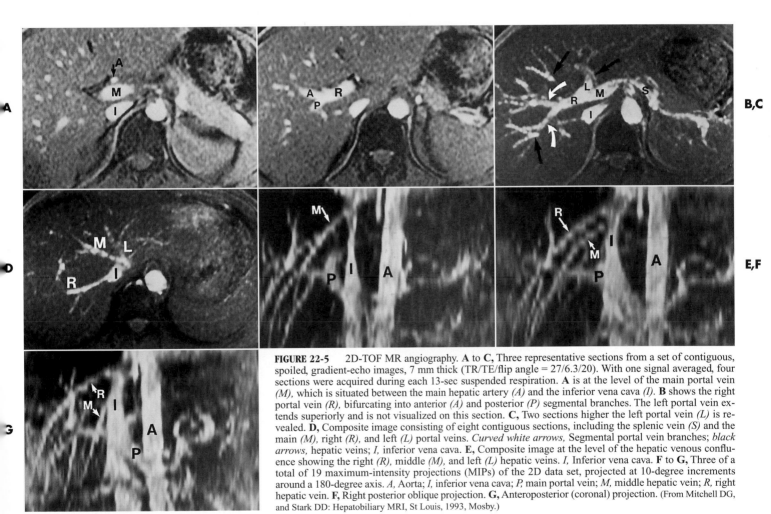

FIGURE 22-5   2D-TOF MR angiography. **A** to **C,** Three representative sections from a set of contiguous, spoiled, gradient-echo images, 7 mm thick (TR/TE/flip angle = 27/6.3/20). With one signal averaged, four sections were acquired during each 13-sec suspended respiration. **A** is at the level of the main portal vein *(M),* which is situated between the main hepatic artery *(A)* and the inferior vena cava *(I).* **B** shows the right portal vein *(R),* bifurcating into anterior *(A)* and posterior *(P)* segmental branches. The left portal vein extends superiorly and is not visualized on this section. **C,** Two sections higher the left portal vein *(L)* is revealed. **D,** Composite image consisting of eight contiguous sections, including the splenic vein *(S)* and the main *(M),* right *(R),* and left *(L)* portal veins. *Curved white arrows,* Segmental portal vein branches; *black arrows,* hepatic veins; *I,* inferior vena cava. **E,** Composite image at the level of the hepatic venous confluence showing the right *(R),* middle *(M),* and left *(L)* hepatic veins. *I,* Inferior vena cava. **F** to **G,** Three of a total of 19 maximum-intensity projections (MIPs) of the 2D data set, projected at 10-degree increments around a 180-degree axis. *A,* Aorta; *I,* inferior vena cava; *P,* main portal vein; *M,* middle hepatic vein; *R,* right hepatic vein. **F,** Right posterior oblique projection. **G,** Anteroposterior (coronal) projection. (From Mitchell DG, and Stark DD: Hepatobiliary MRI, St Louis, 1993, Mosby.)

tion time. Saturation pulses should be used only with caution because many abdominal vessels are tortuous.

Phase-contrast (PC) techniques rely on depicting changes in phase that result from motion.[108] 2D PC techniques can be useful adjuncts for determining the direction and volume of blood flow, acquired either during suspended respiration or using cardiac gating. 3D PC techniques can yield high-quality MR angiograms because of their high resolution and near-total suppression of background tissue; however, these images require more time to acquire. Although not currently available on most systems, flow information on PC images can be depicted in color, similar to methods currently used for color Doppler imaging[231] (Figure 22-6).

Recently, fat-suppressed 3D T1-weighted sequences acquired during or immediately after bolus administration of gadolinium chelates have been used to generate high-quality MR arteriographic images.

Contrast Enhancement

Currently available chelates of gadolinium (Gd), such as gadopentetate dimeglumine, gadoteridol, and gadodiamide, are extracellular space agents. Clinical evaluations for hepatic imaging are in progress for more specific agents that accumulate preferentially in the blood pool (e.g., ultrasmall paramagnetic iron oxide particles)[134] (Figure 22-7) or

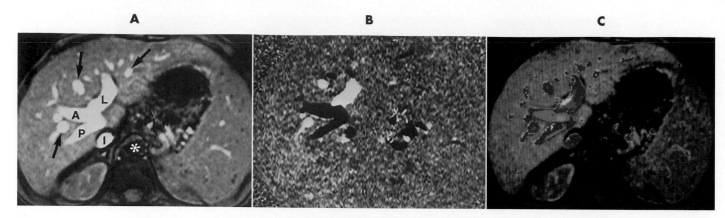

FIGURE 22-6   Color-flow MR angiography produced by unambiguous superimposition of magnitude and phase data from 2D PC images, showing the anterior *(A)* and posterior *(P)* branches of the right portal vein and the left portal vein *(L)*. *I,* Inferior vena cava. A saturation pulse was applied superiorly to eliminate signal from the aorta *(asterisk)*. *Arrows,* Hepatic vein branches. **A,** Magnitude image. **B,** Corresponding phase image. Flow toward the right is black, flow toward the left is white, and background and static tissue are gray. **C,** Color-flow MR image obtained by encoding the phase (flow) data from **B** and superimposing it on the magnitude (static tissue) data from **A.** Magnitude and phase thresholds were used to set the priority between color and gray scale. Blue represents flow toward the right (e.g., right portal vein branches), and red represents flow toward the left (e.g., left portal vein and middle and right hepatic veins). Paler shades of color indicate faster flow along the left-to-right axis. Helical flow in the inferior vena cava resulting from renal vein inflow causes a split-color appearance. (From Mitchell DG, and Stark DD: Hepatobiliary MRI, St Louis, 1993, Mosby.)

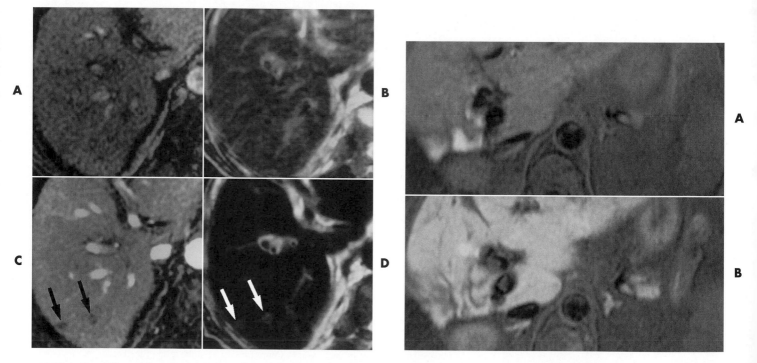

FIGURE 22-7   Ultrasmall superparamagnetic iron oxide particles used as a blood pool agent for depiction of liver metastases from colorectal carcinoma. T1-weighted gradient-echo 120/2.3/90 and T2-weighted multishot FSE 4000/102 images before (**A** and **B**) and after (**C** and **D**) administration of the contrast agent. The lesions *(arrows)* are depicted better after contrast administration, which increases the signal intensity of vessels and uninvolved liver on T1-weighted images (**C**) and decreases the signal intensity of vessels and uninvolved liver on T2-weighted images (**D**).

FIGURE 22-8   Enhancement of the liver, adrenal glands, and stomach relative to spleen and adipose tissue by administration of Mn-DPDP on fat-suppressed, T1-weighted, SE 400/11 images. **A,** Preinjection slices. **B,** After injection of contrast agent. (From Mitchell DG, and Stark DD: Hepatobiliary MRI, St Louis, 1993, Mosby.)

within hepatocytes (e.g., Gd-EOB-DTPA, Gd-DTPA-BOPTA).[64] Mangafodipir trisodium (formerly Mn-DPDP) (Figure 22-8) and ferumoxides (formerly AMI-25) have recently been approved for clinical use, but clinical experience is limited.[44,62,189,263] The use of currently available Gd chelates is emphasized in this chapter.

Extracellular-space contrast agents are distributed initially within the intravascular compartment and diffuse rapidly throughout the ex-

tracellular (vascular plus interstitial) space, similar to water-soluble iodinated contrast agents. Optimal dynamic scanning for detection and characterization of liver lesions is best accomplished if the entire liver can be imaged during a single suspended respiration. The most popular technique for this purpose is the multislice spoiled gradient-echo technique (e.g., fast low-angle shot [FLASH], fast multiplanar spoiled gradient echo [FMPSPGR]) with the longest TR possible

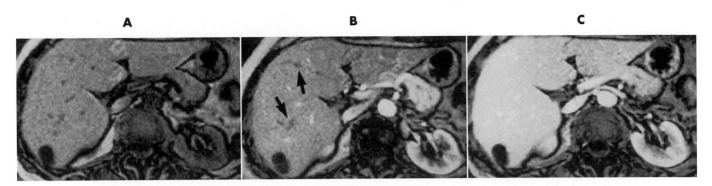

FIGURE 22-9   Hepatic cysts. T1-weighted spoiled gradient-echo 123/2.2/90 images before **(A)** and during capillary **(B)** and portal phases **(C)** after administration of Gd chelate, photographed using identical settings. During the capillary phase **(B)**, the pancreas enhances intensely. Liver enhances minimally, and hepatic veins *(arrows)* are unenhanced. During the portal phase **(C)**, the liver and its veins enhance. (From Mitchell DG: Liver. I. Currently available gadolinium chelates, MRI Clin North Am 4:37, 1996.)

during breath-holding and a flip angle of 90 degrees or slightly less.[47,113,117,198]

We recommend at least four separate sets of images corresponding to four separate physiological phases relative to the dynamic bolus administration of contrast material (Figure 22-9).

1. Baseline precontrast images are essential for determining whether technical quality and anatomical coverage are adequate. Also these images provide a basis of comparison to determine the presence or absence of perfusion, which in turn allows confident differentiation between fluid and tissue.
2. Capillary (arterial or presinusoidal) phase images are especially important for detection of hypervascular malignancies. These images are acquired immediately after a rapid bolus injection of Gd chelate, during which time the patient must be positioned within the magnet bore. Signs of a successful acquisition of arterial phase include intense and approximately equivalent enhancement of the pancreas, spleen, and renal cortex; marked heterogeneity of the spleen; near absence of renal medullary enhancement; and minimal enhancement of liver parenchyma. Contrast material is visible in hepatic arteries and usually in major portal vein branches but not within hepatic veins. Occasionally, part of the medial segment of the left lobe enhances early, probably the result of aberrant drainage of gastric veins to this region.[76]
3. Portal phase images show maximal hepatic enhancement and maximal contrast between liver and hypovascular lesions. These images are acquired approximately 1 min after contrast agent administration. Because most administered contrast material is present throughout the vascular system at this time, these images are similar to blood-pool phase images.
4. Extracellular phase (delayed) images are acquired 2 or more min after injection of contrast material, by which time contrast material has diffused into the interstitium of non–central nervous system (CNS) tissues. These images are quite different from blood-pool phase images. Delayed contrast enhancement is particularly prominent in edematous tissues, such as in neoplasms and areas of inflammation, and within fibrosis. If lipid signal is suppressed via frequency-selective saturation, interstitial enhancement is particularly conspicuous.

NORMAL ANATOMY AND MAGNETIC RESONANCE APPEARANCE

Techniques for resection of hepatic malignancies, including metastases, have improved greatly in the past few years. Sensitivity for additional lesions and their localization within hepatic segments have therefore become increasingly important.[42,56]

Current concepts of surgical anatomy divide the liver into eight segments, each of which can be resected individually or in combination with other segments, provided that enough hepatic tissue remains to preserve hepatic function (Figures 22-10 and 22-11). Segment I is the caudate lobe. The left lobe is divided by the falciform ligament into lateral and medial segments. Segments II and III are the portions of the

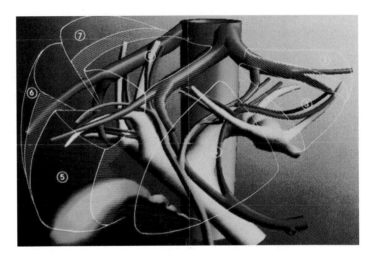

FIGURE 22-10   Functional anatomy of the liver. Three-dimensional representation. *Blue,* Systemic veins; *gray,* portal veins; *red,* hepatic arteries; *green,* bile ducts. (Courtesy Hepatobiliary Surgery and Liver Transplant Unit of Hospital Paul Brousse, Villejuif, France.)

lateral segment that are anterosuperior and posteroinferior, respectively, relative to the plane of the left hepatic vein. Segment IV is the medial segment of the left lobe. The right hepatic lobe is divided into anterior and posterior segments. Each of these two segments of the right lobe is divided into inferior (V and VI) and superior (VII and VIII) segments by the plane of the major branches of the right portal veins.

The vascular anatomy of the liver defines cleavage planes for hepatic surgery. Hepatic arterial, portal venous, and biliary systems are adjacent to each other within intrasegmental hepatic parenchyma, whereas blood drains into hepatic veins between hepatic segments and lobes. The main portal vein branches into the left portal vein, which ascends within the left intersegmental fissure, and the right portal vein, which is horizontal. The left portal vein divides into medial and lateral segmental branches, whereas the right portal vein divides into anterior and posterior segmental branches.

A variety of landmarks define the surgical planes of the liver. The interlobar fissure is defined superiorly by the middle hepatic vein and inferiorly by a line drawn between the inferior vena cava and the gallbladder. The left intersegmental fissure is defined superiorly by the left hepatic vein and inferiorly by the left main portal vein and the falciform ligament. The left intersegmental fissure separates segment IV (medial) from segments II and III (lateral). The right intersegmental fissure, defined superiorly by the right hepatic vein, separates segments V and VIII (anterior right lobe) from segments VI and VII (posterior right lobe). However, there is no consistent anatomical division

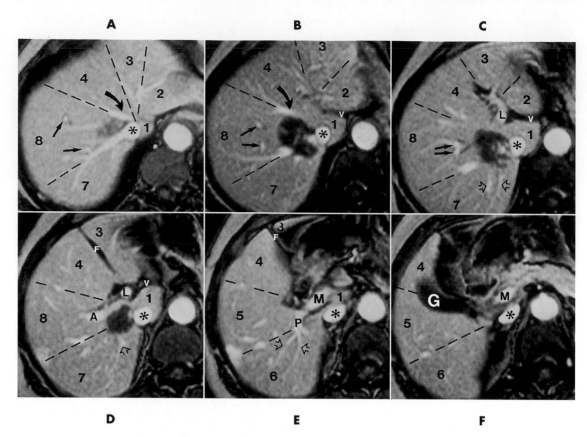

FIGURE 22-11   Hepatic segmental anatomy gradient-echo 84/2.4/90 image after bolus enhancement with Gd chelate. The middle hepatic vein *(curved arrow)* divides the liver into right and left lobes, which are further divided into four sectors by the right and left hepatic veins. The left hepatic vein divides segments 2 and 3 superiorly; inferiorly these segments are defined by branches of the left portal vein that perfuse them. Straight arrows in **A** through **C** indicate tributaries of the anterior branch of the right portal vein *(A)*, whereas open arrows in **C** through **E** indicate tributaries of the posterior branch *(P)*. The ligamentum venosum *(V)* separates segment 2 from segment 1 (caudate lobe). The proximal left portal vein *(L)* and the falciform ligament *(F)* separate segment 3 from segment 4. The level of the bifurcation of the right portal vein into its anterior *(A)* and posterior *(P)* branches, located between the sections in **D** and **E,** defines the transition from the cranial segments 7 and 8 to the caudal segments 5 and 6 of the right lobe. Inferiorly the plane of the gallbladder *(G)* parallels the middle hepatic vein and separates the left and right hepatic lobes. Two cavernous hemangiomas are present (**B** and **C**)—a large one, enhancing peripherally and involving segments 7 and 8 centrally, and a small one (**C** and **D**) located peripherally at the junction of segments 5 through 8. *Asterisk,* Inferior vena cava. (From Mitchell DG, and Stark DD: Hepatobiliary MRI, St Louis, 1993, Mosby.)

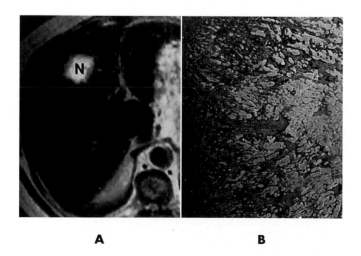

FIGURE 22-12   Central necrosis within colloid carcinoma metastatic from the colon. **A,** SE 2500/80 image depicts central necrosis *(N)* with peripheral intermediate intensity. **B,** Histological section from the center of the tumor showing mucin and debris. (From reference 172.)

of the right lobe, so this division should be considered an approximation at best.[103] The left hepatic vein, within the cephalad portion of the left intersegmental fissure, separates the medial (IV) and lateral (II and III) segments of the left hepatic lobe. The caudate lobe (I), which is perfused and drained by branches of the left and right hepatic vessels as well as its own accessory vessels, is situated medial to the right lobe, between the inferior vena cava and the fissure for the ligamentum venosum.

FOCAL LESIONS

At most centers, suspected focal pathology is the major indication for hepatic imaging. Success at this endeavor depends on high spatial resolution, high contrast between lesion and hepatic parenchyma, and the ability to distinguish between significant and insignificant pathology. Although the spatial resolution of computed tomography (CT) remains superior, MRI has higher contrast resolution and is more capable of detecting and characterizing focal lesions.[198] In this section we examine the MR features of various focal lesions and how they differ from each other.

On T1-weighted images the liver (like the pancreas) has higher signal intensity than most other nonfatty tissues in the abdomen. The short

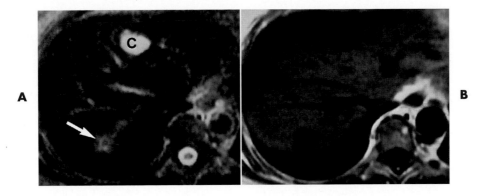

FIGURE 22-13 Metastasis and cyst. **A,** SE 2500/100 image. The cyst *(C)* is isointense with CSF, whereas the metastasis *(arrow)* is less intense. The borders are distinct for the cyst but indistinct for the metastasis. **B,** SE 400/12 image. (From Mitchell DG, and Stark DD: Hepatobiliary MRI, St Louis, 1993, Mosby.)

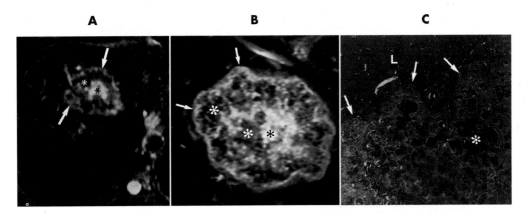

FIGURE 22-14 Peripheral halo. **A,** SE 2500/80 image shows a heterogeneous tumor that has low signal *(white asterisk)* except for the center *(black asterisk)* and a peripheral rim *(arrows)*. **B,** SE 2500/80 image of left lobectomy specimen shows the same characteristics. **C,** Histological section of tumor *(trichrome stain)* shows advancing cellular tumor rime *(arrows)*. Areas of low signal on MR images correspond to coagulative necrosis *(white asterisk)*, which stains dark red, and fibrosis, which stains blue. *L,* Liver. (From reference 172.)

T1 relaxation time of these two organs, which are active in protein synthesis, may be the result of a combination of the large surface area of the endoplasmic reticulum and high manganese content within mitochondria.[20] Thus even though the signal intensity on T1-weighted images of malignant lesions may resemble that of other solid organs, there is usually abundant contrast between liver and lesion.

Differential diagnosis between different focal liver lesions is best accomplished by using a combination of clinical history, signal intensity, and morphology on heavily T2-weighted images, as well as a pattern of enhancement on a series of rapid images obtained after bolus administration of Gd chelates.

Hepatic Metastases

Initial screening for patients at risk for hepatic metastases can be accomplished effectively by either MRI or CT, provided that the appropriate technique is used. In selected patients, such as potential candidates for surgical resection of hepatic metastases, CT with arterial portography (CTAP) is sometimes performed to exclude additional lesions. Although MRI with arterial portography is feasible and at least as sensitive as CTAP,[43,216] few centers have any experience with this technique. Most reports indicate that CTAP is more sensitive but less specific than current MR techniques; however, it is too expensive and invasive for initial screening, and false-positive results are common.[212]

Superparamagnetic iron oxide contrast agents are now available for clinical use. Initial results suggest that specific labeling of Kupffer's cells within nonmalignant liver tissue provides a sensitivity for detection of hepatic metastases comparable to or greater than that of CTAP, potentially rendering obsolete this latter invasive technique.[201]

With heavily T2-weighted pulse sequences, solid tumors, such as metastases, show decreased signal intensity relative to fluid, such as cerebrospinal fluid (CSF) (Figures 22-12 and 22-13). Most metastases have signal intensity similar to that of the spleen on T1- and T2-weighted pulse sequences.[221] In contrast, hemangiomas and cysts have higher signal intensity on T2-weighted images.

Many metastases develop central necrosis. This finding is often manifested as a central increase in signal intensity on T2-weighted images and decreased signal intensity on T1-weighted images.[15,172,261] The centers of necrotic tumors may be liquid and thus have signal intensity as high as that of cavernous hemangiomas or cysts. However, necrotic tumors nearly always have irregular internal morphology, mural nodules, a solid tissue rim, or an indistinct interface with adjacent liver, distinguishing them from hemangiomas or cysts.

Some metastases, especially those of colorectal origin, develop coagulative necrosis centrally, which has signal intensity nearly isointense to that of liver on T2-weighted images. The high signal intensity of the viable tumor tissue surrounding the low–signal intensity coagulative necrosis produces an appearance of a bright peripheral halo resembling peritumoral edema[172] (Figure 22-14). True peritumoral edema may occur, however, if the tumor causes vascular or biliary obstruction.[75,112] Appearances such as these, involving discrepant signal features between the central and peripheral portions of a mass, are rarely seen in hemangiomas or cysts and are therefore strong indicators of malignancy. On occasion, wedge-shaped peritumoral edema may obscure small tumors on unenhanced MR images and therefore be the only visible manifestation of metastases.[57]

Improper photography that compresses the dynamic range for depiction of high-signal tissues can interfere with differential diagnosis.

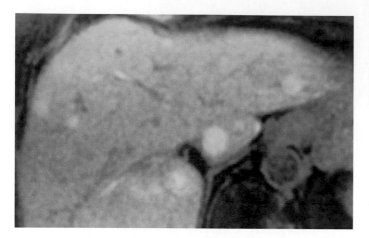

FIGURE 22-15   Malignant melanoma metastases depicted as high signal intensity on T1-weighted gradient-echo 120/2.3 (fat-suppressed) image.

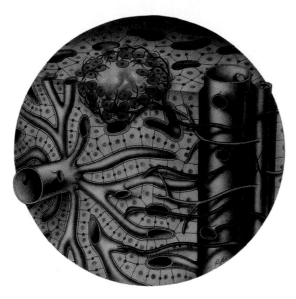

FIGURE 22-16   Extracellular spaces of the liver and a metastasis. *Pink,* Hepatocytes; *red,* hepatic arteries; *purple,* portal vein branches and hepatic sinusoids; *blue,* central veins and hepatic veins; *yellow,* interstitial space; *green,* bile ducts.

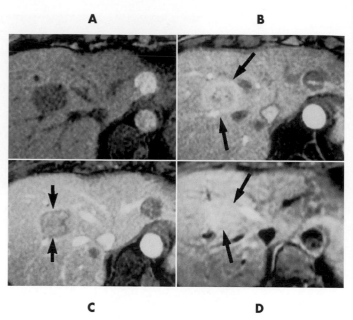

FIGURE 22-17   Primary malignant hepatic carcinoid tumor. T1, spoiled gradient-echo 118/2.3/90 image **(A)** before administration of Gd chelate, and capillary **(B)** and portal **(C)** phases after administration of Gd chelate. **D** is a delayed-phase image using SE 600/18 technique with fat suppression. Prominent rim enhancement *(arrows)* surrounds the mass during the capillary phase, with peripheral wash-out *(arrows)* noted during the portal phase. On the delayed-phase image, contrast material has accumulated throughout the mass *(arrows),* rendering it more intense than the hepatic parenchyma. A cavernous hemangioma lies posterolateral to the IVC (From Mitchell DG: Liver. I. Currently available gadolinium chelates, MRI Clin North Am 4:37, 1996.)

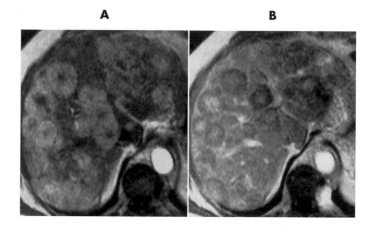

FIGURE 22-18   Hepatic metastases from a carcinoid tumor during the capillary **(A)** and delayed **(B)** phases. In **A,** prominent rim enhancement indicates hypervascular, viable tissue at the periphery of the metastases. In **B** there is peripheral wash-out from the viable tissue but increased enhancement of the interstitium of the partially necrotic centers of the tumors. (From reference 172.)

Images should be photographed so high-signal masses are bright but not absolutely white. Rarely, solid metastases, such as endocrine tumors, can have extremely high signal intensity and therefore mimic hemangiomas on unenhanced images. Dynamic imaging may help in these cases by showing early enhancement, particularly of the rim of the tumor.[100,258]

Metastases from malignant melanoma may be hyperintense on T1-weighted images and hypointense on T2-weighted images[85] (Figure 22-15). Studies with melanoma metastatic to brain indicate that the paramagnetic effects of melanin are an important cause of this unusual signal pattern.[5] Hemorrhage within melanomas and within other tumors also may produce foci of high signal on T1-weighted images.

Dynamic scanning after administration of Gd chelates provides additional parameters that can increase the accuracy of focal hepatic mass characterization.[113,116,148,196,258] Hepatic malignancies are perfused almost entirely by hepatic arteries, compared with the liver, which is perfused primarily by portal veins (Figure 22-16). Therefore on capillary-phase images most malignant tumors enhance more than hepatic parenchyma. This early enhancement of malignancies is typically most pronounced at the periphery of lesions, producing rim enhancement, which is a particularly important sign of malignancy (Figures 22-17 and 22-18). Capillary-phase images are particularly important for detection of hypervascular malignant lesions.[195]

Portal-phase images often help depict tumors as having lower signal intensity than liver parenchyma. Even hypervascular tumors, which are supplied almost entirely by hepatic arteries, usually have less blood-pool than the liver, which receives approximately two thirds of its perfusion from the portal vein.[65,113,139,148]

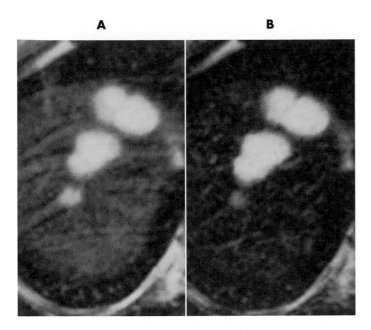

A   **B**

FIGURE 22-19   Ultralong TE for characterization of benign liver lesions. **A,** Multishot FSE 3000/96 image with ETL of 16. Several high-signal lesions are seen in the dome of the liver. **B,** FSE 4000/168 image. Edges are sharper, and motion artifacts are less prominent. (From reference 144.)

On images obtained during or after the portal phase, the periphery of a tumor may have less signal intensity than either its center or adjacent liver parenchyma, producing a "peripheral wash-out sign," which is a strong predictor of a metastatic lesion[116] (Figures 22-17 and 22-18). Although the peripheral wash-out sign may be noted during the portal phase, it is usually most conspicuous shortly after the portal phase.

On extracellular phase (delayed) images, contrast enhancement is based on combined blood-pool and interstitial space enhancement. Some malignant tumors show diffusely increased tumor enhancement, probably because of a combination of greater capillary permeability, larger interstitial space, and slower venous drainage than hepatic parenchyma. This increased enhancement of tumor tissue can occur at the periphery or at the center of metastases and throughout small lesions.

Ovarian carcinoma spreads to the liver primarily via the peritoneum. Therefore the periphery of the liver should be scrutinized, with special attention directed to the right hemidiaphragm and liver capsule where metastases are especially frequent.[6]

After chemotherapy for treatment of metastases, tumors may decrease markedly in size and result in distortion of the liver shape and architecture, especially in patients with breast carcinoma. The residual scarring and distortion may produce an appearance resembling cirrhosis.[268]

Cavernous Hemangioma

Cavernous hemangioma is the most common benign hepatic neoplasm, with an autopsy incidence between 0.4% and 20%.[33,83] The incidence of cavernous hemangiomas appears to be less in patients with cirrhosis.[1] Cavernous hemangiomas are composed primarily of large vascular lakes and channels. Some of these channels undergo thrombosis and fibrous organization.[150] Most lesions change little, if at all, over time.[153] Complications are rare and occur only when large lesions bleed or rupture. The major hazard of cavernous hemangiomas is their incidental discovery and potential misclassification on abdominal sonograms, CT scans, or scintigrams obtained for other reasons, complicating patient management.

Scintigraphy with technetium-labeled erythrocytes (blood-pool study) allows a specific diagnosis of cavernous hemangioma.[1,16] Unfortunately, the blood-pool study adds time and cost beyond that of the initial screening examination and provides no additional information if cavernous hemangioma is not diagnosed. Additionally, blood-pool scintigraphy cannot differentiate between metastases and cysts. Occasionally, false-negative results may be obtained for giant hemangiomas because of the nonperfused central scar that is common in these large lesions.[68]

We recommend blood-pool scintigraphy only for cases that satisfy all of the following criteria: (1) solitary or multiple lesions, each of which are at least 2 cm in diameter; (2) features on other imaging modalities that suggest cavernous hemangiomas; and (3) no other indication for comprehensive hepatic imaging, such as a known primary neoplasm or abnormal liver function tests. Conversely, we recommend MRI for (1) small lesions; (2) lesions with findings suggestive of malignancy, such as ill-defined borders; or (3) patients who would benefit from hepatic MRI of the remainder of the liver, even if the lesion in question proves to be a hemangioma. For instance, a patient with a recently diagnosed malignancy and a 2-cm hemangioma detected by sonography or CT may have small metastases visible only by MRI.

MRI is more sensitive than other imaging methods and is more specific for diagnosing cavernous hemangiomas.[12,16,71,219,248] Cavernous hemangiomas differ from all other hepatic masses in that they are essentially a cluster of lakes of slowly flowing blood. The high intensity of cavernous hemangiomas is due to the extremely long T2 relaxation time of the abundant free fluid in blood.[244] Reported T2 values vary depending on several different parameters of in vitro measurement but are generally in the range of 90 to 200 ms.[58,111,164,219] These values are less than those of simple cysts, which can have T2 values in excess of 300 ms.[58,109]

Some investigators have found signal intensity ratios relative to normal liver tissue useful for distinguishing cavernous hemangiomas from metastases. However, using normal liver as a reference may lead to errors because intensity and T2 time of liver may vary depending on its content of fat, iron, or edema. Near isointensity with CSF on T2-weighted SE images is a simple, practical criterion for diagnosis of cavernous hemangiomas; metastases are rarely as bright as CSF on heavily T2-weighted images, except for central necrosis. However, it may be difficult to avoid mistakes when the high–signal intensity centers of necrotic tumors are measured. Once an MR user has acquired sufficient experience, visual analysis is probably preferable to signal-intensity measurements because morphological features of the lesions can be considered.

Standard TEs of approximately 100 ms are sometimes useful in distinguishing cavernous hemangioma from solid neoplasms, but there may be substantial overlap. However, higher TEs, such as 160 ms or more, generally provide more consistent discrimination between benign and malignant lesions.[49,133,219] On heavily T2-weighted images with TR greater than 4000 ms and TE greater than 160 ms, it is possible to virtually eliminate T1 contrast (Figure 22-19). Breath-hold images with very long TE also eliminate motion-induced partial volume averaging, which is especially significant at the dome of the liver because of averaging between the lesion and air.[7,26] On these images, hemangiomas are not as bright as CSF because the T2 relaxation time of hemangiomas is not as long as that of the simple fluid in CSF. On heavily T2-weighted FSE images with TE greater than 160 ms, hemangiomas have signal intensity intermediate between that of CSF and spleen or kidney, whereas metastases have signal intensity much closer to that of these solid organs. Although the simple criterion of isointensity with CSF does not apply to heavily T2-weighted FSE images, their strong T2 contrast provides better discrimination between solid and nonsolid lesions.

Cavernous hemangiomas, cysts, and malignancies have significantly different T1 relaxation times.[15,58,173] However, depiction of the morphology of lesions is generally poor on unenhanced T1-weighted images because of the low signal intensity of lesions on these images. Therefore unenhanced T1-weighted images are less helpful than T2-weighted images for characterizing most hepatic lesions.

Morphological criteria must be examined to supplement evaluation of relative intensity.[15,261] Cavernous hemangiomas are well circumscribed and tend to be homogeneous, whereas cancers are more commonly heterogeneous, with ill-defined margins or rings. Cavernous hemangiomas are commonly lobulated, but their borders should never be irregular, spiculated, or indistinct.

Hemangiomas do not have low-signal capsules or intermediate-intensity zones of edema, as are often present at the periphery of malignant lesions. Rarely, however, liver tissue adjacent to hemangiomas may show transient increased enhancement during the capillary phase, presumably because of associated alterations in portal circulation.

Cavernous hemangiomas frequently show complex internal architecture, such as low–signal intensity fibrous strands or central scars, particularly within giant cavernous hemangiomas.[26,183,228] However, virtually all cavernous hemangiomas are primarily hyperintense on heavily T2-weighted images, and the borders should always be distinct. Rarely, heavily fibrotic hemangiomas overlap the appearance of metastases, causing ambiguous MR features in only 5% or less of cases.[125,219] Central scars are common in giant hemangiomas, but these scars frequently have a high water content and in fact may have even higher signal intensity than the remainder of the hemangioma on heavily T2-weighted images.

The differences between cavernous hemangiomas and solid malignant tumors are depicted with greater clarity on FSE images than on conventional SE, T2-weighted images. One reason for this is that FSE images tend to be acquired with longer TR and TE and with higher spatial resolution because of more efficient data acquisition. Additionally the signal intensity of solid tissue is decreased on FSE images because of the greater influence of magnetization-transfer (MT) contrast on these images compared with conventional SE images.

Most difficulties distinguishing between cavernous hemangiomas and metastases occur with small lesions, especially those less than 1 cm in diameter.[80,148,196,244] This can be a difficult clinical problem, as other modalities are even less successful at characterizing these lesions. One approach is to obtain an additional heavily T2-weighted sequence with extremely long TR and TE and thin (5 mm or less) sections to reduce the influence of partial volume effects. If possible, obtaining heavily T2-weighted images during suspended respiration using FSE or echo planar techniques may help by eliminating motion-induced partial volume averaging, which is a cause of artifactually decreased signal intensity of hemangiomas. That is, if the lesion moves outside the image section during portions of image acquisition, signal intensity may be decreased.

Dynamic MRI after administration of contrast material will usually confirm the diagnosis of hemangioma if T2-weighted images are equivocal.[148,196,258] Cavernous hemangiomas show sharply marginated nodular enhancement immediately after a bolus of Gd chelate, but the remainder of the lesion usually requires more time to fill in. The initial nodular enhancement is usually peripheral, but occasionally it can be eccentric or even central. The different patterns of initial enhancement of hemangiomas may be related to the variable size and location of feeding vessels. A central appearance occasionally may result on images through the top or bottom of a hemangioma with superior or inferior large feeding vessels, respectively. Initial enhancement centrally or eccentrically is more unusual with metastases than with hemangiomas because the vascularity of metastases is either homogeneous or greatest at the periphery, not eccentrically or at the center. The morphology of the early and late enhancement of a focal lesion is far more important than its central versus peripheral location.

Fill-in of cavernous hemangiomas on sequential images after administration of contrast material is usually clumplike as a result of the large intercommunicating vascular lakes. Most hemangiomas fill in completely within 5 to 30 min. Persistent hyperintensity 15 min after administration of gadopentetate chelates is typical of hemangiomas; however, this can be seen in some metastases with large interstitial spaces and is therefore not a reliable sign. Because of the highly characteristic appearance of the early clumplike enhancement on high-quality breath-hold images, acquisition of delayed images to show complete fill-in is usually unnecessary.

Some subcentimeter cavernous hemangiomas seem to have relatively high flow, manifested as rapid complete enhancement on capillary-phase images with rapid wash-out to isointensity on portal-phase images and delayed images.[196,258] This pattern resembles that seen with many hypervascular metastases. In most cases high signal intensity and high conspicuity on heavily T2-weighted images may confirm the benign diagnosis. However, in some cases high-flow hemangiomas can be particularly difficult to distinguish from solid hypervascular lesions, and follow-up examination may be necessary.

It must be remembered that currently available gadolinium chelates are extracellular space agents, similar to iodinated vascular contrast, rather than a blood-pool agent. Delayed images after administration of Gd chelates depict the combination of blood-pool and interstitial enhancement and are therefore less specific than red blood cell scintigraphy. For this reason, tumors with large interstitial spaces, such as edem-

atous and hypervascular tumors, can mimic the enhancement pattern of hemangiomas. Additionally, large hemangiomas with scar tissue may not fill in completely.

Finally, the importance of clinical history must be emphasized. Small lesions in patients without a known primary malignancy are usually benign. However, in patients with cirrhosis, hemangiomas are quite rare.

Cysts

Cysts of the liver are less common than cavernous hemangiomas and are seldom if ever symptomatic. Cysts are usually discovered incidentally during sonographic or CT examinations. Unlike cavernous hemangiomas, cysts are quite common in patients with cirrhosis, usually arising in association with nearby bile ducts. Although sonographic features are highly diagnostic, small cysts can be confused with malignant lesions by CT.

Simple cysts have even longer T1 and T2 relaxation times than hemangiomas (Figure 22-9). Heavily T2-weighted images show most cysts as isointense with CSF and more intense than cavernous hemangiomas. However, the intensity of cysts on T1-weighted or intermediate images can vary if protein, hemorrhage, or both are present within cyst fluid. These materials can shorten T1 and therefore cause hyperintensity. On T1-weighted or intermediate images, cysts are often less intense than hemangiomas. These two benign lesions can be differentiated unambiguously by administering contrast material, although this is not clinically important.

Multiple cysts of variable intensity, presumably caused by multiple episodes of intracystic hemorrhage, have been described in patients with polycystic liver disease.[37] In some patients all cysts may have low intensity.

Hepatocellular Carcinoma

Hepatocellular carcinoma (HCC) is the most common hepatic malignancy in Asia because of the prevalence of hepatitis B and C.[10,84] HCC is usually associated with chronic liver disease such as cirrhosis, chronic active hepatitis, or hemochromatosis. In one Asian prospective series of patients with cirrhosis, HCC developed within 6 years in more than 50% of patients with viral hepatitis and in 22% of patients without viral hepatitis who drank excessively.[168] Many HCCs develop in a step-wise fashion from dysplastic regenerative nodules, although some tiny HCCs do not appear to be associated with dysplastic nodules.

Early HCCs are usually small and well differentiated and classified as Edmondson grades I or II. The best differentiated HCCs (Edmondson grade I) may have vascularity similar to that of the adjacent liver.[86,91,159,210,267] These small lesions are often missed by diagnostic tests, including MRI, CT, ultrasound, and angiography.[66,210,224-227,229] Arterial portography and intraarterial injection of iodized oil improve the sensitivity of CT (94% and 82%, respectively, in one series),[163] but even these techniques are relatively insensitive for small daughter lesions (38% and 50%).[163,269] Serum α-fetoprotein levels are usually normal with small HCC lesions.[168]

Early HCC is frequently surrounded by a fibrous capsule.[45,79,184] Large HCC lesions are usually hypervascular, often with prominent arteriovenous shunting. Advanced tumors commonly have necrosis and hemorrhage or invasion of hepatic and portal veins. Bile duct obstruction is less common than is venous obstruction, but it can occur.[215]

Solitary HCC (50% of cases) can be treated by surgical resection if the patient's hepatic functional reserve is sufficient. When HCCs less than 3 cm in diameter are resected, the cumulative intrahepatic recurrence rate has been reported as 12% after 1 year and 57% after 3 years.[2] Important indicators of poor prognosis are male gender, low albumin, high alanine aminotransferase levels, and active hepatic parenchymal inflammation, whereas tumor factors, such as size, histological grade, α-fetoprotein levels, and width of resection margin, are less important.[2,123,161] For multinodular or diffuse HCCs or HCCs in patients who are not operative candidates, alternative treatments include chemoembolization, percutaneous injection of ethanol or hot saline, or hepatic transplantation.[67,203,230] Hepatic transplantation should be considered only for small solitary tumors in patients with end-stage hepatic disease.

The reported sensitivity for image-guided percutaneous biopsy of

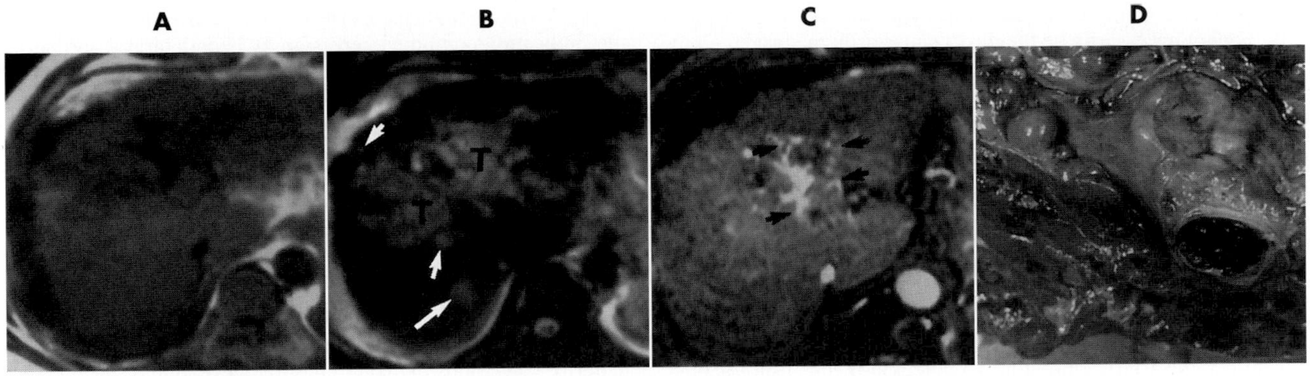

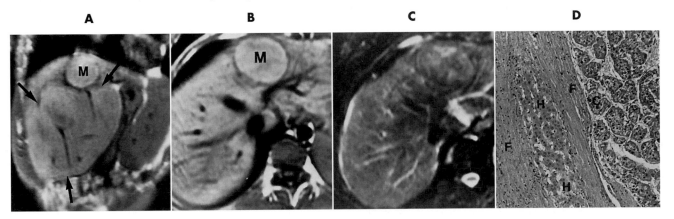

FIGURE 22-20   Multifocal HCC with portal vein invasion. **A,** SE 600/20 image depicts liver nodularity consistent with cirrhosis. There is no distinct mass, but the portal bifurcation is obliterated. **B,** SE 2500/100 image reveals high-signal tumor *(T)* in the expected position of the portal bifurcation, with additional nodules peripherally *(arrows).* **C,** Gradient-echo 25/13/20 image fails to detect the mass, but collateral portal vessels *(arrows)* are depicted. **D,** Tumor thrombus is seen within the portal vein. Nodular surface of the liver indicates cirrhosis. (From Mitchell DG, and Stark DD: Hepatobiliary MRI, St Louis, 1993, Mosby.)

FIGURE 22-21   Encapsulated solitary HCC. **A,** Coronal SE 500/20 image reveals a hyperintense mass *(M)* superiorly in the medial segment of the left lobe and a large isointense mass *(arrows)* inferiorly. **B,** Axial SE 400/20 image reveals a hyperintense encapsulated mass *(M)* between the medial and left hepatic veins. **C,** SE 3000/100 image shows minimally hyperintense mass. **D,** Histological section *(H & E stain)* shows that **C** is a well-differentiated carcinoma with no fatty change. The capsule is composed of hepatocytes *(H)* and abundant fibrous tissue *(F).* (From reference 145.)

HCC ranges from 69% to 90%.[14,17] In one report,[181] 12 of 62 focal lesions detected by ultrasound were diagnosed as regenerative nodules based on negative guided biopsy. On follow-up examination, however, 10 of these 12 lesions were found to be HCC lesions. Some of these cases may represent HCC developing within regenerative nodules, whereas others may have been false-negative biopsy results because of the similarity between well-differentiated HCC and normal hepatic tissue.[91,159]

Advanced HCC is usually hypointense on T1-weighted images and hyperintense on T2-weighted images, similar to metastases[29,72,164] (Figure 22-20). The signal intensity of HCC is more variable than that of other tumors, however. Well-differentiated HCC is usually hyperintense or isointense on T1-weighted images and subtle or isointense on T2-weighted images[46,90,145,156,185] (Figures 22-21 and 22-22).

Hyperintense HCC lesions sometimes contain abundant intracellular triglyceride.[45,122,187,266] Fat is more common in small, well-differentiated HCCs than in large, undifferentiated tumors, probably because of the defective release of fat produced within partially functioning malignant hepatocytes. CSI can provide confirming evidence of intratumoral fat by demonstrating a decrease in tumor signal intensity on an opposed-phase or fat-suppressed image compared with an in-phase image with comparable T1-weighting. Fat is extremely rare within metastases or other malignancies but is an occasional finding in benign hepatocellular masses, such as hepatic adenoma, focal nodular hyperplasia, and regenerative nodules. In most instances, hyperintensity of HCC on T1-weighted images is not the result of fat, although the reason for this is unknown.[85,145] Suggested factors include protein, glycogen, copper, or other unspecified paramagnetic substances. Intra-

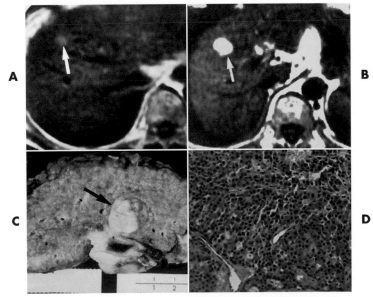

FIGURE 22-22   Solitary HC *(arrows).* **A,** The liver is heterogeneous and abnormally hypointense. **B,** Nine months later the mass *(arrow)* has grown, and ascites has increased. **C,** Cut section shows a pale, encapsulated mass *(arrow)* within a cirrhotic liver. **D,** Microscopic section, demonstrating a well-differentiated HCC with no fat. (From reference 145.)

tumoral copper is commonly increased in hyperintense HCC,[46,90] although it may not necessarily be the direct cause of high signal.

In addition to being hyperintense on T1-weighted images, HCC is commonly subtle on T2-weighted images.[79,156] As with high signal on T1-weighted images, low to intermediate signal on T2-weighted images is especially likely with small, well-differentiated tumors. HCCs are often subtle on nonenhanced MR images, both because well-differentiated tumors can have MR signal features resembling those of normal liver and because the surrounding abnormal liver may have altered morphology, decreased signal intensity of T1-weighted images, and increased signal intensity on T2-weighted images.

Because HCCs are so commonly subtle on unenhanced images, dynamic imaging after bolus injection of contrast agents is particularly important for detecting HCCs.[77,100,117] The blood supply of HCCs is primarily from hepatic arteries, providing a potential mechanism for improved detection and characterization. Therefore, like most metastases, HCC is usually markedly more intense than liver on capillary phase images after a bolus of contrast material. Early enhancement of HCC is usually diffuse, multinodular, or heterogeneous, unlike metastases that commonly show early ringlike enhancement. HCC is usually less intense than liver on portal-phase images, but this finding is less consistent than with metastases because the portal blood supply of cirrhotic liver is often reduced relative to normal liver. On delayed images HCC is usually isointense to surrounding liver, but fibrous capsules surrounding focal HCC are often hyperintense because of the large interstitial space of fibrous tissue. CTAP is especially effective at enhancing liver more than HCC,[128] but its utility is reduced in patients with severely decreased portal flow because of massive portosystemic shunting. CTAP is likely to be ineffective in patients with reversed portal vein flow.

Extremely well-differentiated (Edmonson grade I) HCCs are particularly difficult to detect because of their close histological and functional similarity to benign hepatic parenchyma. On CTAP and CT with direct injection into hepatic arteries, many early HCCs are isoattenuating, indicating combined perfusion by hepatic artery and portal vein similar to that of benign parenchyma.[229]

MRI is diagnostic of HCC more often than CT, sonography, or scintigraphy because of its demonstration of characteristic morphological features. T2-weighted images may show a mosaic or nodules-in-nodule pattern of signal intensity, produced by multiple centers of growth interspersed with areas of low-signal coagulative necrosis, noncancerous regenerative liver tissue, or both.[29] Internal heterogeneity is an important feature for distinguishing HCC from regenerative nodule and adenomatous hyperplasia.

A 0.5- to 3-mm thick capsule often can be identified on T1-weighted MR images.[45,72,79] T2-weighted MR images may not demonstrate the capsule but are more likely to depict the mosaic or nodules-in-nodule patterns. Cavernous hemangiomas and cysts do not form capsules or contain intratumoral nodules. Rarely, metastases or hepatic adenomas may have a capsule. Early enhancement features, as described previously, are helpful in distinguishing HCCs from metastases, particularly in tumors larger than 3 cm in diameter. The most important factor in distinguishing HCCs from hepatic metastases is clinical history; a malignant lesion in a cirrhotic patient without a known primary cancer is almost invariably a primary hepatic malignancy, whereas a malignant lesion in a noncirrhotic liver is more likely to be a metastasis, especially if there is a known primary extrahepatic tumor.

In some cases HCC arises within a dysplastic nodule[4,27,110,127,217] hyperplasia (see next section). The presence of a small HCC tumor within a large siderotic, regenerative nodule causes a particularly characteristic MR appearance, consisting of one or more foci of intermediate intensity within a low-signal nodule[4,147,234] (Figure 22-23). This appearance should be considered strongly suggestive of early HCC, even if α-fetoprotein is normal and biopsy does not reveal tumor. In many cases these small foci of cancer grow rapidly, so aggressive follow-up or treatment should be considered when these small foci are initially detected.[188]

MRI is highly sensitive for detecting intrahepatic vascular invasion. However, interpretation of MR images can be difficult when tumors compress vessels and cause slow flow. Careful comparison between dark-blood and bright-blood MR images may be necessary. When vascular invasion is detected, the diagnosis of HCC should be favored because metastases and other hepatic tumors rarely invade vessels.

After therapeutic embolization, MRI may show increased intensity secondary to necrosis, as well as decreased size.[167] Gas bubbles are also common within 2 weeks of embolization.[52,167] MRI appears promising for tracking HCC after ethanol injection because signal intensity after successful treatment decreases on T2-weighted images and increases on T1-weighted images. Unsuccessful ethanol ablation is manifested as unchanged signal intensity of the tumor.[176,209] Dynamic imaging after administration of Gd chelates appears especially helpful for viewing tumors after nonsurgical treatment; a successfully treated tumor does not enhance on images obtained 1 min or less after injection, whereas

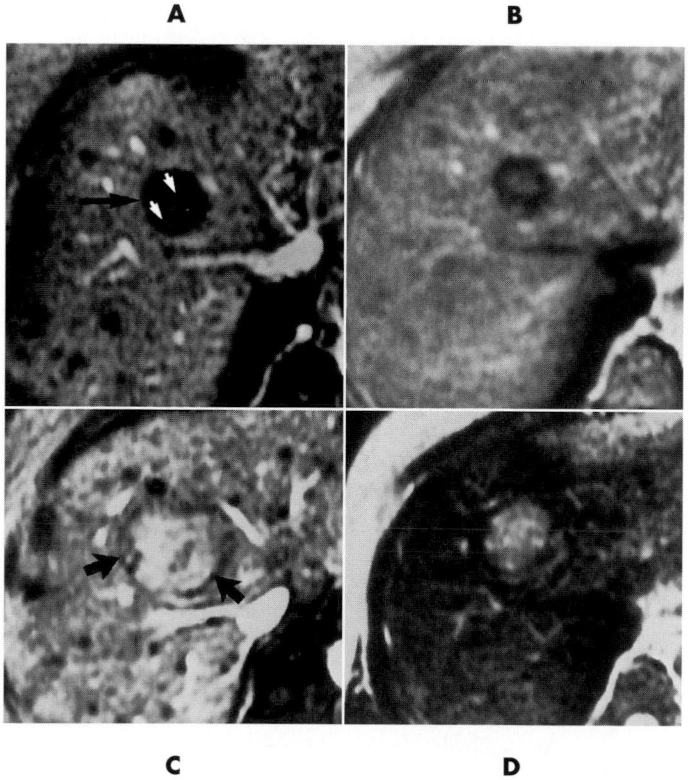

FIGURE 22-23   Small HCC within a large siderotic regenerative nodule (nodules-in-nodule) with rapid growth after negative biopsy. **A,** A 25/13/20 image shows a 2-cm low-signal nodule *(black arrow)* within the anterior segment of the right lobe, containing two isointense foci *(white arrows).* There are numerous other siderotic regenerative nodules. **B,** SE 2500/50 image shows heterogeneity consistent with cirrhosis. **C,** Nine months later, with identical technique, the mass *(arrows)* measures 4.5 cm in diameter and is hyperintense with a dark peripheral capsule. **D,** SE 2500/100 image. (From reference 147.)

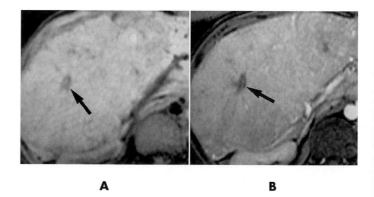

FIGURE 22-24   Fibrolamellar HCC in an 18-year-old man with no prior history of liver disease. **A,** Fat-suppressed SE 500/13 image shows a large mass replacing most of the right lobe. Low signal–intensity scar *(arrow).* **B,** Gradient-echo 85/2.2/90 image after administration of Gd chelate shows enhancement of the mass with no enhancement of the scar.

early enhancement indicates persistent or recurrent tumor.[9,39,155] However, hyperperfusion of hepatic parenchyma has been noted adjacent to HCCs treated with percutaneous ethanol injection.[78]

Fibrolamellar Hepatocellular Carcinoma

Fibrolamellar HCC is an uncommon HCC with characteristics different than those of other forms.[211,246] Fibrolamellar HCC has a nearly equal gender distribution and has been described primarily in American and European patients. Moreover, it is frequently encountered in younger individuals, typically those in the third through fifth decades. Unlike most HCCs, fibrolamellar tumors are typically solitary and are found in patients without underlying cirrhosis. This lesion is not clearly associated with viral or any other etiologies. Elevated levels of serum α-fetoprotein and paraneoplastic syndromes are uncommon.[211]

Most fibrolamellar tumors are well circumscribed, although the periphery may be scalloped or irregular (Figure 22-24). Punctate calcifications and a hypovascular central scar may be present.[13] On microscopy, fibrolamellar tumors are characterized by well-differentiated polygonal hepatocytes filled with granular eosinophilic material and the presence of hypocellular layers of fibrosis.

Fibrolamellar HCC frequently has a central fibrous scar.[13,186,242] Fibrous scars usually have low signal intensity on T1- and T2-weighted images. Vascular scars, common in focal nodular hyperplasias, typically have high intensity on T2-weighted images because of increased free water.[186]

Fibrolamellar HCC tends to be larger, more heterogeneous, and have more lobulated borders than focal nodular hyperplasia (FNH). Calcifications are common with fibrolamellar HCC but rare with FNH. Unlike FNH, fibrolamellar HCC appears to enhance heterogeneously, with persistent nonenhanced regions even on delayed images.[32] In spite of these differences, definitive differential diagnosis is often difficult.

The prognosis of patients with fibrolamellar HCC is more favorable than with other types of HCC. This improved survival probably reflects the greater likelihood of resectability of these tumors at the time of diagnosis rather than a more benevolent natural history or increased responsiveness to chemotherapy. Tumors do progress and metastasize, however, and patients sometimes die of malignant disease.[223]

Dysplastic Nodule

Some large regenerative nodules have dysplastic histology. These nodules are sometimes referred to as *adenomatous hyperplasia*.[4,27,110,127,217] Discrete foci of dysplasia or frank malignancy have been noted within these atypical regenerative nodules.* In one series, each of 12 large regenerative nodules, diagnosed by benign histology on initial aspiration, were enlarged on follow-up examination. Malignancy was eventually diagnosed in 10 of the 12.[181] Experience has shown that many of the tiny foci within dysplastic nodules grow rapidly.[188] Because of the potential for hepatocellular tumors to grow within dysplastic nodules, some investigators recommend aggressive treatment of large dysplastic nodules.[105,110]

Dysplastic nodules that accumulate iron appear to have greater malignant potential than other nodules.[234,236] This may result from the tumor-enhancing effects of iron or to the rapid growth associated with regeneration. One autopsy series noted malignant foci within 19 of 26 (73%) large, iron-accumulative, regenerative nodules. Large, fatty, benign nodules also can exhibit rapid growth and potential for malignancy.[237]

Dysplastic nodules commonly have high signal intensity on T1-weighted MR images, although the cause of the high intensity has not been determined.[127] Because HCCs may also be hyperintense on T1-weighted images, these signal characteristics are not specific. This is consistent with the histological similarity between dysplastic nodules and well-differentiated HCCs.

On T2-weighted images, dysplastic nodules usually appear hypointense or isointense relative to surrounding benign liver tissue; nodules are rarely if ever hyperintense on T2-weighted images. In contrast, HCC is usually isointense to hyperintense.[127] High signal intensity on

T2-weighted images should therefore be considered highly suspicious for HCC. However, HCCs occasionally have low signal intensity on T2-weighted images, particularly well-differentiated Edmondson grade I HCCs.[46,127] Internal foci of high signal intensity on T2-weighted images, or of low signal intensity on T1-weighted images, suggest centers of more rapid growth and thus indicate a high likelihood of malignancy within adenomatous hyperplasia. Other signs of malignancy include capsules and irregular margins; dysplastic nodules have smooth margins and generally lack capsules. Enhancement patterns also tend to differ. Dysplastic nodules are supplied primarily by the portal vein, similar to the remainder of the liver, whereas HCCs are supplied almost exclusively by the hepatic artery. Thus dysplastic nodules usually enhance similar to the remainder of the liver, and HCC usually enhances more than the liver during the capillary phase and less than the liver during the early portal venous phase after a bolus of contrast material. Arterial portography is even more reliable for making this differentiation.[128] This distinction is not absolute, however, because Edmondson grade I HCC often retains some portal perfusion and dysplastic nodules may have relatively increased arterial perfusion.

Large regenerative nodules and dysplastic nodules should be examined carefully for internal foci. If such lesions are found, it might be prudent to proceed directly to surgery if the patient is considered a good surgical risk and no other lesions are evident. Alternatively, percutaneous treatment may be considered. Other potential causes of a high–signal intensity focus within a low–signal intensity nodule, such as an intranodular cyst, are extremely unlikely. Because small HCCs are usually well differentiated, biopsy of nodules such as these may fail to disclose tumor, and serological markers for HCC, such as α-fetoprotein, are usually normal in patients with small tumors.[156,227]

Confluent Fibrosis and Masslike Hypertrophy

When liver is severely damaged, signal intensity may be reduced on T1-weighted images and increased on T2-weighted images. Segmental atrophy may manifest as a wedge-shaped region with abnormal signal intensity, the apex of which should be examined for a tumor or other obstruction.[75,112] In severely damaged livers, areas of scarred liver, sometimes called *focal confluent fibrosis*, may resemble a focal mass with abnormal signal intensity and abnormal enhancement.[165]

Masslike hepatic regeneration may occur as a response to lobar atrophy or severe heterogeneous hepatic disease.[112,146] Regenerative liver may mimic a mass, but it should have signal characteristics similar to those of normal hepatic parenchyma, and hepatic vessels may be visible within it. The surrounding hepatic parenchyma may have grossly abnormal signal as a result of inflammation, necrosis, or fibrosis. Awareness of the normal signal of hepatic parenchyma, which is higher than spleen on T1-weighted images and only slightly higher than muscle on T2-weighted images, should allow differentiation between malignancy and regenerative masses. Identification of the most abnormal-appearing liver tissue is particularly important so that if hepatic biopsy is performed, the most appropriate liver tissue can be sampled. There does not appear to be increased potential for malignancy of masslike hepatic hypertrophy, and these lesions should not be confused with dysplastic nodules.

Focal Nodular Hyperplasia

FNH is a rare benign tumor of the liver that contains hepatocytes, bile duct elements, Kupffer's cells, and fibrous tissue[87] (Figure 22-25). The distinction between FNH and hepatocellular adenoma (HA) is important because FNH can be treated conservatively, whereas HA is often resected because of its propensity for hemorrhage.

Scintigraphy can support the diagnosis of FNH when areas of normal or increased technetium Tc 99m sulfur colloid uptake are identified within the mass, indicating intratumoral Kupffer's cells. Unfortunately, many FNH lesions show decreased activity of Kupffer's cells and therefore cannot be distinguished from cancer. Additionally, large regenerative nodules also may have increased uptake of sulfur colloid relative to surrounding cirrhotic parenchyma, and HA may contain Kupffer's cells and therefore accumulate sulfur colloid. Surgical exploration is frequently necessary because of nonspecific imaging findings.[87,260]

MRI demonstrates FNH by its mass effect and displacement of hepatic vessels, as well as by subtle differences in signal intensity

---

*References 4, 48, 53, 147, 159, 188, 234, 236, 249.

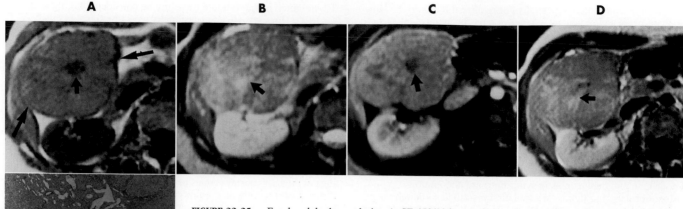

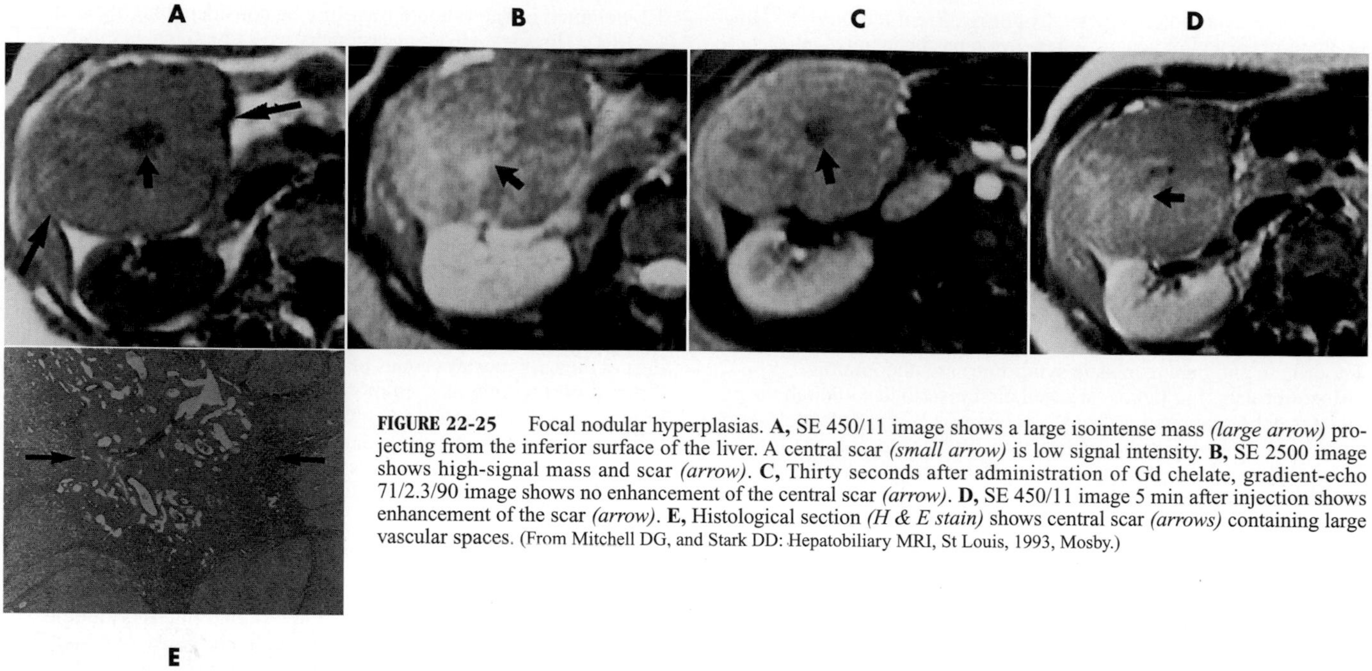

A **B** **C** **D**

E

FIGURE 22-25 Focal nodular hyperplasias. **A,** SE 450/11 image shows a large isointense mass *(large arrow)* projecting from the inferior surface of the liver. A central scar *(small arrow)* is low signal intensity. **B,** SE 2500 image shows high-signal mass and scar *(arrow)*. **C,** Thirty seconds after administration of Gd chelate, gradient-echo 71/2.3/90 image shows no enhancement of the central scar *(arrow)*. **D,** SE 450/11 image 5 min after injection shows enhancement of the scar *(arrow)*. **E,** Histological section *(H & E stain)* shows central scar *(arrows)* containing large vascular spaces. (From Mitchell DG, and Stark DD: Hepatobiliary MRI, St Louis, 1993, Mosby.)

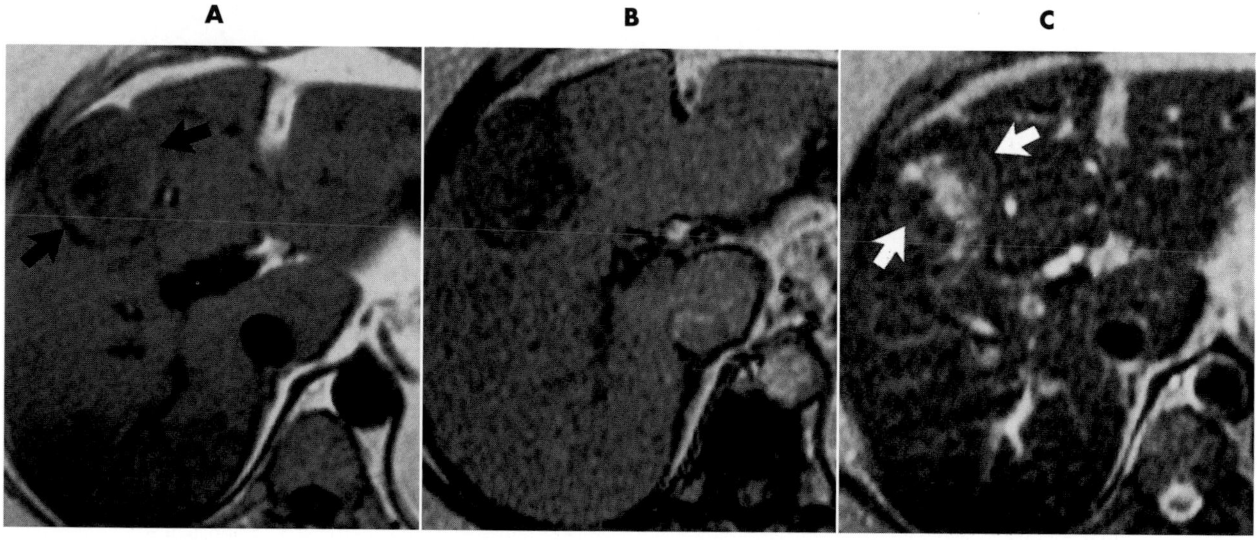

A **B** **C**

FIGURE 22-26 Hepatic adenoma containing lipid and heterogeneous signal intensity on T2-weighted images. **A,** SE 500/11 image shows a mass *(arrows)* that has low signal intensity centrally but is otherwise isointense relative to liver. Note that the liver is much more intense than the spleen. **B,** Opposed-phase gradient-echo 107/2.4/90 image. Liver and spleen are now isointense, indicating diffuse fatty infiltration. The periphery of the mass now has lower signal intensity than the liver, similar to the center of the tumor. This indicates the presence of more lipid than that contained within hepatic parenchyma. **C,** SE 3000/100 image shows a heterogeneous mass *(arrows)*. (From Mitchell DG: Hepatic imaging: techniques and unique applications of magnetic resonance imaging, Magn Reson Q 9:84, 1993.)

compared with adjacent liver. In general, FNH has a signal intensity similar to liver because both tissues consist of normal hepatocytes and Kupffer's cells.[18,102,124,132,191] In most cases, however, FNH is slightly hypointense on T1-weighted images and slightly hyperintense on T2-weighted images, similar to malignant tumors. Because HCC also may be nearly isointense with liver on T1- or T2-weighted images, the overlap between these two lesions prevents definitive diagnosis of FNH in many cases. Features of FNH that facilitate distinction from hepatic adenoma include lack of internal hemorrhage and lack of fat, both of which are common in adenomas. However, fat may rarely be observed within FNH, particularly in patients with fatty infiltration.[145]

FNH often contains a central stellate scar, which usually is bright on T2-weighted images and dark on T1-weighted images. This is because the scar is usually composed of vascular and myxoid tissue, both of which are rich in free water. The presence of edema within the scar correlates with high signal intensity on T2-weighted images.[247] Unfortunately, the presence and characteristics of the scar on unenhanced images do not allow reliable differential diagnosis, and histological diagnosis remains necessary in most cases.[102,186]

The peripherally radiating septa of FNH contain large vascular channels and bile ducts. FNH frequently shows a homogeneous tumor blush on capillary phase postgadolinium images, with rapid fading to isointensity with surrounding liver tissue.[115] Dynamic postgadolinium imaging frequently depicts central scars in FNH that are not seen on unenhanced images. Delayed and persistent enhancement of the scar, similar to that seen with cavernous hemangiomas, is common after administration of Gd chelates (Figure 22-25).

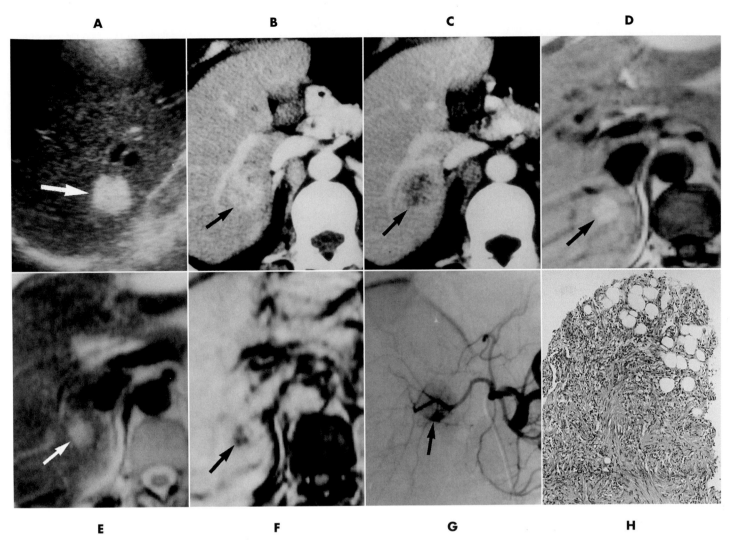

FIGURE 22-27   Angiomyolipoma in a patient with chronic hepatitis B. **A,** Ultrasound shows a well-defined hyperechoic mass with slightly increased transmission of sound consistent with cavernous hemangioma. **B and C,** CT shows immediate heterogeneous enhancement during the capillary phase (**B**) with rapid wash-out during the portal phase (**C**), findings more consistent with HCC than with cavernous hemangioma. SE 650/17 (**D**) and FSE 3200/90 (**E**) MR images show a high signal–intensity mass. **F,** Opposed-phase gradient-echo 153/7 image shows low signal intensity of the mass, indicating fat content. **G,** Celiac arteriography shows a well-defined hypervascular mass *(arrows).* **H,** H & E stain shows a mixture of muscle and adipose tissue. (Courtesy Dr. Joon Koo Han, Seoul National University Hospital.)

Hepatocellular Adenoma

The incidence of HA is greatest in women of childbearing age, especially those who use oral contraceptives. Pathologically the typical features of HA are a thin pseudocapsule; intracellular glycogen, lipid, and bile deposition; lack of architecture; paucity of mature bile ducts; and degenerative necrosis.[87] Necrosis and hemorrhage are common causes of pain, and life-threatening hemorrhage into the peritoneum can occur. Malignant potential has not been established, but if HA fails to regress after cessation of oral contraceptive use, surgical excision is indicated depending on its location. Occasionally, central adenomas adjacent to the confluence of hepatic veins are left alone, with periodic follow-up obtained to exclude persistent growth.

As with FNH, MR tissue characteristics vary, and HA may be difficult to distinguish from malignant tumors. As with other hepatocellular masses, HA may be hyperintense on T1-weighted images relative to liver.[54,175] Many hepatic adenomas have substantial fat, with intratumoral lipid typically distributed homogeneously except for within regions of hemorrhage[175] (Figure 22-26). HA typically has high signal intensity on T2-weighted images, although hemorrhage typically manifests as heterogeneous areas of low signal intensity.[30,175] Rarely, T1-weighted MR images may show low-intensity pseudocapsules, similar to HCC. HA typically does not have a central scar, although this can oc-

cur as a result of earlier central hemorrhage.[186] After hemorrhage, HA may calcify, which manifests as low signal intensity on T2-weighted images. Central foci suggesting separate internal centers of growth, as seen with HCC, are not expected to occur with HA.

Like FNH, HA is typically hypervascular except for areas of hemorrhage or calcification. Thus it shows more enhancement than liver on images obtained immediately after injection of Gd chelates.

Angiomyolipoma

Angiomyolipoma is an uncommon mass in the liver consisting of muscle tissue, fat, and vessels[73] (Figure 22-27).

Peripheral Cholangiocarcinoma

Most cases of cholangiocarcinomas arise from central branches of the biliary system and cause painless jaundice. Some cholangiocarcinomas arise from peripheral intrahepatic ducts and cause liver masses. In these cases clinical presentation and imaging features may overlap those of HCCs and hepatic metastases.

Peripheral cholangiocarcinomas have low signal intensity on T1-weighted images and high signal intensity on T2-weighted images (Figures 22-28 and 22-29). Unlike HCCs, cholangiocarcinomas do not have high signal intensity on T1-weighted images or peritumoral capsules, and invasion and distension of hepatic and portal veins are unusual. However, segmental portal venous obstruction via encasement is common.[28,213] Enhancement features vary, with cellular portions enhancing early and fibrous portions enhancing late.[114,154]

Lymphoma

Primary hepatic lymphoma is rare, but secondary involvement occurs in 20% of patients with Hodgkin's disease.[240,272] Non-Hodgkin's lymphoma may involve the liver in as many as 50% of patients evaluated at autopsy. Because patchy periportal infiltration is common, percutaneous biopsy is unreliable.

Although focal lymphoma has been detected by unenhanced MRI, these lesions may be isointense.[182,255,257] This probably depends on the proportion of lymphoma cells and edema relative to liver tissue (Figure 22-30).

Detection of diffuse lymphoma has been even more elusive. In some cases the lymphoma may incite an inflammatory response, causing a nonspecific diffuse or periportal signal increase on T2-weighted images. Contrast agents that are taken up selectively by liver tissue are likely to improve the accuracy of MRI for detecting hepatic lymphoma.[256]

Hemorrhage

Acute parenchymal or perihepatic hemorrhage usually has low signal intensity on T1- and T2-weighted images because of heterogeneous susceptibility produced by intracellular deoxyhemoglobin (Figures 22-31 and 22-32). A hyperintense rim may be noted on T1- and T2-weighted images, consistent with extracellular methemoglobin.[63] With time, signal intensity increases within the center of the lesion as red blood cells continue to lyse and deoxyhemoglobin is oxidized, forming methemoglobin The signal intensity may vary in different components of the hemorrhage because of gravity and variable effects of motion on red blood cell lysis and clot retraction.

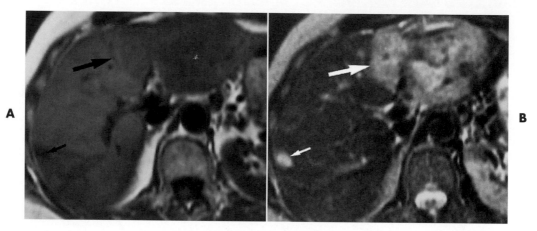

FIGURE 22-28 Cholangiocarcinoma and benign cyst. **A,** SE 400/20 image. The mass in the left lobe *(large arrow)* is slightly hypointense to liver. The smaller mass in the right lobe *(small arrow)* is darkest. **B,** SE 2500/100 image. The mass in the left lobe is hyperintense and heterogeneous. The peripheral lesion, a surgically proven benign cyst with clear fluid, has higher signal intensity and sharp borders.

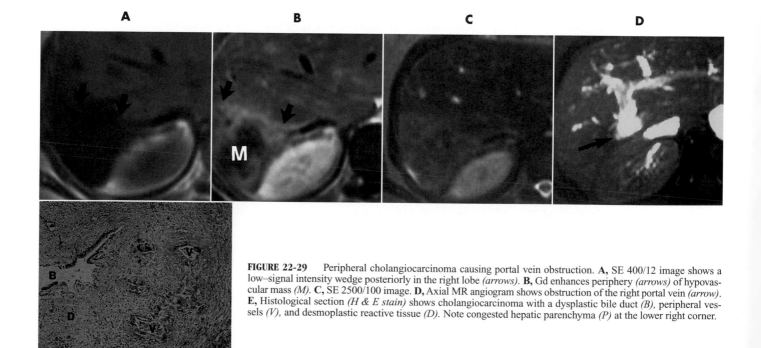

FIGURE 22-29 Peripheral cholangiocarcinoma causing portal vein obstruction. **A,** SE 400/12 image shows a low–signal intensity wedge posteriorly in the right lobe *(arrows)*. **B,** Gd enhances periphery *(arrows)* of hypovascular mass *(M)*. **C,** SE 2500/100 image. **D,** Axial MR angiogram shows obstruction of the right portal vein *(arrow)*. **E,** Histological section *(H & E stain)* shows cholangiocarcinoma with a dysplastic bile duct *(B)*, peripheral vessels *(V)*, and desmoplastic reactive tissue *(D)*. Note congested hepatic parenchyma *(P)* at the lower right corner.

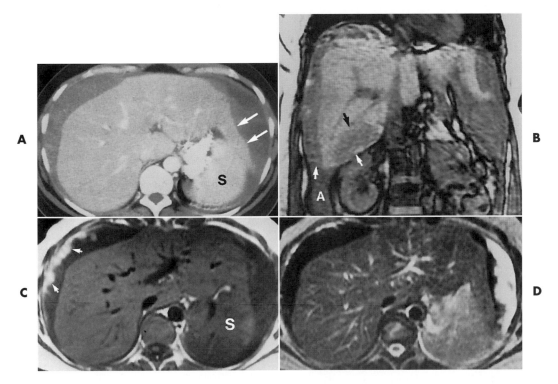

FIGURE 22-30   Primary intrahepatic lymphoma in a patient with acquired immunodeficiency syndrome (AIDS). **A,** SE 400/12 image. **B,** SE 2500/10 image. A low-intensity pseudocapsule *(arrows)* is present. **C,** H & E stain demonstrates well-differentiated lymphoma.

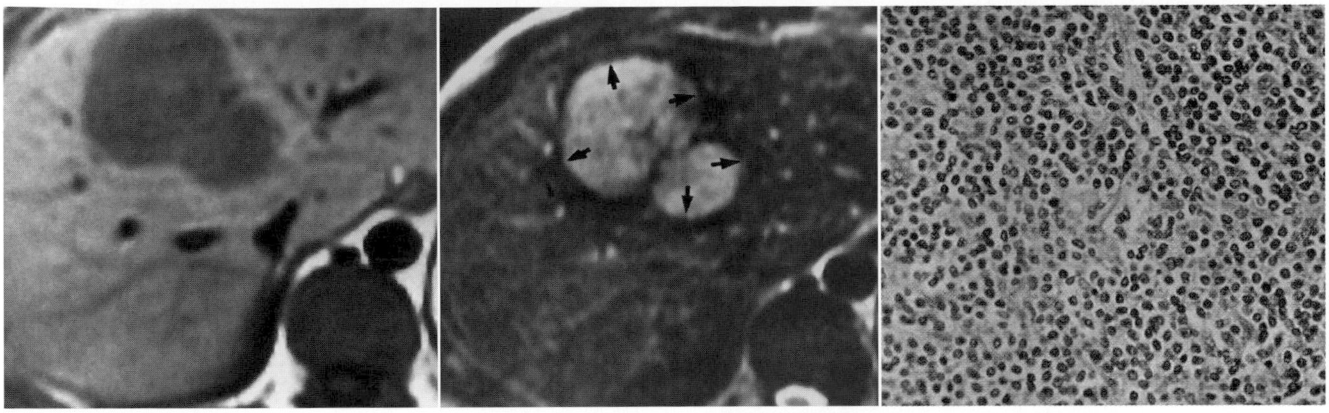

FIGURE 22-31   Massive acute perihepatic subcapsular hemorrhage in a woman with eclampsia. **A,** CT scan demonstrates perihepatic fluid. Note that the left lobe *(arrows)* extends lateral to the spleen *(S)*. **B,** Coronal 101/2.3/90 image distinguishes intermediate-signal subcapsular fluid *(small arrows)* and low-signal ascites *(A)*. **C,** SE 550/12 image shows high signal from methemoglobin loculated anterolaterally *(arrows)*. **D,** SE 3000/100 image shows blood surrounding the right lobe as low signal intensity (short T2) because of intact red blood cells. Blood lateral to the left lobe has high signal intensity (short T1, methemoglobin) indicating lysis of red blood cells. (From Mitchell DG, and Stark DD: Hepatobiliary MRI, St Louis, 1993, Mosby.)

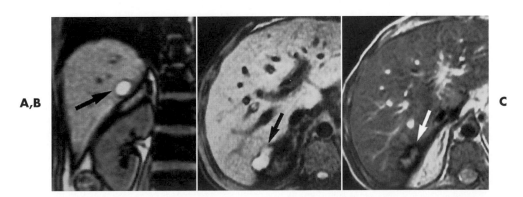

FIGURE 22-32   Perihepatic hematoma secondary to hepatic transplantation. **A,** Coronal T1-weighted gradient-echo 103/2.3/90 image shows a focal high-signal collection *(arrow)* with a dark rim. **B,** SE 400/14 image with fat suppression. **C,** SE 2500/50 image shows the hematoma as high signal, with increased thickness of the short T2 hemosiderotic rim. (From Mitchell DG, and Stark DD: Hepatobiliary MRI, St Louis, 1993, Mosby.)

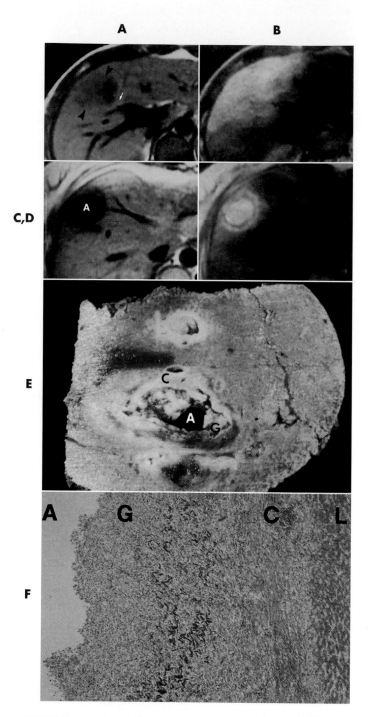

FIGURE 22-33   Amebic liver abscess. **A,** Pretreatment SE 500/28 image at 0.6 T shows a heterogeneous ill-defined mass *(arrowheads)* in the anterior segment, right hepatic lobe. Note deviation of the portal vein *(arrow)*. **B,** SE 2000/84 pulse sequence shows a large area of hepatic edema associated with the abscess. **C,** Follow-up SE 500/28 scan obtained after 2 weeks of antibiotic therapy shows maturation of the abscess. The abscess cavity *(A)* is now a homogeneous low signal intensity. The abscess wall shows concentric rings representing granulation tissue and a thick rim of collagen. **D,** SE 2000/84 sequence confirms resolution of hepatic edema and shows the mural rings characteristic of a healing amebic liver abscess. **E,** Pathological specimen from another patient who died after 4 days of antibiotic therapy. Abscess cavity *(A)* is surrounded by a broad sclerotic rim *(C)*. A thick band of granulation tissue *(G)* is seen in a region of active inflammation. **F,** Histological section through the wall of the partially treated abscess. The liquefied abscess cavity contents *(A)* have been lost in processing. Granulation tissue *(G)* and a bond of collagen *(C)* separate the abscess cavity from liver tissue. The liver parenchyma adjacent to the abscess wall shows sinusoidal dilatation, characteristic of edema. (Courtesy G. Elizondo.)

Postpartum perihepatic hemorrhage can occur in association with preeclampsia. Hemorrhage may be massive, but these patients, especially young primiparas, can be managed nonoperatively.[119] This hemorrhage may be part of the HELLP (*h*emolysis, *e*levated *l*iver enzymes, *l*ow *p*latelet count) syndrome. Hepatic infarction, manifested as a segmental zone of low signal on T1-weighted images and high signal on T2-weighted images, may be seen in these patients.[94]

Hepatic infarction is otherwise rare because of the dual blood supply of the liver via hepatic arteries and portal veins. Additionally there are extensive collateral anastomoses for both of these vascular systems between lobes and segments. Occasionally, infarctions can occur as a result of occlusion of portal veins and hepatic arteries by different pathologies or extensive malignant involvement of portal tracts.

Hepatic Infections

Pyogenic hepatic abscesses are usually associated with recent surgery, Crohn's disease, appendicitis, and diverticulitis.[11] Abscesses typically have high central signal intensity and intermediate peripheral signal intensity. Characteristic contrast-enhanced MR findings are centrally nonenhancing lesions with an enhancing capsule.[136] Abscesses typically have perilesional enhancement with indistinct outer margins on immediate postgadolinium images because of a hyperemic response in adjacent liver. The higher sensitivity of MRI to Gd chelates than of CT to iodinated agents suggests that dynamic Gd-enhanced MRI may be a useful technique for patients in whom distinction between simple cysts and multiple abscesses cannot be made on the basis of CT examination. Metastases may mimic the appearance of hepatic abscesses because both may have prominent rim enhancement.

Amebic abscess occurs in patients who live in or have traveled to tropical climates. Presenting features include pain, fever, weight loss, nausea and vomiting, diarrhea, and anorexia.[180] Lesions are usually solitary, and there is a tendency for invasion of the diaphragm with development of an empyema.[98] Lesions are encapsulated and demonstrate increased enhancement of the capsule on Gd-enhanced images, providing differentiation from liver cysts (Figure 22-33).

Echinococcus granulosus is the causative organism for hydatid cysts and is the form of *Echinococcus* species found in North America. The classic appearance is an intrahepatic encapsulated multicystic lesion with daughter cysts arranged peripherally within the larger cyst (Figure 22-34). Satellite cysts located exterior to the fibrinous membrane of the main hepatic cyst are common. A 16% incidence of satellite cysts was noted in one series of 185 patients with hydatid cysts.[82] The fibrous capsule and internal septations are shown well on contrast-enhanced T1- and T2-weighted images. Lesions are frequently complex, with mixed low signal intensity on T1-weighted images and mixed high signal intensity on T2-weighted images because of the presence of proteinaceous and cellular debris. Calcification of the cyst wall and internal calcification are frequently identified on CT images; however, on MRI, calcification cannot be distinguished from the fibrous tissue of the capsule.

Fungal microabscesses are observed with increasing frequency as a complication of immunosuppression or an immunocompromised state.[107,204] Patients on medical therapy for acute myelogenous leukemia (AML) are the group of patients most susceptible. The most common infecting organism is *Candida albicans*. Acute hepatosplenic candidiasis typically involves the liver and spleen with other organs, such as the kidneys, occasionally involved. Patient survival depends on early diagnosis. Liver lesions are frequently less than 1 cm in size and subcapsular in location. The small size and peripheral nature of these lesions make them difficult to detect with standard SE sequences. Patients with AML undergo multiple blood transfusions, so the liver and spleen usually have low signal intensity.[25,97,199] T2-weighted, fat-suppressed SE images may be of particular importance in detecting these lesions because of the high conspicuity of this sequence for small lesions and the absence of chemical-shift artifact, which may mask small peripheral lesions. STIR images have a similar high conspicuity for lesions.[97] MRI using T2-weighted fat suppression and dynamic Gd-chelate–enhanced FLASH images is more sensitive for detecting these lesions than is contrast-enhanced CT.[199] MRI is also better able to detect lesions that have responded to antifungal therapy.

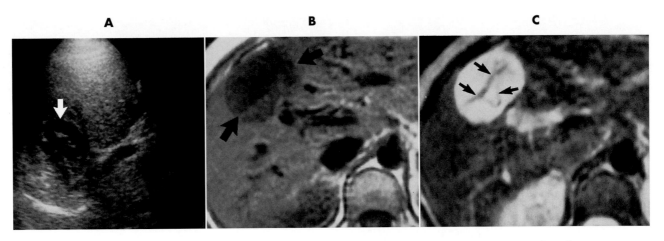

FIGURE 22-34 Echinococcal abscess. **A,** Transverse ultrasound shows a complex mass with strong through transmission. **B,** SE 300/15 image shows a low signal–intensity mass *(arrows).* **C,** SE 3000/100 image shows a cystic mass with an internal membrane *(arrows).* (Courtesy Dr. Jay Lehrman, Garden City, NY.)

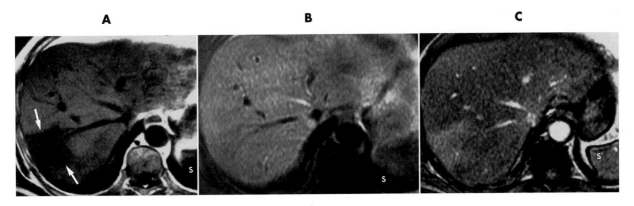

FIGURE 22-35 Fatty liver with wedge-shaped sparing of uncertain cause. **A,** Standard (in-phase) SE 500/11 image shows a wedge of decreased signal intensity *(arrows)* relative to the remainder of the liver. **B,** Fat-suppressed SE 500/12 image shows the wedge isointense with the remainder of the liver, consistent with sparing in an otherwise fatty liver. **C,** Opposed-phase gradient-echo 58/2.4/90 image shows wedge as bright relative to the liver. *S,* Spleen. (See Figure 22-8, *B.*) (From reference 140.)

DIFFUSE AND VASCULAR DISEASE
Fatty Liver

Fat (primarily triglyceride) may accumulate within hepatocytes in patients with diabetes mellitus, obesity, or malnutrition or after exposure to ethanol or other chemical toxins. Fatty change may be patchy or even focal, sometimes because of regional differences in perfusion. For example, areas of decreased portal flow tend to accumulate less fat than better-perfused areas.[3,50,129] This is particularly true near the gallbladder because of aberrant gastric venous drainage, which replaces portal venous flow.[129] Areas of fatty liver may also have relatively decreased portal flow, resulting in false-positive defects on CTAP.[174]

Fatty liver can interfere with detection or exclusion of focal liver masses by CT or ultrasound.[93,265] A suspicious zone of decreased attenuation seen on a CT scan is likely to represent focal fatty infiltration if it appears normal on T2-weighted SE MR images because conventional SE images are relatively insensitive to mild or moderate fatty infiltration. In such cases the suspicious area may have slightly increased signal intensity on T1-weighted images or non–fat-suppressed T2-weighted images. The level of confidence for diagnosing focal fat is increased greatly by the use of chemical-shift MR techniques.

The most effective technique for detecting regions of fatty liver is a comparison of opposed-phase (water − fat) and in-phase (water + fat) images[140,142] (Figures 22-35 and 22-36). Although most tissues appear similar on in- and opposed-phase images, fatty liver will have lower signal intensity on opposed-phase images. Fat saturation images may also be helpful in cases of moderate or severe fatty infiltration, but signal from fatty liver is not reduced as much as on opposed-phase im-

ages. Initially, opposed-phase images were implemented using SE techniques,[41,106,190] but these pulse sequences have never been widely available. Gradient-echo images with appropriate TE (between 2 to 3 ms or 6 to 7 ms at 1.5 T) produce an effective opposed-phase effect during suspended respiration on most clinical MR units.[141,254]

The morphology of focal fatty infiltration must be examined to differentiate it from fat within tumors,[73] such as HCC, HA, FNH, regenerative nodule, or lipomatous masses. Although some well-differentiated HCCs contain lipid, most HCCs with high signal intensity on T1-weighted images do not.[145] Hemorrhage, melanin, copper, and other factors may be associated with nonfatty masses with high signal intensity on T1-weighted images, but CSI should allow distinction between these tumors and lipid-containing masses or focal fatty infiltration. Even if HCC contains lipid, this tumor tends to be better defined than focal fatty infiltration, is often encapsulated, and usually contains some elements with high signal intensity on fat-suppressed T2-weighted images.

Iron Overload

Because of the liver's important functions as a digestive and reticuloendothelial organ, iron is deposited in the liver via several mechanisms. Iron overload within tissues reduces T2 and T2* relaxation times significantly, allowing MRI to be sensitive and specific for iron overload and for its regional distribution[207] (Figure 22-37). Because normal liver is more intense than skeletal muscle on virtually all pulse sequences and because skeletal muscle is unaffected by iron overload, skeletal muscle is a suitable reference tissue for detecting and quantifying de-

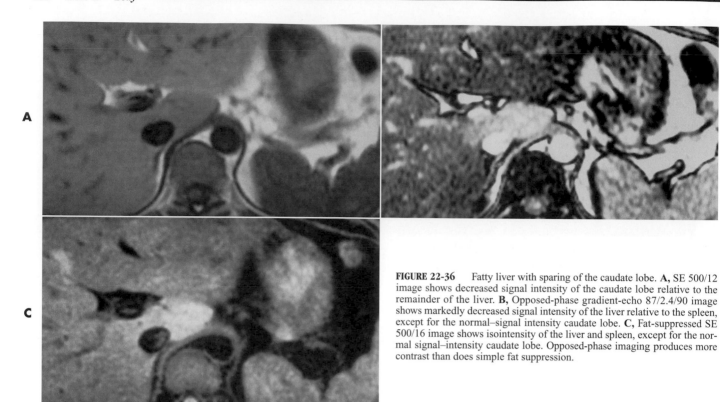

FIGURE 22-36   Fatty liver with sparing of the caudate lobe. **A,** SE 500/12 image shows decreased signal intensity of the caudate lobe relative to the remainder of the liver. **B,** Opposed-phase gradient-echo 87/2.4/90 image shows markedly decreased signal intensity of the liver relative to the spleen, except for the normal–signal intensity caudate lobe. **C,** Fat-suppressed SE 500/16 image shows isointensity of the liver and spleen, except for the normal signal–intensity caudate lobe. Opposed-phase imaging produces more contrast than does simple fat suppression.

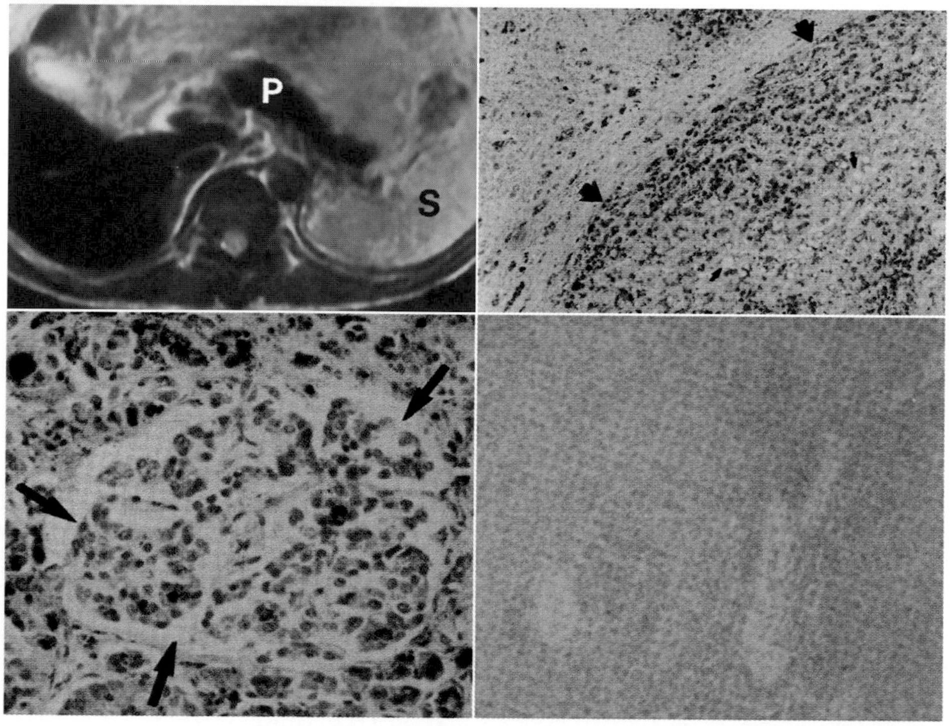

FIGURE 22-37   Hemochromatosis progressing over 6 months. Multisystem iron overload was confirmed at autopsy. **A,** SE 2500/50 image at the level of the pancreatic body *(P).* The pancreas and liver are signal voids, but the spleen *(S)* has normal intensity. **B,** Histological section, Prussian blue stain for iron. A regenerative nodule *(thick arrows)* with abundant iron and moderate fatty change *(small arrows)* is noted, surrounded by fibrotic parenchyma, which also contains abundant iron. **C,** Iron stain of pancreas depicts marked iron deposition *(blue)* within acinar cells. Pancreatic islets are relatively spared *(arrows),* except for B cells. **D,** Iron stain of spleen reveals no iron. (From Mitchell DG, and Stark DD: Hepatobiliary MRI, St Louis, 1993, Mosby.)

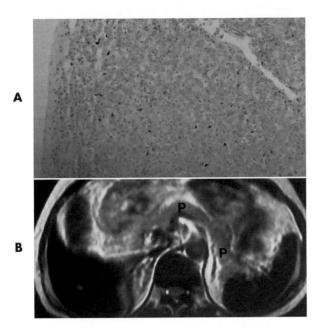

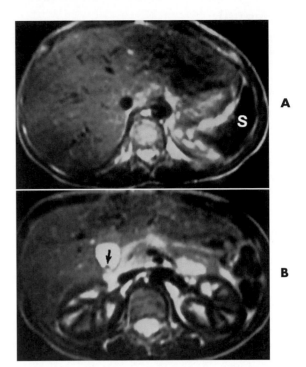

FIGURE 22-38   Transfusional iron overload after surgery for renal transplantation. **A,** Prussian blue stain for iron. Iron overload is severe and involves hepatocytes as well as Kupffer's cells. Systemic iron overload cannot be excluded, so MRI was recommended by the pathologist. **B,** Axial SE 2500/50 image at 1.5 T reveals decreased hepatic and splenic intensity but normal intensity of the pancreas *(P).* The findings are thus consistent with transfusional siderosis. (From Mitchell DG, and Stark DD: Hepatobiliary MRI, St Louis, 1993, Mosby.)

FIGURE 22-39   Intravascular hemolysis in a patient with sickle cell anemia. **A,** SE 2500/40 image depicts a small spleen with absent signal *(S).* The liver has normal signal intensity, however. **B,** SE 2500/40 image showing absent renal cortical signal bilaterally. Arrow indicates gallbladder calculi. (From Mitchell DG and Stark DD: Hepatobiliary MRI, St Louis, 1993, Mosby.)

creased hepatic signal intensity.[24] If images with sufficiently short TE can be obtained, estimation of T2 relaxation time may help quantify iron overload, providing a useful parameter for monitoring response to therapeutic phlebotomy or chelation.[59,89,241] Conditions that may be associated with increased hepatic iron, and therefore decreased hepatic signal intensity, include hemochromatosis, transfusional iron overload, hemolytic anemias, and cirrhosis. For uncertain reasons, segmental iron deposition is sometimes related to focally deficient portal perfusion.[81]

Hemochromatosis involves increased absorption and parenchymal accumulation of dietary iron.[135] Toxic levels of iron accumulate in the liver, pancreas, heart, and other organs. Common causes of death in these patients include cirrhosis, HCC, diabetes mellitus, and congestive cardiomyopathy. In advanced stages of hemochromatosis, decreased signal intensity of the liver and pancreas and normal signal intensity of the spleen are observed on T2- and T2*-weighted images. If phlebotomy therapy is instituted before malignancy or irreversible tissue damage occurs, life expectancy may be returned to normal. Preclinical hemochromatosis, a stage in which diagnosis and treatment are especially important, often manifests on MR images as decreased signal intensity restricted to the liver, which does not show signs of cirrhosis.[206]

Coexisting fat and iron deposition can be reliably detected by using gradient-echo MR images with multiple TEs. In the presence of iron the signal intensity of liver will decrease steadily as TE increases as a result of T2* effects. At opposed-phase TEs both higher and lower than the TE for in-phase images, a disproportionate drop of liver signal intensity will occur relative to spleen because of fat-water phase cancellation.

Many patients with HCC have previously unsuspected hemochromatosis.[207] Tumor cells do not contain excess iron,[234,235] causing especially high contrast relative to iron-overloaded liver on MR images. The use of long TEs does not improve depiction of HCC on long-TR images, and it may obscure small lesions because the heterogeneous magnetic field caused by hepatic parenchymal iron may reduce the signal intensity of small nodules. However, heavily T2-weighted images help differentiate malignant tumors from benign lesions, such as a hemangioma or cyst. If a nonsiderotic nodule in a patient with hemochromatosis is not a hemangioma or cyst, HCC is the most likely diagnosis

because regenerative nodules in these patients contain iron. Adenomatous hyperplasias in patients with increased hepatic iron may contain more or less iron than surrounding hepatic parenchyma.

Hemochromatosis should not be confused with iron overload from multiple transfusions, in which iron accumulates primarily within reticuloendothelial cells of the liver and spleen, sparing hepatocytes, pancreas, and other parenchyma. Although hemochromatosis cannot be differentiated from reticuloendothelial overload based solely on hepatic signal intensity, examination of pancreatic and splenic signal intensity can usually make this distinction. This distinction is clinically important because reticuloendothelial iron overload is less toxic than hepatocellular overload. Signal intensity of the spleen is usually normal with hemochromatosis, whereas signal intensity of the pancreas is normal in most cases of transfusional overload (Figure 22-38). However, if transfusional iron overload is especially massive (e.g., >100 units), the reticuloendothelial system may be saturated, and systemic (including hepatocellular and pancreatic) iron overload may develop.[207]

Hepatic signal intensity in patients with hemolytic anemia is variable, depending on the rate of redistribution of iron toward the bone marrow, the rate of absorption of oral iron, and the patient's transfusional overload history. Patients with thalassemia vera have increased absorption of oral iron and therefore develop erythrogenic hemochromatosis even in the absence of any blood transfusions.[205] Patients with sickle cell anemia have rapid turnover of hepatic iron and will have normal hepatic signal intensity unless they have received recent blood transfusions.[205] Renal cortical signal intensity may be decreased because of filtration and tubular absorption of free hemoglobin, the magnitude of which is not dependent on transfusional history (Figure 22-39). Iron overload in the liver and renal cortex is typically seen in patients with paroxysmal nocturnal hemoglobinuria (Figure 22-40).[207]

Hepatocellular iron is often mildly or moderately increased in patients with cirrhosis, especially those with cirrhosis secondary to ethanol abuse. In some instances iron deposition in the pancreas may be present. Hemochromatosis should not be suggested as the cause for a patient's cirrhosis unless the hepatic iron overload is severe and the pancreas is involved.

Viral Hepatitis

Viral hepatitis can produce significant acute morbidity. Hepatitis B and C viruses are transmitted parenterally and can cause chronic hepatitis and cirrhosis, as well as acute disease. Hepatitis C has been a particular problem in recipients of blood transfusions because screening for hepatitis of donated blood has been instituted only recently.[95] Non-A, non-B, non-C hepatitis is now referred to as *hepatitis-delta.*

Acute hepatitis can be diagnosed by clinical and serological studies, and imaging is not part of the standard initial work up. However, in patients with chronic hepatitis, imaging studies can be used to detect cirrhosis or ascites and to exclude HCC. On T2-weighted images of patients with acute or chronic active hepatitis, a collar of high signal intensity can often be seen surrounding portal vein branches, corresponding to inflammation; however, this finding is nonspecific.[130] In some patients with acute or chronic active hepatitis with focal inflammatory changes or fibrosis, diffuse or regional high signal intensity can be identified on T2-weighted MR images.[74,220]

Enlarged periportal lymph nodes are common in patients with viral hepatitis. These nodes may be discrete or confluent, but the portal vein and other structures usually maintain their shape and are not compressed (Figure 22-41).

Radiation-Induced Hepatitis

Portions of the liver are often included in radiation portals for a variety of malignancies. Within 6 months of radiation injury, edema can be noted, depicted as decreased intensity on T1-weighted and increased intensity on T2-weighted images.[245,264] In patients with fatty liver, fat is usually decreased within the radiation portal,[34,55] presumably because of decreased delivery of triglycerides caused by diminished portal flow.

Sarcoidosis

Focal involvement of the liver and spleen with sarcoidosis can be shown on MR images. Granulomas are small (<1 cm) and hypovascular, which accounts for their MR appearance. Sarcoid granulomas are typically low in signal intensity on T1- and T2-weighted images and enhance in a diminished, delayed fashion on Gd-enhanced spoiled gradient-echo (SGE) images.[88,253] On occasion, signal reversal of liver and spleen are noted on T2-weighted images, with the liver higher in signal than a low–signal intensity spleen[88] (Figure 22-42).

Sclerosing Cholangitis

Sclerosing cholangitis can produce severe damage to liver parenchyma and progress to end-stage cirrhosis. Intense inflammatory fibrosis involves the intrahepatic and extrahepatic biliary system, expanding portal tracts.[23,101,194,259] Enlarged portal lymph nodes are common (Figure 22-43). The hepatic parenchyma may be normal, even in patients with liver failure and portal hypertension. Unlike primary biliary cirrhosis, which predominates in women, approximately 70% of patients with sclerosing cholangitis are men.

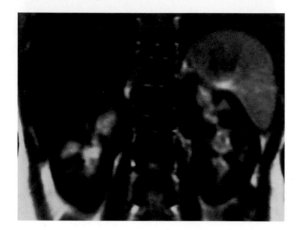

FIGURE 22-40 Paroxysmal nocturnal hemoglobinuria with hepatic and renal parenchymal iron overload from intravascular hemolysis. Coronal SE 2500/40 image reveals absent signal of the liver and renal cortex but normal signal of the spleen. (From reference 207.)

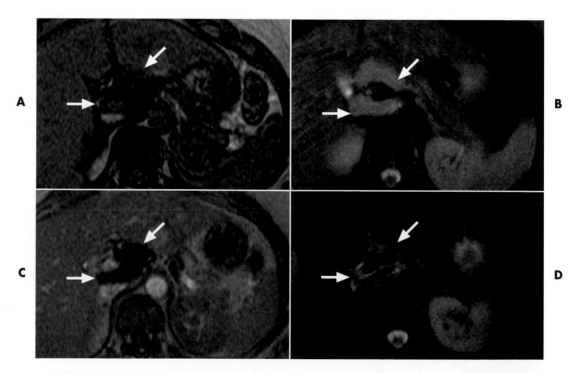

FIGURE 22-41 Benign reactive lymphadenopathy in a patient with hepatitis B, before (**A** and **B**) and 24 hours after (**C** and **D**) administration of ultrasmall superparamagnetic iron oxide particles. Concentration of the contrast agent within lymph nodes confirms benignity of the enlarged nodes. **A,** Gradient-echo 120/2.2 image. The lymph nodes *(arrows)* have signal intensity similar to that of the spleen. **B,** FSE 3633/104 image with fat suppression. The lymph nodes *(arrows)* have high signal intensity. **C,** Gradient-echo 120/4.2/90 image. **D,** FSE 3633/104 images 24 hours after ultrasmall iron oxide contrast agent administration show markedly decreased signal intensity of the lymph nodes.

The etiology of primary sclerosing cholangitis is not known, although many patients have inflammatory bowel disease, particularly ulcerative colitis. Secondary sclerosing cholangitis may occur as a sequela of biliary surgery or choledocholithiasis, or after hepatic arterial 5-fluorouracil deoxyribonucleoside (FUDR) chemotherapy.[202,259]

Cholangiographic findings include beaded dilatation of intrahepatic and extrahepatic bile ducts, with similar findings noted by contrast-enhanced CT.[179,193,233] Bile-duct thickening has been viewed on CT images, although it is uncertain if bile-wall thickening can be distinguished from periportal inflammation.

MR findings include scattered areas of biliary dilatation, peripheral zones of altered signal intensity and early enhancement, and periportal inflammation (Figure 22-43). Biliary dilatation can be distinguished from periportal inflammation on heavily T2-weighted images with sufficient spatial resolution and SNR, on which it is depicted as fluid-equivalent signal paralleling portal vein branches. Periportal inflammation is manifested as low signal intensity on T1-weighted images and signal intermediate between that of liver and bile on T2-weighted images. In many cases this abnormal tissue is more apparent on T1-weighted images. Periportal inflammation may also be depicted on postgadolinium images as enhancing tissue along both sides of the bile ducts. This inflammatory tissue is most conspicuous on delayed images with fat suppression. These findings can be seen at the hepatic hilum and within intrahepatic portal tracts, where they cause a collar surrounding portal vein branches. This high-signal collar is not seen surrounding branches of hepatic veins. However, there is some overlap between the periportal inflammation seen with sclerosing cholangitis and other conditions, such as biliary obstruction, hepatitis, allograft rejection, and periportal malignancy.[130] Segmental atrophy is a common finding in patients with sclerosing cholangitis.[61]

Cirrhosis

Cirrhosis involves irreversible hepatic fibrosis bridging the spaces between portal tracts, destroying the underlying hepatic architecture.[178] Many cirrhotic livers have prolonged T1, T2, or both, presumably secondary to hepatocellular damage or inflammation.[104,121] Mild iron deposition also occurs in many cirrhotic livers, potentially decreasing hepatic signal intensity. Tiny peribiliary cysts are common in cirrhotic livers.[8,69,238] The distorted hepatic architecture and presence of regenerative nodules in cirrhosis increases the difficulty of detecting focal malignant lesions.[138] Portosystemic shunting also decreases the effectiveness of CTAP for detecting focal lesions.[169]

Regenerative nodules result from grossly distorted hepatic architecture, heterogeneous regeneration, and hepatocellular dysplasia. MR images can depict regenerative nodules with greater clarity than other

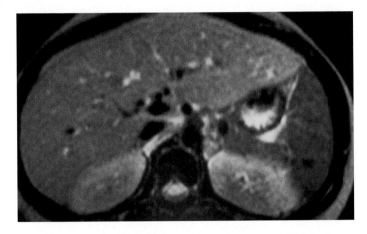

FIGURE 22-42 Hepatic sarcoidosis with liver-spleen "intensity flip-flop" on an SE 3000/100 image. No individual nodules were identified. Liver signal intensity is increased, spleen is normal.

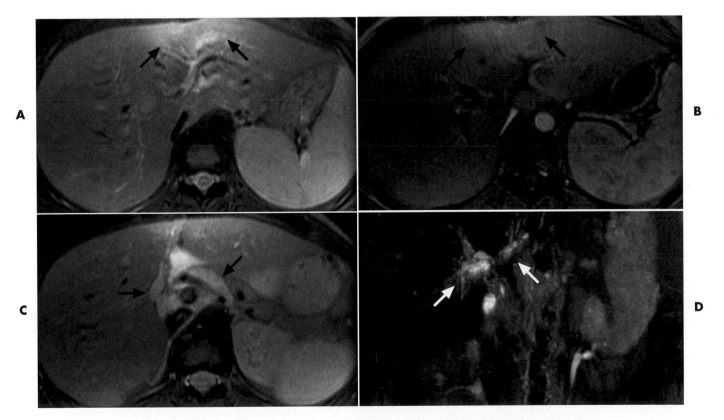

FIGURE 22-43 Primary sclerosing cholangitis. **A,** FSE 2000/52 image shows a zone of high signal intensity in the medial segment of the left lobe *(arrows)*. **B,** Gd-DTPA–enhanced image. **C,** Dilated intrahepatic ducts are visible. Arrows indicate enlarged lymph nodes. **D,** Coronal MR cholangiogram (TR/TE = 12000/256) shows irregularly dilated intrahepatic ducts *(arrows)* and small size and poor definition of the common bile duct.

imaging modalities. On T2-weighted images, regenerative nodules often have low signal intensity relative to high–signal intensity inflammatory fibrous septa or damaged liver.[166] Approximately 25% of regenerative nodules accumulate iron more than the surrounding hepatic parenchyma, facilitating their identification as low signal on T2-weighted SE images and rendering them visible on T2*-weighted gradient-echo images[236] (Figure 22-44). Because biopsy of regenerative nodules may disclose normal hepatic architecture and cause a false-negative diagnosis in patients with suspected cirrhosis, avoidance of these nodules by MR-guided biopsy might be useful. When regenerative nodules are not clearly visible, cirrhosis may be detected by noting irregular linear high-signal abnormalities on a T2-weighted image.[143] Conventional T2-weighted images with a TE of 50 to 70 ms are particularly effective in detecting regenerated nodules. In livers with fatty infiltration, regenerative nodules may have lower signal intensity than do intervening fibrotic septations, especially after injection of Gd chelates. In cirrhosis resulting from schistosomiasis japonica, thick fibrotic bands containing dilated blood vessels may be depicted by MRI as high signal on T2-weighted images with gradient-moment nulling and on Gd-enhanced images.[151]

Atrophy of cirrhotic livers tends to affect the anterior segment of the right lobe and the medial segment of the left lobe most severely. This often leads to expansion of the gallbladder fossa, causing extrahepatic fat to fill the space between the left and right hepatic lobes. This pattern of atrophy may be the result of thrombosis and obliteration of small- and medium-sized portal and hepatic veins.[252] Areas of hyper-

plasia near the gallbladder can be caused by relative sparing resulting from aberrant gastric venous drainage.[131]

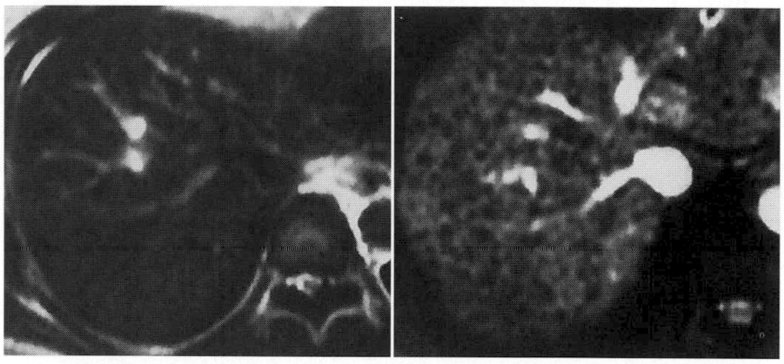

Portal hypertension can result from obstruction at postsinusoidal (e.g., hepatic vein), sinusoidal (e.g., cirrhosis), or presinusoidal (e.g., portal vein) levels.[60] The most common cause is cirrhosis. Portal hypertension causes or exacerbates complications of cirrhosis, such as variceal bleeding, ascites, and splenomegaly. Portosystemic shunts are identified well by 2D TOF techniques (Figures 22-45 and 22-46). Additional information can be gained by determining the direction of flow using 2D PC techniques.

During the early stages of portal hypertension, the portal system dilates but flow is maintained. Later, substantial portosystemic shunting develops, reducing the volume of flow to the liver and decreasing the size of the portal vein. With advanced portal hypertension, portal flow may actually become reversed.

Portal varices, caused by increased portal pressure, shunt portal blood into systemic veins, bypassing hepatic parenchyma. Nutrients absorbed from the gastrointestinal tract are thus metabolized less effectively, and hepatic function decreases. Additionally, toxic metabolites, such as ammonia, accumulate in the blood, producing clinical manifestations, such as hepatic encephalopathy. Because diminished portal flow to the liver parenchyma is an important factor in the production of liver atrophy and prevention of regeneration,[222] it is likely that portosystemic shunting plays a role in the development of hepatic atrophy in advanced cirrhosis. The presence of esophageal varices is particularly deleterious because they may rupture through the esophageal mucosa and produce life-threatening hemorrhage. Flow-sensitive gradient-echo images appear to be at least as sensitive as contrast angiography and endoscopy for detecting varices.[51]

Esophageal varices are usually supplied by a dilated coronary vein, which in normal subjects drains inferiorly toward the confluence of the splenic and superior mesenteric veins. In patients with esophageal varices, the flow in this vein reverses, an alteration that can be depicted using PC imaging or 2D TOF images with superior presaturation pulses. Reversed flow in the coronary vein indicates increased risk for hemorrhage from esophageal varices.

Recently, PC MR measurement of portal venous flow corrected for hepatic mass, also measured by MRI, was found to correlate significantly with increasing severity of clinical disease in patients with cirrhosis.[96]

Nodular Regenerative Hyperplasia

Nodular regenerative hyperplasia, a cause of noncirrhotic portal hypertension, is believed to be a nonspecific response to diffuse small-

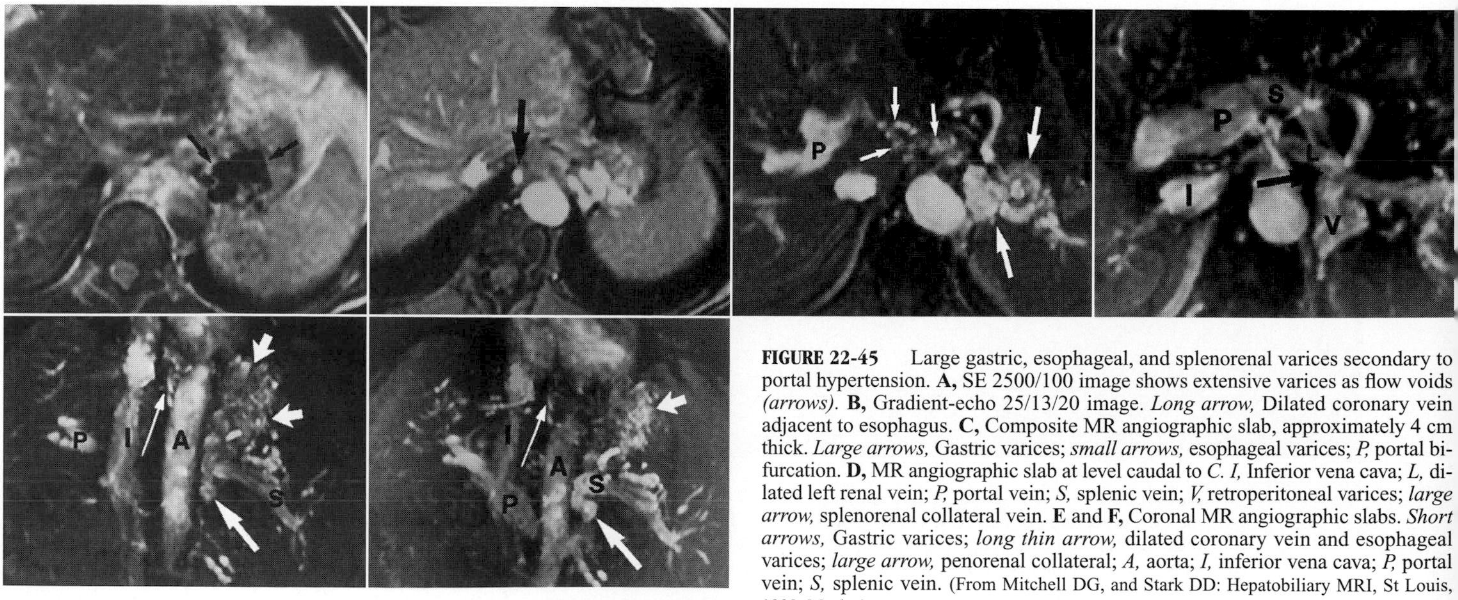

FIGURE 22-44   Cirrhosis with siderotic regenerative nodules. **A,** SE 2500/50 image shows a subtle nodular pattern. **B,** Gradient-echo 25/13/20 image shows obvious nodules. (From Mitchell DG, and Stark DD: Hepatobiliary MRI, St Louis, 1993, Mosby.)

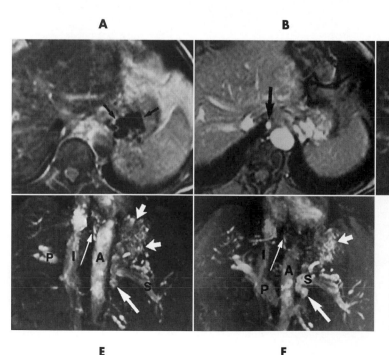

FIGURE 22-45   Large gastric, esophageal, and splenorenal varices secondary to portal hypertension. **A,** SE 2500/100 image shows extensive varices as flow voids *(arrows).* **B,** Gradient-echo 25/13/20 image. *Long arrow,* Dilated coronary vein adjacent to esophagus. **C,** Composite MR angiographic slab, approximately 4 cm thick. *Large arrows,* Gastric varices; *small arrows,* esophageal varices; *P,* portal bifurcation. **D,** MR angiographic slab at level caudal to *C. I,* Inferior vena cava; *L,* dilated left renal vein; *P,* portal vein; *S,* splenic vein; *V,* retroperitoneal varices; *large arrow,* splenorenal collateral vein. **E** and **F,** Coronal MR angiographic slabs. *Short arrows,* Gastric varices; *long thin arrow,* dilated coronary vein and esophageal varices; *large arrow,* penorenal collateral; *A,* aorta; *I,* inferior vena cava; *P,* portal vein; *S,* splenic vein. (From Mitchell DG, and Stark DD: Hepatobiliary MRI, St Louis, 1993, Mosby.)

vessel vasculopathy, usually of the portal venules.* Predisposing conditions include hepatological disorders such as polycythemia vera, Budd-Chiari syndrome, and collagen vascular diseases. Areas of the liver that receive decreased blood flow atrophy, whereas those that receive adequate flow enlarge and form nodules. The result is a liver that consists of numerous regenerative nodules without substantial inflammation or intervening fibrosis. MR findings resemble those of cirrhosis, although there should be no areas of abnormally decreased signal intensity on T1-weighted images or increased signal intensity on T2-weighted images,[208] findings that are common in cirrhosis because of areas of inflammation, fibrosis, or hepatocellular damage.[140,165] Most

of these nodules are less than 3 mm in diameter and therefore are not depicted on imaging studies. Occasionally, focal nodules are noted that are hyperintense on T1-weighted images and isointense on T2-weighted images, findings similar to those of many regenerative nodules and adenomatous hyperplastic nodules. Occasionally the nodules may contain fat.[208] There is no evidence of increased incidence of malignancy in patients with nodular regenerative hyperplasia.

Portal Thrombosis

SE and gradient-echo images are usually effective for depicting obstruction or patency of the main portal vein and its major branches (Figure 22-47).[92] Additionally, lobar or segmental portal vein obstruction by tumor may cause discrete wedge-shaped regions of increased inten-

---

*References 31, 35, 158, 208, 243, 250, 251.

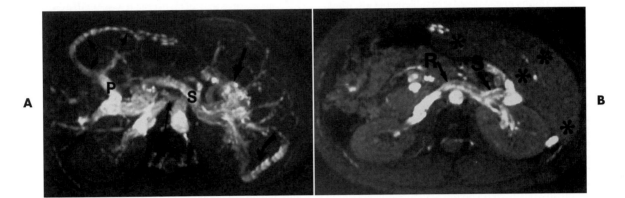

FIGURE 22-46   Portosystemic shunting from splenorenal and retroperitoneal collaterals and a patent paraumbilical vein in a patient with portal hypertension. **A,** Axial MR angiogram (gradient-echo 25/13/20 image) shows the patent paraumbilical vein *(small arrows)* arising from the left portal vein *(P)*. Splenic collateral veins *(large arrow)* can be seen, but the splenorenal shunt, between the splenic vein *(S)* and left renal vein *(R)*, is obscured. Portosystemic collateral veins can be seen posterior to the spleen *(curved arrow)*. **B,** Limited MR angiogram with most of the liver excluded, demonstrating the spontaneous splenorenal collateral *(S)* joining a dilated left renal vein *(R)*. The spleen is enlarged. **C,** Coronal MR angiogram depicts the splenorenal and retroperitoneal collaterals. The patent paraumbilical vein is anterior to this slab.

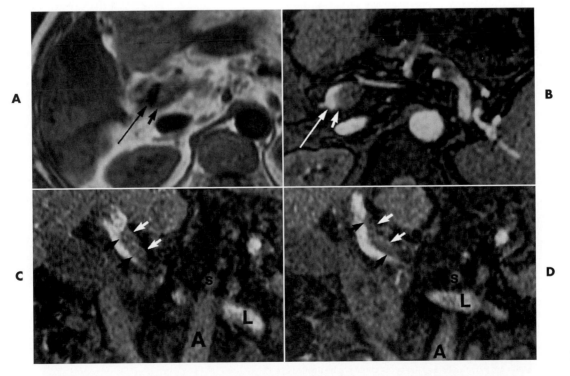

FIGURE 22-47   Nonocclusive thrombosis in a patient with cirrhosis. The lateral portion of the portal vein is patent *(long arrow)*, with thrombus present along the medial border *(short arrow)*. **A,** SE 400/12 image. **B,** Gradient-echo 27/7.4/20 image. **C** and **D,** Coronal gradient-echo 27/7.4/20 images. Arrows indicate portal thrombus. *A,* Aorta; *L,* left renal vein; *S,* superior mesenteric artery origin. (From Mitchell DG, and Stark DD: Hepatobiliary MRI, St Louis, 1993, Mosby.)

sity on T2-weighted images and Gd-enhanced images.* Obstruction of the portal vein also can cause atrophy, with compensatory hypertrophy of other segments.[75,140] Collateral periportal veins may maintain portal perfusion when the main portal vein is thrombosed. With time this network of collateral venous channels dilates and the thrombosed portal vein retracts, producing cavernous transformation.[38,160] After administration of intravenous contrast material, MR images may show increased enhancement of hepatic parenchyma in the areas with decreased portal perfusion most pronounced during the dynamic enhancement or equilibrium phases. This paradoxical increased enhancement of hepatic parenchyma distal to an obstructed portal vein branch may largely reflect increased hepatic arterial supply. Hepatic arterial perfusion is increased to parenchyma deprived of portal blood flow, which may therefore enhance more because there is less dilution of contrast material in hepatic arteries than in portal veins. In addition, decreased blood supply results in decreased size of hepatocytes, which increases the proportion of liver volume occupied by the vascular and interstitial spaces.

Budd-Chiari Syndrome

Budd-Chiari syndrome results from obstruction of venous outflow from the sinusoid bed of the liver, resulting in portal hypertension, ascites, and progressive hepatic failure. In most cases hepatic venous outflow is not completely eliminated because a variety of accessory hepatic veins may drain above or below the principal site of obstruction. In some instances obstruction may even be segmental or subsegmental. Although major hepatic veins may be nonvisualized or thrombosed, demonstration of patent central hepatic veins does not exclude Budd-Chiari syndrome because small- or intermediate-sized veins may be involved.[137] Regions with completely obstructed hepatic venous outflow tend to drain via shunting of blood from hepatic veins and arteries to portal veins, producing reversed portal venous flow.[70,126,157,177] These regions

*References 21, 70, 75, 112, 140, 192.

of the liver will thus be deprived of portal vein supply. Hepatic regeneration, hypertrophy, and atrophy depend in part on the degree of portal perfusion.[222] Budd-Chiari syndrome is typically associated with atrophy of peripheral liver, which has especially severe venous obstruction, and hypertrophy of the caudate lobe and central liver, which are relatively spared (Figure 22-48).

On dynamic iodine-enhanced CT images or Gd-enhanced MR images, the peripheral atrophic liver in Budd-Chiari syndrome may enhance to a greater or lesser extent than normal or hypertrophied liver. Increased enhancement is presumably the result of a combination of decreased portal perfusion (see earlier discussion) and dilatation of hepatic sinusoids. The hypertrophied central liver, if enhanced less than the peripheral atrophied liver, may thus resemble a focal mass.

Massive hypertrophy of the caudate lobe may compress an otherwise patent inferior vena cava and displace the porta hepatis anteriorly. MR images also may demonstrate regional differences in signal intensity because of atrophy, congestion, or iron deposition. The caudate lobe may resemble a focal mass as a result of contrast with the abnormal signal intensity of the peripheral liver.

Chronic hepatic venous obstruction produces hepatic ischemia, which in turn may lead to the development of nodular regenerative hyperplasia.[22,118] The nodules in these livers are typically round, of variable size, and have high signal intensity on T1-weighted images and intermediate or low signal intensity on T2-weighted images, similar to adenomatous hyperplastic nodules.[214]

Hepatic Transplantation

Orthotopic liver transplantation has become the treatment of choice for irreversible liver failure in appropriate candidates. MRI is an outstanding method for comprehensive preoperative evaluation of candidates for liver transplantation. With one examination, patency of the inferior vena cava (IVC), portal vein, hepatic artery, and common bile duct can be confirmed, and early or advanced malignancy can be detected[51,162] (Figure 22-49). If early HCC is detected, the priority for urgent trans-

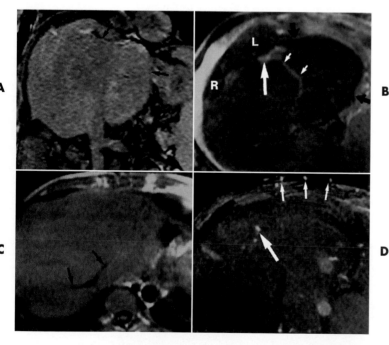

FIGURE 22-48 Budd-Chiari syndrome with patent central hepatic veins. **A,** Coronal gradient-echo 101/2.3/90 image shows massive hypertrophy of the caudate lobe *(arrows).* **B,** Axial SE 2500/50 image shows decreased signal of the liver. The caudate lobe *(short, thick arrows)* is markedly enlarged, and the left *(L)* and right *(R)* lobes are atrophied. *Large arrow,* Porta hepatis; *small arrows,* portal branch to caudate. **C,** SE 400/12 image at the level of the central hepatic veins *(arrows),* two of which are patent. The hepatic veins could not be imaged peripheral to this. *Long arrows,* Hepatic veins; *short arrows,* abdominal wall collateral veins. **D,** MR angiographic slab corresponding to **B.** *Large arrow,* Small portal vein; *small arrows,* body wall collateral veins. (From Mitchell DG, and Stark DD: Hepatobiliary MRI, St Louis, 1993, Mosby.)

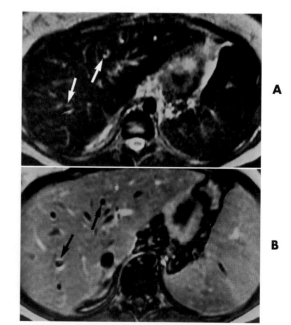

FIGURE 22-49 Periportal edema and transfusional siderosis after hepatic transplantation. **A,** SE 2500/100 image reveals increased signal surrounding portal vein branches *(arrows).* Hepatic signal intensity is decreased because of siderosis from the surgery. **B,** SE 400/12 image after administration of Gd chelate demonstrates periportal enhancement. (From Mitchell DG, and Stark DD: Hepatobiliary MRI, St Louis, 1993, Mosby.)

plantation can be increased, or alternatively the HCC can be treated by percutaneous ethanol ablation or chemoembolization as a temporizing measure while the patient awaits transplantation.[218]

Rejection is the most common cause of early liver-graft failure, and early diagnosis is essential to allow modification of immunosuppressive therapy.[40] Unfortunately, the differential diagnosis of rejection is complex and includes biliary obstruction, cholangitis, ischemic injury, viral infection, and drug toxicity.

MRI often shows periportal abnormalities in transplanted livers. A collar of tissue with long T1 and T2 relaxation times can extend from the porta hepatis along the branching portal tracts out into the liver periphery.[99] In many cases this represents lymphocytic infiltration from rejection but may also be caused by dilated lymphatics resulting from impaired drainage after surgery.[120] Similar nonspecific periportal changes can be observed with acute hepatitis or after biliary surgery for benign or malignant disease or with portal adenopathy.[130] Thus far no MR findings have been useful for diagnosing transplant rejection.

Vascular complications, such as portal vein or IVC thrombosis or hepatic artery stenosis, are important causes of graft failure.[262] Portal vein and IVC patency can be diagnosed reliably by MRI[36] (Figure 22-50). Hepatic artery stenosis is far more important because it can cause biliary complications and graft failure.[170] Hepatic artery patency can be documented by MRI in most cases. Hepatic artery stenosis can sometimes be depicted using optimized techniques (Figure 22-51), although stenosis cannot be excluded by using current techniques.

Fluid collections, especially small HCCs, are common after hepatic transplantation (Figures 22-32 and 22-52). Bile leaks may occur, sometimes associated with biliary strictures. Mucocele of the cystic duct

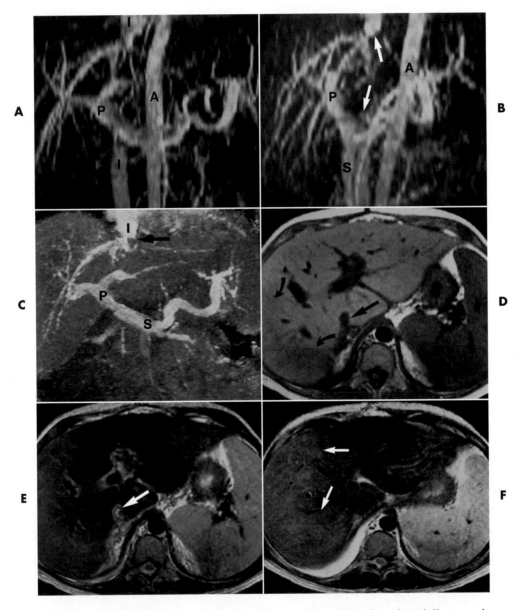

FIGURE 22-50 IVC thrombosis and nonuniform hepatic signal abnormalities after orthotopic liver transplantation. **A,** Coronal reformatted MRA from axial gradient-echo 27/7.4/20 image. Native portions of the inferior vena cava *(I)* are patent, but there is no flow between the inferior and superior anastomoses. *A,* Aorta; *P,* main portal vein. **B,** Right anterior oblique projection demonstrating the sites of obstruction *(arrows). A,* Aorta; *P,* portal vein; *S,* superior mesenteric vein. **C,** Composite slab from coronal gradient-echo 30/7.4/20 image. Spatial presaturation has been applied superiorly and inferiorly, eliminating signal from the aorta and inferior portion of the IVC. *I,* Suprahepatic IVC; *P,* main portal vein; *S,* splenic vein; *arrow,* superior edge of thrombus. **D,** SE 500/12 image at the level of the left portal vein. *Straight arrow,* Thrombus in the IVC. *Curved arrows,* A zone of abnormal signal intensity in the right hepatic lobe. **E,** FSE 4200/102 image. *Straight arrow,* Thrombus in the IVC. The parenchymal abnormality indicated in **D** has slightly increased signal intensity. **F,** Same image as in **E** but higher. The peripheral portion of the right lobe *(arrows)* has abnormally increased signal intensity. (From Mitchell DG, and Stark DD: Hepatobiliary MRI, St Louis, 1993, Mosby.)

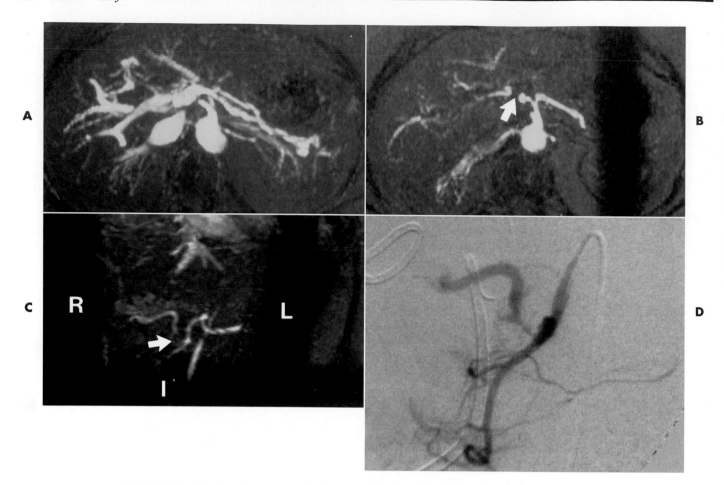

FIGURE 22-51   Hepatic artery stenosis after liver transplantation, depicted by multiple 2D TOF techniques acquired during suspended respirations. **A,** An 8-cm slab of collapsed data from 20 contiguous 4-mm axial sections gradient-echo 40/7.7/45 image. Arterial anatomy is obscured by venous structures. **B,** A 3.2-cm slab from 16 contiguous 2-mm thick sections is more sensitive to slow flow because of decreased section thickness. A saturation band positioned inferior to the slab has removed signal intensity entering the portal vein from the superior mesenteric vein, and a saturation band along the left side of the image has removed signal intensity from the splenic vein. Arrow indicates a stenosis at the origin of the proper hepatic artery. **C,** A 2.4-cm slab collapsed from 12 contiguous 2-mm thick coronal sections acquired anterior to the aorta and IVC. Saturation bands eliminate signal inferiorly *(I)* from the superior mesenteric vein, on the left *(L)* from the splenic vein, and on the right *(R)* from right hepatic veins. Note the superior mesenteric artery penetrating into the inferior saturation band. *Arrow,* Stenotic segment of the proper hepatic artery. **D,** Invasive hepatic arteriogram confirms the hepatic artery stenosis. (From Mitchell DG: Hepatic imaging: techniques and unique applications of magnetic resonance imaging, Magn Reson Q 9:84, 1993.)

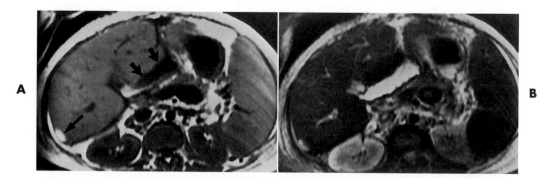

FIGURE 22-52   Perigraft hemorrhage after liver transplantation. **A,** SE 400/12 image reveals hyperintense fluid at the posterior tip of the liver *(long arrow)* consistent with methemoglobin. A larger collection is seen posterior to the medial segment of the left lobe *(short arrows).* This collection has predominantly low signal, except for the dependent portion *(curved arrow).* **B,** SE 2500/50 image. Both collections have high signal intensity. Splenic and hepatic signal intensity are reduced as a result of transfusions given during surgery. (From Mitchell DG, and Stark DD: Hepatobiliary MRI, St Louis, 1993, Mosby.)

remnant is also a recognized complication of hepatic transplantation, manifested as a focal fluid collection adjacent to the hepatic duct.[270] MRI can help distinguish between hematomas and other fluid collections in hepatic allograft recipients.

On occasion, heterotopic liver transplantation is performed on poor operative candidates with fulminant acute hepatitis. In this procedure the hepatic allograft is placed inferior to the native liver with end-to-side anastomosis of vessels and biliary duct.[152,239,271] Banding of the native vessels may be necessary to ensure adequate flow to the graft. After recovery from the acute illness, some hepatic function of the native liver may be regained. Recovery of the native liver may manifest as increasing size and recovery of normal signal characteristics, whereas concomitant graft failure may be depicted as decreasing size and abnormal signal.

REFERENCES

1. Achong D, and Oates E: Hepatic hemangioma in cirrhotics with portal hypertension: evaluation with Tc-99m red blood cell SPECT, Radiology 191:115, 1994.
2. Adachi E, Maeda T, Matsumata T, et al: Risk factors for intrahepatic recurrence in human small hepatocellular carcinoma, Gastroenterology 108:768, 1995.
3. Arai K, Matsui O, Takashima T, et al: Focal spared areas in fatty liver caused by regional decreased portal flow, Am J Roentgenol 151:300, 1988.
4. Arakawa M, Kage M, Sugihara S, et al: Emergence of malignant lesions within an adenomatous hyperplastic nodule in a cirrhotic liver, Gastroenterology 91:198, 1986.
5. Atlas S, Braffman B, LoBrutto R, et al: Human malignant melanomas with varying degrees of melanin content in nude mice: MR imaging, histopathology, and electron paramagnetic resonance, J Comput Assist Tomogr 14:547, 1990.
6. Bagley C Jr, Young R, Schein P, et al: Ovarian carcinoma metastatic to the diaphragm frequently undiagnosed at laparotomy, Am J Obstet Gynecol 116:397, 1973.
7. Barish M, Yucel EK, Soto J, et al: MR cholangiopancreatography: efficacy of three-dimensional turbo spin-echo technique, Am J Roentgenol 165:295, 1995.
8. Baron R, Campbell W, and Dodd G: Peribiliary cysts associated with severe liver disease: imaging-pathologic correlation, Am J Roentgenol 162:631, 1994.
9. Bartolozzi C, Lencioni R, Caramelia D, et al: Treatment of hepatocellular carcinoma with percutaneous ethanol injection: evaluation with contrast-enhanced MR imaging, Am J Roentgenol 162:827, 1994.
10. Benvegnu L, Fattovich G, Noventa F, et al: Concurrent hepatitis B and C virus infection and risk of hepatocellular carcinoma in cirrhosis: a prospective study, Cancer 74:2442, 1994.
11. Bertel CK, Van Heerden JA, and Sheedy PF: Treatment of pyogenic hepatic abscesses, Arch Surg 121:554, 1986.
12. Birnbaum BA, Weinreb JC, Meigibow AJ, et al: Blinded retrospective comparison of MR imaging and Tc-99m–labeled red blood cell SPECT for definitive diagnosis of hepatic hemangiomas, Radiology 173:270, 1989.
13. Brandt DJ, Johnson CD, Stephens DH: Imaging of fibrolamellar hepatocellular carcinoma, Am J Roentgenol 151:295, 1988.
14. Bret PM, Labadie M, Bretangnolle M, et al: Hepatocellular carcinoma: diagnosis by percutaneous fine needle biopsy, Gastrointest Radiol 13:253, 1988.
15. Brown J, Lee JM, Lee JK, et al: Focal hepatic lesions: differentiation with MR imaging at 0.5T, Radiology 179:675, 1991.
16. Brown RKJ, Gomes A, King W, et al: Hepatic hemangiomas: evaluation by magnetic resonance imaging and technetium-99m red blood cell scintigraphy, J Nuc Med 28:1683, 1987.
17. Bru C, Maroto A, Bruix J, et al: Diagnostic accuracy of fine-needle aspiration biopsy in patients with hepatocellular carcinoma, Dig Dis Sci 34:1765, 1989.
18. Butch RJ, Stark DD, and Malt RA: MR imaging of hepatic focal nodular hyperplasia, J Comput Assist Tomogr 10:874, 1986.
19. Butts K, Riederer SJ, and Ehman RL: The effect of respiration on the contrast and sharpness of liver lesions in MRI., Magn Reson Med 33:1, 1995.
20. Cameron IL, Ord WVA, and Fullerton GD: Characterization of proton NMR relaxation times in normal and pathological tissues by correlation with other tissue parameters, Magn Reson Imag 2:97, 1984.
21. Carr D, Hadjis N, Banks L, et al: Computed tomography of hilar cholangiocarcinomas: a new sign, Am J Roentgenol 145:53, 1985.
22. Castellano G, Canga F, Solis-Herruzo J, et al: Budd-Chiari syndrome associated with nodular regenerative hyperplasia of the liver, J Clin Gastroenterol 11:698, 1989.
23. Chapman RWG, Marborgh BA, Rhodes JM, et al: Primary sclerosing cholangitis: a review of its clinical features, cholangiography, and hepatic histology, Gut 21:870, 1980.
24. Chezmar J, Nelson R, Malko J, et al: Hepatic iron overload: diagnosis and quantification by noninvasive imaging, Gastrointest Radiol 15:27, 1990.
25. Cho JS, Kim EE, Varma DGK, et al: MR imaging of hepatosplenic candidiasis superimposed on hemochromatosis, J Comput Assist Tomogr 14:774, 1990.
26. Choi B, Han MC, Park JH, et al: Giant cavernous hemangioma of the liver: CT and MR imaging in 10 cases, Am J Roentgenol 152:1221, 1989.
27. Choi B, Takayasu K, and Han MC: Small hepatocellular carcinomas and associated nodular lesions of the liver: pathology, pathogenesis, and imaging findings, Am J Roentgenol 160:1177, 1993.
28. Choi BI, Han JK, Shin YM, et al: Peripheral cholangiocarcinoma: comparison of MRI with CT, Abdom Imaging 20:357, 1995.
29. Choi BI, Lee GK, Kim ST, et al: Mosaic pattern of encapsulated hepatocellular carcinoma: correlation of magnetic resonance imaging and pathology, Gastrointest Radiol 15:238, 1990.
30. Chung KY, Mayo-Smith W, Saini S, et al: Hepatocellular adenoma: MR imaging features with pathologic correlation, Am J Roentgenol 165:303, 1995.
31. Colina F, Alberti N, Solis JA, et al: Diffuse nodular regenerative hyperplasia of the liver (DNRH): a clinicopathologic study of 24 cases, Liver 9:253, 1989.
32. Corrigan K, and Semelka RC: Dynamic contrast-enhanced MR imaging of fibrolamellar hepatocellular carcinoma, Abdom Imaging 20:122, 1995.
33. Craig J, Peters R, and Edmondson H: Tumors of the liver and intrahepatic bile ducts. In Hartmann H, and Sobin L, eds: Atlas of tumor pathology, vol 2, Washington, DC, 1989, Armed Forces Institute of Pathology.
34. Cutillo DP, Swayne LC, Cucco J, et al: CT and MR imaging in cystic abdominal lymphangiomatosis, J Comput Assist Tomogr 13:534, 1989.
35. Dachman AH, Ros PR, Goldman Z, et al: Nodular regenerative hyperplasia of the liver: clinical and radiologic observations, Am J Roentgenol 148:717, 1987.
36. Dalen N, Day DL, Ascher NL, et al: Imaging of vascular complications after hepatic transplantation, Am J Roentgenol 150:1285, 1988.
37. Davis PL, Kanal E, Farnum GN, et al: MR imaging of multiple hepatic cysts in a patient with polycystic liver disease, Magn Reson Imaging 5:407, 1987.
38. De Gaetano AM, Lafortune M, Patriquin H, et al: Cavernous transformation of the portal vein: patterns of intrahepatic and splanchnic collateral circulation detected with Doppler sonography, Am J Roentgenol 165:1151, 1995.
39. de Santis M, Torricelli P, Cristani A, et al: MRI of hepatocellular carcinoma before and after transcatheter chemoembolization, J Comput Assist Tomogr 17:901, 1993.
40. Demetris AJ, Lasky S, VanThiel DH, et al: Pathology of hepatic transplantation: a review of 62 adult allograft recipients immunosuppressed with a cyclosporine steroid regimen, Am J Pathol 118:151, 1985
41. Dixon W: Simple proton spectroscopic imaging, Radiology 153:189, 1984.
42. Dodd GD: An American's guide to Cuinaud's numbering system, Am J Roentgenol 161:574, 1993.
43. Dravid VS, Shapiro MJ, Mitchell DG, et al: MR portography: preliminary comparison with CT portography and conventional MR imaging, J Magn Reson Imag 4:767,1994.
44. Duda SH, Laniado M, Kopp AF, et al: Superparamagnetic iron oxide: detection of focal liver lesions at high-field strength MR imaging, J Magn Reson Imaging 4:309, 1994.
45. Ebara M, Ohio M, Watanabe Y, et al: Diagnosis of small hepatocellular carcinoma: correlation of MR imaging and tumor histologic studies, Radiology 159:371, 1986.
46. Ebara M, Watanabe S, Kita K, et al: MR imaging of small hepatocellular carcinoma: effect of intratumoral copper content on signal intensity, Radiology 180:617, 1991.
47. Edelman RR, Siegel JB, Singer A, et al: Dynamic MR imaging of the liver with Gd-DTPA: initial clinical results, Am J Roentgenol 153:1213, 1989.
48. Edmondson HA: Benign epithelial tumors and tumorlike lesions of the liver. In Okuda J, and Peters RL, eds: Hepatocellular carcinoma, New York, 1976, John Wiley & Sons.
49. Egglin TK, Rummeny E, and Stark DD: Hepatic tumors: quantitative tissue characterization with MR imaging, Radiology 176:107, 1990.
50. Fernandez M, and Bernardino M: Hepatic pseudolesion: appearance of focal low attenuation in the medial segment of the left lobe at CT arterial portography, Radiology 181:809, 1991.
51. Finn J, Edelman R, Jenkins R, et al: Liver transplantation: MR angiography with surgical validation, Radiology 179:265, 1991.
52. Furui S, Ohtomo K, Itai Y, et al: Hepatocellular carcinoma treated by transcatheter arterial embolization: progress evaluated by computed tomography, Radiology 150:773, 1984.
53. Furuya K, Nakamura M, Yamamoto Y, et al: Macroregenerative nodule of the liver: a clinicopathologic study of 345 autopsy cases of chronic liver disease, Cancer 61:99, 1988.
54. Gabata T, Matsui O, Kadoya M, et al: MR imaging of hepatic adenoma, Am J Roentgenol 155:1009, 1990.
55. Garra BS, Shawker TH, Chang R, et al: The ultrasound appearance of radiation-induced hepatic injury, J Ultrasound Med 7:605, 1988.
56. Gazelle GS, and Haaga JR: Hepatic neoplasms: surgically relevant segmental anatomy and imaging techniques, Am J Roentgenol 158:1015, 1992.
57. Giovagnoni A, Terilli F, Ercolani P, et al: MR imaging of hepatic masses: diagnostic significance of wedge-shaped areas of increased signal intensity surrounding the lesion, Am J Roentgenol 163:1093, 1994.
58. Goldberg M, Hahn P, Saini S, et al: Value of T1 and T2 relaxation time from echoplanar MR imaging in the characterization of focal hepatic lesions, Am J Roentgenol 160:1011, 1993.
59. Gomori JM, Horev G, Tamary H, et al: Hepatic iron overload: quantitative MR imaging, Radiology 179:367, 1991.
60. Groszmann R, and Atterbury C: The pathophysiology of portal hypertension: a basis for classification, Semin Liver Dis 2:177, 1982.
61. Hadjis NS, Adam A, Blenkharn I, et al: Primary sclerosing cholangitis associated with liver atrophy, Am J Surg 158:43, 1989.
62. Hagspiel K, Neidl K, Eichenberger A, et al: Detection of liver metastases: comparison of superparamagnetic iron oxide—enhanced and unenhanced MR imaging at 1.5T with dynamic CT, intraoperative US, and percutaneous US, Radiology 196:471, 1995.
63. Hahn P, Stark D, and Weissleder R: The differential diagnosis of ringed hepatic lesions in MR imaging, Am J Roentgenol 154:287, 1990.
64. Hamm B, Staks T, Muhler A, et al: Phase I clinical evaluation of Gd-EOB-DTPA as a hepatobiliary MR contrast agent: safety, pharmacokinetics, and MR imaging, Radiology 195:785, 1995.
65. Hamm B, Thoeni RFL, Gould RG, et al: Focal liver lesions: characterization with nonenhanced and dynamic contrast material-enhanced MR imaging, Radiology 190:417, 1994.
66. Hayashi N, Yamamoto K, Tamaki N, et al: Metastatic nodules of hepatocellular carcinoma: detection with angiography, CT, and US, Radiology 165:61, 1987.
67. Honda N, Guo Q, Uchida H, et al: Percutaneous hot saline injection therapy for hepatic tumors: an alternative to percutaneous ethanol injection therapy, Radiology 190:53, 1994.

68. Intenzo C, Kim S, Madsen M, et al: Planar and SPECT Tc-99m red blood cell imaging in hepatic cavernous hemangiomas and other hepatic lesions, Clin Nucl Med 15:504, 1988.

69. Itai Y, Ebihara R, Tohno E, et al: Hepatic peribiliary cysts: multiple tiny cysts within the larger portal tract, hepatic hilum, or both, Radiology 191:107, 1994.

70. Itai Y, Murata S, and Kurosaki Y: Straight border sign of the liver: spectrum of CT appearances and causes, Radiographics 15:1089, 1995.

71. Itai Y, et al: Noninvasive diagnosis of small cavernous hemangioma of the liver: advantage of MRI, Am J Roentgenol 145:1195, 1985.

72. Itai Y, Ohtomo K, Furui S, et al: MR imaging of hepatocellular carcinoma, J Comput Assist Tomogr 10:963, 1986.

73. Itai Y, Ohtomo K, Kokubo T, et al: CT and MR imaging of fatty tumors of the liver, J Comput Assist Tomogr 11:253, 1987.

74. Itai Y, Ohtomo K, Kokubo T, et al: CT and MR imaging of postnecrotic liver scars, J Comput Assist Tomogr 12:971, 1988.

75. Itai Y, Ohtomo K, Kokubo T, et al: Segmental intensity differences in the liver on MR images: a sign of intrahepatic portal flow stoppage, Radiology 167:17, 1988.

76. Ito K, Choji T, Fujita F, et al: Early-enhancing pseudolesion in medial segment of left hepatic lobe detected with multisection dynamic MR, Radiology 187:695, 1993.

77. Ito K, Choji T, Nakada T, et al: Multislice dynamic MRI of hepatic tumors, J Comput Assist Tomogr 17:390, 1993.

78. Ito K, Honjo K, Fujita T, et al: Enhanced MR imaging of the liver after ethanol treatment of hepatocellular carcinoma: evaluation of areas of hyperperfusion adjacent to the tumor, Am J Roentgenol 164:1413, 1995.

79. Itoh K, Nishimura K, Togashi K, et al: Hepatocellular carcinoma: MR imaging, Radiology 164:21, 1987.

80. Itoh K, Saini S, Hahn PF, et al: Differentiation between small hepatic hemangiomas and metastases on MR images: importance of size-specific quantitative criteria, Am J Roentgenol 155:61, 1990.

81. Kadoya M, Matsui O, Kitagawa K, et al: Segmental iron deposition in the liver due to decreased intrahepatic portal perfusion: findings at MR imaging, Radiology 193:671, 1994.

82. Kalovidouris A, Voros D, Gouliamos A, et al: Extracapsular (satellite) hydatid cysts, Gastrointest Radiol 17:353, 1993.

83. Karhunen P: Benign hepatic tumours and tumour-like conditions in men, J Clin Pathol 39:183, 1986.

84. Kato Y, Nakata K, Omagari K, et al: Risk of hepatocellular carcinoma in patients with cirrhosis in Japan: analysis of infectious hepatitis viruses, Cancer 74:2234, 1994.

85. Kelekis N, Semelka R, and Woosley J: Malignant lesions of the liver with high signal intensity on T1-weighted MR images, J Magn Reson Imag 6:291, 1996.

86. Kenmochi K, Sugihara S, and Kojiro M: Relationship of histologic grade of hepatocellular carcinoma (HCC) to tumor size, and demonstration of tumor cells of multiple different grades in single small HCC, Liver 7:18, 1987.

87. Kerlin P, Davis GL, McGill DB, et al: Hepatic adenoma and focal nodular hyperplasia. clinical, pathologic and radiologic features, Gastroenterology 84:994, 1983.

88. Kessler A, Mitchell D, Israel H, et al: Hepatic and splenic sarcoidosis: US and MR imaging, Abdom Imaging 18:159, 1993.

89. Kim I, Mitchell D, Vinitski S, et al: MR imaging of hepatic iron overload in rat, J Magn Reson Imag 3:67, 1993.

90. Kitagawa K, Matsui O, Kadoya M, et al: Hepatocellular carcinomas with excessive copper accumulation: CT and MR findings, Radiology 180:623, 1991.

91. Kondo Y, Niwa Y, Akikusa B, et al: A histopathologic study of early hepatocellular carcinoma, Cancer 52:687, 1983.

92. Kraus BB, Ros PR, Abbitt PL, et al: Comparison of ultrasound, CT and MR imaging in the evaluation of candidates for TIPS, J Magn Reson Imag 5:571, 1995.

93. Kreft B, Tanimoto A, Baba Y, et al: Diagnosis of fatty liver with MR imaging, J Magn Reson Imag 2:463, 1992.

94. Kronthal AJ, Fishman EK, Kuhlman JE, et al: Hepatic infarction in preeclampsia, Radiology 177:726, 1990.

95. Kuo G, Choo QL, Alter HJ, et al: An assay for circulating antibodies to major etiologic virus of human non-A, non-B hepatitis, Science 244:362, 1989.

96. Kuo PC, Li K, Alfrey J, et al: Magnetic resonance imaging and hepatic hemodynamics: correlation with metabolic function in liver transplantation candidates, Surgery 117:373, 1995.

97. Lamminen A, Anttila V-J, Bondestam S, et al: Infectious liver foci in leukemia: comparison of short-inversion-time inversion recovery, T1-weighted spin-echo, and dynamic gadolinium enhanced MR imaging, Radiology 191:539, 1994.

98. Landy MJ, Setiawan H, Hirsch G, et al: Hepatic and thoracic amebiasis, Am J Roentgenol 135:449, 1980.

99. Lang P, Schnarkowski P, Grampp S, et al: Liver transplantation: significance of the periportal collar on MRI, J Comput Assist Tomogr 19:580, 1995.

100. Larson RE, Semelka RC, Bagley AS, et al: Hypervascular malignant liver lesions: comparison of various MR imaging pulse sequences and dynamic contrast enhanced CT, Radiology 192:393, 1994.

101. LaRusso NF, Wiesner RH, Ludwig J, et al: Medical intelligence: primary sclerosing cholangitis, N Engl J Med, 310:899, 1984.

102. Lee MJ, Saini S, Hamm B, et al: Focal nodular hyperplasia of the liver: MR findings in 35 proved cases, Am J Roentgenol 156:317, 1991.

103. Leeuwen MS, Noordzij J, Fernandez MA, t al: Portal venous and segmental anatomy of the right hemiliver: observations based on three-dimensional spiral CT renderings, Am J Roentgenol 163:1395, 1994.

104. Lehmann B, Fanucci E, Gigli F, et al: Signal suppression of normal liver tissue by phase corrected inversion recovery: a screening technique, J Comput Assist Tomogr 13:650, 1989.

105. Lencioni R, Bartolozzi C, Caramella D, et al: Management of adenomatous hyperplastic nodules in the cirrhotic liver: U.S. follow-up or percutaneous alcohol ablation? Abdom Imaging 18:50, 1994.

106. Levenson H, Greensite F, Hoefs J, et al: Fatty infiltration of the liver: quantification with phase-contrast MR imaging at 1.5T vs biopsy, Am J Roentgenol 156:307, 1991.

107. Lewis JH, Patel HR, and Zimmerman HJ: The spectrum of hepatic candidiasis, Hepatology 2:479, 1982.

108. Li KCP, Hopkins KL, Dalman RL, et al: Simultaneous measurement of flow in the superior mesenteric vein and artery with cine phase-contrast MR imaging: value in diagnosis of chronic mesenteric ischemia, Radiology 194:327, 1995.

109. Li W, Nissenbaum M, Stehling M, et al: Differentiation between hemangiomas and cysts of the liver with nonenhanced MR imaging: efficacy of T2 values at 1.5T, J Magn Reson Imag 3:800, 1993.

110. Livraghi T, Sangalli G, and Vettori C: Adenomatous hyperplastic nodules in the cirrhotic liver: a therapeutic approach, Radiology 170:155, 1989.

111. Lombardo DM, Baker ME, Spritzer CE, et al: Hepatic hemangiomas vs metastases: MR differentiation at 1.5T, Am J Roentgenol 155:55, 1990.

112. Lorigan JG, Charnsangavej C, Carrasco CH, et al: Atrophy with compensatory hypertrophy of the liver in hepatic neoplasms: radiologic findings, Am J Roentgenol 150:1291, 1988.

113. Low RN, Francis IR, Sigeti JS: Abdominal MR imaging using T2-weighted fast and conventional spin-echo, and contrast-enhanced fast multiplanar spoiled gradient-recalled imaging, Radiology 186:803, 1993.

114. Low RN, Sigeti JS, Francis IR, et al: Evaluation of malignant biliary obstruction: efficacy of fast multiplanar spoiled gradient-recalled MR imaging CT, and cholangiography, Am J Roentgenol 162:315, 1994.

115. Mahfouz A, Hamm B, Taupitz M, et al: Hypervascular liver lesions: differentiation of focal nodular hyperplasia from malignant tumors with dynamic gadolinium-enhanced MR imaging, Radiology 186:133, 1993.

116. Mahfouz A, Hamm B, Wolf KJ, et al: Peripheral washout: a sign of malignancy on dynamic gadolinium- enhanced MR imaging of focal liver lesions, Radiology 190:49, 1994.

117. Mahfouz AE, Hamm B, Wolf KJ, et al: Dynamic gadopentetate dimeglumine–enhanced MR imaging of hepatocellular carcinoma, Eur Radiol 3:453, 1993.

118. Maia deSouza JM, Portmann B, and Williams R: Nodular regenerative hyperplasia of the liver and the Budd-Chiari syndrome: case report: review of the literature and reappraisal of pathogenesis, J Hepatol 12:28, 1991.

119. Manas KJ, Welsh JD, Rankin RA, et al: Hepatic hemorrhage without rupture in preeclampsia, N Engl J Med 312:424, 1985.

120. Marincek B, Barbier PA, Becker CD, et al: CT appearance of impaired lymphatic drainage in liver transplants, Am J Roentgenol 147:519, 1986.

121. Marti-Bonmati L, Talens A, del Olmo J, et al: Chronic hepatitis and cirrhosis: evaluation by means of MR imaging with histologic correlation, Radiology 188:37, 1993.

122. Martin J, Sentis M, Zidan A, et al: Fatty metamorphosis of hepatocellular carcinoma: detection with chemical shift gradient-echo MR imaging, Radiology 195:125, 1995.

123. Masutani S, Sasaki Y, Imaoka S, et al: The prognostic significance of surgical margin in liver resection of patients with hepatocellular carcinoma, Arch Surg 129:1025, 1994.

124. Mathieu D, Rahmouni A, Anglade MC, et al: Focal nodular hyperplasia of the liver: assessment with contrast-enhanced turbo-FLASH MR imaging, Radiology 180:25, 1991.

125. Mathieu D, Rahmouni A, Vasile N, et al: Sclerosed liver hemangioma mimicking malignant tumor at MR imaging: pathologic correlation, J Magn Reson Imag 4:506, 1994.

126. Mathieu D, Vasile N, Menu Y, et al: Budd-Chiari syndrome: dynamic CT, Radiology 165:409, 1987.

127. Matsui O, Kadoya M, Kameyama T, et al: Adenomatous hyperplastic nodules in the cirrhotic liver: differentiation from hepatocellular carcinoma with MR imaging, Radiology 173:123, 1989.

128. Matsui O, Kadoya M, Kameyama T, et al: Benign and malignant nodules in cirrhotic livers: distinction based on blood supply, Radiology 178:493, 1991.

129. Matsui O, Kadoya M, and Takahashi S: Focal sparing of segment IV in fatty livers shown by sonography and CT: correlation with aberrant gastric venous drainage, Am J Roentgenol 164:1137, 1995.

130. Matsui O, Kadoya M, Takashima T, et al: Intrahepatic periportal abnormal intensity on MR images: an indication of various hepatobiliary diseases, Radiology 171:335, 1989.

131. Matsui O, Kadoya M, Yoshikawa J, et al: Aberrant gastric venous drainage in cirrhotic livers: imaging findings in focal areas of liver parenchyma, Radiology 197:345, 1995.

132. Mattison GR, Glazer GM, Quint LE, et al: MR imaging of hepatic focal nodular hyperplasia: characterization and distinction from primary malignant hepatic tumors, Am J Roentgenol 148:711, 1987.

133. McFarland E, Mayo-Smith W, Saini S, et al: Hepatic hemangiomas and malignant tumors: improved differentiation with heavily T2-weighted conventional spin-echo MR imaging, Radiology 193:43, 1994.

134. McLachlan SJ, Morris MR, Lucas MA, et al: Phase I clinical evaluation of a new iron oxide MR contrast agent, J Magn Reson Imag 4:301, 1994.

135. McLaren G, Muir W, and Kellermeyer R: Iron overload disorders: natural history, pathogenesis, diagnosis, and therapy, Crit Rev Clin Lab Sci 19:205, 1984.

136. Mendez RJ, Schiebler ML, Outwater EK, et al: Hepatic abscesses: MR imaging findings, Radiology 190:431, 1994.

137. Miller W, Federle M, Straub W, et al: Budd-Chiari syndrome: imaging with pathologic correlation, Abdom Imaging 18:329, 1993.

138. Miller WJ, Baron RL, Dodd GD, et al: Malignancies in patients with cirrhosis: CT sensitivity and specificity in 200 consecutive transplant patients, Radiology 193:645, 1994.

139. Mirowitz SA, Lee JKT, Gutierrez E, et al: Dynamic gadolinium-enhanced rapid acquisition spin-echo MR imaging of the liver, Radiology 179:371, 1991.

140. Mitchell DG: Focal manifestations of diffuse liver disease at MR imaging, Radiology 185:1, 1992.

141. Mitchell DG, Crovello M, Matteucci T, et al: Benign adrenocortical masses: diagnosis with chemical shift MR imaging, Radiology 185:345, 1992.

142. Mitchell DG, Kim I, Chang TS, et al: Fatty liver: chemical shift saturation and phase-difference MR imaging techniques in animals, phantoms and humans, Invest Radiol 26:1041, 1991.

143. Mitchell DG, Lovett KE, Hann HWL, et al: Cirrhosis: multi-observer analysis of hepatic MRI findings in a heterogeneous population, J Magn Reson Imaging 3:313, 1993.

144. Mitchell DG, Outwater EK, and Vinitsky S: Hybrid RARE: implementations for abdominal MRI, J Magn Reson Imaging 4:109, 1994.

145. Mitchell DG, Palazzo J, Hann H-WYL, et al: Hepatocellular tumors with high signal on T1 weighted MR images: chemical shift MRI and histologic correlation, J Comput Assist Tomogr 15:762, 1991.

146. Mitchell DG, Plazzo J, Hann HYL, et al: Mass-like hepatic hypertrophy: MRI findings with histologic correlation, Magn Reson Imaging 10:541, 1992.

147. Mitchell DG, Rubin R, Siegelman E, et al: Hepatocellular carcinoma within siderotic regenerative nodules: the "nodule-within-nodule" sign on MR images, Radiology 178:101, 1991.

148. Mitchell DG, Sanjay SS, Weinreb J, et al: Hepatic metastases and cavernous hemangiomas: distinction by standard and triple dose gadoteridol-enhanced MRI, Radiology 193:49, 1994.

149. Mitchell DG, Vinitski S, Saponaro S, et al: The liver and pancreas: improved spin-echo T1 contrast by shorter TE and fat suppression at 1.5 Tesla, Radiology 178:67, 1991.

150. Mitsuodo K, Watanabe Y, Saga T, et al: Nonenhanced hepatic cavernous hemangioma with multiple calcifications: CT and pathologic correlation, Abdom Imag 20:459, 1995.

151. Monzawa S, Ohtomo K, Oba H, et al: Septa in the liver of patients with chronic hepatic schistosomiasis japonica: MR appearance, Am J Roentgenol 162:1347, 1994.

152. Moritz MJ, Jarrell BE, Armenti V, et al: Heterotopic liver transplantation for fulminant hepatic failure—a bridge to recovery, Transplantation 50:524, 1990.

153. Mungovan J, Cronan J, and Vacarro J: Hepatic cavernous hemangiomas: lack of enlargement over time, Radiology 191:111, 1994.

154. Murakami T, Nakamura H, Tsuda K, et al: Contrast-enhanced MR imaging of intrahepatic cholangiocarcinoma: pathologic correlation study, J Magn Reson Imaging 5:165, 1995.

155. Murakami T, Nakamura H, Tsuda K, et al: Treatment of hepatocellular carcinoma by chemoembolization: evaluation with 3DFT MR imaging, Am J Roentgenol 160:295, 1993.

156. Muramatsu Y, Nawano S, Takayasu K, et al: Early hepatocellular carcinoma: MR imaging, Radiology 181:209, 1991.

157. Murata S, Itai Y, Hisashi K, et al: Effect of temporary occlusion of the hepatic vein on dual blood supply in the liver: evaluation with spiral CT, Radiology 197:351, 1995.

158. Naber AHJ, Van Haelst U, and Yap SH: Nodular regenerative hyperplasia of the liver: an important cause of portal hypertension in non-cirrhotic patients, Hepatology 12:94, 1991.

159. Nakanuma Y, Ohta G, Sugiura H, et al: Incidental solitary hepatocellular carcinomas smaller than 1 cm in size found at autopsy: a morphologic study, Hepatology 6:631, 1986.

160. Nakao N, Miura K, Takahashi H, et al: Hepatic perfusion in cavernous transformation of the portal vein: evaluation by using CT angiography, Am J Roentgenol 152:985, 1989.

161. Ng IOL, Ng MMT, Lai ECS, et al: Better survival in female patients with hepatocellular carcinoma: possible causes from a pathologic approach, Cancer 75:18, 1995.

162. Nghiem HV, Winter TC, III, Mountford MC, et al: Evaluation of the portal venous system before liver transplantation: value of phase-contrast MR angiography, Am J Roentgenol 164:871, 1995.

163. Ohishi H, Uchida H, Yoshimura H, et al: Hepatocellular carcinoma detected by iodized oil, Radiology 154:25, 1985.

164. Ohtomo D, Itai Y, Yoshida H, et al: MR differentiation of hepatocellular carcinoma from cavernous hemangioma: complementary roles of FLASH and T2 values, Am J Roentgenol 152:505, 1989.

165. Ohtomo K, Baron R, Dodd G, et al: Confluent hepatic fibrosis in advanced cirrhosis: evaluation with MR imaging, Radiology 189:871, 1993.

166. Ohtomo K, Itai Y, Ohtomo Y, et al: Regenerating nodules of liver cirrhosis: MR imaging with pathologic correlation, Am J Roentgenol 154:505, 1990.

167. Ohtomo K, Itai Y, Yoshikawa K, et al: MR imaging of hepatoma treated by embolization, J Comput Assist Tomogr 10:973, 1986.

168. Oka H, Kurioka N, Kim K, et al: Prospective study of early detection of hepatocellular carcinoma in patients with cirrhosis, Hepatology 12:680, 1990.

169. Oliver JH, III, Baron RL, Dodd GD, et al: Does advanced cirrhosis with portosystemic shunting affect the value of CT arterial portography in the evaluation of the liver? Am J Roentgenol 164:333, 1995.

170. Orons PD, Sheng R, and Zajko AB: Hepatic artery stenosis in liver transplant recipients: prevalence and cholangiographic appearance of associated biliary complications, Am J Roentgenol 165:1145, 1995.

171. Outwater EK: MR cholangiography with a fast spin-echo sequence, J Magn Reson Imaging 3:131, 1993.

172. Outwater EK, Tomaszewski JE, Daly JM, et al: Hepatic colorectal metastases: correlation of MR imaging and pathologic findings, Radiology 180:327, 1991.

173. Patrizio G, Pavone P, Testa A, et al: MR characterization of hepatic lesions by t-null inversion recovery sequence, J Comput Assist Tomogr 14:96, 1990.

174. Paulson E, Baker M, Spritzer C, et al: Focal fatty infiltration: a cause of nontumorous defects in the left hepatic lobe during CT arterial portography, J Comput Assist Tomogr 17:590, 1993.

175. Paulson EK, McClellan JS, Washington K, et al: Hepatic adenoma: MR characteristics and correlation with pathologic findings, Am J Roentgenol 163:113, 1994.

176. Phillips JJ, Chang SL, Vargus HI, et al: MR and CT imaging of ethanol treated liver tumors in an animal model, Magn Reson Imaging 9:201, 1991.

177. Pollard JJ, and Nebesar RA: Altered hemodynamics in the Budd-Chiari syndrome demonstrated by selective hepatic and selective splenic angiography, Radiology 89:236, 1967.

178. Popper H: Pathologic aspects of cirrhosis: a review, Am J Pathol 87:228, 1977.

179. Rahn NH III, Koehler RE, Weyman PJ, et al: CT appearance of sclerosing cholangitis, Am J Roentgenol 141:549, 1983.

180. Ralls PW, Henley DS, Colletti PR, et al: Amebic liver abscess: MR imaging, Radiology 165:801, 1987.

181. Rapaccini GL, Ponpili M, Caturelli E, et al: Focal ultrasound lesions in liver cirrhosis diagnosed as regenerating nodules by fine-needle biopsy: follow-up of 12 cases, Dig Dis Sci 35:422, 1990.

182. Richards MA, Webb JAW, Reznek RH, et al: Detection of spread of malignant lymphoma to the liver by low field strength magnetic resonance imaging, Br Med J 293:1126, 1996.

183. Ros PR, Lubbers PR, Olmsted WW, et al: Hemangioma of the liver: heterogeneous appearance on T2 weighted images, Am J Roentgenol 149:1167, 1987.

184. Ros PR, Murphy BJ, Buck JE, et al: Encapsulated hepatocellular carcinoma: radiologis findings and pathologic correlation, Gastrointest Radiol 15:233, 1990.

185. Rosenthal RE, and Davis PL: MR imaging of hepatocellular carcinoma at 1.5T, Gastrointest Radiol 17:49, 1992.

186. Rummeny E, Weissleder R, Sironi S, et al: Central scars in primary liver tumors: MR features, specificity, and pathologic correlation, Radiology 171:323, 1989.

187. Rummeny EJ, Weissleder R, Stark DD, et al: Primary liver tumors: diagnosis by MR imaging, Am J Roentgenol 152:63, 1989.

188. Sadek AG, Mitchell DG, Siegelman ES, et al: Early hepatocellular carcinoma that develops within macroregenerative nodules: growth rate depicted at serial MR imaging, Radiology 195:753, 1995.

189. Saini S, Edelman RR, Sharma P, et al: Blood-pool MR contrast material for detection and characterization of focal hepatic lesions: initial clinical experience with ultrasmall superparamagnetic iron oxide (AMI- 227), Am J Roentgenol 164:1147, 1995.

190. Schertz L, Lee J, Heiken J, et al: Proton spectroscopic imaging (Dixon method) of the liver: clinical utility, Radiology 173:401, 1989.

191. Schiebler ML, Kressel HY, Saul SH, et al: MR imaging of focal nodular hyperplasia of the liver, J Comput Assist Tomogr 11:651, 1987.

192. Schlund JF, Semelka RC, Kettritz U, et al: Transient increased segmental hepatic enhancement distal to portal vein obstruction on dynamic gadolinium-enhanced gradient echo MR images, J Magn Reson Imaging 4:375, 1995.

193. Schulte S, Baron R, Teffey S, et al: CT of the extrahepatic bile ducts: wall thickness and contrast enhancement in normal and abnormal ducts, Am J Roentgenol 154:79, 1990.

194. Schwartz SI: Primary sclerosing cholangitis: a disease revisited, Surg Clin North Am 53:1161, 1973.

195. Semelka RC, Bagley AS, Brown ED, et al: Malignant lesions of the liver identified on T1- but not T2-weighted MR images at 1.5T, J Magn Reson Imaging 4:315, 1994.

196. Semelka RC, Brown ED, Ascher SM, et al: Hepatic hemangiomas: a multi-institutional study of appearance on T2- weighted and serial gadolinium-enhanced gradient echo MR images, Radiology 192:401, 1994.

197. Semelka RC, Chew W, Hricak H, et al: Fat-saturation MR imaging of the upper abdomen, Am J Roentgenol 155:1111, 1990.

198. Semelka RC, Shoenut JP, Ascher SM, et al: Solitary hepatic metastasis: comparison of dynamic contrast-enhanced CT and MR imaging with fat-suppressed T2-weighted, breath-hold T1-weighted FLASH, and dynamic gadolinium-enhanced FLASH sequences, J Magn Reson Imaging 4:319, 1994.

199. Semelka RC, Shoenut PM, Greenberg HM, et al: Detection of acute and treated lesions of hepatosplenic candidiasis: comparison of dynamic contrast enhanced CT and MR imaging, J Magn Reson Imaging 2:341, 1992.

200. Semelka RC, Simm FC, Recht M, et al: T1-weighted sequences of the liver: comparison of three techniques for single breath whole volume acquisition at 1.0T and 1.5T, Radiology 180:629, 1991.

201. Senéterre E, Vergnes C, Taorel P, et al: CT arterial portography (CTAP) versus superparamagnetic iron oxide enhanced MR imaging for screening of hepatic metastases, Nice, France, 1995, Society of Magnetic Resonance, Third Scientific Meeting and Exhibition.

202. Shea J, W.J., Demas BE, et al: Sclerosing cholangitis associated with hepatic arterial FUDR chemotherapy: radiographic-histologic correlation, Am J Roentgenol 146:717, 1986.

203. Shiina S, Tagawa L. Niwa Y, et al: Percutaneous ethanol injection therapy for hepatocellular carcinoma: results in 146 patients, Am J Roentgenol 160:1023, 1993.

204. Shirkhoda A, Lopez-Beresstein G, Holbert JM, et al: Hepatosplenic fungal infection: CT and pathologic evaluation after treatment with liposomal amphotericin B, Radiology 159:349, 1986.

205. Siegelman E, Outwater E, Hanau CA, et al: Abdominal iron distribution in sickle cell disease: MR findings in transfusion and non-transfusion dependent patients, J Comput Assist Tomogr 18:63, 1994.

206. Siegelman ES, Mitchell DG, Outwater E, et al: Idiopathic hemochromatosis: spectrum of MR findings in cirrhotic and precirrhotic patients, Radiology 188:637, 1993.

207. Siegelman ES, Mitchell DG, Rubin R, et al: Parenchymal versus reticuloendothelial iron overload in the liver: distinction with MR imaging, Radiology 179:361, 1991.

208. Siegelman ES, Outwater EK, Schnall MD, et al: MRI of hepatic nodular regenerative hyperplasia, J Magn Reson Imaging 5:730, 1995.

209. Sironi S, Livraghi T, and DelMaschio A: Small hepatocellular carcinoma treated with percutaneous ethanol injection: MR imaging findings, Radiology 180:333, 1991.

210. Sonoda T, Shirabe K, Takenaka K, et al: Angiographically undetected hepatocellular carcinoma: clinicopathologic characteristics, follow-up and treatment, Hepatology 10:1003, 1989.

211. Soreide O, Czerniak A, Bradpiece H, et al: Characteristics of fibrolamellar hepatocellular carcinoma, Am J Surg 151:518, 1986.

212. Soyer P, Bluemke DA, and Fishman EK: CT during arterial portography for the preoperative evaluation of hepatic tumors: how, when, and why? Am J Roentgenol 163:1325, 1994.

213. Soyer P, Bluemke DA, Sibert A, et al: MR imaging of intrahepatic cholangiocarcinoma, Abdom Imaging 20:126, 1995.

214. Soyer P, Lacheheb D, Caudrom C, et al: MRI of adenomatous hyperplastic nodules of the liver in Budd-Chiari syndrome, J Comput Assist Tomogr 17:86, 1992.

215. Soyer P, Laissy JP, Bluemke DA, et al: Bile duct involvement in hepatocellular carcinoma: MR demonstration., Abdom Imaging 20:118,1995.

216. Soyer P, Laissy JP, Sibert A, et al: Hepatic metastases: detection with multisection FLASH MR imaging during gadolinium chelate-enhanced arterial portography, Radiology 189:401, 1993.

217. Soyer P, Laissy JP, Sibert A, et al: Focal hepatic masses: comparison of detection during arterial portography with MR imaging and CT, Radiology 190:737, 1994.

218. Spreafico C, Marchiamo A, Regalia E, et al: Chemoembolization of hepatocellular carcinoma in patients who undergo liver transplantation, Radiology 192:687, 1994.

219. Stark DD, Felder R, Wittenberg J, et al: Magnetic resonance imaging of cavernous hemangioma of the liver: tissue specific characterization, Am J Roentgenol 145:213, 1985.

220. Stark DD, Goldberg HI, Moss AA, et al: Chronic liver disease: evaluation by magnetic resonance, Radiology 150:149, 1984.

221. Stark DD, Wittenberg J, Edelman RR, et al: Detection of hepatic metastases: analysis of pulse sequence performance in MR imaging, Radiology 159:365, 1986.

222. Starzl T, Halgrimson C, Francavilla F, et al: The origin, hormonal nature and action of hepatotropic substances in portal venous blood, Surg Gynecol Obstet 137:179, 1973.

223. Stevens WR, Johnson CD, Stephens DH, et al: Fibrolamellar hepatocellular carcinoma: stage at presentation and results of aggressive surgical management, Am J Roentgenol 164:1153, 1995.

224. Sumida M, Ohio M, Ebara M, et al: Accuracy of angiography in the diagnosis of small hepatocellular carcinoma, Am J Roentgenol 147:531, 1986.

225. Takayasu K, Furukawa H, Wakao F, et al: CT diagnosis of early hepatocellular carcinoma: sensitivity, findings, and CT-pathologic correlation, Am J Roentgenol 164:885, 1995.

226. Takayasu K, Makuuchi M, and Takayama T: Computed tomography of a rapidly growing hepatic hemangioma, J Comput Assist Tomogr 14:143, 1990.

227. Takayasu K, Moriyama N, Muramatsu Y, et al: The diagnosis of small hepatocellular carcinomas: efficiency of various imaging procedures in 100 patients, Am J Roentgenol 155:49, 1990.

228. Takayasu K, Moriyama N, Shima Y, et al: Atypical radiographic findings in hepatic cavernous hemangioma: correlation with histologic features, Am J Roentgenol 146:1149, 1986.

229. Takayasu K, Muramatsu Y, Furukawa H, et al: Early hepatocellular carcinoma: appearance at CT during arterial portography and CT arteriography with pathologic correlation, Radiology 194:101, 1995.

230. Takayasu K, Shima Y, Muramatsu Y, et al: Hepatocellular carcinoma: treatment with intraarterial iodized oil with and without chemotherapeutic agents, Radiology 162:345, 1987.

231. Tasciyan TA, Mitchell DG, and Spritzer CE: Color flow-encoded MR imaging, J Magn Reson Imaging 1:715, 1991.

232. Taupitz M, Hamm B, Speidel A, et al: Multisection FLASH: method for breath-hold MR imaging of the entire liver, Radiology 183:73, 1992.

233. Teefey S, Baron R, Rohrmann C, et al: Sclerosing cholangitis: CT findings, Radiology 169:635, 1988.

234. Terada T, Kadoya M, Nakanuma Y, et al: Iron-accumulating adenomatous hyperplastic nodule with malignant foci in the cirrhotic liver, Cancer 65:1994, 1990.

235. Terada T, and Nakanuma Y: Iron-negative foci in sideroic macroregenerative nodules in human cirrhotic liver, Arch Pathol Lab Med 113:916, 1989.

236. Terada T, and Nakanuma Y: Survey of iron-accumulative macroregenerative nodules in cirrhotic livers, Hepatology 10:851, 1989.

237. Terada T, Nakanuma Y, Hoso M, et al: Fatty macroregerative nodule in non-steatotic liver cirrhosis: a morphologic study, Arch Pathol Anat 415:131, 1989.

238. Terayama N, Matsui O, Hoshiba K, et al: Peribiliary cysts in liver cirrhosis: US, CT, and MR findings, J Comput Assist Tomogr 19:419, 1995.

239. Terpstra OT, Metselaar HJ, Hesselink EJ, et al: Auxiliary partial liver transplantation for acute and chronic liver disease, Transplant Proc 22:1564, 1990.

240. Thomas JL, Bernardino ME, Vermess M, et al: EOE-13 in the detection of hepatosplenic lymphoma, Radiology 145:629, 1982.

241. Thomsen C, Wiggers P, Larsen H, et al: Identification of patients with hereditary hemochromatosis by magnetic resonance imaging and spectroscopic relaxation time measurements, Magn Reson Imag 10:867, 1992.

242. Titelbaum DS, Hatabu H, Schiebler ML, et al: Fibrolamellar hepatocellular carcinoma: MR appearance, J Comput Assist Tomogr 12:588, 1988.

243. Trauner M, Stepan KM, Resch M, et al: Diagnostic problems in nodular regenerative hyperplasia (nodular transformation) of the liver, J Gastroenterol 30:187, 1992.

244. Tung G, Vaccaro J, Cronan J, et al: Cavernous hemangioma of the liver: pathologic correlation with high field MR imaging, Am J Roentgenol 162:1113, 1994.

245. Unger EC, Lee JKT, and Weyman PJ: CT and MR imaging of radiation hepatitis, J Comput Assist Tomogr 11:264, 1987.

246. Vecchio F: Fibrolamellar carcinoma of the liver: a distinct entity within the hepatocellular tumors, Appl Pathol 6:139, 1988.

247. Vilgrain V, Flejou JF, Arrive L, et al: Focal nodular hyperplasia of the liver: MR imaging and pathological correlation in 37 patients, Radiology 184:699, 1992.

248. Vlachos L, Trakadas S, Gouliamos A, et al: Comparative study between ultrasound, computed tomography, intra-arterial digital subtraction angiography, and magnetic resonance imaging in the differentiation of tumors of the liver, Gastrointest.Radiol 15:102, 1990.

249. Wada K, Kondo F, and Kondo Y: Large regenerative nodules and dysplastic nodules in cirrhotic livers, Hepatology 8:1684, 1988.

250. Wanless IR: Micronodular transformation (nodular regenerative hyperplasia) of the liver: a report of 64 cases among 2500 autopsies and a new classification of benign hepatocellular nodules, Hepatology 11:787, 1990.

251. Wanless IR, Allen F, and Feder A: Nodular regenerative hyperplasia of the liver in hematologic disorders: a possible response for obliterative disorders, Medicine 59:367, 1980.

252. Wanless IR, Wong F, Blendis LM, et al: Hepatic and portal vein thrombosis in cirrhosis: possible role in development of parenchymal extinction and portal hypertension, Hepatology 21:1238, 1995.

253. Warshauer D, Semelka R, and Ascher S: Nodular sarcoidosis of the liver and spleen: appearance on MR images, J Magn Reson Imaging 4:553, 1994.

254. Wehrli F, Perkins T, Shimakawa A, et al: Chemical shift-induced amplitude modulations in images obtained with gradient refocusing, Magn Reson Imag 5:157, 1987.

255. Weinreb JC, Brateman L, and Maravilla KR: Magnetic resonance imaging of hepatic lymphoma, Am J Roentgenol 143:1211, 1984.

256. Weissleder R, Stark DD, Compton CC, et al: Ferrite-enhanced MR imaging of hepatic lymphoma: an experimental study in rats, Am J Roentgenol 149:1161, 1987.

257. Weissleder R, Stark DD, Elizondo G, et al: MRI of hepatic lymphoma, Magn Reson Imaging 6:675, 1988.

258. Whitney WS, Herfkens RJ, Jeffrey RB, et al: Dynamic breath-hold multiplanar spoiled gradient-recalled MR imaging with gadolinium enhancement for differentiating hepatic hemangiomas from malignancies at 1.5T, Radiology 190:417, 1993.

259. Wiesner RH, and LaRusso NF: Clinicopathologic features of the syndrome of primary sclerosing cholangitis, Gastroenterology 79:200, 1980.

260. Wilbur AC, and Gyi B: Hepatocellular carcinoma: MR appearance mimicking focal nodular hyperplasia, Am J Roentgenol 149:721, 1987.

261. Wittenberg J, Stark D, Forman B, et al: Differentiation of hepatic metastases from hepatic hemangiomas and cysts by using MR imaging, Am J Roentgenol 151:79, 1988.

262. Wozney P, Zajko AB, Bron KM, et al: Vascular complications after liver transplantation: a 5-year experience, Am J Roentgenol 147:657, 1986.

263. Yamamoto H, Yamashita Y, Yoshimatsu S, et al: Hepatocellular carcinoma in cirrhotic livers: detection with unenhanced and iron oxide-enhanced MR imaging, Radiology 195:106, 1995.

264. Yankelevitz D, Henschke CI, Chu F, et al: Serial MR imaging evaluation of effects of radiation therapy on bone marrow and liver, Radiology 177:274, 1989.

265. Yates C, and Streight R: Focal fatty infiltration of the liver simulating metastatic disease, Radiology 159:83, 1986.

266. Yoshikawa J, Matsui O, Takashima T, et al: Fatty metamorphosis in hepatocellular carcinoma: radiologic features in 10 cases, Am J Roentgenol 151:717, 1988.

267. Yoshimatsu S, Inouse Y, Ibukuro K, et al: Hypovascular hepatocellular carcinoma undetected at angiography and CT with iodized oil, Radiology 171:343, 1989.

268. Young ST, Paulson EK, Washington D, et al: CT of the liver in patients with metastatic breast carcinoma treated by chemotherapy: findings simulating cirrhosis, Am J Roentgenol 163:1385, 1994.

269. Yumoto Y, Jinno K, Tokuyama K, et al: Hepatocellular carcinoma detected by iodized oil, Radiology 154:19, 1985.

270. Zajko AB, Bennett MJ, Campbell WL, et al: Mucocele of the cystic duct remnant in eight liver transplant recipients: findings at cholangiography, CT and US, Radiology 177:691, 1990.

271. Zonderland HM, Lameris JS, Terpstra OT, et al: Auxiliary partial liver transplantation: imaging evaluation in 10 patients, Am J Roentgenol 153:981, 1989.

272. Zornoza J, and Ginaldi S: Computed tomography in hepatic lymphoma, Radiology 138:405, 1981.

23 Biliary System, Pancreas, Spleen, and Alimentary Tract

Peter F. Hahn

✓ KEY POINTS

- MRC agrees with endoscopic cholangiography in 90% of cases.
- MRCP is noninvasive, eliminating risk of aspiration, perforation, pancreatitis, bleeding, sepsis, and pain associated with ERCP.
- MRCP can be performed with a variety of T2-weighted techniques reconstructed using angiographic MIP algorithms.
- CT remains the procedure of choice for diagnosis and staging of nonhepatic intraabdominal infections and tumors.
- Iron-oxide enhanced MRI of the spleen can improve detection of lymphoma and metastases.

The biliary system, spleen, pancreas, and alimentary tract are familiar from liver imaging studies, but targeted magnetic resonance (MR) techniques provide new information about them. Specialized pulse sequences, three-dimensional (3D) image processing, and new contrast agents have helped to establish MR as a primary imaging tool for these organs.

Important technical advances have introduced new applications for pancreaticobiliary magnetic resonance imaging (MRI). These advances include new pulse sequences and a better understanding of the use of contrast agents. During its first decade, MRI reliably depicted only the overall pancreatic contour and detected only gross disturbance of pancreatic and biliary morphology. Experience with the MR appearance of the pancreas and biliary structures came largely from their inclusion on hepatic MR images, and the goal seemed to be imitation of the cross-sectional anatomy seen on x-ray computed tomography (CT). Introduction of fast gradient-echo and echo-planar imaging (EPI), development of the fast (turbo) spin echo (FSE), more widespread use of enhancement with gadolinium (Gd) chelates, and development of MR cholangiopancreatography (MRCP) and visceral MR angiography

(MRA) have permitted MRI to play an increasingly important clinical role in evaluating patients with known or suspected pancreatic or biliary disease. Techniques developed for MRI, such as contrast enhanced–dual phase pancreatic imaging and 3D workstation reconstructions of planar images have been exported back to CT for use on helical scanners.

MRI of the spleen and alimentary tract also has been advanced by some of the newer techniques. Motion-artifact suppression and better appreciation of the role of contrast agents have improved the diagnostic information available from MRI. Equally important, acceptance of MRI as a first-line abdominal diagnostic modality has produced imaging of a widening range of pathology related to the spleen and to the bowel, and dissemination of this experience has contributed new understanding about the MR imaging of these organs.

BILIARY SYSTEM
MR Cholangiopancreatography

MR cholangiography (MRC) and MRCP comprise a body of MR imaging techniques only recently reaching a level of clinical utility. MRC and MRCP refer to the generation of projectional MR images of the biliary tree and pancreatic ducts achieved in such a way as to mimic projectional radiographs obtained by contrast injection during percutaneous transhepatic cholangiography (THC) or endoscopic retrograde cholangiopancreatography (ERCP). By noninvasively providing a set of projectional images of the pancreaticobiliary tree, MRCP has the potential to limit the use of THC and ERCP to only those cases in which the diagnostic component of these invasive procedures is preliminary to percutaneous or endoscopic therapeutic intervention. MRCP has gained rapid acceptance by endoscopists and surgeons because of the familiar projectional image format. MRCP is less useful if performed after endoscopic or percutaneous procedures because air, clot, spasm of the ampullary sphincter of Oddi, or stents may artifactually influence the ductal appearance.

The fundamental concept of MRCP is straightforward. Bile and pancreatic duct fluid are static and have long T2 times. Therefore high-resolution, heavily T2-weighted images display these important structures as areas of high signal intensity against solid parenchymal organs and flowing blood with a shorter T2 or rapid dephasing. Three-dimensional (3D) reconstruction algorithms familiar from MRA can then be applied to produce images of the entire biliary tree or pancreatic duct.

Several different techniques have been investigated for MRCP. These techniques include both gradient-echo steady state free precession (SSFP)[53,62,91,150] and FSE pulse sequences* for acquiring raw data. Echo-planar methods also are being developed.[21] With various tech-

*References 11, 43, 44, 108, 123, 135, 141.

niques, data may be acquired during either suspended respiration or free breathing, on two-dimensional (2D) (slice) or 3D (slab) matrices, and with either body coils or local multicoils. Moreover, ray-tracing, shaded-surface display, and maximum-intensity projection (MIP) algorithms have been used for reconstructions. However, all of the available methods have several important common attributes. They use heavy T2 weighting to distinguish the fluid contents of the pancreaticobiliary tree from adjacent solid structures, they are noninvasive, and they acquire images of the biliary and pancreatic structures in their native configuration, without the pressure distension associated with injection of contrast agents.[99,79] Agreement in more than 90% of cases between MRC and contrast cholangiography has been reported.[11] The development of MRCP incorporates into MRI a large body of knowledge developed from interpretation of transhepatic cholangiograms and ERCPs.[103]

Anatomy of the Biliary Tree

The common hepatic duct is formed by the confluence of right and left bile ducts in the porta hepatis (Figure 23-1). The right and left ducts, visualized in more than 90% of MRCs, are themselves formed from segmental ducts that comprise, with portal vein and hepatic artery branches, the portal triad. Segmental ducts are demonstrated in at least 80% of MRCs.[75] The cystic duct, identified by the characteristic spiral valves of Heister, arises from the neck of the gallbladder and joins the common hepatic duct to form the common bile duct. The common hepatic duct and common bile duct are sometimes collectively called the *common duct.* The common bile duct passes through the pancreatic head and empties into the duodenum at the ampulla of Vater. The normal common hepatic duct measures less than 7 mm in diameter in the porta hepatis, and the normal common bile duct diameter is up to 10 mm in diameter.[137] There is considerable variation in intrahepatic ductal anatomy. Tiny ducts of Luschka from the right lobe rarely may drain directly into the gallbladder, a variant that would not be reliably demonstrated on MRCs with currently available spatial resolution. Bile ducts surgically decompressed via hepaticojejunostomy empty into the jejunum through an anastomosis with the common hepatic duct or sometimes through separate anastomoses of the right and left hepatic ducts.

Biliary Dilatation

Dilatation of the bile ducts occurs most frequently as the result of obstruction. Obstruction to biliary outflow can occur at any level, in-

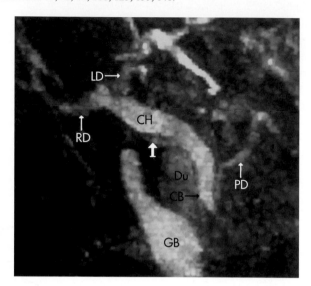

FIGURE 23-1   Single breath-hold echo-planar MRCP showing mild pancreaticobiliary dilatation from ampullary stenosis. Confluence of the right *(RD)* and left *(LD)* intrahepatic bile ducts form the common hepatic duct *(CH)*. Confluence of the common hepatic duct and cystic duct *(stemmed arrow)* from the gallbladder *(GB)* form the common bile duct *(CB)*. Common bile duct and pancreatic duct *(PD)* empty through the ampulla of Vater into the duodenum *(Du)*. Coronal source images were projected along a ray oriented obliquely 30 degrees from anteroposteriorly to avoid overlap of anatomical structures.

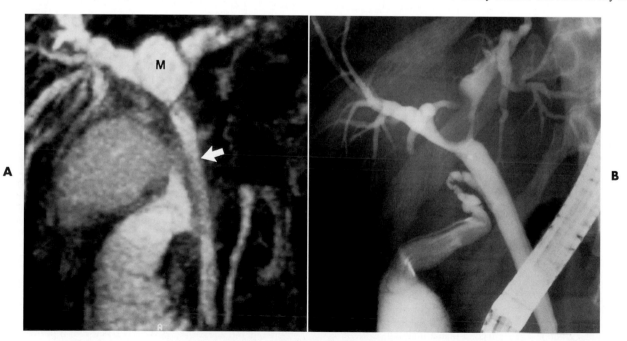

FIGURE 23-2   Biliary cystadenocarcinoma. **A,** MRCP using FSE 3D slab technique shows a normal common duct *(arrow)*. Intrahepatic ducts are obstructed at their confluence by a cystic mass *(M)*. **B,** ERCP shows mass effect and stricture caused by a malignant tumor, but the tumor itself is unopacified. (From reference 11.)

cluding in the bowel. Obstruction of the common duct produces proximal dilatation, which is reliably demonstrated on MRC. Multifocal intrahepatic ductal obstruction, as may occur along with multifocal strictures in inflammatory diseases (such as sclerosing cholangitis), and attenuation of the intrahepatic ducts associated with cirrhosis are conditions more difficult to identify with current technology.

Obstruction at the portal confluence often is secondary to a tumor (Klatskin's tumor) arising in the bile ducts. Cholangiocarcinoma is the most frequent type, but other histologies can produce the same appearance. The stricture is usually short and abrupt, and there may be an overhanging edge visible at the proximal margin. Distally the duct is of normal caliber. If the stricture involves the confluence itself, the right and left ducts are obstructed separately (Figure 23-2). Metastases in the porta can produce an obstruction similar in cholangiographic appearance to Klatskin's tumor (Figure 23-3), but there is often more mass effect, and on high-resolution cholangiograms the strictured duct is usually smoother. MRC is equivalent to ERCP in determining the level of ductal obstruction and in distinguishing benign strictures from malignant ones.[70]

Obstruction of bile ducts distal to the porta may be secondary to intrinsic tumor, but other causes of obstruction are more common. These causes include iatrogenic strictures of the mid-common duct, common bile duct obstruction caused by pancreatic carcinoma, and obstruction at the ampulla of Vater caused by stones, tumors, or inflammatory strictures. Sclerosing cholangitis and cholangitis in AIDS patients produce multifocal strictures alternating with dilatation. Rarely, processes arising in the gallbladder may obstruct the bile ducts; obstruction caused by inflammation associated with a gallstone impacted in the neck of the gallbladder is called *Mirizzi's syndrome.* Benign strictures tend to be longer, smoother, and more gradual than malignant ones. For evaluation of a distal stricture, MRCP should be combined with an axial imaging evaluation of the pancreas (see later discussion).

Choledochal cysts comprise a group of developmental abnormalities resulting in focal dilatation of the biliary tree. Todani's modification of Alonso-Lej's classification[145] is used to describe individual cases (Box 23-1). MRC readily demonstrates the relationship of the common duct to these lesions (Figure 23-4), which are often resected because of the risk of malignancy. Conventional T2-weighted axial images show the multiple foci of saccular intrahepatic ductal dilatation in Caroli's disease (Figure 23-5). This entity should be distinguished from peribiliary cysts sometimes arrayed in strings along the portal structures in advanced liver disease.[13]

Biliary Filling Defects

Filling defects in the biliary tree include stones, sludge, clots, and parasites. Stones appear on MRC as filling defects that may be round or faceted. Biliary calculi are more readily identified in dilated ducts (Figure 23-6). Reliable demonstration of common duct stones 6 mm or larger has been reported, but stones smaller than 4 mm are rarely identified with MRC.[43,44] Thin-section source images more sensitively detect stones than MIP or thick-section slab images.[160] Clots may form a cast of the entire biliary tree. T1 shortening makes hemobilia evident on conventional MR images as T1 hyperintensity, but clots may not be apparent on MRC unless there is concomitant T2 shortening. MRC findings in parasitic infestation have not been reported. Large worms of ascariasis likely would be identified, whereas tiny liver flukes would not.

MR Cholangiography Versus Direct X-Ray Cholangiography

Direct x-ray cholangiography is an invasive procedure requiring either percutaneous transhepatic or endoscopic access to the biliary tree. Because MRC is noninvasive, complications of THC (pain, hemorrhage, hemobilia, pneumothorax, and sepsis) and ERCP (aspiration, perforation, pancreatitis, and sepsis) do not occur with MRC. Conversely, MRC does not offer the options for therapeutic intervention, including biliary decompression and stone extraction, that can be performed once percutaneous or endoscopic access has been achieved.

BOX 23-1
Choledochal Cyst Classification

Type I	Fusiform dilatation of the common duct
Type II	Saccular outpouching from the common duct
Type III	Choledochocele
Type IVa	Multiple cysts in the intrahepatic and extrahepatic ducts
Type IVb	Multiple cysts in the extrahepatic ducts
Type V	Single or multiple intrahepatic bile duct cysts (includes Caroli's disease)

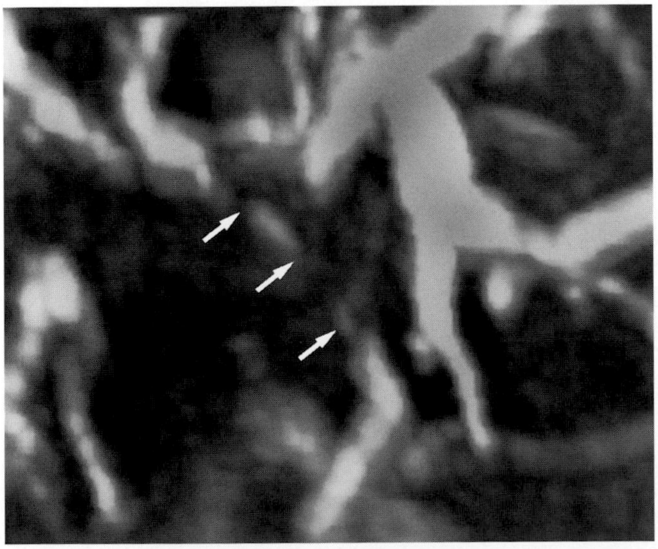

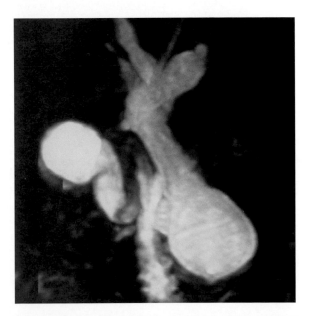

FIGURE 23-3 Biliary obstruction secondary to breast cancer metastases. Non–breath-hold coronal FSE MRCP shows long, nonuniform stricture *(arrows)* involving the common hepatic duct and the confluence of the right and left hepatic ducts. The intrahepatic ducts are markedly distended.

FIGURE 23-4 Type IVa choledochal cyst. MIP image made from serial breath-hold FSE acquisitions shows fusiform dilatation of both the common duct and intrahepatic bile ducts. (Courtesy K. Chung, Boston.)

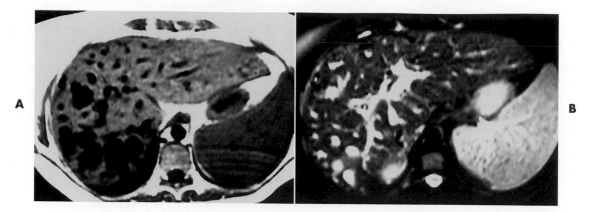

FIGURE 23-5   Caroli's disease. Axial T1-weighted (SE 300/12) **(A)** and slightly caudal T2-weighted (SE 2200/80) **(B)** images show irregular saccular dilatation of the intrahepatic bile ducts.

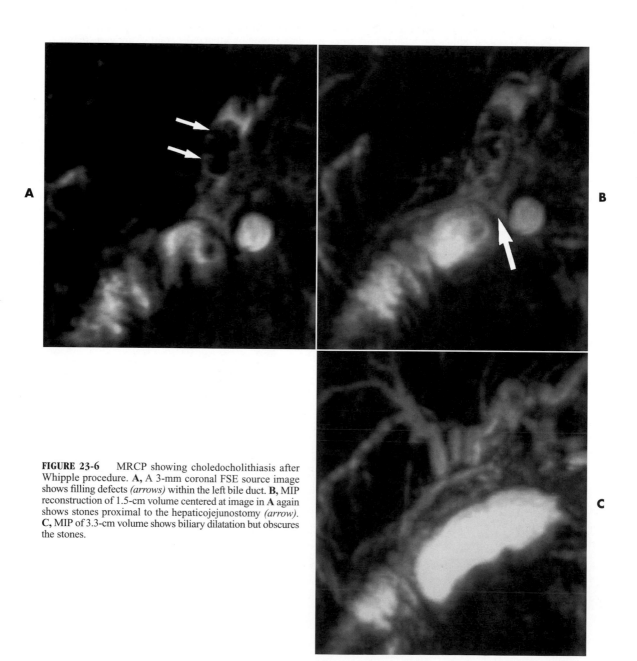

FIGURE 23-6   MRCP showing choledocholithiasis after Whipple procedure. **A,** A 3-mm coronal FSE source image shows filling defects *(arrows)* within the left bile duct. **B,** MIP reconstruction of 1.5-cm volume centered at image in **A** again shows stones proximal to the hepaticojejunostomy *(arrow).* **C,** MIP of 3.3-cm volume shows biliary dilatation but obscures the stones.

In high-grade biliary obstruction the endoscopic and MR cholangiographic views may be complementary. Retrograde opacification shows the distal end of a stricture but may fail to demonstrate the ductal anatomy proximal to the stricture and may not indicate whether intrahepatic duct branches are separately obstructed. This limitation also applies to THC, in which multiple needle punctures may be necessary to show all obstructed segments. If the duct is decompressed beyond an obstruction, MRC will not provide a detailed image of the distal end of the stricture as compared with a contrast-distended view during ERCP. Because MRC images can be rotated in three dimensions, MRC is not limited as direct cholangiography is to the projections obtained while the patient is on the table.

MRC images have a lower spatial resolution than x-ray cholangiograms. This limits the reliability of MRC to detect small filling defects (see Biliary Filling Defects). However, small filling defects also may be obscured during x-ray cholangiograms, particularly in ducts distended with high-density iodinated contrast. Filling of a periductal structure, such as a cyst or pseudocyst, during direct contrast cholangiography proves that there is communication with the duct injected. Any cystic structure close to the pancreaticobiliary tree will appear on MRCP whether or not it communicates (Figure 23-2).

MRC provides a set of noninvasive projectional images of the bile ducts. MRC is therefore indicated when diagnostic information gained from the examination would be likely to obviate direct x-ray cholangiography, either because a normal examination would be considered sufficient to exclude pathology or because the next step would likely be surgery. MRC is indicated for diagnostic evaluation of patients in whom endoscopic cholangiography is impossible.[136] This includes many patients with hepaticojejunostomy or Billroth II gastrojejunostomy, patients with gastric outlet obstruction, and some with ampullary strictures or diverticula. In these patients MRC can be useful even if there is compelling evidence (e.g., cholangitis or advanced jaundice) that transhepatic biliary drainage is required because MRC helps to map a transhepatic approach.

Biliary System on Conventional MRI

Normal intrahepatic bile ducts are not visible on conventional MR pulse sequences designed to evaluate the liver. Rephased (bright) signal from blood vessels should not be confused with long T2 of dilated intrahepatic ducts. The distal common bile duct can be demonstrated in up to 70% of studies.[137]

The gallbladder is readily visualized in the interlobar fissure using either T1- or T2-weighted pulse sequences. T2-weighted pulse sequences with long echo delays routinely show gallbladder bile with high signal intensity similar to other fluids, such as gastric contents and cerebrospinal fluid. The appearance of gallbladder bile varies on T1-weighted images, depending on gallbladder function and bile concentration.

Unconcentrated bile has a water content of approximately 95% and shows a low signal intensity on T1-weighted images, consistent with the long T1 of water. With reabsorption of water and increased solute (cholesterol and bile salt) concentration, water content falls to approximately 84%, and the T1 relaxation time decreases.[28,72] Therefore the appearance of bile on T1-weighted images varies from hypointense to hyperintense to liver and sometimes exhibits a gradient with concentrated bile layering dependently. Failure of the gallbladder to concentrate bile is a feature of gallbladder disease, and long T1 bile in fasting subjects is a sign of acute cholecystitis.[105] Unfortunately, T1-hyperintense bile also appears in suppurative and hemorrhagic cholecystitis, and impaired liver function can lead to reduced gallbladder bile concentration. A single examination showing uniform bile does not imply gallbladder disease. It may be possible to establish gallbladder function by imaging patients in both the nonfasting and fasting states.[58] Concentration of bile in the fasting state, determined by increasing signal intensity on T1-weighted images, would indicate normal gallbladder function.

Gallstones are frequently encountered in routine MRI as a signal void surrounded by high-intensity bile when T2-weighted images are obtained. It is worthwhile to recognize gallstones when they are incidentally discovered, but because of limited spatial resolution, MRI is less sensitive than ultrasound for detecting cholelithiasis. Although most gallstones appear as a signal void in vivo, in vitro T1-weighted imaging categorizes stones as dark (35%), rimmed (40%), laminated

(14%), homogeneously bright (5%), or homogeneously faint (7%) based on cross-sectional structure.[12] T1 shortening in intrahepatic ductal calculi has been reported, and T1 shortening within gallbladder calculi can be observed occasionally.

Thickening of the gallbladder wall occurs in both neoplastic and inflammatory diseases and is particularly pronounced when caused by severe liver dysfunction. Thickening of the gallbladder wall, fluid in the gallbladder fossa, or fluid within the gallbladder wall itself can occasionally be detected on T2-weighted MR images. When present, these signs furnish more specific evidence of gallbladder disease than that provided by analysis of the relaxation times of bile.[152] Enhancement of the inflamed gallbladder wall with intravenous Gd chelates has been reported.[24] Regular concentric rings in a thickened gallbladder wall diminish the likelihood of malignancy.[96] Invasion of adjacent liver tissue by a process in the gallbladder can occur as a result of inflammation, especially xanthogranulomatous cholecystitis, or of gallbladder cancer.

Gallbladder carcinoma usually occurs in the setting of chronic cholecystitis with cholelithiasis. It is an incidental discovery in about 1% of cholecystectomies. When the presentation suggests neoplasm, the tumor is usually advanced, appearing as a mass extensively involving the gallbladder, porta, head of the pancreas, and liver, and survival is poor. Although it is the fifth most common malignancy arising from the gastrointestinal tract, carcinoma of the gallbladder has been the subject of few reports in the MR literature.[2,113] The mass is seen on T2-weighted images thickening a portion of the gallbladder wall (Figure 23-7), hypointense relative to the very long T2 of gallbladder bile. Usually the lesion has longer T2 than adjacent liver tissue, although a very desmoplastic hypointense gallbladder carcinoma has been reported.[156]

Prospective differentiation of gallbladder carcinoma from inflammatory thickening of the gallbladder wall or from tumors of the liver crossing the interlobar fissure may be difficult because the signal characteristics are similar. Moreover, after cholecystectomy, loops of bowel in the gallbladder fossa could simulate the appearance of a mass. Early

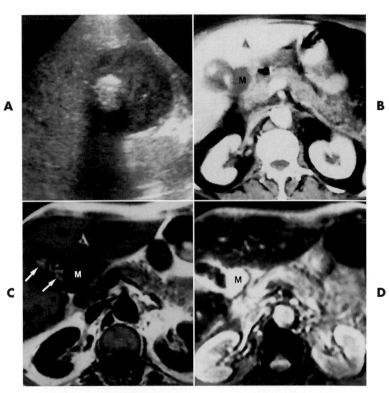

FIGURE 23-7   Adenocarcinoma of the gallbladder. **A,** Sonogram demonstrates a shadowing echogenic gallstone with an adjacent soft tissue mass. Doppler demonstrated flow within the mass. **B,** CT scan shows low-density mass *(M)* with adjacent calcified gallstones. **C,** Axial T1-weighted (SE 300/12) image shows that the mass *(M)* has a long T1 value. Laterally, foci with short T1 values are present within several gallstones *(arrows).* **D,** T2-weighted (SE 2000/80) image shows the long T2 value of the carcinoma *(M)* in the gallbladder fossa. Gallstones appear as low signal intensity.

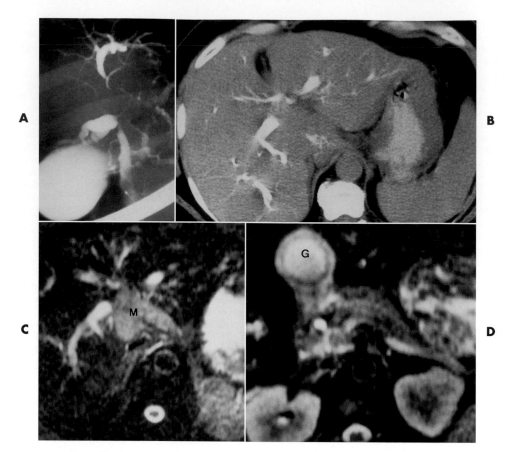

FIGURE 23-8   Klatskin's tumor with carcinoid histology. **A,** Endoscopic cholangiogram shows multisegmental obstruction; gallbladder is distended. **B,** CT after ERCP shows contrast in intrahepatic ducts obstructed by an isodense mass in the porta hepatis. **C,** FSE T2-weighted image shows a tumor with a relatively long T2 value *(M)* readily distinguished from dilated ducts and normal liver. **D,** On a section caudal to **C** the gallbladder *(G)* is distended, and the gallbladder wall is thickened.

dynamic post–Gd chelate imaging has been proposed for differentiating malignant gallbladder-wall thickening from chronic cholecystitis and adenomyomatosis. Early enhancement of carcinoma is focal and pronounced, correlating with the depth of histological invasion into the liver.[27] However, wall enhancement is greatest in acute cholecystitis, which may be accompanied by pericholecystic hepatic enhancement that should be distinguished from tumor invasion.[73]

Peripheral tumors of the bile ducts present differently from those arising centrally. Central tumors, such as cholangiocarcinoma and granular cell myoblastoma, produce jaundice. The tumor itself may be difficult to identify on MR images because of partial volume averaging with nearby portal vessels and dilated bile ducts.[114] Cholangiocarcinoma tracking along the portal tracts can cause an increase in tissue water sufficient to produce zones of long T2 from hepatic congestion and bile stasis. Occasionally, Klatskin's tumors reach sufficient size to be visible on conventional imaging of the liver (Figure 23-8). Peripheral cholangiocarcinomas are best regarded in the differential diagnosis of other primary liver tumors and are considered in Chapter 24.

Biliary cystadenoma and biliary cystadenocarcinoma (Figure 23-2) constitute less than 5% of intrahepatic cysts of biliary origin. Many pathologists consider biliary cystadenomas to be premalignant. Septations may occur in either (Figure 23-9), but nodularity suggests malignancy.[19]

PANCREAS
Normal Pancreas

On axial images the pancreas appears as a thick, transversely oriented linear structure in the midline, surrounded by retroperitoneal fat. The head of the gland, bordered on the right by the descending (second and third) and posteriorly by the transverse (fourth) portions of the duo-

denum, is thicker and more rounded than the neck, body, and tail. The body and tail usually appear on sections cephalad to the head, so the long axis of the pancreas makes an angle of 27 to 30 degrees with the axial plane. Posterior to the neck, the superior mesenteric vein passes cephalad to join the splenic vein, forming the portal vein at the splenoportal junction. The splenic vein marks the posterior margin of the body and tail. Anterior to the pancreas is the lesser sac of the peritoneal cavity. The common bile duct passes posterior to the second portion of the duodenum, entering the head of the pancreas to empty into the duodenum via the ampulla of Vater. The pancreatic duct passes centrally within the pancreas from left to right, carrying exocrine secretions into the duodenum. Most commonly the pancreatic duct also drains through the ampulla of Vater via the duct of Wirsung, but it may have a branch from the dorsal primordium emptying into the duodenum through a more proximal opening at the lesser ampulla.

In younger individuals the pancreas has a smooth contour. With aging there is frequently atrophy, with replacement of the gland by fat. The pancreas then takes on a more serrated contour as individual lobules become visible.

The signal-intensity characteristics of the pancreas depend on the MR technique used to obtain the image. On conventional T1-weighted images the pancreas is of intermediate signal intensity similar to the liver and hypointense to surrounding retroperitoneal fat. However, with fat suppression the relative signal intensity of the pancreas increases dramatically so that the pancreas is the brightest soft tissue structure in the upper abdomen and is clearly demarcated from darker fat. In most individuals the normal pancreas is hyperintense to liver on FSE T1-weighted images, although with advancing age the normal pancreas signal intensity may diminish to equality with that of the liver.[158] On proton density–weighted and T2-weighted images the pancreas also is

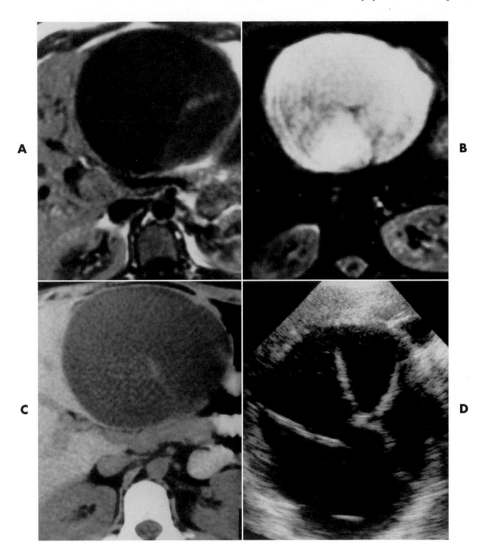

FIGURE 23-9   Biliary cystadenoma. **A** and **B,** T1- and T2-weighted MR images show a large cyst with linear internal septations. There is no discernible wall. **C,** CT shows similar findings. **D,** Ultrasound provides further definition of internal septations. These should not be confused with daughter cysts in hydatid disease. (Courtesy L.-G. Viçi, Caracas, Venezuela.)

similar in signal intensity to the liver or is slightly hyperintense.[148] Fat around the pancreas may be similar in signal intensity to the pancreas on conventional T2-weighted images or markedly higher or lower when FSE images are obtained with or without fat suppression. Like most abdominal fluids, bile and exocrine pancreatic secretions have a T2 value that is much longer than adjacent soft tissue structures, a property exploited in MRCP (see later discussion).

The pancreas enhances before the liver after bolus intravenous administration of Gd chelates. Maximal enhancement of the pancreas occurs soon after peak aortic enhancement and remains high during the later portal phase of liver enhancement. By 1 min after injection, both the pancreas and liver have reached peak signal intensity and are isointense.[83] Over the first 5 min the pancreas diminishes in signal intensity less rapidly than other organs of the upper abdomen.

Because of its central location in the upper abdomen, the pancreas presents special problems for MRI. Noise from respiration, peristalsis, and vascular pulsation may obscure fine detail. Several strategies have been applied to improve the diagnostic quality of pancreatic MR images.[87] These strategies include signal averaging, respiratory compensation, software-motion compensation, presaturation, antiperistaltic medication, local receiver multicoils, and fast imaging. Most pancreatic protocols use some combination of these techniques. Oral contrast materials may be used to distinguish stomach and small bowel from pancreas and peripancreatic processes.

Adenocarcinoma of the Pancreas

Pancreatic adenocarcinoma is an important clinical problem, accounting for 27,000 new cases and 5% of all cancer-related deaths each year. Tumors of the body and tail tend to grow insidiously, presenting late with ill-defined symptoms, such as back pain. Tumors in the head of the gland frequently come to attention when they obstruct the bile duct, producing jaundice. Some pancreatic carcinomas present with pancreatitis. They can be particularly difficult to diagnose because both pancreatitis and pancreatic carcinoma can enlarge the gland and produce similar-appearing changes in the pancreas and peripancreatic tissues.

Pancreatic carcinoma has a T1 slightly longer than a healthy pancreas and T2 equal to or slightly longer than pancreatic tissue. The T2 of pancreatic carcinoma rarely is sufficiently prolonged for ready detection of pancreatic carcinoma on T2-weighted images unless there is substantial necrosis. Carcinoma may appear as an area of reduced signal intensity on T1-weighted images, but optimum detection based on T1 requires use of fat saturation on T1-weighted SE images. On FSE T1-weighted images, pancreatic tumor is hypointense to a normal pancreas. In patients with chronic pancreatitis, pancreatic T1 may be reduced so that tumors are inconspicuous,[36] but noncontrast MRI is at least competitive with contrast-enhanced CT in detection of pancreatic carcinoma.[61,148]

Gd chelate injection followed immediately by dynamic imaging, such as with breath-holding T1-weighted gradient echoes, is the most reliable widely available method of detecting or excluding small pancreatic and ampullary carcinomas with MRI.[40,125] Dynamic imaging with Gd chelates compares favorably with helical CT, especially in equivocal cases.[60,122] The tumor appears distinctly hypointense to the pancreas only during the first 1 to 2 min after injection, when the pancreas is maximally enhanced (Figure 23-10). Thereafter, leakage of contrast into the extracellular fluid compartment of the tumor reduces tumor-pancreas contrast and compromises tumor conspicuity. As this contrast leakage continues, the tumor appears isointense to hyperintense on fat-saturated T1-weighted images 5 to 10 min after contrast injection.

Ductal strictures occur in almost all pancreatic carcinomas. Carcinomas of the pancreatic head present with jaundice and occlusion of both the common bile duct and pancreatic duct. This "double duct" pattern of obstruction detected on MRCP (Figure 23-11) strongly suggests the presence of a pancreatic or ampullary carcinoma, even if the tumor itself is not detected. Large masses of the pancreatic head region not causing obstruction of the ducts usually are some other histology, including metastases or lymphoma in the peripancreatic lymph nodes or focal pancreatitis. Carcinomas of the body and tail present without jaundice and with focal stricture or obliteration of only the pancreatic duct on MRCP.

At centers where whole-body EPI is available, single-shot EPI offers another approach to motion noise reduction for detection of small pancreatic cancers.[109] Heavily T2-weighted images can be obtained in less

than 100 ms, and corresponding short TI inversion recovery (STIR) images in 150 ms. With these methods the pancreas has very low signal intensity, and small pancreatic tumors are seen as distinct hyperintense foci (Figure 23-12). The snapshot rapidity of image acquisition permits use of a long-T2 aqueous contrast material to demonstrate the duodenum (see the following section). The principal penalty for single-shot imaging to date has been reduced spatial resolution of approximately 1.5×3 mm, which limits assessment of local invasion.

Staging of pancreatic carcinoma involves detection of both local and remote spread of the tumor. Size is not a reliable indicator of stage because more than 50% of patients with tumors of 2 cm or smaller in size have lymph node metastases, serosal invasion, retroperitoneal implants, or vascular invasion.[147] Metastases to the liver or peritoneum render a tumor unresectable. Contiguous spread of the tumor to the mesentery, particularly if the mesenteric vessels are involved, also may lead to unresectability or may indicate use of preoperative chemotherapy or radiation therapy. T1-weighted SE images without fat saturation both before and after Gd chelates show peripancreatic tumor well.[134] Contact with tumor on both sides of a vessel, such as the superior mesenteric vein or portal vein, correlates with vascular encasement. Alternatively, time-of-flight MRA can be used to demonstrate narrowing or displacement of the mesenteric vessels (Figure 23-10). Careful attention to the source images and the reconstructed MRA is important to correlate segments of suspected vascular abnormality with anatomical location of the tumor. In a small series, Gd-enhanced vascular MRI is more accurate than

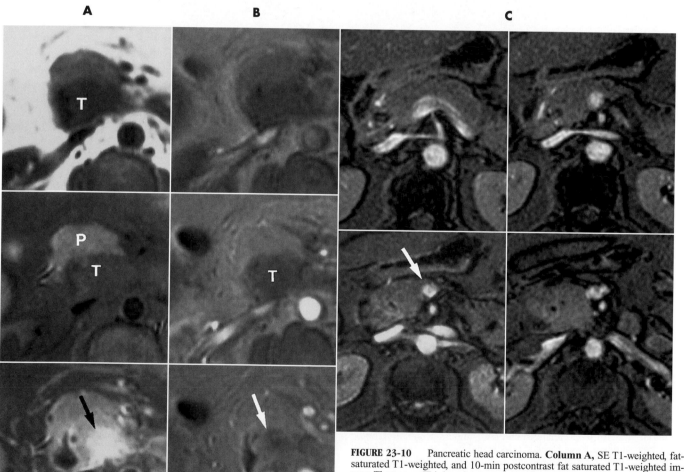

A   **B**   **C**

FIGURE 23-10 Pancreatic head carcinoma. **Column A,** SE T1-weighted, fat-saturated T1-weighted, and 10-min postcontrast fat saturated T1-weighted images. The tumor *(T)* is hypointense to normal pancreas on both precontrast images but is better distinguished from pancreas *(P)* with fat saturation because of the compressed dynamic range. However, with fat saturation the tumor is isointense to retroperitoneal fat. After the delay, part of the tumor has become hyperintense *(arrow)* to the pancreas. **Column B,** Dynamic gradient-echo images (120/2.5/80 degrees) precontrast, arterial phase, and portal phase. The tumor *(T)* is hypointense to pancreas, becoming more conspicuous as the pancreas enhances during the arterial phase. Leakage of contrast into tumor during the portal phase partially obscures the tumor *(arrow).* **Column C,** Four time-of-flight source images (top left highest, bottom right lowest) after Gd-chelate injection. Tumor contacts the superior mesenteric vein, but only normal pancreatic tissue extends around it *(arrow,* lower left). This tumor was completely resected after adjuvant therapy.

angiography in predicting nonresectability of pancreatic carcinoma based on venous involvement.[78]

The accuracy of cross-sectional imaging in staging pancreatic adenocarcinoma remains a subject of controversy. A major effort to define the role of both CT and MRI in staging pancreatic carcinoma was recently reported by the Radiology Diagnostic Oncology Group.[80] This multicenter trial compared contrast-enhanced axial CT and four MR pulse sequences (T1, T2, STIR, and gradient-recalled echo [GRE]) with the ultimate surgical findings in more than 100 patients, examining vascular invasion, lymph node involvement, liver metastases, and overall predicted resectability. Positive findings on either CT or MRI strongly indicated nonresectability, with the positive predictive value of both MRI and CT measured at 0.88 to 0.89. Both modalities fairly accurately excluded patients with liver metastases, with a negative predictive value of 0.89 for MRI and 0.87 for CT. However, neither modality reliably detected local extrapancreatic spread. Negative predictive value for vascular invasion was 0.23 (MRI) and 0.28 (CT), and for lymph nodes it was 0.56. Moreover, results were not improved by use of both modalities together. Readers at different centers performed with varying accuracy in this study, which enrolled patients from 1990 to 1992. Technical advances in both CT (dual-phase helical protocols, CT angiography) and MR (fat saturation, dynamic imaging with Gd chelates, MRA) have not as yet been subjected to the same rigorous evaluation but will likely improve performance of both modalities for staging pancreatic carcinoma.

An additional problem in staging of pancreatic carcinoma is peritoneal seeding. Of patients with apparently resectable tumor by preoperative imaging, 40% will be unresectable because of peritoneal seeding.[33] Half of these patients have macroscopic implants of tumor on the capsule of the liver, detectable during laparoscopy. It is not known whether wider use of oral and intravenous MR contrast agents will permit MRI to detect some of these patients preoperatively.

The MR imaging approach to a patient with known or suspected pancreatic tumor depends on the clinical history and the information required from the examination. Although MRI is the only imaging modality capable of detecting and staging the local, biliary, vascular, and hepatic manifestations of pancreatic carcinoma,[88] it is often unnecessary to apply in one case all of the available techniques. For example, many patients present for cross-sectional imaging after biliary decompression. In such patients an MRC would be of little clinical benefit. Conversely, careful local staging of pancreatic adenocarcinoma by MRA would not be indicated when the tumor is already metastatic to the liver. A specific MR protocol should be tailored for a given patient after review of prior imaging and clinical history and only with an understanding of the information required by the treating physician. For staging after insertion of a biliary endoprosthesis, there are differences in ferromagnetic properties among different models of metallic stents.[39]

Islet Cell Tumors

Islet cell tumors of the pancreas present differently depending on whether they produce a hormonally active peptide (functioning tumors)

or do not (nonfunctioning tumors). Nonfunctioning tumors typically are larger at presentation, often arising from the pancreatic tail. These tumors come to attention because of mass effect or metastases. They are hypointense to pancreas on T1-weighted images, hyperintense on T2-weighted images, and enhance rapidly with Gd-chelate injection.

Functioning pancreatic endocrine neoplasms are clinically apparent in 50% to 80% of patients with the classic multiple endocrine neoplasia syndrome, type I (MEN I), along with primary hyperparathyroidism and pituitary adenomas. Functioning islet cell tumors also occur in type IIa von Hippel-Lindau disease in association with pheochromocytoma[22] and in a newer MEN syndrome, including duodenal somatostatinomas, pheochromocytomas, and neurofibromatosis.[93]

The Zollinger-Ellison syndrome of fulminant peptic ulcer disease is caused by excess secretion of gastrin by one or more islet cell tumors. Of patients with Zollinger-Ellison syndrome, 20% to 40% have MEN I. Gastrinoma is the most frequent islet cell tumor in patients with

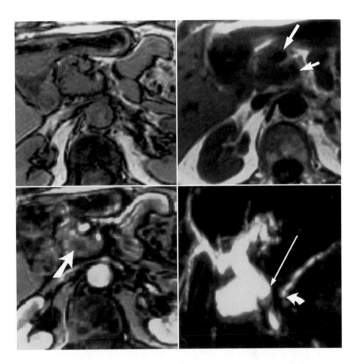

FIGURE 23-11   Pancreatic carcinoma. *Top,* Unenhanced gradient-recalled echo (GRE) and SE T1-weighted images show focal enlargement of the pancreatic head. There is abnormal tissue partially enveloping the superior mesenteric vein *(long arrow)* and superior mesenteric artery *(short arrow). Bottom,* Dynamic postcontrast image shows focal hypoperfusion in the pancreatic head *(oblique arrow),* indicating presence of tumor. MRCP shows "double duct" sign, simultaneous occlusion of the bile *(long arrow)* and pancreatic *(curved arrow)* ducts. (From reference 72.)

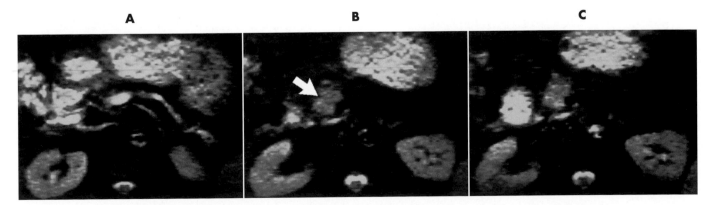

FIGURE 23-12   Pancreatic carcinoma, demonstrated by single-shot EPI. **A,** Instascan TE 50-ms SE image shows dilated pancreatic duct just cephalad to tumor. **B,** 1.25-cm caudal to **A,** a mass with a long T2 value *(arrow)* is seen surrounded by dark, fat-replaced gland. **C,** Instascan STIR (TI, 100 ms) image at same level as **B.** (From reference 109.)

MEN I. Compared with patients without MEN I, gastrinomas in patients with MEN I are more likely to be multiple and more likely to be found outside of the pancreas.[93] Of gastrinomas, 20% to 40% are multicentric, and 60% are malignant, with 80% of these already metastatic at presentation. Metastasis is usually to the liver but sometimes to peripancreatic nodes or even to the lung. Ninety percent of gastrinomas are found in the anatomical triangle whose vertices are the cystic duct confluence, the junction of the pancreatic neck and body, and the junction of the second and third portions of duodenum[138]; 54% are in the pancreatic head.

Because of potential malignancy and multicentricity of gastrinomas, preoperative imaging is important in evaluating patients with Zollinger-Ellison syndrome. Gastrinomas are distinctly hypointense to the pancreas on fat-saturation T1-weighted images, are hyperintense on T2-weighted FSE images,[86] and may be cystic (Figure 23-13). There is ring enhancement on GRE images after Gd chelate bolus injection.[120] Most gastrinomas are 2 cm or more in diameter when clinically apparent. Although several authors have described successful localization of these tumors, careful surgical palpation and intraoperative ultrasound may identify additional foci, particularly in patients with MEN I.

In contrast to gastrinomas, 90% of insulinomas are benign; 90% of patients with insulinomas have only one, and insulinomas are uniformly distributed throughout the pancreas. Detection of multiple insulinomas should instigate a search for other features of MEN syndromes.[93] Of insulinomas, 70% are less than 1.5 cm in diameter. Although detection of local invasion or metastasis is the only reliable indicator of malignancy, malignant insulinomas tend to be larger and occur more frequently in men.

Several MR techniques have been reportedly successful in preoperative localization of insulinomas, which are usually smaller at presentation than are gastrinomas. Insulinomas appear as tiny, well-circumscribed hypointense foci on fat-saturation T1-weighted images (Figures 23-14 and 23-15) and markedly hyperintense on STIR images.[67,120] Marked uniform enhancement in the arterial phase after Gd chelate injection helps to identify lesions that might be overlooked, particularly those located at the pancreatic margins.[52,120] MRI is superior to CT for localization of small functioning islet cell tumors.[120] Sonography and MRI have complementary roles, together localizing 97% of insulinomas in a series of 28 cases.[4] However, some argue that the preoperative imaging search for insulinoma, whether by CT, MRI, endoscopic ultrasound, or venous sampling, is unnecessary, given the high combined accuracy of intraoperative ultrasound and palpation by an experienced surgeon.[6]

Rare functioning islet cell tumors include glucagonoma, vipoma, and somatostatinoma. Each has a distinctive clinical presentation. Glucagonomas and vipomas of the pancreas occur most frequently in the body and tail, whereas most somatostatinomas arise in the head.[93] However, a significant number of somatostatinomas occur in peripancreatic tissues or small bowel (Figure 23-16). Glucagonomas and somatostatinomas tend to be larger at presentation than vipomas, but more than 50% of all three types of pancreatic tumors are malignant and metastatic at presentation. Irregular enhancement of two glucagonomas after Gd-chelate administration has been described.[120]

Pancreatic Cysts and Cystic Tumors

True pancreatic cysts are rare but may occur in conjunction with systemic congenital disease, including cystic fibrosis and polycystic disease. Typical of cysts elsewhere, true pancreatic cysts have a uniform long T2 and a thin wall, and they fail to enhance with contrast. Retention cysts arise from progressive dilatation of the pancreatic duct behind an obstruction; occurring in chronic pancreatitis, they may be impossible to distinguish from a chronic pseudocyst, even histologically.[107]

The term *pancreatic pseudocyst* refers to a collection of pancreatic juice without a true cyst lining, contained within a fibrous capsule, and

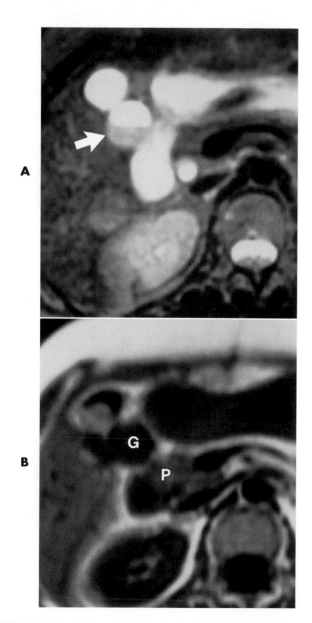

FIGURE 23-13 Cystic gastrinoma. **A,** FSE image (5500/104; ET 16) shows fluid level in lesion *(arrow)* between the gallbladder and duodenal bulb. **B,** On T1-weighted image (300/11) the lesion *(G)* is contiguous to the pancreatic head, from which it arose by a short pedicle.

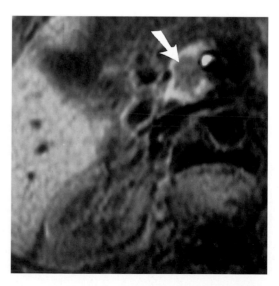

FIGURE 23-14 Insulinoma. Fat-saturated T1-weighted SE image (400/10) shows a well-demarcated hypointense lesion *(arrow)* in the head of the pancreas.

complicating pancreatic inflammation or trauma. During acute pancreatitis, fluid collections may appear in the peripancreatic tissues. Such collections are ill defined and changeable in appearance on cross-sectional imaging and often resolve spontaneously. Chronic pseudocysts (Figure 23-17), those that appear or have failed to resolve more than 3 weeks after an episode of acute pancreatitis, rarely resolve spontaneously and usually arise within the substance of the pancreas.

Microcystic adenomas of the pancreas are cystic neoplasms. They are thin walled, with single (Figure 23-18) or more commonly multiple small cyst spaces containing clear fluid and lined by cuboidal epithelial cells with glycogen-rich cytoplasm. Consequently, microcystic adeno-

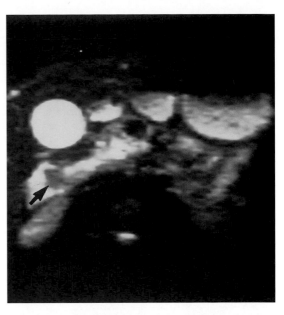

FIGURE 23-16   Somatostatinoma arising from the ampulla of Vater. Single-shot EPI (infinity/100) shows a hypointense mass *(arrow)* projecting into the duodenum. Aqueous oral contrast was administered to distend the duodenum.

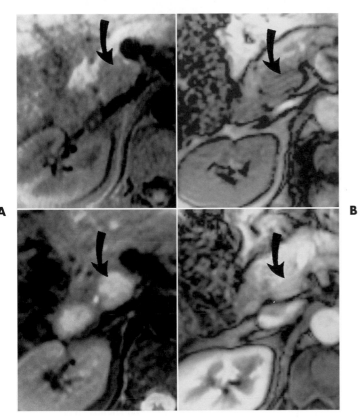

FIGURE 23-15   Insulinoma. **A,** Fat-saturated SE (500/10) and FSE (5000/108) images show a focal lesion *(arrow)* in the pancreatic head. Both the T1 and T2 values are distinctly longer than in the pancreas. **B,** Before and immediately after 0.1 mmol/kg Gd-chelate administration, FMP-SPGR (80/2.5/80 degrees) breath-hold images reveal that the lesion enhances markedly *(arrow)*. Images were obtained with a phased-array multicoil at 1.5 T.

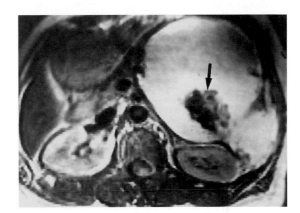

FIGURE 23-17   Pancreatic pseudocyst. Axial T2-weighted image (SE 1600/70) shows a large, high–signal intensity lesion with a thin wall and dependent necrotic debris *(arrow)*. (Courtesy Y. Itai.)

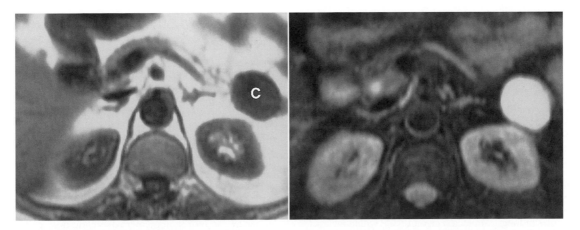

FIGURE 23-18   Unilocular serous cystadenoma of the pancreas. T1-weighted *(left)* and FSE T2-weighted *(right)* images show cyst *(C)* arising from atrophic pancreatic tail. Pancreatic signal intensity was normal on fat-saturated T1-weighted image (not shown).

A   **B**   **C**

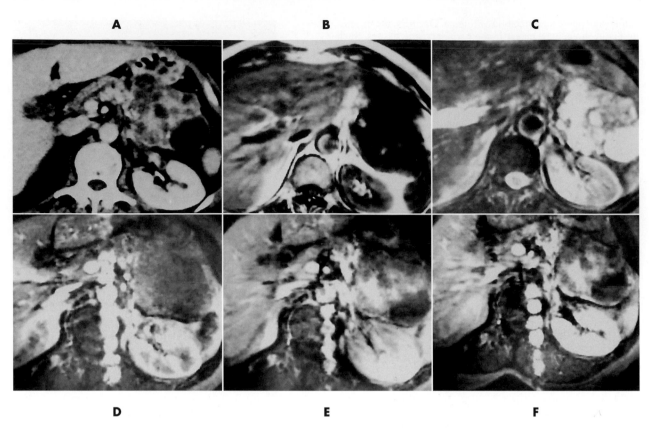

D   **E**   **F**

FIGURE 23-19   Serous cystadenoma. **A,** Bolus contrast CT shows complex mass in the tail of the pancreas. Low-attenuation cysts are set in a matrix of enhancing solid tissue. **B,** SE (600/17) image (1.5 T) shows a low–signal intensity mass in the tail of the pancreas. Small foci of high signal intensity indicate bleeding within two small cysts, a relatively unusual occurrence in this histology. **C,** Corresponding T2-weighted image (SE 2000/75) shows multiple cysts with long T2 values and high signal intensity. **D** to **F,** Gradient-echo images (FLASH19/12/90 degrees) before, 10 sec after, and 4 min after intravenous Gd chelate, 0.05 mmol/kg. Enhancement of the solid portions of the tumor corresponds closely to the enhancement pattern of CT. (Courtesy Y. Itai.)

mas are often called *serous cystadenomas.* These tumors are considered benign. They occur in women more than men, by a ratio of 6 to 1, usually in the sixth and seventh decades of life.[107] Microcystic tumors are lobulated, with thin walls and thin internal septations. Signal intensity usually is homogeneous, with long T2. Bleeding into microcystic tumors, which is less common than in mucinous tumors, can occur, leading to variation in signal intensity. Some microcystic adenomas consist of multiple tiny cysts in a solid-appearing matrix that enhances with Gd chelate injection (Figure 23-19). Pancreatic cysts and microcystic adenomas occur commonly in patients with von Hippel-Lindau disease (Figure 23- 20), but the frequency varies widely among families.[22]

Mucinous pancreatic lesions comprise a spectrum of malignant and premalignant neoplastic conditions of the pancreas characterized by production of mucus. Patients are usually women, typically presenting in middle age. Tumors may be unilocular or multilocular, often with thick walls and papillary projections (Figure 23-21). Cyst contents usually have a long T2, but T1 shortening resulting from hemorrhage or high protein content may be present. Enhancement with Gd chelates may show thick walls and septations or frank nodules of malignant tumor (Figure 23-22). However, cystic tumors may be impossible to distinguish from pancreatic pseudocysts by imaging. When clinical history is inconclusive, aspiration biopsy or surgery is required to establish the diagnosis.[34] In mucinous ductal ectasia (MDE) the mucin-producing cells of a mucinous cystic neoplasm communicate with the pancreatic duct, producing marked distension. MRI and MR pancreatography readily display the ductal distension. MR pancreatography usually fails to demonstrate globules of long T2 mucus seen on ERCP within the duct.[29]

Solid and epithelial neoplasms of the pancreas comprise a rare type of pancreatic tumor, typically presenting in young women as a solitary mass in the pancreas.[98,104,20] Grossly the tumor may be entirely solid or entirely cystic but most commonly is composed of components. The

solid tissue is isointense to slightly hypointense relative to surrounding normal pancreas on T1-weighted images and slightly hyperintense on T2-weighted images. A frequent finding is hemorrhage within the cystic components, which are then hyperintense on T1-weighted images and may be hypointense on T2-weighted images. There can be a hypointense capsule. The diagnosis can be suggested from MR appearance with discovery of a mixed-type hemorrhagic tumor in a young woman. Without a capsule, the more solid tumors resemble islet cell neoplasms, and the purely cystic ones cannot be distinguished from mucinous cystic neoplasms, which can also hemorrhage.

Pancreatitis

Because of the powerful digestive enzymes that can be liberated from the pancreas, acute inflammation of the pancreas is a potentially devastating disease. The hallmark of acute pancreatitis is hyperamylasemia. Other causes of hyperamylasemia include bowel obstruction, perforation, or ischemia; ectopic pregnancy; aortic dissection; renal failure; and macroamylasemia. The two most common causes of acute pancreatitis are alcohol abuse and gallstone pancreatitis, but trauma (including ERCP),[142] heritable defects, viral infection, ischemia, malnutrition, and drug therapy are among less frequent causes. In some patients no precipitating cause or risk factor is identified.[23] The grading scale of Balthazar (Table 23-1) is widely used for assessing severity of pancreatitis on cross-sectional images. Developed for use with contrast-enhanced CT, the Balthazar severity index is based on a combination of changes in pancreatic morphology, peripancreatic fluid collections, and mapping of pancreatic necrosis detected by contrast media hypoperfusion.[10] Patients with a high severity index (7 to 10) were found to have 92% morbidity and 17% mortality, versus 2% and 0% for patients with a low severity index (0 to 2).

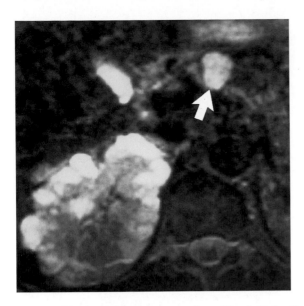

FIGURE 23-20   Pancreatic serous cystadenoma in von Hippel–Lindau disease. T2-weighted FSE image shows lobulated cystic lesion *(arrow)* in the pancreatic head. There are multiple right renal cysts after left nephrectomy for multiple renal cell carcinomas.

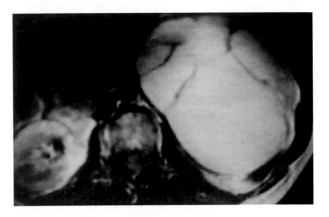

FIGURE 23-21   Mucinous cystadenoma. SE 2000/22 image shows a cystic mass with incomplete septations. (Courtesy Y. Itai.)

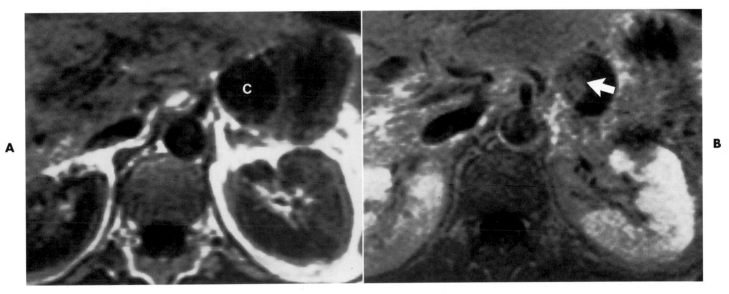

FIGURE 23-22   Mucinous cystic neoplasm. **A,** Noncontrast T1-weighted SE image (300/11) shows a smooth, low signal–intensity cyst *(C)* in the pancreatic tail. **B,** After administration of Gd chelate, an enhancing mural nodule is visible *(arrow).* The nodule contained adenocarcinoma. (Courtesy D.S. Lu, Los Angeles.)

Morphological changes of pancreatitis have been described based on CT findings.[143] Fast scans obtained during breath-holding more consistently mirror CT findings. In mild forms of pancreatitis, no morphological changes are perceptible, particularly because there is considerable variability in gland size in normal subjects. Enhancement after injection of Gd chelates will likewise be prompt and uniform.[18] With increasing severity, there is gland swelling, which sometimes is focal. Strands of inflammation extend from the gland and are best seen on fast scans that emphasize signal intensity of peripancreatic fat, such as T1-weighted gradient echo and non–fat-saturated proton density–weighted FSE images. Small fluid collections may appear in the lesser peritoneal sac anterior to the body and tail or in the anterior pararenal space of the retroperitoneum and are best detected on T2-weighted images made with fat saturation (Figure 23-23). In severe pancreatitis, focal areas of increased T1 and T2 values appear within the pancreas itself; T1 shortening in these areas corresponds to hemorrhagic necrosis (Figure 23-24). Devascularized portions of the gland fail to enhance on

Table 23-1   Acute Pancreatitis Severity Index

POINTS	GRADE	MORPHOLOGY
0	A	Normal pancreas
1	B	Focal or diffuse gland enlargement
2	C	Intrinsic abnormality with peripancreatic strands or blurring
3	D	Single ill-defined peripancreatic collection
4	E	Multiple collections or extraluminal gas
Add points for necrosis		
0	—	Necrosis absent
2	—	Necrosis in ⅓ of pancreas
4	—	Necrosis in ½ of pancreas
6	—	Necrosis in >½ of pancreas

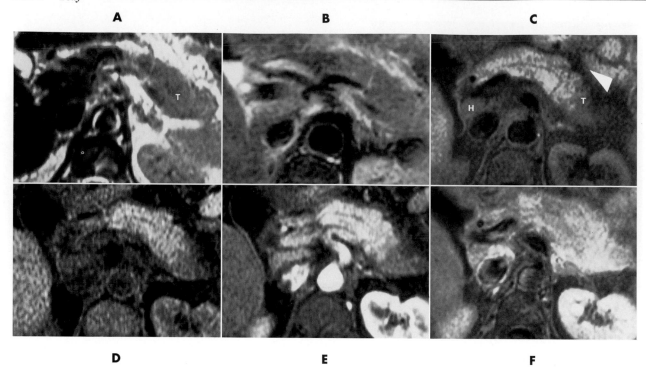

FIGURE 23-23   Acute pancreatitis. **A,** Breath-hold FSE image (3500/102, ET 16) shows a swollen pancreatic tail *(T),* with strands of inflammation invading the anterior peripancreatic fat. **B,** FSE image (4000/102, ET 8) shows high-signal edema in the peripancreatic fat. **C,** On fat-saturated T1-weighted image (600/11) the signal intensity of the pancreatic head *(H)* and tail *(T)* is diminished, and the body is heterogeneous. **D** and **E,** FS-FMP-SPGR images (150/2.6/75 degrees) before and immediately after Gd-chelate injection. There is diminished enhancement of pancreatic tissue in the head and tail. Fat at the SMA origin is normal. **F,** Repeat fat-saturated T1-weighted image 6 min postcontrast shows enhancement of the inflamed peripancreatic tissue. (Courtesy G.T. Sica, Boston.)

FIGURE 23-24   Hemorrhagic pancreatitis. T1-weighted FMP-SPGR (77/2.6/80 degrees) **(A)** and T2-weighted FSE (3550/85, ET 8) **(B)** images show pancreatic swelling and disorganization. High signal intensity *(arrow* in **A**) within the pancreas in **A** indicates hemorrhagic necrosis.

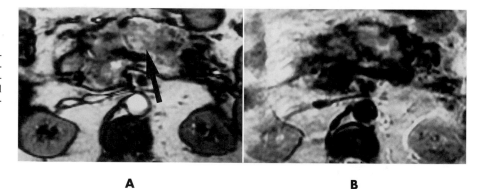

dynamic Gd chelate images, but these hypoperfused intrapancreatic zones, as well as peripancreatic inflammation, can enhance on delayed images. MRI appears to be considerably more sensitive than CT for detection of hypoperfusion after injection of intravenous contrast.[131]

Formation of acute and chronic peripancreatic fluid collections, abscess, and hemorrhage are complications of acute pancreatitis. Evaluation of peripancreatic fluid is an important goal in cross-sectional imaging of acute pancreatitis. Detection of extraluminal gas is a specific but not very sensitive sign of infection, usually indicating early operative intervention. It may be difficult to distinguish areas of liquefactive peripancreatic necrosis from more solid phlegmon. Homogeneous long T2; absence of short T1 hemorrhage or contrast enhancement; presence of rounded, well-defined contours; and development of a capsule are features suggesting that a peripancreatic fluid collection might be amenable to drainage, as opposed to debridement.[90]

Vascular complications of pancreatitis include venous thrombosis and arterial pseudoaneurysm formation. Pseudoaneurysms complicate up to 10% of severe cases. Most commonly the splenic artery is involved (Figure 23-25). Pseudoaneurysms must be distinguished from pancreatic fluid collections and from incidental atherosclerotic aneurysms because pseudoaneurysm rupture is associated with a high mortality, whereas atherosclerotic aneurysms rarely hemorrhage.

Signs of chronic pancreatitis on imaging studies include atrophy of the gland, changes in signal characteristics of pancreatic parenchyma, irregular dilatation of the pancreatic duct, pancreatic calcifications, and chronic pseudocysts. Focal enlargement of the pancreas may be present, simulating the appearance of a neoplasm. Superimposed acute pancreatitis, with focal or diffuse pancreatic swelling and peripancreatic stranding and fluid, may complicate the appearance of chronic pancreatitis when patients present for imaging. Obstruction of the pancreatic duct can result in chronic pancreatitis distal to (to the left of) a pancreatic neoplasm. Diminished signal intensity on fat-saturation T1-weighted images has been attributed to fibrosis reducing the concentration of soluble proteins that shorten T1 values of the healthy gland.[18] In advanced cases of chronic pancreatitis all of the findings can be discerned on conventional images, with diminished parenchymal thickness, prolonged T1 times, marked ductal dilatation, and sometimes focal signal voids caused by parenchymal calcifications. In patients with significant fibrosis, there is also reduced enhancement in the arterial phase after bolus injection of Gd chelates.[121]

MRCP demonstrates ductal changes that appear in milder forms of chronic pancreatitis, including segmental dilatation and narrowing, concretions, and, less reliably, beading or dilatation of ductal side branches.[141] Pseudocysts in or near the pancreas are demonstrated by

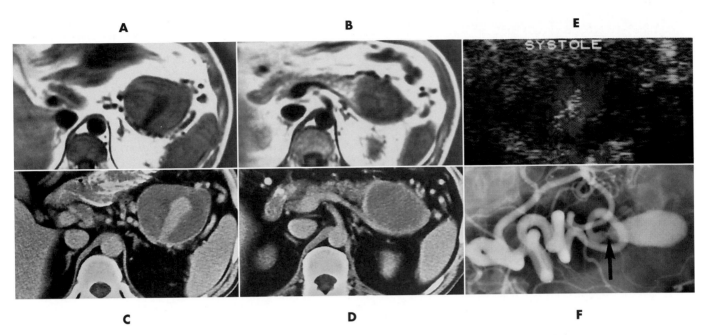

FIGURE 23-25   Splenic artery pseudoaneurysm complicating pancreatitis. **A** and **B,** T1-weighted MR images through the tail of the pancreas show a mass of intermediate signal intensity anterior to the splenic vein. Centrally there is a zone of low signal intensity. **C** and **D,** Corresponding CT sections show contrast opacification of the lumen of the aneurysm surrounded by clot. **E,** Transverse color Doppler image shows flow within the center of the lesion. Flow was pulsatile. **F,** Celiac arteriogram shows lumen of the aneurysm supplied through a narrow neck *(arrow)* by the splenic artery. The aneurysm was treated by surgical resection. (From Mitchell D**G,** et al: Radiographics 10:366, 1990.)

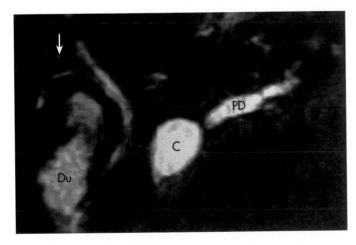

FIGURE 23-26   FSE MRCP showing pancreatic duct changes of chronic pancreatitis. The proximal pancreatic duct *(PD)* in the tail is dilated, terminating at a large pseudocyst *(C).* The distal pancreatic duct in the pancreatic head is thin, irregular, and poorly seen, and it proved to be obstructed on ERCP. In this MIP image the gallbladder has been removed by postprocessing, and part of the common hepatic duct is posterior to the imaged volume. Aberrant right hepatic duct *(arrow)* drains directly into the common hepatic duct. (Courtesy E. Cortell, Boston.)

MRCP whether or not they communicate with the duct (Figure 23-26). MRCP can be useful in identifying predominant drainage of the main pancreatic duct via the lesser ampulla through the dorsal duct of Santorini.[17,57,135] This condition, called *pancreas divisum* (Figure 23-27), is considered by some to be a risk factor for pancreatitis. MRCP performed before and after secretin injection can show abnormal persistent poststimulatory dilatation, a sign of ampullary dysfunction.[76]

Metabolic Disorders

The pancreas is among the exocrine glands affected by cystic fibrosis (CF), and malabsorption secondary to pancreatic insufficiency is a common clinical feature of this familial disease. Impaired anion transport

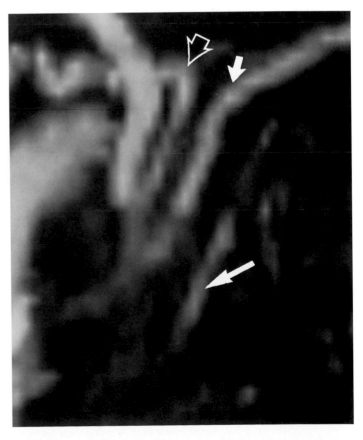

FIGURE 23-27   Pancreas divisum. Coronal section from respiratory-triggered FSE 3D slab shows the main pancreatic duct joining the duct of Santorini *(short arrow)* to drain into the duodenum via the minor ampulla. A smaller duct of Wirsung *(long arrow)* drains through the major ampulla with the common bile duct. Note low insertion of the cystic duct *(open arrow),* a common variant. (From reference 135.)

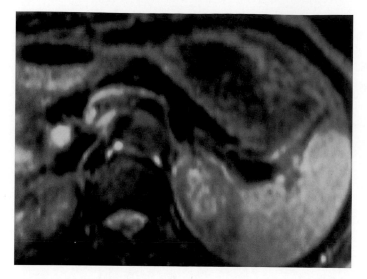

FIGURE 23-28   Hereditary hemochromatosis. T2-weighted SE (3000/80) image shows markedly diminished pancreatic signal intensity and normal spleen.

leads to low water content of ductal fluid, which in turn results in precipitation of protein, obstructing small pancreatic ducts. The MR appearance of the pancreas in young adults with CF is variable; four abnormal patterns have been described.[35,144] In most CF patients with pancreatic insufficiency, signal intensity on T1-weighted images is increased because of fatty replacement. The gland may be either swollen or small and atrophic. Less commonly the pancreas is atrophic, without obvious T1 shortening. This pattern resembles atrophy in chronic pancreatitis. Rarely the CF pancreas is completely replaced by cysts. Abnormal morphology correlates well in CF patients with clinical pancreatic insufficiency.

Pancreatic atrophy is accelerated in patients with diabetes mellitus. It has been suggested based on CT morphology that atrophy of the diabetic gland is nonuniform, occurring first in the body and tail and sparing until late the posterior aspect of the head, which is derived embryologically from the ventral primordium. The pancreas is larger in obese patients whether diabetic or not.[38]

In patients with hemochromatosis, pancreatic iron overload can result in pancreatic islet cell atrophy and diabetes. MRI shows a decreased intensity of iron-overloaded pancreatic tissue that is most marked on gradient-echo and T2-weighted SE sequences (Figure 23-28). The mechanism has been studied most thoroughly in the liver and spleen, where the decreased signal intensity results from paramagnetic

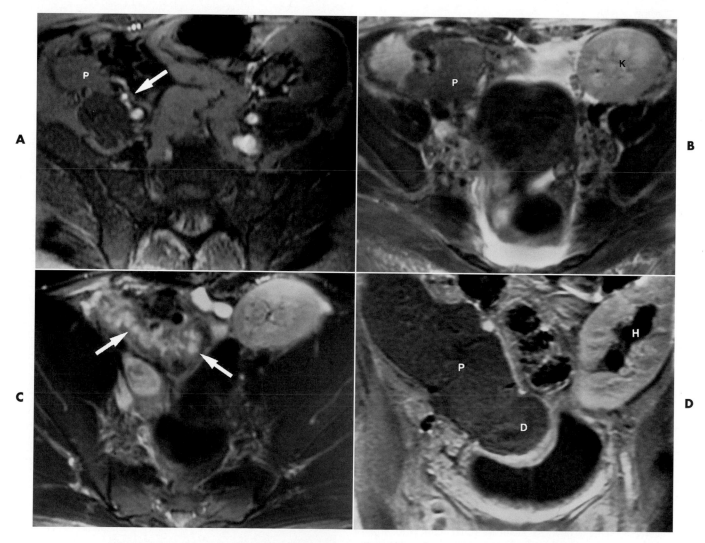

FIGURE 23-29   Pancreatic allografts. **A,** Axial GRASS (50/8/45 degrees) image shows normal graft *(P)* with flow-related enhancement of main arterial and venous pedicles *(arrow).* **B,** Axial T2-weighted FSE image shows another normal allograft *(P). K,* Contralateral renal graft. **C,** Biopsy-proven severe rejection. Axial T2-weighted FSE image shows multiple foci with long T2 values *(arrows).* **D,** In a fourth case, a coronal dynamic Gd-enhanced FMP-SPGR (150/4.2/60 degrees) image demonstrates a swollen, nonenhancing duodenum *(D)* and graft *(P),* found to be infarcted at explantation. The left renal allograft is hydronephrotic *(H).* (**A** and **D,** From reference 69; **B** and **C,** courtesy T.L. Krebs, Baltimore.)

susceptibility effects of intracellular iron particles.[42,139] Although both T1 and T2 relaxation enhancement is observed, the 15 times greater T2 relaxivity compared with T1 relaxivity produces a net decrease in signal intensity. Changes in the pancreas resemble but are less marked than changes in the liver and are proportional to the expected pancreatic iron levels. MRI therefore is useful in detecting pancreatic iron overload and assessing the risk for diabetes in patients with hemochromatosis.[64]

Pancreatic Allografts

Pancreatic transplantation in conjunction with renal transplantation is used to treat selected cases of type 1 diabetes mellitus. Complications include sepsis, rejection, pancreatitis, and graft-vessel thrombosis.[69] The current bladder-drained technique places the allograft in the iliac fossa, with arterial supply from the external iliac artery to both the donor superior mesenteric artery and splenic artery via a Y-shaped jump graft. The splenic vein drains via the donor portal vein into the external iliac vein, and the exocrine secretions drain into the bladder via a transplanted segment of duodenum.

Clinical and laboratory assessment of pancreatic allografts is limited. Therefore imaging plays an important role in management of pancreatic allografts. Because of the superficial location, pancreatic allografts are well imaged, especially with a local multicoil. On static MR images, signs of edema associated with graft dysfunction are swelling and parenchymal T2 lengthening, which often is focal[162] (Figure 23-29). Patchy areas of hemorrhage appear as T1 shortening. These findings are common immediately after transplantation but should regress after 4 weeks. Recent studies indicate the value of Gd chelates for detecting and characterizing graft dysfunction. Weak, delayed enhancement on GRE images suggests rejection. Virtually no enhancement is seen in areas of infarction.[32] Additional information can be obtained by MRA, which has been found to be better than 90% accurate for diagnosis of acute vascular compromise.[69]

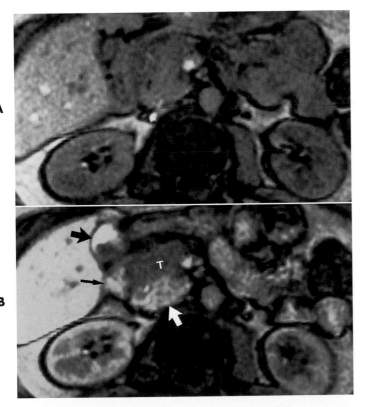

FIGURE 23-30   Enhanced detection of pancreatic carcinoma with Mn-DPDP. **A,** Gradient-echo image (80/2.8/80 degrees) before contrast shows no focal abnormality in the pancreas. **B,** Fifteen minutes after Mn-DPDP injection, normal pancreatic tissue *(white arrow)* is enhanced, but anterior tumor *(T)* is not, improving tumor conspicuity. Note also the enhancement of gallbladder bile *(black arrow)* and duodenal contents *(small black arrow)* from enhanced bile excreted into the lumen.

Mn-DPDP–Enhanced Imaging

Increased signal intensity of the pancreas has been detected on T1-weighted images within 3 min after injection of the paramagnetic hepatobiliary contrast agent manganese-dipyridoxal diphosphate (Mn-DPDP). Marketing of this agent in the United States began in 1998. Peak enhancement of normal pancreatic tissue occurs after about 90 min.[37] Pancreatic tumors do not exhibit prolonged enhancement, so Mn-DPDP increases tumor–pancreas contrast on delayed postinjection images (Figure 23-30). The imaging window for Mn-DPDP enhancement of the pancreas is several hours, and both breath-hold and non–breath-hold T1-weighted images may be used to acquire images of the pancreas after Mn-DPDP injection.

SPLEEN
Normal Spleen

The spleen is an intraperitoneal organ with a smooth serosal surface and is attached to the retroperitoneum by fatty ligaments containing its vascular pedicle. The spleen is a unique immunological organ with a large fractional blood content and relatively long T1 and T2 relaxation times. Consequently the spleen appears considerably lower in signal intensity than liver on conventional T1-weighted images and higher on T2-weighted images. The MR tissue characteristics of normal splenic tissue (hydrogen density, T1, T2, and chemical shift) are indistinguishable from the average tissue characteristics of cancer metastatic to the liver.[49,133] Vessels arborizing within the spleen cannot be traced beyond the central third. The infant spleen has a shorter T2 and longer T1 than the spleen of older children and adults, attributed to the smaller amount of white pulp in immature spleens. Thus the spleen may normally be isointense to liver on either T1- or T2-weighted images during the first year of life.[30]

Like MR images of the pancreas, images of the spleen are degraded by motion artifacts. Transmitted cardiac pulsation, bowel peristalsis, and respiratory excursion all contribute to the noise. Motion of the spleen itself during data acquisition can lead to phase displacement of signal arising from the spleen, artifactually reducing the spleen signal intensity and further degrading the image. Development of motion-suppression techniques has improved splenic imaging. These techniques include signal averaging, respiratory compensation, gradient-moment nulling, and breath-holding. Gradient-moment nulling (flow compensation) prevents phase displacement of splenic signal and provides a more accurate measure of spleen signal intensity on T2-weighted images.[84]

The low signal-to-noise ratio and poor contrast available with gradient-echo and other forms of fast imaging have led to the use of dynamic Gd chelate–enhanced imaging to evaluate the spleen. On fast T1-weighted images the normal spleen enhances in a heterogeneous, arciform, or serpentine fashion (Figure 23-31) during the first 30 to 60 sec after bolus administration of Gd chelate.[82,119] This enhancement pattern, found occasionally in CT, is far more frequent during MRI because of the

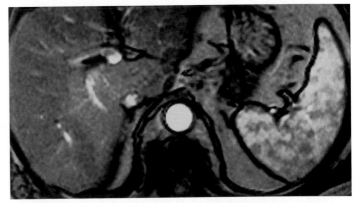

FIGURE 23-31   Normal splenic enhancement. FMP-SPGR (77/2.6/80) image immediately after bolus injection of 0.1 mmol/kg Gd chelate shows serpentine enhancement not apparent 15 sec later (not shown). Patient has fatty liver secondary to insulinoma.

tighter bolus of paramagnetic contrast administered rather than because of differences in pharmacokinetics between MR and CT contrast agents. The serpentine enhancement is thought to represent differing blood flow rates between splenic sinuses and splenic chords or between red pulp and white pulp.[119] After 60 sec the spleen has a uniformly increased signal intensity and is isointense to liver, maintaining more than twice the precontrast baseline signal intensity for at least 5 min but gradually returning toward baseline.[83]

Detection of Splenic Abnormalities

Unenhanced MRI is insensitive for detection of splenic abnormality. The relaxation times of most solid pathological tissue are prolonged relative to those of the liver. Because splenic relaxation times are similarly prolonged, conventional MRI often fails to detect abnormal tissue present in the spleen.[49] Additional difficulties are the variable size and shape of the spleen and the effects of motion and noise on images of the left upper quadrant.

Some factors, including necrosis, focally prolonging T2, and hemorrhage that shortens T1, promote detection of splenic abnormalities. Splenic iron overload, seen after multiple blood transfusions,[132,161] reduces the signal intensity of the spleen on T2-weighted and gradient-echo images. Because iron deposition occurs in reticuloendothelial system (RES) cells, abnormal tissue lacking RES appears as focal areas of higher signal intensity.

Intravenous administration of Gd chelates has been advocated to increase the sensitivity of MRI for detection of splenic pathology. Recognition that the normal splenic enhancement pattern is initially heterogeneous will avoid misinterpretation. Absence of early heterogeneous enhancement is abnormal but may reflect a "downstream" neoplastic or inflammatory process, especially in the pancreas or in the liver, rather than indicating disease in the spleen itself. However, it has been argued that diffuse infiltration of the spleen is excluded by detection of the normal enhancement.[18] Moreover, as discussed later, improved detection of focal lesions has been reported from dynamic use of Gd chelates.

An alternative strategy for evaluating the spleen is to use RES-targeted contrast agents. Superparamagnetic iron oxide (SPIO) particles are taken up by RES in the spleen and liver. By producing local distortion of the magnetic field, these particles reduce signal intensity, producing a map of normal RES function. Acting like transfusional iron overload, contrast agents of this type identify focal abnormalities as islands of undiminished signal intensity. Diffuse abnormalities are detected when the expected postcontrast loss of splenic signal does not occur. The first SPIO contrast agent, ferumoxides iv, was approved for marketing in the United States in 1996. The recommended 10 µmol/kg dose for liver imaging is likely to be too low for optimum detection of splenic disease.

Hematological Malignancy

Lymphoma is the most common malignancy involving the spleen. Spleen size is an unreliable indicator of involvement by lymphoma because reactive hyperplasia or congestion accounts for up to 30% of cases of splenomegaly in lymphoma patients.[126] Approximately one third of patients with Hodgkin's disease or non–Hodgkin's lymphoma have splenic involvement. Although splenic lymphoma is usually considered a diffuse disease, lymphoma often presents in the spleen with nodules that are visible on gross inspection. In Hodgkin's disease, nodules larger than 1 cm are present in 33% to 64% of involved spleens, and lymphomatous nodules larger than 5 mm were found in one third of splenectomies for non–Hodgkin's lymphoma.[1] Leukemic involvement of the spleen is almost always diffuse, with splenomegaly and prolonged T2; focal leukemic infiltration (chloroma) is very rare (Figure 23-32). Therefore MR evaluation of lymphoma and leukemia requires detection of both diffuse infiltration and focal lesions, and in distinguishing the latter from infarction, opportunistic infections, and extramedullary hematopoiesis (Figure 23-33).

Unfortunately, lymphoid tissues have similar MR tissue characteristics, whether or not cells are malignant.[95] Large lymphomatous masses involving the spleen and adjacent organs may occur. Focal splenic lesions have been detected, according to the principles discussed earlier, associated with necrosis, hemorrhage, iron overload, or perhaps fibrosis (Figure 23-34). Dynamic Gd images may show focal hypointense defects or merely nonspecific absence of early heterogeneous enhancement.

In patients with diffuse infiltration by lymphoma, neoplastic tissue with diminished or absent RES cells reduces the phagocytic capacity per unit volume of spleen. As a result, the signal loss after SPIO injection is less in infiltrated spleens than in normal spleens. Moreover, in patients with splenomegaly caused by passive congestion rather than neoplastic infiltration, phagocytic capacity is maintained. These spleens avidly take up iron particles and lose signal ac-

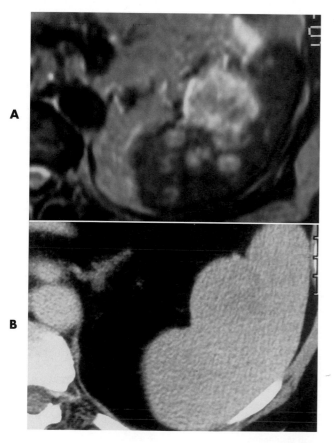

FIGURE 23-32 Acute leukemia. **A,** T2-weighted SE image (3000/80) shows multiple hyperintense lesions. **B,** Only the largest lesion is visible on contrast CT. Diagnosis of chloroma not histologically proved but suspected because of absence of infection and proven leukemic infiltration of other organs.

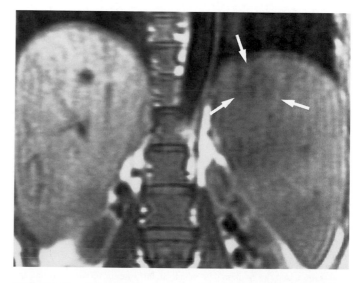

FIGURE 23-33 Polycythemia vera. Coronal T1-weighted image shows marked splenomegaly. Subtle lesion of mixed signal intensity *(arrows)* was subsequently proved by percutaneous biopsy to represent extramedullary hematopoiesis.

cordingly. In a small series, postcontrast signal loss permits differential diagnosis of patients with lymphomatous and benign splenomegaly[155] (Figure 23-35).

Metastases

Metastases to the spleen are uncommon except in advanced disease. However, discovery of a splenic metastasis sometimes is the only indication of disease recurrence or unresectability. Splenic metastases most commonly result from melanoma, but lung, breast, ovarian, and gastrointestinal primaries also metastasize to the spleen. Melanoma metastases can sometimes be diagnosed specifically because of homogeneous T1 shortening associated with tumor pigment, resulting in lesions that are T1 hyperintense to spleen (Figure 23-36). Both Gd chelate and SPIO contrast agents have been used to detect splenic metastases (Figures 23-37 and 23-38). Dynamic imaging should be used with Gd chelates because metastases that are initially hypointense may become isointense within 2 min of bolus administration.[82]

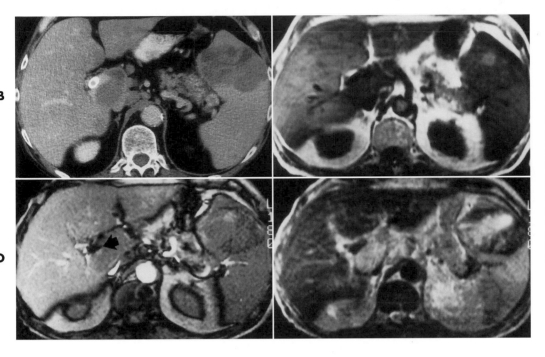

FIGURE 23-34   Hepatosplenic lesions of diffuse large cell lymphoma. **A,** CT scan shows a large low-attenuation splenic lesion anteriorly and a caudate liver lesion. Note metallic biliary endoprosthesis. **B** and **C,** T1-weighted SE (300/12) and FMP-SPGR (39/2.6/80 degrees) images show focal hemorrhage in the splenic lesion. **D,** In this T2-weighted SE image (3000/90) the splenic lesion is hypointense to spleen except for an extensive area of central necrosis. Note minimal image distortion associated with metallic biliary stent (*arrow* in **C**).

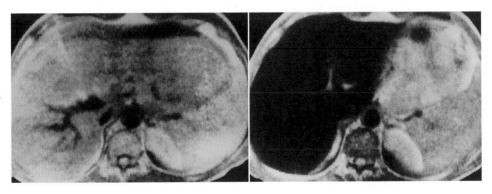

FIGURE 23-35   Iron oxide–enhanced detection of splenic lymphoma. **A,** SE (1500/42) image at 0.3 T shows normal splenic configuration and signal intensity. **B,** Same pulse sequence after administration of 40 μmol/kg of superparamagnetic iron oxide (AMI-25) shows marked hepatic signal loss. Diffuse infiltration by Hodgkin's disease prevents iron particle phagocytosis by the spleen, resulting in very little signal decrement compared with the unenhanced image. In benign splenomegaly, phagocytosis is preserved, resulting in marked splenic signal loss. (From reference 153.)

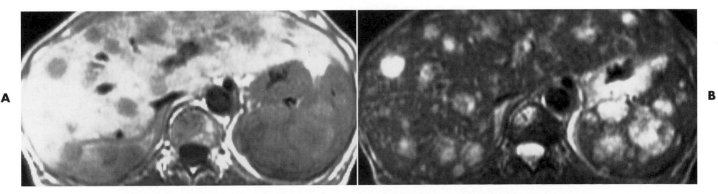

FIGURE 23-36   Melanoma metastatic to liver, spine, and spleen. **A,** SE T1-weighted (300/12) image shows that liver lesions are hypointense to liver, whereas splenic lesions are slightly hyperintense to spleen. **B,** On T2-weighted (3100/80) image, all of the lesions are hyperintense.

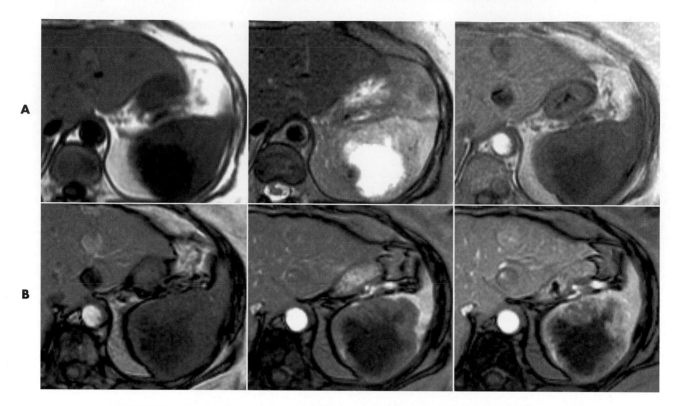

FIGURE 23-37   Ovarian carcinoma metastatic to spleen. **Row A,** SE T1-weighted (300/12), FSE T2-weighted (5000/104), and in-phase GRE (91/4.2 ms) images. These images show only the central necrotic part of the lesion. **Row B,** Dynamic opposed-phase GRE (88/2.6 ms) sequence, precontrast and during arterial and portal phases after injection of Gd chelate. Maximum tumor–spleen contrast is seen on the arterial-phase image because contrast material subsequently leaks into the tumor. In- and opposed-phase images perform similarly for splenic imaging because the spleen does not contain fat.

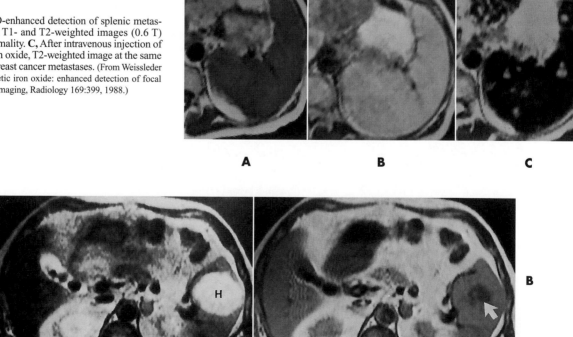

FIGURE 23-38   SPIO-enhanced detection of splenic metastases. **A** and **B,** Axial T1- and T2-weighted images (0.6 T) show no splenic abnormality. **C,** After intravenous injection of superparamagnetic iron oxide, T2-weighted image at the same level shows multiple breast cancer metastases. (From Weissleder R, et al: Superparamagnetic iron oxide: enhanced detection of focal splenic tumors with MR imaging, Radiology 169:399, 1988.)

A   **B**   **C**

FIGURE 23-39   Cavernous hemangioma of the spleen. **A,** SE (2000/100) image shows round hyperintense lesion *(H)* that is isointense to gallbladder bile. Low–signal intensity gallstones are present. **B,** On SE (2091/20) image, lesion is only slightly hyperintense. There is a central stellate low–signal intensity scar *(arrow).*

Benign Splenic Lesions

Cysts are the most common benign tumors of the spleen. These cysts may be congenital (true cysts, 20%) or traumatic (false cysts, 80%). Cysts may be multiple and should not be confused with abscesses, pseudocysts, and parasitic lesions. Cysts have smooth borders and homogeneous long T1 and very long T2 signal characteristics.

Splenic hemangiomas follow cysts as the second most common benign tumor in the spleen. These hemangiomas have MR features similar to hemangiomas elsewhere, with long T1 and distinctively long T2 (Figures 23-39 and 23-40). Therefore, on heavily T2-weighted images, hemangiomas, like cysts, are smoothly marginated, well-defined, homogeneous, and hyperintense relative to the surrounding spleen. As in the liver, giant hemangiomas in the spleen can be heterogeneous, with hemorrhage, thrombosis, fibrosis, and hemosiderin deposition.[71,112,153] Because of the relatively longer T2 of spleen compared with liver, splenic hemangiomas may be more difficult to recognize solely on the basis of high signal intensity on T2-weighted images. This finding has led to efforts to characterize splenic hemangiomas with injection of Gd chelates. In the largest series reported to date,[106] 19 of 22 splenic hemangiomas showed peripheral enhancement on dynamic enhanced images, whereas the others enhanced unevenly. Unlike hepatic hemangiomas, enhancement was less often nodular than ringlike and of variable thickness. Most of the lesions initially enhancing in the periphery subsequently filled in with contrast. Because enhancement of metastases and lymphomas to hyperintensity relative to spleen has not been reported, peripheral enhancement is likely to be a highly specific sign of benignity in patients evaluated for metastatic disease. Because of the highly selective nature of the available series, however, the sensitivity of peripheral enhancement has not been determined. Caution also should be exercised in diagnosis of patients who might have a pri-

mary malignancy because the MRI characteristics of few angiosarcomas have been described. Many splenic angiosarcomas present with focal internal hemorrhage, recognition of which should cast doubt on a diagnosis of splenic hemangioma.[45]

The third most common benign splenic tumor is the lymphangioma. The spleen may be involved as part of a diffuse abdominal lymphangiomatosis, or the spleen may be the primary site of involvement. In the cystic form the lesions appear as clusters of cysts (Figure 23-41). These clusters may imitate simple cysts, with homogeneously long T1 and long T2 values,[149] or may have varying signal intensity from protein content or hemorrhage.[25] Splenic lymphangiomas with tiny cysts are known; their MR appearance has not been studied.

Splenic infarcts usually arise as focal lesions because infarction of the entire spleen is rare. Total infarction can occur with torsion when the ligamentous attachments of the spleen are lax or incomplete. Infarcts occur most often in the blood dyscrasias, such as sickle-cell disease or myeloproliferative disorders, or in systemic embolism from endocarditis or septum defects. Only one third of infarcts are peripheral, wedge-shaped lesions; other configurations are multiple heterogeneous (42%) or massive (25%) lesions replacing normal splenic tissue.[8] Infarcts are visible on MR images most commonly in association with iron overload of the spleen, such as in patients with sickle-cell disease and lymphoma. In this setting the infarct appears as a zone of high signal intensity against the low–signal intensity background of iron-overloaded spleen. Focal areas of low and high signal reported on gradient-echo images presumably are related to hemorrhage.[54]

Hamartomas are benign focal splenic lesions consisting of normal splenic tissue without trabeculae or follicles.[146] Hamartomas are usually solid but may contain cysts and calcifications. Hamartomas have been reported to be isointense on T1-weighted images and hyperintense on T2-weighted images, with a characteristic prolonged enhancement after Gd chelate injection.[97,106]

Siderotic nodules, also called *Gamna-Gandy bodies,* are brown, organized foci of hemorrhage present in the spleen of patients with portal hypertension. The lesions appear as areas of low signal intensity and may be single or multiple. Signal loss is caused by hemosiderin deposition and is best seen in gradient-echo images, but it also may be seen on T2-weighted SE images, especially at high field strength. Because of the sensitivity to field inhomogeneity, MRI is more sensitive than CT or ultrasound in detecting these nodules[81,115] (Figure 23-42).

Gaucher's disease is a hereditary disorder caused by deficiency in the enzyme glucocerebrosidase resulting in accumulation of the glycolipid glucocerebroside in macrophages (Gaucher cells) of many organs, including the spleen. Because of marrow replacement, extramedullary hematopoiesis also occurs. These factors lead to massive splenomegaly, with focal lesions associated with collections of Gaucher cells, extramedullary hematopoiesis, infarction, and fibrosis.[55] Unless hemorrhagic, the focal lesions of Gaucher's disease are best seen on T2-weighted images, where their signal intensity can be either hypointense or hyperintense to surrounding tissue (Figure 23-43).

Sarcoidosis involves the spleen in 25% of cases, but imaging findings are encountered less frequently. There may be only splenomegaly, but occasionally the spleen contains numerous hypointense nodules

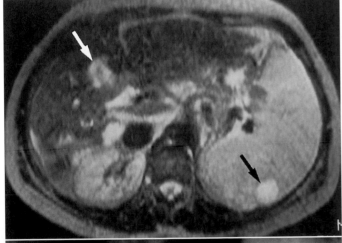
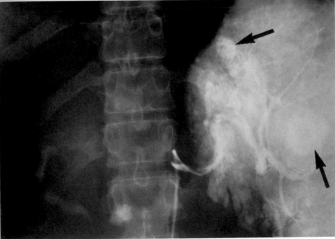

FIGURE 23-40 Cavernous hemangiomas. **A,** SE (2350/180) image shows hyperintense lesions *(arrows)* in liver and spleen. **B,** Selective splenic arteriogram shows multiple hypervascular splenic tumors *(arrows).*

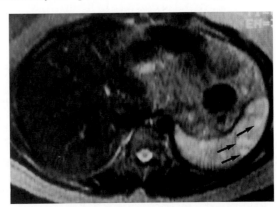

FIGURE 23-41 Lymphangiomatosis with splenic involvement. SE (2350/180) image shows multiple hyperintense foci, indicating lymphangiomatous cysts within the spleen. Other levels showed extensive retroperitoneal cysts and channels.

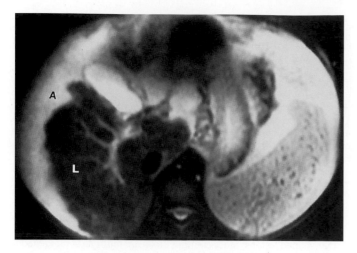

FIGURE 23-42 Advanced cirrhosis with siderotic nodules in the spleen. T2-weighted image (fat-saturation SE 2200/80) shows nodular, shrunken liver *(L)* surrounded by ascites *(A)*. The spleen contains multiple foci of low signal intensity from siderotic deposits (Gamna-Gandy bodies).

(Figure 23-44). These nodules may be visible discretely on either T1- or T2-weighted images, or they may confer a subtle mottled appearance.[66] Dynamic Gd imaging improves detection of these lesions, which do not enhance.[151]

Numerous infectious diseases can involve the spleen. Although bacterial abscesses can be encountered, opportunistic infections in immunocompromised hosts are being imaged more frequently. These include mycobacterial infections, fungal microabscesses, *Pneumocystis carinii* infection, and bacillary angiomatosis. In chronically ill patients, blood transfusions may make these lesions easier to detect because the overall splenic T2 is diminished. The MR appearance of *Candida* organism microabscesses has been described, consisting of multiple focal lesions relatively hyperintense to spleen (Figure 23-45), with improved detection after dynamic splenic enhancement with Gd chelate.[118]

Splenic Hemorrhage

Splenic hemorrhage can be either subcapsular or intraparenchymal. Subcapsular hematoma occurs most commonly as the result of trauma. Subcapsular hematomas appear as crescentic abnormalities immediately adjacent to splenic parenchyma. Like space-occupying hematomas elsewhere in the body, splenic subcapsular hematomas undergo a complex series of biochemical transformations that determine the

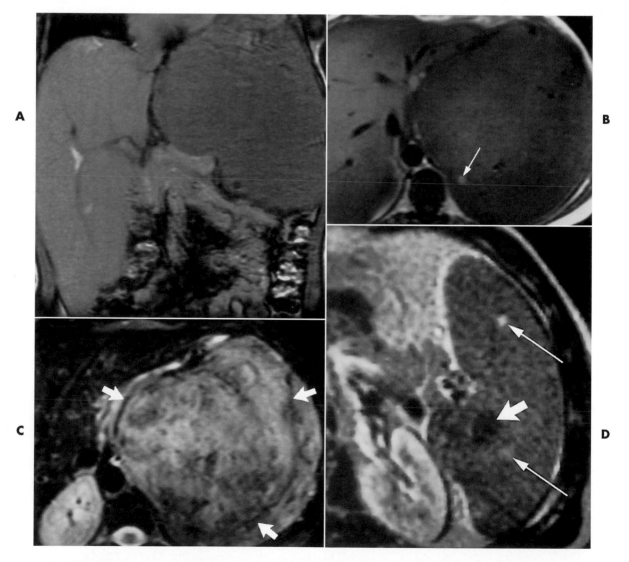

FIGURE 23-43 Gaucher's disease. Coronal GE (76/2.6/80 degrees) **(A)** and axial SE (350/12) T1-weighted **(B)** images show massive splenomegaly with a small medial focus of hemorrhage *(arrow* in **B)**. T2-weighted FSE (4500/104) image **(C)** shows large heterogeneous nodule *(arrows)*. Typical changes of Gaucher's disease with scarring were found at partial splenectomy. SE (3000/80) image **(D)** showing another case of Gaucher's disease, with both hypointense *(short arrow)* and hyperintense *(long arrows)* focal splenic lesions. Mild iron overload reduces splenic signal intensity.

imaging appearance as a function of time (see Bowel Wall Hematoma section). Parenchymal bleeding is often associated with tumors, infarcts, or coagulopathy. Even in trauma, parenchymal hemorrhage rarely presents as a space-occupying collection of extravasated blood. In splenic laceration, T1-weighted MR images show bright streaks of short T1 across the spleen (Figure 23-46). Usually there is associated hemorrhage outside the spleen.

ALIMENTARY TRACT

MRI is not the primary imaging modality for screening patients with suspected pathological conditions of the gastrointestinal (GI) tract. Except in the esophagus and rectum, there is no natural plane for sectioning the gut; bowel loops course into and out of any imaging section. In addition, spatial resolution of submillimeter magnitude is needed to image the characteristic mucosal patterns of malabsorption, early adenocarcinoma, or superficial ulceration. Barium fluoroscopy is an interactive, projective modality superior to MRI and CT in these respects, and it is the preferred imaging modality for detecting and characterizing mucosal abnormalities. Nevertheless, development of contrast materials, specialized pulse sequences, and local coil technology has gradually improved MRI of the GI tract. Wider use of this technology will undoubtedly lead to more frequent MRI of bowel pathology, both as an incidental finding and as the primary indication for the study.

Normal Anatomy

Signal is contributed to an MR image by the bowel mesentery, the bowel wall, and the luminal contents. The appearance of these structures and their contribution to the image depend on the technique used to perform the examination. The factors most important are the pulse sequence and whether T1 or T2 tissue differences are emphasized.

On SE images, individual loops of bowel may be demonstrated but are not sharply defined. The stomach is routinely visible. Gas in the lumen produces a signal void on all pulse sequences. Luminal fluid con-

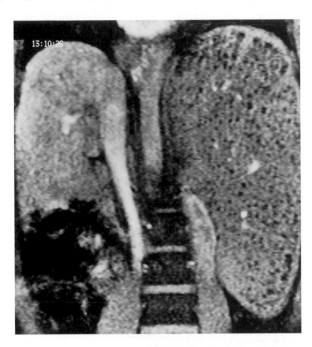

FIGURE 23-44   Splenic sarcoid. Coronal gradient-echo image (57/12/30) shows marked splenomegaly with myriad tiny foci of signal loss. (From reference 146.)

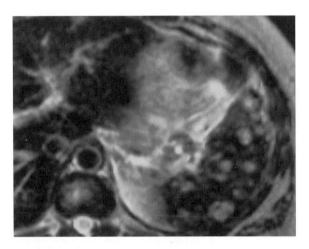

FIGURE 23-45   *Candida* organism microabscesses. T2-weighted image (2100/90) shows multiple hyperintense 1- to 2-cm focal splenic lesions. Lesions are well seen because splenic T2 is reduced by excess iron. (From reference 146.)

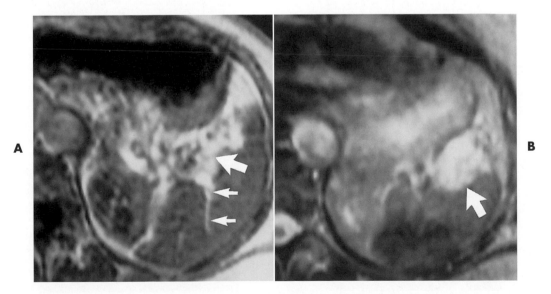

FIGURE 23-46   Splenic laceration. **A,** T1-weighted breath-hold image (MPGR 150/5/90 degrees) image shows straight linear hyperintense defect *(small arrows)* incompletely bisecting the spleen and extending medially into a hematoma *(large arrow)*. **B,** More cephalad T2-weighted (SE 3000/80) image reveals blood *(arrow)* anterior to the spleen.

tents, which are usually aqueous, have long-T1 and long-T2 tissue characteristics. Dietary products such as infant formula, green tea, and blueberry juice can result in T1 shortening. On T1-weighted images the gastric wall may be resolved as a region of signal intermediate between gastric fluid and surrounding fat. When a short-T1 oral contrast material is used, individual gastric folds often can be observed near the gastroesophageal junction, outlined by the high signal intensity of lumen contents. Individual jejunal folds can sometimes be demonstrated on breath-hold images. On fat-saturation T1-weighted images the bowel wall is hyperintense to surrounding fat and enhances moderately after intravenous Gd chelate. On breath-holding half-Fourier single-shot turbo spin echo (HASTE) and ultrafast (less than 100 ms) T2-weighted EPI, aqueous bowel contents are distinctly hyperintense to bowel wall,[14] but this difference is difficult to appreciate on conventional T2-weighted images because of motion-associated blurring. Analysis of motion artifacts suggests that aqueous bowel contents contribute significantly to overall image noise.[140] This observation has led some centers to use pharmacological suppression of peristalsis with glucagon or butylscopolamine bromide routinely for abdominal and pelvic MRI.

Contrast Agents for the Gastrointestinal Tract

An orally administered material was the first MR contrast agent to be used in a human.[16] Dozens of substances have been proposed as GI tract MR contrast agents.[102] However, none has been universally adopted as meeting the complex requirements for safety, effectiveness, patient acceptance, and moderate cost. Moreover, the regulatory processes of various countries have lead to different agents being commercially available in Europe, Japan, and the United States.

GI tract contrast agents are classified as positive or negative, depending on whether they are intended to increase or decrease signal intensity of bowel lumen contents relative to bowel wall. Most oral agents for CT are positive contrast agents. Positive MR contrast agents include gadopentetate dimeglumine[65] and ferric ammonium citrate.[101,154] Perflubron (perfluoro-octyl bromide; see later discussion), dense barium[9] or barium-antacid mixtures,[31] and most superparamagnetic iron oxide particles[50,7] are negative contrast agents (Figure 23-47). The terminology is complicated by the need to specify the pulse sequence used. Many substances that shorten both the T1 and T2 of water are mixed positive and negative agents, bright on T1 and dark on T2. Examples are paramagnetic substances like manganese chloride,[15] diamagnetic clay minerals,[85] and ultrasmall preparations of superparamagnetic iron oxides.[111] Water and other aqueous materials may be regarded as positive contrast agents on T2-weighted images, but they contribute excessive noise unless used in conjunction with ultrafast imaging[51] (Figure 23-48).

The most important function of a GI tract contrast agent is to mark the bowel. Bowel marking delineates anatomical landmarks, such as the pancreatic head, and avoids confusing bowel loops for lymphadenopathy or mesenteric masses. Bowel distension also is desirable because it permits assessment of bowel wall thickness. An additional potential benefit of negative agents on T2-weighted images is reduced overall noise contributed by high–signal intensity fluid,[56] but this reduction may be offset by changes in respiration and peristalsis caused by the sensation of fullness. Rigorous clinical proof is lacking that any oral contrast material permits detection of conditions not otherwise diagnosable. This very difficult problem has slowed the regulatory approval of oral MR contrast agents and led to off-label local use of many common substances as oral MR contrast agents.[68]

In 1995 perflubron became the first oral MR contrast material approved for marketing in the United States. This perfluorocarbon is a neat (chemically homogeneous) liquid that contains no hydrogen atoms. When perflubron replaces bowel contents, the gut is distended and the lumen has no signal on either T1- or T2-weighted images[77] (Figure 23-49). Rapid intestinal transit of perflubron makes optimum gastric distension short-lived (less than 10 min) but confers an advantage for eval-

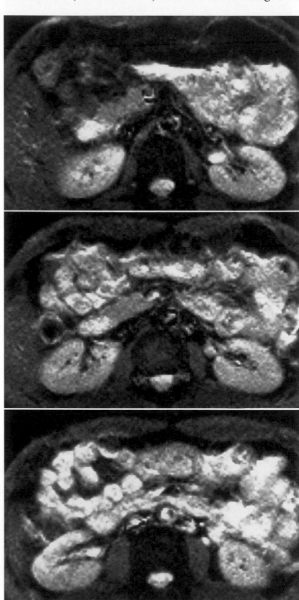

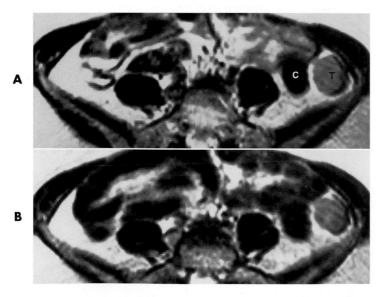

FIGURE 23-47 Mesenteric lymphoma defined by iron oxide particle oral contrast agent (OMP, Nycomed). **A,** On T2-weighted FSE image, tumor *(T)* is isointense to fluid-filled small bowel loops. *C,* Descending colon. **B,** After oral contrast, small bowel loops have low signal intensity, permitting easier identification of the nonbowel nature of the mass.

FIGURE 23-48 Aqueous oral contrast with ultrafast imaging. Two-shot EPIs through the pancreas and duodenum in a normal subject, showing the bright-bowel CT-like effect produced by water when motion is limited by ultrafast image acquisition.

uating pelvic pathology and suspected small bowel obstruction.[3] Significant cost limits acceptance of perflubron.

Two years after the introduction of perflubron the superparamagnetic iron oxide, ferumoxil oral suspension, became the second oral MR contrast agent marketed in the United States. Like perflubron, ferumoxil is a negative contrast agent on both T1- and T2-weighted pulse sequences. As a suspension of iron particles, ferumoxil mixes with gut contents, and its transit time is slower than that of perflubron. During clinical trials, ferumoxil-enhanced images were shown to be competitive with oral contrast CT for detecting abnormalities of the GI tract.[63] It is too soon to determine whether the lower cost of ferumoxil will result in widespread use.

It is expected that GI MR contrast agents representing several different classes just discussed will become available for clinical use during the next few years, and oral contrast administration will gradually become routine. The choice of which agent to use may have to be tailored to the individual clinical presentation.

Gastrointestinal Tract Neoplasms

Ordinarily, bowel tumors must attain considerable size[124] or produce gross wall thickening[157] before they can be identified on MR scans (Figure 23-50). MRI is not a reliable screening test for mucosal alimentary tract cancers. Moreover, complete screening of the entire abdomen and pelvis is time consuming unless performed entirely with fast scanning. Virtual colonoscopy using interior surface display of thin-section MR images of the Gd-distended colon has been proposed but is not yet clinically validated.[117]

Most tumors of the bowel are of moderately long T1 and T2 and thus are difficult to distinguish from bowel wall (Figures 23-51 and 23-52). Exceptions are lipomas, with characteristic short T1 of fat; melanoma metastases (Figure 23-53), which sometimes have T1 shortening from tumor pigments; and some very desmoplastic infiltrating cancers (Figure 23-54). After intravenous administration of Gd chelates, most bowel tumors exhibit heterogeneous enhancement.[129]

Staging of colorectal mucosal tumors involves determining depth of invasion, involvement of local and regional lymph nodes, and detecting remote metastases, especially to the liver. The recent Radiology Diagnostic Oncology Group (RDOG) multicenter trial was conducted to determine the accuracy of MRI with CT for staging colorectal carcinoma, using surgical stage as the gold standard.[163] In this study, conducted over several years, contrast-enhanced CT was compared with

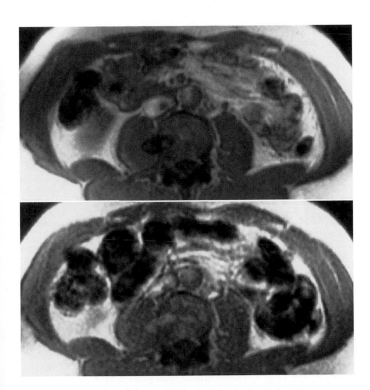

FIGURE 23-49   Perflubron oral contrast agent. T1-weighted breath-hold gradient-echo images before *(top)* and after *(bottom)* contrast ingestion. There is uniform small bowel darkening without distortion of the surrounding tissues.

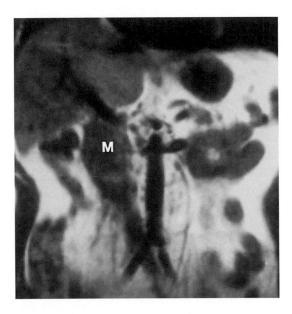

FIGURE 23-51   Duodenal adenocarcinoma. Coronal T1-weighted image at the level of the porta hepatis and descending duodenum demonstrates an oblong mass *(M)* with major axis in the cephalocaudal dimension.

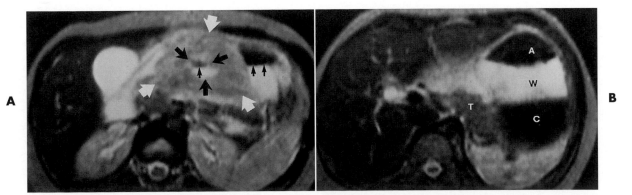

FIGURE 23-50   Gastric outlet obstruction from ulcerating gastric lymphoma. **A,** T2-weighted image (SE 2000/80) shows large gastric mass *(white arrows)* with central ulceration *(large black arrows)*. Air-fluid level extends into ulcer crater *(small black arrows)*. **B,** Lesion obstructs the gastric fundus, where air *(A)*, aqueous fluid *(W)*, and sedimented barium sulfate *(C)* form three distinct layers. A nodule of tumor *(T)* is outlined by the aqueous fluid and barium. (Courtesy F. Hoffer, Boston.)

unenhanced MRI images obtained with a body coil. The RDOG trial showed that neither MRI nor CT accurately predicts the presence of transmural disease, and neither can detect the relatively frequent occurrence of tumor in normal-sized lymph nodes. However, some have argued that Gd contrast enhancement used with fat-saturated T1-weighted images makes transmural invasion easier to detect,[127] so a final answer on the utility of body-coil MRI in staging colorectal cancer remains unattainable.

About one third of colorectal cancers occur in the rectum. Risk of rectal carcinoma recurrence is directly related to the depth of tumor invasion (Table 23-2). Although T1 and T2 tumors recur locally with a frequency of 5% to 10%, the local recurrence rate after transmural invasion is 25%.[94] Patients with transmural disease are candidates for

preoperative therapy, such as radiation, to shrink the extent of disease, but clinical staging is inaccurate at predicting patients who would benefit. Unfortunately, results of the recent RDOG trial found body-coil MRI even less effective than CT in predicting transmural invasion in rectal carcinoma.[163]

Use of an endorectal local coil offers the best possibility of improved spatial resolution. In analogy with endorectal coil imaging of the prostate, better spatial resolution offers the possibility of improved definition of the tumor and of local structures in relation to it. Initial attempts to use a prostate coil in patients with rectal carcinoma were disappointing because the balloon fixation device tended to efface the tumor. More recently a purpose-built soft endorectal coil has been marketed specifically for rectal cancer staging, and preliminary results of its use are encouraging.

In high-resolution endorectal coil imaging, both T2-weighted FSE images and T1-weighted images are obtained. T2-weighted images display the annular layers of the rectal wall. T1-weighted images show the interface between muscular bowel wall and fat and are best suited for showing extramural tumor and lymph nodes.[116] On T2-weighted images the high signal intensity inner layer represents lumen fluid and mucus. Surrounding this layer is a low signal associated with mucosa and muscularis mucosa, then a high–signal intensity submucosa and low–signal intensity muscularis propria. Beyond the rectal wall is perirectal fat, normally seen as high signal intensity on FSE images. Disruption of the mural structures by intermediate–signal intensity rectal carcinoma has been found to correlate well with histopathological depth of invasion (T stage) determined at surgery (Figure 23-55).

The ability of MRI to characterize presacral masses after anteroposterior resection for rectosigmoid carcinoma has been the subject of numerous studies and reports. Initially it was hoped that the prolonged T2 associated with highly cellular tumor would differentiate tumor re-

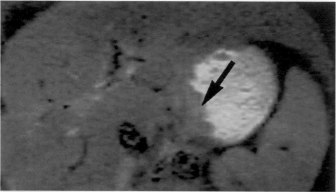

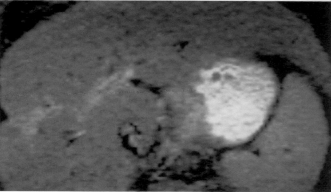

FIGURE 23-52 Gastric carcinoma. Single-shot SE *(top)* and STIR *(bottom)* EPIs show tumor *(arrow)* at the gastroesophageal junction. Orally administered dilute barium suspension used as "thick water" provides gastric distension and improves contrast between tumor and lumen contents.

Table 23-2   TNM Staging System for Rectal Carcinoma

STAGE	LEVEL OF INVOLVEMENT
Tumor	
T1	Limited to mucosa and submucosa
T2	Extension into but not through muscularis propria
T3	Invasion of perirectal fat
T4	Invasion of adjacent structures
Nodes	
N0	No involved lymph nodes
N1	Fewer than four regional nodes positive for tumor
N2	More than four regional nodes positive for tumor
N3	Central nodes positive for tumor metastases
Metastases	
M0	No metastases
M1	Distant metastases

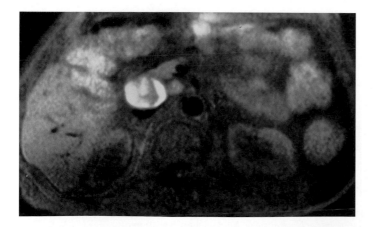

FIGURE 23-53 Peripancreatic metastasis from melanoma. Fat-saturation T1-weighted image shows markedly hyperintense mass obscuring the pancreatic head.

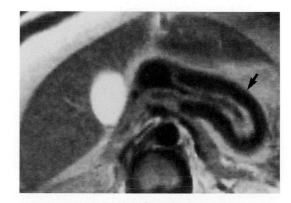

FIGURE 23-54 Infiltrating gastric carcinoma. SE 2000/60 image shows diffuse concentric thickening of the gastric wall *(arrow)* with short T2 caused by fibrotic reaction induced by the tumor. (From reference 157.)

currence from benign fibrosis.[92] MRI is now known to be limited in this capacity. Immature fibrous tissue during at least the first 6 months can have a long T2 and can enhance with intravenous Gd chelates for 1 year after surgery.[127] Moreover, zones of nonneoplastic inflammation and edema can persist for much longer periods, and tumor recurrence may be as dark as fibrosis on T2-weighted images.[26] Serial MR studies showing a previously short T2 area developing long T2 characteristics are the most specific finding in evaluating a presacral mass for rectosigmoid carcinoma recurrence. In patients with presacral pain or a rounded presacral mass, tumor recurrence should be suspected regardless of the MR tissue characteristics.

The most significant contribution made by MRI in the evaluation of patients with bowel tumors is in searching for remote disease. MRI is a sensitive noninvasive test for metastatic deposits in the liver and provides an effective means of distinguishing metastases from cavernous hemangioma (see Chapter 24).

Inflammatory Diseases of the Bowel

Inflammation of the bowel can be the result of primary bowel abnormalities or secondary involvement, as in pancreatitis or cholecystitis. Increased thickness and rigidity of the bowel wall and changes in the mesenteric, retroperitoneal, omental, or perirectal fat suggest the presence of inflammation.

Several strategies for obtaining images of bowel-wall inflammation have been suggested. One approach uses an oral or rectal contrast material to distend the bowel lumen. If a T1-shortening agent is used, then T1-weighted images show low-signal bowel wall distinguished between bright lumen and bright fat (Figure 23-56). With this approach, suspected inflammation of the perirectal fat appears as reduced signal and can be confirmed by detecting abnormal increased signal intensity with fat-saturated T2-weighted images.

An alternative approach is to use intravenous enhancement with Gd chelate to detect and stage bowel-wall inflammation. Focally excessive enhancement of the bowel is best appreciated on fat-saturated T1-weighted images, which also show enhancement of the extramural fat (Figure 23-57). Several studies have reported successful staging of inflammatory bowel disease using this approach.[128,130,159] In the colon, intense submucosal or transmural enhancement occurs in Crohn's disease, whereas ulcerative colitis tends to exhibit sparing of a thin margin of submucosa parallel to the markedly hyperintense inflamed mucosa. Severity of disease has been correlated with the percent of contrast en-

hancement. With this strategy, marking of bowel lumen with a positive (T1-shortening) contrast agent would be undesirable because the lumen contents might obscure the degree of enhancement in the bowel wall. Precontrast imaging remains important because ischemia can produce bowel-wall thickening while prolonging T1 relaxation time[41] (Figure 23-58).

MRI has been shown to be a useful technique for evaluating perianal fistulas and abscesses, such as occur as a complication of Crohn's disease.[74,46] Reliable demonstration of these lesions in multiple planes, using external devices, and without ionizing radiation are important features unique to MRI. FSE T2-weighted imaging is performed in both axial and coronal planes; fat saturation helps to distinguish fluid from perirectal fat. T1-weighted images are obtained to identify anatomical features[5,59] (Figure 23-59). Both body and pelvic phased-array coils have been used successfully. Some authors recommend insertion of a plastic enema tip to distend the lumen. Large matrices, at least 256 × 256 pixels, and sections no more than 5-mm thick are recommended to detect perianal fistulas and abscesses.

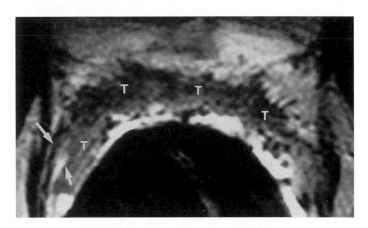

FIGURE 23-55   Endoluminal coil imaging of rectal carcinoma. Axial T2-weighted image (fat-saturation FSE 4000/144, 3-mm thickness) shows marked thickening of the mucosal layer by tumor *(T)*. Anteriorly the high–signal intensity submucosa *(short arrow)* and low–signal intensity muscularis propria *(long arrow)* are disrupted, confirming transmural invasion by this T3 lesion. (From reference 116.)

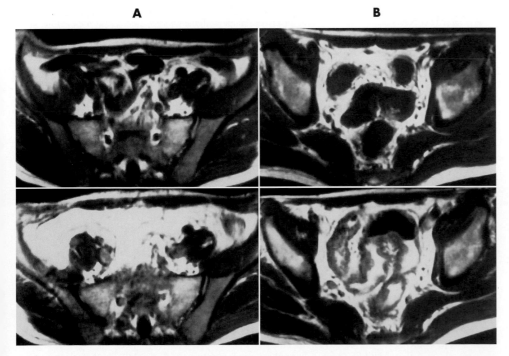

FIGURE 23-56   Gd-DTPA oral contrast agent in a patient with ulcerative colitis. **A** and **B,** T1-weighted images through the pelvis before contrast. **C** and **D,** After gadopentetate dimeglumine/mannitol administration, both the small bowel and colon are distended with bright bowel contrast. Normal small bowel wall is thin and almost imperceptible **(C)**, whereas colon wall in thickened by inflammation **(D)**. Scopolamine was given to reduce peristalsis. (Courtesy M. Laniado, Tubingen.)

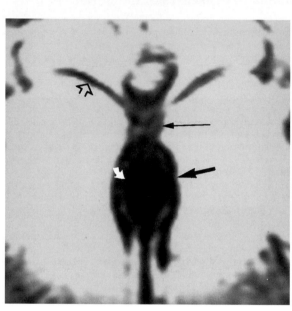

FIGURE 23-57 Periduodenal inflammation enhanced by Gd chelate injection. **A,** Precontrast T1-weighted image shows thick, indistinct wall of descending duodenum *(D)*. **B,** Postcontrast fat-saturation T1-weighted image shows enhancement of the duodenal wall and surrounding tissues *(arrow)*. An inflamed cystic duct remnant was found at surgery.

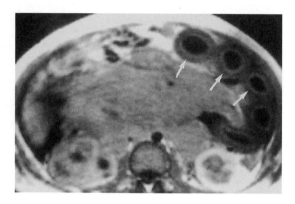

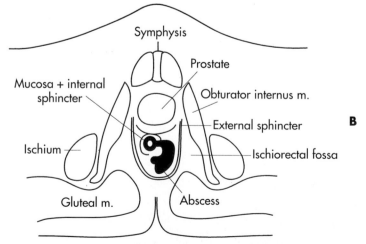

FIGURE 23-58 Small bowel ischemia. On this T1-weighted image, several segments of the small bowel are dilated and have thickened walls *(arrows)*. The mucosa of the affected segments has high signal intensity. A large lymphomatous mass obstructs the mesenteric veins. (Courtesy H.I. Goldberg, San Francisco.)

FIGURE 23-59 Anatomy of the anus. Coronal T1-weighted image of a 50-year-old woman without related complaints. The levator ani muscles *(open arrow)* form an inverted triangle with the puborectalis muscle *(thin arrow)* at its apex, below which the external anal sphincter *(thick arrow)* arises to surround the intersphincteric space and the internal sphincter *(curved white arrow)*. The intersphincteric space contains thin strands of longitudinal muscle fibers. The ischiorectal fossa is lateral and inferior to the levator ani muscles. The supralevator space lies superiorly.

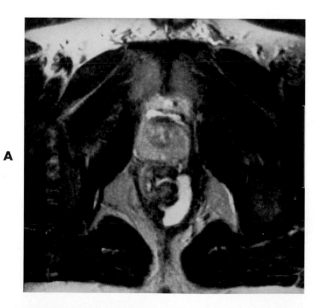

FIGURE 23-60 Intersphincteric perianal fistula. **A,** Axial SE (2500/90) multi-coil image shows a fistula with a long T2 value fistula extending from the anal canal through the internal sphincter into the intersphincteric space. **B,** Line drawing indicates the anatomy in this case. (From Skalej M, et al: Magnetic resonance imaging in perianal Crohn's disease, Dtsch Med Wschr 118:1791, 1993.)

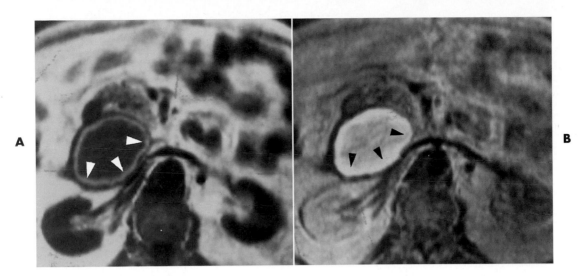

FIGURE 23-61 Duodenal hematoma. SE (310/20) **(A)** and SE (2350/60) **(B)** images show a round mass in the wall of the duodenum. The concentric hyperintense short T1 ring *(arrowheads)* permitted diagnosis of hematoma not obvious from clinical history. The lesion gradually diminished to complete resolution. (From reference 47.)

On fat-saturation T2-weighted images, fistulas and abscesses appear as hyperintense linear or round structures in the perirectal fat or muscle. Fistulas communicate with the lumen and pass to the skin, whereas sinus tracts retain no enteric communication, and abscesses are fluid collections that may have no cutaneous communication. A fistula may stay limited to the plane between the internal and external anal sphincters (intersphincteric) (Figure 23-60), penetrate through the external sphincter into the ischiorectal fossa (transsphincteric), arch across the levator into the ischiorectal fossa (suprasphincteric), or extend from the rectum to the perianal skin with or without penetrating the sphincter mechanism (extrasphincteric). Abscesses may form in the ischiorectal fossa, supralevator space, or levator ani muscle itself. In equivocal cases, fat-saturated T1-weighted images after Gd chelate enhancement can help to distinguish inflamed soft tissue from liquefied abscess. Preoperative staging of fistula-in-ano as provided by MRI can effectively guide treatment, avoiding, for example, iatrogenic conversion of a suprasphincteric fistula into an extrasphincteric one, which usually then requires a temporary colostomy.[100]

Bowel Wall Hematoma

Hemorrhage into the bowel wall appears similar to intramuscular hemorrhage elsewhere.[47,48] When the hematoma forms a space-occupying mass, the appearance undergoes a characteristic evolution to assume a distinctive appearance because of magnetically active iron-containing hemoglobin degradation products. In the acute period the hematoma appears as a typical aqueous material with high protein content, with a long T2 and intermediate T1. Over days, the T1 falls as hemoglobin is oxidized to methemoglobin within the mass. There may be a fluid-fluid level (with short-T1, short-T2 material dependent), or there may be bright streaks. Over several weeks, the short-T1 material coalesces at the periphery to form a bright ring around the lesion. Often the bright ring is itself rimmed by a pseudocapsule with very low effective T2 that has been attributed to hemosiderin taken up in phagocytes (Figure 23-61). On high-field systems (1 T and above) the center of an early hematoma is intensely dark, an effect seen on intermediate systems using gradient-echo pulse sequences. Because intraabdominal hemorrhage may present as an occult mass without clear history of trauma or coagulopathy, this MR appearance can be valuable in characterizing the lesion and distinguishing it from neoplasm. When a subacute hematoma is recognized, evidence of other injuries should be sought on the images.

REFERENCES

1. Ahmann DL, Kiely JM, Harrison EG, et al: Malignant lymphoma of the spleen: a review of 49 cases in which the diagnosis was made at splenectomy, Cancer 19:461, 1966.
2. Albertini RG, di Girolamo M, Cardone M, et al: Magnetic resonance in gallbladder carcinoma: its diagnostic reliability, Radiol Med (Torino) 87:96, 1994.
3. Anderson CM, Brown JJ, Balfe DM, et al: MR imaging of Crohn disease: use of perflubron as a gastrointestinal contrast agent, J Magn Reson Imaging 4:491, 1994.
4. Angeli E, Vanzulli A, Castrucci M, et al: Value of abdominal sonography and MR imaging at 0.5 T in preoperative detection of pancreatic insulinoma: a comparison with dynamic CT and angiography, Abdom Imaging 22:295, 1997.
5. Aronson MP, Lee RA, and Berquist TH: Anatomy of anal sphincters and related structures in continent women studied with magnetic resonance imaging, Obstet Gynecol 76:846, 1990.
6. Axelrod L: Insulinoma: cost-effective care in patients with a rare disease, Ann Intern Med 123:311, 1995.
7. Bach-Gansmo T, Dupas B, Gayet-Delacroix M, et al: Abdominal MRI using a negative contrast agent, Br J Radiol 66:420, 1993.
8. Balcar I, Seltzer SE, Davis S, et al: CT patterns of splenic infarction: a clinical and experimental study, Radiology 151:723, 1984.
9. Ballinger JR, and Ros PR: High density barium sulfate suspension for MRI: optimization of concentration for bowel opacification, Magn Reson Imaging 10:637, 1992.
10. Balthazar EJ, Robinson DL, Megibow AJ, et al: Acute pancreatitis: value of CT in establishing prognosis, Radiology 174:331, 1990.
11. Barish MA, Yucel EK, Soto JA, et al: MR cholangiography: efficacy of three-dimensional turbo spin-echo technique, Am J Roentgenol 165:295, 1995.
12. Baron RL, Shuman WP, and Lee SP: MR appearance of gallstones in vitro at 1.5 T: correlation with chemical composition, Am J Roentgenol 153:497, 1989.
13. Baron RL, Campbell WL, and Dodd GD III: Peribiliary cysts associated with severe liver disease: imaging-pathologic correlation, Am J Roentgenol 162:631, 1994.
14. Beall DP, and Regan F: MRI of bowel obstruction using the HASTE sequence, J Comput Assist Tomogr 20:823, 1996.
15. Bernardino ME, Weinreb JC, Mitchell DG, et al: Safety and optimum concentration of a manganese chloride-based oral MR contrast agent, J Magn Reson Imaging 4:872, 1994.
16. Bottomley PA, Hardy CJ, Argersinger RE, et al: A review of 1H nuclear magnetic resonance relaxation in pathology: are T1 and T2 diagnostic? Med Phys 14:1, 1987.
17. Bret PM, Reinhold C, Taourel P, et al: Pancreas divisum: evaluation with MR cholangiopancreatography, Radiology 199:99, 1996.
18. Brown ED, and Semelka RC: Magnetic resonance imaging of the spleen and pancreas, Top Magn Reson Imaging 7:82, 1995.
19. Buetow PC, Buck JL, Pantongrag-Brown L, et al: Biliary cystadenoma and cystadenocarcinoma: clinical-imaging-pathologic correlation with emphasis on the importance of ovarian stroma, Radiology 196:805, 1995.
20. Buetow PC, Buck JL, Pantongrag-Brown L, et al: Solid and papillary epithelial neoplasm of the pancreas: imaging-pathologic correlation on 56 cases, Radiology 199:707, 1996.
21. Buff BL, Zuo C, Jenkins RL, et al: Steps in the evolution of MR cholangiography, Radiology 197(P):510, 1995.
22. Choyke PL, Glenn GM, Walther MM, et al: von Hippel-Lindau disease: genetic, clinical, and imaging features, Radiology 194:629, 1995.
23. Clemens JA, and Cameron JL: The pathogenesis of acute pancreatitis. In Carter DC, and Warshaw AL, eds: Pancreatitis, Edinburgh, 1989, Churchill Livingstone.
24. Curati WL, Halevy A, Gibson RN, et al: Ultrasound, CT, and MRI comparison in primary and secondary tumors of the liver, Gastrointest Radiol 13:123, 1988.
25. Cutillo DP, Swayne LC, Cucco J, et al: CT and MR imaging in cystic abdominal lymphangiomatosis, J Comput Assist Tomogr 13:534, 1989.
26. de Lange EE, Fechner RE, and Wanebo HJ: Suspected recurrent rectosigmoid carcinoma after abdominoperineal resection: MR imaging and histopathologic findings, Radiology 170:323, 1989.
27. Demachi H, Matsui O, Hoshiba K, et al: Dynamic MRI using a surface coil in chronic cholecystitis and gallbladder carcinoma: radiologic and histopathologic correlation, J Comput Assist Tomogr 21:643, 1997.

28. Demas BE, Hricak H, Moseley M, et al: Gallbladder bile: an experimental study in dogs using MR imaging and proton MR spectroscopy, Radiology 157:453, 1985.

29. Dohke M, Watanabe Y, Saga T, et al: High-resolution MR cholangiopancreatography, Radiology 197(P):513, 1995.

30. Donnelly LF, Emery KH, Bove KE, et al: Normal changes in the MR appearance of the spleen during early childhood, Am J Roentgenol 166(3):635, 1996.

31. Ernst O, Sergent G, and L'Hermine C: Oral administration of a low-cost negative contrast agent: a three-year experience in routine practice, J Magn Reson Imaging 7:495, 1997.

32. Fernandez MP, Bernadino ME, Neylan JF, et al: Diagnosis of pancreatic transplant dysfunction: value of gadopentetate dimeglumine-enhanced MR imaging, Am J Roentgenol 156:1171, 1991.

33. Fernandez-del Castillo C, and Warshaw AL: Laparoscopy for staging in pancreatic carcinoma, Surg Oncol 2(S)1:25, 1993.

34. Fernandes-del Castillo C, and Warshaw AL: Cystic tumors of the pancreas, Surg Clin North Am 75:1001, 1995.

35. Ferrozzi F, Bova D, Campodonico F, et al: Cystic fibrosis: MR assessment of pancreatic damage, Radiology 198:875, 1996.

36. Gabata T, Matsui O, Kadoya M, et al: Small pancreatic adenocarcinomas: efficacy of MR imaging with fat suppression and gadolinium enhancement, Radiology 193:683, 1994.

37. Gehl HB, Vorwerk D, Klose KC, et al: Pancreatic enhancement after low-dose infusion of Mn-DPDP, Radiology 180:337, 1991.

38. Gilbeau J-P, Poncelet V, Libon E, et al: The density, contour, and thickness of the pancreas in diabetics: CT findings in 57 patients, Am J Roentgenol 159:527, 1992.

39. Girard MJ, Hahn PF, Saini S, et al: Wallstent metallic biliary endoprosthesis: MR imaging characteristics, Radiology 184:874, 1992.

40. Gohde SC, Toth J, Krestin GP, et al: Dynamic contrast-enhanced FMPSPGR of the pancreas: impact on diagnostic performance, Am J Roentgenol 168:689, 1997.

41. Picanza J: Transrectal coil moves MR ahead in GI tract, Radiol Today 7:1, 1990.

42. Gomori JM, Grossman RI, and Drott HR: MR relaxation times and iron content of thalassemic spleens: an in vitro study, Am J Roentgenol 150:567, 1988.

43. Guibaud L, Bret PM, Reinhold C, et al: Diagnosis of choledocholithiasis: value of MR cholangiography, Am J Roentgenol 163:847, 1994.

44. Guibaud L, Bret PM, Reinhold C, et al: Bile duct obstruction and choledocholithiasis: diagnosis with MR cholangiography, Radiology 197:109, 1995.

45. Ha HK, Kim HH, Kim BK, et al: Primary angiosarcoma of spleen: CT and MR imaging, Acta Radiol 35:455, 1994.

46. Haggett PJ, Moore NR, Shearman JD, et al: Pelvic and perineal complications of Crohn's disease: assessment using magnetic resonance imaging, Gut 36:407, 1995.

47. Hahn PF, Stark DD, Vici L-G, et al: Duodenal hematoma: the ring sign in MR imaging, Radiology 159:379, 1986.

48. Hahn PF, Saini S, Stark DD, et al: Intraabdominal hematoma: the concentric ring sign in MR imaging, Am J Roentgenol 148:115, 1987.

49. Hahn PF, Weissleder R, Stark DD, et al: MR imaging of focal splenic tumors, Am J Roentgenol 150:823, 1988.

50. Hahn PF, Stark DD, Lewis JM, et al: First clinical trial of a new superparamagnetic iron oxide for use as an oral gastrointestinal MR contrast agent, Radiology 175:695, 1990.

51. Hahn PF, Saini S, Cohen MS, et al: An aqueous gastrointestinal contrast agent for use in echo-planar MR imaging, Magn Reson Med 25:380, 1992.

52. Hahn PF, Saini S, Goldberg MA, et al: Echo-planar MR imaging of abdominal neuroendocrine tumors, Radiology 189(P):282, 1993.

53. Hall-Craggs MA, Allen CM, Owens CM, et al: MR cholangiography: clinical evaluation in 40 cases, Radiology 189:423, 1993.

54. Hess CF, Griebel J, Schmiedl U, et al: Focal lesions of the spleen: preliminary results with fast MR imaging at 1.5T, J Comput Assist Tomogr 12:569, 1988.

55. Hill SC, Damaska BM, Ling A, et al: Gaucher disease: abdominal MR imaging findings in 46 patients, Radiology 184:561, 1992.

56. Hirohashi S, Hirohashi R, Uchida H, et al: MR cholangiopancreatography and MR urography: improved enhancement with a negative oral contrast agent, Radiology 203:281, 1997.

57. Hirohashi S, Hirohashi R, Uchida H, et al: Pancreatitis: evaluation with MR cholangiopancreatography in children, Radiology 203:411, 1997.

58. Hricak H, Filly RA, Margulis AR, et al: Work in progress: nuclear magnetic resonance imaging of the gallbladder, Radiology 147:481, 1983.

59. Hussain SM, Stoker J, and LamÈris JS: Anal sphincter complex: endoanal MR imaging of normal anatomy, Radiology 197:671, 1995.

60. Ichikawa T, Haradome H, Hachiya J, et al: Pancreatic ductal adenocarcinoma: preoperative assessment with helical CT versus dynamic MR imaging, Radiology 202:655, 1997.

61. Irie H, Honda H, Kaneko K, et al: Comparison of helical CT and MR imaging in detecting and staging small pancreatic adenocarcinoma, Abdom Imaging 22:429, 1997.

62. Ishizaki Y, Wakayama T, Okada Y, et al: Magnetic resonance cholangiography for evaluation of obstructive jaundice, Am J Gastroenterol 88:2072, 1993.

63. Johnson WK, Stoupis C, Torres GM, et al: Superparamagnetic iron oxide (SPIO) as an oral contrast agent in gastrointestinal (GI) magnetic resonance imaging (MRI): comparison with state-of-the-art computed tomography (CT), Magn Reson Imaging 14:43, 1996.

64. Johnston DL, Rice L, Vick GW III, et al: Assessment of tissue iron overload by nuclear magnetic resonance imaging, Am J Med 87:40, 1989.

65. Kaminsky S, Laniado M, Gogoll M, et al: Gadopentetate dimeglumine as a bowel contrast agent: safety and efficacy, Radiology 178:503, 1991.

66. Kessler A, Mitchell DG, Israel HL, et al: Hepatic and splenic sarcoidosis: US and MR imaging, Abdom Imaging 18:159, 1993.

67. Kier R, and Kinder B: Insulinomas: MR imaging with STIR sequences and motion suppression, Am J Roentgenol 158:457, 1992.

68. Kraus BB, Rappaport DC, and Torres GM: Evaluation of oral contrast agents for abdominal magnetic resonance imaging, Magn Reson Imaging 12:847, 1994.

69. Krebs TL, Daly B, Wong JJ, et al: Vascular complications of pancreatic transplantation: MR evaluation, Radiology 196:793, 1995.

70. Lee MG, Lee HJ, Kim MH, et al: Extrahepatic biliary diseases: 3D MR cholangiopancreatography compared with endoscopic retrograde cholangiopancreatography, Radiology 202:663, 1997.

71. Levine E, Wetzel LH, and Neff JR: MR imaging and CT of extrahepatic cavernous hemangiomas, Am J Roentgenol 147:1299, 1986.

72. Loflin TG, Simeone JF, Mueller PR, et al: Gallbladder bile in cholecystitis: in vitro MR evaluation, Radiology 157:457, 1985.

73. Loud PA, Semelka RC, Kettritz U, et al: MRI of acute cholecystitis: comparison with the normal gallbladder and other entities, Magn Reson Imaging 14:349, 1996.

74. Lunniss PJ, Armstrong P, Barker PG, et al: Magnetic resonance imaging of anal fistulae, Lancet 340:394, 1992.

75. Macaulay SE, Schulte SJ, Sekijima JH, et al: Evaluation of a non-breath-hold MR cholangiography technique, Radiology 196:27, 1995.

76. Matos C, Metens T, Deviere J, et al: Pancreatic duct: morphologic and functional evaluation with dynamic MR pancreatography after secretin stimulation, Radiology 203:435, 1997.

77. Mattrey RF, Trambert MA, Brown JJ, et al: Perflubron as an oral contrast agent for MR imaging: results of a phase III clinical trial, Radiology 191:841, 1994.

78. McFarland EG, Kaufman JA, Saini S, et al: Preoperative staging of cancer of the pancreas: value of MR angiography versus conventional angiography in detecting portal venous invasion, Am J Roentgenol 166:37, 1996.

79. Meakem TJ III, and Schnall MD: Magnetic resonance cholangiography, Gastroenterol Clin North Am 24:221, 1995.

80. Megibow AJ, Zhou XH, and Rotterdam H: Pancreatic adenocarcinoma: CT versus MR imaging in the evaluation of resectability—report of the Radiology Diagnostic Oncology Group, Radiology 195:327, 1995.

81. Minami M, Itai Y, Ohtomo K, et al: Siderotic nodules in the spleen: MR imaging of portal hypertension, Radiology 172:681, 1989.

82. Mirowitz SA, Brown JJ, Lee JKT, et al: Dynamic gadolinium-enhanced MR imaging of the spleen: normal enhancement patterns and evaluation of splenic lesions, Radiology 179:681, 1991.

83. Mirowitz SA, Gutierrez E, Lee JK, et al: Normal abdominal enhancement patterns with dynamic gadolinium-enhanced MR, Radiology 180:637, 1991.

84. Mitchell DG, Vinitski S, Burk DL Jr, et al: Motion artifact reduction in MR imaging of the abdomen: gradient moment nulling versus respiratory-sorted phase encoding, Radiology 169:155, 1988.

85. Mitchell DG, Vinitski S, and Mohamed FB: Comparison of Kaopectate with barium for negative and positive enteric contrast at MR imaging, Radiology 181:475, 1991.

86. Mitchell DG, Cruvella M, Eschelman DJ, et al: MRI of pancreatic gastrinomas, J Comput Assist Tomogr 16:583, 1992.

87. Mitchell DG, Shapiro M, Schuricht A, et al: Pancreatic disease: findings on state-of-the-art MR images, Am J Roentgenol 159:533, 1992.

88. Mitchell DG: Diagnosis and staging of pancreatic tumors. In Myers M, ed: Diagnosis and staging of neoplasms of the digestive tract, New York, 1996, JB Lippincott.

89. Miyazaki T, Yamashita Y, Tsuchigame T, et al: MR cholangiopancreatography using HASTE (half-Fourier acquisition single-shot turbo spin-echo) sequences, Am J Roentgenol 166:1297, 1996.

90. Morgan DE, Baron TH, Smith JK, et al: Pancreatic fluid collections prior to intervention: evaluation with MR imaging compared with CT and US, Radiology 203:773, 1997.

91. Morimoto K, Shimoi M, Shirakawa T, et al: Biliary obstruction: evaluation with three-dimensional MR cholangiography, Radiology 183:578, 1992.

92. Moss AA: Imaging colorectal carcinoma, Radiology 170:308, 1989.

93. Mozell E, Woltering EA, Stenzel P, et al: Functional endocrine tumors of the pancreas: clinical presentation, diagnosis, and treatment, Curr Probl Surg 27:309, 1990.

94. Newland RC, Chapuis PH, Pheils MT, et al: The relationship of survival to staging and grading of colorectal carcinoma: a prospective study of 503 cases, Cancer 47:1424, 1981.

95. Nyman R, Rehn S, Glimelius B, et al: Magnetic resonance imaging, chest radiography, computed tomography and ultrasonography in malignant lymphoma, Acta Radiol 28:253, 1987.

96. Ohgi K, Kohno A, and Shigeta A: Acute cholecystitis: MR evaluation of thickened gallbladder wall, Radiology 181(P):94, 1991.

97. Ohtomo K, Fukuda H, Mori K, et al: CT and MR appearances of splenic hamartoma, J Comput Assist Tomogr 16:425, 1992.

98. Ohtomo K, Furui S, Onue M, et al: Solid and papillary epithelial neoplasm of the pancreas: MR imaging and pathologic correlation, Radiology 184:567, 1992.

99. Outwater EK, and Gordon SJ: Imaging the pancreatic and biliary ducts with MR, Radiology 192:19, 1994.

100. Parks AG, Gordon PH, and Hardcastle JD: A classification of fistula-in-ano, Br J Surg 63:1, 1976.

101. Patten RM, and Moss AA: OMR, a positive bowel contrast agent for abdominal and pelvic MR imaging: safety and imaging characteristics, J Magn Reson Imaging 2:25, 1992.

102. Pels Rijcken TH, Davis MA, and Ros PR: Intraluminal contrast agents for MR imaging of the abdomen and pelvis, J Magn Reson Imaging 4:291, 1994.

103. Pott G, and Schrameyer B: ERCP Atlas, Toronto, 1989, BC Decker.

104. Procacci C, Graziani R, Bicego E, et al: Papillary cystic neoplasm of the pancreas: radiological findings, Abdom Imaging 20:554, 1995.

105. Pu Y, Yamamoto F, Igimi H, et al: A comparative study usefulness [sic] of magnetic resonance imaging in the diagnosis of acute cholecystitis, J Gastroenterol 29:192, 1994.
106. Ramani M, Reinhold C, Semelka RC, et al: Splenic hemangiomas and hamartomas: MR imaging characteristics of 28 lesions, Radiology 202:166, 1997.
107. Rattner DW, and Warshaw AL: Pancreatic pseudocysts, cystic neoplasms and fistulas. In Carter DC, and Warshaw AL, eds: Pancreatitis, Edinburgh, 1989, Churchill Livingstone.
108. Regan F, Smith D, Khazan R, et al: MR cholangiography in biliary obstruction using half-Fourier acquisition, J Comput Assist Tomogr 20:627, 1996.
109. Reimer P, Saini S, Hahn PF, et al: Techniques for high-resolution echo-planar MR imaging of the pancreas, Radiology 182:175, 1992.
110. Reinhold C, and Bret PM: Current status of MR cholangiopancreatography, Am J Roentgenol 166:1285, 1996.
111. Rogers J, Lewis J, and Josephson L: Use of AMI-227 as an oral MR contrast agent, Magn Reson Imaging 12:631, 1994.
112. Ros PR, Moser RP Jr, Dachman AH, et al: Hemangioma of the spleen: radiologic-pathologic correlation in 10 cases, Radiology 162:73, 1987.
113. Rossman MD, Friedman AC, Radecki PD, et al: MR imaging of gallbladder carcinoma, Am J Roentgenol 148:143, 1987.
114. Rummeny E, Weissleder R, Stark DD, et al: Primary liver tumors: diagnosis by MR imaging, Am J Roentgenol 152:63, 1989.
115. Sagoh T, Itoh K, and Togashi K, et al: Gamna-Gandy bodies of the spleen: evaluation with MR imaging, Radiology 172:685, 1989.
116. Schnall MD, Furth EE, Rosato EF, et al: Rectal tumor stage: correlation of endorectal MR imaging and pathologic findings, Radiology 190:709, 1994.
117. Schoenenberger AW, Bauerfeind P, Krestin GP, et al: Virtual colonoscopy with magnetic resonance imaging: in vitro evaluation of a new concept, Gastroenterology 112:1863, 1997.
118. Semelka RC, Shoenut JP, Greenberg HM, et al: Detection of acute and treated lesions of hepatosplenic candidiasis: comparison of dynamic contrast-enhanced CT and MR imaging, J Magn Reson Imaging 2:341, 1992.
119. Semelka RC, Shoenut JP, Lawrence PH, et al: Spleen: dynamic enhancement patterns on gradient-echo MR images enhanced with gadopentetate dimeglumine, Radiology 185:479, 1992.
120. Semelka RC, Cummings M, Shoenut JP, et al: Islet cell tumors: a comparison of detection by dynamic contrast-enhanced CT and MRI with dynamic gadolinium-enhanced imaging and fat suppression, Radiology 186:799, 1993.
121. Semelka RC, Shoenut JP, Kroeker MA, et al: Chronic pancreatitis: MR imaging features before and after administration of gadopentetate dimeglumine, J Magn Reson Imaging 3:79, 1993.
122. Semelka RC, Kelekis NL, Molina PL, et al: Pancreatic masses with inconclusive findings on spiral CT: is there a role for MRI? J Magn Reson Imaging 6:585, 1996.
123. Semelka RC, Kelekis NL, Thomasson D, et al: HASTE MR imaging: description of technique and preliminary results in the abdomen, J Magn Reson Imaging 6:698, 1996.
124. Semelka RC, John G, Kelekis NL, et al: Small bowel neoplastic disease: demonstration by MRI, J Magn Reson Imaging 6:855, 1996.
125. Semelka RC, Kelekis NL, John G, et al: Ampullary carcinoma: demonstration by current MR techniques, J Magn Reson Imaging 7:153, 1997.
126. Shirkhoda A, Ros PR, Farah J, et al: Lymphoma of the solid abdominal viscera, Radiol Clin North Am 28:785, 1990.
127. Shoenut JP, Semelka RC, Silverman R, et al: Magnetic resonance imaging evaluation of the local extent of colorectal mass lesions, J Clin Gastroenterol 17:2248, 1993.
128. Shoenut JP, Semelka RC, Silverman R, et al: Magnetic resonance imaging in inflammatory bowel disease, J Clin Gastroenterol 17:73, 1993.
129. Shoenut JP, Semelka RC, Silverman R, et al: The gastrointestinal tract. In Semelka RC, Shoenut JP, eds: MRI of the abdomen with CT correlation, New York, 1993, Raven Press.
130. Shoenut JP, Semelka RC, Magro CM, et al: Comparison of magnetic resonance imaging and endoscopy in distinguishing the type and severity of inflammatory bowel disease, J Clin Gastroenterol 19:31, 1994.
131. Sica GT, Chai JL, Polger MR, et al: MR imaging of pancreatitis: evaluation of findings on unenhanced and contrast-enhanced images, Radiology 197(P):244, 1995.
132. Siegelman ES, Mitchell DG, Outwater E, et al: Idiopathic hemochromatosis: MR imaging findings in cirrhotic and precirrhotic patients, Radiology 188:637, 1993.
133. Siewert B, Muller MF, Foley M, et al: Fast MR imaging of the liver: quantitative comparison of techniques, Radiology 193:37, 1994.
134. Sironi S, De Cobelli F, Zerbi A, et al: Pancreatic adenocarcinoma: assessment of vascular invasion with high-field MR imaging and a phased-array coil, Am J Roentgenol 167:997, 1996.
135. Soto JA, Barish MA, Yucel EK, et al: Pancreatic duct: MR cholangiopancreatography with a three-dimensional fast spin-echo technique, Radiology 196:459, 1995.
136. Soto JA, Yucel EK, Barish MA, et al: MR cholangiopancreatography after unsuccessful or incomplete ERCP, Radiology 199:91, 1996.
137. Spritzer C, Kressel HY, Mitchell D, et al: MR imaging of normal extrahepatic bile ducts, J Comput Assist Tomgr 11:248, 1987.
138. Stabile BE, Morrow DJ, and Passaro E: The gastrinoma triangle: operative implications, Am J Surg 147:25, 1984.
139. Stark DD, Moseley ME, Bacon BR, et al: Magnetic resonance imaging and spectroscopy of hepatic iron overload, Radiology 154:137, 1985.
140. Stark DD, Hendrick RE, Hahn PF, et al: Motion artifact reduction with fast spin echo imaging, Radiology 164:183, 1987.
141. Takehara Y, Ichijo K, Tooyama N, et al: Breath-hold MR cholangiopancreatography with a long-echo-train fast spin-echo sequence and a surface coil in chronic pancreatitis, Radiology 192:73, 1994.
142. Thoeni RF, Fell SC, and Goldberg HI: CT detection of asymptomatic pancreatitis following ERCP, Gastrointest Radiol 15:291, 1990.
143. Thoeni RF, and Blankenberg F: Pancreatic imaging: computed tomography and magnetic resonance imaging, Radiol Clin North Am 31:1085, 1993.
144. Tjon A, Tham RTO, Heyerman HGM, et al: Cystic fibrosis: MR imaging of the pancreas, Radiology 179:183, 1991.
145. Todani T, Watanaabe Y, Narusue M, et al: Congenital bile duct cysts: classification, operative procedures, and review of thirty-seven cases including cancer arising from choledochal cyst, Am J Surg 134:263, 1977.
146. Torres GM, Terry NL, Mergo P, et al: MR imaging of the spleen, MRI Clin North Am 3:39, 1995.
147. Tsuchiya R, Noda T, Harada N, et al: Collective review of small carcinomas of the pancreas, Ann Surg 203:77, 1986.
148. Vellet AD, Romano W, Bach DB, et al: Adenocarcinoma of the pancreatic ducts: comparative evaluation with CT and MR imaging at 1.5T, Radiology 183:87, 1992.
149. Wadsworth DT, Newman B, Abramson SJ, et al: Splenic lymphangiomatosis in children, Radiology 202:173, 1997.
150. Wallner BK, Schumacher KA, Weidenmaier W, et al: Dilated biliary tract: evaluation with MR cholangiography with a T2-weighted contrast-enhanced fast sequence, Radiology 181:805, 1991.
151. Warshaue DM, Semelka RC, and Ascher SM: Nodular sarcoidosis of the liver and spleen: appearance on MR images, J Magn Reson Imaging 4:553, 1994.
152. Weissleder R, Stark DD, Compton C, et al: Cholecystitis: diagnosis by MR imaging, Magn Res Imaging 6:345, 1988.
153. Weissleder R, Elizondo G, Stark DD, et al: The diagnosis of splenic lymphoma by MR imaging: value of superparamagnetic iron oxide, Am J Roentgenol 152:175, 1989.
154. Weissleder R, and Stark DD: MR atlas of the abdomen, London, 1989, Martin Dunitz.
155. Wesbey GE, Brasch RC, Engelstad BL, et al: Nuclear magnetic resonance contrast enhancement study of the gastrointestinal tract of rats and a human volunteer using nontoxic oral iron solutions, Radiology 149:175, 1983.
156. Wilbur AC, Gyi B, and Renigers SA: High-field MRI of primary gallbladder carcinoma, Gastrointest Radiol 13:142, 1988.
157. Winkler ML, Hricak H, and Higgins CB: MR imaging of diffusely infiltrating gastric carcinoma, J Comput Assist Tomogr 11:337, 1987.
158. Winston CB, Mitchell DG, Outwater EK, et al: Pancreatic signal intensity on T1-weighted fat saturation MR images: clinical correlation, J Magn Reson Imaging 5:267, 1995.
159. Worawattanakul S, Semelka RC, Kelekis NL, et al: MR findings of intestinal graft-versus-host disease, Magn Reson Imaging 14:1221, 1996.
160. Yamashita Y, Abe Y, Tang Y, et al: In vitro and clinical studies of image acquisition in breath-hold MR cholangiopancreatography: single-shot projection technique versus multislice technique, Am J Roentgenol 168:1449, 1997.
161. Yoon DY, Choi BI, Han JK, et al: MR findings of secondary hemochromatosis: transfusional vs erythropoietic, J Comput Assist Tomogr 18:416, 1994.
162. Yuh WTC, Hunsicker LG, Nghiem DD, et al: Pancreatic transplants: evaluation with MR imaging, Radiology 170:171, 1989.
163. Zerhouni EA, Rutter C, Hamilton SR, et al: CT and MR imaging in the staging of colorectal carcinoma: report of the Radiology Diagnostic Oncology Group II, Radiology 200:443, 1996.

24 Adrenal Glands

Sharon S. Burton and Pablo R. Ros

 KEY POINTS

- CT is preferred for localization of small, functional adrenocortical tumors (Cushing's or Conn's syndrome).
- Pheochromocytoma, extraadrenal paraganglioma, and vascular invasion by adrenal carcinoma are best imaged with MRI.
- Adrenal adenomas can be distinguished from primary or metastatic cancer because 80% of adenomas contain fat detectable by unenhanced CT (HU <0) or chemical-shift (opposed-phase) MRI.

Magnetic resonance imaging (MRI) is recommended for characterization of incidental adrenal masses, pheochromocytoma localization, preoperative planning for adrenal carcinoma, and imaging of patients with prior iodinated-contrast reaction, poor renal function, or artifact caused by surgical clips.* Computed tomography (CT) is otherwise the preferred imaging study for adrenal disorders because of its lower cost, greater availability, and higher spatial resolution compared with MRI.[24,27,58]

A primary challenge of adrenal imaging is differentiation of benign adenomas from malignant tumors. Conventional spin-echo (SE) techniques have limited utility for characterizing adrenal masses because of a 21% to 31% overlap of signal characteristics in benign and malignant lesions.[36,73] Noncontrast CT can separate adenomas from malig-

*References 15, 18, 28, 50, 58, 64, 86.

nant lesions based on attenuation values, but it has low sensitivity.[57] Chemical shift MRI, using in- and opposed-phase breath-hold sequences, is the most promising MR technique available for identifying lipid-containing adrenal adenomas.[58,61,63] Noncontrast CT and chemical-shift imaging (CSI) are expected to play a key role in management of cancer patients with incidental adrenal masses.[25,58,63]

MAGNETIC RESONANCE IMAGING TECHNIQUES

Adrenal MRI is performed in axial and coronal planes using 5- to 10-mm sections with a 0- to 2-mm interslice gap. Sagittal views are helpful for differentiating large masses of adrenal origin from hepatic and renal lesions.[64,80] A body coil is preferred to allow imaging of adjacent organs, such as the liver and spleen, which are used as a reference for comparison with adrenal lesions. Surface coils improve the signal-to-noise ratio and spatial resolution, but the limited field of view is not optimum for routine use.[26,27,95]

Protocols for adrenal MRI have traditionally used SE techniques with T1-weighted images (repetition time [TR] 300 to 600, echo time [TE] 10 to 30 ms, 32-cm field of view, 256 × 128 matrix, four signals averaged, respiratory and flow compensation) for contrast and anatomical definition (Figure 24-1, *A*).[28] Dual-echo T2-weighted images (TR 2000 to 3000, TE 20/80 to 100 ms, two signals averaged, 256 × 128 matrix) have been used to characterize lesions (Figure 24-1, *B*).[28] Current adrenal protocols include techniques to optimize image quality and enhance tissue characterization.[58] The most important of these are fat suppression, fast SE T2-weighted imaging, and in- and opposed-phase chemical-shift sequences. Gradient-echo imaging with dynamic gadolinium enhancement has been evaluated but is less useful than CSI for characterizing adrenal masses.[51,52,54,78] Echo-planar imaging has the potential for characterizing masses based on calculated T2 values but is not widely available at this time.[78]

Fat Suppression

Fat suppression is performed in SE sequences by applying a frequency-selective radiofrequency pulse before the 90-degree excitation pulse. This saturates triglyceride magnetization and reduces signal intensity in fat. Fat suppression reduces respiratory motion artifact, eliminates chemical-shift artifact, enhances image sharpness, and reduces noise. It also decreases the dynamic range of contrast, making subtle differences in contrast more apparent.[58,79] This technique can be used in T1- and T2-weighted sequences and is beneficial for imaging the adrenal glands, liver, pancreas, and kidneys. Drawbacks of fat suppression are a 15% reduction in number of slices per acquisition and artifact caused by inhomogeneity in fat suppression.[79]

Fast Spin-Echo Imaging

The primary advantage of fast SE T2-weighted sequences (4000/104, echo-train length of 16, receive bandwidth of 32 kHz, and 256 × 192 matrix) is a significant reduction in scanning time compared with conventional T2-weighted imaging.[58] Fast SE T2 images improve spatial resolution and decrease blurring but have the disadvantage of decreased tissue contrast compared with conventional T2-weighted images.[11]

Chemical-Shift Imaging

CSI takes advantage of the fact that protons in water and lipid precess at a different frequency within a magnetic field. By choosing a TE appropriate for the magnetic field strength, images are obtained in which

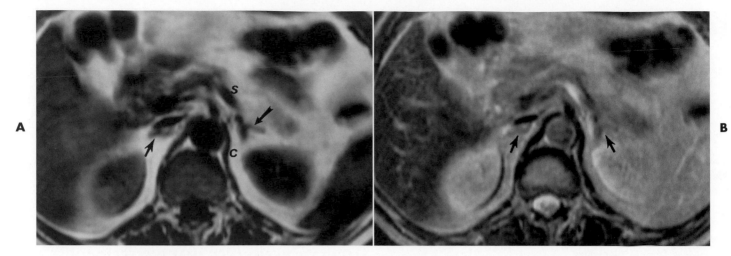

FIGURE 24-1 Normal adrenal glands. **A,** SE T1-weighted image (600/20). The left adrenal gland *(arrow)* is shaped like an inverted Y and is hypointense compared with perinephric fat. It is located posterior to the splenic vein *(s)* and lateral to the aorta and diaphragm crus *(c)*. The right adrenal gland is posterior to the inferior vena cava and has a linear configuration *(arrow)*. **B,** SE T2-weighted image (2500/80). The adrenal glands *(arrows)* remain isointense with liver and are not as clearly delineated from the perinephric fat in comparison with T1-weighted images.

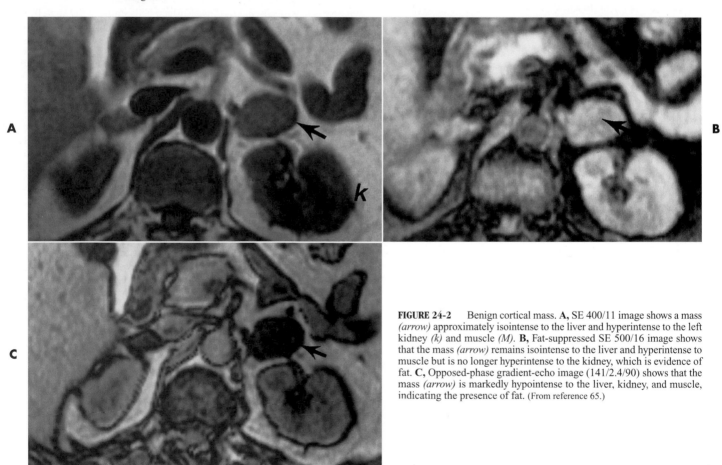

FIGURE 24-2 Benign cortical mass. **A,** SE 400/11 image shows a mass *(arrow)* approximately isointense to the liver and hyperintense to the left kidney *(k)* and muscle *(M)*. **B,** Fat-suppressed SE 500/16 image shows that the mass *(arrow)* remains isointense to the liver and hyperintense to muscle but is no longer hyperintense to the kidney, which is evidence of fat. **C,** Opposed-phase gradient-echo image (141/2.4/90) shows that the mass *(arrow)* is markedly hypointense to the liver, kidney, and muscle, indicating the presence of fat. (From reference 65.)

fat and water are maximally in phase or out of phase. Structures that contain both water and fat, such as lipid-containing adrenal adenomas, show a reduction in signal intensity on opposed-phase images in comparison with in-phase images (Figure 24-2). Metastases, pheochromocytomas, cysts, hemorrhage,[70] and up to 20% of adenomas do not contain sufficient lipid to show signal loss on CSI. This rapid magnetic resonance (MR) technique has very high specificity for detection of benign adenomas.

The technical parameters described for chemical-shift sequences vary based on the magnetic field strength. The first report by Mitchell et al at 1.5 Tesla (T) compared T1-weighted opposed-phase images (TR 59 to 142, TE 2.3 to 2.5, flip angle of 90 degrees, one signal averaged) with standard T1-weighted images (TR 400 to 600, TE 11 to 22).[65] Subsequent authors[58,63,70] recommend identical breath-hold gradient-echo sequences for both in- and opposed-phase images, except for the variance in TE. In-phase images (TR 117, TE 4.6, 80-degree flip angle, 256 × 192 matrix, one signal, 10-mm thickness) are compared with opposed-phase images (TR 117, TE 2.3). At 1.5 T a TE of 5 and 7 ms can be used for in-phase and opposed-phase images, respectively, although the chemical-shift effect is optimized using the lowest TE possible.[58,70] At 0.5 T, opposed-phase gradient-echo sequences (142/6.3, 90-degree flip angle) have been compared with conventional T1-weighted images (TR 550, TE 20).[7] Chemical-shift images have been analyzed using quantitative measurements[7,63,88] and qualitative visual assessment.[54,61] The technique is recommended for adrenal lesions greater than 1 cm in diameter to avoid error caused by volume averaging.

ANATOMY AND IMAGING PITFALLS

The adrenal glands are located in the perirenal space, where they are attached to the anteromedial and superior aspect of Gerota's fascia.[66] In axial images the right adrenal gland is posterior to the inferior vena cava (IVC) and superior to the upper pole of the right kidney. It typically has a linear or inverted V configuration. The left adrenal gland is anteromedial to the upper pole of the kidney and posterior to the pancreas. It is often triangular in shape but may appear as an inverted T, Y, or V on axial images.[51,67] Normal adrenals range from less than 5 mm in thickness to a maximum of 10 mm in thickness and are 2 to 4 cm in length. The left adrenal is more easily identified because it is surrounded by a more prominent fat pad than is the right adrenal gland.

On conventional SE images, the adrenal glands have homogeneous, low signal intensity in contrast with the high intensity of perinephric fat (Figure 24-1). They are isointense or hypointense relative to liver on SE T1- and T2-weighted images.[28,36] With fat suppression, the adrenals appear hyperintense in comparison with adjacent fat and liver on both imaging sequences.[58] In opposed-phase chemical-shift images, there is signal loss at the periphery of the adrenal glands at the interface with adjacent fat.

Pitfalls in adrenal imaging may be seen because of variations in patient anatomy. Absence of sufficient retroperitoneal fat makes it more difficult to identify normal adrenal glands.[12] Adrenal pseudomasses from adjacent structures have been documented in CT[5] and may appear in MRI. These include a fluid-filled gastric fundus or diverticulum,[83] prominent splenic lobulation, tortuous splenic vessels, and varices of the left inferior phrenic vein.[9] Masses arising in the kidneys or tail of the pancreas may also simulate a mass of adrenal origin.[5] With MRI, multiplanar imaging helps to clarify the origin of masses, and vascular structures are less likely to be confused with solid adrenal nodules because of flow phenomena.[9] Use of an oral contrast agent has been helpful in CT for identifying pseudomasses of gastrointestinal (GI) tract origin,[5] although the benefit of oral contrast for adrenal MRI has not been definitely proved.

FUNCTIONAL ADRENAL DISORDERS

The adrenal cortex and medulla are two separate functional units with different embryonic origins, which unite within a single capsule during fetal life.[66] The cortex arises from mesodermal tissues of the urogenital ridge and differentiates into three histological zones. The outer cortical zone is the zona glomerulosa, which produces aldosterone. The middle and inner zones are the zona fasciculata and zona reticularis, which are responsible for glucocorticoid and adrenal androgen production. Ectodermal cells from the neural crest form the primitive sympathetic ganglia and adrenal medulla. They have two lines of differentiation—chromaffin cells (pheochromocytes), which produce epinephrine and norepinephrine, and autonomic ganglion cells.

Although the cortex, medulla, and their subzones are not distinguishable by MRI,[12] an understanding of the histological regions and their hormonal functions provides a framework for classifying adrenal lesions. Adrenal disorders can be categorized based on hormonal function into diseases that cause adrenocortical or medullary hyperfunction, adrenocortical insufficiency, and lesions associated with normal adrenal function.

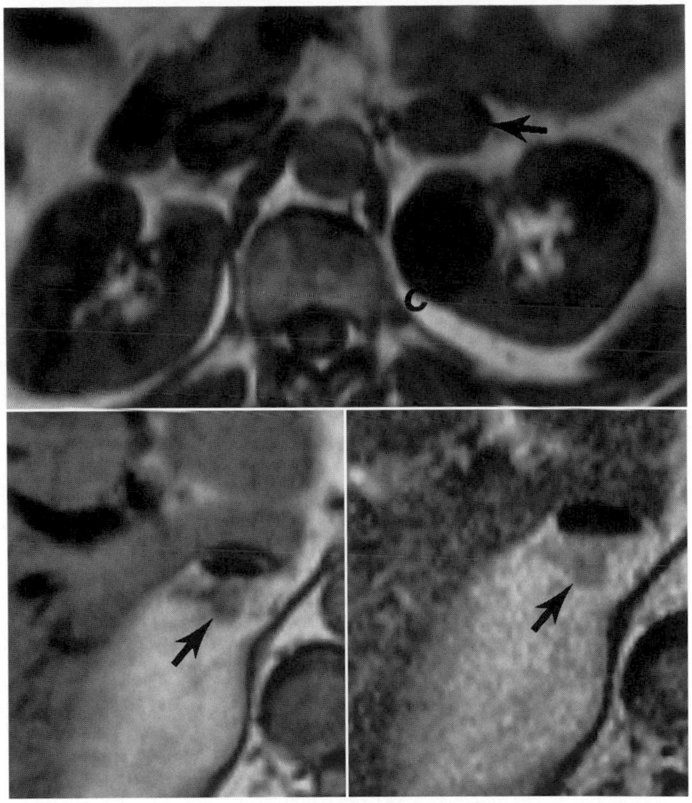

FIGURE 24-3   Primary hyperaldosteronism. **A,** SE 500/15 image. Solitary 2.5-cm left adrenal mass *(arrow)*. Incidentally noted is a cyst in the left kidney *(c)*. **B** and **C,** SE T1- and T2-weighted images demonstrate a small nodule in the right adrenal gland *(arrow)*. Based on results of adrenal vein sampling, the patient was treated medically for nodular hyperplasia.

Adrenocortical Hyperfunction

Primary Hyperaldosteronism. This syndrome is characterized by excessive mineralocorticoid production of adrenal origin. Clinical manifestations include hypertension, hypokalemia, fluid retention, weakness, and cardiac dysrhythmias. Elevated plasma aldosterone level and decreased plasma renin activity are diagnostic laboratory findings.[96] Approximately 75% to 85% of patients with primary hyperaldosteronism have a benign, aldosterone-producing adenoma (Conn's syndrome) and are treated by surgical resection. Adrenal hyperplasia accounts for 20% to 25% of cases and is treated medically because bilateral adrenalectomy may not alleviate the clinical findings.[2,92] Excessive aldosterone production by adrenocortical carcinoma occurs rarely but is associated with profound hypokalemia and marked elevation in plasma aldosterone.[30]

Adrenal gland images must be obtained using thin sections (1.5 to 5 mm) because these tumors are small. In a study of 23 aldosterone-producing tumors, the average diameter was 1.5 cm with a range of 0.5 to 3.5 cm. The sensitivity of CT for diagnosis of aldosteronoma has ranged from 75% to 88%.[33,43] In a small series of patients studied by MRI, aldosteronomas have been isointense or hyperintense to liver on T2-weighted images (Figure 24-3, *A*).[75]

In primary hyperaldosteronism caused by adrenal hyperplasia, the adrenal glands may appear normal on imaging studies. Pathologically, bilateral nodules are found, varying in size from 0.25 to 1 cm and occasionally up to 2 to 3 cm.[43] Hyperplasia with a dominant nodule may be mistaken for a single adenoma unless imaging resolution is sufficient to show nodularity in the contralateral gland (Figure 24-3, *B* and *C*). In four patients with hyperaldosteronism caused by nodular hyperplasia, MRI identified only the dominant nodule in three of four patients.[43] In the abdomen, CT generally has higher spatial resolution than MRI and is recommended for evaluation of patients with suspected

Conn's syndrome.[37,43,58] Alternative diagnostic procedures for primary aldosteronism include selective adrenal vein sampling, which has a 96% accuracy rate,[33] and I-131 NP-59 scintigraphy.[12,43]

Cushing's Syndrome. Cushing's syndrome results from glucocorticoid excess and is characterized by truncal obesity, hirsutism, abdominal striae, muscle wasting, osteoporosis, hypertension, and hypercortisolism.[96] Glucocorticoid excess most often is due to exogenous steroids used in medical therapy. Endogenous sources of Cushing's syndrome include cortisol-producing adrenal adenoma (20%), adrenocortical carcinoma (10%), and adrenocortical hyperplasia from excess adrenocorticotropic hormone (ACTH) production (70%).[24,96] Ninety percent of patients with excess ACTH have Cushing's syndrome caused by a hyperfunctioning pituitary adenoma. Ten percent of patients have ectopic ACTH production associated with neoplasms, such as oat cell carcinoma, bronchial carcinoid, pheochromocytoma, and tumors of the ovary, pancreas, thymus, and thyroid.[23]

Cortisol-producing adenomas are easily demonstrated with CT or MRI because they are usually larger than 2 cm in diameter and are surrounded by abundant retroperitoneal fat. The contralateral adrenal gland is normal or atrophic as a result of suppression of ACTH production by autonomous cortisol secretion.[21] Using SE imaging, the signal intensity of adenomas is variable. In a series of 30 adenomas, 71% were isointense to liver, 19% were hyperintense, and 10% were hypointense to liver on SE T2-weighted images.[75] Rarely, adenomas are very hyperintense on SE T2-weighted images, making them indistinguishable from metastatic disease or adrenal carcinoma.[4] There are no imaging features that can differentiate between nonhyperfunctioning and hyperfunctioning adenomas.[75] CSI can confirm a diagnosis of lipid-containing adenoma in Cushing's syndrome because the mass shows reduction in signal intensity on opposed-phase images (Figure 24-4).

Adrenal hyperplasia in Cushing's syndrome has a variable appearance.[24] Up to 50% of patients have normal-appearing adrenal glands.

Diffuse unilateral or bilateral enlargement and macronodular hyperplasia may occur (Figure 24-5). When a dominant nodule is found and the contralateral gland is nodular, this most likely reflects nodular cortical hyperplasia. Recognition of this will prevent unnecessary adrenalectomy for a dominant nodule in patients with nodular hyperplasia. Petrosal venous sampling for ACTH may be needed to confirm a diagnosis of ACTH-producing pituitary microadenoma causing nodular adrenal hyperplasia when the pituitary MR examination is normal.[21,24]

A rare variant of Cushing's syndrome that occurs in children and young adults is known as *primary pigmented nodular adrenocortical disease* (PPNAD).[22] Patients have short stature and profound osteoporosis. Associated findings include spotty skin pigmentation, calcified Sertoli cell tumors of the testes, and cardiac and soft tissue myxomas (Carney complex). Pathologically, PPNAD is characterized by multiple pigmented nodules of hyperplastic cells and atrophy of normal tissue between the nodules. With high-resolution CT and MR techniques, multiple nodules ranging from 5 to 10 mm in size can be documented in these patients.[22] Using CT, the nodules have low attenuation. In SE images the nodules show low signal intensity on both T1- and T2-weighted images. Treatment for PPNAD is bilateral adrenalectomy followed by hormone-replacement therapy.

Adrenocortical Carcinoma. Primary adrenocortical carcinoma is a rare malignancy with an incidence of 1 to 2 per million persons.[24,86] Hormonal hyperfunction occurs in 50% of patients. Depending on the hormones produced, clinical findings may include Cushing's syndrome, virilization, feminization, and rarely hyperaldosteronism. Hormonally active tumors are smaller at the time of diagnosis than are nonfunctioning tumors,[32] which tend to remain clinically silent until their large size produces local mass effect or metastatic disease develops. Metastases involve regional and paraaortic lymph nodes, lung, liver, and vascular invasion into the IVC.[86] Surgical excision is performed by en-bloc resection, but the prognosis is poor.

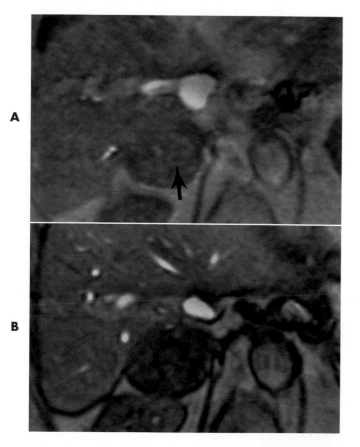

FIGURE 24-4   Cushing's adenoma. **A,** In-phase axial FMP-SPGR 45/4.2/60 image shows intermediate signal intensity (143, arbitrary scale) in the right adrenal mass *(arrow)* **B,** Out-of-phase axial FMP-SPGR 45/3.1/60 image shows reduction in signal intensity (94, same scale as **A**) in the right adrenal mass, confirming the presence of lipid. (Courtesy E. Siegelman.)

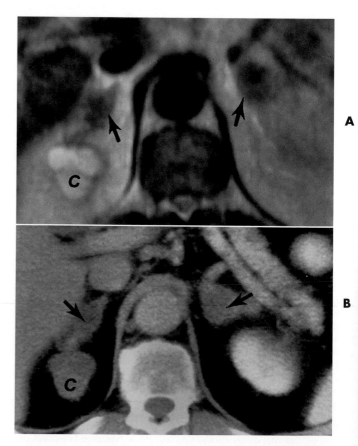

FIGURE 24-5   Adrenal hyperplasia. **A,** FSE T2-weighted image shows bilateral adrenal enlargement *(arrows)* with signal intensity equivalent to liver. Septated cyst *(c)* in the right kidney. **B,** CT scan.

Adrenocortical carcinomas are typically large masses, up to 20 cm in diameter, with inhomogeneous enhancement and central necrosis (Figure 24-6, *A* and *B*).[37] Calcifications occur in 30% of cases and are better demonstrated on CT than MRI. The MR signal characteristics reported for adrenocortical carcinoma resemble those seen with metastatic disease: They are hypointense relative to liver on T1-weighted images and hyperintense on SE T2-weighted sequences.[86] Central necrosis, peripheral nodules of enhancement, and internal hemorrhage are common MR features.[76] Small carcinomas less than 5 cm can be homogeneous without necrosis,[32] simulating a benign adenoma[35] in SE imaging.

In vitro studies using MR spectroscopy have shown a small lipid component (1.5%) in adrenal carcinomas compared with a lipid content of 17.5% for benign adenomas.[59] By in vivo MR spectroscopy the mean percentage of lipid in masses larger than 1.5 cm was 13.4% for adenomas and 3.5% for carcinomas.[60] Experience with CSI in adrenal carcinoma is limited. However, two tumors have shown localized areas of signal-intensity loss on opposed-phase images because of fat content within the tumor.[76] This is unlike the homogeneous signal-intensity loss seen in opposed-phase imaging in benign lipid-containing adenomas.

Although CT is often the initial imaging study in patients with adrenal carcinoma, multiplanar MRI is more accurate than CT in determining the site of origin of large masses, involvement of the liver, and invasion of the adrenal vein and IVC (Figure 24-6, *C*).[80,82,86] The renal corticomedullary differentiation provided by MRI helps define intrarenal or extrarenal origin of tumors.[80] MRI accurately localizes the extent and level of vena cava involvement, which in turn determines the need for cardiopulmonary bypass during surgery. MRI with intravenous contrast enhancement has been used to differentiate bland thrombus from tumor thrombus invading the IVC.[29] Based on these advantages, MRI has been recommended for preoperative staging before surgical resection of adrenocortical carcinomas.[50]

Adrenomedullary Hyperfunction

Pheochromocytoma. Paragangliomas are rare neuroendocrine tumors that arise within the adrenal medulla or from paraganglionic tissue extending from the base of the skull to the pelvis. Approximately 85% to 90% of paragangliomas arise in the adrenal gland and are called *pheochromocytomas*. They occur in the fourth and fifth decades of life, predominantly in women.[94] Pheochromocytomas are usually hormonally active, producing both norepinephrine and epinephrine. Symptomatic patients have sustained or paroxysmal hypertension and episodic attacks of anxiety, headache, visual blurring, sweating, and vasomotor changes caused by transient elevations in catecholamine levels. Paragangliomas of the urinary bladder produce symptoms with micturition.

Several familial syndromes are associated with pheochromocytoma.[96] These include (1) multiple endocrine neoplasia (MEN) IIa (pheochromocytoma, medullary carcinoma of the thyroid, and parathyroid hyperplasia); (2) MEN IIb (pheochromocytoma, medullary carcinoma of the thyroid, and mucocutaneous disorders, including mucosal neuromas); (3) neurofibromatosis; (4) von Hippel-Lindau syndrome (pheochromocytoma, renal cell carcinoma, cystic disease of the kidney and pancreas, and hemangioblastoma of the central nervous system [CNS]); and (5) familial pheochromocytoma. Patients with MEN syndromes are frequently asymptomatic (50%) and tend to have bilateral tumors, which are almost always intraadrenal.[14,24]

Extraadrenal paragangliomas arising from the sympathetic chain and retroperitoneal ganglia tend to occur in the second and third decades in both men and women.[94] They are less often hormonally active and secrete norepinephrine.[90] Common sites of extraadrenal paragangliomas are the superior paraaortic region near the renal hilum (46%), the inferior paraaortic region at the organ of Zuckerkandl (29%), the thoracic paraspinal region (10%), and the wall of the urinary bladder (10%).[94] Extraadrenal tumors are multicentric in 15% to 25% of cases and are more likely to be malignant (up to 40%) than are adrenal pheochromocytomas (2% to 11%).[90,94] Pheochromocytomas occurring in childhood are more often extraadrenal and multicentric and are less likely to be malignant than those occurring in adulthood.[94]

Laboratory diagnosis of pheochromocytoma is based on elevated plasma and urinary levels of catecholamines or their metabolites, including norepinephrine, vanillylmandelic acid (VMA), and metanephrine. Once a clinical diagnosis of pheochromocytoma is made, imaging studies are performed to localize the tumor. Initial screening of the adrenal glands is performed with CT or MRI, which detect 90% of cases. If no adrenal mass is found, a complete examination of the abdomen and pelvis is warranted to localize extraadrenal tumors. If this is also normal, MRI of the chest is recommended.

Adrenal pheochromocytomas are usually larger than 3 cm at the time of diagnosis and are readily diagnosed by CT or MRI. MRI has the advantage of improved tissue characterization over that obtainable with CT (Figure 24-7, *A*). On SE T2-weighted images the majority of pheochromocytomas have very high signal intensity (Figure 24-7, *B*).[64] Larger tumors tend to be inhomogeneous, containing central necrosis, calcification, or hemorrhage (Figures 24-8 and 24-9). Quantitative measurements using adrenal mass or liver signal-intensity ratios[31,74] and

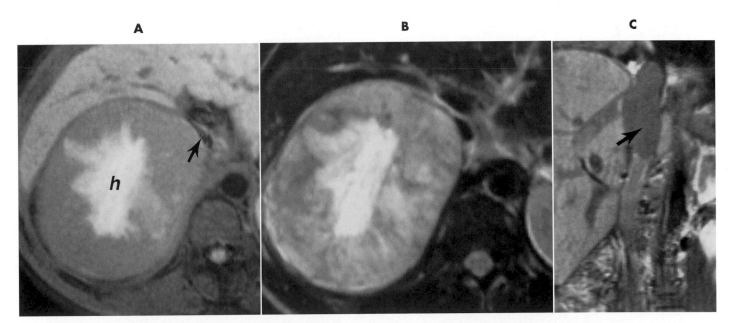

FIGURE 24-6   Adrenocortical carcinoma. **A,** Fat-suppressed T1-weighted image shows a large right adrenal mass with internal hemorrhage *(h)* compressing and displacing the IVC anteriorly. **B,** T2-weighted image. **C,** Coronal section from postoperative examination shows extensive thrombosis *(arrow)* of the IVC to the level of the right atrium, with extension into the hepatic vein.

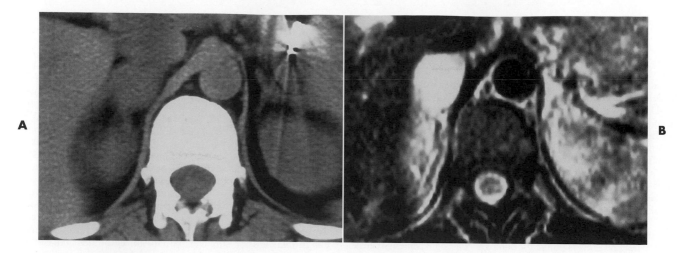

FIGURE 24-7   Pheochromocytoma. **A,** CT scan in patient with episodic hypertension. There is a small right adrenal mass *(arrow)* that has a nonspecific appearance. Note clip artifacts. **B,** T2-weighted image. Right adrenal mass has extremely high signal intensity, which is typical of most pheochromocytomas.

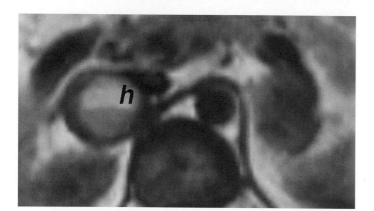

FIGURE 24-8   T1-weighted image shows bilateral adrenal masses *(arrows)* in a 29-year-old man with MEN IIb. Layering of high signal intensity indicates hemorrhage *(h)* in the right adrenal mass.

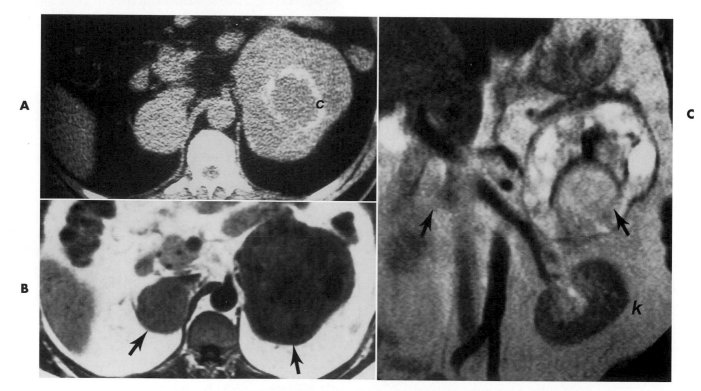

FIGURE 24-9   CT scan **(A)** shows bilateral adrenal masses with calcifications *(c)*. T1-weighted **(B)** and coronal T2-weighted **(C)** images show the bilateral masses *(arrows)* with heterogeneous signal intensity. The coronal image nicely shows the depression of the left kidney *(k)* by the large adrenal mass. Calcifications are not well shown in MR images.

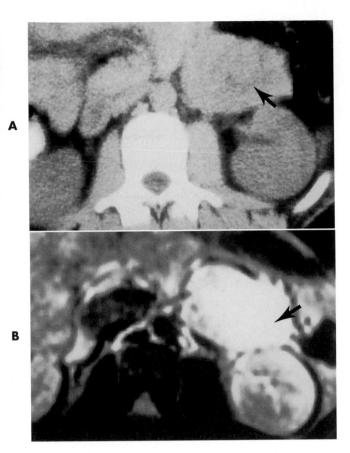

FIGURE 24-10 Extraadrenal paraganglioma. **A,** Unenhanced CT shows a mass *(arrow)* that is difficult to diagnose because it resembles poorly opacified bowel. **B,** T2-weighted image demonstrates very high signal intensity.

calculated T2 values[4] show the majority of pheochromocytomas as separate and distinct from other adrenal masses. Some pheochromocytomas, however, do not show the hyperintense appearance on T2-weighted imaging, causing them to be misclassified as adenomas based on SE techniques.[58] CSI may help with this differentiation because pheochromocytomas do not show the signal intensity loss on opposed-phase images that is found in most lipid-containing adenomas.

For extraadrenal paragangliomas, MRI is superior to CT because of improved tissue characterization and multiplanar imaging capabilities (Figure 24-10).[90] MRI is especially useful for paragangliomas arising in a juxtacardiac location, in the wall of the urinary bladder (Figure 24-11), in the retroperitoneum, and adjacent to surgical clips.[24,72] An alternative to MRI for detection of extraadrenal paragangliomas is iodine-131 metaiodobenzylguanidine (^{131}I MIBG) scintigraphy.[72] This study is not available in many institutions and has a 13% false-negative rate because of insufficient uptake of radiotracer by the neoplasm.[81] When available, ^{131}I MIBG scintigraphy can be used to localize recurrent or metastatic lesions in extraadrenal sites and serve as a guide for further imaging with MRI for precise anatomical localization.[72]

Neuroblastoma. Pheochromocytomas in childhood are very rare. Neuroblastoma is the primary neoplasm producing adrenomedullary hyperfunction in children and the most common extracranial malignant tumor in children.[93] Most arise from the adrenal gland, but they may develop from any tissue of neural crest cell origin. Neuroblastoma is usually a poorly defined tumor that is often calcified. MRI is superior to CT and ultrasound for staging neuroblastoma because it excels at defining the origin of the mass, characterizing the tumor, depicting vascular encasement, and demonstrating intraspinal extension of tumor. MRI is also useful in postoperative assessment because there are fewer artifacts from surgical clips than on CT studies, and residual or recurrent tumor is more reliably differentiated from fibrosis on T2-weighted images than it is by CT.[18] Hemorrhagic neuroblastoma may be difficult to

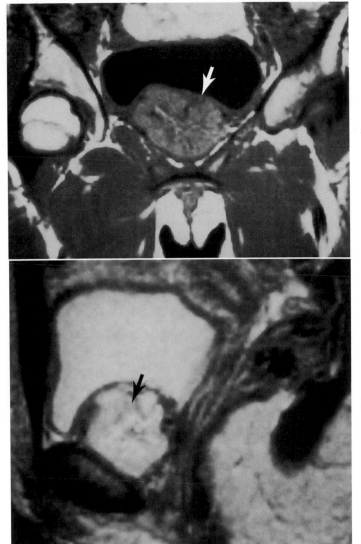

FIGURE 24-11 Paraganglioma in urinary bladder in patient with micturition headache. Coronal T1-weighted **(A)** and parasagittal T2-weighted **(B)** images show heterogeneous, hyperintense mass. (Courtesy C. Powers.)

differentiate from traumatic adrenal hemorrhage in neonates, even with MRI. Urinary catecholamine screening and sonographic follow-up are recommended to ensure resolution of the hemorrhage and exclude a hemorrhagic neuroblastoma.[93]

Adrenocortical Insufficiency

Chronic adrenocortical insufficiency (Addison's disease) is caused by progressive destruction of the adrenal cortices. Clinical findings include weakness, fatigue, anorexia, increased skin pigmentation, and hypotension. Laboratory assessment shows low levels of plasma cortisol and elevated levels of plasma ACTH.[96]

The most common cause of Addison's disease is idiopathic atrophy. This is probably an autoimmune disorder and manifests as severe atrophy of the adrenal glands on imaging studies.[20,24] Tuberculosis is the second most common cause, accounting for one third of cases. Histoplasmosis, blastomycosis, and fungal disease rarely involve the adrenal glands.[97] Tuberculosis can cause enlargement of the adrenal glands with preservation of the normal configuration. In later stages the adrenals are often calcified. Active tuberculosis also may produce bilateral adrenal enlargement with high signal intensity on T2-weighted images, mimicking malignant disease.[3]

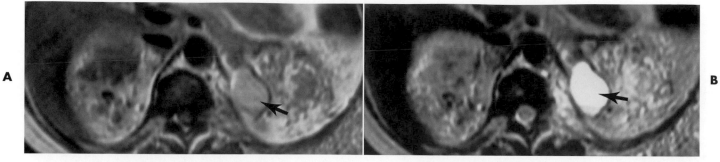

FIGURE 24-12   Adrenal hemorrhage in a patient with extensive subcutaneous hemangioma (Klippel-Trenaunay syndrome). **A,** T1-weighted image shows a moderately high signal intensity in left adrenal mass indicative of methemoglobin. Also shown are multiple vessels of the hemangioma involving the perinephric space, left subcutaneous tissues, and abdominal musculature. **B,** T2-weighted image shows uniform high signal intensity in the hemorrhagic left adrenal gland.

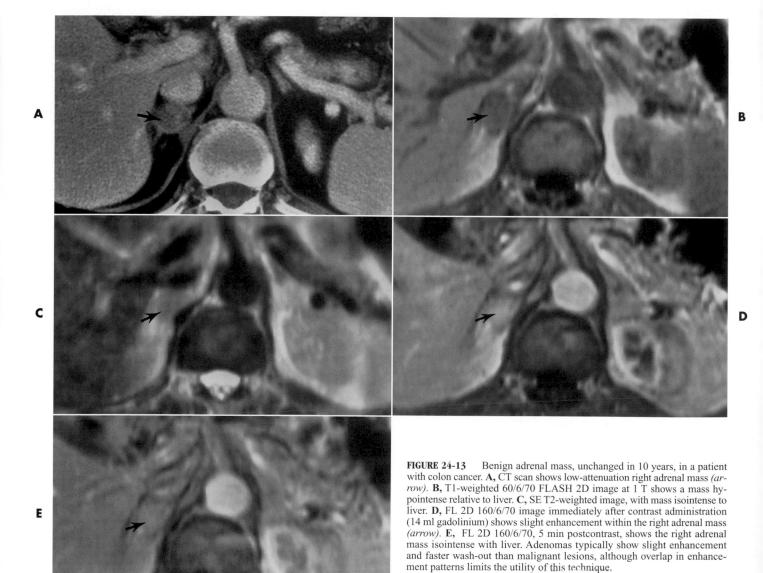

FIGURE 24-13   Benign adrenal mass, unchanged in 10 years, in a patient with colon cancer. **A,** CT scan shows low-attenuation right adrenal mass *(arrow)*. **B,** T1-weighted 60/6/70 FLASH 2D image at 1 T shows a mass hypointense relative to liver. **C,** SE T2-weighted image, with mass isointense to liver. **D,** FL 2D 160/6/70 image immediately after contrast administration (14 ml gadolinium) shows slight enhancement within the right adrenal mass *(arrow)*. **E,** FL 2D 160/6/70, 5 min postcontrast, shows the right adrenal mass isointense with liver. Adenomas typically show slight enhancement and faster wash-out than malignant lesions, although overlap in enhancement patterns limits the utility of this technique.

Bilateral adrenal hemorrhage is another cause of adrenocortical insufficiency. In adults, hemorrhage is associated with coagulopathy from a bleeding disorder or anticoagulation or is due to stress from surgery, sepsis, trauma, or hypotension.[51] In neonates, hemorrhage most often is due to trauma and seldom results in adrenocortical insufficiency. Using CT, acute hemorrhage produces hyperdense adrenal masses that decrease in density with time, later forming pseudocysts with rim calcification. On MRI in the subacute phase, areas of high signal intensity caused by blood products, including methemoglobin, can be seen on T1-weighted images (Figure 24-12).[28]

Metastatic disease is an uncommon cause of adrenocortical insufficiency because adrenal function is maintained until greater than 90% of the glands are destroyed or replaced.[24] Breast and lung tumors most often give rise to adrenal metastasis. Non-Hodgkin's lymphoma involves the adrenals in a small percentage of patients, occurring in 4% of 173 patients in one series, and may produce adrenocortical insufficiency when extensive bilateral involvement occurs.[71] The MR characteristics of metastatic lesions are discussed in the following section.

ADRENAL MASSES WITH NORMAL FUNCTION
Adenoma

Nonhyperfunctioning adenomas of the adrenal gland are such common findings that they have been called "incidentalomas."[37] In a series of 9866 consecutive autopsies, cortical adenomas greater than 3 mm in diameter were found in 2.9% of patients.[16] If macroscopic and microscopic nodules found at autopsy are included, the incidence of adenomas is as high as 64.5%.[19] By CT examination, small nonhyperfunctioning adrenal masses are found in approximately 1% of patients[34] and are more commonly seen with increasing age and in patients with hypertension and diabetes.[39]

Most adenomas are less than 3 cm in size with low attenuation on CT (Figure 24-13, *A*). Calcifications are uncommon and are usually central when they occur.[47] Noncontrast CT is one means of differentiating benign adenomas from other masses based on attenuation values. The presence of lipid-rich cells in many adrenal adenomas accounts for their low attenuation on unenhanced CT.[53] Lee et al[57] found a mean attenuation coefficient of -2.2 Hounsfield units (HU) +/- 16 in 38 adenomas in comparison with a mean attenuation coefficient of 28.9 HU +/- 10.6 in 28 malignant masses. They suggest that an adrenal mass with CT attenuation values of less than 0 HU can be considered a benign lesion, and further follow-up is unnecessary. Van Erkel et al[89] proposed a CT attenuation value of 15 HU as the discriminating point between benign and malignant masses. A threshold of 10 HU gives a sensitivity of 74% and a specificity of 96% for diagnosis of adenoma.[55] Early delayed CT has proved useful in characterizing adenomas, although the precise threshold for benign lesions has not been established in a large series.[8,87] A conservative approach, using 0 HU as the upper limit for benign lesions, reduces the likelihood of misdiagnosing a low-density metastasis as a benign lesion.[57,58,63] Noncontrast CT for adrenal mass characterization is a key component of the algorithmic approach to adrenal imaging presented at the end of this chapter.

Using SE techniques, adenomas commonly have signal intensity similar to liver on T1- and T2-weighted images (Figure 24-13, *B* and *C*). Metastases and adrenal carcinomas are typically hyperintense relative to liver on T2-weighted images. Early MRI researchers were hopeful that signal-intensity ratios could reliably differentiate benign from malignant adrenal lesions.[13,35,73] Unfortunately, the signal characteristics of adenomas are variable because of hemorrhage, necrosis, and calcifications (Figure 24-14, *A* and *B*).[3] Likewise, all metastatic lesions and pheochromocytomas do not fit the "typical" patterns.[36,37,58] Because of these factors, the success of SE imaging in classifying adrenal masses has been limited. Using mid field–strength magnets and a variety of signal-intensity ratios, 21% to 31% of adrenal masses fall into an indeterminate range in which benign and malignant adrenal lesions overlap.[35-37,74] Calculated T2 relaxation time is more useful in distinguishing adrenal masses at 1.5 T,[4] but there is still overlap between benign and malignant lesions using this technique.[49]

Use of dynamic gadolinium enhancement during fast gradient-echo imaging was initially thought to improve the accuracy of adrenal mass characterization (Figure 24-13, *D* and *E*). In a study of 38 adrenal masses[56] using intravenous gadolinium injection and dynamic scanning, adenomas showed less enhancement and faster wash-out than

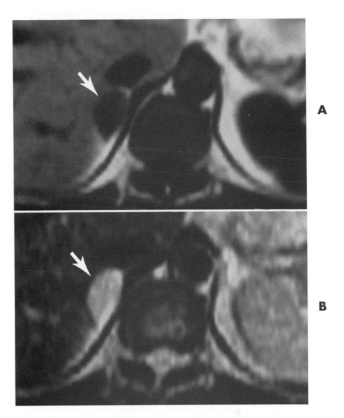

FIGURE 24-14   Atypical adrenal adenoma by SE imaging. **A,** T1-weighed SE 275/14 image at 0.5 T shows a small right adrenal adenoma *(arrow)*. **B,** T2-weighted SE 2350/120 image shows adenoma *(arrow)* hyperintense relative to the liver, simulating a metastasis. (From reference 58.)

metastases and pheochromocytomas. Accuracy of characterizing adrenal masses was 90% when dynamic gadolinium perfusion studies were used. Ichikawa et al[42] found the pattern of enhancement to be helpful in separating adrenal masses at 1.5 T. Other investigators[54,58] have not, however, found dynamic enhancement to be useful because of overlap in enhancement and wash-out patterns between benign and malignant lesions.

Of all MRI techniques to date, CSI is the most promising method of identifying benign adrenocortical masses. Mitchell et al[65] found reduction in signal intensity on chemical-shift images in comparison with standard images in 26 of 27 benign cortical masses and two myelolipomas. Twelve metastases, three hemorrhages, and one cyst had no loss of signal relative to standard images. Korobkin et al[54] evaluated 35 adenomas and 16 nonadenomas in 43 patients using qualitative visual inspection. They compared the signal intensity of the mass relative to liver on opposed- and in-phase images. Only adenomas showed a decrease in relative signal-intensity ratio (specificity, 100%; sensitivity, 81%), although 6 of 35 adenomas did not show signal loss on opposed-phase images because of lack of sufficient lipid within the mass (Figures 24-15 and 24-16). Schwartz et al[77] studied 23 malignant and 45 benign masses in 68 patients with known malignancy at 1.5 T. Using an adrenal-mass-to-spleen ratio of 0.55, sensitivity of CSI for benign lesions was 80%, and specificity was 100%. Use of the spleen as a reference for comparison avoided error caused by fatty change in the liver (Figure 24-16). Visual inspection by experienced observers was as accurate as quantitative measures for assessing chemical-shift sequences.[52,54,57]

Although most studies of CSI have been performed at 1.5 T, the work by Bilbey et al[7] performed at 0.5 T supports these results. Use of the spleen as a reference standard provided complete separation in signal-intensity ratios for adenomas and nonadenomas with no overlap. Further testing of nonadenomatous masses is needed to better define the true specificity of this technique,[52] but CSI appears to be a promising tool for diagnosis of benign lipid-containing adenomas.

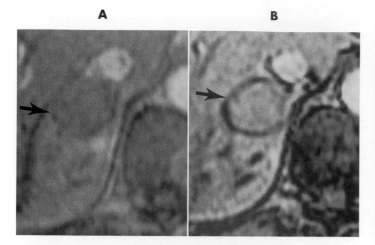

FIGURE 24-15 Benign adrenal lesion without fat. In-phase **(A)** and opposed-phase **(B)** fast multiplanar spoiled gradient-recalled echo MR images show a right adrenal mass *(arrow)* slightly hyperintense to spleen on both sequences, indicating no significant lipid content. Lesion was stable on serial CT examinations for 4½ years. (From reference 70.)

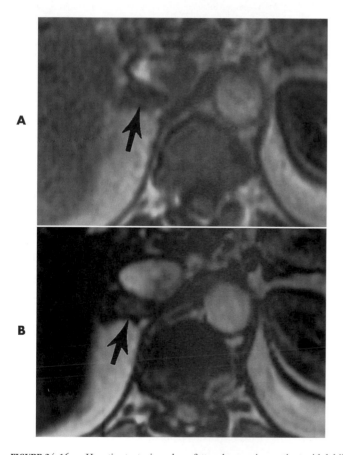

FIGURE 24-16 Hepatic steatosis and nonfatty adenoma in a patient with labile hypertension. **A,** In-phase 150/4.2 gradient-echo image shows a small right adrenal nodule *(arrow)* behind the IVC. **B,** Opposed-phase 150/2.6 image shows no loss in signal intensity within the adrenal nodule. This was suspected to be a pheochromocytoma but proved to be a benign adenoma. Note the reduction in intensity of the fatty liver on the opposed-phase image, making the spleen a better (nonfatty) standard for comparison. (Courtesy E. Siegelman.)

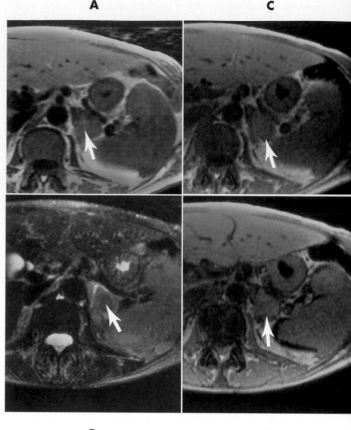

FIGURE 24-17 Metastasis from lung cancer. **A,** SE 450/10 image shows a 3.5-cm left adrenal mass *(arrow)*. **B,** FSE 4500/36 image with fat suppression shows a mass hyperintense *(arrow)* relative to liver. **C,** In-phase T1-weighted FMP-SPGR 180/120/4.2 image shows a mass isointense to muscle and spleen. **D,** Opposed-phase gradient-echo 120/6.3 image shows no evidence of fat cancellation within the metastasis. (Courtesy E. Siegelman.)

There is a high correlation between CT attenuation and chemical-shift measurements, and neither is more accurate in characterizing adrenal masses.[69] Identification of lipid in an adrenal mass, using either non-contrast CT or CSI, eliminates the need for sequential imaging follow-up or biopsy to confirm a benign condition.

Metastasis

The adrenal glands are a common site of metastatic disease, representing the fourth most commonly involved organ after lung, liver, and bone.[51] In an autopsy study of 1000 patients with epithelial cancers, 27% had metastatic disease in the adrenal glands.[1] The primary tumors most often involved include lung, breast, thyroid, colon, and melanoma.[51] In lung cancer, adrenal metastases occur in patients with a large tumor burden and clinical indications of widespread disease.[85]

Although metastatic disease occurs commonly in patients with malignancies, an isolated adrenal mass in a cancer patient is still most likely to be benign disease. Among 25 patients with non–small-cell bronchogenic carcinoma of the lung who underwent biopsies of solitary adrenal masses, 32% had metastasis and 68% had adenomas.[68] Percutaneous biopsy of adrenal masses in another series of cancer patients showed adenomas in 43%.[45]

On imaging studies, adrenal metastasis is seen as rounded or oval soft tissue masses or diffuse enlargement of the adrenal glands. Attenuation values of metastatic lesions on noncontrast CT are usually greater than 20 HU.[57,58,89] On MRI (Figure 24-17, *A* and *B*) the majority of metastatic lesions are hyperintense relative to liver on T2-weighted images. Uncommonly, metastatic lesions may show low intensity on T2-weighted images. This finding has been reported in

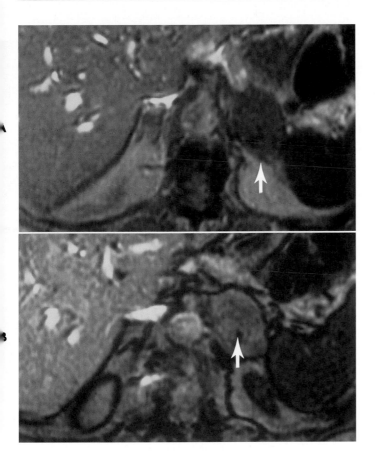

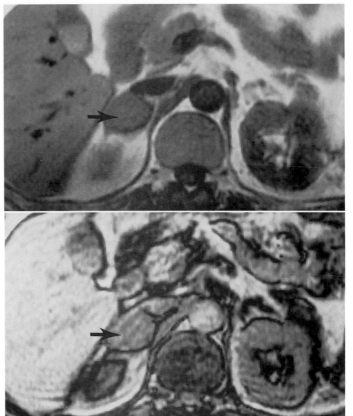

A

B

FIGURE 24-18   Metastasis from lung cancer. **A,** In-phase GRE 150/5/90 image shows a large left adrenal lesion *(arrow)* that is isointense relative to muscle, slightly hyperintense relative to the spleen, and hypointense relative to the liver. **B,** Opposed-phase GRE 150/7/90 image shows no evidence of fat cancellation within the lesion, which is consistent with the biopsy-proved diagnosis of an adrenal metastasis. (From reference 58.)

FIGURE 24-19   Metastasis from renal cell carcinoma. T1-weighted SE **(A)** and opposed-phase T1-weighted GRE **(B)** images show a right adrenal mass *(arrow)* with no signal loss relative to spleen on opposed-phase image, suggestive of metastasis. Lesion showed growth in parallel with bone metastasis on serial studies 4 months apart. (From reference 70.)

metastatic lesions arising from lung, colon, and carcinoid tumors,[36] as well as in lymphoma.[4] Such lesions simulate the appearance of a benign adenoma on SE images.

CSI is a valuable addition to SE imaging in this regard because no metastatic lesion evaluated to date has shown loss of signal intensity that would mimic a benign adenoma (Figures 24-17, *C* and *D*; 24-18; and 24-19). Several primary tumors may contain lipid, including hepatocellular carcinoma, renal cell carcinoma, and liposarcoma,[41] but no metastatic lesion containing lipid has been encountered in CSI thus far.

The differential diagnosis for an adrenal mass that does not show signal loss on opposed-phase imaging includes adenoma without lipid, metastasis, pheochromocytoma, cyst, hemorrhage, or adrenocortical carcinoma.[70] Other imaging features may help differentiate these possibilities. However, in a patient with malignancy, percutaneous biopsy of an adrenal mass may be required to confirm the histological diagnosis of metastatic disease if the diagnosis will alter treatment.[6,58,63] Elderly or debilitated patients who are not candidates for surgical therapy and patients with widespread evidence of metastatic disease need not be subjected to adrenal biopsy. When biopsy of an adrenal mass is required, clinical and biochemical screening for pheochromocytoma is indicated because biopsy of a pheochromocytoma can induce a hypertensive crisis and death.[62] Complications from percutaneous adrenal biopsy occur in up to 9% of patients[84] and include pain, pneumothorax, hemothorax, and bleeding.

Myelolipoma

This uncommon, benign neoplasm of the adrenal gland contains both fat and myeloid (bone marrow) elements. The mass may be primarily

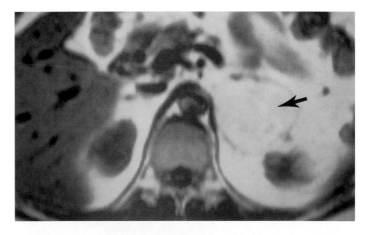

FIGURE 24-20   Adrenal myelolipoma. T1-weighted image shows signal intensity within the left adrenal mass *(arrow)* is nearly equal to that of perinephric fat.

lipomatous or solid in appearance with small foci of fat. CT is sufficient for diagnosis of myelolipoma, although MRI can also demonstrate fat density or fat signal intensity within the tumor (Figure 24-20, *A*).[24,64] Documentation of fat in an adrenal mass is diagnostic of myelolipoma because other retroperitoneal fat-containing tumors, including teratoma, lipoma, or liposarcoma, rarely involve the adrenal gland. In patients with a known malignancy, adrenal masses containing only a small

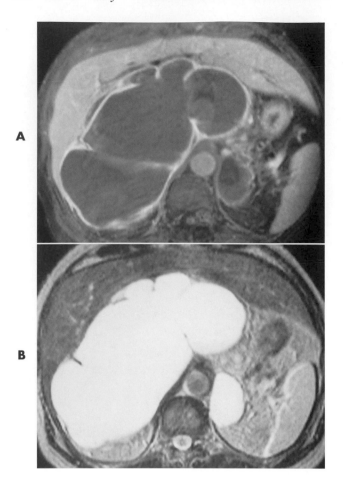

FIGURE 24-21   Bilateral adrenal lymphangiomas in a patient with basal cell nevus syndrome. **A,** SE T1-weighted image with fat suppression and gadolinium enhancement showing bilateral, cystic adrenal masses *(arrows)* with internal septations and peripheral enhancement caused by rich vascular supply. **B,** SE T2-weighted image.

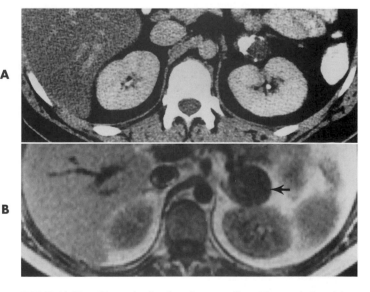

FIGURE 24-22   Hemorrhagic adrenal cyst confirmed by surgical excision. **A,** CT scan shows low-density left adrenal mass with peripheral calcifications. **B,** T1-weighted image shows no evidence of hemorrhage or calcifications.

quantity of fat or peripherally located fat can represent metastasis with engulfment of surrounding perirenal fat.[38] Percutaneous biopsy may be considered in these cases, and aspiration of myeloid elements is confirmatory for myelolipoma.

Cysts

Cysts of the adrenal gland rarely occur, with a reported incidence of 0.06% in 14,000 autopsies.[91] Endothelial cysts are most common, accounting for 45% of adrenal cysts, and are most commonly lymphangiomatous (Figure 24-21). Pseudocysts represent 39% of adrenal cysts and are the most common to be diagnosed clinically. They probably result from hemorrhage within the adrenal gland and have a fibrous wall with linear calcifications[47] and internal septations (Figure 24-22). Epithelial cysts make up 9% of adrenal cysts, and parasitic cysts account for 7%. Most of these are asymptomatic because of their small size.[44,46]

The MR appearance of adrenal cysts depends on the content of the cyst. Most cysts are hypointense relative to liver on T1-weighted images and very hyperintense to liver on T2-weighted images. If hemorrhage is present, increased signal intensity can be present within the cyst on T1-weighted images.

MANAGING THE INCIDENTAL ADRENAL MASS

When an adrenal mass is discovered incidentally on imaging studies, the following two questions should be asked: (1) Is it hormonally active, and (2) is it benign or malignant?[4,40]

In the absence of clinical symptoms of hormonal hyperfunction, limited laboratory evaluation may be warranted to exclude subclinical hyperfunction.[40] In a series of 342 patients with incidental adrenal masses, the frequency of functional adrenal tumors was 2%. Limited laboratory evaluation (24-hour urine metanephrine level, serum potassium level, and 1 mg overnight dexamethasone suppression test) was recommended in patients with adrenal nodules larger than 1 cm to identify functional tumors that should be treated surgically.[40]

To assess whether a nonhyperfunctioning mass is benign or malignant, the size of the mass and clinical history of the patient must be considered. In 39 patients with extraadrenal malignancy, 89% of masses smaller than 3 cm were benign, and 95% of masses larger than 3 cm were malignant.[10] Absolute size criteria are not reliable, however, because metastases and adrenocortical carcinomas can be small initially, and not all large adrenal masses are malignant. Among 45 patients with adrenal masses larger than 5 cm,[48] 30 had benign lesions, including 16 pheochromocytomas, 6 adrenocortical adenomas, 4 cysts, 2 myelolipomas, 1 hematoma, and 1 ganglioneuroma. The 15 malignant masses included 5 metastases, 7 adrenocortical carcinomas, and 3 lymphomas. Although the exact size criterion is debated, most authorities recommend that masses larger than 4[40] or 5 cm[17] be surgically excised. This is primarily because the possibility of carcinoma is increased in large lesions, and differentiation of benign adenoma from carcinoma cannot be reliably made by the pathologist based on percutaneous biopsy.

The clinical history of the patient is the most critical factor influencing management of the incidental adrenal mass. An adrenal mass found in a patient with no history of malignancy is far more likely to be a nonhyperfunctioning adenoma than an occult metastasis or adrenocortical carcinoma. Standard management of these patients formerly included imaging follow-up with serial CT or MR scans obtained at 3 months, 6 months, and 1 year. If the mass was stable at 1 year, it was considered benign and no further follow-up was required.[24,51]

On the other hand, an adrenal mass found incidentally in a patient with malignancy may represent a nonhyperfunctioning adenoma or metastasis. Imaging follow-up is not feasible in this case if the presence of a metastatic lesion will significantly alter the choice of therapy. Many of these patients formerly underwent adrenal biopsy if the diagnosis of metastasis would change their management.

An algorithmic approach to characterizing adrenal masses in patients with cancer was recently proposed[63] and relies on the presence of lipid in benign lesions. In Step I of the algorithm, the density of the adrenal lesion is measured on noncontrast CT. If it is less than 0 HU, the lesion is benign and no further investigation is required. If the density by CT is greater than 20 HU, the lesion is probably malignant.

Table 24-1   Adrenal Imaging Summary

TYPE OF LESION	PREFERRED IMAGING STUDY	CT MORPHOLOGY	T1WI	T2WI	CHEMICAL SHIFT*
Nonhyperfunctioning adenoma	Noncontrast CT Chemical shift if HU >0 and <20	<3-cm hypodense mass, HU <0	Isointense to liver	Most isointense but variable	Homogeneous signal loss†
Adenoma, Conn's syndrome	CT	Small, mean 1.5-cm diameter	Isointense to liver	Variable	Homogeneous signal loss
Adrenal hyperplasia	CT	Normal, diffuse enlargement or multinodular	Isointense	Variable	Homogeneous signal loss
Adenoma, Cushing's syndrome	CT	>2-cm nodule	Isointense to liver	Variable	Homogeneous signal loss
Pheochromocytoma	MRI	Adrenal mass (90%) or extraadrenal lesion	Isointense to liver	Typically very hyperintense	No signal loss
Adrenal carcinoma	CT MRI for IVC invasion, preoperative planning	Large mass with necrosis	Heterogeneous, hemorrhagic	Heterogeneous, hyperintense	Heterogeneous; may have focal areas of signal loss
Metastasis	CT Chemical shift if HU >0 and <20	Focal or diffuse enlargement; HU >20	Most hypointense	Most hyperintense but variable	No signal loss
Myelolipoma	CT	Fat contained in tumor	Regions of high intensity caused by fat	Variable with evidence of fat	Fatty regions show signal loss
Hemorrhage	CT MRI for subacute hemorrhage	Unilateral or bilateral enlargement, hyperdense early, hypodense in chronic phase	Variable with stage of hemorrhage	Variable	No signal loss

T1WI, T1-weighted image; *T2WI,* T2-weighted image; *HU,* Hounsfield units; *IVC,* inferior vena cava.
*Appearance on opposed-phase images relative to in-phase images.
†80% of adenomas.

Biopsy is performed only if the diagnosis of malignancy will change patient management.

Step II is performed if the density by noncontrast CT is 0 to 20 HU. In this range the lesion is indeterminate, and chemical-shift MRI is performed. In- and opposed-phase images are performed using identical parameters except for variance in TE.

The adrenal-spleen ratio (ASR) is calculated by the following formula and reflects the percentage drop-off in signal of the adrenal lesion relative to the internal standard of the spleen on opposed-phase images:

(EQ. 1)

$$ASR = \frac{SI \text{ lesion (opposed phase)}/SI \text{ spleen (opposed phase)}}{SI \text{ lesion (in phase)}/SI \text{ spleen (in phase)}} \times 100$$

If ASR is less than 70, meaning that the signal intensity (SI) in the lesion is decreased relative to the spleen on opposed-phase images, the lesion can be regarded as benign and no further investigation is needed.

SUMMARY

The role of MRI in adrenal disorders continues to evolve as new techniques are developed and evaluated in clinical trials. Table 24-1 provides a summary of current recommendations on imaging strategy and findings in common adrenal disorders.

REFERENCES

1. Abrams HL, Spiro R, and Goldstein N: Metastases in carcinoma. Analysis of 1000 autopsied cases, Cancer 3:74, 1950.
2. Auda SA, et al: Evolution of the surgical management of primary aldosteronism, Ann Surg 191:1, 1980.
3. Baker ME, et al: Benign adrenal lesions mimicking malignancy on MR imaging: report of two cases, Radiology 163:669, 1987.
4. Baker ME, et al: MR evaluation of adrenal masses at 1.5 T, Am J Roentgenol 153:307, 1989.
5. Berliner L, Bosniak MA, and Megibow A: Adrenal pseudotumors on computed tomography, J Comput Assist Tomogr 6(2):281,1982.
6. Bernardino ME: Management of the asymptomatic patient with a unilateral adrenal mass, Radiology 166:121, 1988.
7. Bilbey JH, et al: MR imaging of adrenal masses: value of chemical-shift imaging for distinguishing adenomas from other tumors, Am J Roentgenol 164:637, 1995.
8. Boland GW et al: Adrenal masses: characterization with delayed contrast-enhanced CT, Radiology 202:693, 1997.
9. Brady TM, et al: Adrenal pseudomasses due to varices: angiographic-CT-MRI-pathologic correlations, Am J Roentgenol 145:301, 1985.
10. Candel AG, et al: Fine-needle aspiration biopsy of adrenal masses in patients with extraadrenal malignancy, Surgery 114:1132, 1993.
11. Catasea JV, and Mirowitz SA: T2-weighted MR imaging of the abdomen: fast spin-echo vs. conventional spin-echo sequences, Am J Roentgenol 162:61, 1994.
12. Chang A, et al: Adrenal gland: MR imaging, Radiology 163:123, 1987.
13. Chezmar JL, et al: Adrenal masses: characterization with T1-weighted MR imaging, Radiology 166:357, 1988.
14. Cho KJ, et al: Adrenal medullary disease in multiple endocrine neoplasia type II, Am J Roentgenol 134:23, 1980.
15. Choyke PL: Invited commentary, Radiographics 14(5):1029, 1994.
16. Commons RR, and Callaway CP: Adenomas of the adrenal cortex, Arch Intern Med 81:37, 1948.
17. Copeland PM: The incidentally discovered adrenal mass, Ann Intern Med 98:940, l983.
18. Daneman A: Adrenal neoplasms in children, Semin Roentgenol 23:205, 1988.
19. Dobbie JW: Adenocortical nodular hyperplasia: the aging adrenal, J Pathol 99(1):1, 1969.
20. Doppman JL, et al: CT findings in Addison disease, J Comput Assist Tomogr 6:757, 1982.
21. Doppman JL, et al: Macronodular adrenal hyperplasia in Cushing disease, Radiology 166:347, l988.
22. Doppman JL, et al: Cushing syndrome due to primary pigmented nodular adrenocortical disease: findings at CT and MR imaging, Radiology 172:415, 1989.
23. Doppman JL, et al: Ectopic adrenocorticotropic hormone syndrome: localization studies in 28 patients, Radiology 172:115, 1989.
24. Dunnick NR: Adrenal imaging: current status, Am J Roentgenol 154:927, 1990.
25. Dunnick NR, Korobkin M, and Francis I: Adrenal radiology: distinguishing benign from malignant adrenal masses, Am J Roentgenol 167:861, 1996.
26. Edelman RR, et al: Surface coil MR imaging of the abdominal viscera. I. Theory, technique, and initial results, Radiology 157:425, 1985.
27. Egglin TK, Hahn PF, and Stark DD: MRI of the adrenal glands, Semin Roentgenol 23(4):280, 1988.
28. Falke THM, et al: Magnetic resonance imaging of the adrenal glands, Radiographics 7(2):343, 1987.
29. Falke THM, et al: Gadolinium-DTPA enhanced MR imaging of intravenous extension of adrenocortical carcinoma, J Comput Assist Tomogr 12(2):331, 1988.
30. Farge D, et al: Isolated clinical syndrome of primary aldosteronism in four patients with adrenocortical carcinoma, J Am Med 83:635, 1987.
31. Fink IJ, et al: MR Imaging of pheochromocytomas, J Comput Assist Tomogr 9(3):454, 1985.
32. Fishman EK, et al: Primary adrenocortical carcinoma: CT evaluation with clinical correlation, Am J Roentgenol 148:531, 1987.
33. Geisinger MA, et al: Primary hyperaldosteronism: comparison of CT, adrenal venography, and venous sampling, Am J Roentgenol 141:299, 1983.
34. Glazer HS, et al: Nonfunctioning adrenal masses: incidental discovery on computed tomography, Am J Roentgenol 139:81, 1982.
35. Glazer GM, et al: Adrenal tissue characterization using MR imaging, Radiology 158:73, 1986.

36. Glazer GM: MR imaging of the liver, kidneys, and adrenal glands, Radiology 166:303, 1988.
37. Glazer GM, Francis IR, and Quint LE: Progress in clinical radiology: imaging of the adrenal glands, Invest Radiol 23:3, 1988.
38. Green KM, Brantly PN, and Thompson WR: Adenocarcinoma metastatic to the adrenal gland simulating myelolipoma: CT evaluation, J Comput Assist Tomogr 9(4):820, 1985.
39. Hedeland H, et al: On the prevalence of adrenocortical adenomas in an autopsy material in relation to hypertension and diabetes, Acta Med Scand 184:211, 1968.
40. Herrera MF, et al: Incidentally discovered adrenal tumors: an institutional perspective, Surgery 110:1014, 1991.
41. Hertzler G, et al: The adrenal gland. In Someren A, ed: Urologic pathology with clinical and radiologic correlations, New York, 1989, Macmillan.
42. Ichikawa T, et al: Contrast-enhanced dynamic MRI of adrenal masses: classification of characteristic enhancement patterns, Clin Radiol 50:295, 1995.
43. Ikeda DM, et al: The detection of adrenal tumors and hyperplasia in patients with primary aldosteronism: comparison of scintigraphy, CT, and MR imaging, Am J Roentgenol 153:301, 1989.
44. Johnson CD, Baker ME, and Dunnick NR: CT demonstration of an adrenal pseudocyst, J Comput Assist Tomogr 9(4):817, 1985.
45. Katz RL, and Shirkhoda A: Diagnostic approach to incidental adrenal nodules in the cancer patient: results of a clinical, radiologic, and fine needle aspiration study, Cancer 55:1995, 1985.
46. Kearney GP, et al: Functioning and nonfunctioning cysts of the adrenal cortex and medulla, Am J Surg 134:363, 1977.
47. Kenney PJ, and Stanley RJ: Calcified adrenal masses, Urol Radiol 9:9, 1987.
48. Khafagi FA, et al: Clinical significance of the large adrenal mass, Br J Surg 78:828, 1991.
49. Kier R, and McCarthy S: MR characterization of adrenal masses: field strength and pulse sequence considerations, Radiology 171:671, 1989.
50. King BF: Editorial comment, Urology 43(6):873, 1994.
51. Korobkin M: Overview of adrenal imaging/adrenal CT, Urol Radiol 11:221, 1989.
52. Korobkin M, and Dunnick NR: Characterization of adrenal masses, Am J Roentgenol 164:643, 1995.
53. Korobkin M, et al: Adrenal adenomas: relationship between histological lipid and CT and MR findings, Radiology 200:743, 1996.
54. Korobkin M, et al: Characterization of adrenal masses with chemical shift and gadolinium-enhanced MR imaging, Radiology 197:411, 1995.
55. Korobkin M, et al: Differentiation of adrenal adenomas from nonadenomas using CT attenuation values, Am J Roentgenol 166:531, 1996.
56. Krestin BP, Steinbrich W, and Friedmann G: Adrenal masses: evaluation with fast gradient-echo MR imaging and Gd-DTPA-enhanced dynamic studies, Radiology 171:675, 1989.
57. Lee MJ, et al: Benign and malignant adrenal masses: CT distinction with attenuation coefficients, size and observer analysis, Radiology 179:415, 1991.
58. Lee MJ, et al: State-of-the-art MR imaging of the adrenal gland, Radiographics 14:1015, 1994.
59. Leroy-Willig A, et al: In vitro adrenal cortex lesions characterized by NMR spectroscopy, Magn Reson Imaging 5:339, 1987.
60. Leroy-Willig A, et al: In vivo MR spectroscopic imaging of the adrenal glands: distinction between adenomas and carcinomas larger than 15 mm based on lipid content, Am J Roentgenol 153:771, 1989.
61. Mayo-Smith WW, et al: Characterization of adrenal masses (<5 cm) by use of chemical shift MR imaging: observer performance versus quantitative parameters, Am J Roentgenol 165:91, 1995.
62. McCorkell SJ, and Niles NL: Fine-needle aspiration of catecholamine-producing adrenal masses: a possibly fatal mistake, Am J Roentgenol 145:113, 1985.
63. McNicholas MMJ, et al: An imaging algorithm for the differential diagnosis of adrenal adenomas and metastasis, Am J Roentgenol 165:1453, 1995.
64. Mezrich R, Banner MP, and Pollack HM: Magnetic resonance imaging of the adrenal glands, Urol Radiol 8:127, 1986.
65. Mitchell DG, et al: Benign adrenocortical masses: diagnosis with chemical shift MR imaging, Radiology 185:345, 1992.
66. Mitty HA: Embryology, anatomy, and anomalies of the adrenal gland, Semin Roentgenol 23(4):271, 1988.
67. Montagne J, et al: Computed tomography of the normal adrenal glands, Am J Roentgenol 130:963, 1978.
68. Oliver TW, et al: Isolated adrenal masses in nonsmall-cell bronchogenic carcinoma, Radiology 153:217, 1984.
69. Outwater EK, et al: Adrenal masses: correlation between CT attenuation value and chemical shift ratio at MR imaging with in-phase and opposed-phase sequences, Radiology 200:749, 1996.
70. Outwater EK, et al: Distinction between benign and malignant adrenal masses: value of T1-weighted chemical-shift MR imaging, Am J Roentgenol 165:579, 1995.
71. Paling MR, and Williamson BRJ: Adrenal involvement in Non-Hodgkin lymphoma, Am J Roentgenol 141:303, 1983.
72. Quint LE: Pheochromocytoma and paraganglioma: comparison of MR imaging with CT and I-131 MIBG scintigraphy, Radiology 165:89, 1987.
73. Reinig JW, et al: MRI of indeterminate adrenal masses, Am J Roentgenol 147:493, 1986.
74. Reinig JW, et al: Adrenal masses differentiated by MR, Radiology 158:81, 1986.
75. Remer EM, et al: Hyperfunctioning and nonhyperfunctioning benign adrenal cortical lesions: characterization and comparison with MR imaging, Radiology 171:681, 1989.
76. Schlund JF, et al: Adrenocortical carcinoma: MR imaging appearance with current techniques, J Magn Reson Imaging 5:171, 1995.
77. Schwartz LH, et al: Echoplanar MR imaging for characterization of adrenal masses in patients with malignant neoplasms: preliminary evaluation of calculated T2 relaxation values, Am J Roentgenol 164:911, 1995.
78. Schwartz LH, et al: Adrenal masses in patients with malignancy: prospective comparison of echo-planar, fast spin-echo, and chemical shift MR imaging, Radiology 197:421, 1995.
79. Semelka RC, et al: Fat-saturation MR imaging of the upper abdomen, Am J Roentgenol 155:1111, 1990.
80. Semelka RC, et al: Evaluation of adrenal masses with gadolinium enhancement and fat-suppressed MR imaging, J Magn Reson Imaging 3:337, 1993.
81. Shapiro B, et al: Iodine-131 metaiodobenzylguanidine for the locating of suspected pheochromocytoma: experience in 400 cases, J Nucl Med 26:576, 1985.
82. Siegelbaum MH, et al: Use of magnetic resonance imaging scanning in adrenocortical carcinoma with vena caval involvement, Urology 43(6):869, 1994.
83. Silverman PM: Gastric diverticulum mimicking adrenal mass: CT demonstration, J Comput Assist Tomogr 10(4):709, 1986.
84. Silverman SG: Predictive value of image-guided adrenal biopsy: analysis of results of 101 biopsies, Radiology 187:715, 1993.
85. Silvestri GA, et al: The relationship of clinical findings to CT scan evidence of adrenal gland metastases in the staging of bronchogenic carcinoma, Chest 102:1748, 1992.
86. Smith SM: Magnetic resonance imaging of adrenal cortical carcinoma, Urol Radiol 11:1, 1989.
87. Szolar DH, and Kammerhuber F: Quantitative CT evaluation of adrenal gland masses: a step forward in the differentiation between adenomas and nonadenomas? Radiology 202:517, 1997.
88. Tsushima Y, Ishizaka H, and Matsumoto M: Adrenal masses: differentiation with chemical shift, fast low-angle shot MR imaging, Radiology 186:705, 1993.
89. van Erkel AR, et al: CT and MR distinction of adenomas and nonadenomas of the adrenal glands, J Comp Assist Tomogr 18(3):432, 1994.
90. van Gils APG: MR imaging and MIBG scintigraphy of pheochromocytomas and extraadrenal functioning paragangliomas, Radiographics 11:37, 1991.
91. Wahl HR: Adrenal cysts, Am J Pathol 27:798, 1951.
92. Weinberger MH, et al: Primary aldosteronism: diagnosis, localization and treatment, Ann Intern Med 90:386, 1979.
93. Westra SJ, et al: Imaging of the adrenal gland in children, Radiographics 14:1323, 1994.
94. Whalen RK, Althausen AF, and Daniels GH: Extra-adrenal pheochromocytoma, J Urol 147:1, 1992.
95. White EM, et al: Surface coil MR imaging of the abdominal viscera. II. The adrenal glands, Radiology 157:431, 1985.
96. Williams TC: Functional disorders of the adrenal glands: an overview, Semin Roentgenol 23(4):304, 1988.
97. Wilson, et al: Histoplasmosis of the adrenal glands studied by CT, Radiology 150:779, 1984.

CHAPTER

25 Kidney

Gladys M. Torres and Pablo R. Ros

 KEY POINTS

- CT and ultrasound remain the primary techniques for diagnosis.
- MRI is helpful for diagnosing venous invasion by renal carcinoma.
- MRI is improving but not yet competitive with catheter angiography.
- MR urography using T2-weighted MIP techniques is under development. CT is superior to MRI for detecting ureteral calculi.

Multiplanar capability and angiographic capabilities have made magnetic resonance imaging (MRI) a useful method for evaluating the kidneys. Prominent drawbacks are artifacts resulting from physiological motions of respiration, intestinal peristalsis, and heartbeat. MRI also shows limited contrast between renal masses and the kidney. Computed tomography (CT) and ultrasound are powerful, inexpensive competitors.[39,74]

Fast imaging sequences reduce motion artifacts. Gadolinium diethylene-triamine-pentaacetic acid (Gd-DTPA) permits assessment of parenchymal perfusion and renal excretory function. Like the iodinated urographic agents used in CT scanning, Gd-DTPA is freely filtered by the kidney; its excretion reflects the glomerular filtration rate and tubular absorption of water.*

The principal indications for renal MRI are evaluation and characterization of renal masses and fluid collections, accurate staging of renal cancer, semiquantitative evaluation of renal function using contrast-enhanced dynamic studies, and evaluation of renal vessels using magnetic resonance angiography (MRA). It can also be used as an alternative imaging modality to CT for patients allergic to iodine or patients with an inconclusive CT study.[45]

TECHNIQUES

Initial localization may be performed in the coronal plane with a fast gradient-echo technique and suspended respiration. The fundamental MR technique is the T1-weighted spin-echo (SE) sequence in the transverse plane analogous to CT scanning. SE or fast SE, single- or double-echo images complete the routine examination.

If there is a pathological condition involving the vessels, gradient-echo images are performed to visualize blood flow. Multiple overlapping axial scans are performed using typical abdominal MRA sequences (see Chapters 19 and 48). Gd-DTPA–enhanced perfusion studies allow the evaluation of renal masses in conjunction with fast imaging after an intravenous bolus injection.[42]

Fat-suppression techniques[76] based on selective chemical-shift suppression imaging, especially with the use of Gd-DTPA, are useful for diagnosing and characterizing small renal lesions and helping to visualize perirenal and pararenal extension of disease.[8]

NORMAL ANATOMY

Differences in water content between the cortex and medulla provide good contrast.[39,56,60,61] Compared with the medulla, the renal cortex has a lower water content, a shorter T1 relaxation time, and therefore a higher signal intensity on T1-weighted images. The medulla appears as central triangular regions of lower signal intensity. Renal sinus fat is identified within the hilum of the kidney and has high signal intensity on both T1- and T2-weighted images. The renal pelvis and calyxes, if distended, are delineated by the low signal intensity of urine with long T1 values. Renal arteries and veins are best shown on gradient-echo images. The high signal intensity of flowing blood allows the demonstration of vascular patency.[47] Corticomedullary boundaries are less well differentiated on T2-weighted images. Gd-DTPA renography is performed with a fast T1-sensitive technique, such as turbo-FLASH (fast low-angle shot). The first image is obtained immediately before injection of Gd-DTPA. The signal intensity of renal cortex increases 5 to 20 sec after intravenous Gd-DTPA injection. The signal intensity in the medulla increases to a level similar to that in the cortex after 20 to 30 sec, when the contrast agent passes into the calyxes.[45]

BENIGN RENAL MASSES
Cysts

Simple Cysts. Simple cyst, the most frequent renal mass in adults, is often detected incidentally. Cysts are simply and accurately characterized as such by ultrasound. MRI has a minor role in the evaluation of

---

*References 6, 7, 12, 13, 45, 46, 65, 72.

A   B   C

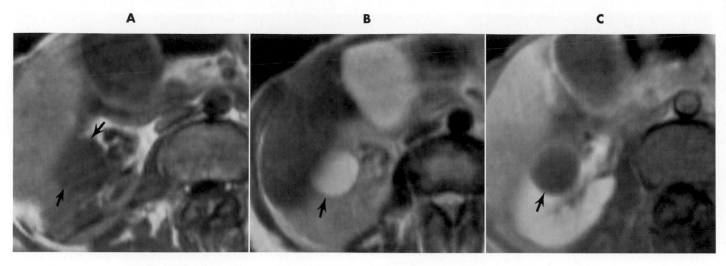

FIGURE 25-1   Simple cyst. **A,** T1-weighted SE image shows a hypointense homogeneous mass arising within the right kidney. The gallbladder has a similar signal intensity. **B,** T2-weighted image shows an increase in the signal intensity of the cyst relative to the renal cortex and often shows solid organs. **C,** Gd-enhanced image demonstrates lack of enhancement and smooth cyst borders.

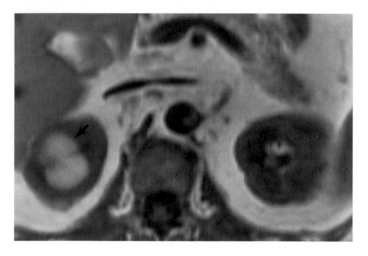

FIGURE 25-2   Hemorrhagic cyst. T1-weighted SE image shows a heterogeneous mass with a higher signal intensity than renal cortex.

cystic masses that cannot be categorized as confidently as simple renal cysts by CT or ultrasonography.

The MR characteristics of a renal cyst vary depending on the composition of the fluid within the cyst and the pulse sequence used.[26,58] Simple cysts have homogeneous low signal intensity (clear fluid) on T1-weighted images and high signal intensity on T2-weighted images[3,26,33,45,58] (Figure 25-1, *A* and *B*).

Cysts can be better defined after the administration of urographic contrast agents such as Gd-DTPA.[10] Contrast-enhanced, fat-suppressed T1-weighted images and breath-holding gradient-echo images provide higher sensitivity than CT in detecting cystic lesions.[78] As with CT, the diagnostic criteria for a simple cyst are lack of enhancement, smooth borders, and homogeneous content (Figure 25-1, *C*).

Complicated Cysts. Complicated cysts account for approximately 5% of renal masses[1] and have irregular borders, wall calcification, septations, or internal hemorrhage or contain high concentration of protein or milk of calcium. The differential diagnosis of a necrotic (cystic) neoplasm may be difficult[39] (Figure 25-2).

Elevated concentrations of proteinaceous material or blood products in the internal fluid of a cyst variably increase the signal intensity on T1-weighted images. High signal intensity is generally maintained

on T2-weighted images. Hemorrhagic cysts vary in appearance, depending on the amount and age of the blood products within them[26,33,38,57] (Figure 25-2). Paramagnetic hemoglobin-degradation products within hemorrhagic cysts decrease both T1 and T2 values below those measured for simple cysts. Fluid and blood cell levels can also be seen in hemorrhagic cysts.[26,57]

Cyst wall calcification is poorly detected by MRI. The inability to detect calcifications causes some complicated cysts to appear as simple cysts.

Adult Polycystic Kidney Disease

Adult polycystic kidney disease is an autosomal dominant disease in which the kidneys are markedly enlarged and replaced by multiple cysts of variable signal intensities, depending on whether they are simple, hemorrhagic, or infected[26,33,53] (Figure 25-3). Although hemorrhagic fluid has a characteristic signal intensity on MRI, imaging with MRI, CT, and ultrasound cannot reliably differentiate among infected, hemorrhagic, and malignant cysts.

Multilocular Cystic Nephromas

Multilocular cystic nephroma is an uncommon benign neoplasm composed of noncommunicating cysts and fibrous stroma.[3] The cystic components of this neoplasm may have varying signal intensity, depending on the composition of the fluid.[16,44] The fibrous capsule and septa can appear as low–signal intensity structures on T2-weighted images.

Angiomyolipomas

Angiomyolipoma (AML) is the most frequent renal mass of mesenchymal origin. It is an unencapsulated hamartomatous tumor composed of thick-walled vessels and smooth muscle fibers as well as lipocytes in different proportions. AMLs present as spontaneous solitary tumors in women ranging in age from 40 to 60 years and as multiple, bilateral lesions in patients with tuberous sclerosis (Bourneville's disease). Some 20% of all AMLs are multiple, bilateral, and associated with tuberous sclerosis, whereas 5% are multiple and bilateral and have no association with tuberous sclerosis.[5,85] AMLs can become very large, measuring up to 20 cm in diameter.

The MR appearance depends on the composition of the tumor. Most contain a portion of grossly visible fat and appear with high signal intensity on T1- and T2-weighted images (Figures 25-4 and 25-5). Some may show low, inhomogeneous signal intensity on gradient-recalled

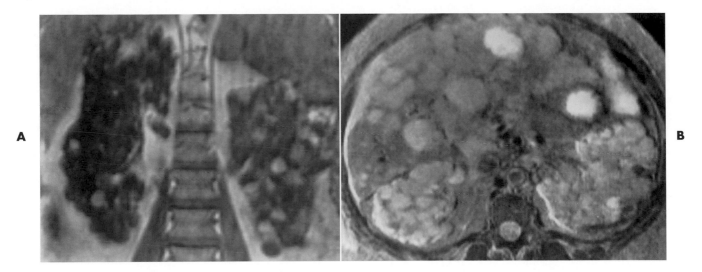

FIGURE 25-3   Adult polycystic kidney disease. **A,** Coronal T1-weighted SE image demonstrates bilateral enlarged kidneys with multiple cysts of varying signal intensity (lowest signal intensity, uncomplicated cysts; high signal intensity, hemorrhagic cysts). **B,** T2-weighted SE image of the same patient with enlarged kidneys with multiple high–signal intensity cysts. Multiple cysts are also seen in the liver.

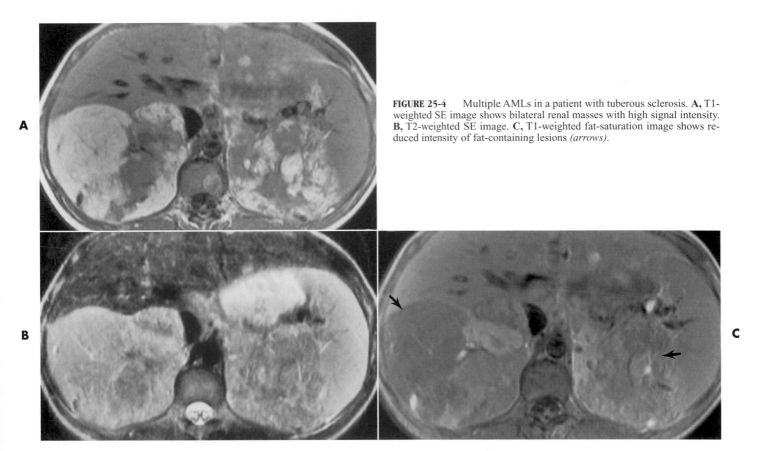

FIGURE 25-4   Multiple AMLs in a patient with tuberous sclerosis. **A,** T1-weighted SE image shows bilateral renal masses with high signal intensity. **B,** T2-weighted SE image. **C,** T1-weighted fat-saturation image shows reduced intensity of fat-containing lesions *(arrows).*

echo images, probably as a result of susceptibility artifacts and chemical-shift effects caused by iron-containing hemoglobin derivatives and dephasing between fat and water protons.[5,85] Fat-suppressed images allows the discrimination of fat within the lesion from hemorrhagic lesions. If smooth muscle predominates, these lesions cannot be differentiated from solid tumors such as renal cell carcinoma (RCC).

Other Benign Neoplasms

Hemangioma, lymphangioma, leiomyoma, lipoma, and juxtaglomerular tumors show no diagnostic morphology or specific tissue character-

istics. Lipoma shows high signal intensity on T1-weighted SE images equal to retroperitoneal fat.

POTENTIALLY MALIGNANT NEOPLASMS
Oncocytomas

Oncocytoma is a rare form of renal adenoma composed of eosinophilic cells. It is a frequently asymptomatic mass, and therefore it is discovered incidentally. Oncocytoma is usually a single tumor, although it may be multifocal or bilateral. It is well circumscribed and frequently displays a central star-shaped scar composed of white fibrous tissue.[2,62]

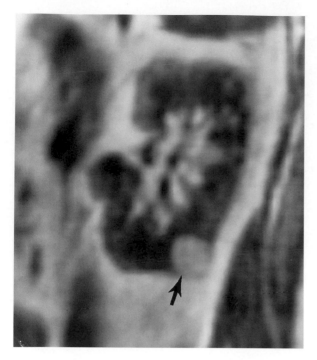

FIGURE 25-5 AML. Sagittal T1-weighted SE image shows a small high-intensity lesion at the lower pole of the kidney *(arrow).*

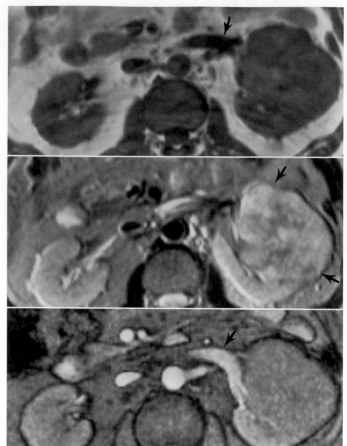

FIGURE 25-7 RCC. **A,** T1-weighted SE image shows a mixed-intensity left renal mass. The left renal vein is patent *(arrow).* **B,** T2-weighted SE image shows a heterogeneous mass *(arrows).* **C,** Gradient-recalled echo image demonstrates flow within the left renal vein *(arrow).*

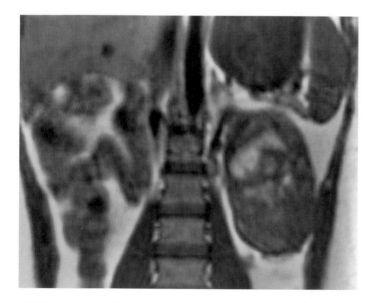

FIGURE 25-6 Left RCC has areas of hemorrhage, which are identified by high–signal intensity areas with all echo sequences. This is a coronal T1-weighted image.

Oncocytomas were historically considered benign tumors, but evidence now indicates that they may contain foci of malignant cells and should be reclassified as low-grade renal malignancies.[54,66,88]

On nonenhanced MR scans, oncocytomas generally display the same signal intensity as the surrounding renal parenchyma and may be visualized only because of their mass effect.[10] The central scar most often seen in large oncocytomas is often dark on T2-weighted images, reflecting fibrous tissue with short T2 values. In one reported case the scar had high signal intensity apparently because of increased water content.[68] Oncocytoma may simulate an RCC if there are central necrosis and hemorrhage, resulting in mixed signal intensity.[81] Dense calcifications in oncocytomas may appear as signal voids. After Gd-DTPA

administration, oncocytomas demonstrate intense enhancement.[18] The central scar usually does not enhance; however, this finding is unreliable in the diagnosis of oncocytoma.[2,81]

Adenomas

Renal adenomas may not be clearly distinguished from RCC by histological examinations. The conventional wisdom is that adenomas larger than 3 cm in diameter must be considered malignant. However, adenomas smaller than 2 cm in size have been reported to metastasize, whereas larger ones do not necessarily spread.[51]

On MRI, adenomas are reported to be isointense with renal parenchyma on T1-weighted images. The signal intensity is high on T2-weighted images.[10]

MALIGNANT NEOPLASMS
Renal Cell Carcinomas

RCC is the most common malignant tumor of the kidney, with an overall incidence rate of about 2% of all cancers in adults. Approximately 10,300 people die of RCC each year. RCCs are slow-growing tumors and in the early stages are silent. Symptoms usually denote more advanced tumor. Typical presenting signs and symptoms are hematuria, which occurs when the collecting system is invaded; pain, which occurs when the renal capsule is stretched; and a palpable mass and fever, which occur when there is calyceal or pelvic obstruction.[28,59] About

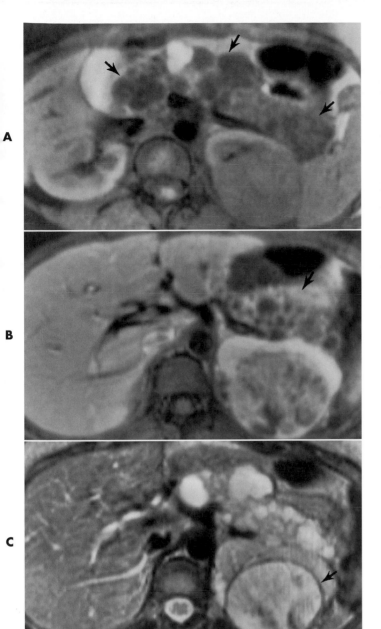

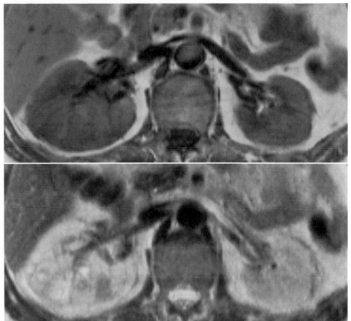

FIGURE 25-9   RCC of the right kidney is isointense with renal parenchyma. **A,** T1-weighted image. **B,** T2-weighted image. The right kidney is enlarged, and the corticomedullary boundaries are ill defined.

FIGURE 25-8   RCC in a patient with von Hippel-Lindau syndrome. Fat-suppression images before **(A)** and after **(B)** Gd-DTPA enhancement reveal a well-encapsulated enhancing lesion with central areas of necrosis within the left kidney. Note the multiple pancreatic cysts *(arrows)*. Hyperintense mass with low–signal intensity capsule *(arrow)* is seen on T2-weighted SE image **(C).** There is an increase in the signal of the pancreatic cysts.

Table 25-1	Robson's Classification of RCC
STAGE	**EXTENT**
I	Tumor confined to the kidney
II	Tumor spread to the perinephric fat but within Gerota's fascia
IIIA	Tumor spread to the renal vein or inferior vena cava
IIIB	Tumor spread to local lymph nodes
IIIC	Tumor spread to local veins and lymph nodes
IVA	Tumor spread to adjacent organs (including adrenal gland)
IVB	Distant metastases

From reference 71.

15% of RCCs are cystic as a result of hemorrhage, tumor necrosis, or cystic growth.[45]

Improvement in the quality of excretory urography and nephrotomography, ultrasound, CT, and MRI has significantly increased the early detection of asymptomatic unsuspected RCC.[28] The accuracy of current imaging methods in detection of RCC approaches 100%.[89]

The MR signal intensity of RCC is variable.[33,38,52,67,80] Furthermore, there are no specific morphological findings specifically diagnostic of RCC. On T1-weighted images, the signal intensity is frequently lower than that of the normal cortex. Hemorrhagic or necrotic RCCs have mixed signal intensity and may have areas of high signal intensity on T1- and T2-weighted images (Figures 25-6 to 25-8). Iron deposition within the tumor cells may produce low signal intensities.[84] Large RCCs are well visualized on T2-weighted images and appear as heterogeneous masses with frequent low–signal intensity bands corre-

sponding to fibrotic strands that give RCCs a lobulated and nodular appearance.[67] RCCs may be isointense with renal parenchyma and may be distinguished only by contour changes or renal enlargement[9,38] (Figure 25-9). The size of the smallest RCC detected by unenhanced MRI is around 2 cm,[22,38] with only a 63% tumor detection rate when the lesions are smaller than 3 cm.[34]

Gd-DTPA administration in conjunction with rapid scanning may improve small tumor detection.[45,50,78,79] Gd-DTPA enhancement in conjunction with fat suppression also improves detection.[28] Fat suppression is important for minimizing motion artifacts, and fast scanning allows scanning during the arterial phase of injection.[89] Patterns of tumor enhancement vary from homogeneous (typical for small solid lesions) to heterogeneous and purely peripheral with absent central enhancement (typical for cystic necrotic lesions)[18] (Figures 25-8 to 25-12).

Assessment of tumor spread is relevant to establishing a prognosis and treatment plan (Table 25-1). The hematogenous spread of RCC occurs early and commonly involves the lungs and mediastinum, liver, bone, brain, adrenal glands, or contralateral kidney. Infiltration of the surrounding structures, particularly the renal veins and inferior vena cava (IVC), is also common (Figures 25-10 and 25-11). Lymphatic spread involves the paraaortic lymph nodes.

Improved 5-year survival is seen after radical nephrectomy for patients with stage I (60% to 75%) and stage II (47% to 65%) disease.[71] Although ultrasonography and venacavography can be used, staging of RCC requires CT or MRI. The reported accuracy of both techniques is similar, ranging from 67% to 96%.[34,36,37] The major advantages of MRI

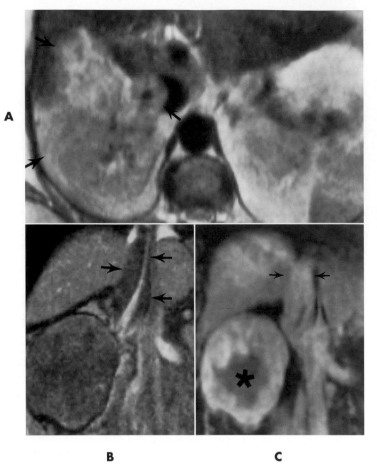

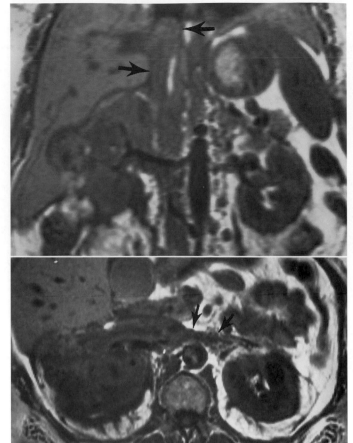

FIGURE 25-10   RCC with venous extension in a patient with stage IIIa disease. **A,** T2-weighted SE image demonstrates a hyperintense right renal mass with tumor extension to the renal vein and inferior vena cava *(arrows).* **B,** Coronal gradient-recalled echo image. Tumor thrombus from primary RCC fills the distended inferior vena cava *(arrows)* and extends to the intrahepatic portion. **C,** Coronal Gd-DTPA-enhanced fat-suppression image. Enhancing RCC with a central area of necrosis *(asterisk)* and an enhancing tumor thrombus into the intrahepatic inferior vena cava *(arrows).*

FIGURE 25-11   Extracapsular extension of RCC of the right kidney (stage IIIc). Coronal **(A)** and transverse **(B)** T1-weighted SE images. Large mixed-intensity mass with extracapsular extension to the perinephric fat and to the soft tissues anterior and to the left of the aorta *(arrows* in **A)** with paraaortic adenopathy. There is extensive tumor thrombus involving the inferior vena cava to the level of the origin of the right atrium *(arrows* in **B).**

include direct imaging in the sagittal and coronal planes, the ease of distinguishing tumor thrombus within the venous system from flowing blood, the lack of injection of iodinated contrast material with known nephrotoxicity, and the ability to discriminate between tumor and bland thrombus in the IVC.[89]

The multiplanar capability of MRI facilitates evaluation of the extent of the tumor (Figure 25-11). Invasion of perinephric fat by tumor may be indistinguishable from changes in the perirenal fat resulting from lymphatic or venous edema.[45]

Screening for invasion of the renal vein, IVC, or right atrium is one of the most important uses of MRI[27,29,38] (Figures 25-10 and 25-11). Tumor thrombus can be directly visualized within the renal vein and IVC, which normally are devoid of signal. In a study by Rubidoux et al,[75] the sensitivity of gradient-recalled echo MRI was 100% for thrombi in the IVC and 80% for intraatrial tumor spread. Involvement of the renal vein could be predicted with 80% sensitivity and 75% specificity.[75] MRI of the IVC can be limited in the presence of bulky lymphadenopathy or bulky RCC because they can abut and deform the IVC.[29] In these cases, inferior venacavography can be used as a complementary technique to MRI. When both techniques are combined, the accuracy for the evaluation of IVC thrombus is reported to be 100%.[29]

Evaluation of the lymph nodes is limited for both MRI and CT because size remains the only criterion for the diagnosis of malignant involvement. There are no reliable signal characteristics to differentiate reactive nodes from malignant ones[18,45] (Figure 25-11).

Metastatic RCC, like all other cancers, usually has the same T1 and T2 relaxation times as the primary tumor.[64] RCC metastases are generally hypervascular and enhance with Gd-DTPA.

Lymphomas and Leukemia

Because of the lack of lymphoid tissue within the kidney, primary lymphoma of the kidney is very rare or is merely occult secondary involvement. Normal lymphatics are present in the collecting system, and therefore lymphoma grows from the calyxes into the parenchyma. Lymphomatous involvement of the kidney is usually the result of hematogenous involvement or contiguous growth from retroperitoneal lymphadenopathy.[69] Postmortem studies demonstrated that one third of patients with non-Hodgkin's lymphoma have renal involvement.[30] Renal lymphoma may be diffuse or may be manifested as a focal or multiple mass lesions. MRI shows focal renal lymphoma as it would any other solid neoplasm and does not permit histological differentiation. Diffuse lymphomatous or leukemic infiltration of the kidney results in generalized enlargement of the kidney with indistinctness (or loss) of the corticomedullary junction[38,55,58] (Figure 25-13). Perirenal lymphadenopathy can be found in half of patients.[30] On unenhanced MRI, lymphoma has the same signal intensity as the surrounding renal parenchyma. Paramagnetic contrast administration helps differentiate between renal infiltration by contiguous growth and nodular intrarenal spread.[45]

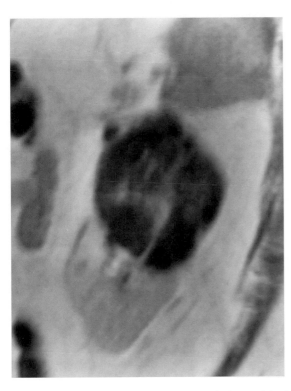

FIGURE 25-12   Cystic RCC. Gd-DTPA-enhanced sagittal T1-weighted image demonstrates a large nonenhancing hypointense mass with internal areas of septation in the upper pole of the kidney. Complicated cysts and cystic neoplasms may be difficult to differentiate.

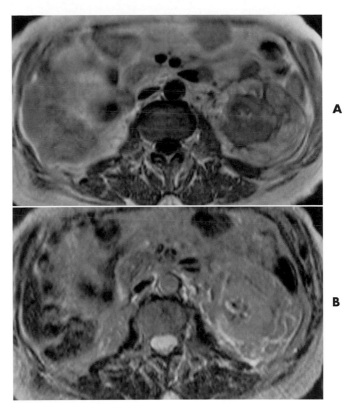

FIGURE 25-13   A 78-year-old man with history of Burkitt's lymphoma. Axial T1-weighted **(A)** and axial T2-weighted **(B)** images show a lymphomatous mass surrounding the left kidney.

Transitional Cell Carcinomas

Transitional cell carcinoma is the second most frequent renal malignancy in adulthood and the most common tumor arising from the urothelium. It is often multifocal; more than 40% of the tumors arising in the renal pelvis have associated urothelial neoplasms in the ipsilateral ureter or bladder.[70] The most sensitive imaging modality for detecting and delineating tumors in the renal pelvis is retrograde pyelography. These tumors are detected by CT or MRI only if there is an association with a dilated collecting system. With hydronephrosis a tumor is well depicted as a solid mass against the urine-filled renal pelvis.

Larger infiltrating transitional cell carcinomas are readily detectable with MRI; however, they are indistinguishable from other renal neoplasms. The main role of MRI may be in the detection of extrapelvic and extrarenal tumor spread (Figure 25-14). Transitional cell carcinomas occasionally extend into the renal vein.[45]

Metastatic Neoplasms

Metastasis is the most common multifocal renal neoplasm. Renal metastases most commonly arise from primary tumors of the lung, colon, melanoma, head and neck, and breast.[11] Metastases are indistinguishable from primary neoplasms of the kidney when they are imaged. Existence of a known extrarenal malignancy or imaging evidence of spread to other organs may suggest metastatic involvement in the renal mass or masses. The MR appearance is variable, generally resembling that of the primary tumor (Figure 25-15).

INFLAMMATORY DISEASE

The spectrum of inflammatory disease involving the kidney includes acute uncomplicated pyelonephritis, focal bacterial nephritis, and intrarenal or perinephric abscess. In acute bacterial nephritis or acute glomerulonephritis, the kidney is usually diffusely enlarged (edematous) with loss of corticomedullary differentiation.[52,58] In acute focal disease the inflamed area produces lower or mixed signal intensity on T1-weighted images[24] (Figure 25-15). Focal bacterial infectious lesions show poor Gd-DTPA enhancement and may be identified as focal areas of low signal intensity.[8] A renal abscess appears as a localized fluid collection with peripheral rim enhancement.

A specific MR diagnosis of abscess versus other focal lesions is not possible, since necrotic renal neoplasms may cause similar findings (Figure 25-16). In acute tubular necrosis, the medulla may appear swollen and the corticomedullary boundary less well demarcated than in normal kidney.[52]

Paroxysmal nocturnal hemoglobinuria[63] is characterized by secondary hemosiderin deposition in the proximal tubular cells of the renal cortex. This produces a decrease of cortical signal intensity resulting from the paramagnetic effect of iron.

Sickle cell nephropathy[49] similarly shows a decrease of signal intensity in the cortex, particularly on T2-weighted images. This reflects iron deposition in the glomerular epithelium of the renal cortex.

In chronic pyelonephritis and glomerulonephritis, the kidneys are usually small, and the corticomedullary boundaries are blurred or absent[52] (Figure 25-17). Renal sinus fat is abundant, and the remaining

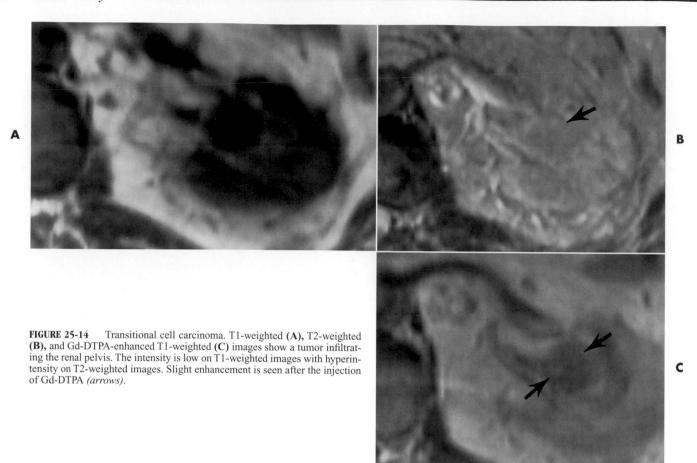

FIGURE 25-14 Transitional cell carcinoma. T1-weighted **(A)**, T2-weighted **(B)**, and Gd-DTPA-enhanced T1-weighted **(C)** images show a tumor infiltrating the renal pelvis. The intensity is low on T1-weighted images with hyperintensity on T2-weighted images. Slight enhancement is seen after the injection of Gd-DTPA *(arrows)*.

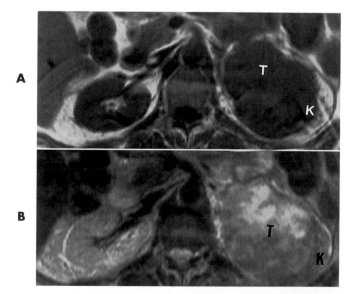

FIGURE 25-15 Metastatic squamous cell carcinoma of the lung. Tumor *(T)* is not distinguishable from any of the primary renal neoplasms. **A,** On a T1-weighted image, the tumor is isointense with the remaining renal parenchyma. **B,** On a T2-weighted image, the tumor is better delineated and demonstrates higher signal intensity than that of the kidney *(K)*. (From reference 39.)

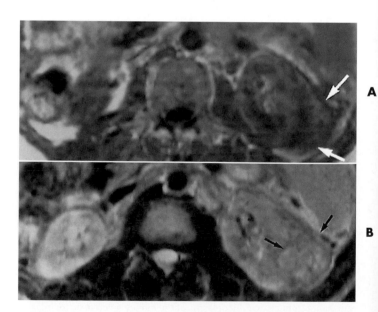

FIGURE 25-16 Renal abscess in a 44-year-old man with diabetes. In T1-weighted **(A)** and T2-weighted **(B)** images, a heterogeneous–signal intensity mass is seen in the left kidney. (From reference 39.)

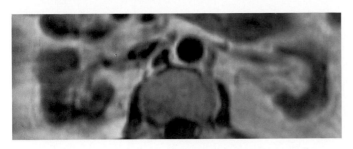

FIGURE 25-17   Chronic pyelonephritis on a T1-weighted SE image. Both kidneys are small and scarred, and signal intensity is reduced. Renal sinus fat is abundant.

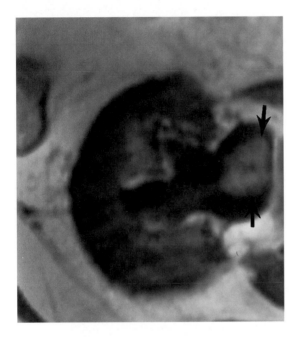

FIGURE 25-18   Hydronephrosis on an axial T1-weighted SE image. The dilated renal pelvis and calyxes have low signal intensity. A clot of increased signal intensity is seen in the renal pelvis *(arrows).*

renal parenchyma may have low signal intensity. Focal scarring may be demonstrated in chronic pyelonephritis as decreased intensity both on T1- and on T2-weighted images.

Xanthogranulomatous pyelonephritis is manifested as a mass lesion associated with obstructive stone disease. The inflammatory mass demonstrates mixed signal intensity and may simulate a neoplasm.[19,55] The diagnosis is aided by the signal void caused by the renal calculus. The disease process may extend beyond the renal capsule.[19]

HYDRONEPHROSIS

The diagnosis of hydronephrosis is readily made using MRI of the dilated collecting system in both axial and coronal projections, preferably on T1-weighted images[32,40,52,58,77] (Figure 25-18). In acute obstruction the corticomedullary demarcation is preserved, whereas in chronic obstruction the demarcation is often absent. Parenchymal atrophy resulting from chronic obstruction is well identified with MRI and with CT or ultrasound. In acute obstruction, after the administration of Gd-DTPA, the renal cortex shows enhancement similar to that shown in a normal kidney, but medullary enhancement is greater and sustained.[77] In chronic obstruction, cortical enhancement is lower than in the normal kidney, and the tubular phase is prolonged.[77]

TRAUMA AND HEMORRHAGE

Patients who have undergone extracorporeal shock wave lithotripsy show loss of corticomedullary demarcation. This is attributed to renal edema.[41,42]

The MR appearance of renal or perirenal hemorrhage depends on the time of examination, the presence of intact or lysed red blood cells, and the oxidation state of hemoglobin in different areas of hemorrhage. The intensity of a T1-weighted image generally increases with the age of the hematoma when clotting or organization has occurred[39,41,42] (Figure 25-19). Acute renal or perirenal hematomas either are isointense to renal cortex or have mixed intensity on T1-weighted images and have a greater relative signal intensity on T2-weighted images. Subcapsular hemorrhage is well outlined against the parenchyma and is surrounded by the renal capsule.[41,42]

ATRAUMATIC VASCULAR DISEASES
Arteriovenous Fistulas and Aneurysms

Renal vascular abnormalities include congenital or spontaneous arteriovenous fistulas and renal artery aneurysms. Small vascular lesions are usually occult on MRI but can be detected invasively with angiography or noninvasively with Doppler ultrasound. Larger lesions show

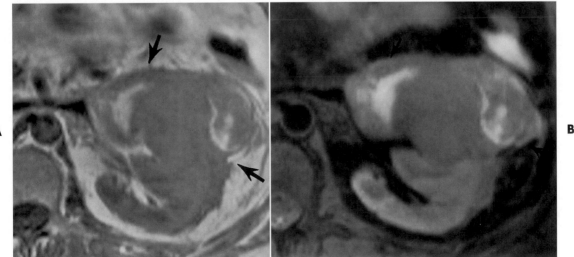

FIGURE 25-19   Spontaneous left renal and perirenal hematoma in a 44-year-old man. A T1-weighted image **(A)** and a T1-weighted image with fat suppression **(B)** show a hyperintense renal hematoma extending to the perirenal space *(arrows).*

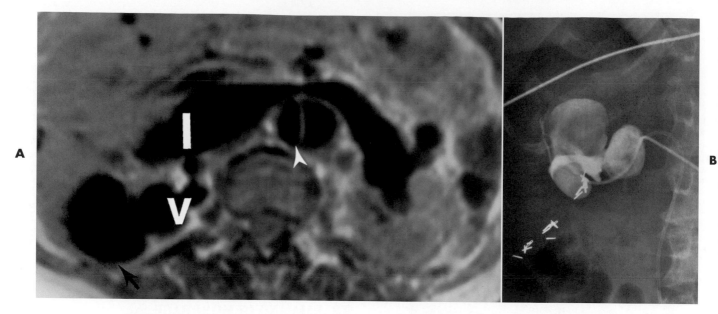

FIGURE 25-20   Spontaneous arteriovenous fistula in a 74-year-old woman with heart failure. **A,** In this T1-weighted image the right kidney has a large area of signal void *(arrow)*. The right renal vein *(v)* and inferior vena cava *(I)* are dilated. Aortic dissection is seen *(arrowhead)*. **B,** Renal arteriogram demonstrates a large arteriovenous fistula with immediate filling of the inferior vena cava.

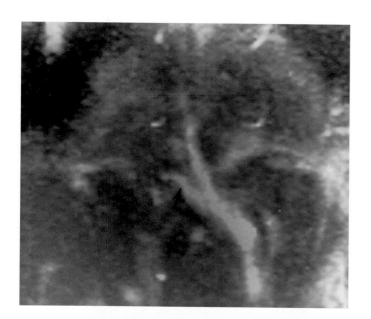

FIGURE 25-21   Hypertension in a 24-year-old man. Coronal two-dimensional time-of-flight MRA shows stenosis of the proximal right renal artery *(arrow)*.

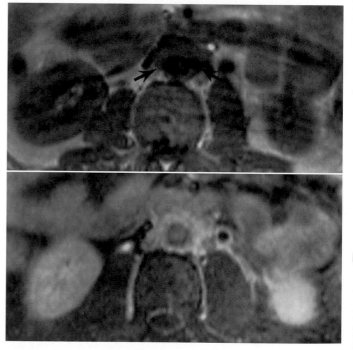

FIGURE 25-22   Idiopathic retroperitoneal fibrosis. **A,** T1-weighted image shows a rim of tissue surrounding the aorta *(arrows)*. This tissue has signal intensity similar to muscle. **B,** Gd-DTPA fat-suppressed image shows enhancement of the abundant capillary network.

nonspecific features on MR images (Figure 25-20). Differential diagnosis include hemorrhagic masses or cyst.

Renal Vein Thrombosis

Acute renal vein occlusion causes venous congestion and increases parenchymal free water, resulting in increased T1 and T2 relaxation times. Enlargement of the kidney may also be seen.

Renal Artery Stenosis

Renovascular disease is the cause of hypertension in up to 5% of the 60 million Americans with increased blood pressure.[25] It is important to diagnose renal artery stenosis because with adequate treatment, it is potentially correctable. Although angiography and radionuclide angiography are accurate for the diagnosis of renovascular hypertension,[14] these tests expose patients to the added risk of an invasive procedure, radioactivity, and nephrotoxic agents.

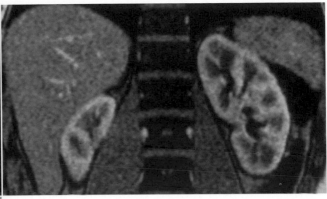

FIGURE 25-23   Coronal T1-weighted turbo-fast low-angle shot (turbo-FLASH) images obtained 5 sec **(A)**, 15 sec **(B)**, and 45 sec **(C)** after the injection of Gd-DTPA in a volunteer show dynamic changes in signal intensity in both kidneys. Early glomerular clearance of contrast material increases the signal intensity of the renal cortexes seen 5 sec after injection. At 45 sec, Gd-DTPA has been transported from the glomeruli to the tubules, and signal intensities are equally high in the cortexes and medulla of both kidneys. (From reference 72.)

MRA has been shown to be feasible for the evaluation of renal artery stenosis (Figure 25-21) (see Chapter 21). The sensitivity (87%) and specificity (97%) of these tests compare favorably with those of conventional angiography.[15] However, the severity of stenosis is overestimated in one third of cases.[15] MRA image quality is too often unpredictable because it is degraded by respiratory motion and aortic pulsation.[43] Spatial resolution achieved with routine MRA methods and body radiofrequency coils may be adequate only for evaluating the proximal renal arteries.

PERIRENAL DISEASE

Retroperitoneal fibrosis rarely involves the perirenal space directly. Fibrotic retroperitoneal masses more commonly obstruct the ureter. These masses have low signal intensity on T2-weighted images[87] (Figure 25-22).

Perirenal hemorrhage is usually associated with trauma to the kidney; however, hypervascular renal tumors may rupture and hemorrhage into the space (Figure 25-19). Perirenal abscesses are most often associated with acute renal infections.

RENAL TRANSPLANTATION

Functioning renal transplant allografts show signal characteristics identical to those of normal kidneys. In early publications, reduced or absent corticomedullary demarcation was reported to be a diagnostic feature of acute or chronic rejection,[23,31] whereas acute tubular necrosis could be distinguished by the presence of corticomedullary demarcation.[23] The loss of corticomedullary demarcation may be a rather sensitive indicator for renal transplant dysfunction, but its specificity in regard to the causes of transplant failure is low.[3,17,82] Corticomedullary demarcation also may be lost in cases of infarction and ischemia.[35] On the other hand, the corticomedullary boundary is preserved in some cases of rejection,[3] acute tubular necrosis, or cyclosporin toxicity.[83]

Ureteral obstruction resulting in hydronephrosis, perirenal fluid collections such as lymphocele, perirenal hemorrhage, or abscess and space-occupying lesions are easily demonstrated by MRI. However, ultrasound and CT are more cost-effective imaging methods.

MAGNETIC RESONANCE RENOGRAPHY

Like technetium 99m DTPA, Gd-DTPA is eliminated by glomerular filtration and excreted into the collecting system.[20,21] Approximately 5 sec after intravenous administration of Gd-DTPA, early glomerular clearance of contrast causes a discernible increase in the signal intensity of the renal cortex (Figure 25-23, *A*). A total of 15 sec after contrast injection, there is increased signal intensity in the renal cortex with minimal enhancement of the medulla (Figure 25-23, *B*). Between 20 and 30 sec after injection, the contrast has been transported from the glomeruli into the tubules, and signal intensity is equally bright in the renal cortex and medulla (Figure 25-23, *C*).

Dynamic examinations can be quantitatively evaluated by plotting the signal intensity values in the renal cortex and medulla as a function of time.[45,48,86] Dynamic functional MRI allows the evaluation of renal excretory function even in patients with diffuse functional impairment.[45,73]

REFERENCES

1. Balfe DM, et al: Evaluation of renal masses considered indeterminate on computed tomography, Radiology 142:421, 1982.
2. Ball DS, et al: Scar sign of renal oncocytoma: magnetic resonance imaging appearance and lack of specificity, Urol Radiol 8:46, 1986.
3. Baumgartner BR, and Chezmar JL: Magnetic resonance imaging of the kidneys and adrenal glands, Semin Ultrasound CT MR 10:43, 1989.
4. Baumgartner BR, et al: MR imaging of renal transplant, Am J Roentgenol 147:949, 1986.
5. Bret PM, Bretagnolle M, Gaillard D, et al: Small, asymptomatic angiomyolipomas of the kidney, Radiology 153:181, 1984.
6. Carvlin MJ, et al: Acute tubular necrosis: use of gadolinium-DTPA and fast MR imaging to evaluate renal function, J Comput Assist Tomogr 11:488, 1987.
7. Carvlin MJ, et al: Use of Gd-DTPA and fast gradient-echo and spin-echo MR imaging to demonstrate renal function in the rabbit, Radiology 170:705, 1989.
8. Choyke PL: MR imaging of the kidneys and retroperitoneum. In MR imaging syllabus, Chicago, 1991, Radiological Society of North America.
9. Choyke PL: MR imaging of renal cell carcinoma, Radiology 169:572, 1988.
10. Choyke PL, and Pollack HM: The role of MRI in diseases of the kidney, Radiol Clin North Am 26:617, 1988.
11. Choyke PL, et al: Renal metastases: clinicopathologic and radiologic correlation, Radiology 162:359, 1987.
12. Choyke PL, et al: Dynamic Gd-DTPA enhanced MR imaging of the kidney: experimental results, Radiology 170:713, 1989.

13. Choyke PL, et al: Determination of glomerular filtration rate with gadolinium clearance, Radiology 177(P):110, 1990.

14. Davidson RA, and Wilcox CS: Newer tests for the diagnosis of renovascular disease, JAMA 268:3353, 1992.

15. Debatin JF, et al: Imaging of the renal arteries: value of MR angiography, Am J Roentgenol 157:981, 1991.

16. Dikengil A, et al: MRI of multilocular cystic nephroma, Urol Radiol 10:95, 1988.

17. Dunbar KR, et al: Loss of corticomedullary demarcation on magnetic resonance imaging: an index of biopsy proven acute renal transplant dysfunction, Am J Kidney Dis 12:200, 1988.

18. Eilenberg SS, et al: Renal masses: evaluation with gradient-echo Gd-DTPA-enhanced dynamic MR imaging, Radiology 176:333, 1990.

19. Feldberg MAM, et al: Xantogranulomatous pyelonephritis: comparison of extent using computed tomography and magnetic resonance in one case, Urol Radiol 10:92, 1988.

20. Frank JA, et al: Gadopentetate dimeglumine clearance in renal insufficiency rabbits, Invest Radiol 25:1212, 1990.

21. Frank JA, et al: Functional MR of the kidney, Magn Reson Med 22:319, 1991.

22. Fritzsche PJ: Current state of MRI in renal mass diagnosis and staging of RCC, Urol Radiol 11:210, 1989.

23. Geisinger MA, et al: Magnetic resonance imaging of the renal transplants, Am J Roentgenol 143:1229, 1984.

24. Hamlin DJ, et al: Magnetic resonance imaging of renal abscess in an experimental model, Acta Radiol Diagn 26:315, 1985.

25. Hillman BJ: Imaging advances in the diagnosis of renovascular hypertension, Am J Roentgenol 153:5, 1989.

26. Hilpert PL, et al: MRI of hemorrhagic renal cysts in polycystic kidney disease, Am J Roentgenol 146:1167, 1986.

27. Hockley NM, et al: Use of magnetic resonance imaging to determine surgical approach to renal cell carcinoma with caval extension, Urology 36:55, 1990.

28. Holleb AI, Fink DJ, and Murphy GP, editors: American Cancer Society Textbook of Clinical Oncology, Atlanta, 1991, American Cancer Society.

29. Horan JJ, et al: The detection of renal cell carcinoma extension into the renal vein and the inferior vena cava: a prospective comparison of venacavography and magnetic resonance imaging, J Urol 142:943, 1989.

30. Horii SC, et al: Correlation of CT and ultrasound in the evaluation of renal lymphoma, Urol Radiol 5:69,1983.

31. Hricak H, Terrier F, and Demas B: Renal allografts: evaluation by MR imaging, Radiology 159:435, 1986.

32. Hricak H, et al: Nuclear magnetic imaging of the kidney, Radiology 146:425, 1983.

33. Hricak H, et al: Nuclear magnetic resonance imaging of the kidneys: renal masses, Radiology 147:765, 1983.

34. Hricak H, et al: Detection and staging of renal neoplasms: a reassessment of MR imaging, Radiology 166:643, 1988.

35. Ishakawa I, et al: Magnetic resonance imaging in renal infarction and ischemia, Nephron 51:99, 1989.

36. Johnson CD, et al: Renal adenocarcinoma CT staging of 100 tumors, Am J Roentgenol 148:59, 1987.

37. Kabala JE, et al: Magnetic resonance imaging in the staging of renal cell carcinoma, Br J Radiol 64:683, 1991.

38. Kaude JV, and Kinard RE: Magnetic resonance imaging of renal mass lesions. In Lohr E, and Leder LD, eds: Renal and adrenal tumors, ed 2, Berlin, 1987, Springer-Verlag.

39. Kaude J, and Torres GM: Kidney. In Ros PR, and Bidgood WD, eds: Abdominal magnetic resonance imaging, St Louis, 1993, Mosby.

40. Kaude JV, et al: Imaging of unilateral hydronephrosis in an experimental animal model: with special reference to magnetic resonance, Acta Radiol Diagn 25:501, 1984.

41. Kaude JV, et al: Renal morphology and function immediately after extracorporeal shock wave lithotripsy, Am J Roentgenol 145:305, 1985.

42. Kaude JV, et al: Magnetic resonance imaging of the kidney after ESWL. In Gravenstein JS, and Peter K, eds: Extracorporeal shock-wave lithotripsy for renal stone disease: technical and clinical aspects, Boston, 1986, Butterworths.

43. Kim D, et al: Abdominal aorta and renal artery stenosis: evaluation with MR angiography, Radiology 174:727, 1990.

44. Kim SH, et al: Multilocular cystic nephroma: MR findings, Am J Roentgenol 153:1317, 1989.

45. Krestin GP: Magnetic resonance imaging of the kidneys: current status, Magn Reson Q 10:2, 1994.

46. Krestin GP: Morphologic and functional MR of the kidneys and adrenal glands, Philadelphia, 1990, Field and Wood.

47. Krestin GP, et al: Fast ME imaging of renal and adrenal tumors: the value of dynamic studies with Gd-DTPA, Radiology 165(P):272, 1987.

48. Krestin GP, et al: Functional dynamic MR imaging, pharmacokinetics and safety of gadolinium-DTPA in patients with impaired renal function, Eur Radiol 2:16, 1992.

49. Lande IM, et al: Sickle cell nephropathy: MR imaging, Radiology 158:379, 1986.

50. Laniado M, et al: Gd-DTPA in imaging of renal tumors, Radiology 157(P):276, 1985.

51. Leder L-D, and Richter HJ: Pathology of renal and adrenal neoplasms. In Lohr E, and Leder L-D, eds: Renal and adrenal tumors, ed 2, Berlin, 1987, Springer-Verlag.

52. Leung AW-L, et al: Magnetic resonance imaging of the kidneys, Am J Roentgenol 143:1215, 1984.

53. Levine E, and Granthamm JJ: Perinephric hemorrhage in autosomal dominant polycystic kidney disease: CT and MR findings, J Comput Assist Tomogr 11:108, 1987.

54. Lieber MM, Tomera KM, and Farron GM: Renal oncocytoma, J Urol 125:481, 1981.

55. LiPuma JP: Magnetic resonance imaging of the kidney, Radiol Clin North Am 22:925, 1984.

56. Love L, et al: Computed tomography of extraperitoneal spaces, Am J Roentgenol 136:781, 1981.

57. Marotti M, et al: Complex and simple renal cysts: comparative evaluation with MR imaging, Radiology 162:679, 1987.

58. Marotti M, et al: MRI in renal disease, Magn Reson Med 5:160, 1987.

59. Marshall FF, and Walsh PC: Extrarenal manifestations of renal cell carcinoma, J Urol 117:439, 1977.

60. Marx WJ, and Patel SK: Renal fascia: its radiographic importance, Urology 13:1, 1979.

61. Meyers MA: Dynamic radiology of the abdomen in normal and pathologic anatomy, Heidelberg, 1987, Springer-Verlag.

62. Mooring FJ, Kaude JV, and Wajsman Z: Bilateral renal oncocytomas, J Med Imaging 3:27, 1989.

63. Mulopolus GP, et al: MRI of the kidneys in paroxysmal nocturnal hemoglobinuria, Am J Roentgenol 146:51, 1986.

64. Pettersson H, et al: Magnetic resonance imaging and tissue characterization of a renal cell carcinoma and its osseous metastases, Acta Radiol Diagn 26:193, 1985.

65. Price PR, et al: Gd-DTPA kinetics in an excised kidney model with use of snapshot FLASH MR imaging, Radiology 177(P):110, 1990.

66. Psiluramis KE, et al: Further evidence that renal oncocytoma has malignant potential, J Urol 139:585, 1988.

67. Quint LE, et al: In vivo and in vitro MR imaging of renal tumors: histopathologic correlation and pulse sequence optimization, Radiology 169:359, 1988.

68. Remark PR, et al: Magnetic resonance imaging of renal oncocytoma, Urology 31:176, 1988.

69. Richmond J, et al: Renal lesions associated with malignant lymphomas, Am J Med 32:184, 1962.

70. Riches EW, Griffiths IH, and Thackeray AC: New growths of the kidney and ureter, Br J Urol 23:297, 1951.

71. Robson CJ, Churchill BM, and Anderson W: The results of radical nephrectomy for renal cell carcinoma, J Urol 101:297, 1969.

72. Ros PR, et al: Diagnosis of renal artery stenosis: feasibility of combining MR angiography, MR renography, and gadopentetate-based measurement of glomerular filtration rate, Am J Roentgenol 165:1447, 1995.

73. Rothpearl A, et al: MR urography: technique and application, Radiology 194:125, 1995.

74. Roubidoux MA: MR imaging of hemorrhage and iron deposition in the kidney, Radiographics 14:1033, 1994.

75. Roubidoux MA, et al: Renal carcinoma: detection of venous extension with gradient echo MR imaging, Radiology 182:269, 1992.

76. Semelka RC, et al: Improved MR imaging in the upper abdomen with fat saturation imaging technique, Radiology 173(P):388, 1989.

77. Semelka RC, et al: Obstructive nephropathy: evaluation with dynamic Gd-DTPA-enhanced MR imaging, Radiology 175:797, 1990.

78. Semelka RC, et al: Combined gadolinium-enhanced and fat saturation MR imaging of renal masses, Radiology 178:803, 1991.

79. Semelka RC, et al: Renal lesions: controlled comparison between CT and 1.5 T MR imaging with nonenhanced and gadolinium-enhanced fat-suppressed spin-echo and breath-hold FLASH techniques, Radiology 182:425, 1992.

80. Singer J, and McClennan BL: The diagnosis, staging, and follow-up of carcinomas of the kidney, bladder, and prostate: the role of cross-sectional imaging, Semin Ultrasound CT MR 10:481, 1989.

81. Sohn HK, Kim SY, and Seo HS: MR imaging of a renal oncocytoma, J Comput Assist Tomogr 11:1085, 1987.

82. Steinberg HV, et al: Renal allograft rejection: evaluation by Doppler US and MR imaging, Radiology 162:337, 1987.

83. Strake L, et al: Magnetic resonance imaging of renal transplants: its value in the differentiation of acute rejection and cyclosporin A nephrotoxicity, Clin Radiol 39:220, 1988.

84. Sussman SK, Glikstein MF, and Krymowski GA: Hypointense renal cell carcinoma: MR imaging with pathologic correlation, Radiology 177:495, 1990.

85. Vas W, et al: MRI of an angiomyolipoma, Magn Reson Imaging 4:485, 1986.

86. von Schulthess GK, et al: Semiautomated ROI analysis in dynamic MR studies. II. Application to renal function examination, J Comput Assist Tomogr 15:733, 1991.

87. Yancey JM, and Kaude JV: Diagnosis of perirenal fibrosis by MR imaging, J Comput Assist Tomogr 12:335, 1988.

88. Young RH, Dunn J, and Dickersin R: An unusual oncocytic renal tumor with sarcomatoid foci and osteogenic differentiation, Arch Pathol Lab Med 112:937, 1988.

89. Zagoria RJ, et al: CT features of renal cell carcinoma with emphasis on relation to tumor size, Invest Radiol 25:261, 1990.

26 Peritoneum, Mesentery, and Retroperitoneum

Evan S. Siegelman and Pablo R. Ros

 KEY POINTS

- CT remains the procedure of choice for imaging tumors and fluid collections.
- MRI is helpful for staging tumors extending to the paraspinous region.

Computed tomography (CT) is considered the initial imaging modality of choice for evaluation of diseases of the peritoneum, mesentery, and retroperitoneum. However, because of its better soft tissue characterization, direct multiplanar capabilities, and lack of ionizing radiation, current state-of-the-art magnetic resonance imaging (MRI) is useful when contrast CT is relatively contraindicated or not defini-

tive.[89] This chapter reviews the pathophysiology and magnetic resonance (MR) findings of the most common focal and diffuse processes involving the peritoneum, mesentery, and retroperitoneum encountered in clinical practice. The imaging of the normal anatomy of the peritoneum and retroperitoneum and descriptions of the "dynamic" pathway of spread of pathological processes have been extensively reviewed elsewhere and are not discussed here.*

PERITONEUM AND MESENTERY
Cystic Lesions

Lymphangioma. Lymphangiomas (Figure 26-1) are developmental benign neoplasms that arise from sequestered lymphatics that lack normal communications with the remainder of the lymphatic system. Between one half and two thirds of lymphangiomas occur in the head, neck, and axilla.[93] The majority of these tumors occur by the age of 2 years. Even though it is not common in this location, lymphangioma is the most common cystic mass of the mesentery and omentum.[299] Although 60% of abdominal lymphangiomas appear in childhood, a significant number of cases are seen in adults.[93,104] Patients can often have acute symptoms caused by bowel ischemia or obstruction.[93] Surgical removal is recommended.

Imaging shows a multiseptated, cystic mass centered in the mesentery or omentum. Lesions can contain areas of simple fluid, fluid with fat, or hemorrhagic components, or both.†

Pancreatic lymphangioma may be difficult to distinguish from cystic pancreatic neoplasms.[271,276] Angiomatosis and hemangiomatosis may have imaging features similar to those of lymphangioma.[67,72,224,251]

Peritoneal Pseudocyst (Peritoneal Inclusion Cyst). A subtype of nonpancreatic pseudocysts occurs in the pelvis of women who have had prior surgical procedures.[136,169,193,336] Peritoneal pseudocysts characteristically adhere to the ovaries without invasion.[155,217] Serous fluid contained in these lesions is derived from the ovaries. However, unlike normal women, these patients have extensive adhesions that prevent normal resorption of this fluid and a pseudocyst results. Direct multiplanar MR images show an irregularly shaped unilocular or multilocular pelvic fluid collection with boundaries formed by normal pelvic structures.[46,335]

Peritoneal pseudocysts and other peritoneal cystic masses can be distinguished from peritoneal cystic mesothelioma. The latter is a benign mesenchymal neoplasm that often involves the peritoneal surfaces of the pelvic viscera in middle-aged women. With peritoneal cystic mesotheliomas, with the benign form there is no association with asbestos exposure. MRI will demonstrate a multiloculated pelvic mass in a middle-aged women whose T1 and T2 signal characteristics follow that of simple fluid.[128,235,299]

Pseudomyxoma Peritonei. Pseudomyxoma peritonei (Figure 26-2) is an uncommon condition characterized by the presence of mucinous ascites or implants in the peritoneal cavity. Most cases are caused by low-grade mucinous adenocarcinomas of the appendix (Figure 26-3).[247] Women with pseudomyxoma peritonei can also have well-differentiated or borderline mucinous neoplasms of the ovaries.[326] Most investigators believe that the appendiceal tumor is the primary site and the ovarian disease and peritoneal mucin result from implanted mucus-

---

*References 14, 15, 20, 58, 77, 80, 165, 179, 202-207, 209, 234, 253, 254, 269, 309, 325.
†References 97, 132, 135, 139, 143, 182, 300.

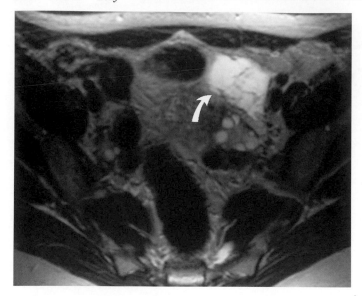

FIGURE 26-1 Complex left adnexal mass in a 36-year-old woman. Fast spin-echo (TR 4000/TE 108) image shows a nonaggressive, septated, cystic mass *(arrow)* that is separate from the left ovary and does not have the appearance of a hydrosalpinx. Laparoscopic removal confirmed the diagnosis of lymphangioma.

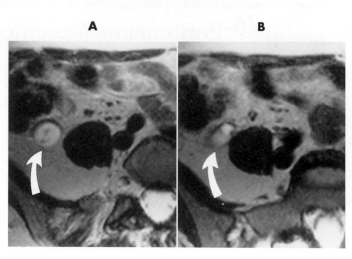

FIGURE 26-3 **A** and **B,** Appendiceal mucinous adenocarcinoma. Fast spin-echo (5000/105) image in a 48-year-old woman shows a heterogeneous high–signal intensity appendix that is enlarged *(arrow).* Pseudomyxoma peritonei and ovarian metastases were also present (not shown).

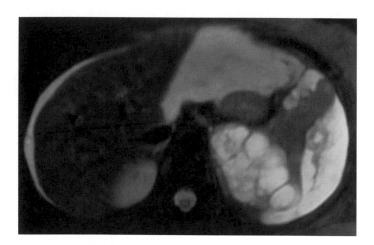

FIGURE 26-2 Pseudomyxoma peritonei. Fast spin-echo (4000/72) image in a 59-year-old woman shows complex ascites that deforms the lateral and medial surfaces of the spleen. Surgery confirmed ovarian mucinous cystadenocarcinoma of low malignant potential with peritoneal extension.

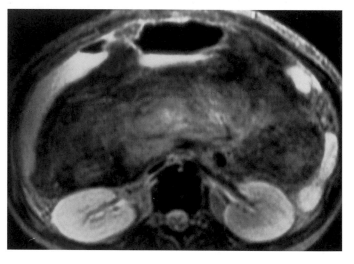

FIGURE 26-4 Fibromatosis. A 17-year-old young woman with a history of Gardner's syndrome, prior colectomy, and abdominal mass. Conventional spin-echo image (2500/80) shows an infiltrative low–signal intensity mass of the retroperitoneum and mesentery.

producing epithelial cells.[162,168,255,265] However, the Armed Forces Institute of Pathology believes that the ovarian and appendiceal lesions are of independent origin.[278]

Pseudomyxoma peritonei is treated by aggressive surgical debridement along with intraperitoneal chemotherapy.[264,283,302,303] The appendix should be removed at the time of surgery; occult low-grade mucinous adenocarcinomas have been found in appendices that were "normal" at surgical inspection and palpation.[247] Patients who do not have epithelial cells present within the peritoneal mucin deposits have an indolent course and a better prognosis.[44,119,247,264,324] Necrosis and calcification can occur after chemotherapy.[191]

Solid Neoplasms

Fibromatosis. Superficial (fascial) fibromatosis involves the palmar aponeurosis (Dupuytren's disease), plantar aponeurosis (lederhosen

disease), and the penis (Peyronie's disease).[93] Deep (musculoaponeurotic) fibromatosis involves extraabdominal, abdominal wall (desmoid tumor), and intraabdominal sites (Figure 26-4).

Intraabdominal fibromatosis (IAF) is the most common tumor of the mesentery[52,85] but is still uncommon, with an annual incidence of approximately 4 cases per million.[256] IAF occurs with frequencies ranging from 3% to 30% in familial adenomatous polyposis (FAP).[33,52,120] It has been estimated that persons with FAP have more than 800 times the comparative risk of developing IAF of the general population.[120] The prevalence of FAP in series of patients with IAF varies from 13% to 92%.[42,85] Although IAFs are not considered malignant, they are aggressive neoplasms that have recurrence rates varying between 5% and 75% (Figure 26-5).[195,259] Although surgery is often successful as the primary treatment modality for extraabdominal fibromatosis, there is significant morbidity associated with IAFs, and surgery is suggested only for symptomatic lesions.[195] In cases of IAFs associated with FAP,

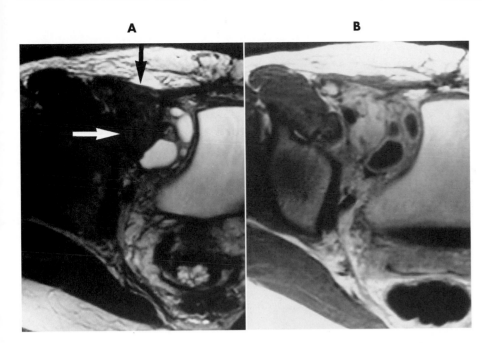

FIGURE 26-5   Recurrent fibromatosis. A 25-year-old woman with a history of two prior surgical excisions of fibromatosis and right lower-quadrant fullness. Fast spin-echo (4000/144) **(A)** and contrast-enhanced T1-weighted **(B)** images show a short T2 signal intensity, enhancing infiltrative process (*arrows* in **A**) located between the right ovary medially and the external iliac vessels laterally.

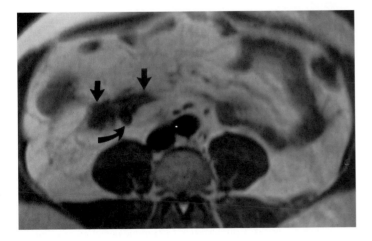

FIGURE 26-6   Mesenteric metastatic carcinoid tumor. Spin-echo (500/12) image shows a spiculated, mesenteric mass *(straight arrows)* that surrounds the anterior portion of a dilated ureter *(curved black arrow)*. Note standing of surrounding mesenteric fat. Such "misty mesentery" is not specific for carcinoid tumor but can be present in a variety of inflammatory and neoplastic disease processes that involve the mesentery. (From reference 213.)

large mesenteric masses (>10 cm), bilateral hydronephrosis, multiple mesenteric masses, and small bowel encasement are poor prognostic signs.[33]

Early reports of soft tissue fibromatosis suggested that low signal intensity on T2-weighted images was characteristic, corresponding to decreased cellularity and increased collagen.[3,127,249,306,316] However, more recent studies have shown that a short T2 time is neither sensitive nor specific[166] because fibromatosis may have heterogeneous intermediate to high signal intensity on T2-weighted images.* Furthermore, neither signal intensity nor contrast enhancement correlates with biological behavior.[262] Because of the infiltrative nature of this tumor and its proclivity for invading neurovascular structures,[131] MRI is the ideal imaging modality for detection and delineation.[233]

Carcinoid (Gastrointestinal Neuroendocrine Tumors).

Obendorfer[232] first used the term *karzinoide* to describe a distinct morphological subset of gastrointestinal tumors that had less aggressive behavior than typical adenocarcinoma. Because carcinoids (Figure 26-6) produce substances such as serotonin that are also found in the central nervous system (CNS), it has been suggested that they be reclassified as neuroendocrine tumors.[49] Most (more than 85%) carcinoid tumors occur in the gastrointestinal tract, with the appendix and ileum being the two most common locations.[113,189] Appendiceal carcinoids are usually incidental, small (<2 cm) lesions that are cured with appendectomy.[70,178,189,215] Carcinoids of the ileum have variable but more aggressive behavior. Approximately two thirds of patients with ileal carcinoids have metastatic disease at presentation,[90] and up to 20% of ileal tumors of less than 1 cm in size have metastatic disease.[178]

Patients with localized carcinoid tumors are often asymptomatic. Patients with liver and mesenteric metastases can have carcinoid syndrome or nonspecific pain and weight loss, respectively. The prognosis of patients with carcinoid tumors is better than that of patients with adenocarcinoma, as initially observed by Obendorfer.[232] The mean survival of patients with metastatic carcinoid tumor is 8 years.[214] Primary treatment consists of surgical removal of the primary bowel tumor, any ischemic or obstructed bowel segments, and mesenteric masses and potential curative removal of liver metastatic disease.[178] Symptomatic patients with stable metastatic disease benefit from somatostatin therapy, which decreases both the flushing and the diarrhea that occur with carcinoid syndrome.[11,171] Occasional regression of metastatic disease has also been reported with somatostatin therapy.[71,328] Patients with persistent symptoms or unfavorable prognostic signs can also benefit from transcatheter hepatic artery embolization and chemoembolization.[50,243,313]

Metastatic mesenteric carcinoid masses are often larger than the primary bowel tumor itself,[178] and the latter is often not identified on cross-sectional imaging studies.[65,244] One study found 1 of 52 midgut carcinoid tumors on CT.[334] The most common reported CT findings have been mesenteric masses (calcified in 40% to 70%) with associated radiating soft tissue spokes, adenopathy, and liver metastases.* Serotonin secreted by the tumor is likely to be responsible for the fibrosis, stranding, and desmoplastic reaction present in the mesentery in patients with metastatic carcinoid. Metastatic carcinoid has been reported as a cause of malignant retroperitoneal fibrosis.[118]

---

*References 52, 96, 131, 166, 233, 249.

*References 39, 65, 128, 240, 244, 334.

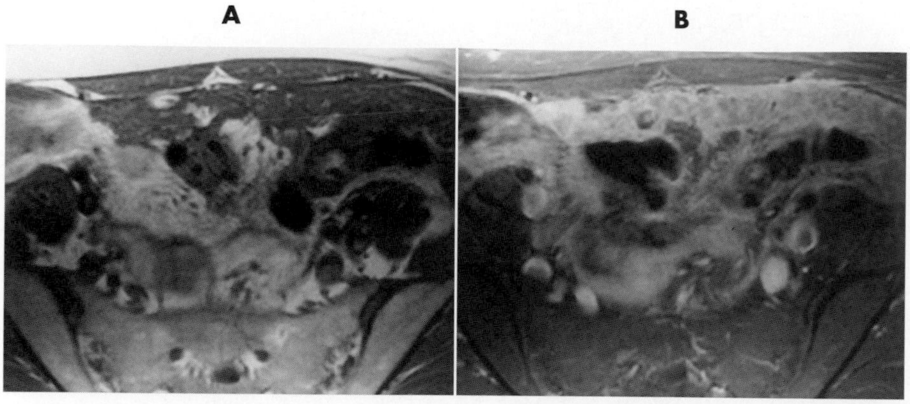

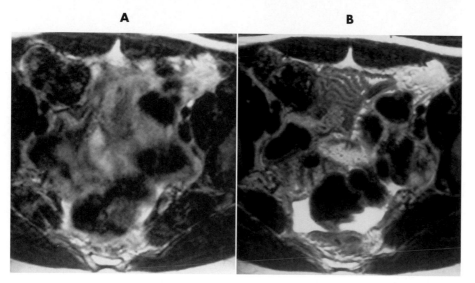

FIGURE 26-7 Omental cake in a 43-year-old woman with ovarian carcinoma who was suboptimally debulked on subsequent laparotomy. Axial T1-weighted pelvic-coil images obtained before **(A)** and after **(B)** contrast enhancement and fat suppression show an irregular enhancing rind of soft tissue anterior to the bowel and subjacent to the rectus muscles.

FIGURE 26-8 Importance of glucagon in evaluating for peritoneal disease. Axial pelvic-coil fast spin-echo images (5000/108, FOV 20) obtained before **(A)** and after **(B)** intramuscular injection of glucagon. Bowel peristalsis limits evaluation of the bowel and peritoneal structures. After glucagon, cul-de-sac fluid, bowel, and peritoneal surfaces are well seen. When bowel motion is adequately suppressed, native fluid, gas, and stool within the bowel segments are readily identified and should not be confused with adenopathy or other masses.

Peritoneal Carcinomatosis. Malignancies arising from intraabdominal organs can metastasize to the peritoneal surfaces. Precise detection of the size and number of peritoneal metastases helps the surgeons and oncologists determine the appropriate therapy.[299,301] For example, in women with ovarian cancer, CT or MRI can help identify those with advanced tumor burden who may not benefit from initial cytoreductive surgery (Figure 26-7).* In patients who have had initial surgical treatment and chemotherapy for ovarian carcinoma, accurate determination of residual or recurrent disease could help determine whether additional debulking or a "second-look" surgery is needed.[21,318]

Multiple studies have shown that contrast-enhanced CT has limited sensitivity for detecting implants in women with ovarian carcinoma.† Subcentimeter implants and implants without surrounding ascites have been particularly difficult to detect on CT.[145,229,270] The intraperitoneal administration of either air or iodinated contrast can improve the sensitivity of CT for detecting smaller peritoneal implants.[51,109,126,147] However, such invasive procedures can still miss the majority of lesions in the greater omentum and small bowel mesentery, which are areas that tend to have the highest frequency of metastases.[229]

MRI also has the ability to detect peritoneal metastatic disease.‡ When one is imaging for subtle peritoneal disease, two techniques are strongly encouraged. First, whenever possible, a phased-array pelvic coil should be used to increase signal-to-noise ratio and allow smaller field-of-view images to be acquired to increase spatial resolution.[47,290,291] Second, glucagon should routinely be given before imaging to decrease bowel peristalsis and limit motion artifact from bowel (Figure 26-8). Enhanced fat-suppressed breath-hold spoiled gradient-echo imaging outperforms CT for distinguishing peritoneal disease from ovarian cancer.[180,285] CT outperforms MRI in the detection of calcified peritoneal metastases from serous carcinomas of the ovary.[212,230]

Nonneoplastic Peritoneal Disease

Endometriosis. Endometriosis is characterized by the presence of endometrial glands and stroma outside the uterus.[37] The MR appearance of typical endometrial cysts has been well described as multifocal, multilocular, high T1 signal intensity, intermediate to low T2 signal intensity adnexal masses.*

Occasional solid masses of endometriosis can be identified on MRI that are predominantly low signal on T2-weighted images and have punctate areas of high T1 signal intensity; the latter represents foci of hemorrhage, and the former reflects the abundant acellular fibrosis that is present in these lesions.[285] These MR findings are unusual for peritoneum-based malignancy and should not be confused as such. Such lesions have been imaged in the abdominal wall (Figure 26-9) and cul-de-sac, around the sciatic nerve, and along the undersurface of the diaphragm.† The presence of endometriosis in the abdominal wall of hysterectomy scars in patients who have no intraperitoneal endometriosis suggests direct implantation as the cause of ectopic endometrial tissue.

*References 100, 137, 201, 228, 275, 279.
†References 45, 63, 126, 197, 229, 286.
‡References 57, 59, 60, 134, 149, 246, 280.

*References 12, 122, 236, 304, 307, 314, 341.
†References 78, 230, 245, 285, 332, 339.

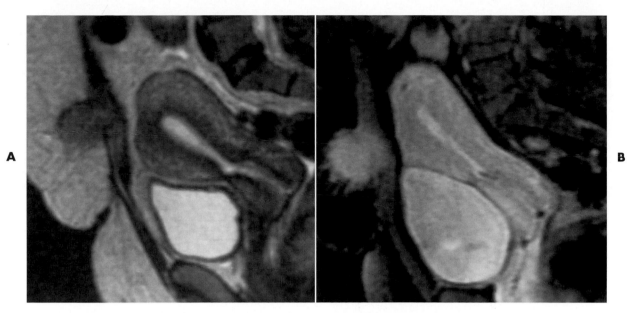

FIGURE 26-9   Endometriosis in a transverse incision scar. Sagittal fast spin-echo (4000/85) **(A)** and fat-saturated, T1-weighted, spoiled gradient-echo (TR 150/TE 2.9, FA 80 degrees) **(B)** images show a spiculated lesion of the anterior abdominal wall. A low transverse incision from a prior cesarean section is present in the anterior uterine wall. A desmoid tumor could have a similar appearance. Endometriosis, likely implanted at the time of cesarean section, was found at surgery.

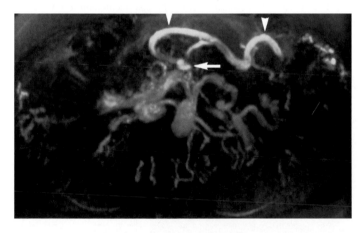

FIGURE 26-10   Enlarged gastrocolic trunk. Maximum intensity projection (MIP) image of an axially acquired MR angiogram obtained without saturation bands (37/8, FA 45 degrees) shows an enlarged collateral vessel that empties into the superior mesenteric vein *(arrows)*. No splenic vein is identified. Other images (not shown) confirmed encasement and thrombosis of the splenic vein and encasement of portions of the superior mesenteric vein and artery.

Mesenteric Vascular Abnormalities

Gastrocolic Trunk. Veins from the stomach (gastroepiploic vein), duodenum, and pancreas normally drain into the gastrocolic trunk (GCT), which empties into the superior mesenteric vein at the level of the uncinate process of the pancreas 1.5 cm below the splenomesenteric confluence.[184,344] The normal GCT measures up to 4.7 mm.[68,218] MRI can visualize an enlarged GCT with either routine spin-echo images or MR angiographic sequences (Figure 26-10). The gastroepiploic vein and GCT often dilate in cases of splenic vein thrombosis, which is a useful sign for evaluation of staging of pancreatic disease.[186-188] However, an enlarged GCT is not specific for pancreatic malignancy, having been seen in more than 13% of 266 patients with chronic pancreatitis or pseudocyst.[22]

Superior Mesenteric Vessel Inversion. Numerous imaging reports have documented inversion of the normal relationship between the superior mesenteric artery and vein in cases of midgut malrotation.[107,181,282] The presence of inversion is not sensitive enough to justify screening for this imaging finding when malrotation is the suspected diagnosis.[343] In addition, large hepatic and retroperitoneal masses can cause a pseudoinversion caused by displacement of the superior mesenteric vein (Figure 26-12, *B*).[342] MRI can easily demonstrate the abnormal relationship between these two vessels on axial spin-echo or time-of-flight images and suggest a primary (malrotation) or secondary (displacement by adjacent mass) origin.

RETROPERITONEUM
Retroperitoneal Sarcomas

Retroperitoneal sarcomas are rare. They make up 0.15% of all malignant lesions and 15% of the 4500 soft tissue sarcomas diagnosed in the United States each year.[194,298,333] Retroperitoneal sarcomas occur in men and women in equal numbers and usually occur in the fifth or sixth decades of life. These slow-growing tumors are often large when they appear as a palpable mass, with minimal or nonspecific symptoms.[55,194,297] In descending order, liposarcoma, leiomyosarcoma, and malignant fibrous histiocytoma account for the great majority of encountered lesions.*

Retroperitoneal sarcomas are staged by the American Joint Commission on Cancer (AJCC) classification system. Interestingly, tumor histology is not part of the classification scheme. Tumors are staged according to size, histological grade, and the presence or absence of nodes or metastatic disease.[17] The treatment of choice for retroperitoneal sarcomas is an aggressive operative attempt at complete surgical resection.[73,115,267,297] With modern surgical techniques, more than 90% of retroperitoneal sarcomas are resectable.[150] Unfortunately, 50% to 90% of patients who have undergone surgical resection have local recurrences and usually die of complications of local disease.[73,194,297] Unlike the results obtained with soft tissue sarcomas of the extremities, postoperative chemotherapy of retroperitoneal sarcomas does not improve survival and has significant morbidity.[111,288,289] Neither preoperative nor postoperative radiation therapy prevents local recurrences or improves survival to any significant degree.[53,288] Favorable prognosis is associated with low histological grade, lack of tumor invasion into surround-

---

*References 53, 73, 130, 267, 297, 298.

ing retroperitoneal structures, and complete surgical resection with negative margins.[53,194,267,289] Patients who have complete resections can have 10-year survival rates of up to 45%.[55,194] Neither tumor subtype nor tumor size is independently related to prognosis.[55,298]

Retroperitoneal Liposarcoma. Liposarcoma is the most common retroperitoneal sarcoma (Figure 26-11). It commonly occurs in middle age and has a mild predilection for women. From 15% to 20% of liposarcomas occur in the retroperitoneum, which is the second most common site for liposarcoma after the extremity.[93] Treatment is surgical. Recurrence rate of tumor is high.[151,159] In one series of 34 retroperitoneal liposarcomas, all tumors recurred after surgery.[159] The 5-year survival rate for retroperitoneal liposarcoma is approximately 40% (extremity liposarcomas have a 70% 5-year survival rate).[93,159]

Pathologically there are four subtypes of liposarcomas: well differentiated, myxoid, pleomorphic, and round cell. Round-cell and pleo-

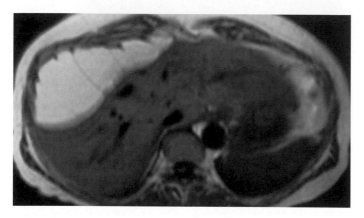

FIGURE 26-11 Well-differentiated liposarcoma. SE 550/12 image shows a lobular, septated, fat-containing mass in the right superior subhepatic space.

morphic tumors tend to be more aggressive and have a worse prognosis than the myxoid and well-differentiated subtypes. However, because patients with the latter tumors tend to live longer, they have a higher number of reported occurrences. The most common subtypes in the retroperitoneum include the well-differentiated and pleomorphic subtypes.[167] Usually, only the well-differentiated liposarcomas show macroscopic fat on T1-weighted images.[158] The majority of retroperitoneal liposarcomas that we have seen have been well-differentiated lesions that have fat signal intensity on T1-weighted images. MRI can help distinguish between atypical lipomas and well-differentiated liposarcomas. The former have thin, nonenhancing fibrous septa, whereas the latter tend to have thick, enhancing septa that contain skeletal muscle.[138] Some myxoid tumors resemble cystic masses; contrast enhancement may be necessary to establish the solid nature of these tumors.[158]

Primary Leiomyosarcoma. Leiomyosarcoma (LMS) is the second most common retroperitoneal sarcoma in the adult population after liposarcoma.[130] Half of soft tissue LMSs occur in the retroperitoneum, which is the most common location for LMS.[93,284] Two thirds of LMSs occur in women, and the mean age is the sixth decade of life. Two thirds of LMSs are totally extravascular (Figure 26-12), whereas one third of LMSs have components that are intravascular (Figure 26-13). The mean size is 16 cm at the time of diagnosis.[284] Central necrosis is a common feature; fat and calcification typically are not present.[10,130,173,196]

When LMS has a partial or complete intravascular component, the tumor can be smaller at the time of diagnosis because of early symptoms from either intrinsic or extrinsic compression on the inferior vena cava (IVC) (Figure 26-13). Symptoms typical of Budd-Chiari syndrome can occur when tumor involves the suprarenal or intrahepatic IVC (the most common location).[242] Nephrotic syndrome can occur with renal vein tumor, and lower extremity swelling can occur with tumor of the infrarenal IVC.[130]

MRI of LMS shows an aggressive, infiltrative lesion. The coronal or sagittal plane is ideal for showing the relationship of the tumor to the IVC and other vital retroperitoneal structures. The mass is usually heterogeneous and of low to intermediate signal intensity on T1-weighted

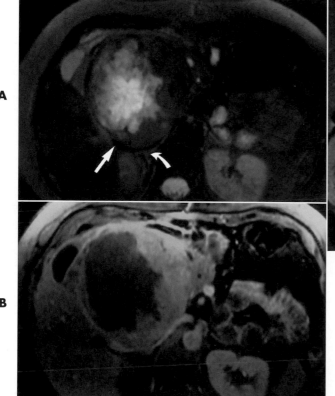

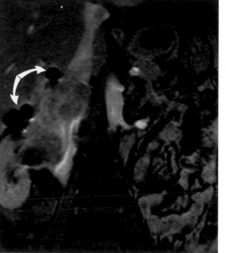

FIGURE 26-12 A 57-year-old woman referred for further evaluation after exploratory laparotomy showed an unexpected mass. An axial fat-suppressed body-coil, fast spin-echo image (3500/85) **(A)** shows a 12- × 11-cm mass with a centrally necrotic center. The mass compresses and displaces the IVC posteriorly *(straight white arrow)* and displaces the gallbladder laterally and the pancreatic head medially. The right adrenal gland *(curved white arrow)* is normal and is located behind the IVC. Axial **(B)** and sagittal **(C)** breath-hold, pelvic-coil, fat-saturated, spoiled gradient-echo images (100/2.6, FA 80 degrees) show central nonenhancement and superior mesenteric artery and vein inversion resulting from mass effect and long extension of tumor in the pericaval location. Note foci of magnetic susceptibility from the ferromagnetic surgical clip *(curved white arrows in **C**)*. The central necrosis and pericaval location are both typical for leiomyosarcoma, which was confirmed at surgery.

images and heterogeneous and of intermediate to high signal intensity on T2-weighted images. Any well-differentiated smooth muscle within the tumor should be of low to intermediate T2 signal intensity (as in uterine leiomyomas and benign smooth muscle located elsewhere in the body). Intratumoral necrosis is evident as a high T2 signal intensity central zone of the tumor that shows no enhancement. No fat or calcium should be present.

Malignant Fibrous Histiocytoma.

Malignant fibrous histiocytoma (MFH) is the most common soft tissue sarcoma in adults, with the majority of these tumors localized to the extremities.[92] However, the retroperitoneum is the second most common location. Most lesions occur in middle- to late-age men. The MRI findings of MFH have been described.[170,185,208,223,239] A large retroperitoneal mass that contains neither fat components nor central necrosis is suggestive of the diagnosis. Foci of very high T2 signal intensity that show some enhancement suggest a diagnosis of myxoid MFH, which is the second most common subtype after storiform pleomorphic[92,223] (Figure 26-14).

Other Solid Neoplasms

Intravenous Leiomyomatosis.

Intravenous leiomyomatosis (IVL) is a rare condition that is characterized by the intravenous growth of benign smooth muscle tumor.[90,164] IVL is the progression of the microscopic precursor condition of leiomyomas with vascular invasion. If the latter condition results in hematogenous spread of tumor cells, benign metastasizing leiomyoma results.[48] The majority of cases of IVL arise from leiomyoma of the uterus; however, some cases appear to arise directly from smooth muscle cells of extrapelvic veins.[117] Symptoms are related to either uterine fibroids[221] or compression of the pelvic veins or IVC. Unusual cases of extension to the right atrium resulting in syncope or sudden death have been reported.[226,260,294] The treatment of choice is hysterectomy and removal of any intravascular tumor. Up to 30% of surgically treated patients develop new masses, presumably resulting from regrowth of intravenous tumor.[64]

Because of its direct multiplanar capability and superb contrast resolution, MRI is an ideal imaging modality to diagnose IVL and other processes involving the IVC. IVL should be considered when MRI shows enhanced soft tissue in multiple dilated pelvic veins or within the IVC in a woman with uterine fibroids.[153,268]

With the advent of dynamic CT scanning and the use of power injectors, radiologists had to learn how to properly identify and disregard the "pseudothrombus" that occurs in the suprarenal IVC.[94] This pseudothrombus is rarely an issue in MRI, where typical findings on spin-echo and gradient-echo images confirm vessel patency.[27,29,30] In cases of true venous thrombus, MRI has the ability to distinguish between bland and malignant etiologies; the latter will be enhanced, whereas the former will not (Figure 26-15).[107]

Extragonadal Germ Cell Tumors.

Extragonadal germ cell tumors (EGCTs) (Figure 26-16) represent between 1% and 5% of all germ cell tumors.[43,61,125,295] The retroperitoneum is the second most common location of EGCTs, after the mediastinum. EGCTs are believed to arise from midline primordial germ cells that had an arrested caudal migration during embryogenesis.[25,231] EGCTs occur in similar age groups (third to fourth decades) and have histological subtypes similar to those of primary testicular carcinoma.[125] Recent studies show that survival of EGCT is equivalent to that of primary testicular neoplasms with bulky adenopathy.[121,125]

Extragonadal seminomas usually do not have elevated tumor markers and are treated primarily by radiation therapy.[125,161] Seminomas larger than 5 cm are also treated with cisplatin-based chemotherapy, as are nonseminomatous EGCTs.[231] Nonseminomatous EGCTs often have

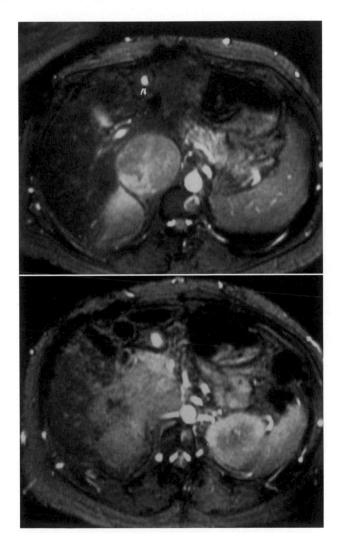

FIGURE 26-13 Leiomyosarcoma of the IVC. T2*-weighted gradient-echo images (25/13, FA 30 degrees) show a heterogeneous, high-signal, infiltrative mass that replaces and extends through the intrahepatic IVC. Note the multiple abdominal wall and paraspinal collateral vessels. An aggressive tumor of the IVC suggests leiomyosarcoma, which was confirmed at surgery.

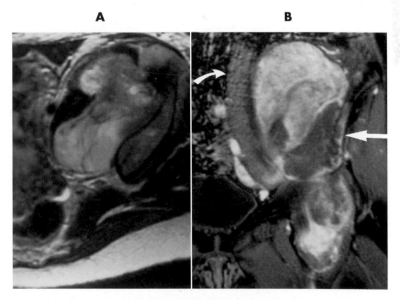

FIGURE 26-14 Myxoid malignant fibrous histiocytoma. **A,** Fast spin-echo (4700/80) image shows a large, heterogeneous, high-signal mass that has replaced the left iliacus muscle and displaced the psoas muscle anteromedially. **B,** Coronal fat-suppressed, gradient-echo (160/2.6, FA 90 degrees), contrast-enhanced image shows the displaced psoas muscle *(curved white arrow),* an abnormally enhancing left iliac bone *(straight white arrow),* and the extent of tumor extension into the anterior compartment of the thigh. Enhanced components are typical for myxomatous tissue.

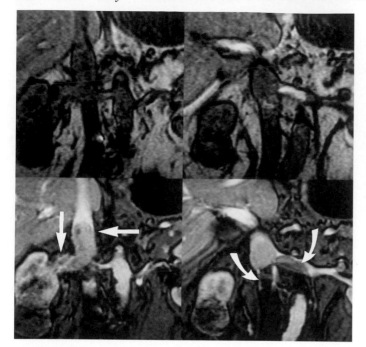

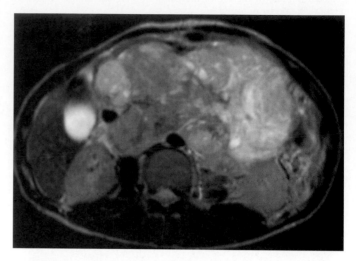

FIGURE 26-15   Distinction between benign and malignant tumor thrombus. Coronal, breath-hold, pelvic-coil, spoiled T1-weighted gradient-echo images (85/2.9, FA 80 degrees) obtained before *(top row)* and after *(bottom row)* contrast enhancement show right lower-pole renal cell carcinoma with enhanced malignant tumor thrombus in the right renal vein and infrahepatic IVC *(straight white arrows)*. On precontrast images there is high-signal thrombus (caused by methemoglobin) in the left renal vein and the infrarenal IVC that shows no enhancement *(curved white arrows)* postcontrast, which correlates with a bland clot that formed because of stasis.

FIGURE 26-16   Germ cell tumor. A 26-year-old man who felt a mass after falling at work. Axial fast spin-echo image (7700/102) shows a large heterogeneous midline retroperitoneal mass. Biopsy confirmed malignant germ cell tumor. Mass has markedly decreased in size with cisplatin-based chemotherapy. High-resolution scrotal ultrasound examinations both before and after therapy were entirely normal.

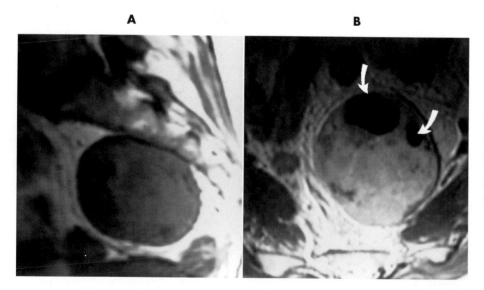

A

B

FIGURE 26-17   Benign schwannoma in a 57-year-old woman with low back pain. Sagittal (500/11) **(A)** and enhanced axial (700/13) **(B)** T1-weighted spin-echo images obtained with a dedicated spine coil shows a well-circumscribed, intensely enhancing presacral mass with foci of nonenhanced cystic degeneration *(arrows)* that were of fluid signal intensity on T2-weighed images (not shown).

elevated serum levels of alpha-fetoprotein (AFP) and human chorionic gonadotropin (hCG) that are useful in both the diagnosis and the monitoring of therapy. An elevated AFP or hCG in a young man with a large midline retroperitoneal mass is considered so typical of EGCT that some investigators will treat empirically with chemotherapy without an open biopsy.[125,231]

Thorough evaluation of the testes of patients with presumed EGCT is clinically important. Physical palpation of the testes is insensitive for detecting some occult primary tumors. Thus before the era of high-resolution cross-sectional imaging, many occult primary testicular tumors with retroperitoneal or mediastinal adenopathy were misclassi-

fied as EGCTs. Surprisingly, some clinicians still use palpation as the sole means to exclude a testicular primary carcinoma.[112] In a study of 39 EGCTs, bilateral testicular biopsies showed carcinoma in situ in greater than 40% of patients[75]; some positive biopsies occurred in testes with normal ultrasound examinations. Occasionally, only a focal scar is identified on testicular biopsy and is considered to be a "burned out" carcinoma. The retroperitoneal malignancy could represent either true metastases or a metachronous second primary tumor.[61,75] Chemotherapeutic agents can have decreased access to the testicle because of the blood-testis barrier.[25,281] The testes can harbor residual tumor even after successful treatment of extratesticular disease.[116] For all of the afore-

A   **B**

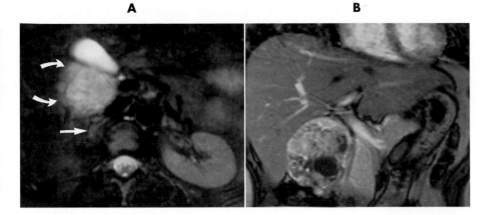

FIGURE 26-18 Retroperitoneal paraganglioma. **A**, Coronal, pelvic-coil, dynamic, contrast-enhanced, breath-hold, spoiled gradient-echo image (150/2.5, FA 80). **B**, Axial, fat-suppressed, fast spin-echo image (4800/85) through the superior portion of the mass (*curved arrows* in **A**) shows a heterogeneously hypervascular neoplasm that is separate from the adrenal gland (*straight arrow* in **A**) and has high signal intensity on T2-weighted images. Low-signal, linear, intrahepatic structures present in **A** represent unopacified hepatic veins that were enhanced on delayed images (not shown). LMS or nerve sheath tumor could have a similar appearance, although this would be an atypical location for the latter. The fact that the patient had no clinical or chemical evidence of catecholamine excess excludes the diagnosis of extraadrenal pheochromocytoma.

mentioned reasons, orchiectomy should be considered if there is suspicion of intratesticular disease.[25]

CT and MR findings of EGCT typically show a large midline heterogeneous mass with low attenuation and high T2-weighted signal-intensity components within that correspond to necrosis and hemorrhage on histological examination.[24,273] Retroperitoneal masses of metastatic adenopathy from primary testicular germ cell neoplasms have a similar MR appearance but tend not to be centered in the midline.

Nerve Sheath Tumors. Most benign nerve sheath tumors represent either schwannoma (neurilemoma) or neurofibroma (Figure 26-17).[91] Schwannomas are often encapsulated, are not associated with neurofibromatosis, and are benign. Neurofibromas are usually unencapsulated, can be associated with neurofibromatosis, and can degenerate into a neurofibrosarcoma. Benign nerve sheath tumors occur equally in both genders, mostly in the third to fifth decades of life. Although most lesions occur along the flexor surfaces of the extremities and in the head and neck, retroperitoneal tumors have been described.[91]

The MR appearance of peripheral nerve tumors has been well described.* Benign lesions are well-defined, spherical or fusiform masses with smooth margins. Most are isointense to muscle on T1-weighted images, are very hyperintense to muscle on T2-weighted images, and show intense contrast enhancement. The presence of a low-signal capsule is more suggestive of a schwannoma than of a neurofibroma.[54] Some studies have shown a characteristic target sign on both T2-weighted and contrast-enhanced images of both neurofibromas and schwannomas.[305,320] The high T2 signal, enhanced peripheral component of the tumor represents myxomatous tissue, whereas the central low T2 signal, hypovascular area represents fibrous and collagenous material.[320] This zonal pattern does not correlate histologically with the proportion of Antoni-A and Antoni-B type tissue present.[101] Retroperitoneal schwannomas are often found in a presacral location.[156]

Paraganglioma. Paragangliomas are tumors of the extraadrenal paraganglion system. Some authors use the term *extraadrenal pheochromocytoma* only when the tumors are functioning.[40,327] Most paragangliomas occur in the retroperitoneum between the diaphragm and the lower pole of the kidneys and are functioning. Extraadrenal pheochromocytomas represent at least 15% of pheochromocytomas in the adult population, and up to 40% can be malignant. Paragangliomas are part of Carney's triad syndrome (along with pulmonary chondroma and gastric smooth muscle neoplasms).[40,327] The treatment of choice is surgical removal of the primary tumor with medical therapy for unresectable, symptomatic, residual disease.[327] The MR findings of paragangliomas have been described[261,312,319] and are similar to the MR findings of adrenal pheochromocytoma.† Lesions are of high T2 signal intensity (Figure 26-18). Heterogeneity is caused by intratumoral cyst formation or hemorrhage and is more common in larger lesions. Signal intensity alone cannot distinguish between benign and malignant tu-

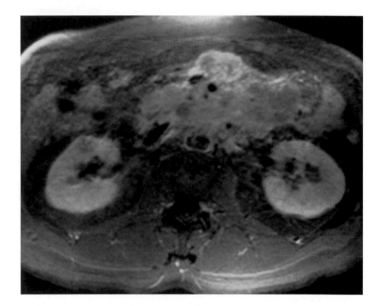

FIGURE 26-19 Non-Hodgkin's lymphoma. Fat-suppressed, T1-weighted spin-echo (500/10), contrast-enhanced image shows a conglomerate-enhanced mass of adenopathy surrounding the mesenteric vessels.

mors.[192] Lesions with lower T2 signal intensity tend to have less catecholamine production.[310] Because these lesions are not related to the cells of the adrenal cortex, they do not contain intracellular lipid and therefore will not lose signal intensity with chemical-shift imaging.

Lymphoma and Adenopathy. Lymphoma can involve any nodal chain in the body.[99] Lymphoma, and particularly non-Hodgkin's lymphoma (Figure 26-19), commonly involves both retroperitoneal and mesenteric lymph nodes. Conglomerate retroperitoneal masses can surround or invade the kidneys.*

Although some studies have shown different T1[237,252] or T2 values[329] in malignant adenopathy, most investigators believe that quantitative T1 or T2 measurements are of limited utility.[74,81,110,157] The empirical observation that many malignancies tend to follow the signal intensity of spleen (which can be thought of simplistically as benign lymphoid tissue) also suggests a limited discriminatory value in evaluating the signal intensity of nodes.

Enteric contrast agents may occasionally facilitate the distinction of bowel from adenopathy.† Injection of glucagon by itself may be helpful (Figure 26-8). Ultrasmall superparamagnetic iron oxide particles

*References 54, 69, 163, 292, 305, 320, 322.
†References 19, 26, 95, 142, 192, 310.

*References 66, 86, 98, 248, 257, 258.
†References 23, 84, 180, 213, 227, 311, 315.

have been used as MR lymph node contrast agents[8,9,321] to differentiate between benign and malignant nodes. Benign nodes accumulate the iron and lose signal on T2-weighted images, whereas nodes replaced by malignancy do not. Several studies have documented that evaluating the T2 signal intensity of lymphomatous nodal masses after therapy is useful; masses with low T2 signal intensity have high negative predictive value for nonviable tumor.* Most of the patients in the series studied had treated mediastinal masses of Hodgkin's disease. Nonneoplastic masses with high T2 signal intensity (caused by edema, granulation tissue, hemorrhage, or immature fibrosis) may persist up to 12 months after therapy,[1,250] and therefore it is recommended that MRI be performed 1 year after treatment.

Nonneoplastic Processes

Retroperitoneal Fibrosis. Retroperitoneal fibrosis (RPF) is an uncommon fibrotic and inflammatory process that is characteristically centered in the caudal retroperitoneum at the L4-L5 level (Figure 26-20). RPF is more common in men and usually occurs in the fifth or sixth decades of life, although it has been described in children.[6,35,152] Most cases are idiopathic. Idiopathic RPF is very closely related to inflammatory abdominal aortic aneurysm. With the exception of aortic size, there are no significant clinical or pathological differences between the two conditions,[105,241] which may be caused by an autoallergic reaction resulting from leakage of lipid material from arthrosclerotic plaque into the periaortic soft tissues.[5,133,154,317] In the older literature the most common known cause of RPF was methysergide, a medicine that was

---

*References 1, 88, 106, 134, 225, 250.

prescribed for headaches.[87] Other cases have been attributed to various infections and malignancies.

Cellular components and inflammatory cells accompany fibrosis,[105,241] causing variable, heterogeneous signal intensity on MRI.* Anterior displacement of the aorta is not specific but may occur in RPF, malignancy,[34] mesenteric adenopathy, and subjacent osseous destruction.[32,76]

Ovarian Vein Thrombosis. Ovarian vein thrombosis (OVT) occurs most often in the postpartum period, where it has an incidence of 1 in 600 to 2000 births.[56,287] Women with OVT usually have fever and pain between 3 and 20 days after delivery.[330] The differential diagnosis includes endometritis, appendicitis, pyelonephritis, torsion, and tuboovarian abscess.[287,330] Most cases of OVT involve the right side. Many theories have been proposed to explain this empirical observation. First, the uterus tends to be dextroverted in pregnancy, which would favor compression of the right ovarian vein. Second, the right ovarian vein is longer and has more competent valves. Third, the right ovarian vein crosses the ureter at the level of the pelvic brim. All of these findings foster stasis.[56,287] Treatment of OVT consists of intravenous antibiotics and heparin. A clinical response may occur only after 48 hours and should not exclude a diagnosis of OVT that has been established based on clinical and imaging findings.[82,330] OVT has been detected on imaging studies in patients receiving chemotherapy[144] and persons with acute inflammation of the gastrointestinal tract.[146] Many of these patients had no symptoms referable to their OVT, and the thrombosis resolved without treatment.

---

*References 5, 6, 13, 83, 105, 129, 133, 160, 174, 176, 220, 263, 293, 317, 323, 338, 340.

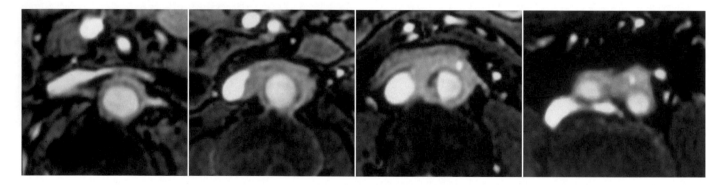

FIGURE 26-20   Stable retroperitoneal fibrosis in a 69-year-old man. Contrast-enhanced, fat-suppressed, spoiled gradient-echo images (68/2.3, FA 80 degrees, FOV 26) show an enhanced circumaortic rind of soft tissue. Despite high T2 signal intensity (not shown) and moderate enhancement after contrast, this process is benign and has been stable for several years.

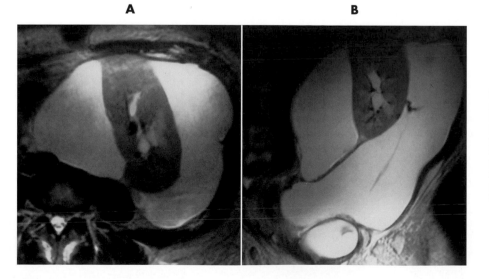

A   **B**

FIGURE 26-21   Retroperitoneal lymphocele. Fast spin-echo (4000/19) transverse **(A)** and coronal **(B)** images show complex, septated fluid collection that surrounds the left lower-quadrant renal transplant placed 2 months before imaging. Contrast study (not shown) demonstrated normal transplant enhancement and excretion. Presence of septations, lack of hemorrhagic components, and normal transplant function all suggest that this fluid collection is a lymphocele and not a hematoma or urinoma.

Before the era of cross-sectional imaging, the diagnosis was usually suspected when a tubular structure extending superolaterally from the uterus was palpated and confirmed by laparotomy. Now, MRI can establish the diagnosis in a noninvasive fashion.[38,140,190,211,272] Both spin-echo and gradient-echo techniques can be used to establish the lack of flow in an enlarged ovarian vein that courses through the retroperitoneum from the adnexa to the renal vein (left) or IVC (right).[12,112,122,161,236] Ultrasound can be limited in these patients because of bowel gas and abdominal tenderness, and established cases of OVT have been missed with this modality.[287]

Lymphocele. Retroperitoneal lymphoceles occur after gynecological or urological pelvic surgery.[200] Lymphoceles are most commonly seen after renal transplantation, when the incidence is between 1% and 20% (Figure 26-21). Lymphoceles form because of disruption of afferent lymphatics along the iliac vessels, transplant hilum, or transplant capsule.[4,18,41] Most lymphoceles are small and asymptomatic, and they usually resorb over time. Larger lymphoceles can become symptomatic because of local mass effect and cause lower extremity swelling or obstructive uropathy 2 weeks to 6 months after transplantation. Treatment options include percutaneous drainage with or without a sclerosing agent[108] or peritoneal marsupialization through either an open or a laparoscopic approach.[141,219] MRI shows a well-circumscribed fluid collection located between the renal transplant and the bladder. Septations are common, very high T1-weighted signal-intensity components caused by methemoglobin are usually absent, and there should be no irregular rim enhancement. These characteristics should help distinguish a lymphocele from a urinoma, hematoma, and abscess, respectively.

Hematoma. Paramagnetic effects of blood products dramatically influence MR signal intensity (see Chapter 58).* The concentric ring sign is extremely helpful in establishing a diagnosis of maturing hematoma (Figure 26-22)[123] in the retroperitoneum. Untreated "masses" that contain a component of very high signal intensity on T1-weighted images (representing methemoglobin) are usually benign hematomas rather than hemorrhagic neoplasms. In addition, when MRI is used to follow known malignancies during treatment, it can establish that an enlarging mass represents benign intratumoral hemorrhage rather than growing viable tumor.[239] The most common processes affecting the iliopsoas compartment are hematomas, abscesses, and neoplasms.[175,198] Unlike MRI, CT is unable to distinguish among hematomas, abscesses, and neoplasms of the iliopsoas muscles.[175]

Abscess. There have been limited published reports to date concerning the appearance of retroperitoneal and abdominal or pelvic abscesses (Figure 26-23).[148,177,274,296] However, findings in this portion

---

*References 16, 28, 36, 62, 79, 123, 124, 277, 308, 337.

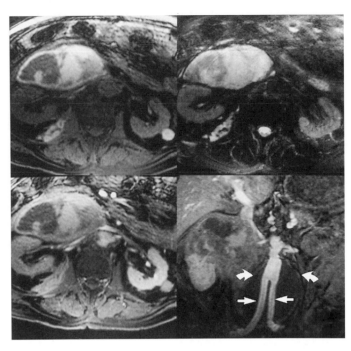

FIGURE 26-22 Complex hematoma in a 73-year-old man after aneurysm repair. Fat-suppressed, spoiled gradient-echo image (100/2.6) shows a large collection in the right anterior pararenal space, which has both low– and high–signal intensity components. A smaller hemorrhagic collection lies adjacent to the right psoas muscle.

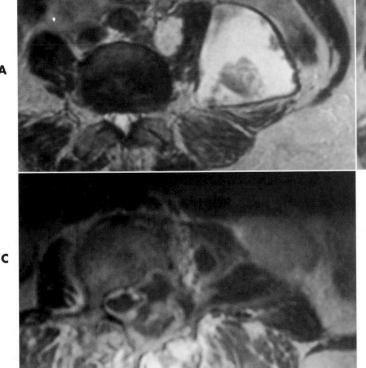

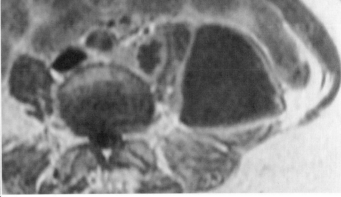

A B C

FIGURE 26-23 Tuberculous abscess in a 67-year-old woman with increasing chronic back pain. **A,** Axial fast spin-echo image (4000/102) through the midabdomen demonstrates complex fluid collections that surround and distort the left psoas muscle. **B,** Axial T1-weighted spin-echo images (600/12) obtained postcontrast show rim enhancement. **C,** Postcontrast T1-weighted spin-echo image obtained at a level caudal to **A** and **B** shows tuberculous involvement of the psoas muscle, left pedicle, and posterior elements of L3 and the epidural space. Osseous involvement, extensive psoas collection, and only mild, chronic symptoms are all suggestive of tuberculosis. (From reference 114.)

of the body do not differ from findings regarding the appearance of abscesses in the liver or musculoskeletal system.[199,222] Specifically, abscesses appear as complex fluid collections that show rim enhancement after contrast enhancement. Depending on location and extent, treatment consists of antibiotics or percutaneous or open drainage.[102,172,183,331]

REFERENCES

1. Abrahamsen AF, Lien HH, Aas M, et al: Magnetic resonance imaging and 67gallium scan in mediastinal malignant lymphoma: a prospective pilot study, Ann Oncol 5:433, 1994.
2. Acha T, Picazo B, Garcia-Martin FJ, et al: Carney's triad: apropos of a new case, Med Pediatr Oncol 22:216, 1994.
3. Aisen AM, Martel W, Braunstein EM, et al: MRI and CT evaluation of primary bone and soft-tissue tumors, Am J Roentgenol 146:749, 1986.
4. Amante AJ, and Kahan BD: Technical complications of renal transplantation, Surg Clin North Am 74:1117, 1994.
5. Amis ES, Jr: Retroperitoneal fibrosis [see comments], Am J Roentgenol 157:321, 1991.
6. Amis ES, Jr: Retroperitoneal fibrosis, Urol Radiol 12:135, 1990.
7. Anonymous: Case records of the Massachusetts General Hospital: weekly clinico-pathological exercises, Case 12-1989, A 24-year-old Haitian man with right flank pain and recent fever, N Engl J Med 320:790, 1989.
8. Anzai Y, Blackwell KE, Hirschowitz SL, et al: Initial clinical experience with dextran-coated superparamagnetic iron oxide for detection of lymph node metastases in patients with head and neck cancer [see comments], Radiology 192:709, 1994.
9. Anzai Y, McLachlan S, Morris M, et al: Dextran-coated superparamagnetic iron oxide, an MR contrast agent for assessing lymph nodes in the head and neck, Am J Neuroradiol 15:87, 1994.
10. Arakawa A, Yasunaga T, Yano S, et al: Radiological findings of retroperitoneal leiomyoma and leiomyosarcoma: report of two cases, Comput Med Imaging Graph 17:125, 1993.
11. Arnold R, Frank M, and Kajdan U: Management of gastroenteropancreatic endocrine tumors: the place of somatostatin analogues, Digestion 55:107, 1994.
12. Arrive L, Hricak H, and Martin MC: Pelvic endometriosis: MR imaging, Radiology 171:687, 1989.
13. Arrive L, Hricak H, Tavares NJ, et al: Malignant versus nonmalignant retroperitoneal fibrosis: differentiation with MR imaging, Radiology 172:139, 1989.
14. Auh YH, Rubenstein WA, Markisz JA, et al: Intraperitoneal paravesical spaces: CT delineation with US correlation, Radiology 159:311, 1986.
15. Auh YH, Rubenstein WA, Schneider M, et al: Extraperitoneal paravesical spaces: CT delineation with US correlation, Radiology 159:319, 1986.
16. Barkovich AJ, and Atlas SW: Magnetic resonance imaging of intracranial hemorrhage, Radiol Clin North Am 26:801, 1988.
17. Beahrs OH, Hemson DE, Hutter RVP, et al: Manual for staging of cancer, ed 4, Philadelphia, 1992, Lippincott.
18. Becker JA, Choyke PL, Hill M, et al: Imaging the transplanted kidney. In Pollack HM, ed: Clinical urography, vol 3, Philadelphia, 1990, WB Saunders.
19. Beland SS, Vesely DL, Arnold WC, et al: Localization of adrenal and extra-adrenal pheochromocytomas by magnetic resonance imaging, South Med J 82:1410, 1989.
20. Bennett HF, and Balfe DM: MR imaging of the peritoneum and abdominal wall, MRI Clin North Am 3:99, 1995.
21. Berek JS: Interval debulking of ovarian cancer—an interim measure, N Engl J Med 332:675, 1995 (editorial comment).
22. Bernades P, Baetz A, Levy P, et al: Splenic and portal venous obstruction in chronic pancreatitis: a prospective longitudinal study of a medical-surgical series of 266 patients [see comments], Dig Dis Sci 37:340, 1992.
23. Bernardino ME, Weinreb JC, Mitchell DG, et al: Safety and optimum concentration of a manganese chloride–based oral MR contrast agent, J Magn Reson Imaging 4:872, 1994.
24. Blomlie V, Lien HH, Fossa SD, et al: CT in primary malignant germ cell tumors of the retroperitoneum, Acta Radiol 32:155, 1991.
25. Bohle A, Studer UE, Sonntag RW, et al: Primary or secondary extragonadal germ cell tumors? J Urol 135:939, 1986.
26. Boland GW, and Lee MJ: Magnetic resonance imaging of the adrenal gland, Crit Rev Diagn Imaging 36:115, 1995.
27. Bradley WG Jr: Flow phenomena in MR imaging. Carmen lecture, Am J Roentgenol 150:983, 1988.
28. Bradley WG Jr: MR appearance of hemorrhage in the brain [see comments], Radiology 189:15, 1993.
29. Bradley WG Jr, and Waluch V: Blood flow: magnetic resonance imaging, Radiology 154:443, 1985.
30. Bradley WG Jr, Waluch V, Lai KS, et al: The appearance of rapidly flowing blood on magnetic resonance images, Am J Roentgenol 143:1167, 1984.
31. Brice P, Rain JD, Frija J, et al: Residual mediastinal mass in malignant lymphoma: value of magnetic resonance imaging and gallium scan, Nouv Rev Fr Hematol 35:457, 1993.
32. Brooks AP: Computed tomography of idiopathic retroperitoneal fibrosis ('periaortitis'): variants, variations, patterns and pitfalls, Clin Radiol 42:75, 1990.
33. Brooks AP, Reznek RH, Nugent K, et al: CT appearances of desmoid tumours in familial adenomatous polyposis: further observations, Clin Radiol 49:601, 1994.
34. Brooks AP, Reznek RH, and Webb JA: Aortic displacement on computed tomography of idiopathic retroperitoneal fibrosis, Clin Radiol 40:51, 1989.
35. Brooks MT, Magill HL, Hanna SL, et al: Case of the day. Pediatric. Idiopathic retroperitoneal fibrosis, Radiographics 10:1096, 1990.
36. Brooks RA, Di Chiro G, and Patronas N: MR imaging of cerebral hematomas at different field strengths: theory and applications, J Comput Assist Tomogr 13:194, 1989.
37. Brosens IA: The endometrial implant. In Thomas E, and Rock J, eds: Modern approaches to endometriosis, Boston, 1991, Kluwer.
38. Brown CE, Lowe TW, Cunningham FG, et al: Puerperal pelvic thrombophlebitis: impact on diagnosis and treatment using x-ray computed tomography and magnetic resonance imaging, Obstet Gynecol 68:789, 1986.
39. Buck JL, and Sobin LH: Carcinoids of the gastrointestinal tract, Radiographics 10:1081, 1990.
40. Buckley KM, and Whitman GJ: Diaphragmatic pheochromocytoma, Am J Roentgenol 165:260, 1995.
41. Burgos FJ, Teruel JL, Mayayo T, et al: Diagnosis and management of lymphoceles after renal transplantation, Br J Urol 61:289, 1988.
42. Burke AP, Sobin LH, Shekitka KM, et al: Intra-abdominal fibromatosis: a pathologic analysis of 130 tumors with comparison of clinical subgroups [see comments], Am J Surg Pathol 14:335, 1990.
43. Buskirk SJ, Evans RG, Farrow GM, et al: Primary retroperitoneal seminoma, Cancer 49:1934, 1982.
44. Buy JN, Malbec L, Ghossain MA, et al: Magnetic resonance imaging of pseudomyxoma peritonei, Eur J Radiol 9:115, 1989.
45. Buy JN, Moss AA, Ghossain MA, et al: Peritoneal implants from ovarian tumors: CT findings, Radiology 169:691, 1988.
46. Caldamone AA, Snyder HMD, and Duckett JW: Ureteroceles in children: follow-up of management with upper tract approach, J Urol 131:1130, 1984.
47. Campeau NG, Johnson CD, Felmlee JP, et al: MR imaging of the abdomen with a phased-array multicoil: prospective clinical evaluation, Radiology 195:769, 1995.
48. Canzonieri V, D'Amore ES, Bartoloni G, et al: Leiomyomatosis with vascular invasion: a unified pathogenesis regarding leiomyoma with vascular microinvasion, benign metastasizing leiomyoma and intravenous leiomyomatosis, Virchows Arch 425:541, 1994.
49. Capella C, Heitz PU, Hofler H, et al: Revised classification of neuroendocrine tumors of the lung, pancreas and gut, Digestion 55:11, 1994.
50. Carrasco CH, Charnsangavej C, Ajani J, et al: The carcinoid syndrome: palliation by hepatic artery embolization, Am J Roentgenol 147:149, 1986.
51. Caseiro-Alves F, Goncalo M, Abraul E, et al: Induced pneumoperitoneum in CT evaluation of peritoneal carcinomatosis, Abdom Imaging 20:52, 1995.
52. Casillas J, Sais GJ, Greve JL, et al: Imaging of intra- and extraabdominal desmoid tumors, Radiographics 11:959, 1991.
53. Catton CN, O'Sullivan B, Kotwall C, et al: Outcome and prognosis in retroperitoneal soft tissue sarcoma, Int J Radiat Oncol Biol Phys 29:1005, 1994.
54. Cerofolini E, Landi A, DeSantis G, et al: MR of benign peripheral nerve sheath tumors, J Comput Assist Tomogr 15:593, 1991.
55. Chang AE, and Sondak VK: Clinical evaluation and treatment of soft tissue tumors. In Enzinger FM, and Weiss SW, eds: Soft tissue tumors, ed 3, St Louis, 1995, Mosby.
56. Chawla K, Mond DJ, and Lanzkowsky L: Postpartum ovarian vein thrombosis, Am J Emerg Med 12:82, 1994.
57. Chou CK, Chen LT, Sheu RS, et al: MRI manifestations of gastrointestinal wall thickening [see comments], Abdom Imaging 19:389, 1994.
58. Chou CK, Liu GC, Chen LT, et al: MRI demonstration of peritoneal ligaments and mesenteries, Abdom Imaging 18:126, 1993.
59. Chou CK, Liu GC, Chen LT, et al: MRI manifestations of peritoneal carcinomatosis, Gastrointest Radiol 17:336, 1992.
60. Chou CK, Liu GC, Su JH, et al: MRI demonstration of peritoneal implants, Abdom Imaging 19:95, 1994.
61. Choyke PL, Hayes WS, and Sesterhenn IA: Primary extragonadal germ cell tumors of the retroperitoneum: differentiation of primary and secondary tumors, Radiographics 13:1365, 1993.
62. Clark RA, Watanabe AT, Bradley WG Jr, et al: Acute hematomas: effects of deoxygenation, hematocrit, and fibrin-clot formation and retraction on T2 shortening, Radiology 175:201, 1990.
63. Clarke-Pearson DL, Bandy LC, Dudzinski M, et al: Computed tomography in evaluation of patients with ovarian carcinoma in complete clinical remission: correlation with surgical-pathologic findings, JAMA 255:627, 1986.
64. Clement PB: Intravenous leiomyomatosis of the uterus, Pathol Annu 23:153, 1988.
65. Cockey BM, Fishman EK, Jones B, et al: Computed tomography of abdominal carcinoid tumor, J Comput Assist Tomogr 9:38, 1985.
66. Cohan RH, Dunnick NR, Leder RA, et al: Computed tomography of renal lymphoma, J Comput Assist Tomogr 14:933, 1990.
67. Cohen MD, Rougraff B, and Faught P: Cystic angiomatosis of bone: MR findings, Pediatr Radiol 24:256, 1994.
68. Crabo LG, Conley DM, Graney DO, et al: Venous anatomy of the pancreatic head: normal CT appearance in cadavers and patients, Am J Roentgenol 160:1039, 1993.
69. Cretella JP, Rafal RB, McCarron JP, Jr, et al: MR imaging in the diagnosis of a retroperitoneal schwannoma, Comput Med Imaging Graph 18:209, 1994.
70. Creutzfeldt W: Historical background and natural history of carcinoids, Digestion 55:3, 1994.
71. Creutzfeldt W, Bartsch HH, Jacubaschke U, et al: Treatment of gastrointestinal endocrine tumours with interferon-alpha and octreotide, Acta Oncol 30:529, 1991.
72. Cutillo DP, Swayne LC, Cucco J, et al: CT and MR imaging in cystic abdominal lymphangiomatosis, J Comput Assist Tomogr 13:534, 1989.
73. Dalton RR, Donohue JH, Mucha P Jr, et al: Management of retroperitoneal sarcomas, Surgery 106:725, 1989.
74. Damadian R, Zaner K, Hor D, et al: Human tumors detected by nuclear magnetic resonance, Proc Natl Acad Sci USA 71:1471, 1974.
75. Daugaard G, Rorth M, von der Maase H, et al: Management of extragonadal germ-cell tumors and the significance of bilateral testicular biopsies, Ann Oncol 3:283, 1992.
76. Degesys GE, Dunnick NR, Silverman PM, et al: Retroperitoneal fibrosis: use of CT in distinguishing among possible causes, Am J Roentgenol 146:57, 1986.
77. DeMeo JH, Fulcher AS, and Austin RF: Anatomic CT demonstration of the peritoneal spaces, ligaments, and mesenteries: normal and pathologic processes, Radiographics 15:755, 1995.

78. Descamps P, Cottier JP, Barre I, et al: Endometriosis of the sciatic nerve: case report demonstrating the value of MR imaging, Eur J Obstet Gynecol Reprod Biol 58:199, 1995.

79. Di Cesare E, Di Renzi P, Pavone P, et al: Evaluation of hematoma by MRI in follow-up of aorto-femoral bypass, Magn Reson Imaging 9:247, 1991.

80. Dodds WJ, Darweesh RM, Lawson TL, et al: The retroperitoneal spaces revisited, Am J Roentgenol 147:1155, 1986.

81. Dooms GC, Hricak H, Moseley ME, et al: Characterization of lymphadenopathy by magnetic resonance relaxation times: preliminary results, Radiology 155:691, 1985.

82. Dunnihoo DR, Gallaspy JW, Wise RB, et al: Postpartum ovarian vein thrombophlebitis: a review, Obstet Gynecol Surv 46:415, 1991.

83. Ebner F, Kressel HY, Mintz MC, et al: Tumor recurrence versus fibrosis in the female pelvis: differentiation with MR imaging at 1.5 T, Radiology 166:333, 1988.

84. Einstein DM, Singer AA, Chilcote WA, et al: Abdominal lymphadenopathy: spectrum of CT findings, Radiographics 11:457, 1991.

85. Einstein DM, Tagliabue JR, and Desai RK: Abdominal desmoids: CT findings in 25 patients, Am J Roentgenol 157:275, 1991.

86. Eisenberg PJ, Papanicolaou N, Lee MJ, et al: Diagnostic imaging in the evaluation of renal lymphoma, Leuk Lymphoma 16:37, 1994.

87. Elkind AH, Friedman AP, Bachman A, et al: Silent retroperitoneal fibrosis associated with methysergide therapy, JAMA 206:1041, 1968.

88. Elkowitz SS, Leonidas JC, Lopez M, et al: Comparison of CT and MRI in the evaluation of therapeutic response in thoracic Hodgkin disease, Pediatr Radiol 23:301, 1993.

89. Engelton JD, and Ros PR: Retroperitoneal MR imaging, Magn Reson Imaging Clin N Am 5:165, 1997.

90. Enzinger FM, and Weiss SM: Benign tumors of smooth muscle. In Enzinger FM, and Weiss SW: Soft tissue tumors, ed 3, St Louis, 1995, Mosby.

91. Enzinger FM, and Weiss SW: Benign tumors of peripheral nerves. In Enzinger FM, and Weiss SW, eds: Soft tissue tumors, ed 3, St Louis, 1995, Mosby.

92. Enzinger FM, and Weiss SW: Malignant fibrohistiocytic tumors. In Enzinger FM, and Weiss SW, eds: Soft tissue tumors, ed 3, St Louis, 1995, Mosby.

93. Enzinger FM, and Weiss SW: Tumors of lymph vessels. In Enzinger FM, and Weiss SW, eds: Soft tissue tumors, ed 3, St Louis, 1995, Mosby.

94. Fagelman D, Lawrence LP, Black KS, et al: Inferior vena cava pseudothrombus in computed tomography using a contrast medium power injector: a potential pitfall, J Comput Assist Tomogr 11:1042, 1987.

95. Falke TH, van Gils AP, van Seters AP, et al: Magnetic resonance imaging of functioning paragangliomas, Magn Reson Q 6:35, 1990.

96. Feld R, Burk DL Jr, McCue P, et al: MRI of aggressive fibromatosis: frequent appearance of high signal intensity on T2-weighted images, Magn Reson Imaging 8:583, 1990.

97. Feldberg MA, Hendriks AV, Van Leeuwen MS, et al: Retroperitoneal cystic lymphangioma section imaging in two cases, and review of the literature, Clin Imaging 14:26, 1990.

98. Ferry JA, Harris NL, Papanicolaou N, et al: Lymphoma of the kidney: a report of 11 cases, Am J Surg Pathol 19:134, 1995.

99. Fishman EK, Kuhlman JE, and Jones RJ: CT of lymphoma: spectrum of disease, Radiographics 11:647, 1991.

100. Forstner R, Chen M, and Hricak H: Imaging of ovarian cancer, J Magn Reson Imaging 5:606, 1995.

101. Friedman DP, Tartaglino LM, and Flanders AE: Intradural schwannomas of the spine: MR findings with emphasis on contrast-enhancement characteristics, Am J Roentgenol 158:1347, 1992.

102. Fry DE: Noninvasive imaging tests in the diagnosis and treatment of intra-abdominal abscesses in the postoperative patient, Surg Clin North Am 74:693, 1994.

103. Gaines PA, Saunders AJ, and Drake D: Midgut malrotation diagnosed by ultrasound, Clin Radiol 38:51, 1987.

104. Galifer RB, Pous JG, Juskiewenski S, et al: Intraabdominal cystic lymphangiomas in childhood, Prog Pediatr Surg 11:173, 1978.

105. Gans RO, Hoorntje SJ, Rauwerda JA, et al: The inflammatory abdominal aortic aneurysm: prevalence, clinical features and diagnostic evaluation, Neth J Med 43:105, 1993.

106. Gasparini MD, Balzarini L, Castellani MR, et al: Current role of gallium scan and magnetic resonance imaging in the management of mediastinal Hodgkin lymphoma, Cancer 72:577, 1993.

107. Gehl HB, Bohndorf K, and Klose KC: Inferior vena cava tumor thrombus: demonstration by Gd-DTPA enhanced MR, J Comput Assist Tomogr 14:479, 1990.

108. Gilliland JD, Spies JB, Brown SB, et al: Lymphoceles: percutaneous treatment with povidone-iodine sclerosis, Radiology 171:227, 1989.

109. Giunta S, Tipaldi L, Diotellevi F, et al: CT demonstration of peritoneal metastases after intraperitoneal injection of contrast media, Clin Imaging 14:31, 1990.

110. Glazer GM, Orringer MB, Chenevert TL, et al: Mediastinal lymph nodes: relaxation time/pathologic correlation and implications in staging of lung cancer with MR imaging [see comments], Radiology 168:429, 1988.

111. Glenn J, Sindelar WF, Kinsella T, et al: Results of multimodality therapy of resectable soft-tissue sarcomas of the retroperitoneum, Surgery 97:316, 1985.

112. Gonzalez-Vela JL, Villalona-Calero MA, Torkelson JL, et al: Extragonadal abdominal germ cell cancers, Am J Clin Oncol 15:308, 1992.

113. Goodwin JD: Carcinoid tumors: an analysis of 2,837 cases, Cancer 36:560, 1975.

114. Graves VB, and Schreiber MH: Tuberculous psoas muscle abscess, J Can Assoc Radiol 24:268, 1973.

115. Greiner RH, Munkel G, Blattmann H, et al: Conformal radiotherapy for unresectable retroperitoneal soft tissue sarcoma, Int J Radiat Oncol Biol Phys 22:333, 1992.

116. Greist A, Einhorn LH, Williams SD, et al: Pathologic findings at orchiectomy following chemotherapy for disseminated testicular cancer, J Clin Oncol 2:1025, 1984.

117. Grella L, Arnold TE, Kvilekval KH, et al: Intravenous leiomyomatosis, J Vasc Surg 20:987, 1994.

118. Gupta A, Saibil F, Kassim O, et al: Retroperitoneal fibrosis caused by carcinoid tumour, Q J Med 56:367, 1985.

119. Gupta S, Gupta RK, Gujral RB, et al: Peritoneal mesothelioma simulating pseudomyxoma peritonei on CT and sonography, Gastrointest Radiol 17:129, 1992.

120. Gurbuz AK, Giardiello FM, Petersen GM, et al: Desmoid tumours in familial adenomatous polyposis, Gut 35:377, 1994.

121. Gutierrez Delgado F, Tjulandin SA, and Garin AM: Long term results of treatment in patients with extragonadal germ cell tumours, Eur J Cancer 29A:1002, 1993.

122. Ha HK, Lim YT, Kim HS, et al: Diagnosis of pelvic endometriosis: fat-suppressed T1-weighted vs conventional MR images, Am J Roentgenol 163:127, 1994.

123. Hahn PF, Saini S, Stark DD, et al: Intraabdominal hematoma: the concentric-ring sign in MR imaging, Am J Roentgenol 148:115, 1987.

124. Hahn PF, Stark DD, Vici LG, et al: Duodenal hematoma: the ring sign in MR imaging, Radiology 159:379, 1986.

125. Hainsworth JD, and Greco FA: Extragonadal germ cell tumors and unrecognized germ cell tumors, Semin Oncol 19:119, 1992.

126. Halvorsen RA Jr, Panushka C, Oakley GJ, et al: Intraperitoneal contrast material improves the CT detection of peritoneal metastases, Am J Roentgenol 157:37, 1991.

127. Hamlin DJ, Paige R, Pettersson H, et al: Magnetic resonance characteristics of an abdominal desmoid tumor, Comput Radiol 10:11, 1986.

128. Hamrick-Turner JE, Chiechi MV, Abbitt PL, et al: Neoplastic and inflammatory processes of the peritoneum, omentum, and mesentery: diagnosis with CT, Radiographics 12:1051, 1992.

129. Harreby M, Bilde T, Helin P, et al: Retroperitoneal fibrosis treated with methylprednisolon pulse and disease-modifying antirheumatic drugs, Scand J Urol Nephrol 28:237, 1994.

130. Hartman DS, Hayes WS, Choyke PL, et al: From the archives of the AFIP: leiomyosarcoma of the retroperitoneum and inferior vena cava: radiologic-pathologic correlation, Radiographics 12:1203, 1992.

131. Hartman TE, Berquist TH, and Fetsch JF: MR imaging of extraabdominal desmoids: differentiation from other neoplasms, Am J Roentgenol 158:581, 1992.

132. Hayami S, Adachi Y, Ishigooka M, et al: Retroperitoneal cystic lymphangioma diagnosed by computerized tomography, magnetic resonance imaging and thin needle aspiration, Int Urol Nephrol 28:21, 1996.

133. Higgins PM, Bennett-Jones DN, Naish PF, et al: Non-operative management of retroperitoneal fibrosis, Br J Surg 75:573, 1988.

134. Hill M, Cunningham D, MacVicar D, et al: Role of magnetic resonance imaging in predicting relapse in residual masses after treatment of lymphoma, J Clin Oncol 11:2273, 1993.

135. Hoeffel JC: CT differentitiation of large abdominal lymphangiomas from ascites, Pediatr Radiol 24:152, 1994.

136. Hoffer FA, Kozakewich H, Colodny A, et al: Peritoneal inclusion cysts: ovarian fluid in peritoneal adhesions, Radiology 169:189, 1988.

137. Hoskins WJ, McGuire WP, Brady MF, et al: The effect of diameter of largest residual disease on survival after primary cytoreductive surgery in patients with suboptimal residual epithelial ovarian carcinoma, Am J Obstet Gynecol 170:974, 1994.

138. Hosono M, Kobayashi H, Fujimoto R, et al: Septum-like structures in lipoma and liposarcoma: MR imaging and pathologic correlation, Skeletal Radiol 26:150, 1997.

139. Hovanessian LJ, Larsen DW, Raval JK, et al: Retroperitoneal cystic lymphangioma: MR findings, Magn Reson Imaging 8:91, 1990.

140. Huch Boni RA, Heusler RH, Hebisch G, et al: [CT and MRI in inflammations of female genital organs], Radiologe 34:390, 1994.

141. Iselin CE, Rochat CH, Morel P, et al: Laparoscopic drainage of postoperative pelvic lymphocele, Br J Surg 81:274, 1994.

142. Ishii K, Yoshida Y, Matsui R, et al: [MRI of pheochromocytoma], Rinsho Hoshasen 35:1021, 1990.

143. Iyer R, Eftekhar F, Varma D, etal: Cystic retroperitoneal lymphangioma: CT, ultrasound and MR findings, Peditr Radiol 23:305, 1993.

144. Jacoby WT, Cohan RH, Baker ME, et al: Ovarian vein thrombosis in oncology patients: CT detection and clinical significance, Am J Roentgenol 155:291, 1990.

145. Jacquet P, Jelinek JS, Steves MA, et al: Evaluation of computed tomography in patients with peritoneal carcinomatosis, Cancer 72:1631, 1993.

146. Jain KA, and Jeffrey RB Jr: Gonadal vein thrombosis in patients with acute gastrointestinal inflammation: diagnosis with CT, Radiology 180:111, 1991.

147. Jeffrey RB Jr: Imaging of the peritoneal cavity, Curr Opin Radiol 3:471, 1991.

148. Johnson PL, Nguyen M, Dautenhahn J, et al: The magnetic resonance appearance of extraperitoneal bowel perforation: a case report, J Okla State Med Assoc 86:217, 1993.

149. Kainz C, Prayer L, Gitsch G, et al: The diagnostic value of magnetic resonance imaging for the detection of tumor recurrence in patients with carcinoma of the ovaries, J Am Coll Surg 178:239, 1994.

150. Karakousis CP, Kontzoglou K, and Driscoll DL: Resectability of retroperitoneal sarcomas: a matter of surgical technique? Eur J Surg Oncol 21:617, 1995.

151. Karanikas I, Liakakos T, Koundourakis S, et al: Surgical management of primary retroperitoneal liposarcomas, Acta Chir Belg 93:177, 1993.

152. Kasales CJ, and Hartman DS: Genitourinary case of the day: retroperitoneal fibrosis, Am J Roentgenol 162:1454, 1994.

153. Kawakami S, Sagoh T, Kumada H, et al: Intravenous leiomyomatosis of uterus: MR appearance, J Comput Assist Tomogr 15:686, 1991.

154. Keith DS, and Larson TS: Idiopathic retroperitoneal fibrosis, J Am Soc Nephrol 3:1748, 1993.

155. Kim JS, Lee HJ, Woo SK, et al: Peritoneal inclusion cysts and their relationship to the ovaries: evaluation with sonography, Radiology 204:481, 1997.

156. Kim SH, Choi BI, Han MC, et al: Retroperitoneal neurilemoma: CT and MR findings, Am J Roentgenol 159:1023, 1992.

157. Kim SH, Kim SC, Choi BI, et al: Uterine cervical carcinoma: evaluation of pelvic lymph node metastasis with MR imaging, Radiology 190:807, 1994.

158. Kim T, Murakami T, Oi H, et al: CT and MR imaging of abdominal liposarcoma, Am J Roentgenol 166:829, 1996.

159. Kinne DW, Chu FCH, Huvos AG, et al: Treatment of primary and recurrent retroperitoneal liposarcoma: twenty-five year experience at Memorial Hospital, Cancer 31:53, 1973.

160. Kitamura M, Miyanaga T, Sato Y, et al: [A case of retroperitoneal fibrosis with special emphasis on diagnosis using the magnetic resonance imaging], Hinyokika Kiyo 39:253, 1993.

161. Klepp O: Serum tumour markers in testicular and extragonadal germ cell malignancies, Scand J Clin Lab Invest Suppl 206:28, 1991.

162. Klutke CG, and Siegel CL: Functional female pelvic anatomy, Urol Clin North Am 22:487, 1995.

163. Kobayashi H, Kotoura Y, Sakahara H, et al: Schwannoma of the extremities: comparison of MRI and pentavalent technetium-99m-dimercaptosuccinic acid and gallium-67-citrate scintigraphy, J Nucl Med 35:1174, 1994.

164. Konrad P, and Mellblom L: Intravenous leiomyomatosis, Acta Obstet Gynecol Scand 68:371, 1989.

165. Korobkin M, Silverman PM, Quint LE, et al: CT of the extraperitoneal space: normal anatomy and fluid collections, Am J Roentgenol 159:933, 1992.

166. Kransdorf MJ, Jelinek JS, and Moser RP, Jr: Imaging of soft tissue tumors, Radiol Clin North Am 31:359, 1993.

167. Kransdorf MJ, Moser RP Jr, Meis JM, et al: Fat-containing soft-tissue masses of the extremities, Radiographics 11:81, 1991.

168. Kraus BB: Anatomy of the pelvis. In Ros PR, and Bidgood WD, eds: Abdominal magnetic resonance imaging, St Louis, 1993, Mosby.

169. Kurachi H, Murakami T, Nakamura H, et al: Imaging of peritoneal pseudocysts: value of MR imaging compared with sonography and CT, Am J Roentgenol 161:589, 1993.

170. Kuroda H, Kishimoto T, Yasunaga Y, et al: [Retroperitoneal giant malignant fibrous histiocytoma: report of a case], Hinyokika Kiyo 38:1143, 1992.

171. Kvols LK, Brown ML, O'Conner MK, et al: Treatment of the malignant carcinoid syndrome: evaluation of a long-acting somatostatin analogue, N Engl J Med 315:663, 1986.

172. Lambiase RE: Percutaneous abscess and fluid drainage: a critical review, Cardiovasc Intervent Radiol 14:143, 1991.

173. Lane RH, Stephens DH, and Reiman HM: Primary retroperitoneal neoplasms: CT findings in 90 cases with clinical and pathologic correlation, Am J Roentgenol 152:83, 1989.

174. Lee JK, and Glazer HS: Controversy in the MR imaging appearance of fibrosis, Radiology 177:21, 1990 (editorial comment).

175. Lenchik L, Dovgan DJ, and Kier R: CT of the iliopsoas compartment: value in differentiating tumor, abscess, and hematoma, Am J Roentgenol 162:83, 1994.

176. Leseche G, Schaetz A, Arrive L, et al: Diagnosis and management of 17 consecutive patients with inflammatory abdominal aortic aneurysm, Am J Surg 164:39, 1992.

177. Lev-Toaff AS, Baka JJ, Toaff ME, et al: Diagnostic imaging in puerperal febrile morbidity, Obstet Gynecol 78:50, 1991.

178. Loftus JP, and van Heerden JA: Surgical management of gastrointestinal carcinoid tumors, Adv Surg 28:317, 1995.

179. Love L, Meyers MA, Churchill RJ, et al: Computed tomography of extraperitoneal spaces, Am J Roentgenol 136:781, 1981.

180. Low RN, Carter WD, Saleh F, et al: Ovarian cancer: comparison of findings with perfluorocarbon-enhanced MR imaging, In-111-CYT-103 immunoscintigraphy, and CT, Radiology 195:391, 1995.

181. Loyer E, and Eggli KD: Sonographic evaluation of superior mesenteric vascular relationship in malrotation, Pediatr Radiol 19:173, 1989.

182. Lugo-Oliviera CH, and Taylor GA: CT differentiation of large abdominal lymphangioma from ascites, Pediatr Radiol 23:129, 1993.

183. MacGillivray DC, Valentine RJ, and Johnson JA: Strategies in the management of pyogenic psoas abscesses, Am Surg 57:701, 1991.

184. Maeda T: [Clinical significance of CT in evaluation of the gastrocolic trunk and its tributaries], Nippon Igaku Hoshasen Gakkai Zasshi 53:419, 1993.

185. Mahajan H, Kim EE, Wallace S, et al: Magnetic resonance imaging of malignant fibrous histiocytoma, Magn Reson Imaging 7:283, 1989.

186. Marn CS, Edgar KA, and Francis IR: CT diagnosis of splenic vein occlusion: imaging features, etiology and clinical manifestations, Abdom Imaging 20:78, 1995.

187. Marn CS, and Francis IR: CT of portal venous occlusion, Am J Roentgenol 159:717, 1992.

188. Marn CS, Glazer GM, Williams DM, et al: CT-angiographic correlation of collateral venous pathways in isolated splenic vein occlusion: new observations, Radiology 175:375, 1990.

189. Marshall JB, and Bodnarchuk G: Carcinoid tumors of the gut: our experience over three decades and review of the literature, J Clin Gastroenterol 16:123, 1993.

190. Martin B, Mulopulos GP, and Bryan PJ: MRI of puerperal ovarian-vein thrombosis (case report), Am J Roentgenol 147:291, 1986.

191. Matsuoka Y, Ohtomo K, Itai Y, et al: Pseudomyxoma peritonei with progressive calcifications: CT findings, Gastrointest Radiol 17:16, 1992.

192. Maurea S, Cuocolo A, Reynolds JC, et al: [Role of magnetic resonance in the study of benign and malignant pheochromocytomas: quantitative analysis of the intensity of the resonance signal], Radiol Med (Torino) 85:803, 1993.

193. McFadden DE, and Clement PB: Peritoneal inclusion cysts with mural mesothelial proliferation: a clinicopathological analysis of six cases, Am J Surg Pathol 10:844, 1986.

194. McGrath PC: Retroperitoneal sarcomas, Semin Surg Oncol 10:364, 1994.

195. McKinnon JG, Neifeld JP, Kay S, et al: Management of desmoid tumors, Surg Gynecol Obstet 169:104, 1989.

196. McLeod AJ, Zornoza J, and Shirkhoda A: Leiomyosarcoma: computed tomographic findings, Radiology 152:133, 1984.

197. Megibow AJ, Bosniak MA, Ho AG, et al: Accuracy of CT in detection of persistent or recurrent ovarian carcinoma: correlation with second-look laparotomy, Radiology 166:341, 1988.

198. Mendez G, Jr, Isikoff MB, and Hill MC: Retroperitoneal processes involving the psoas demonstrated by computed tomography, J Comput Assist Tomogr 4:78, 1980.

199. Mendez RJ, Schiebler ML, Outwater EK, et al: Hepatic abscesses: MR imaging findings, Radiology 190:431, 1994.

200. Metcalf KS, and Peel KR: Lymphocele, Ann R Coll Surg Engl 75:387, 1993.

201. Meyer JI, Kennedy AW, Friedman R, et al: Ovarian carcinoma: value of CT in predicting success of debulking surgery, Am J Roentgenol 165:875, 1995.

202. Meyers MA: Distribution of intra-abdominal malignant seeding: dependency on dynamics of flow of ascitic fluid, Am J Roentgenol Radium Ther Nucl Med 119:198, 1973.

203. Meyers MA, ed: Dynamic radiology of the abdomen, ed 4, New York, 1994, Springer-Verlag.

204. Meyers MA: Intraperitoneal spread of malignancies and its effect on the bowel, Clin Radiol 32:129, 1981.

205. Meyers MA: Metastatic seeding along the small bowel mesentery: roentgen features, Am J Roentgenol Radium Ther Nucl Med 123:67, 1975.

206. Meyers MA: The spread and localization of acute intraperitoneal effusions, Radiology 95:547, 1970.

207. Meyers MA, Oliphant M, Berne AS, et al: The peritoneal ligaments and mesenteries: pathways of intraabdominal spread of disease, Radiology 163:593, 1987.

208. Miller TT, Hermann G, Abdelwahab IF, et al: MRI of malignant fibrous histiocytoma of soft tissue: analysis of 13 cases with pathologic correlation, Skeletal Radiol 23:271, 1994.

209. Mindell HJ, Mastromatteo JF, Dickey KW, et al: Anatomic communications between the three retroperitoneal spaces: determination by CT-guided injections of contrast material in cadavers, Am J Roentgenol 164:1173, 1995.

210. Mindelzun RE, Jeffrey RB, Jr, Lane MJ, et al: The misty mesentery on CT: differential diagnosis, Am J Roentgenol 167:61, 1996.

211. Mintz MC, Levy DW, Axel L, et al: Puerperal ovarian vein thrombosis: MR diagnosis, Am J Roentgenol 149:1273, 1987.

212. Mitchell DG, Hill MC, Hill S, et al: Serous carcinoma of the ovary: CT identification of metastatic calcified implants, Radiology 158:649, 1986.

213. Mitchell DG, Vinitski S, Mohamed FB, et al: Comparison of Kaopectate with barium for negative and positive enteric contrast at MR imaging, Radiology 181:475, 1991.

214. Moertel CG, Sauer WG, Dockerty MB, et al: Life history of the carcinoid tumor of the small intestine, Cancer 14:901, 1961.

215. Moertel CG, Weiland LH, Nagorney DM, et al: Carcinoid tumor of the appendix: treatment and prognosis, N Engl J Med 317:1699, 1987.

216. Montgomery SP, Guillot AP, and Barth RA: MRI of disseminated neonatal hemangiomatosis: case report, Pediatr Radiol 20:204, 1990.

217. Moran RE, Older RA, De Angelis GA, et al: Genitourinary case of the day: peritoneal inclusion cyst in a patient with a history of prior pelvic surgery, Am J Roentgenol 167:247, 1996.

218. Mori H, McGrath FP, Malone DE, et al: The gastrocolic trunk and its tributaries: CT evaluation, Radiology 182:871, 1992.

219. Mulgaonkar S, Jacobs MG, Viscuso R, et al: Laparoscopic internal drainage of lymphocele in renal transplant, Am J Kidney Dis 19:490, 1992.

220. Mulligan SA, Holley HC, Koehler RE, et al: CT and MR imaging in the evaluation of retroperitoneal fibrosis, J Comput Assist Tomogr 13:277, 1989.

221. Mulvany NJ, Slavin JL, Ostor AG, et al: Intravenous leiomyomatosis of the uterus: a clinicopathologic study of 22 cases, Int J Gynecol Pathol 13:1, 1994.

222. Munk PL, Vellet AD, Hilborn MD, et al: Musculoskeletal infection: findings on magnetic resonance imaging, Can Assoc Radiol J 45:355, 1994.

223. Murphey MD, Gross TM, and Rosenthal HG: From the archives of the AFIP: musculoskeletal malignant fibrous histiocytoma: radiologic-pathologic correlation, Radiographics 14:807 1994.

224. Murphy MD, Fairbairn KJ, Parman LM, et al: Musculoskeletal angiomatous lesions: radiologic-pathologic correlation, Radiographics 15:893, 1995.

225. Musumeci R, and Tesoro-Tess JD: New imaging techniques in staging lymphomas, Curr Opin Oncol 6:464, 1994.

226. Nakayama Y, Kitamura S, Kawachi K, et al: Intravenous leiomyomatosis extending into the right atrium, Cardiovasc Surg 2:642, 1994.

227. Negendank WG, al-Katib AM, Karanes C, et al: Lymphomas: MR imaging contrast characteristics with clinical-pathologic correlations [see comments], Radiology 177:209, 1990.

228. Nelson BE, Rosenfield AT, and Schwartz PE: Preoperative abdominopelvic computed tomographic prediction of optimal cytoreduction in epithelial ovarian carcinoma, J Clin Oncol 11:166, 1993.

229. Nelson RC, Chezmar JL, Hoel MJ, et al: Peritoneal carcinomatosis: preoperative CT with intraperitoneal contrast material, Radiology 182:133, 1992.

230. Nguyen BD, Georges NP, Hamper UM, et al: Primary cervicovaginal endometriosis: sonographic findings with MR imaging correlation, J Ultrasound Med 13:809, 1994.

231. Nichols CR, and Fox EP: Extragonadal and pediatric germ cell tumors, Hematol Oncol Clin North Am 5:1189, 1991.

232. Obendorfer S: Ueber die kleinen Dunndarmcarcinome, Verh Dtsch Ges Pathol 11:1213, 1907.

233. O'Keefe F, Kim EE, and Wallace S: Magnetic resonance imaging in aggressive fibromatosis, Clin Radiol 42:170, 1990.

234. Oliphant M, Berne AS, and Meyers MA: Spread of disease via the subperitoneal space: the small bowel mesentery, Abdom Imaging 18:109, 1993.

235. O'Neil JD, Ros PR, Storm BL, et al: Cystic mesothelioma of the peritoneum, Radiology 170:333, 1989.

236. Outwater E, Schiebler ML, Owen RS, et al: Characterization of hemorrhagic adnexal lesions with MR imaging: blinded reader study, Radiology 186:489, 1993.

237. Padwal AJ, Trivedi PN, Talwalkar GV, et al: Role of 'cell type' in proton relaxation in normal and neoplastic lymph nodes characterized by pulsed NMR spectroscopy, Physiol Chem Phys Med NMR 20:79, 1988.

238. Pandolfo I, Blandino A, Gaeta M, et al: Calcified peritoneal metastases from papillary cystadenocarcinoma of the ovary: CT features, J Comput Assist Tomogr 10:545, 1986.

239. Panicek DM, Casper ES, Brennan MF, et al: Hemorrhage simulating tumor growth in malignant fibrous histiocytoma at MR imaging, Radiology 181:398, 1991.

240. Pantongrag-Brown L, Buetow PC, Carr NJ, et al: Calcification and fibrosis in mesenteric carcinoid tumor: CT findings and pathologic correlation, Am J Roentgenol 164:387, 1995.

241. Parums DV: The spectrum of chronic periaortitis, Histopathology 16:423, 1990.

242. Peh WC, Cheung DL, and Ngan H: Smooth muscle tumors of the inferior vena cava and right heart, Clin Imaging 17:117, 1993.

243. Pentecost MJ: Transcatheter treatment of hepatic metastases, Am J Roentgenol 160:1171, 1993.

244. Picus D, Glazer HS, Levitt RG, et al: Computed tomography of abdominal carcinoid tumors, Am J Roentgenol 143:581, 1984.

245. Posniak HV, Keshavarzian A, and Jabamoni R: Diaphragmatic endometriosis: CT and MR findings, Gastrointest Radiol 15:349, 1990.

246. Prayer L, Kainz C, Kramer J, et al: CT and MR accuracy in the detection of tumor recurrence in patients treated for ovarian cancer, J Comput Assist Tomogr 17:626, 1993.

247. Prayson RA, Hart WR, and Petras RE: Pseudomyxoma peritonei: a clinicopathologic study of 19 cases with emphasis on site of origin and nature of associated ovarian tumors, Am J Surg Pathol 18:591, 1994.

248. Prince MR, and Chew FS: Renal lymphoma, Am J Roentgenol 158:570, 1992.

249. Quinn SF, Erickson SJ, Dee PM, et al: MR imaging in fibromatosis: results in 26 patients with pathologic correlation, Am J Roentgenol 156:539, 1991.

250. Rahmouni A, Tempany C, Jones R, et al: Lymphoma: monitoring tumor size and signal intensity with MR imaging, Radiology 188:445, 1993.

251. Ramon F, Degryse H, and De Schepper A: Vascular soft tissue tumors: medical imaging, J Belge Radiol 75:303, 1992.

252. Ranade SS, Trivedi PN, and Bamane VS: Mediastinal lymph nodes: relaxation time/pathologic correlation and implications in staging of lung cancer with MR imaging, Radiology 174:284, 1990 (letter; comment).

253. Raptopoulos V, Lei QF, Touliopoulos P, et al: Why perirenal disease does not extend into the pelvis: the importance of closure of the cone of the renal fasciae, Am J Roentgenol 164:1179, 1995.

254. Raval B, and Lamki N: CT demonstration of preferential routes of the spread of pelvic disease, Crit Rev Diagn Imaging 27:17, 1987.

255. Reinig JW: MR imaging differentiation of adrenal masses: has the time finally come? Radiology 185:339, 1992 (editorial comment).

256. Reitamo JJ, Scheinin TM, and Hayry P: The desmoid syndrome: new aspects in the cause, pathogenesis and treatment of the desmoid tumor, Am J Surg 151:230, 1986.

257. Reznek RH, Mootoosamy I, Webb JA, et al: CT in renal and perirenal lymphoma: a further look [published erratum appears in Clin Radiol 43(4):289, 1991], Clin Radiol 42:233, 1990.

258. Richards MA, Mootoosamy I, Reznek RH, et al: Renal involvement in patients with non-Hodgkin's lymphoma: clinical and pathological features in 23 cases, Hematol Oncol 8:105, 1990.

259. Rodriguez-Bigas MA, Mahoney MC, Karakousis CP, et al: Desmoid tumors in patients with familial adenomatous polyposis, Cancer 74:1270, 1994.

260. Roman DA, and Mirchandani H: Intravenous leiomyoma with intracardiac extension causing sudden death, Arch Pathol Lab Med 111:1176, 1987.

261. Romano CC, Munk PL, Vellet AD, et al: Magnetic resonance imaging of a giant nonfunctioning retroperitoneal paraganglioma, Can Assoc Radiol J 44:466, 1993.

262. Romero JA, Kim EE, Kim CG, et al: Different biological features of desmoid tumors in adult and juvenile patients: MR demonstration, J Comput Assist Tomogr 19:782, 1995.

263. Rominger MB, and Kenney PJ: Perirenal involvement by retroperitoneal fibrosis: the usefulness of MRI to establish diagnosis, Urol Radiol 13:173, 1992.

264. Ronnett BM, Kurman RJ, Zahn CM, et al: Pseudomyxoma peritonei in women: a clinicopathologic analysis of 30 cases with emphasis on site of origin, prognosis, and relationship to ovarian mucinous tumors of low malignant potential, Hum Pathol 26:509, 1995.

265. Ronnett BM, Shmookler BM, Diener-West M, et al: Immunohistochemical evidence supporting the appendiceal origin of pseudomyxoma peritonei in women, Int J Gynecol Pathol 16:1, 1997.

266. Ros PR, Olmsted WW, Moser RP Jr, et al: Mesenteric and omental cysts: histologic classification with imaging correlation, Radiology 164:327, 1987.

267. Rossi CR, Nitti D, Foletto M, et al: Management of primary sarcomas of the retroperitoneum, Eur J Surg Oncol 19:355, 1993.

268. Rotter AJ, and Lundell CJ: MR of intravenous leiomyomatosis of the uterus extending into the inferior vena cava, J Comput Assist Tomogr 15:690, 1991.

269. Rubenstein WA, and Whalen JP: Extraperitoneal spaces, Am J Roentgenol 147:1162, 1986.

270. Saida Y, Tsunoda HS, Itai Y, et al: Peritoneal implants without ascites: preoperative CT diagnosis in colon carcinoma patients, Radiat Med 12:221, 1994.

271. Salimi Z, Fishbein M, Wolverson MK, et al: Pancreatic lymphangioma: CT, MRI, and angiographic features, Gastrointest Radiol 16:248, 1991.

272. Savader SJ, Otero RR, and Savader BL: Puerperal ovarian vein thrombosis: evaluation with CT, US, and MR imaging, Radiology 167:637, 1988.

273. Scatarige JC, Fishman EK, Kuhajda FP, et al: Low attenuation nodal metastases in testicular carcinoma, J Comput Assist Tomogr 7:682, 1983.

274. Schutter EM: [Psoas abscess in pregnancy: a case report], Geburtshilfe Frauenheilkd 51:489, 1991.

275. Schwartz PE, Chambers JT, and Makuch R: Neoadjuvant chemotherapy for advanced ovarian cancer, Gynecol Oncol 53:33, 1994.

276. Scotte M, Majerus B, Laquerriere A, et al: [Cystic lymphangiomas of the pancreas: three new cases], Ann Chir 46:359, 1992.

277. Seelos KC, Funari M, Chang JM, et al: Magnetic resonance imaging in acute and subacute mediastinal bleeding, Am Heart J 123:1269, 1992.

278. Seidman JD, Elsayed AM, Sobin LH, et al: Association of mucinous tumors of the ovary and appendix: a clinicopathologic study of 25 cases [see comments], Am J Surg Pathol 17:22, 1993.

279. Seifer DB, Kennedy AW, Webster KD, et al: Outcome of primary cytoreduction surgery for advanced epithelial ovarian carcinoma, Cleve Clin J Med 55:555, 1988.

280. Semelka RC, Lawrence PH, Shoenut JP, et al: Primary ovarian cancer: prospective comparison of contrast-enhanced CT and pre- and postcontrast, fat-suppressed MR imaging, with histologic correlation, J Magn Reson Imaging 3:99, 1993.

281. Setchell BP: The functional significance of the blood-testis barrier, J Androl 1:3, 1980.

282. Shatzkes D, Gordon DH, Haller JO, et al: Malrotation of the bowel: malalignment of the superior mesenteric artery-vein complex shown by CT and MR, J Comput Assist Tomogr 14:93, 1990.

283. Shelton MW, Morian JP, and Radford DM: Pseudomyxoma retroperitonei associated with appendiceal cystadenoma, Am Surg 60:958, 1994.

284. Shmookler BM, and Lauer DH: Retroperitoneal leiomyosarcoma: a clinicopathologic analysis of 36 cases, Am J Surg Pathol 7:269, 1983.

285. Siegelman ES, Outwater E, Wang T, et al: Solid pelvic masses caused by endometriosis: MR imaging features, Am J Roentgenol 163:357, 1994.

286. Silverman PM, Osborne M, Dunnick NR, et al: CT prior to second-look operation in ovarian cancer, Am J Roentgenol 150:829, 1988.

287. Simons GR, Piwnica-Worms DR, and Goldhaber SZ: Ovarian vein thrombosis, Am Heart J 126:641, 1993.

288. Sindelar WF, Kinsella TJ, Chen PW, et al: Intraoperative radiotherapy in retroperitoneal sarcomas: final results of a prospective, randomized, clinical trial, Arch Surg 128:402, 1993.

289. Singer S, Corson JM, Demetri GD, et al: Prognostic factors predictive of survival for truncal and retroperitoneal soft-tissue sarcoma, Ann Surg 221:185, 1995.

290. Smith RC: Magnetic resonance imaging of the female pelvis: technical considerations, Top Magn Reson Imaging 7:3, 1995.

291. Smith RC, Reinhold C, McCauley TR, et al: Multicoil high-resolution fast spin-echo MR imaging of the female pelvis, Radiology 184:671, 1992 (comment).

292. Soderlund V, Goranson H, and Bauer HC: MR imaging of benign peripheral nerve sheath tumors, Acta Radiol 35:282, 1994.

293. Spillane RM, and Whitman GJ: Treatment of retroperitoneal fibrosis with tamoxifen, Am J Roentgenol 164:515, 1995 (letter).

294. Stancanelli B, Seminara G, Vita A, et al: Extension of a pelvic tumor into the right atrium, N Engl J Med 333:1013, 1995.

295. Steiner MS, Goldman SM, Smith DP, et al: Extragonadal germ cell tumor originating in iliac fossa, Urology 41:575, 1993.

296. Stephenson CA, Seibert JJ, Golladay ES, et al: Abscess of the iliopsoas muscle diagnosed by magnetic resonance imaging and ultrasonography, South Med J 84:509, 1991.

297. Storm FK, and Mahvi DM: Diagnosis and management of retroperitoneal soft-tissue sarcoma, Ann Surg 214:2, 1991.

298. Storm FK, Sondak VK, and Economou JS: Sarcomas of the retroperitoneum. In Eilber FR, Morton DL, Sondak VK, et al, eds: The soft tissue sarcomas, New York, 1987, Grune & Stratton.

299. Stoupis C, Ros PR, Abbitt PL, et al: Bubbles in the belly: imaging of cystic mesenteric or omental masses, Radiographics 14:729, 1994.

300. Stoupis S, Ros PR, Williams JL, et al: Hemorrhagic lymphangioma mimicking hemoperitoneum: MR imaging diagnosis, J Magn Reson Imaging 3:541, 1993.

301. Sugarbaker PH: Surgical treatment of peritoneal carcinomatosis: 1988 Du Pont lecture, Can J Surg 32:164, 1989.

302. Sugarbaker PH, Kern K, and Lack E: Malignant pseudomyxoma peritonei of colonic origin: natural history and presentation of a curative approach to treatment, Dis Colon Rectum 30:772, 1987.

303. Sugarbaker PH, Zhu BW, Sese GB, et al: Peritoneal carcinomatosis from appendiceal cancer: results in 69 patients treated by cytoreductive surgery and intraperitoneal chemotherapy, Dis Colon Rectum 36:323, 1993.

304. Sugimura K, Okizuka H, Imaoka I, et al: Pelvic endometriosis: detection and diagnosis with chemical shift MR imaging, Radiology 188:435, 1993.

305. Suh JS, Abenoza P, Galloway HR, et al: Peripheral (extracranial) nerve tumors: correlation of MR imaging and histologic findings, Radiology 183:341, 1992.

306. Sundaram M, McGuire MH, and Schajowicz F: Soft-tissue masses: histologic basis for decreased signal (short T2) on T2-weighted MR images, Am J Roentgenol 148:1247, 1987.

307. Takahashi K, Okada S, Ozaki T, et al: Diagnosis of pelvic endometriosis by magnetic resonance imaging using "fat-saturation" technique, Fertil Steril 62:973, 1994.

308. Takahashi N, Murakami J, Murayama S, et al: MR evaluation of intrapulmonary hematoma, J Comput Assist Tomogr 19:125, 1995.

309. Takeda H, Matsunaga N, Fukuda T, et al: [X-ray computed tomography and magnetic resonance imaging of the retroperitoneal space and the pelvic extraperitoneal space], Rinsho Hoshasen 34:1277, 1989.

310. Takeda M, Katayama Y, Takahashi H, et al: [MRI of pheochromocytoma—comparison with CT, ^{131}I-MIBG, urinary catecholamine level and operative findings], Nippon Hinyokika Gakkai Zasshi 83:33, 1992.

311. Tart RP, Li KC, Storm BL, et al: Enteric MRI contrast agents: comparative study of five potential agents in humans, Magn Reson Imaging 9:559, 1991.

312. Terk MR, de Verdier H, and Colletti PM: Giant extra-adrenal pheochromocytoma: magnetic resonance imaging with gadolinium-DTPA enhancement, Magn Reson Imaging 11:47, 1993.

313. Therasse E, Breittmayer F, Roche A, et al: Transcatheter chemoembolization of progressive carcinoid liver metastasis, Radiology 189:541, 1993.

314. Togashi K, Nishimura K, Kimura I, et al: Endometrial cysts: diagnosis with MR imaging, Radiology 180:73, 1991.

315. Torres GM, Erquiaga E, Ros PR, et al: Preliminary results of MR imaging with superparamagnetic iron oxide in pancreatic and retroperitoneal disorders, Radiographics 11:785, 1991.

316. Tung GA, and Davis LM: The role of magnetic resonance imaging in the evaluation of the soft tissue mass, Crit Rev Diagn Imaging 34:239, 1993.

317. van Bommel EF, van Spengler J, van der Hoven B, et al: Retroperitoneal fibrosis: report of 12 cases and a review of the literature, Neth J Med 39:338, 1991.

318. van der Burg ME, van Lent M, Buyse M, et al: The effect of debulking surgery after induction chemotherapy on the prognosis in advanced epithelial ovarian cancer. Gynecological Cancer Cooperative Group of the European Organization for Research and Treatment of Cancer [see comments], N Engl J Med 332:629, 1995

319. van Gils AP, Falke TH, van Erkel AR, et al: MR imaging and MIBG scintigraphy of pheochromocytomas and extraadrenal functioning paragangliomas, Radiographics 11:37, 1991.

320. Varma DG, Moulopoulos A, Sara AS, et al: MR imaging of extracranial nerve sheath tumors, J Comput Assist Tomogr 16:448, 1992.

321. Vassallo P, Matei C, Heston WD, et al: AMI-227-enhanced MR lymphography: usefulness for differentiating reactive from tumor-bearing lymph nodes, Radiology 193:501, 1994.

322. Verstraete KL, Achten E, De Schepper A, et al: Nerve sheath tumors: evaluation with CT and MR imaging, J Belge Radiol 75:311, 1992.

323. Watanabe H, Morioka M, Kohama Y, et al: [Magnetic resonance imaging for retroperitoneal fibrosis: report of two cases], Nippon Hinyokika Gakkai Zasshi 81:626, 1990.

324. Weigert F, Lindner P, and Rohde U: Computed tomography and magnetic resonance of pseudomyxoma peritonei, J Comput Assist Tomogr 9:1120, 1985.

325. Weill F, Watrin J, Rohmer P, et al: Ultrasound and CT of peritoneal recesses and ligaments: a pictorial essay, Ultrasound Med Biol 12:977, 1986.

326. Wertheim I, Fleischhacker D, McLachlin CM, et al: Pseudomyxoma peritonei: a review of 23 cases, Obstet Gynecol 84:17, 1994.

327. Whalen RK, Althausen AF, and Daniels GH: Extra-adrenal pheochromocytoma, J Urol 147:1, 1992.

328. Wiedenmann B, Rath U, Radsch R, et al: Tumor regression of an ileal carcinoid under the treatment with the somatostatin analogue SMS 201-995, Klin Wochenschr 66:75, 1988.

329. Wiener JI, Chako AC, Merten CW, et al: Breast and axillary tissue MR imaging: correlation of signal intensities and relaxation times with pathologic findings, Radiology 160:299, 1986.

330. Witlin AG, and Sibai BM: Postpartum ovarian vein thrombosis after vaginal delivery: a report of 11 cases, Obstet Gynecol 85:775, 1995.

331. Wittich GR: Radiologic treatment of abdominal abscesses with fistulous communications, Curr Opin Radiol 4:110, 1992.

332. Wolf GC, and Kopecky KK: MR imaging of endometriosis arising in cesarean section scar, J Comput Assist Tomogr 13:150, 1989.

333. Wood WC, and Tepper J: Retroperitoneal and abdominal wall sarcomas. In Raaf JH, ed: Soft tissue sarcomas, St Louis, 1993, Mosby.

334. Woodard PK, Feldman JM, Paine SS, et al: Midgut carcinoid tumors: CT findings and biochemical profiles, J Comput Assist Tomogr 19:400, 1995.

335. Yaegashi N, and Yajima A: Multilocular peritoneal inclusion cysts (benign cystic mesothelioma): a case report, J Obstet Gynaecol Res 22:129, 1996.

336. Yamashita N, Toyoda N, and Sugaya K: [A case of huge abdominal unilocular peritoneal inclusion cyst], Nippon Sanka Fujinka Gakkai Zasshi 45:1433, 1993.

337. Yamashita Y, Torashima M, Harada M, et al: Postpartum extraperitoneal pelvic hematoma: imaging findings, Am J Roentgenol 161:805, 1993.

338. Yancey JM, and Kaude JV: Diagnosis of perirenal fibrosis by MR imaging, J Comput Assist Tomogr 12:335, 1988.

339. Yu CY, Perez-Reyes M, Brown JJ, et al: MR appearance of umbilical endometriosis, J Comput Assist Tomogr 18:269, 1994.

340. Yuh WT, Barloon TJ, Sickels WJ, et al: Magnetic resonance imaging in the diagnosis and followup of idiopathic retroperitoneal fibrosis, J Urol 141:602, 1989.

341. Zawin M, McCarthy S, Scoutt L, et al: Endometriosis: appearance and detection at MR imaging, Radiology 171:693, 1989.

342. Zerin JM, and DiPietro MA: Mesenteric vascular anatomy at CT: normal and abnormal appearances, Radiology 179:739, 1991.

343. Zerin JM, and DiPietro MA: Superior mesenteric vascular anatomy at US in patients with surgically proved malrotation of the midgut, Radiology 183:693, 1992.

344. Zhang J, Rath AM, Boyer JC, et al: Radioanatomic study of the gastrocolic venous trunk, Surg Radiol Anat 16:413, 1994.

27 Urinary Bladder

Evan S. Siegelman and Mitchell D. Schnall

 KEY POINTS

- Multiplanar capabilities give MRI an advantage over CT for staging tumors.
- Effective bowel-marking contrast agents make CT the more reliable imaging method.

BLADDER CANCER
Epidemiology and Rationale for Imaging

There were 50,000 cases of bladder cancer in the United States in 1995 that accounted for more than 11,000 deaths.[126] Bladder carcinoma is the fourth most common cancer in men (prostate, lung, and colon are the top three) and accounts for 5% and 3% of all cancer deaths in men and women, respectively.[20,126]

Two systems have been used to stage bladder cancer: the tumor-node-metastasis (TNM[47]) and the Jewett-Strong-Marshall[54,71] classifications (Table 27-1 and Figure 27-1). Both prognosis and treatment depend on the stage of the tumor. The clinical staging of bladder carcinoma includes cystoscopy and biopsy with supplementary examination under anesthesia, intravenous urography, or both types of examination.[98] Studies performed before the era of cross-sectional imaging report clinical staging accuracies of less than 50%.[57,71,93,96,98] More recent studies show that stage T2 and T3 tumors, especially those with higher grade, are understaged in up to a third of cases.[48,125] Superficial

lesions are less often overstaged. A potential cause of overstaging is misinterpretation of the smooth muscle fibers in the lamina propria as true detrusor muscle on a biopsy specimen.[1]

It is important to accurately stage bladder cancer because treatment is based in part on the depth of invasion of the tumor into the bladder wall. Superficial bladder cancer (TNM stage T1) is treated and often cured by transurethral resection alone.[20,77] The role of any imaging technique for suspected superficial bladder tumors in such patients is to ensure that there is no invasion by tumor into the underlying detrusor muscle. Treatment for invasive carcinoma (TNM stage T2) is often cystectomy, preoperative radiation therapy, or the use of both. The role of imaging of invasive lesions is to confirm persistent tumor deep to the submucosa (some minimally invasive tumors are totally removed at initial cystoscopic resection) and to accurately determine tumor extent. Some invasive tumors can be treated with partial cystectomy. If an imaging modality could accurately detect sufficient normal detrusor muscle deep to a lesion, some surgeons would attempt a curative endoscopic resection.[55]

Technique Optimization

Although routine body-coil imaging may be adequate to confirm gross extravesicular tumor, it is insensitive for detecting small tumors and subtle muscle invasion. Initial magnetic resonance (MR) studies using standard, nonenhanced, body-coil imaging failed to show tumors measuring less than 1.5 cm[18,33] and were unable to document muscle invasion in the absence of extravesicular tumor.[4,16] The use of phased-array external surface coils and endoluminal surface coils allows the acquisition of images with higher signal-to-noise ratios obtained with smaller fields of view, with resultant higher spatial resolution.[67,73,88,97,103] Both techniques have been successfully applied to the imaging of bladder carcinoma.[11,74,105] Some form of phased-array coil should be used, if available, when bladder cancer is staged. Endorectal coil imaging should be considered if the tumor is known to be located in the posterior bladder wall, bladder base, or bladder neck.[105,108]

Most investigators have used the three standard orthogonal planes to image bladder cancer. Ideally, one would want to image in a plane that is perpendicular to the tumor–bladder wall interface to avoid volume averaging and potential overstaging.[77] We recommend the routine intramuscular injection of 1 mg of glucagon to decrease the noise from bowel peristalsis and allow the accurate diagnosis of bowel invasion, especially for tumors of the posterior wall or bladder dome[77] (see Figure 26-8). The bladder should be emptied 1 to 3 hours before scanning to avoid significant underdistension or overdistension that could alter diagnostic accuracy.[12,13,114]

Bladder Carcinoma

On T2-weighted images, transitional cell carcinoma tends to have an intermediate signal intensity that is greater than normal detrusor muscle. Thus preservation of the low-signal bladder wall subjacent to the epicenter of the tumor on T2-weighted images would suggest that the tumor is stage T1 or less. On precontrast T1-weighted images, the bladder wall and tumor have similar low to intermediate signal intensity that is greater than urine and lower than perivesicular fat. Gross soft tissue extension into the perivesicular fat should accurately predict stage T3b disease[6,13,43] (Figures 27-2 and 27-3). The recently developed techniques of "MR urography"* can be used to detect and characterize

Modified in part from Siegelman ES, and Schnall MD: Contrast-enhanced MR imaging of the bladder and prostate, Magn Reson Imaging Clin North Am 4:153, 1996.

*References 2, 30, 50, 64, 85, 92, 112.

a distal ureteral obstruction from involvement by aggressive extramural bladder cancers (Figure 27-2, *A*).

Gadolinium enhancement can improve the accuracy of the staging of bladder cancer.[102] Dynamic, enhanced studies can confirm the lack of invasion into the detrusor muscle in suspect superficial lesions (Figure 27-4), determine the depth of tumor penetration into the detrusor muscle (Figure 27-5), characterize a soft tissue abnormality of the perivesicular fat as tumor or nonneoplastic tissue (Figure 27-6), and establish invasion into adjacent organs (Figure 27-7).

In 1989, Neuerburg et al[79] imaged 48 bladder tumors with gadolinium and found that tumor enhanced immediately and intensely compared with the uninvolved bladder wall, resulting in optimal contrast on T1-weighted images of the tumor and bladder wall. Other studies confirmed that imaging should be performed in the first 90 seconds after contrast injection to optimize tumor–bladder wall contrast.* However, even when other investigators used nondynamic postcontrast im-

ages, there was still improvement in the detection of smaller tumors[81,106] and a modest increase in staging accuracy.[32,106]

Subsequent reports used body-coil imaging and dynamic spin-echo (repetition time = 100, single-slice acquisition in 15 sec)[111,113] or gradient-echo enhanced[78,104] imaging for bladder tumor staging. The latter studies showed significant improvement in staging accuracy (85%) compared with contrast-enhanced computed tomography (CT) (55%) and conventional magnetic resonance imaging (MRI) (58%).[113] The tumors of patients enrolled in these studies were imaged before the

---

*References 7, 10, 12, 13, 79, 111, 119.

Table 27-1	Bladder Cancer Staging: TNM and Jewett-Strong-Marshall Systems	
JEWITT-STRONG-MARSHALL	**TNM**	**PATHOLOGY**
O	T0	No tumor
O	Tis	Carcinoma in situ
O	Ta	Superficial papillary tumor
A	T1	Submucosa invasion
B1	T2	Superficial muscle invasion
B2	T3a	Deep muscle invasion
C	T3b	Perivascular fat invasion
D1	T4	Adjacent organ invasion
D1	N1-N3	Positive pelvic nodes
D2	N4	Positive nodes above aortic bifurcation
D2	M1	Distant metastases

Modified from references 47, 54, and 71.

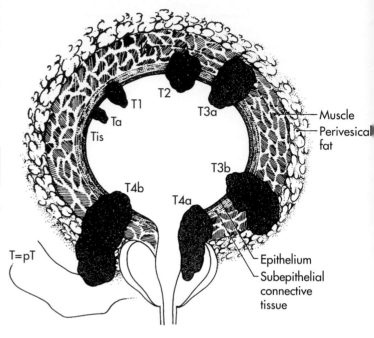

FIGURE 27-1 Pictorial demonstration of the TNM staging system of bladder carcinoma. (From reference 12.)

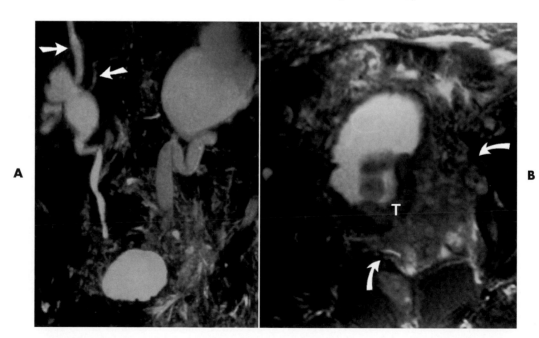

FIGURE 27-2 MR urogram shows asymmetrical bilateral hydronephrosis and hydroureter. **A,** Coronal fast spin-echo 12,000/256 repetition time/echo time image obtained with fat saturation shows a mildly dilated common bile duct and a normal pancreatic duct detected in the same imaging volume *(arrows).* **B,** Transverse fat-saturated fast spin-echo 4000/136 image confirms the presence of a primary bladder tumor of the left ureterovesical junction *(T)* and marked extravesicular spread of tumor into the left hemipelvis *(arrows).*

initial biopsy or resection. Although it was once believed to be "impossible"[12] to differentiate between tumor and recent postbiopsy changes of the bladder wall, recent studies have shown that dynamic postgadolinium imaging shows promise in this distinction. Tumor will enhance before nonneoplastic edema, and granulation tissue[7,10,105] (Figures 27-2 and 27-3) and bland blood clots should not enhance.[45] Still, when contrast-enhanced MRI is performed, false-positive diagnoses can still occur in cases of active inflammation, sterile radiation change, or cystitis (Figure 27-8), although less frequently when compared with CT and unenhanced MR pulse sequences.[45,56,58,105] Fast gradient-echo sequences acquired at least once every 2 sec can distinguish bladder cancer from postbiopsy changes with greater accuracy than routine dynamic scanning. On average, viable bladder cancer enhanced 6.5 sec after contrast enhancement and postbiopsy inflammation and granulation tissue enhanced 13.6 sec after contrast.[9] Thus use of such a "fast dynamic" technique can decrease the number of false-positive MR scans.

Bladder Diverticula

Because of urinary stasis and chronic inflammation, there is a 3% to 7% incidence of carcinoma that develops within bladder diverticula.[31,96]

A narrow diverticular neck or unusual location can preclude adequate visualization at cystoscopy. By definition the detrusor muscle is absent in diverticula, and therefore tumors often have invaded the perivesical fat at the time of diagnosis (Figure 27-9).

Adenopathy

Patients with lymph nodes positive for transitional cell carcinoma have a worse prognosis, and the majority do not benefit from cystectomy.[98] CT and MRI have equivalent accuracies of approximately 90% when either the short- or the long-axis dimensions of the nodes are used as criteria for malignancy.[12] Two studies have shown that unenhanced, three-dimensional, magnetization prepared–rapid acquisition gradient-echo (MP-RAGE) images improved the staging accuracy of bladder carcinoma, in part because of improved detection of suspicious lymph nodes.[8,52] There is significant overlap of both T1 and T2 values of reactive and neoplastic lymph nodes. Lymphotropic contrast agents have been developed that may distinguish between benign and malignant adenopathy. One family of agents, ultrasmall superparamagnetic iron oxide (USPIO) particles, has been shown to accumulate in benign nodes but not in malignant nodes.[123] This class of contrast agents has the potential to improve the staging of bladder cancer.

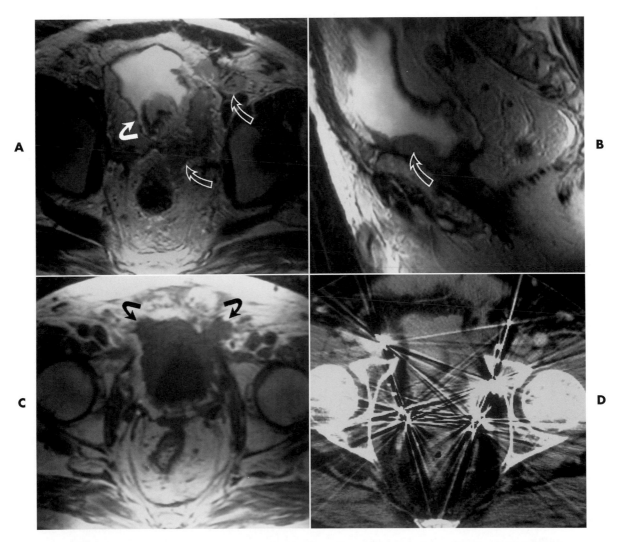

FIGURE 27-3   Recurrent transitional cell carcinoma after continent Indiana pouch reconstruction. Axial **(A)** and sagittal **(B)** fast spin-echo 5000/102 images show a portion of distal ilial segment used for bladder reconstruction *(solid curved arrow)*. Gross recurrent tumor is present in the reconstructed bladder base, sigmoid mesentery, and left external iliac nodes *(open curved arrows)*. Axial T1-weighted spin-echo image **(C)** through the bladder base shows tumor involvement of perivesicular fat *(curved black arrows)* to better advantage than a corresponding contrast-enhanced computed tomographic scan **(D)**, which is degraded by beam-hardening artifacts from multiple metallic clips that did not affect the MR scan.

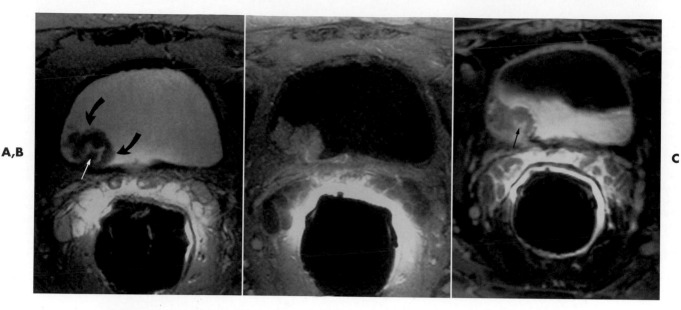

FIGURE 27-4 Superficial papillary transitional cell carcinoma. **A,** Axial endorectal surface-coil fast spin-echo 5000/144 image shows a polypoid mass of the right posterior bladder wall *(black arrows).* A central fibrous core is seen *(thin white arrow).* The soft tissue that is anterolateral to the mass represents another polypoid lesion (seen better on adjacent sections). **B,** Dynamic gadolinium diethylene-triamine-pentaacetic acid-enhanced T1-weighted gradient-echo 68/4.3/60 image shows enhancement of the peripheral portion of the lesion. The fibrous core and underlying detrusor muscle do not enhance. Superficial papillary cancer was removed at cystoscopy hours after imaging. **C,** Delayed T1-weighed, fat-suppressed, gradient-echo 200/2.9/90 image, shows delayed enhancement of the fibrous core (thin black arrow) and subjacent detrusor muscle. Delayed detrusor enhancement is nonspecific and cannot be used to diagnose infiltration by cancer.

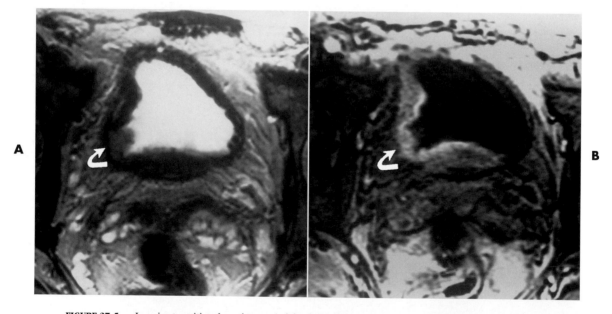

FIGURE 27-5 Invasive transitional carcinoma. Axial pelvic surface-coil, fast spin-echo 4000/144 image **(A)** and dynamic, contrast-enhanced, spoiled gradient-recalled echo 100/3.1/80 image **(B)** show a focal mass of the right ureterovesical junction *(curved white arrow)* that demonstrates full-thickness detrusor invasion. Stage T3a cancer was confirmed at subsequent cystectomy.

Other Neoplasms

Urachal Carcinoma

The majority of urachal carcinomas are mucin-producing adenocarcinomas of the juxtavesical segment of the urachus.[91] The unenhanced MR findings of urachal carcinoma have been described.[60,68,91] Diagnosis is often facilitated by the characteristic location of the mass, which is optimally delineated by imaging in the sagittal and coronal planes. MR detection of solid components or nodular areas of en-

hancement suggests malignant degeneration of a urachal cyst (Figure 27-10).

Nonepithelial Neoplasms

Smooth muscle neoplasms. Leiomyoma is the most common mesenchymal tumor of the bladder and represents less than 1% of all bladder tumors.[44] Like uterine fibroids, most lesions occur in young to middle-aged women. Several MR reports of this unusual tumor have

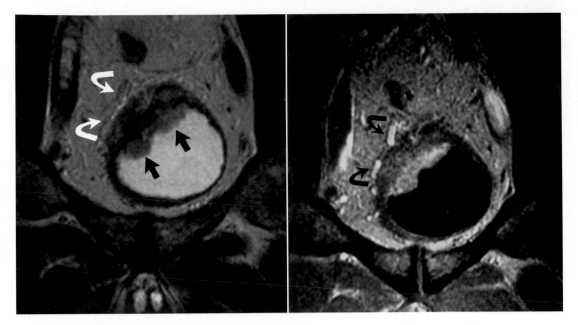

A **B**

FIGURE 27-6 Contrast-enhanced MR image excludes perivesicular (T3b) tumor. **A,** Coronal fast spin-echo 5000/136 image shows a focal mass of the right bladder dome *(black arrows)*. The irregularity of the perivesicular fat *(curved arrows)* suggests stage T3b disease. **B,** Corresponding dynamic, contrast-enhanced GRE 100/4.2/80 image confirms muscle-invasive disease but also shows that the perivesicular abnormalities represent vessels *(curved arrows)*. No perivesicular tumor was detected at cystectomy.

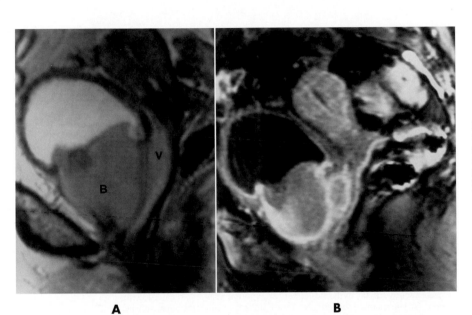

A **B**

FIGURE 27-7 Vaginal invasion by transitional cell carcinoma. **A,** Sagittal fast spin-echo 4000/102 image shows a bladder neck mass *(B)* with probable invasion into the anterior vagina *(V)*. **B,** Dynamic, enhanced, sagittal gradient-echo 140/2.9/80 image shows rim-enhancing tumor of both the bladder neck and the anterior vagina. Vaginal involvement by tumor confirmed surgically.

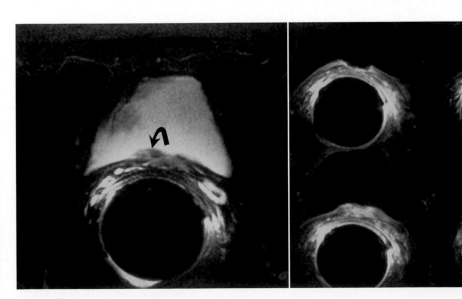

A **B**

FIGURE 27-8 Postbiopsy changes mimicking residual tumor. Biopsy-proven, muscle-invasive transitional cell carcinoma shown 4 weeks before MRI. Axial fat-suppressed fast spin-echo 3000/140 image **(A)** and four consecutive dynamic contrast-enhanced gradient-recalled echo 68/2.9/60 images **(B)** show a high-signal intensity T2 process that involves the trigone *(curved black arrow)*. The enhanced study demonstrates the prior surgical defect *(curved white arrow)* and subjacent enhancement that suggests persistent muscle-invasive tumor. Moderate dysplasia without residual carcinoma was found at subsequent surgery.

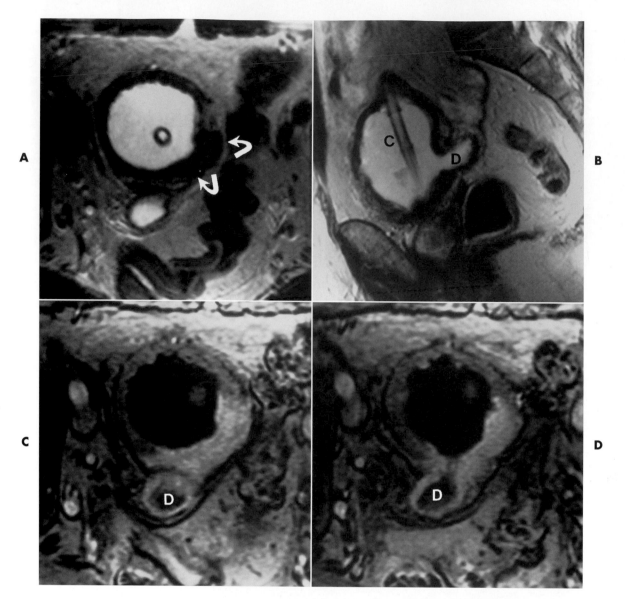

FIGURE 27-9   Transitional cell carcinoma involving a bladder diverticulum. Axial **(A)** and sagittal **(B)** fast spin-echo 5000/108 images of a Foley catheter **(C)**, posterior diverticulum **(D)**, and focal mass of the left lateral bladder wall *(curved white arrows)*. Two consecutive axial dynamic, enhanced, spoiled gradient-recalled echo 120/2.9/60 images **(C** and **D)** show deep muscle invasion of the left lateral wall. Enhancement of the adjacent wall of the diverticulum *(D)* suggests that it is also involved.

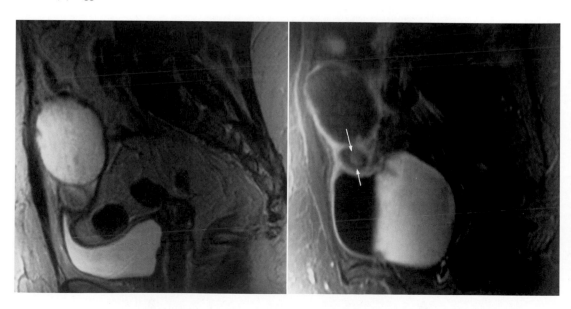

FIGURE 27-10   Urachal carcinoma. Sagittal pelvic surface-coil, fast spin-echo 4000/126 image *(left)* and fat-suppressed, contrast-enhanced, T1-weighted spin-echo 600/11 image *(right)* show a septate cystic mass that originates from the anterosuperior aspect of the bladder. Solid enhancing tissue toward the base of the lesion is suspicious for neoplasm *(thin white arrows)*. Adenocarcinoma of urachal origin was confirmed at subsequent surgery.

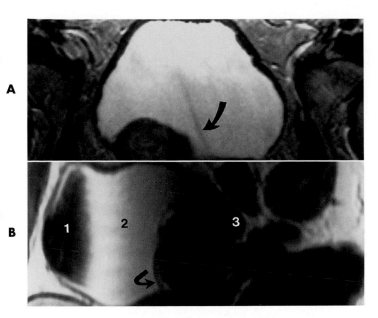

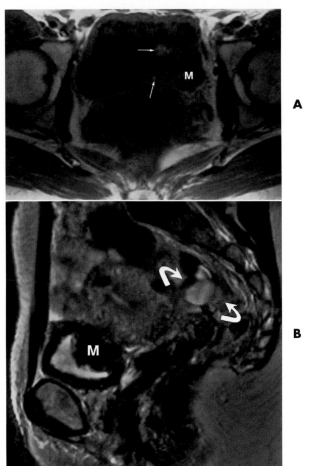

FIGURE 27-11   Well-differentiated leiomyosarcoma originating from the bladder wall. **A,** Axial fast spin-echo 4000/144 image demonstrates a heterogeneous, sharply circumscribed mass of the right ureterovesical junction whose epicenter is located in the detrusor muscle. Note the normal turbulence "jet" from the left ureteral orifice *(curved arrow)*. **B,** Sagittal enhanced, T1-weighted spin-echo 400/17 image shows homogeneous enhancement of the peripheral portion of the tumor and central nonenhancement. The bladder mucosa *(curved arrow)* is uplifted and separate from the tumor, suggesting a submucosal origin of the mass. Three layers of urine are seen. The anterior layer *(1)* represents urine without contrast, with typical long T1 values. The high-signal intensity T1-weighted middle layer *(2)* has low concentrations of paramagnetic contrast, where the effects of the T1 process are dominant. The posterior dependent layer *(3)* contains concentrated paramagnetic contrast, where the effects of the T2 process caused by the concentrated paramagnetic contrast obliterate all signal despite effects of the T1 process.

FIGURE 27-12   Endometriosis of the bladder. Axial, pelvic surface-coil, T1-weighted spin-echo 450/16 image **(A)** and sagittal fast spin-echo 4600/119 image **(B)** show an irregular mass of the left posterior bladder wall *(M)*. The low–signal intensity T2-weighted components suggest fibrosis. Punctate areas of high signal (which did not lose signal on fat-suppressed images) represent hemorrhage *(thin white arrows)*. Endometriosis is also present in the cul-de-sac *(curved white arrows)*. The bladder mass enhanced with contrast (not shown). Solid, enhancing peritoneal masses of endometriosis have been reported and should not be confused with malignancy.

been published.* The MR appearance is similar to that of uterine leiomyoma: a well-circumscribed mass with low– to intermediate–signal intensity T2-weighted areas, which correspond to nondegenerated tumor, and foci of high–signal intensity T2-weighted areas, which correspond to cystic degeneration. Irregular margins,[89] a size larger than 5 cm, or large areas of central necrosis should suggest the even rarer leiomyosarcoma, which typically occurs in middle-aged or elderly men[109] (Figure 27-11).

Pheochromocytoma

Between 10% and 20% of pheochromocytomas occur in an extraadrenal location, and approximately 1% of these ectopic tumors occur in the bladder.[110,115,122] Like pheochromocytomas located elsewhere in the body (see Figure 26-18), bladder pheochromocytomas tend to have heterogeneous high signal intensity on T2-weighted images and enhance intensely after contrast.[17,26,118,122] Metaiodobenzylguanidine (MIBG) scintigraphy has limited diagnostic accuracy in the diagnosis because of normal accumulation of urinary bladder tracer.[118] Preoperative tissue characterization is important to initiate pharmacological adrenergic blockade; massive catecholamine release can occur during anesthesia induction before surgical removal.[124]

NONNEOPLASTIC DISEASES OF THE BLADDER
Endometriosis

Between 1% and 2% of women with pelvic endometriosis have involvement of the urinary tract, and the bladder is most often affected[84,100] (Figure 27-12). Patients can have urinary urgency, frequency, or pain, any of which can be cyclical.† Hematuria is unusual

---

*References 21, 33, 69, 72, 82, 114, 128.
†References 5, 65, 76, 80, 94, 95.

because lesions usually are intramural and do not involve the urothelium.[120] Most cases are associated with extensive pelvic endometriosis, but examples of direct implantation after bladder injury associated with cesarean section or hysterectomy have been reported.[84,120,129] Treatment consists of hormonal therapy combined with laparoscopic or transurethral resection.[34,40,95] Rare cases of malignant transformation into endometrioid carcinoma have been reported.[3,22]

The typical appearance of adnexal endometriomas, consisting of multiple high–signal intensity T1-weighted and low–signal intensity T2-weighted lesions, has been well described.[87,116] We have seen examples of solid masses of bladder-wall endometriosis that are primarily of low signal intensity on both T1- and T2-weighted images. Punctate foci of high signal intensity may be present on the T1-weighted images that represent hemorrhage. The extramucosal location of these lesions, along with the MR findings of typical adnexal endometriosis, should suggest the etiology of a bladder-wall tumor in a young woman.

Ureterocele

A ureterocele is a dilated, cystic terminal segment of the intravesical ureter[24] (Figure 27-13). Ureteroceles are classified as either ectopic (some portion located in the bladder neck or urethra, 75%) or orthotopic (simple, entirely located in an intravesical location, 25%).[24,39] Ectopic ureteroceles are congenital and develop because of deficient surrounding musculature ("poor detrusor backing").[36,107] The majority of

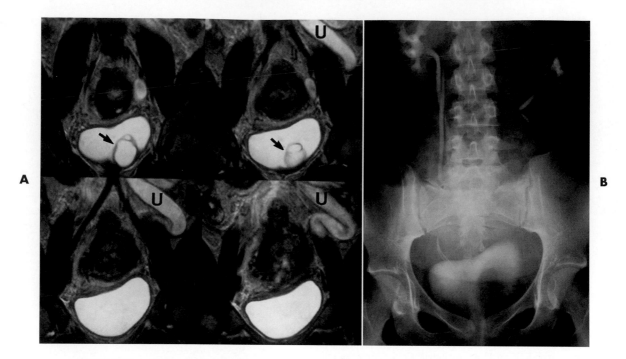

FIGURE 27-13   Bladder mass secondary to an ectopic ureterocele. **A,** Four consecutive coronal, pelvic surface-coil fast spin-echo 4500/119 images show a septate cystic lesion in the region of the left ureterovesical junction and bladder neck *(black arrow)*. Note the dilated, fluid-filled mid-left ureter *(U)*. **B,** Subsequent intravenous urogram confirms a nonfunctional left upper pole and a filling defect of the left bladder base, all diagnostic of a duplex collecting system with an obstructed upper pole. MRI best demonstrates the dilated dysfunctional left upper pole, whereas the intravenous urogram better shows the nondilated duplicated left lower pole and the duplicated right collecting system.

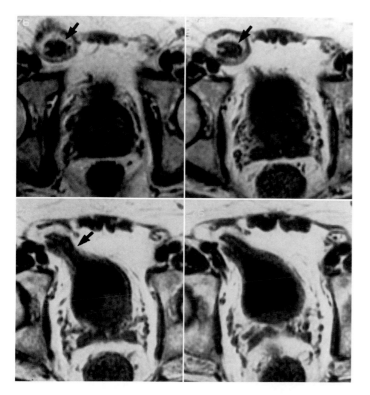

FIGURE 27-14   Bladder hernia in a 63-year-old man being evaluated for prostate cancer. Four consecutive axial spin-echo 600/20 images filmed from inferior to superior show herniation of the right inferior bladder into the right inguinal canal *(black arrow)*.

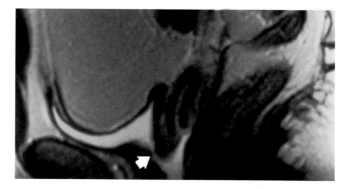

FIGURE 27-15   Low vesicovaginal fistula in a 23-year-old woman after surgical repair of a vaginal septum. Sagittal fast spin-echo 4700/140 image shows the direct communication of the bladder neck with the proximal vagina *(white arrow)*.

ureteroceles are present in the female pediatric population, in whom they are usually ectopic and associated with the upper pole of a duplex collecting system. Patients have recurrent urinary tract infections; the obstructed upper-pole collecting system may be palpated as a mass on physical examination.[19] In cases detected early, endoscopic incision is the treatment of choice to prevent reflux and loss of function of the ipsilateral upper pole.[25]

Simple ureteroceles are most often encountered in adults and may be acquired secondary to inflammatory or traumatic narrowing of the distal ureteral orifice.[25,36] The majority of simple ureteroceles are asymptomatic; occasionally larger lesions can obstruct the bladder neck or result in hydronephrosis.[36]

Heavily T2-weighted MR images ("MR urography") can optimally demonstrate the dilated intravesicular cystic mass and the proximal hydroureter without the use of ionizing radiation or of contrast material.

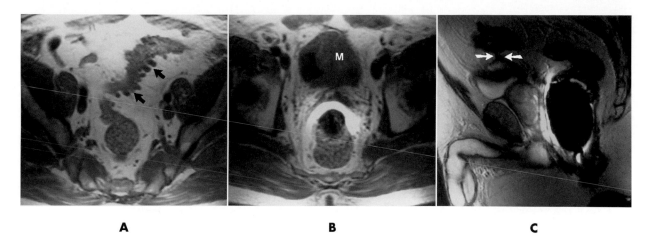

A   **B**   **C**

FIGURE 27-16   Vesicoenteric fistula secondary to diverticulitis in a 66-year-old man with dysuria, a bladder mass, and a prior biopsy that showed inflammatory change without tumor. **A** and **B,** Axial T1-weighted spin-echo 500/12 images at the level of the sigmoid colon and bladder dome show sigmoid diverticulosis *(black arrows)* and a bladder mass *(M)*. **C,** Sagittal fast spin-echo 3700/138 image shows a low-signal tract *(arrows)* from the bladder dome to the thickened sigmoid colon. A focal high-signal fluid collection is present in the outer bladder wall. No suspicious bladder mucosal lesion is present. Diverticulitis with fistulous communication to the bladder was confirmed clinically.

Hernia

Approximately 2% of hernias include a segment of bladder.[28] The majority of bladder hernias occur in an inguinal location (Figure 27-14). Segments of bladder are present in up to 10% of larger inguinal hernias in middle-aged to elderly men.[49,51] The majority of bladder hernias are asymptomatic,[28,117] but some are associated with reflux or stone formation.[66,83] Perhaps the greatest morbidity associated with this condition is inadvertent bladder injury that occurs during hernia repair when the surgeon was not aware that a segment of bladder was associated with the hernia sac.[23,29]

Fistula

Because of its superb soft tissue contrast, direct multiplanar imaging capability, and exquisite sensitivity for detecting fluid, MRI has been used to evaluate fistula tracts in many parts of the body.*

Vesicovaginal Fistula. Vesicovaginal fistulas are the most commonly encountered fistula in the genitourinary tract.[38] Worldwide, the most common etiology is obstetric trauma, whereas in the United States injury during gynecologic procedures (Figure 27-15) (particularly hysterectomy) is most often encountered.[61,62,70] Fistulas caused by the spread of cervical or bladder carcinoma can occur, often after treatment with radiation therapy. Affected women have constant urinary incontinence. The majority of cases are treated surgically through a vaginal approach.[70]

Enterovesical Fistula. The majority of enterovesical fistulas (Figure 27-16) are secondary to diverticulitis, pelvic malignancy, or Crohn's disease.[41,42,90] Some 5% of cases arise from unusual presentations of appendicitis.[35,37] CT has been shown to be the imaging modality of choice and outperforms cystoscopy and barium enema in the diagnosis of colovesical fistula.[53] However, with appropriate technique we have found that MRI can identify the fistula and correctly categorize the underlying pathological condition as malignant or inflammatory in the majority of cases.

Rare cases of vesicouterine fistula have been reported after cesarean sections or uterine biopsy.[27,63,75,121] Patients can have urinary incontinence or menstruation through the bladder (menouria).

REFERENCES

1. Abel PD, Henderson D, Bennet MK, et al: Differing interpretations by pathologists of the pT category and grade of transitional cell cancer of the bladder, Br J Urol 62:339, 1988.

2. Aerts P, Van Hoe L, Bosmans H, et al: Breath-hold MR urography using the HASTE technique, Am J Roentgenol 166:543, 1996.

3. al-Izzi MS, Horton LW, Kelleher J, et al: Malignant transformation in endometriosis of the urinary bladder, Histopathology 14:191, 1989.

4. Amendola MA, Glazer GM, Grossman HB, et al: Staging of bladder carcinoma: MRI-CT-surgical correlation, Am J Roentgenol 146:1179, 1986.

5. Arap Neto W, Lopes RN, Cury M, et al: Vesical endometriosis, Urology 24:271, 1984.

6. Banson ML: Normal MR anatomy and techniques for imaging of the male pelvis, Magn Reson Imaging Clin North Am 4:481, 1996.

7. Barentsz JO, Erning LJv, Rujis JH, et al: Dynamic turboFLASH substraction MR imaging: perfusion of pelvic tumors, Radiology 185(P):340, 1992.

8. Barentsz JO, Jager G, Mugler JP, et al: Staging of urinary bladder cancer: value of T1-weighted three-dimensional magnetization prepared-rapid gradient-echo and two-dimensional spin-echo sequences, Am J Roentgenol 164:109, 1995.

9. Barentsz JO, Jager GJ, van Vierzen PB, et al: Staging urinary bladder cancer after transurethral biopsy: value of fast dynamic contrast-enhanced MR imaging, Radiology 201:185, 1996.

10. Barentsz JO, Jaher GJ, Witjes F, et al: Dynamic substraction FLASH MR imaging in staging urinary bladder cancer after transurethral resection and chemotherapy, Radiology 193(P):167, 1994.

11. Barentsz JO, Lemmens JAM, Ruijs SHJ, et al: Carcinoma of the urinary bladder: MR imaging with a double surface coil, Am J Roentgenol 151:107, 1988.

12. Barentsz JO, Ruijs SH, Strijk SP: The role of MR imaging in carcinoma of the urinary bladder, Am J Roentgenol 160:937, 1993.

13. Barentsz JO, Ruijs SH, van Erning LJ: Magnetic resonance imaging of urinary bladder cancer: an overview and new developments, Magn Reson Q 9:235, 1993.

14. Blomlie V, Rofstad EK, Trope C, et al: Critical soft tissues of the female pelvis: serial MR imaging before, during, and after radiation therapy, Radiology 203:391, 1997.

15. Boudghene F, Aboun H, Grange JD, et al: [Magnetic resonance imaging in the exploration of abdominal and anoperineal fistulas in Crohn's disease], Gastroenterol Clin Biol 17:168, 1993.

16. Bryan PJ, Butler HE, LiPuma JP, et al: CT and MR imaging in staging bladder neoplasms, J Comput Assist Tomogr 11:96, 1987.

17. Buckley KM, Whitman GJ, and Chew FS: Diaphragmatic pheochromocytoma (clinical conference), Am J Roentgenol 165:260, 1995.

18. Buy JN, Moss AA, Guinet C, et al: MR staging of bladder carcinoma: correlation with pathologic findings, Radiology 169:695, 1988.

19. Caldamone AA, Snyder HMD, and Duckett JW: Ureteroceles in children: follow-up of management with upper tract approach, J Urol 131:1130, 1984.

20. Catalona WJ: Urothelial tumors of the urinary tract. In Walsh PC, Retik AB, Stamey TA, et al, eds: Campbellís urology, vol 2, ed 6, Philadelphia, 1992, WB Saunders.

21. Chen M, Lipson SA, and Hricak H: MR imaging evaluation of benign mesenchymal tumors of the urinary bladder, Am J Roentgenol 168:399, 1997.

22. Chor PJ, Gaum LD, and Young RH: Clear cell adenocarcinoma of the urinary bladder: report of a case of probable mullerian origin, Mod Pathol 6:225, 1993.

23. Colodny AH: Bladder injury during herniorrhaphy manifested by ascites and azotemia, Urology 3:89, 1974.

24. Conlin MJ, Skoog SJ, and Tank ES: Current management of ureteroceles, Urology 45:357, 1995.

25. Coplen DE, and Duckett JW: The modern approach to ureteroceles, J Urol 153:166, 1995.

26. Crecelius SA, and Bellah R: Pheochromocytoma of the bladder in an adolescent: sonographic and MR imaging findings, Am J Roentgenol 165:101, 1995.

27. Crimail P, and Lymperopoulou-Dodou A: [Uterine bladder fistula after a cesarean: a case report], J Gynecol Obstet Biol Reprod (Paris) 21:112, 1992.

*References 14, 15, 46, 59, 86, 99, 101, 127.

28. Curry N: Hernias of the urinary tract. In Pollack HM, ed: Clinical urography, vol 3, Philadelphia, 1990, WB Saunders.

29. De Giovanni L, Civello IM, Matei DV, et al: [Inguinal-scrotal hernia of a bladder diverticulum], J Urol (Paris) 100:155, 1994.

30. Di Girolamo M, Pirillo S, Laghi A, et al: [Urography with magnetic resonance: a new method for the study of the renal collecting system in patients without obstructive uropathy], Radiol Med (Torino) 92:758, 1996.

31. Dondalski M, White EM, Ghahremani GG, et al: Carcinoma arising in urinary bladder diverticula: imaging findings in six patients, Am J Roentgenol 161:817, 1993.

32. Doringer E, Joos H, Forstner R, et al: [MRT of bladder carcinoma: tumor staging and gadolinium contrast behavior], Rofo Fortschr Geb Rontgenstr Neuen Bildgeb Verfahr 154:357, 1991.

33. Fisher MR, Hricak H, and Tanagho EA: Urinary bladder MR imaging. II. Neoplasm, Radiology 157:471, 1985.

34. Foster RS, Rink RC, and Mulcahy JJ: Vesical endometriosis: medical or surgical treatment, Urology 29:64, 1987.

35. Fraley EE, Reinberg Y, Holt T, et al: Computerized tomography in the diagnosis of appendicovesical fistula, J Urol 149:830, 1993.

36. Friedland GW, DeVries PA, Nino-Mrucio M, et al: Congenital anomalies of the urinary tract. In Pollack HM, ed: Clinical urography, vol 1, Philadelphia, 1990, WB Saunders.

37. Garb M: Case of the season: appendico-vesical fistula, Semin Roentgenol 29:228, 1994.

38. Gerber GS, and Schoenberg HW: Female urinary tract fistulas [see comments], J Urol 149:229, 1993.

39. Glassberg KI, Braren V, Duckett JW, et al: Suggested terminology for duplex systems, ectopic ureters and ureteroceles, J Urol 132:1153, 1984.

40. Goldstein MS, and Brodman ML: Cystometric evaluation of vesical endometriosis before and after hormonal or surgical treatment, Mt Sinai J Med 57:109, 1990.

41. Goldman SM, Fishman EK, Gatewood OM, et al: CT demonstration of colovesical fistulae secondary to diverticulitis, J Comput Assist Tomogr 8:462, 1984.

42. Goldman SM, Fishman EK, Gatewood OM, et al: CT in the diagnosis of enterovesical fistulae, Am J Roentgenol 144:1229, 1985.

43. Gualdi GF, Volpe A, Polettini E, et al: [A comparison between intraurethral echography, computed tomography and magnetic resonance in the staging of bladder tumors], Clin Ter 141:393, 1992.

44. Hahn D: Neoplasms of the urinary bladder. In Pollack HM, ed: Clinical urography, vol 2, Philadelphia, 1990, WB Saunders.

45. Hawnaur JM, Johnson RJ, Read G, et al: Magnetic resonance imaging with gadolinium-DTPA for assessment of bladder carcinoma and its response to treatment, Clin Radiol 47:302, 1993.

46. Healy JC, Phillips RR, Reznek RH, et al: The MR appearance of vaginal fistulas, Am J Roentgenol 167:1487, 1996.

47. Hermanek P, and Sobin LH: TNM classification of malignant tumors/UICC, International Union Against Cancer, ed 4, New York, 1987, Springer-Verlag.

48. Herr HW, Whitmore WF, Morse MJ, et al: Neoadjuvant chemotherapy in invasive bladder cancer: the evolving role of surgery, J Urol 144:1083, 1990.

49. Holmer P, and Eldrup J: [Inguinal hernias with bladder herniation], Ugeskr Laeger 154:1191, 1992.

50. Hussain S, O'Malley M, Jara H, et al: MR urography, Magn Reson Imaging Clin North Am 5:95, 1997.

51. Iason AH: Repair of urinary bladder herniation, Am J Surg 63:69, 1944.

52. Jager GJ, Barentsz JO, Oosterhof GO, et al: Pelvic adenopathy in prostatic and urinary bladder carcinoma: MR imaging with a three-dimensional TI-weighted magnetization-prepared-rapid gradient-echo sequence, Am J Roentgenol 167:1503, 1996.

53. Jarrett TW, and Vaughan ED, Jr: Accuracy of computerized tomography in the diagnosis of colovesical fistula secondary to diverticular disease, J Urol 153:44, 1995.

54. Jewett HJ, and Strong GH: Infiltrating carcinoma of the bladder: relation of depth of penetration of the bladder wall to incidence of local extension and metastases, J Urol 55:366, 1946.

55. Johnson RJ, Carrington BM, Jenkins JP, et al: Accuracy in staging carcinoma of the bladder by magnetic resonance imaging, Clin Radiol 41:258, 1990.

56. Kaminsky S, Gogoll M, Neumann K, et al: [Bladder tumors—Magnevist-assisted magnetic resonance tomography], Aktuelle Radiol 2:303, 1992.

57. Kenny GM, Hardner GH, and Murphy GP: Clinical staging of bladder tumors, J Urol 104:720, 1970.

58. Kim B, Semelka RC, Ascher SM, et al: Bladder tumor staging: comparison of contrast-enhanced CT, T1- and T2-weighted MR imaging, dynamic gadolinium-enhanced imaging, and late gadolinium-enhanced imaging, Radiology 193:239, 1994.

59. Koelbel G, Schmiedl U, Majer MC, et al: Diagnosis of fistulae and sinus tracts in patients with Crohn disease: value of MR imaging, Am J Roentgenol 152:999, 1989.

60. Krysiewicz S: Diagnosis of urachal carcinoma by computed tomography and magnetic resonance imaging, Clin Imaging 14:251, 1990.

61. Lang EK, and Fritzsche P: Fistulas of the genitourinary tract. In Pollack HM, ed: Clinical urography, Philadelphia, 1990, WB Saunders.

62. Lee RA, Symmonds RE, and Williams TJ: Current status of genitourinary fistula, Obstet Gynecol 72:313, 1988.

63. Lenkovsky Z, Pode D, Shapiro A, et al: Vesicouterine fistula: a rare complication of cesarean section, J Urol 139:123, 1988.

64. Li W, Chavez D, Edelman RR, et al: Magnetic resonance urography by breath-hold contrast-enhanced three-dimensional FISP, J Magn Reson Imaging 7:309, 1997.

65. Lopez ME, Prats LJ, Prera VA, et al: [Bladder endometriosis simulating a bladder tumor], Arch Esp Urol 45:158, 1992.

66. Loup J: [Huge hernia of the bladder causing lithiasis, hematuria and retention], Ann Urol (Paris) 6:191, 1972.

67. Maeda H, Kinukawa T, Hattori R, et al: Detection of muscle layer invasion with submillimeter pixel MR images: staging of bladder carcinoma, Magn Reson Imaging 13:9, 1995.

68. Maeda H, Kinukawa T, Kuhara H, et al: MR findings in urachal carcinoma, Am J Roentgenol 158:1171, 1992 (letter).

69. Marc B, Lebon E, and Mazeman E: [Leiomyoma of the bladder: apropos of a case], J Urol (Paris) 96:45, 1990.

70. Margolis T, and Mercer LJ: Vesicovaginal fistula, Obstet Gynecol Surv 49:840, 1994.

71. Marshall VF: The relation of the preoperative estimate to the pathologic demonstration of the extent of vesical neoplasms, J Urol 68:714, 1952.

72. Maya MM, and Slywotzky C: Urinary bladder leiomyoma: magnetic resonance imaging findings, Urol Radiol 14:197, 1992.

73. McCauley TR, McCarthy S, and Lange R: Pelvic phased array coil: image quality assessment for spin-echo MR imaging, Magn Reson Imaging 10:513, 1992.

74. McGinnis DE, Rifkin MD, and Gomella LG: New MR imaging techniques for staging bladder cancer: endorectal coil and gadolinium image enhancement, J Urol 147:402A, 1992 (abstract).

75. Mercader VP, McGuckin JF Jr, Caroline DF, et al: CT of vesicocorporeal fistula with menouria: a complication of uterine biopsy, J Comput Assist Tomogr 19:324, 1995.

76. Mor Y, Nass D, Ben-Chaim J, et al: [Endometriosis of the bladder], Harefuah 125:79, 127, 1993.

77. Narumi Y, Kadota T, Inoue E, et al: Bladder tumors: staging with gadolinium-enhanced oblique MR imaging, Radiology 187:145, 1993.

78. Neuerburg JM, Bohndorf K, Sohn M, et al: Staging of urinary bladder neoplasms with MR imaging: is Gd-DTPA helpful? J Comput Assist Tomogr 15:780, 1991.

79. Neuerburg JM, Bohndorf K, Sohn M, et al: Urinary bladder neoplasms: evaluation with contrast-enhanced MR imaging, Radiology 172:739, 1989.

80. Nezhat CR, and Nezhat FR: Laparoscopic segmental bladder resection for endometriosis: a report of two cases, Obstet Gynecol 81:882, 1993.

81. Nicolas V, Spielmann R, Maas R, et al: [The diagnostic value of MR tomography following gadolinium-DTPA compared to computed tomography in bladder tumors], Rofo Fortschr Geb Rontgenstr Neuen Bildgeb Verfahr 153:197, 1990.

82. Nishiyama H, Nakamura K, and Nishimura M, et al: [Male bladder leiomyoma: a case report], Hinyokika Kiyo 38:949, 1992.

83. Noble JG, Christmas TJ, Chapple CR, et al: Inguinal bladder hernia associated with vesico-ureteric reflux, Postgrad Med J 68:299, 1992.

84. Older RA: Endometriosis of the genitourinary tract. In Pollack HM, ed: Clinical urography, vol 3, Philadelphia, 1990, WB Saunders.

85. O'Malley ME, Soto JA, Yucel EK, et al: MR urography: evaluation of a three-dimensional fast spin-echo technique in patients with hydronephrosis, Am J Roentgenol 168:387, 1997.

86. Outwater E, and Schiebler ML: Pelvic fistulas: findings on MR images, Am J Roentgenol 160:327, 1993.

87. Outwater E, Schiebler ML, Owen RS, et al: Characterization of hemorrhagic adnexal lesions with MR imaging: blinded reader study, Radiology 186:489, 1993.

88. Outwater EK, and Mitchell DG: Magnetic resonance imaging techniques in the pelvis, MRI Clin North Am 2:481, 1994.

89. Pattani SJ, Kier R, Deal R, et al: MRI of uterine leiomyosarcoma, Magn Reson Imaging 13:331, 1995.

90. Pontari MA, McMillen MA, Garvey RH, et al: Diagnosis and treatment of enterovesical fistulae, Am Surg 58:258, 1992.

91. Rafal RB, and Markisz JA: Urachal carcinoma: the role of magnetic resonance imaging, Urol Radiol 12:184, 1991.

92. Regan F, Bohlman ME, Khazan R, et al: MR urography using HASTE imaging in the assessment of ureteric obstruction, Am J Roentgenol 167:1115, 1996.

93. Richie JP, Skinner DG, and Kaufman JJ: Carcinoma of the bladder: treatment by radical cystectomy, J Surg Res 18:271, 1975.

94. Romero PP, Lobato EJJ, Perez LLA, et al: [Endometriosis of the bladder muscular layer as a cause of acute abdomen], Arch Esp Urol 48:395, 1994.

95. Sampietro CA, Fernandez DAM, Ruiz MR, et al: [Bladder endometriosis: a new case and review of the literature], Arch Esp Urol 48:314, 1995.

96. Schmidt JD, and Weinstein SH: Pitfalls in clinical staging of bladder tumors, Urol Clin North Am 3:107, 1976.

97. Schnall MD, Connick T, Hayes CE, et al: MR imaging of the pelvis with an endorectal-external multicoil array, J Magn Reson Imaging 2:229, 1992.

98. See WA, and Fuller JR: Staging of advanced bladder cancer: current concepts and pitfalls, Urol Clin North Am 19:663, 1992.

99. Semelka RC, Hricak H, Kim B, et al: Pelvic fistulas: appearances on MR images, Abdom Imaging 22:91, 1997.

100. Shook TE, and Nyberg LM: Endometriosis of the urinary tract, Urology 31:1, 1988.

101. Siegelman ES, Banner MP, Ramchandani P, et al: Multicoil MR imaging of symptomatic female urethral and periurethral disease, Radiographics 17:349, 1997.

102. Siegelman ES, and Schnall MD: Contrast-enhanced MR imaging of the bladder and prostate, Magn Reson Imaging Clin North Am 4:153, 1996.

103. Smith RC, Reinhold C, McCauley TR, et al: Multicoil high-resolution fast spin-echo MR imaging of the female pelvis, Radiology 184:671, 1992.

104. Sohn M, Neuerburg J, Teufl F, et al: Gadolinium-enhanced magnetic resonance imaging in the staging of urinary bladder neoplasms, Urol Int 45:142, 1990.

105. Soucek M, Carr JJ, Schnall MD, et al: MR imaging with endorectal surface and multiarray coils in evaluation of lesions of bladder neck, proximal urethra, and posterior bladder wall, Radiology 193(P):167, 1994.

106. Sparenberg A, Hamm B, Hammerer P, et al: [The diagnosis of bladder carcinomas by NMR tomography: an improvement with Gd-DTPA?], Rofo Fortschr Geb Rontgenstr Neuen Bildgeb Verfahr 155:117, 1991.

107. Stephens FD: Aetiology of ureteroceles and effects of ureteroceles on the urethra, Br J Urol 40:483, 1968.

108. Sugimura Y, Hayashi N, Yamashita A, et al: [Endorectal magnetic resonance imaging of the prostate and bladder], Hinyokika Kiyo 40:31, 1994.

109. Swartz DA, Johnson DE, Ayala AG, et al: Bladder leiomyosarcoma: a review of 10 cases with 5-year follow-up, J Urol 133:200, 1985.

110. Sweetser PM, Ohl DA, and Thompson NW: Pheochromocytoma of the urinary bladder, Surgery 109:677, 1991.

111. Tachibana M, Baba S, Deguchi N, et al: Efficacy of gadolinium-diethylenetriamine-pentaacetic acid-enhanced magnetic resonance imaging for differentiation between superficial and muscle-invasive tumor of the bladder: a comparative study with computerized tomography and transurethral ultrasonography, J Urol 145:1169, 1991.

112. Tang Y, Yamashita Y, Namimoto T, et al: The value of MR urography that uses HASTE sequences to reveal urinary tract disorders, Am J Roentgenol 167:1497, 1996.

113. Tanimoto A, Yuasa Y, Imai Y, et al: Bladder tumor staging: comparison of conventional and gadolinium-enhanced dynamic MR imaging and CT, Radiology 85:741, 1992.

114. Teeger S, and Sica GT: MR imaging of bladder diseases, Magn Reson Imaging Clin North Am 4:565, 1996.

115. Thrasher JB, Rajan RR, Perez LM, et al: Pheochromocytoma of urinary bladder: contemporary methods of diagnosis and treatment options, Urology 41:435, 1993.

116. Togashi K, Nishimura K, Kimura I, et al: Endometrial cysts: diagnosis with MR imaging, Radiology 180:73, 1991.

117. Tsujihata M, Yokokawa K, and Nakano E: [A case of inguinal bladder hernia], Hinyokika Kiyo 37:1053, 1991.

118. van Gils AP, Falke TH, van Erkel AR, et al: MR imaging and MIBG scintigraphy of pheochromocytomas and extraadrenal functioning paragangliomas, Radiographics 11:37, 1991.

119. Venz S, Ilg J, Ebert T, et al: [Determining the depth of infiltration in urinary bladder carcinoma with contrast medium enhanced dynamic magnetic resonance tomography: with reference to postoperative findings and inflammation], Urologe A 35:297, 1996.

120. Vermesh M, Zbella EA, Menchaca A, et al: Vesical endometriosis following bladder injury, Am J Obstet Gynecol 153:894, 1985.

121. Vu KK, Brittain PC, Fontenot JP, et al: Vesicouterine fistula after cesarean section: a case report, J Reprod Med 40:221, 1995.

122. Warshawsky R, Bow SN, Waldbaum RS, et al: Bladder pheochromocytoma with MR correlation, J Comput Assist Tomogr 13:714, 1989.

123. Weissleder R, Elizondo G, Wittenberg J, et al: Ultrasmall superparamagnetic iron oxide: an intravenous contrast agent for assessing lymph nodes with MR imaging, Radiology 175:494, 1990.

124. Whalen RK, Althausen AF, and Daniels GH: Extra-adrenal pheochromocytoma, J Urol 147:1, 1992.

125. Wijkstrom H, Edsmyr F, and Lundh B: The value of preoperative classification according to the TNM system, Eur Urol 10:101, 1984.

126. Wingo PA, Tong T, and Bolden S: Cancer statistics, CA Cancer J Clin 45:8, 1995.

127. Yazawa K, Nonomura N, Kokado Y, et al: Vesico-adnexal fistula following endometriosis of an ovary, Br J Urol 79:658, 1997.

128. Yoon IJ, Kim KH, and Lee BH: Leiomyoma of the urinary bladder: MR findings, Am J Roentgenol 161:449, 1993 (letter).

129. Zieba Z, and Kaczmarek J: [Endometriosis of the bladder and vesico-uterine fistula as complications of cesarean section], Ginekol Pol 60:297, 1989.

28 Female Pelvis

Leslie M. Scoutt and Shirley M. McCarthy

 ## KEY POINTS

- Sagittal and transverse T2-weighted (CSE or FSE) images are standard, with matching T1-weighted images obtained in either plane.
- MRI is not used for screening but is often helpful for differential diagnosis.
- MRI is superior to CT and US for delineation of congenital anomalies and staging of tumors.

TECHNIQUE

Both T1-weighted and T2-weighted spin-echo (SE) multiplanar images are essential for imaging of the female pelvis. On T1-weighted images, there is optimal soft tissue contrast between pelvic fat and the normal uterus and ovaries, which appear as homogeneous, low–signal intensity structures. T1-weighted images are also useful for identifying lymph nodes and bowel. In addition, T1-weighted images aid in tissue characterization by identifying lipid and blood products. However, T2-weighted sequences are essential for delineating the normal zonal anatomy of the female reproductive tract as well as pelvic pathology. T2-weighted images should be obtained in at least two imaging planes with either conventional spin-echo (CSE) or fast spin-echo (FSE) se-

quences. FSE imaging allows acquisition of T2-weighted images more than 16 times faster than CSE sequences.

FSE sequences can also be obtained with a very long echo train length (ETL) and half-Fourier transformation, yielding high-quality images in 17 seconds (e.g., fat-saturated half-Fourier single-shot turbo SE sequence, echo time [TE] effective [eff] 82, ETL 128).[98] Shorter imaging time reduces artifacts caused by respiratory motion, vascular pulsations, and bowel peristalsis (Figure 28-1). Thus glucagon is not necessary to reduce bowel peristalsis. In addition, greater T2 weighting can be obtained. A longer repetition time (TR) is generally used, since for a given TR, fewer slice locations can be obtained with FSE imaging. FSE images are superior to CSE images when judged according to image quality, reduction of motion artifact, clarity of pelvic organ definition as well as zonal anatomy, and conspicuity of pathology.[139,184] Imaging characteristics are very similar on CSE and FSE sequences, with the exception that lipid generates higher signal on FSE than on CSE images. Thus lesions surrounded by fat are potentially less conspicuous on FSE images. Complementary T1-weighted images must be obtained in at least one plane.[187]

High-resolution images of the female pelvis may be obtained using a dedicated phased-array multicoil. With such a coil, multiple independent receive-only surface coils input into separate receiver channels, generating individual data sets for each coil, which are then combined and reconstructed into a single composite image. Such multicoil images have the same high signal-to-noise ratio as a surface coil but a larger field of view comparable to the body coil. Several studies have demonstrated that this technique produces excellent image quality with superior depiction of anatomical detail[66,121,185] (Figure 28-2). When combined with FSE imaging, high-resolution images of the pelvis can be obtained in less than 5 minutes. Because respiratory compensation techniques are incompatible with FSE imaging, saturation pulses should be placed within the anterior and posterior subcutaneous fat to diminish ghost artifact.[184,185]

Chemical-shift imaging with fat- or water-suppression techniques is useful for differentiating between lipid and blood products when lesions are high signal intensity on T1-weighted images and isointense to fat on T2-weighted images. Signal from fat is suppressed before the slice-selective pulse of the standard SE sequence by application of a non–slice-selective 90-degree pulse having a narrow bandwidth centered on the precessional frequency of fat, immediately followed by a spoiler gradient. Conversely, if the narrow bandwidth pulse is centered on the precessional frequency of water, signal from water will be suppressed, and lesions containing fat will remain high signal and therefore more conspicuous.[187]

Contrast enhancement after the intravenous administration of 0.1 mmol/kg of gadolinium (Gd) chelate is useful in some clinical situations. Paired T1-weighted sequences with fat suppression before and after Gd enhancement are obtained with short TE (12 to 15 ms) for optimal contrast enhancement. Contrast-enhanced images have been demonstrated to be useful in evaluating the internal architecture of pelvic masses, particularly in differentiating clot and debris from solid components and in identifying cystic/necrotic areas of neoplasms, endometrial polyps, and serosal/peritoneal implants.* Dynamic contrast-enhanced images may also be helpful for the staging of endometrial carcinoma.[85,216,218]

We perform all pelvic MR imaging with a dedicated phased-array multicoil and obtain FSE T2-weighted images. After a fast sagittal short tau inversion recovery sequence, axial T1-weighted and axial plus coro-

---

*References 50, 51, 82, 189, 195, 196, 214.

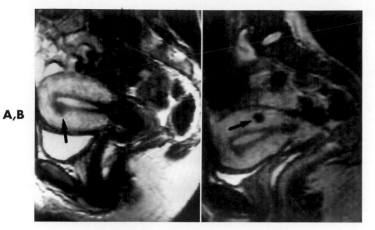

FIGURE 28-1   FSE T2-weighted imaging. **A,** Adenomyosis *(arrow).* **B,** Leiomyoma.

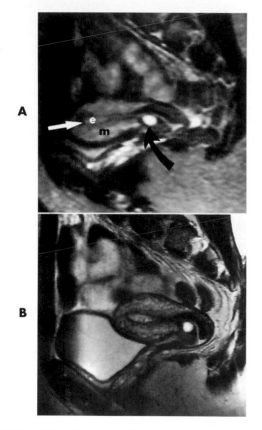

FIGURE 28-2   Nabothian cyst. **A,** Conventional T2-weighted midline sagittal image demonstrating normal uterine zonal anatomy. *e,* Endometrium; *white arrow,* junctional zone; *m,* outer myometrium. The nabothian cyst is near the internal os *(curved black arrow).* Scan time was 9 min, 18 sec. **B,** High-resolution FSE technique using high-resolution matrix and pelvic multicoil provides even sharper detail and soft tissue contrast. Scan time was 4 min, 30 sec.

nal or sagittal T2-weighted sequences are obtained. The field of view is kept as small as possible, usually 20 to 24 cm. Saturation (SAT) pulses are placed based on the sagittal localizer to include the air–subcutaneous fat interface. The T1-weighted sequence is obtained using TR 600 ms/minimum TE, 5-mm section thickness with 2.5-mm gap, 256 × 160 matrix, 1 signal acquired, and respiratory compensation. FSE T2-weighted sequences are acquired with TR/TE 6000/117, ETL 16, 5-mm section thickness with 2-mm gap, 256 × 256 matrix, and 2 signals acquired. If a high–signal intensity lesion is detected on the axial T1-weighted series, fat-suppression and/or water-suppression sequences are obtained.

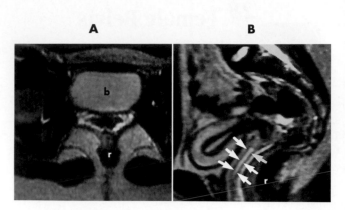

FIGURE 28-3   Normal anatomy of the vagina. **A,** Axial T2-weighted image demonstrates the vaginal fornices. The vaginal wall is low signal intensity, and the lateral margins are sharply angulated or triangular in contour. Surrounding the vaginal fornices are serpiginous channels of increased signal intensity representing the normal venous plexus. *b,* Bladder; *r,* rectum. **B,** Midline sagittal T2-weighted image. The vaginal wall is low signal intensity *(arrows),* whereas mucus within vaginal lumen is of high signal intensity. Note the fat planes between the vagina and rectum *(r)* posteriorly and the vagina and bladder *(arrows)* anteriorly.

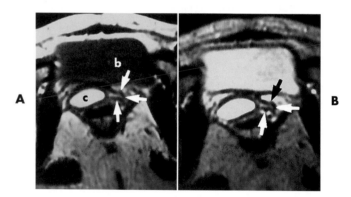

FIGURE 28-4   Axial intermediate-weighted **(A)** and axial T2-weighted **(B)** images demonstrating a Gartner's duct cyst *(c),* which is high signal intensity on both intermediate and T2-weighted images and protrudes into the vaginal lumen. The low-signal intensity vaginal wall *(arrows)* is clearly seen. *b,* Bladder.

VAGINA
Normal Anatomy

The vagina is best evaluated on T2-weighted axial and sagittal images.[72,120] The vaginal epithelium and contents of the vaginal canal are high signal intensity, whereas the vaginal wall is low signal intensity because of the short T2 of smooth muscle (Figure 28-3). The lateral fornices demarcate the upper third of the vagina, and the bladder base and urethra demarcate the lower third. The magnetic resonance (MR) appearance of the vagina depends on the hormonal status of the patient. The central mucus and wall are thickest and of highest signal intensity during the midsecretory phase. However, there is maximal contrast (and therefore optimal visualization) between the vaginal wall and surrounding pelvic fat during the early proliferative or late secretory phase.[72] In postmenopausal women, the central mucous layer is thinned. The vagina is surrounded by a prominent, high–signal intensity venous plexus. A tampon should not be used to localize the vagina because it will obscure detail. The vaginal wall typically enhances after the administration of intravenous (IV) Gd but the intraluminal portion does not in most patients.[71,74]

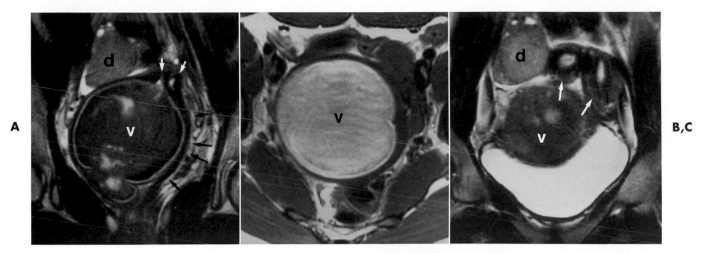

FIGURE 28-5   Duplication of the uterus, cervix, and vagina with obstruction of the right sided vagina. **A,** T2-weighted coronal image demonstrates a distended right vagina *(v)*, normal left side *(black arrows)*, and two endocervical canals *(white arrows)*. Right ovarian intermediate signal mass *(d)* was a dysgerminoma. **B,** High signal intensity within the obstructed right vagina *(v)* on the axial T1-weighted image confirms the presence of blood (hematocolpos). **C,** More anterior T2-weighted coronal image demonstrates the two uterine horns *(white arrows)*.

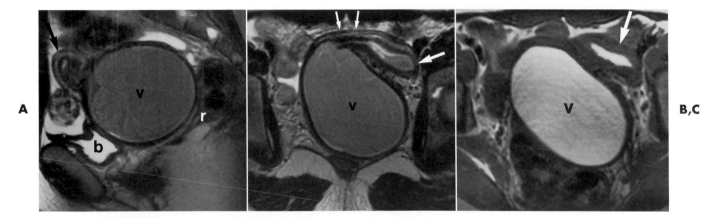

FIGURE 28-6   Distal vaginal atresia. Sagittal T2-weighted **(A)**, axial T2-weighted **(B)**, and axial T1-weighted **(C)** images demonstrate a cystic mass *(v)* with signal intensity consistent with blood displacing the uterus *(long arrow)* anteriorly. *Short arrows,* Cervix. This is a proximal hematocolpos caused by distal vaginal atresia. Note the absence of distal vaginal tissue between the bladder *(b)* and rectum *(r)* on **A.** Signal intensity within endometrial cavity in **B** and **C** is consistent with minimal hematometria.

Gartner's duct cysts arise from remnants of the vaginal portion of the mesonephric ducts. On magnetic resonance imaging (MRI), such cysts appear as cystic structures within the vaginal wall: high signal intensity on T2-weighted images and occasionally high signal intensity on T1-weighted images (Figure 28-4). Bartholin's cysts have a similar appearance but are located more distally in the labia.[91]

Congenital Anomalies

Because the upper two thirds of the vagina derives from fusion of the müllerian ducts and the lower one third develops separately from the urogenital sinus, congenital abnormalities of the vagina can be quite complex and are often associated with anomalies of the uterus, cervix, and kidneys (Figure 28-5). Furthermore, normal-appearing external genitalia do not necessarily predict the presence of normal internal reproductive structures. MRI is the imaging modality of choice for the evaluation of complete or partial vaginal agenesis. The exact distance between the introitus and the blind end of the upper vagina or cervix is extremely important for surgical planning and can be measured easily on MR examination[72,161,203] (Figure 28-6). In addition, the presence or

absence of functional endometrium and cervix is readily demonstrated on MRI[72,161,203] (Figures 28-7 and 28-8). This information is crucial for patient counseling concerning reproductive capability. Hysterectomy is required if functional endometrium is present without a cervix because pregnancy cannot be sustained in the presence of a uterovaginal fistula. Hysterectomy will also prevent the development of endometriosis after spontaneous obliteration of the uterovaginal fistula.[161] Transverse or longitudinal vaginal septations are more difficult to visualize on MRI. Hematocolpos may result from obstructing transverse septations or partial atresia (Figures 28-5 and 28-6).

Vaginal Neoplasms

Squamous cell carcinoma of the vagina accounts for only 1% to 2% of all gynecological malignancies. The peak incidence of vaginal carcinoma occurs in the sixth decade. Patients most often have vaginal bleeding or discharge.[133,169] Human papillomavirus infection may be a significant risk factor for squamous cell carcinoma. Clear cell adenocarcinomas occur in women exposed in utero to diethylstilbestrol (DES) and come to medical attention at an earlier age. Carcinoma of the vagina is staged according to the International Federation of Gynecology and Obstetrics (FIGO) Staging System (Table 28-1). Carcinomas arising from the upper posterior vaginal wall are most common and invade locally with subsequent spread to the obturator, iliac, and hypogastric lymph nodes. Tumors arising from the lower vagina initially metastasize to inguinal lymph nodes. Patients are treated primarily with radiation therapy, and prognosis is related to tumor size and stage at presentation. Tumors arising in the lower vagina have a slightly worse prognosis.[133] The 5-year survival rate is reported to range from 64% to 76% for stage I disease; 37% to 59% for stage II disease; 23% to 36% for stage III disease; and up to 40% for stage IV disease.[133]

Carcinoma of the vagina with full-thickness invasion of the wall (FIGO stage I) appears as a focal area of increased signal intensity on T2-weighted images, disrupting the low signal intensity of the vaginal wall.[25] Once subvaginal extension (FIGO stage II) occurs, the normal high signal intensity of the paravaginal fat/venous plexus will be disrupted by tumor mass (Figure 28-9). Extension to the pelvic wall (FIGO

stage III) may be diagnosed when the relatively high signal intensity of the tumor disrupts the normal low signal intensity of the piriformis and obturator internus muscles on T2-weighted images. Invasion of the bladder or rectum (FIGO stage IV) may be documented when the tumor mass disrupts these structures. Gd-enhanced T1-weighted imaging has not been definitively shown to be useful, although experience is limited.[71]

Recurrence usually occurs within the first 2 years of diagnosis, and differentiation between recurrent disease and radiation fibrosis is extremely important. A mass remaining low signal intensity on both T1- and T2-weighted images most likely represents radiation fibrosis. Recurrent tumor reportedly demonstrates increased signal intensity on T2-weighted sequences.[25] However, this finding is nonspecific, and in a series of 17 patients with clinical suspicion of recurrent disease, Chang et al[25] described two patients with high–signal intensity masses on T2-weighted images in whom only inflammation was found at biopsy.

Metastatic disease, usually from direct invasion of uterine or cervical neoplasms, is more common than primary vaginal carcinoma.[133,169] On MRI a mass with signal characteristics similar to those of the primary neoplasm will be noted to disrupt the low signal intensity of the vaginal wall. However, false-positive diagnoses of tumor invasion may occur as a result of vascular congestion or inflammation, which can

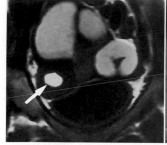
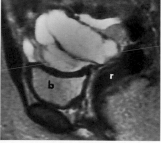

A,B

FIGURE 28-7   Vaginal agenesis. **A,** Coronal T1-weighted image demonstrates hematosalpinx and hematometra *(arrow)*. **B,** Midline sagittal T2-weighted image. Note that only fat is present between the bladder *(b)* and rectum *(r)* and that no vaginal wall or mucosa is seen. This patient had congenital absence of the vagina. The uterus and fallopian tubes were obstructed and filled with blood, which indicates that functional endometrial tissue is present.

Table 28-1   FIGO Staging of Primary Carcinoma of the Vagina

STAGE	PATHOLOGY
I	Carcinoma limited to vaginal wall
II	Carcinoma involves subvaginal tissue without extension to pelvic wall
III	Carcinoma extends to pelvic wall
IV	Carcinoma extends beyond true pelvis, involves bladder or rectal mucosa

From reference 133.

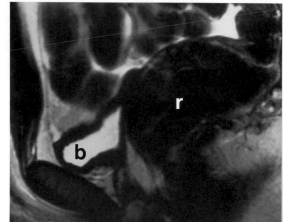
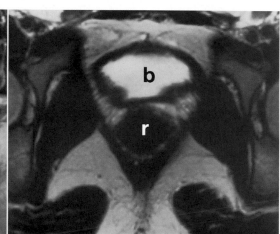
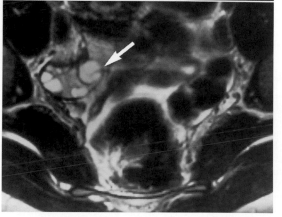

A   **B**   **C**

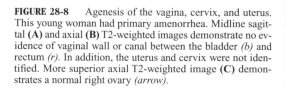

FIGURE 28-8   Agenesis of the vagina, cervix, and uterus. This young woman had primary amenorrhea. Midline sagittal **(A)** and axial **(B)** T2-weighted images demonstrate no evidence of vaginal wall or canal between the bladder *(b)* and rectum *(r)*. In addition, the uterus and cervix were not identified. More superior axial T2-weighted image **(C)** demonstrates a normal right ovary *(arrow)*.

produce focal areas of increased signal intensity.[25] In addition, it may be difficult to differentiate true invasion from compression or thinning of the vaginal wall when prolapsed tumor distends the vaginal cavity.

UTERUS
Normal Anatomy

The uterus is divided into the uterine corpus and uterine cervix at the level of the internal os. The entire posterior surface of the uterus and the anterior surface to the level of the internal os are invested with peritoneum. A total of eight suspensory ligaments hold the uterus in place. Four of these, the paired round ligaments (which initially travel in the broad ligaments then anteriorly toward the abdominal wall) and the paired sacral-uterine ligaments (which arise from the sacrum and pass anteriorly on either side of the rectum to attach near the internal os) are often seen on T1-weighted images. T1-weighted images are optimal for visualization of the uterine contour because of high contrast between fat and soft tissue structures. However, the uterus is of uniformly low signal intensity on T1-weighted images, and no internal anatomy is visualized.

In almost all premenopausal patients, three distinct zones within the uterine corpus can be depicted on T2-weighted images (Figure 28-10). A central high–signal intensity stripe corresponds to the endometrium and secretions within the endometrial cavity.[80,104] This is surrounded by a low–signal intensity band referred to as the *junctional zone (JZ)*. Histological studies have demonstrated that this zone corresponds to the innermost layer of myometrium and has an increased nuclear area compared with the outer myometrium, primarily reflecting increased cellularity.[17,171] Decreased water content in the JZ in comparison with

the outer myometrium has also been documented.[119] The outer layer of myometrium is of intermediate signal intensity. The internal os, which separates the cervix from the uterine body, is recognizable by a constriction in the external contour of the uterus and an accompanying abrupt decrease in the width of the myometrium.[120]

The uterus is a dynamic organ, and its size and appearance are dependent on the hormonal status of the patient. On MRI the average size of the uterine corpus in the premenopausal woman is 4×5 cm,[120] but this increases slightly during the midsecretory stage.[38] The central high–signal intensity stripe is thinnest during menstruation but increases in width during the menstrual cycle as a result of both estrogen and progesterone stimulation.[67,87,120] Thickness may vary from 4 mm early in the proliferative phase to 13 mm in the late secretory phase. Similarly, the outer myometrium may increase slightly in signal intensity and width during the menstrual cycle, reaching a maximum width of 2.5 cm during the midsecretory to late secretory stage.[38,67] The width of the JZ averages 5 mm and does not vary significantly during the menstrual cycle.[67,120]

In postmenopausal women or women taking gonadotropin-releasing hormone (GnRH) analog, the uterine corpus shrinks until it approximates the length of the cervix. The endometrium thins, averaging 3 mm.[38,75] No large series has as yet been published to establish an upper limit in width for the endometrium in postmenopausal women. However, MR measurement of endometrial thickness is usually less than corresponding ultrasound (US) measurements, and recently Lin et al[109] have suggested 8 mm as an upper limit on US examination in asymptomatic postmenopausal women. In women taking exogenous hormonal replacement therapy, endometrial thickness will vary depending on the hormonal regimen. Myometrial signal intensity is diminished in the postmenopausal uterus. Therefore myometrial/JZ contrast is diminished, and the JZ are less easily definable and may not always be present.[38,75] In postmenopausal women on exogenous estrogen replacement therapy the uterus is similar in appearance to the premenopausal uterus.[38] Postmenopausal women taking tamoxifen for breast cancer therapy or prophylaxis show either homogeneous or heterogeneous thickening of the endometrium (mean 1.1 to 1.8 cm), often with associated subendometrial cysts[5] (Figure 28-11). In women taking oral contraceptives the endometrium thins, averaging 2 mm, and does not vary in width. The size of the uterine corpus and width of the JZ is diminished. Myometrial signal intensity is increased relative to women who do not use oral contraceptives, possibly related to increased uterine water content[38,120] (Figure 28-12). Thus MR images of the uterus must be carefully interpreted in light of the patient's menstrual and hormonal history.

Visualization of the uterine zonal anatomy on T1-weighted Gd contrast-enhanced images is quite variable and dependent both on the timing of imaging after injection and on the hormonal status of the patient.[21,71,74] Several patterns of enhancement have been reported with dynamic imaging. Initial enhancement of a thin subendometrial layer followed by myometrial enhancement has been reported in post-

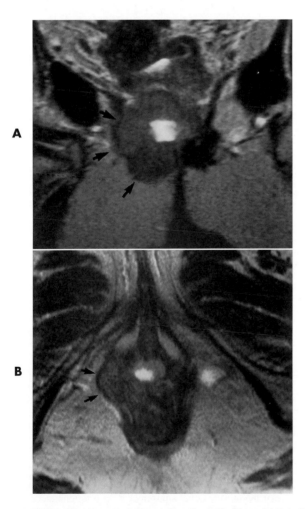

FIGURE 28-9   Carcinoma of the vagina. Coronal **(A)** and axial **(B)** T2-weighted FSE images demonstrating a mass extending through the vaginal wall on the right *(arrows)* in this woman with vaginal carcinoma. The perivaginal venous plexus is obliterated, and the mass invades the surrounding fat.

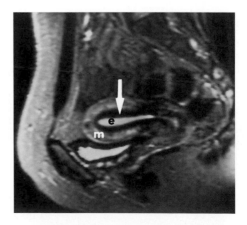

FIGURE 28-10   Normal uterine zonal anatomy. High–signal intensity endometrial stripe *(e)* is surrounded by low–signal intensity junctional zone *(arrow)*. The outer myometrium *(m)* is intermediate signal intensity.

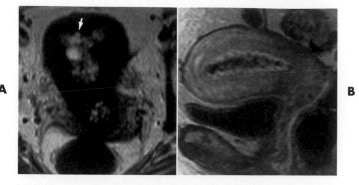

FIGURE 28-11 Benign polyp and subendometrial cysts in a woman taking tamoxifen for breast cancer therapy shown on axial FSE T2-weighted image. **A,** Heterogeneous mass distends the endometrial and endocervical canals. Note the subendometrial area of increased signal intensity *(arrow).* **B,** Sagittal Gd-enhanced, T1-weighted, gradient-recalled echo image demonstrates latticelike enhancement of endometrial mass and no enhancement of subendometrial cysts. (Courtesy Dr. Susan Ascher, Georgetown University.)

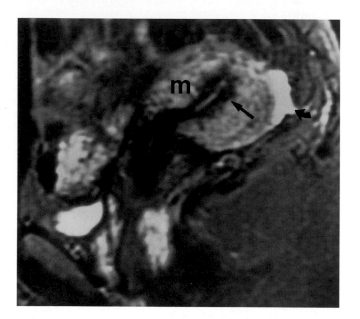

FIGURE 28-12 Oral contraceptives and normal uterine zonal anatomy. The uterine corpus is equal in length to the cervix, the endometrium is thinned, the JZ is present *(straight arrow),* and the outer myometrium *(m)* is slightly increased in signal intensity. Free fluid in the cul-de-sac *(curved arrow).*

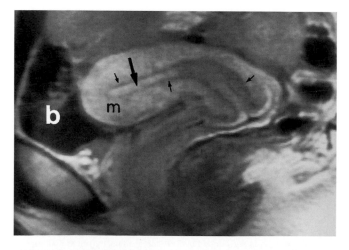

FIGURE 28-13 Gd chelates. Normal endometrium enhances intensely *(long arrow)* with much less enhancement of the JZ and fibrous cervical stroma *(short arrows).* The outer zone *(m)* demonstrates moderate enhancement. *b,* Bladder.

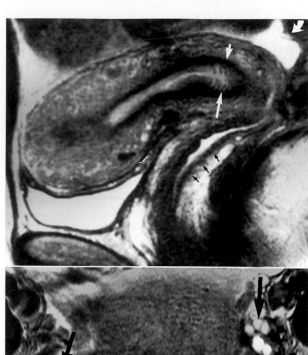
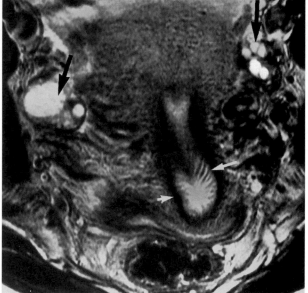

FIGURE 28-14 Normal cervical zonal anatomy. Sagittal **(A)** and axial **(B)** FSE T2-weighted images demonstrate four distinct zones within the cervix. The central high–signal intensity zone represents mucus within the endocervical canal. This is surrounded by an intermediate signal layer, which represents the mucosa. On high-resolution images, mucosal folds *(long white arrow),* the plicae palmatae, can be identified. Subjacent is a band of low signal intensity *(short white arrow),* which is contiguous with the JZ of the uterine corpus. The outermost zone is of intermediate signal intensity and is continuous with the outer myometrium. Note the high–signal intensity fluid within the vaginal canal, the low signal intensity of the vaginal wall *(short black arrows),* and the fluid in the cul-de-sac *(curved arrow)* in **A** and the normal ovaries *(long black arrows)* in **B.**

menopausal women and in women in the proliferative stage of the menstrual cycle.[21] During the secretory stage, initial marked enhancement of the JZ is often observed. During the menstrual phase, enhancement of the entire myometrium, particularly the outer myometrium, may be seen.[21] On delayed (i.e., nondynamic) contrast-enhanced images, enhancement of the endometrium and myometrium with relatively decreased enhancement of the JZ (most likely because of diminished extracellular space within the JZ[171]) has been reported in both premenopausal and postmenopausal women[71] (Figure 28-13). Fluid within the endometrial canal will not enhance. However, great variation in the appearance of the uterine zonal anatomy on contrast-enhanced images has been described, and one study reported that the uterine zonal anatomy was completely obscured in up to 50% of patients on postcontrast images.[74]

With high-resolution multicoil imaging, four distinct zones can be identified within the cervix on T2-weighted images[185] (Figure 28-14). A

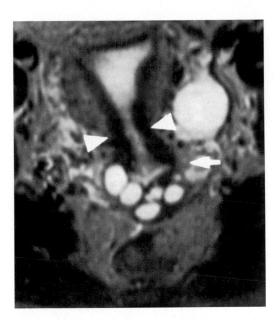

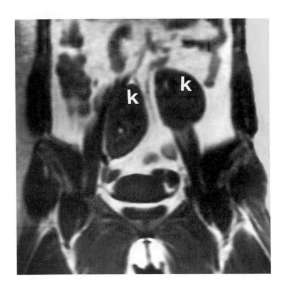

FIGURE 28-15 Nabothian cysts. FSE T2-weighted image reveals five cysts at the external cervical os. The internal os is located at the waist of the uterus *(arrowheads)*. The high signal intensity of the endocervical canal most likely represents mucus and fluid within the endocervical glands and cavity and is continuous with the central endometrial stripe. A cylinder of low signal intensity is continuous with the JZ of the uterus, and an outer zone of intermediate signal intensity *(short arrow)* is continuous with the outer myometrium. A left ovarian cyst *(c)* is present.

FIGURE 28-16 Bilateral pelvic kidneys *(k)* in a patient with a müllerian anomaly. T1-weighted coronal image.

central stripe of high signal intensity represents mucus within the endocervical canal. Immediately subjacent is a zone of intermediate signal intensity, most likely representing the cervical mucosa. Mucosal folds, the plicae palmatae, can often be visualized within this layer. Surrounding this layer is a band of low signal intensity. This band is contiguous with the JZ of the uterine corpus and most likely represents the fibrous cervical stroma. The outermost zone is contiguous with and isointense to the outer zone of the myometrium.[67,80,173] The MR appearance of the cervical zonal anatomy does not appear to be hormonally dependent.[67,120]

After Gd administration, delayed images of the cervix typically reveal marked enhancement of the glandular tissue in the endocervical canal, minor enhancement of the cervical stroma, and enhancement of the outer layer similar to outer myometrial enhancement. In a minority of patients, marked cervical stroma enhancement is observed, which obscures visualization of the normal cervical zonal anatomy.[74]

Nabothian cysts may be identified as cystic areas within the fibrous cervical stroma. They are high signal intensity on T2-weighted images and occasionally also high signal intensity on T1-weighted sequences (Figure 28-15).

Congenital Anomalies

Congenital anomalies of the female reproductive tract occur in 0.1% to 0.5% of all women. However, the incidence is higher, perhaps 9%, in women with infertility or fetal loss. Renal anomalies, particularly renal agenesis or ectopia, are frequently associated[20,21] (Figure 28-16). The fallopian tubes, uterus, cervix, and upper third of the vagina derive from the paired müllerian ducts. During the first two months of fetal life, the müllerian ducts migrate caudally and fuse. By the ninth week the sinovaginal bulb has migrated cephalad, joining the müllerian ducts to complete formation of the vagina, and by the eighteenth week of embryogenesis, recanalization of the female reproductive tract has occurred.[102] The ovaries arise separately from the müllerian ducts. Lack of development, fusion, or recanalization of the müllerian ducts may lead to developmental abnormalities. Because the lower third of the vagina develops separately, the external genitalia may be normal despite anomalous development of the internal female reproductive tract. The most commonly accepted classification of uterine congenital anomalies is presented in Box 28-1.[20] Uterine anomalies may result in infertility, re-

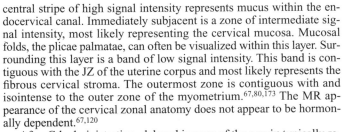

BOX 28-1
Classification of Müllerian Anomalies*

I. Segmental müllerian agenesis or hypoplasia
II. Unicornuate uterus
    A. With rudimentary horn
    B. Without rudimentary horn
III. Uterus didelphys
IV. Bicornuate uterus
    A. Complete (down to internal os)
    B. Partial
    C. Arcuate
V. Septate uterus
    A. Complete (down to internal os)
    B. Partial
VI. Diethylstilbestrol-related

From reference 20.
*Vaginal/cervical/septa or transverse septations causing obstruction may be associated.

peated spontaneous abortion, premature labor, or fetal malpresentation, although patients with uterus didelphys may be completely asymptomatic and without reproductive dysfunction.[20,58] Management of the different uterine anomalies varies considerably, and precise preoperative diagnosis is essential.

Hysterosalpingography (HSG) is routinely used to evaluate the infertile patient because it is the best means of assessing tubal patency and uterine synechiae (Asherman's syndrome). However, HSG is of limited value in classifying uterine anomalies. Neither the external contour of the uterine fundus (the most important feature for distinguishing the septate from bicornuate uterus) nor noncommunicating (obstructed) uterine horns are visualized on HSG (Figures 28-17 and 28-18). Even with endovaginal ultrasound (EVUS) it is not always possible to visualize the contour of the uterine fundus[153]; it is also not possible to evaluate for associated septa in the cervix or vagina. The presence of leiomyoma and/or adnexal masses may also limit US evaluation.[115]

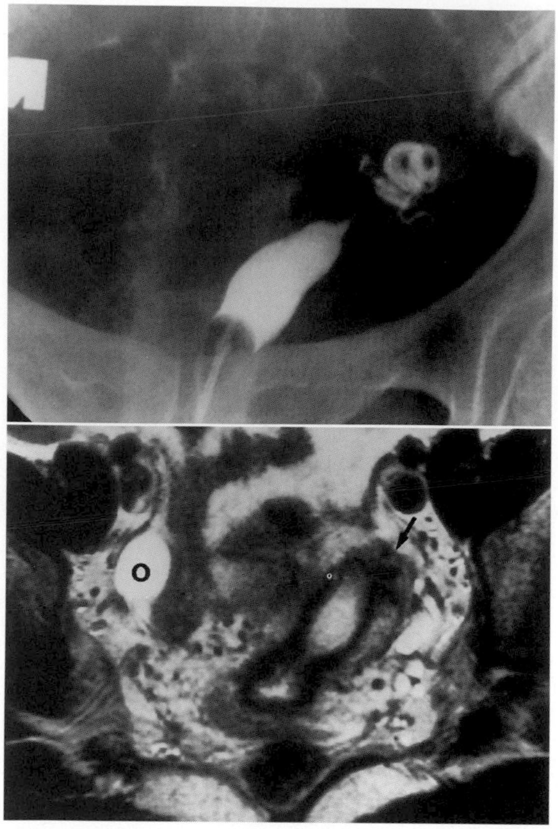

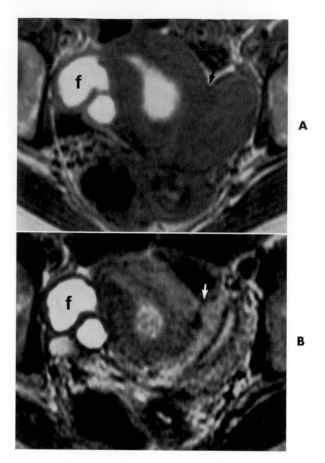

FIGURE 28-17   Unicornuate uterus. **A,** HSG demonstrates a single uterine horn with a patent left fallopian tube. This HSG is compatible with either a unicornuate uterus or a duplicated uterus with unilateral obstruction. **B,** Axial T2-weighted image demonstrates banana-shaped single uterine horn *(arrow). O,* Right ovarian cyst.

FIGURE 28-18   Bicornuate uterus. T1-weighted **(A)** and T2-weighted **(B)** images show an obstructed right horn. In **A,** a cleft *(arrow)* exists between the two uterine horns. The right horn and fallopian tube *(f)* are dilated and obstructed. High signal intensity on both T1- and T2-weighted pulse sequences is consistent with the presence of blood (hematometria and hemosalpinx). Increased signal intensity of the right myometrium in **B** is consistent with edema.

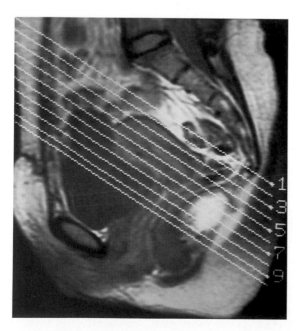

FIGURE 28-19   Oblique coronal images parallel to the long axis of the uterus, as indicated here, should be obtained in all patients when evaluating for suspected uterine anomalies.

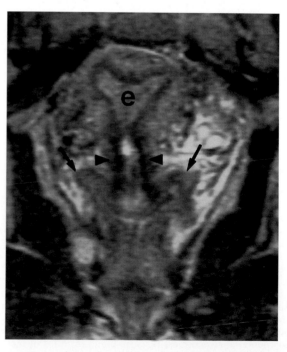

FIGURE 28-20   Arcuate uterus. Coronal image demonstrates heart-shaped endometrial cavity *(e). Arrowheads,* cervix; *arrows,* vaginal fornices.

Both the external contour of the uterus as well as the internal zonal anatomy of the female reproductive tract are well depicted on MRI, enabling highly accurate diagnosis and classification of uterine and vaginal congenital anomalies. In addition, MRI is an excellent means of evaluating other pelvic pathology, such as adenomyosis, leiomyomas, endometriosis, and hydrosalpinx, which may also contribute to reproductive dysfunction. Standard axial and coronal imaging planes should not be used because of the wide variability in uterine flexion. Rather, an oblique "coronal" plane parallel to the long axis of the uterus (endometrial cavity) and an oblique "axial" sequence perpendicular to the long axis of the uterus should be obtained (Figure 28-19). T2-weighted images are required for optimal evaluation of the zonal anatomy, whereas a "coronal" T1-weighted sequence through the uterine fundus is best for evaluating the fundal contour. In addition, a standard T1-weighted coronal sequence through the renal fossa should be obtained to evaluate the possibility of associated renal anomalies.

A unicornuate uterus is diagnosed by its elongated banana shape, quite unlike the triangular shape of the normal uterus[24,129] (Figure 28-17, *B*). MRI is clearly more accurate than EVUS for diagnosing the unicornuate uterus.[105] An arcuate uterus has a heart-shaped endometrial cavity. The fundus may be flattened, and the partial septum contains myometrium[24] (Figure 28-20). Uterus didelphys is diagnosed when two separate uteri and cervixes are visualized. Hematosalpinx or hematometra may develop in any uterine anomaly if segmental hypoplasia or a transverse septation obstructs outflow of blood into the vagina. Obstructed müllerian anomalies have the highest incidence of associated renal anomalies. MRI will demonstrate a dilated uterine horn distended with material, exhibiting signal characteristics consistent with hemorrhage (Figure 28-18). However, it is easy to overlook incomplete septations or longitudinal vaginal septations because of partial voluming.[24,45,129] It may also be difficult to distinguish a double cervix from a cervical septation[128] (Figure 28-21). Vaginal septations are most commonly associated with uterus didelphys.

The external contour of the uterine fundus is the pivotal feature differentiating the septate and bicornuate uterus. A septate uterus has a smooth or minimally indented fundal contour (<1 cm), whereas a definitive fundal notch is present in a bicornuate uterus. In a recent study, HSG was found to have an accuracy of only 55% in distinguishing septate from bicornuate uteri. In this study the diagnosis of a septate uterus was made if the angle of divergence between the two uterine horns was 75 degrees or less. The diagnostic accuracy improved to 90% if US findings were included.[162] Traditionally, laparoscopy has been the only reliable method of differentiating between these two entities. However, several studies have demonstrated that the uterine fundal contour is accurately depicted on MRI, allowing precise diagnosis[24,45,153] (Figures 28-22 and 28-23). Hence preoperative MRI may obviate the need for laparoscopic diagnosis, thereby markedly diminishing health care costs. It should be noted that the composition of the septum between the uter-

ine horns is not a differential feature, since fibrous tissue and/or myometrium may be found in both entities.

Accurate differentiation between the septate and bicornuate uterus is very important for patient management. The septate uterus is associated with a higher rate of reproductive failure (up to 67%)[21] but may be repaired via hysteroscopic metroplasty.[46,205] Although the bicornuate uterus is less often a cause of fetal loss, repair requires a transabdominal approach because of the risk of perforating the myometrium. Advantages to hysteroscopic repair include decreased hospitalization and recovery time, less invasive surgery, and a shorter delay before conception can be safely attempted, as well as the possibility of future vaginal delivery.[46] Recent research suggests that hysteroscopic metroplasty may be safely attempted without significant risk of uterine perforation even in the bicornuate uterus (i.e., a uterus with a fundal notch) if the

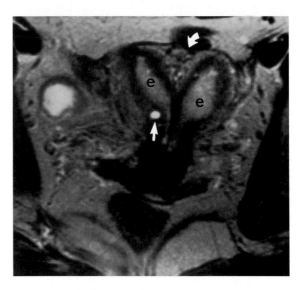

FIGURE 28-22   Septate uterus. The septum *(curved arrow)* between the two uterine horns *(e)* contains tissue isointense to myometrium. The uterine fundal contour is smooth and flat and without indentation *(curved arrow)*. Incidental note is made of a high–signal intensity subendometrial cyst *(straight arrow)*.

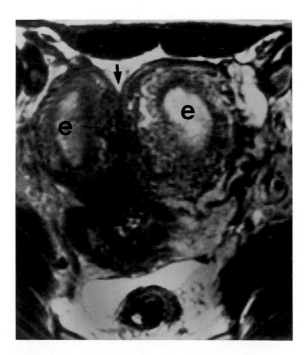

FIGURE 28-23   Bicornuate uterus. Note the cleft *(arrow)* between the two uterine horns on this axial T2-weighted image. *e*, Endometrium.

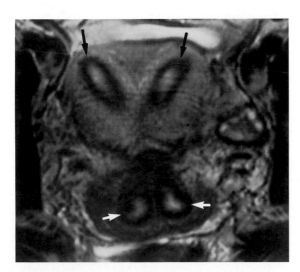

FIGURE 28-21   Septate uterus with two cervixes. There are two uterine horns *(black arrows)* with a smooth, convex uterine fundus. Two cervixes *(white arrows)* are also seen.

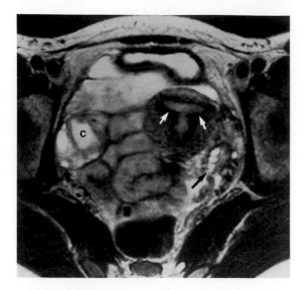

FIGURE 28-24   DES exposure in utero. Note T shape of endometrial canal *(white arrows)* and irregularity of the JZ. *Black arrow,* Left ovary; *c,* dominant cyst in right ovary.

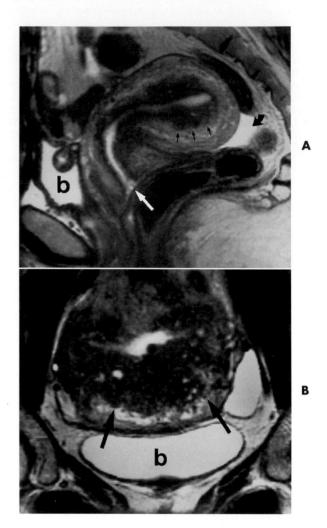

FIGURE 28-25   Diffuse adenomyosis. **A,** T2-weighted sagittal image. Note the diffuse, irregular thickening of the JZ *(small arrows)* with several small focal areas of increased signal intensity. The endocervical canal is well seen *(white arrow). b,* Bladder; *curved arrow,* fluid in cul-de-sac. **B,** Coronal FSE T2-weighted image of a different patient with diffuse adenomyosis. The JZ *(arrows)* is thickened and irregular and contains numerous small high–signal intensity cystic areas. *b,* Bladder.

deepest portion of the cleft is at least 5 mm above a line connecting the tubal ostia.[46]

Uterine anomalies have been reported to be present in up to 50% of women exposed in utero to DES, a synthetic estrogen used until 1970 to prevent miscarriage in women with bleeding in the first trimester. Associated anomalies include hypoplasia, T-shaped uterus, contractions, and marginal irregularities of the endometrial cavity[44] and result in an increased incidence of early reproductive loss.[58] HSG has been the standard imaging modality used to document these abnormalities. However, in a small series, van Gils et al[207] reported that MRI can document all but the subtle margin irregularities associated with DES exposure (Figure 28-24). In their series, focal thickening of the JZ was noted to correspond to the constrictions of the uterine cavity seen on HSG.[207] Renal anomalies are not associated with DES-related uterine malformations. The etiology of Asherman's syndrome, intrauterine endometrial adhesions, is generally considered to be trauma to the postgravid endometrium. An increased incidence of Asherman's syndrome has been reported in women with congenital uterine anomalies, perhaps because of the increased rate of spontaneous abortions.[101] On T2-weighted images, attenuation and irregularity of the endometrium and JZ have been described.[7]

MRI may also be useful in evaluating patients with ambiguous genitalia. Accurate assessment of internal genitalia is an important part of assigning gender and in evaluating the child for corrective surgery. The earlier these decisions are made, the less the psychosocial impact. Localization of the gonads is also important because of the risk of neoplasm. Two series have been reported indicating that MRI is highly accurate in detecting uterus, vagina, testes, and penis in these children. MRI has been less successful in identifying the ovaries because it is difficult to identify small streak ovaries.[161,175]

Adenomyosis

Adenomyosis is defined as the presence of heterotopic endometrium located within the myometrium, most likely a result of direct invasion of the basal endometrium into the myometrium. The cause for this migration is not known. The cyclical hemorrhage of normally functioning endometrium is infrequently observed because the basalis endometrium is typically resistant to hormonal stimulation. The surrounding smooth muscle hypertrophies in a coarse, trabecular pattern and interdigitates with the normal smooth muscle of the myometrium without forming a well-defined border or capsule.[136] Adenomyosis may be microscopic, focal, or diffuse.

Patients most commonly have pelvic pain, menorrhagia, an enlarged uterus,[136] or a combination thereof, although adenomyosis in many is asymptomatic.[160] Although adenomyosis is most frequently diagnosed

in multiparous, premenopausal women, the exact incidence is unknown, with reported estimates ranging from 20% to 65%.[136] The signs and symptoms are nonspecific, mimicking those of leiomyomas or dysfunctional uterine bleeding. However, establishing the correct diagnosis is essential, since the treatment of these three entities differs markedly. The definitive treatment of adenomyosis requires hysterectomy, whereas leiomyomas may be successfully treated with uterus-conserving myomectomy and dysfunctional uterine bleeding with dilatation and curettage (D&C).

Adenomyosis results in thickening, either focal or diffuse, of the JZ on T2-weighted images. The exact width at which the JZ is considered to be abnormal has been variably reported as greater than 5 mm[3,116] and as greater than 12 mm[160] (Figure 28-25). On T2-weighted images, focal adenomyosis appears as an ill-defined, poorly marginated area of low signal intensity within the myometrium but contiguous with the JZ.[3,116,160,198] An ill-defined border is the hallmark of focal adenomyosis, distinguishing adenomyoma from leiomyoma[116,198] (Figure 28-26). However, small leiomyomas (<2 to 3 cm in diameter) may have ill-defined borders,[198] and adenomyomas misclassified as leiomyoma have

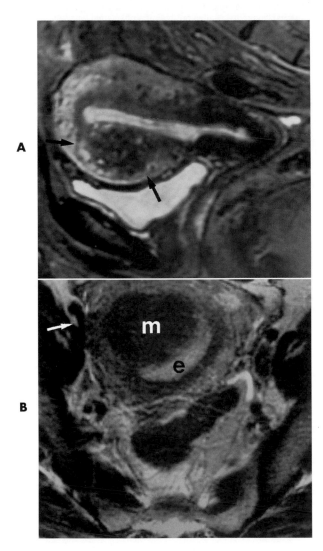

FIGURE 28-26   Focal adenomyosis. **A,** Note focal, irregular thickening of the JZ *(arrows)* on this T2-weighted sagittal image. The outer margin is indistinct. **B,** In comparison an intramural leiomyoma *(m)* deviates the endometrial canal *(e)* on an axial T2-weighted image. The outer margin is sharply demarcated. This patient had swelling of the right leg. Note compression of the right external iliac vein *(white arrow)*.

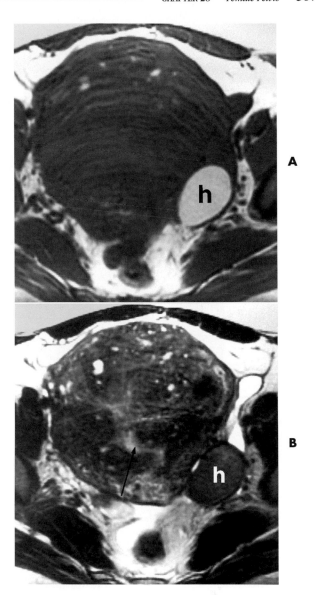

FIGURE 28-27   Diffuse adenomyosis. T1-weighted **(A)** and T2-weighted **(B)** images reveal diffuse, uneven thickening of the JZ and distortion of the endometrial canal *(arrow* in **B**). Punctate areas of high signal intensity on both the T1- and T2-weighted images are small focal areas of hemorrhage. *h,* Left hemorrhagic ovarian cyst.

also been reported.[3] Small punctate areas of increased signal intensity on T2-weighted images may be seen. These have been shown to correspond to small foci of hemorrhage on pathological correlation when also bright on T1-weighted sequences[201] (Figure 28-27). Microscopic foci of adenomyosis are not demonstrable on MRI.[116]

Although diagnostic criteria have differed slightly, several studies have reported that MRI is highly accurate in diagnosing adenomyosis, particularly in symptomatic women or those with uterine enlargement.[3,116,160,198,201] Ascher et al[3] reported that MRI is more accurate than US (*p* <0.02) in identifying women with pathologically proven adenomyosis. Thickening of the JZ more than 5 mm was diagnostic of adenomyosis in this series. However, others report that EVUS is equally sensitive and specific as MRI for diagnosing adenomyosis.[160] Using thickening of the JZ greater than 12 mm as a discriminatory value, MRI had a sensitivity of 86% and a positive predictive value (PPV) of 65%. Most patients were asymptomatic in this series.[160] The ability of MRI to depict the depth of endometrial penetration in women with adenomyosis may help guide patient management. In a small series, patients with superficial adenomyosis had good results with rollerball endome-

trial ablation. The authors postulate that hysterectomy may be required only for deep adenomyosis.[122]

Leiomyomas

Leiomyomas are the most common uterine tumor, occurring in 20% to 30% of premenopausal women, with a significantly increased incidence in black women.[34,136] Leiomyomas are benign, well-circumscribed smooth muscle cell neoplasms and are sharply demarcated from the surrounding myometrium. The smooth muscle cells are arranged in a whorl-like pattern with a variable amount of collagen, extracellular matrix, and fibrous tissue. Leiomyomas may be submucosal, intramural, subserosal, or cervical in location. Rarely, a leiomyoma may be found in the broad ligament or even detached from the uterus, parasitizing its blood supply from another organ or the omentum.[136] Leiomyomas are estrogen-dependent tumors and therefore usually decrease in size after menopause but may increase in size during pregnancy. Leiomyomas often calcify (particularly in postmenopausal women), and large tumors may develop hyaline, myxomatous, cystic, or hemorrhage degenera-

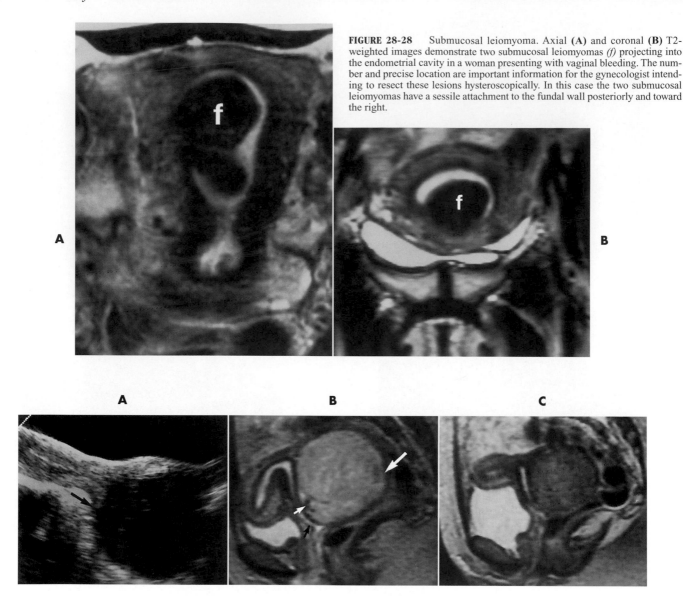

FIGURE 28-28 Submucosal leiomyoma. Axial **(A)** and coronal **(B)** T2-weighted images demonstrate two submucosal leiomyomas *(f)* projecting into the endometrial cavity in a woman presenting with vaginal bleeding. The number and precise location are important information for the gynecologist intending to resect these lesions hysteroscopically. In this case the two submucosal leiomyomas have a sessile attachment to the fundal wall posteriorly and toward the right.

FIGURE 28-29 Cervical leiomyoma. Sagittal US *(black arrow)* **(A)** and MRI *(white arrow)* **(B)** show stalk (small white arrow) and exact relationship to the endocervical canal *(small black arrow)* are well seen on MR. After 6 months of GnRH analog therapy **(C)**, both the cervical leiomyomas and the uterine corpus have decreased in size. (From reference 222.)

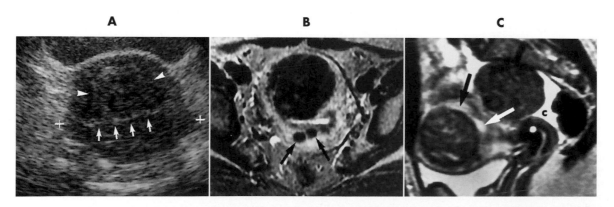

FIGURE 28-30 Leiomyoma. **A,** Axial transabdominal US demonstrates enlarged inhomogeneous uterus. Above the endometrial stripe *(arrows)* is an ill-defined mass within the myometrium *(arrowheads)*. **B,** Axial T2-weighted MRI demonstrates a large intramural leiomyoma in the anterior wall of the uterus. Two small intramural leiomyomas (missed by US) can be seen in the posterior wall *(arrows)*. **C,** Sagittal T2-weighted MRI demonstrates a subserosal leiomyoma arising from the posterior surface of the uterus and an intramural fundal leiomyoma displacing the endometrial stripe *(arrows)* posteriorly. A nabothian cyst is near the internal os, and fluid is in the cul-de-sac *(c)*.

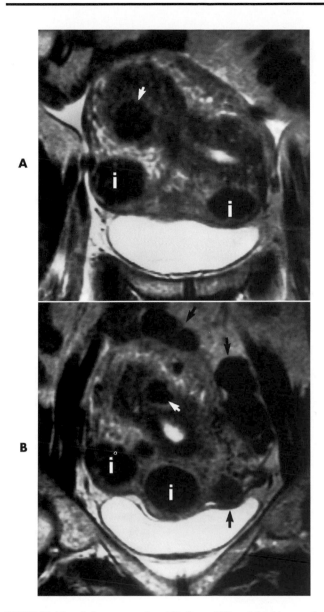

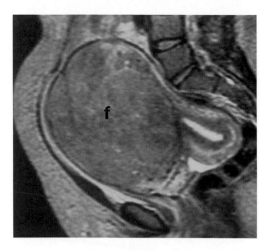

FIGURE 28-32 Cervical leiomyoma *(f)* nearly fills the pelvis on this T2-weighted sagittal image. The uterine corpus is retroverted, and there is a small amount of fluid in the cul-de-sac.

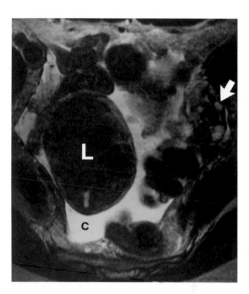

FIGURE 28-31 Leiomyomas. **A** and **B,** Coronal T2-weighted images demonstrating submucosal *(white arrow),* intramural *(i),* and subserosal *(black arrows)* fibroids.

FIGURE 28-33 Broad ligament leiomyoma appears as low–signal intensity right adnexal mass *(L)* on this T2-weighted axial image. This was mistaken for a solid ovarian mass on physical examination. *Arrow,* Left ovary; *c,* fluid in cul-de-sac.

tion. Torsion, infection, and sarcomatous degeneration are infrequent complications.[34,136]

Although intramural leiomyomas are most common, submucosal leiomyomas are most often symptomatic. Menorrhagia, dysmenorrhea, infertility, habitual abortions in the second trimester, and pelvic pain or pressure are the most frequent presenting symptoms. Symptoms are related to location. For example, menorrhagia is most frequently associated with submucosal lesions, whereas a leiomyoma that distorts the endometrial cavity or blocks the oviducts may be the cause of habitual abortion or infertility.[136] A pedunculated subserosal leiomyoma may be mistaken for an ovarian mass or cause pelvic pain and pressure. A cervical leiomyoma may cause dyspareunia or interfere with vaginal delivery.

In patients wishing to preserve fertility, myomectomy is increasingly performed as an alternative to hysterectomy. Submucosal leiomyomas may be resected hysteroscopically, but laparoscopic or transabdominal myomectomy is required for intramural or subserosal lesions. Consequently, knowledge of the exact location and size of these lesions is extremely important for patient management (Figure 28-28). Medical therapy with GnRH analog is also available to shrink leiomyomas[54,222] (Figure 28-29). However, patients may develop osteoporosis after long-term therapy, and leiomyomas may rebound after medication is discontinued.

Ultrasound remains the initial imaging modality of choice for patients with suspected leiomyomas. The diagnostic criteria have been well described and include uterine contour abnormality, uterine enlargement, and focal alterations in echotexture.[61,210] However, US is neither as sensitive nor as specific as MRI.[213,224] Even retrospectively, US may be completely normal in up to 22% of patients with leiomyomas.[61] Also US is generally unable to precisely localize leiomyomas or identify lesions smaller than 2 cm in size. In addition, US may not be able to differentiate leiomyomas from adnexal masses, congenital anomalies, or adenomyosis.[61] Although EVUS increases the sensitivity and specificity of US in both identifying and localizing leiomyomas, the limited field of view on EVUS hampers evaluation of the markedly enlarged uterus.[124]

MRI is the most accurate imaging technique for the detection and localization of leiomyomas.* On T2-weighted images, leiomyomas usually appear as sharply marginated homogeneous areas of decreased signal intensity (Figure 28-30). Lesions as small as 0.3 cm may be identified. Leiomyomas can easily be classified as submucosal, intramural, subserosal, or cervical in location (Figures 28-28 and 28-30 through 38-33). MRI may be used to identify prolapsed submucosal leiomy-

*References 42, 83, 124, 201, 213, 224.

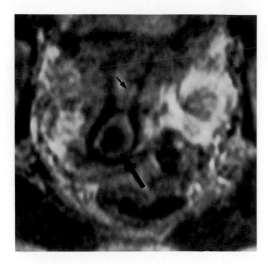

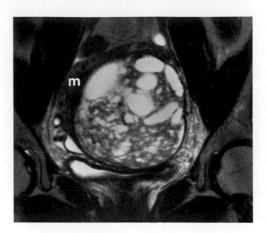

FIGURE 28-34   Prolapsed leiomyoma. Axial T2-weighted image demonstrates a low–signal intensity mass within the endocervical canal *(long arrow)* and attached by a long, thin stalk or pedicle *(short arrow)* to the mucosal surface of the uterine fundus.

FIGURE 28-35   Cystic degeneration of a leiomyoma. Note the focal areas of increased signal intensity. *m,* Myometrium. Coronal T2-weighted image.

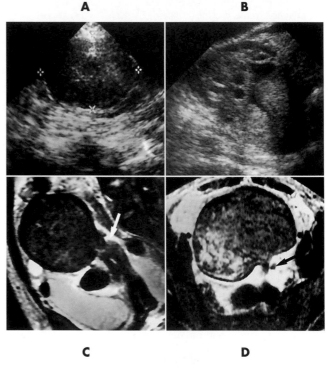

FIGURE 28-36   Acute torsion of pedunculated subserosal leiomyoma. US examination reveals an unremarkable subserosal fundal leiomyoma **(A)** and free pelvic fluid **(B)** in a patient with a known leiomyoma and acute onset of pelvic pain. T2-weighted sagittal **(C)** and axial **(D)** MR scans demonstrate a large pedunculated subserosal leiomyoma, which has undergone torsion around its pedicle *(arrow).* Areas of high signal intensity are consistent with necrosis. A large portion of the leiomyoma was infarcted at the time of surgery.

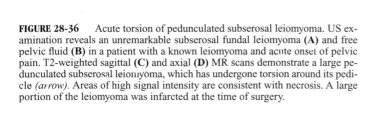

FIGURE 28-37   Acute hemorrhagic necrosis of a uterine leiomyoma. Patient with a known large leiomyoma developed acute postpartum pain. Sagittal US **(A)** demonstrates several hypoechoic areas consistent with fluid and necrosis within a fundal leiomyoma. On MR examination, intramural leiomyoma demonstrates high signal intensity on both axial T1-weighted **(B)** and sagittal T2-weighted **(C)** sequences, which is consistent with the presence of subacute hemorrhage. At surgery, the patient was found to have hemorrhagic necrosis of a large intramural leiomyoma.

omas. Prospective localization of the stalk may aid in hysteroscopic resection[149] (Figure 28-34). A high–signal intensity rim representing a combination of dilated lymphatics, veins, or edema has been reported to surround some intramural leiomyomas.[132] Lesions larger than 3 to 5 cm may have heterogeneous areas of increased signal intensity representing degeneration (Figure 28-35). However, MRI cannot accurately differentiate among hyaline, myxomatous, and cystic degeneration,[83] although areas of hemorrhagic degeneration would be expected to demonstrate increased signal intensity on T1-weighted images. MRI may also be useful in identifying unusual complications of leiomyomas, such as torsion (Figure 28-36), acute hemorrhagic necrosis (Figure 28-37), and increased vascularity (Figure 28-38). The appearance of leiomyomas after the administration of Gd is quite variable. However, most often, leiomyomas heterogeneously (76%) enhance less than the surrounding myometrium (65%) and remain well marginated (67%).[82]

Occasionally, atypical features may be present. Cellular leiomyomas have been reported to demonstrate diffuse, relatively homogeneous increased signal intensity on T2-weighted images[63,145,217] (Figure 28-31). Malignant degeneration occurs rarely (0.1% to 0.6%) but should be suspected if a leiomyoma enlarges suddenly, especially after menopause,[136] or if an indistinct border or irregular contour is noted on MRI.[152]

Endometrial Polyps

Endometrial polyps are found in approximately 10% to 24% of hysterectomy specimens.[136] They may be sessile or pedunculated and are usually attached to the uterine fundus. Endometrial polyps are localized hyperplastic overgrowths of endometrial glands and stroma. They are almost always benign; invasive carcinoma is found in less than 0.6%.[136] Polyps present most commonly in the fourth to sixth decade with vaginal spotting,[136] and there may be an increased incidence of polyp formation in women on tamoxifen therapy.

On T2-weighted images an endometrial polyp may be suspected when the endometrial cavity is distended by an intermediate signal mass, particularly if a linear low-signal area is seen peripherally, most likely representing fibrous tissue within the pedunculated stalk (Figures 28-39 and 28-11). The normal uterine zonal anatomy will be preserved. Contrast enhancement has been reported to improve the sensitivity of MRI for the detection of endometrial polyps[82] (Figure 28-11). Generally, polyps enhance less than the surrounding endometrium. However, these findings are nonspecific, and it is not always possible to differentiate polyps from submucosal leiomyomas or noninvasive endometrial carcinoma.

Endometrial Carcinoma

Endometrial carcinoma is the most common invasive carcinoma of the female reproductive tract and the fourth most common cancer in women in the United States. The American Cancer Society predicts that 36,100 new cases of endometrial carcinoma will be diagnosed in 1998, and that 6300 cancer-related deaths will occur.[151] There has been a threefold increase in the incidence of endometrial carcinoma over the last 30 years. Risk factors include obesity, multiparity, unopposed exogenous estrogen replacement therapy, late-onset menopause, diabetes mellitus, anovulatory cycling, polycystic ovaries, and adenomatous hyperplasia. White upper-class women are also at increased risk. Prolonged estrogen exposure unopposed by progesterone may explain many of these risk factors.[32,169]

Adenocarcinomas account for 90% to 95% of all endometrial carcinomas. Papillary serous carcinomas, adenoacanthomas, adenosquamous carcinomas, and clear cell carcinomas are much less common. Endometrial carcinoma initially invades the myometrium and then the endocervix. After transserosal spread, direct invasion of the parametrium, bladder, or bowel occurs. Lymphangitic spread to pelvic and paraaortic lymph nodes is frequent. Metastases to paraaortic lymph nodes may occur without pelvic lymph node involvement if the tumor spreads via the lymphatics accompanying the ovarian vessels. Hematogenous and intraperitoneal spread is rarer, with the lung and peritoneal surfaces of the upper abdomen being the most frequent sites of distant metastases. Metastases also may occur to liver, bone, and brain.[169] The uterus (if not surgically removed) and vaginal apex are the most common sites of local recurrence, which occurs most often within the first 3 years.[169] Papillary serous and clear cell carcinomas have a worse prognosis than adenocarcinomas. Papillary serous carcinoma has a biological behavior similar to that of ovarian carcinoma.[32]

The peak incidence of endometrial carcinoma occurs between the ages of 55 and 65.[32,169] Most women come to medical attention early in the course of their disease with abnormal or postmenopausal vaginal bleeding, and the condition is rapidly diagnosed using D&C. Endometrial carcinoma is staged according to the FIGO staging system (Table 28-2), which is now a surgical staging system.[35] The prognosis is largely related to the nuclear grade, depth of myometrial invasion, stage of tumor, and presence of lymph node metastases. Both higher nuclear grade and greater than 50% myometrial invasion are associated with an increased incidence of pelvic and paraaortic lymph node metastases as well as relapse.[14,15,32,33] Tumors reaching 5 mm of the serosal surface have also been reported to have a worse prognosis.[113] The 5-year survival rate for stage IA G1 tumors is 95%, and it is 64% for G3 tumors. For stage 1C disease the 5-year survival rate is 33% for G1 and 25% for G3 tumors.[141] Cervical extension, particularly cervical stromal invasion, also worsens the prognosis. The 5-year survival rate is 52% to 83% for stage II tumors, but it is much worse for stage IIB than stage IIA tumors. The overall 5-year survival rate for stage III disease is 30%. The prognosis for stage IV tumors is universally poor.[32]

Although treatment protocols vary across the United States, and the tumors are now surgically staged, some clinicians feel that preopera-

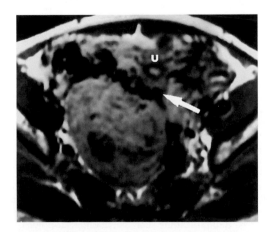

FIGURE 28-38 Vascular leiomyoma. T2-weighted MR scan demonstrates a large subserosal leiomyoma posterior to the uterus *(u)*. A pedicle or connection to the uterus is seen *(arrow)*. Serpiginous channels of low signal intensity anterior to the leiomyoma are consistent with feeding vessels. The surgeon elected to treat the patient for 6 months with GnRH analog therapy to decrease the vascularity and size of the leiomyoma before attempting surgery.

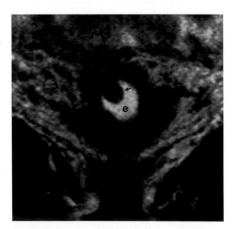

FIGURE 28-39 Endometrial polyp. Coronal T2-weighted MRI reveals a low–signal intensity mass *(arrow)* arising from the endometrium in the lower uterine segment in this woman with irregular vaginal bleeding. *e,* Endometrial cavity.

Table 28-2   FIGO Staging System for Endometrial Carcinoma

STAGE*		PATHOLOGY
I		Carcinoma confined to uterine corpus
	A	Tumor limited to endometrium
	B	Tumor invasion through <50% myometrial thickness
	C	Tumor invasion through >50% myometrial thickness
II		Cervical invasion
	A	Endocervical glandular involvement only
	B	Cervical stromal invasion
III		Invasion of true pelvis
	A	Invasion of serosa, adnexa, or positive peritoneal cytology
	B	Vaginal metastases
	C	Metastases to pelvic or paraaortic lymph nodes
IV		Extension beyond true pelvis
	A	Invasion of bladder or bowel mucosa
	B	Distant metastases, including intraabdominal or inguinal metastases

From reference 35.
*All stages further subdivided by tumor histological grade: G1, G2, or G3.

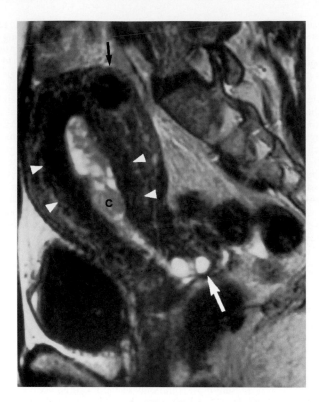

FIGURE 28-40   Stage IA endometrial carcinoma. A heterogeneous mass *(c)* distends the endometrial cavity, including the lower uterine segment, on this sagittal T2-weighted image. However, the JZ *(arrowheads)* is intact. Pathological examination revealed well-differentiated endometrial carcinoma without myometrial invasion. Several nabothian cysts *(white arrow)* are present on the posterior lip of the cervix. *Black arrow,* Intramural leiomyoma.

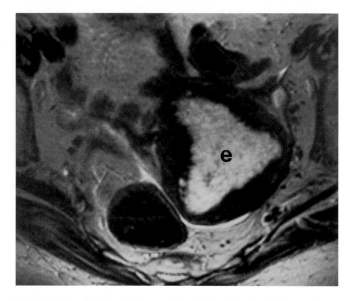

FIGURE 28-41   Endometrial hyperplasia. T2-weighted axial image demonstrates a distended endometrial canal *(e),* but no discrete mass is seen in this patient with endometrial hyperplasia. The JZ is intact.

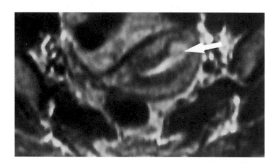

FIGURE 28-42   Stage IB endometrial carcinoma. Axial T2-weighted image demonstrates a mass of intermediate signal intensity focally disrupting the left lateral aspect of the JZ and extending through approximately 40% of the myometrium *(arrow).*

tive knowledge of the depth of myometrial invasion, cervical involvement, or both factors would potentially alter patient management. In the presence of deep (>50%) myometrial or cervical stromal invasion, preoperative intracavity radiation therapy or more extensive paraaortic lymph node sampling could be planned.

On contrast-enhanced computed tomography (CT) the typical appearance of endometrial carcinoma as a hypodense mass within the endometrial cavity is neither sensitive nor specific and can be mimicked by leiomyomas, endometrial polyps, or cervical stenosis.[209] The depth of myometrial invasion cannot be assessed. However, CT accurately demonstrates extrauterine spread of disease.[9,209] Numerous studies have addressed the potential of EVUS to assess the depth of myometrial invasion. The presence of an endometrial mass disrupting the subendometrial halo or extending asymmetrically into the myometrium has been reported to indicate myometrial invasion, whereas an intact subendometrial halo suggests superficial disease.[37,59,211] However, both overdiagnosis and underdiagnosis are reported.[37,59] US is not accurate in assessing cervical or parametrial invasion.

Because most endometrial carcinomas are diagnosed by D&C, the normal appearance of the uterus after this procedure is important. After uncomplicated D&C, clot characteristically appears as a linear area of signal void, and the typical appearance of the uterine zonal anatomy is not disrupted.[6] The MR appearance of noninvasive endometrial carcinoma, stage 1A, is nonspecific. The uterus may appear entirely normal, or the endometrial stripe may appear homogeneously widened (>8 mm in postmenopausal women). Alternatively, a heterogeneous mass may be noted distending the endometrial cavity (Figure 28-40). The JZ or endometrial–myometrial interface will be smooth and intact.[75,107,182,219] Benign lesions such as endometrial polyps, adenomatous hyperplasia, and even hemorrhage have been reported to have a similar appearance[75] (Figure 28-41). Therefore MRI has no role as a screening technique. The accuracy of MR in differentiating noninvasive (stage 1A) from invasive endometrial carcinoma has been reported to range from 74% to 85%.[75,81,182,183] Specificity as high as 97%[183] has been reported, although excluding microscopic invasion is difficult.

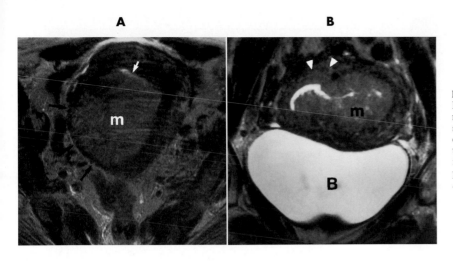

FIGURE 28-43   Stage IC endometrial carcinoma. **A,** Axial FSE T2-weighted image demonstrates a large mass of intermediate signal *(m)* extending to within millimeters of the serosal surface *(black arrows). White arrow,* Endometrial canal. **B,** On a coronal T2-weighted image, a mass *(m)* of intermediate signal intensity is seen within the endometrial cavity on the left in another patient. The JZ is disrupted in several places, with the tumor approaching the serosal surface *(arrowheads). B,* Bladder.

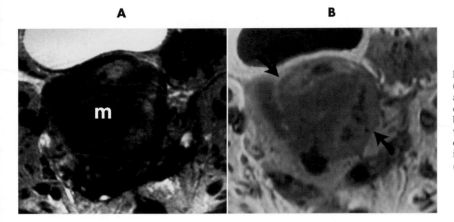

FIGURE 28-44   Invasive (>50%) endometrial carcinoma (stage IC). T2-weighted MRI **(A)** shows that the uterine zonal anatomy is obliterated. Margins of the mass *(m)* are difficult to define, and the exact depth of the myometrial invasion cannot be ascertained. After the administration of intravenous Gd, T1-weighted MRI **(B)** demonstrates heterogeneous enhancement of the uterine mass consistent with necrosis. Deep myometrial invasion nearly to the serosal surface is more easily identified *(arrows).*

When myometrial invasion occurs (stages 1B and 1C), the intermediate–signal intensity tumor will be noted on T2-weighted images to disrupt the JZ or the endometrial–myometrial interface and invade the myometrium.* The percentage of wall thickness invaded by the mass is easily calculated, allowing patients to be separated into those with stage 1B (<50% myometrial wall invasion) disease or those with stage 1C (>50% myometrial wall invasion) disease (Figures 28-42 and 28-43). Studies have indicated that the accuracy of MRI in distinguishing deep invasion (stage 1C) from superficial disease (stages 1A and 1B) ranges from 75% to 95%.† In these studies, an intact JZ has had close to a 100% negative predictive value (NPV) in excluding deep myometrial invasion. However, MRI is considerably less accurate when the myometrium is thinned because of distension of the endometrial cavity by polyp, polypoid tumor, pus, or blood; when the JZ is absent; or when the zonal anatomy is distorted by uterine anomalies or leiomyomas.‡

Several authors have reported that Gd contrast-enhanced T1-weighted images are more sensitive than T2-weighted images for detecting tumor, as well as more accurate for differentiating tumor from debris[74,183] and for assessing the depth of myometrial invasion[183,216] (Figure 28-44). Accuracy in assessing the depth of the myometrial invasion has been reported to be even higher (85% to 91%) with dynamic contrast-enhanced T1-weighted sequences than on T2-weighted or delayed contrast-enhanced sequences because of improved tumor myometrial contrast.[85,218] In general, endometrial carcinomas enhance later than normal endometrium. Hence on early phase-dynamic imaging, endometrial carcinomas will appear hypointense relative to endometrium. Early tumor enhancement may indicate more aggressive pathology.[96] In these series, the preservation of a smooth layer of subendometrial enhancement has been reported to be extremely accurate in excluding deep myometrial invasion.[21,85] However, only a small number of cases have been reported, and studies comparing contrast-enhanced T1-weighted images with FSE T2-weighted images using a dedicated pelvic multicoil have not been performed. MRI is reportedly more accurate than CT or US for detecting myometrial invasion.[92,216]

The superficial spread of endometrial carcinoma to endocervical glands, stage IIA, is indicated on T2-weighted images by distension of the endocervical canal with or without visualization of a mass. Invasion of the cervical stroma, stage IIB, is documented when the relatively high–signal intensity tumor mass disrupts the low signal intensity of the fibrous cervical stroma[12,75,182,219] (Figure 28-45). Although the number of reported cases is small, MRI is reported to be sensitive in detecting cervical invasion, occasionally establishing the diagnosis when physical examination and D&C are negative.[12,75,219] In addition, the NPV of MRI has been reported to be high. This is extremely important because the presence of cervical involvement substantially worsens the prognosis. However, false-positive results may occur when the cervical canal is merely distended with mass, debris, or clot, and false-negative results may occur when microscopic invasion is present. Gd-enhanced MRI is generally not helpful in evaluating cervical stromal involvement by endometrial cancer, since the normal cervical stroma enhances in a pattern indistinguishable from tumor enhancement.[68]

Although experience in the evaluation of stage III and IV disease on MRI is limited (Figure 28-46), extrauterine spread to the parametria, ovaries, bowel, bladder, lymph nodes, and vagina as well as ascites and pelvic implants has been documented.[26,75,219] When parametrial extension occurs, the tumor mass will be seen to penetrate the serosal surface, disrupting the normal signal intensity of the parametrial fat.[75] Ovarian spread is suggested when a mass of indeterminate signal intensity is noted in the ovary and occurs most commonly when the carcinoma is located near the cornua.[26,75] Peritoneal or omental implants are typically intermediate signal on T1-weighted images and high signal intensity on T2-weighted images.[26,75] The signal characteristics of lymph nodes are not predictive of tumor involvement. MRI, like CT,

*References 12, 26, 75, 107, 182, 219.

†References 26, 75, 81, 107, 182, 183.

‡References 107, 170, 182, 183, 216, 219.

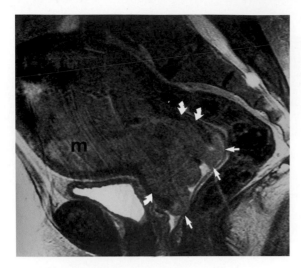

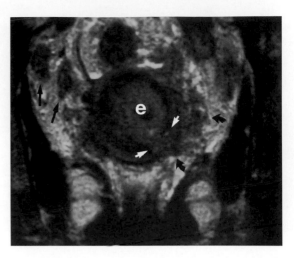

FIGURE 28-45   Stage IIB endometrial carcinoma. Sagittal FSE T2-weighted image demonstrates a large heterogeneous mass *(m)* invading the cervix *(curved arrows)* and prolapsing into the upper vagina *(straight arrows)*.

FIGURE 28-46   Coronal T2-weighted MRI shows a papillary serous carcinoma involving the lower uterine segment. The endometrial mass *(e)* disrupts the JZ *(white arrows)* and extends into the left parametria *(curved black arrows)*. Enlarged pelvic lymph nodes are noted as well *(straight black arrows)*.

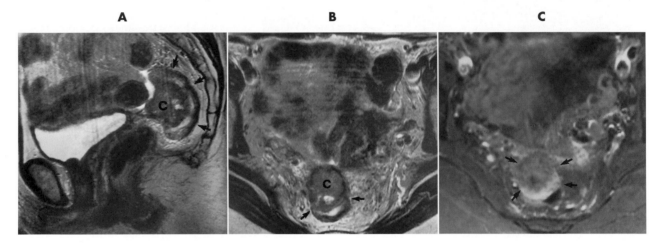

FIGURE 28-47   Recurrent endometrial carcinoma. **A** and **B,** T2-weighted MR images show a heterogeneous mass *(c)* invading the rectum and sigmoid colon *(arrows)*. **C,** T1-weighted, fat-suppressed, Gd-enhanced image shows irregular enhancement of the mass *(arrows)*.

must rely on size criteria, and lymph nodes larger than 1.5 cm are considered abnormal.[26,75,219] It is difficult to assess the PPV of MR findings of advanced endometrial carcinoma given the limited published experience. Certainly, enlarged lymph nodes may result from inflammation. However, MRI appears to have a high NPV in excluding advanced disease, although again, statistical analysis will invariably be skewed by the preponderance of reported cases with limited (stages I and II) disease. Furthermore, neither microscopic spread of disease nor small peritoneal and omental implants (<1 to 2 cm) would be expected to be visualized on MR examination, the latter because of limitations in spatial resolution secondary to motion artifact. MRI may be helpful in identifying recurrent disease (Figure 28-47).

Uterine Sarcomas

Uterine sarcomas account for only 2% to 6% of all uterine cancers. The three most common histological types are malignant mixed müllerian tumor (MMT, 40%), leiomyosarcoma (40%), and endometrial stromal sarcoma (10% to 15%).[112] Some 35% of patients with MMTs have a history of prior pelvic radiation. These are usually large polypoid tumors arising from the endometrial cavity. MMTs are more aggressive than endometrial carcinomas, and deep myometrial invasion is present in most cases.[112] Shapeero et al[177] reported a series of seven

patients with MMT, describing large polypoid tumors with deep myometrial invasion, similar in appearance on MRI to endometrial carcinoma.

Leiomyosarcomas most commonly occur in perimenopausal women and arise either de novo or from sarcomatous degeneration of a leiomyoma. Presenting symptoms are nonspecific: pelvic pain, vaginal bleeding, and pelvic mass. Rapid growth of leiomyoma or uterus, especially in a postmenopausal woman, should raise concern. The diagnosis can be made by D&C only if a component of the tumor is submucosal. Leiomyosarcomas spread first within the myometrium and later invade blood vessels, lymphatics, and contiguous pelvic structures. The lung is the most common site of distant metastases.[112] Experience on MRI is limited, but the presence of a heterogeneous myometrial mass with an indistinct border is worrisome.[152]

Primary lymphoma of the uterus is rare, although diffuse uterine infiltration may occur in advanced stages of generalized disease.[29] The preoperative diagnosis is rarely considered because of its rarity and nonspecific presenting symptoms. In a small series, the presence of diffuse or focal enlargement of the uterus exhibiting hyperintense signal intensity on T2-weighted images with preservation of the endometrium, cervical epithelium, or both structures was speculated to be a characteristic finding.[88] However, if only the cervix is involved, the hyperintense tumor can be indistinguishable from cervical carcinoma.[88]

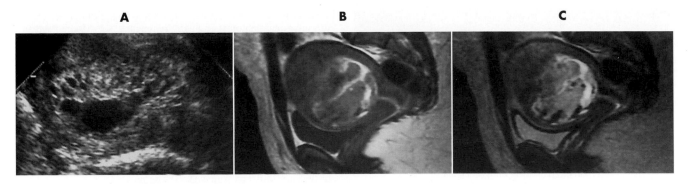

FIGURE 28-48   Hydatidiform mole. **A,** Transvaginal US shows distension of the endometrial cavity by a complex, echogenic mass containing several cystic or vesicular areas in a patient with an elevated serum β-hCG level. **B** and **C,** Heterogeneous high signal intensity on T1- and T2-weighted images indicates blood within the endometrial cavity, as well as the mass.

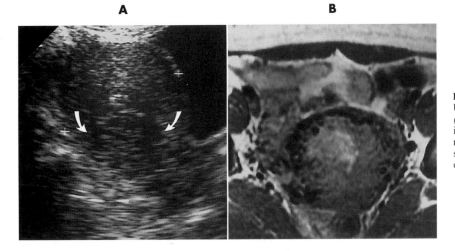

FIGURE 28-49   Persistent GTN. **A,** Sagittal transabdominal US demonstrates an ill-defined mass in the posterior wall *(curved arrows)* of the uterus. **B,** Axial intermediate-weighted image demonstrates increased vascularity within and surrounding the uterus. Centrally there is a mass of intermediate signal intensity with an ill-defined border invading the myometrium.

Gestational Trophoblastic Neoplasia

Gestational trophoblastic neoplasia (GTN) is the result of the excessive proliferation of villous trophoblastic tissue. The disease spectrum includes complete hydatidiform mole, partial hydatidiform mole, invasive mole, and choriocarcinoma. Complete hydatidiform mole is characterized by trophoblastic proliferation without the development of an embryo. Genetic material is entirely paternal. A partial mole generally contains embryonic or fetal tissue, and both mole and fetus exhibit a triploid karyotype with an extra paternal haploid set. Invasive moles are believed to develop from complete moles and are characterized by myometrial invasion. Choriocarcinoma, the most aggressive form of GTN, arises most commonly after a molar pregnancy but may follow any gestational event, including abortion or ectopic or term pregnancy. Metastases to the lung (80%), vagina (30%), pelvis (20%, usually as a result of local extension), liver, and brain may occur.[8,150]

The incidence of hydatidiform mole is 1 in 2000 live births in the United States but is reported to be as high as 1 in 80 live births in southeast Asia.[169] Although some degree of myometrial invasion is present in most hydatidiform moles, evacuation of the molar pregnancy results in cure in 70% to 90% of patients.[8,150] The serum β-human chorionic gonadotropin (β-hCG) level is a sensitive indicator of the presence of disease and has been the mainstay of patient follow-up and treatment planning. A rise or plateau of the serum β-hCG level after evacuation indicates persistent GTN. Patients who have large-for-date uteri, who have bilateral ovarian enlargement (>6 cm because of lutein cysts), who are older than 40 years old, or who have a serum β-hCG titer higher than 100,000 mIu/ml are at greatest risk to develop persistent GTN.[13] However, GTN is very sensitive to chemotherapy, and patients with invasive GTN or choriocarcinoma, even in the presence of metastases, have a cure rate of nearly 100% unless they are in the high-risk category. Liver or brain metastases, multiple metastases, a markedly elevated serum β-hCG titer, older age, and the development of GTN after

a normal pregnancy or 6 to 12 months after the last gestation place the patient in a high-risk category. Cure rates with more aggressive chemotherapy have been reported ranging from 70% to 90% for this group.[8,13]

The diagnosis of hydatidiform mole and persistent GTN is clinically based on abnormally elevated serum β-hCG levels. Nonetheless, imaging has an important role. Initially, US may be performed to exclude a normal intrauterine or ectopic gestation. For example, a pregnancy involving twins may lead to an unexpectedly elevated serum β-hCG level and uterine enlargement. On US the typical appearance of a hydatidiform mole is of a soft tissue mass containing numerous cystic spaces and distending the uterine cavity (Figure 28-48). However, hydropic degeneration of the placenta and missed abortions may have a similar US appearance.[193] In patients with persistently elevated serum β-hCG levels, US may demonstrate focal areas of increased echogenicity in the myometrium, indicating persistent or invasive disease.[23] In this clinical setting, CT is most often used to screen for lung, liver, and brain metastases.[36,135] CT can also document the parametrial spread of disease, a relative contraindication to hysterectomy because of the risk of excessive bleeding.[36] However, neither US nor CT has been shown to be sensitive or specific in demonstrating locally invasive uterine disease.

There are little data regarding the role of MRI in the evaluation of patients with GTN. Complete hydatidiform moles have been described on MRI as heterogeneous masses with vesicular spaces distending the endometrial canal.[11,157] The myometrium should remain intact[157] (Figure 28-48). In patients with persistent or invasive GTN, heterogeneous, predominantly high–signal intensity masses invading the myometrium and distorting the uterine zonal anatomy have been described.[11,76,159] Foci of increased signal intensity on T1-weighted images, suggesting hemorrhage, and increased vascularity have also been noted (Figures 28-49 and 28-50). Similar findings are seen in patients with incomplete abortions.[11] After chemotherapy, uterine size, tumor size, and tumor

Table 28-3 FIGO Staging System for Carcinoma of the Cervix

STAGE		PATHOLOGY
O		Carcinoma
I		Carcinoma is strictly confined to cervix
	Ia1	Microscopic invasion
	Ia2	Measurable invasion: depth of invasion from base of epithelium <5 mm; horizontal spread <7 mm
	Ib1	Lesions of greater dimension than stage Ia2 but ≤4 cm
	Ib2	Lesions >4 cm
II		Carcinoma extends beyond cervix but not to pelvic side wall or lower third of vagina
	IIa	No obvious parametrial involvement
	IIb	Obvious parametrial involvement
III		Carcinoma extends to lower third of vagina or to pelvic side wall
	IIIa	No extension to pelvic side wall; lower third of vagina involved
	IIIb	Extension to pelvic side wall; all cases with hydronephrosis or nonfunctioning kidney unless other cause known
IV		Carcinoma extends beyond true pelvis or involves bladder or rectal mucosa

From reference 207.

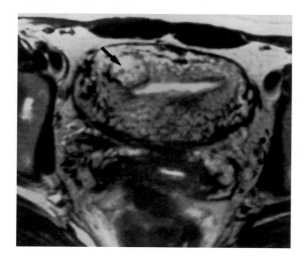

FIGURE 28-50 Invasive GTN. High–signal intensity mass *(arrow)* invades the myometrium.

vascularity decrease. Intralesional hemorrhage may develop, and the uterine zonal anatomy gradually reappears.[76,159] Myometrial invasion may be better appreciated on Gd contrast-enhanced images.[215] Whether MRI will be clinically useful in evaluating patients with primary disease or in assessing residual pelvic or uterine abnormality in patients with plateaued or rising serum β-hCG levels remains to be determined.

Cervical Carcinoma

The American Cancer Society estimates that 13,700 new cases of invasive cervical carcinoma will be diagnosed in the United States in 1998 and that 4900 disease-related deaths will occur.[151] However, early detection with the Papanicolaou smear has led to a significant decrease in the mortality rate since 1953. The peak incidence occurs between the ages of 45 and 55 years. Risk factors include multiple sexual partners, early age of first intercourse, childbearing before age 17, low socioeconomic background, cigarette smoking, and infection with human papillomavirus.[31,169] Cervical epithelia neoplasia (CIN) is considered a precursor lesion and is divided into three grades: CIN grade 1 (minor dysplasia), CIN grade 2 (moderate dysplasia), and CIN grade 3 (severe dysplasia or carcinoma in situ). It is projected that up to 40% of CIN grade 3 lesions would progress to invasive carcinoma if left untreated.[31] Nearly 90% of all cervical carcinomas are squamous cell carcinomas. The rest are adenocarcinomas or adenosquamous carcinomas. Mucin-secreting tumors and adenocarcinomas have a worse prognosis. Other features indicating poor prognosis include young age, lymphatic or vascular invasion, tumor diameter greater than 4 cm, advanced stage, and endometrial extension.[31,73,133,154]

Most cervical carcinomas develop at the squamocolumnar junction, which lies exposed on the vaginal surface of the cervix in women under the age of 35, but regresses to lie within the endocervical canal in older women. Carcinomas arising outside the endocervical canal tend to grow in a polypoid manner. However, carcinomas arising within the endocervical canal expand the canal, giving rise to a barrel-shaped deformity, and tend to be more infiltrative, spreading through the cervical wall. Cervical carcinoma spreads predominately via local extension or lymphangetic spread. Tumor may locally invade the vagina, lower uterine segment, and parametrium to finally reach the pelvic sidewall. The ureters, bladder, and rectum may be invaded as the disease advances. Lymphangitic spread occurs first to the internal and external iliac lymph nodes and later to the common iliac and paraaortic lymph nodes. If the tumor extends to the lower vagina, metastases may occur to inguinal nodes. Hematogenous spread is rare and occurs only with advanced disease, most commonly involving the chest.[19,31,169]

Cervical carcinoma is staged according to the FIGO staging system (Table 28-3). Routine clinical staging incorporates bimanual pelvic examination under anesthesia, chest x-ray, and excretory urography. In symptomatic patients or patients with advanced disease, barium enema, cystoscopy, and proctoscopy are performed. Patients with carcinoma in situ (stage 0) or microinvasive disease (stage Ia1 and Ia2) are usually treated with simple hysterectomy. The 5-year survival rate for these pa-

FIGURE 28-51 Stage I cervical carcinoma. Sagittal **(A)** and coronal **(B)** high-resolution T2-weighted images demonstrate a mass of intermediate signal intensity *(white arrow)* distending the endocervical canal. The low signal fibrous cervical stroma is intact *(black arrows)*. Note intrauterine pregnancy in breech presentation.

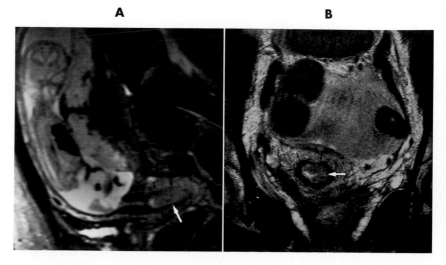

tients is 98%. Patients with invasive carcinoma (stage Ib) or stage IIa disease generally are treated with radical hysterectomy and pelvic lymph node dissection. A patient with a large tumor or a barrel-shaped cervix may be a candidate for adjuvant radiation therapy. Patients with more advanced disease typically are treated with radiation therapy. The 5-year survival rates are estimated as follows: stages Ib, 80% to 85%; stage II, 59%; stage III, 31%; and stage IV, 8%.[169]

Neither carcinomas in situ nor stage 1a tumors will be routinely identified on MRI. However, MRI surpasses clinical examination in detecting stromal invasion below a normal-appearing surface epithelium.[77,94,163,199] Macroinvasive cervical carcinoma (>5 × 7 mm), stage Ib, appears on T2-weighted images as an intermediate signal mass that may expand the endocervical canal, disrupt the low signal intensity of the fibrous cervical stroma, or prolapse into the vagina. The lateral margin of the cervix should be smooth and the parametrial fat undisrupted (Figure 28-51). Togashi et al[199] reported that the detection of macroscopic tumor on MR examination had a 100% PPV for the presence of invasive disease. The NPV of a normal MRI was, however, only 90%. Thus a normal MRI does not exclude invasive disease. Recent studies have reported that MRI has an 88% accuracy for detecting stromal invasion[190] and a 76% to 85% accuracy in assessing depth of stromal invasion.[93,181,190] Researchers have shown a strong correlation between MRI estimates and surgical measurements of tumor size (r = 0.87 to 0.95).[65,84,190] However, when full-thickness stromal invasion occurs, microscopic parametrial extension may be present despite a smooth, lateral cervical margin and the absence of abnormality in the parametrial fat.[65] MRI is not able to discriminate postbiopsy changes from primary tumor.[65,77]

Extension of tumor into the upper vagina, stage IIa, can also be diagnosed on MRI, although prolapse may occur without frank invasion[65,190] (Figure 28-52). However, it is the determination of the presence or absence of parametrial extension that is crucial, since patients with parametrial extension (stage IIb) are not surgical candidates at most medical centers. Parametrial extension is suggested when there is full-thickness invasion of the cervical stroma associated with irregularity or asymmetry of the lateral cervical margin, parametrial mass, or stranding within the parametrial fat (Figure 28-53). Studies have shown that a completely intact ring of low-signal intensity cervical stroma has a near 100% NPV in excluding parametrial invasion[77,93,180,181,199] (Figure 28-54). However, full-thickness disruption of the fibrous cervical stroma by tumor has a PPV for parametrial invasion that is significantly lower than 100%[93,190] (Figure 28-55). One would expect the presence of an obvious parametrial tumor mass to have a high PPV for parametrial invasion, although inflammatory changes or an exophytic stage I tumor can lead to false-positive diagnoses.[181,190] Overall, MRI has been reported to be 67% to 94% accurate in diagnosing parametrial invasion[65,93,108,190] and 94% accurate in identifying operative candidates (stage Ib and minimal stage IIa).[190]

Staging of more advanced disease is also possible on MRI, although statistical analysis of the published experience is limited by the small number of reported cases with surgical correlation. Tumor mass infiltrating the lower vaginal wall, soft tissue stranding, tumor mass extending to the pelvic sidewall, or hydronephrosis identifies patients with stage III disease. Bladder or rectal involvement (stage IV) is suggested by loss of perivesicular/perirectal fat planes, focal disruption of the normal low–signal intensity of the outer wall, or the mucosal signal of these organs, nodular wall thickening, or intraluminal masses (Figure 28-56).

Although not a part of the FIGO staging system, the presence of lymph node metastases adversely affects prognosis, precluding surgical

A   **B**

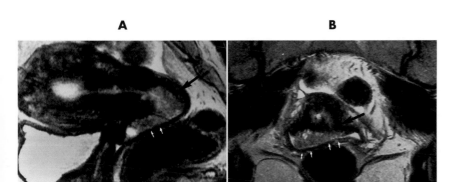

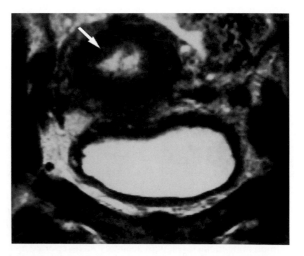

FIGURE 28-52   Stage I cervical carcinoma with prolapse into the vagina. Sagittal **(A)** and coronal **(B)** T2-weighted images reveal an intermediate-signal intensity mass distending the endocervical canal and invading the fibrous cervical stroma *(black arrow)*. The mass is noted to distend the vagina as well. However, on the coronal image **(B)** the intravaginal mass is largely surrounded by fluid, and the vaginal wall appears intact *(white arrows)*.

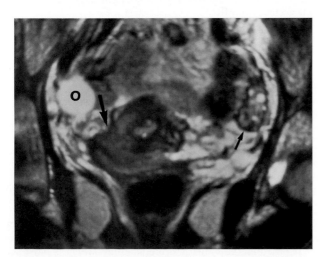

FIGURE 28-53   Parametrial invasion from cervical carcinoma, stage IIB. An intermediate-signal intensity mass disrupts the fibrous cervical stroma and infiltrates the entire cervical wall invading the right parametrium *(long arrow)* (coronal T2-weighted MRI). *O,* Right ovarian cyst; *short arrow,* left ovary.

FIGURE 28-54   Stage I cervical carcinoma. Endocervical mass obliterates the normal mucosal folds *(arrow).* The low-signal fibrous cervical stroma and outer zone are intact.

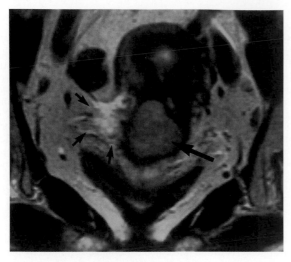

FIGURE 28-55   Cervical carcinoma. The mass invades the fibrous cervical stroma *(long arrow)*. Full-thickness invasion of the fibrous cervical stroma is seen on the right. The lateral cervical margin appears irregular. Edema *(short arrows)* is present in the right parametrium. No parametrial invasion was present at surgery (stage I).

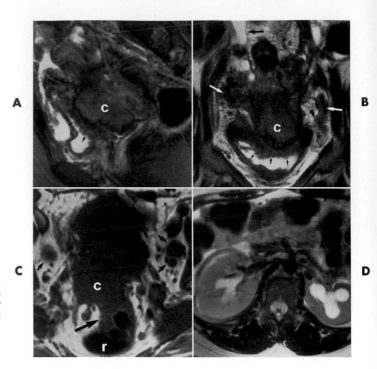

FIGURE 28-56   Extensive cervical carcinomas *(c)*. Nodular mucosal surface of the bladder indicates bladder invasion *(tiny black arrows)* seen on both sagittal **(A)** and coronal **(B)** T2-weighted images. Pelvic lymphadenopathy *(white arrows)* and a dilated right ureter *(black arrow)* is noted on **B**. On a T2-weighted image **(C)**, the mass invades *(long arrow)* the rectum *(r)*, and soft tissue stranding in the parametrium bilaterally suggests tumor invasion. **D,** Bilateral hydronephrosis.

cure and necessitating the extension of radiation ports.[19,73,154,169] Because signal characteristics have not been proved to discriminate between benign and malignant lymph nodes, MRI (like CT) must rely on size criteria.[40,65,77,93,103] Lymph nodes larger than 1.5 cm are considered abnormal, and nodes between 1 and 1.5 cm in size or multiple lymph nodes are considered suspicious (Figure 28-56). Lymph nodes are best depicted on T1-weighted images because of increased soft tissue contrast with the surrounding fat. Flow phenomenon may be used to differentiate lymph nodes from vessels. The accuracy of MRI and CT in diagnosing lymph node metastases is essentially equivalent and has been reported to range from 75% to 93%.[65,93-95,190,199] Neither modality will reveal the presence of microscopic disease in normal-sized lymph nodes, and inflammatory changes may result in false-positive diagnoses.

Clinical staging remains the gold standard by which treatment protocols are designed for patients with invasive cervical carcinoma. However, it is well known that clinical staging is inaccurate (overall 34.2%),[178] particularly in patients with advanced disease and large endophytic tumors. Staging errors are reported ranging from 17% to 32% for stage Ib disease and from 50% to 64% for stage IIa to stage IIIb disease.[99,178,208] In addition, although important both prognostically and for treatment planning, lymph node metastases are not included in clinical staging.[154]

Recent studies suggest that MRI is both an accurate and a cost-effective means of staging invasive cervical carcinoma; it is superior to either CT or clinical staging.[65,70,78,93,190] MRI is clearly more accurate than CT or clinical staging in identifying stromal invasion (88%) and assessing its depth (76% to 85%).[93,181,190] In addition, MRI is reported to be highly accurate in assessing tumor size.[65,70,190] Because a tumor larger than 2 cm is associated with an increased likelihood of parametrial invasion and lymph node metastases,[19,154] this is important prognostic information. In a study comparing MRI, CT, and pelvic examination under anesthesia, the overall staging accuracy of MRI (75%) was much higher than CT (32%) or clinical staging (55%).[70] Similarly, MRI was more accurate in assessing parametrial status: 90% for MRI versus 55% for CT and 82.5% for examination under anesthesia.[70] MRI is more accurate than CT in assessing parametrial invasion (94% versus 76%) and in determining operative candidates (stage Ib and minimal stage IIa) (94% versus 76%), as well as overall staging (90% versus 65%).[190] MRI and CT appear roughly equivalent in identifying lymph node metastases, with accuracy rates reported as high as 86% to 93%.[65,78,95,190] In patients with cervical carcinoma for whom MRI is the initial diagnostic study, studies report that fewer procedures and fewer invasive studies need to be performed, resulting in a net cost savings.[78,165]

A role for Gd-enhanced MRI in staging cervical carcinoma has not yet been proved. Two studies have reported that Gd-enhanced T1-weighted images were less accurate (38% and 57%) than T2-weighted images (76% and 85%, respectively).[74,181] The depth of cervical stromal invasion and invasion of adjacent structures were consistently overestimated after Gd enhancement. However, Yamashita et al[216] have reported in a small series that dynamic Gd-enhanced images are more accurate than either T2-weighted or contrast-enhanced T1-weighted images. Cervical carcinomas may display increased enhancement in the early dynamic phase (30 to 60 seconds) with improved tumor-to-cervix contrast. Fat-suppressed imaging may improve the detection of parametrial spread.[216] Endorectal coil imaging has not been shown to improve the staging accuracy of MRI.[114]

Patients with locally recurrent cervical carcinoma may be candidates for pelvic exenteration, provided that disease does not extend to the pelvic sidewall or outside the true pelvis, including the paraaortic lymph nodes. Clinically, it may be quite difficult to distinguish recurrent disease from radiation fibrosis. On T2-weighted images, recurrent tumor masses, most commonly found near the vaginal apex, are reported to demonstrate increased signal intensity in comparison with T1-weighted images, whereas masses caused by radiation fibrosis remain low–signal intensity if imaged more than 12 months after radiation therapy.[43,79,212] Reappearance of the normal cervical zonal anatomy and homogeneous low signal intensity cervical stroma have been reported to have an NPV of 97% in excluding tumor recurrence. Conversely, a measurable cervical mass has a PPV of 86% in predicting tumor recurrence.[79] Gd-enhanced imaging does not appear to be helpful in differentiating between recurrent tumor and radiation fibrosis except possibly when pelvic sidewall or adnexa is involved.[79]

MRI may prove useful in planning the treatment of four-field pelvic radiation for carcinoma of the cervix, since the design of the lateral fields is based on individual morbid anatomy, which is most accurately depicted on MRI.[194] Furthermore, sequential tumor volumetry using MRI may prove useful in monitoring the patient's response to therapy and possibly by identifying patients at high risk for treatment failure.[118]

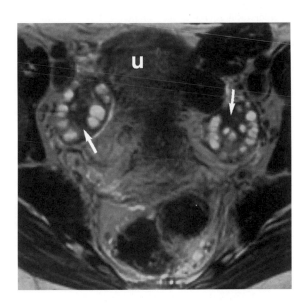

FIGURE 28-57 Normal ovaries. Follicular cysts shown on this FSE T2-weighted axial image. The ovarian stroma *(arrows)* is darker. *u,* Uterus.

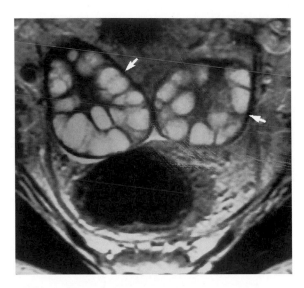

FIGURE 28-58 Polycystic ovarian disease. Numerous peripheral follicular cysts are seen within both ovaries. All cysts are smaller than 1 cm in size. The ovarian capsule is prominent *(arrows).*

OVARY
Normal Anatomy

On T1-weighted images the ovaries appear as homogeneous low–signal intensity oval structures. There is high soft tissue contrast between the ovaries and the surrounding pelvic fat, but the ovaries are less easily distinguished from adjacent loops of bowel or subserosal leiomyoma. On T2-weighted images, fluid within the peripheral follicular cysts becomes high signal intensity, whereas the central ovarian stroma remains low to moderate signal intensity (Figure 28-57). On high-resolution images a low–signal intensity rim corresponding to the fibrous capsule may sometimes be identified.[148] The ovaries are routinely identified on MR examination in 96% of premenopausal women.[224] The ovaries are less frequently identified in postmenopausal women because of atrophy and the absence of follicular cysts.[41]

Ovarian Cysts

Polycystic ovarian disease is the result of acyclic hypothalamic activity, which leads to a persistently elevated ratio of luteinizing hormone to follicular stimulating hormone such that ovulation is not triggered. Multiple chronically stimulated peripheral ovarian cysts, almost always under 1 cm in diameter, are seen under a thick fibrous capsule. Centrally the ovarian stroma is hypertrophied.[27] Women classically have hirsutism, menstrual irregularity, and infertility. However, a broad spectrum of clinical presentation exists, and the diagnosis requires biochemical assay. MR findings include numerous small subcapsular cysts of high signal intensity on T2-weighted images with stromal hypertrophy and sometimes mild ovarian enlargement (Figure 28-58). However, MR findings, although more sensitive than transabdominal ultrasound, are nonspecific.[131]

Simple serous cysts include follicular cysts, corpus luteum cysts, theca lutein cysts, and paratubal cysts. Such cysts on MR examination are homogeneous with signal intensity isointense to urine on all pulse sequences: low signal intensity on T1-weighted images and very high signal intensity on T2-weighted images (Figure 28-59). Cysts filled with proteinaceous fluid may be high signal intensity on both T1- and T2-weighted images. The cyst wall should be thin and smooth. Rarely a cystadenoma or cystic teratoma of the ovary may mimic this appearance.[117,130,172]

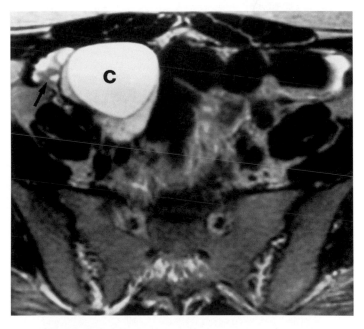

FIGURE 28-59 Simple cyst *(c)* in the right ovary *(arrow)* is high signal intensity on this T2-weighted image.

Hemorrhagic cysts are most often corpus luteal cysts. On MRI, hemorrhagic cysts have variable signal intensity on T1- and T2-weighted images because of the variation in signal intensity of hemorrhage over time. Most commonly, hemorrhagic cysts are intermediate to high signal intensity on T1-weighted images and lower signal intensity on heavily T2-weighted sequences, although cysts of high signal intensity on both T1- and T2-weighted images also may be seen.[41,142,144,172] The cyst wall should be thin and smooth but may demonstrate intense enhancement after the administration of Gd[147] (Figure 28-60). Layering (the hematocrit effect) or debris may also be noted. Contrast-enhanced images may help differentiate adherent clot from a mural nodule because clot will not enhance after the administration of Gd.[147,189,195,196,214]

Hemorrhagic cysts may be difficult to differentiate from other hemorrhagic adnexal lesions, especially endometriomas. However, hemorrhagic cysts tend to be solitary with round or oval configuration and are usually brighter on T2-weighted images than endometriomas, which typically have more profound T2 shortening, manifested or described as shading.[147,172,200]

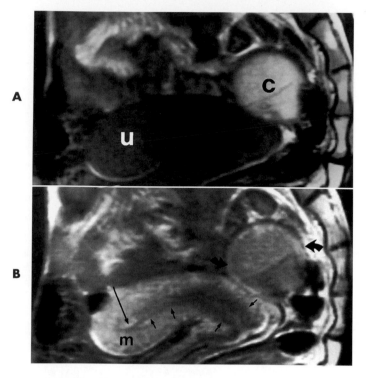

FIGURE 28-60   Hemorrhagic cyst. **A,** T1-weighted sagittal MR image shows high–signal intensity cystic structure *(c)* in the cul-de-sac. *u,* Uterus. **B,** T1-weighted, fat-suppressed, Gd-enhanced sagittal MR image shows enhancement of the cyst wall *(curved arrows)* but no enhancement of cyst contents. Note the normal uterine zonal anatomy. There are moderate enhancement of the outer myometrium *(m),* no enhancement of the JZ or fibrous cervical stroma *(short arrows),* and intense enhancement of the endometrium *(long arrow).*

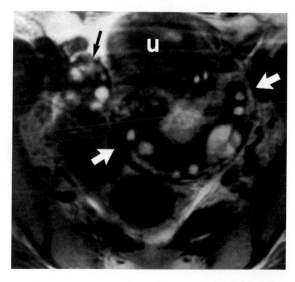

FIGURE 28-61   Ovarian torsion. The left ovary *(white arrows),* located posterior to the uterus *(u),* is enlarged with numerous peripheral cysts (T2-weighted MR image). The high signal intensity of the central ovarian stroma indicates edema. *Black arrow,* Normal right ovary.

Ovarian Torsion

Ovarian torsion occurs most commonly in association with an adnexal mass, usually a dermoid cyst, but may also occur spontaneously. Depending on the degree of torsion, either venous flow alone or both venous and arterial flow will be cut off. The ovary becomes engorged and swollen. Interstitial edema as well as hemorrhage and infarction will develop. On MRI the ovary appears enlarged, with signal behavior consistent with edema as well as hemorrhage. Often peripheral cysts are noted (Figure 28-61). Deviation of the uterus toward the side of torsion, a tubular protrusion at the edge of the mass (believed to represent the twisted tube and blood vessels), and the complete absence of Gd enhancement (if arterial occlusion has occurred) are considered diagnostic of ovarian torsion.[96]

Endometriosis

Endometriosis most commonly presents in middle-aged, upper-class, nulliparous women with pelvic pain, dysmenorrhea, dyspareunia, infertility, or a combination thereof. However, endometriosis may also be an incidental finding and has been reported in up to 35% to 50% of women undergoing major gynecological surgery.[28] *Endometriosis* is defined as the presence of functioning endometrium, the zona functionalis, located outside the uterus. This ectopic endometrium responds to hormonal stimulation and undergoes repeated cycles of hemorrhage, with the resultant development of blood-filled cysts called *endometriomas.* Adhesions, fibrosis, and scarring are common and are believed to be secondary to the irritant effect of blood leaking from the endometriotic cysts. The most frequent sites of implantation of ectopic endometrium in descending order of frequency are ovary, uterosacral ligaments, cul-de-sac, posterior wall of lower uterine segment, fallopian tube, rectovaginal septum, and sigmoid colon.[10,28] However, virtually any intraperitoneal surface may be affected, and endometriosis in distant sites, including the vagina, lymph nodes, lung, skeletal tissue, and bone, has been reported.[10,28] Retrograde menstruation via tubal reflux and coelomic metaplasia are the two most likely causes of endometriosis.[10,28]

Risk factors for the development of endometriosis include advanced maternal age during pregnancy and high socioeconomic class. There is a familial tendency, and recent data suggest that the disease is equally prevalent among black and white women.[28] Although the pelvic pain may be incapacitating, the severity of the pain is not necessarily related to the pathological extent of disease. Diagnosis requires laparoscopy, and patients are staged according to a point system based on the presence, size, and location of endometrial implants and adhesions.[1] Treatment options include surgery or hormonal suppression and depend on the severity of symptoms.[10,28]

US and CT are neither sensitive nor specific in the diagnosis or staging of endometriosis.[30,48,53,55] The classic appearance of an endometrioma on US is of a complex, multiloculated cyst with diffuse low-level echoes. On CT the appearance of endometriomas is quite varied, and sometimes these lesions may even appear solid. Neither US nor CT will accurately identify small implants or adhesions. US has been reported to have a sensitivity of only 11% when used as a screening technique.[55]

MRI has been reported to have a sensitivity of 90% to 92%, a specificity of 91% to 98%, and an accuracy of 91% to 96% for diagnosing endometriomas in women with a clinically suspected adnexal mass.[172,200] On MRI, endometriomas appear most commonly as multiple lesions with signal behavior consistent with hemorrhage of varying age.[2,143,146,200,223] The most specific MR criteria include multiplicity, angular margins or distorted shape, and high signal intensity on T1-weighted sequences with shading or low signal intensity on T2-weighted sequences because of the T1 and T2 shortening of methemoglobin[146,147,200] (Figure 28-62). Small implants may appear as areas of signal void because of the presence of hemosiderin-laden microphages[2,143,146,200,223] or solid, contrast-enhancing lesions of intermediate signal on T1-weighted images with punctate foci of high signal intensity.[179] Other, less specific features include adhesions (obliteration of fat planes between adjacent organs, low signal bands connecting or surrounding pelvic organs, and angulation of bowel loops) and a thick low–signal intensity rim, which may enhance after Gd administration. Hemorrhagic cysts may also have contrast-enhancing rims and similar signal behavior (Figure 28-63). Adhesions are infrequently visualized (Figure 28-64) and may also be seen in patients with ovarian carcinoma or pelvic inflammatory disease or in those who have had prior surgery.

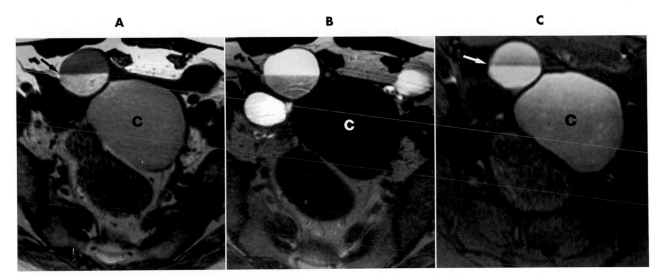

FIGURE 28-62   Endometriosis. T1-weighted **(A)** and T2-weighted **(B)** MR images show several adnexal cystic structures with different combinations of signal intensity *(arrow)*, indicating hemorrhage of varying ages. The low signal intensity on the T2 image **(B)**, irregularity of the cyst wall *(c)*, and multiplicity of lesions are more compatible with the diagnosis of endometriomas than hemorrhagic ovarian cysts. Fat saturation **(C)** does not suppress the signal intensity of hemorrhage as it does fat.

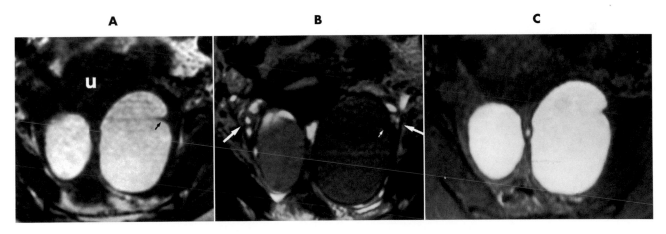

FIGURE 28-63   Hemorrhagic ovarian cysts. **A,** T1-weighted MR image shows two high–signal intensity structures posterior to the uterus *(u)*. **B,** T2-weighted MR image shows these cysts connected to the ovaries *(large arrows)* and decreased in signal intensity. **C,** Cyst signal does not suppress on the fat-saturation image, confirming that hemorrhage, not fat, is present.

Endometriomas may be high signal intensity on both T1-and T2-weighted images, but this signal behavior is nonspecific and more often seen in hemorrhagic or proteinaceous ovarian cysts.[146]

T1-weighted fat-saturated images increase the sensitivity of MRI for the diagnosis of small endometriomas (<1 cm).[4,62,191] The increased sensitivity most likely is due to increased contrast resolution (by narrowing the dynamic range), increased signal-to-noise ratio as signal from pelvic fat is suppressed, and decreased chemical-shift and respiratory artifacts. Outwater et al[146] have suggested that FSE imaging with a phased-array multicoil is also more sensitive than conventional SE imaging because of increased resolution and longer effective TE, which makes T2 dephasing effects more readily appreciable.

Thus, although MRI has been reported to have a high sensitivity and specificity for the diagnosis of endometriomas in patients with adnexal masses,[172,200] differentiation of endometriomas from other hemorrhagic adnexal pathology, especially hemorrhagic cysts, is more difficult.[146] Furthermore, the identification of adhesions, implants, and small (<1 cm) endometriomas remains difficult (sensitivity estimated at 47%)

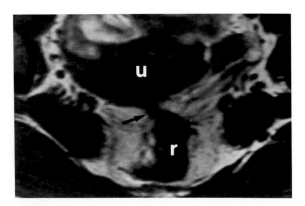

FIGURE 28-64   Adhesions in a patient with endometriosis. Soft tissue strands *(arrow)* connect the posterior surface of the uterus *(u)* to the anterior rectal *(r)* wall.

despite recent advances in imaging technique such as fat-suppression, FSE imaging and high-resolution multicoil imaging.[4,62,148,191] Hence the correlation between MR findings and staging or severity of disease remains inexact. Still, although MRI should not replace laparoscopy as a method of diagnosing and staging endometriosis, it is useful in evaluating patients with adnexal masses after nondiagnostic US examinations, in monitoring patient response to therapy, and in evaluating patients in whom dense adhesions or other contraindications preclude adequate surgical evaluation.[223]

Cystic Teratomas of the Ovary

Cystic teratomas of the ovary, or dermoid cysts, are most commonly diagnosed in women of reproductive age and account for 20% of all ovarian neoplasms.[174] All three germ cell layers are present in these neoplasms, but the ectoderm component predominates. The cystic cavity is usually filled with fatty and sometimes serous fluid. Hair, teeth, a mural nodule (Rokitansky's protuberance), or a combination thereof may be seen. Approximately 12% of dermoid cysts are bilateral; malignant degeneration occurs in less than 2%. Patients are usually asymptomatic but may present with pelvic pain or a pelvic mass. Surgical resection is recommended because of the relatively high incidence of torsion and rupture.[60,174]

A cystic teratoma is infrequently but confidently diagnosed on a plain radiograph of the pelvis when a radiolucent mass containing a focal calcification is seen. On CT the presence of fat (Hounsfield unit numbers, −130 to −90) in an ovarian mass is pathognomonic of a dermoid cyst.[22] US is neither sensitive nor specific. The classic US appearance of a dermoid cyst is a complex, layering (fat/fluid level) cystic adnexal mass with an echogenic component demonstrating good

through transmission, with or without an echogenic mass floating at a fluid–fluid interface, calcification, or mural nodule.[100,167] However, such findings are present in only one third of cases. As many as 23% of dermoids may be missed on US examination because fat within a dermoid may be echogenic and therefore hard to separate from adjacent bowel.[100]

On MR examination the key to diagnosing a dermoid cyst is the identification of fat within an adnexal mass. On SE sequences, lipid within the lesion will be isointense to subcutaneous or pelvic fat on all pulse sequences (i.e., high signal intensity on T1-weighted images and intermediate to high signal intensity on T2-weighted images), and internal or external chemical-shift artifact will be noted at fat–water interfaces along the frequency-encoding gradient. However, hemorrhage and even proteinaceous fluid may be isointense to fat, and chemical-shift artifact may not always be identified, particularly at low field strengths, wider bandwidths, curved interfaces, small fields of view, and thicker slice sections.[186] Chemical-shift imaging is the most definitive way to differentiate fat within a dermoid cyst from a hemorrhagic adnexal lesion, which will also be high signal intensity on T1-weighted images[90,188,191] (Figures 28-65 and 28-66). A frequency-selective fat presaturation sequence (see technique section) will suppress signal from fat, and conversely a water-saturation pulse sequence will suppress signal from water or hemorrhage, whereas fat remains high signal intensity. Morphological features typically observed in dermoid cysts on MRI include fluid/fluid layering, floating debris or hair balls, palm tree-like protrusions, mural nodules (Rokitansky's protuberance), and areas of signal void[202] (Figure 28-67). However, MRI is less sensitive than CT in detecting calcification.

Scoutt et al[172] reported that MRI was 100% sensitive, 99% specific, and 99% accurate in diagnosing dermoid cysts in women with adnexal

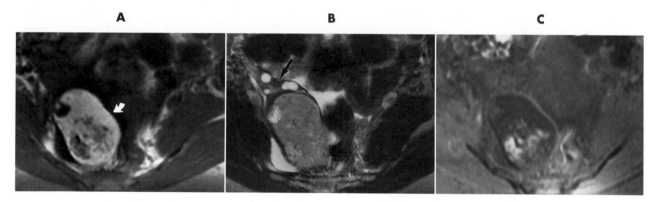

FIGURE 28-65   Cystic teratoma. **A,** T1-weighted MRI shows a bright right adnexal mass *(arrow).* **B,** On T2-weighted MRI the signal intensity of the mass decreases relative to muscle but remains isointense to subcutaneous fat. A small amount of free fluid is seen in the cul-de-sac. *Arrow,* Right ovary. **C,** Fat-saturation MRI suppresses signal from the part of the mass that was high signal intensity on T1-weighted MRI **(A),** confirming the presence of fat within the mass.

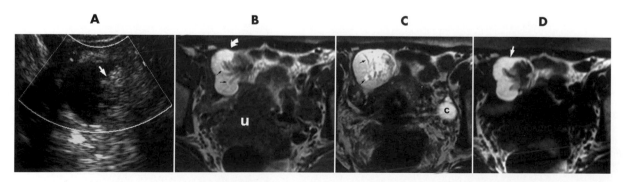

FIGURE 28-66   Cystic teratoma. **A,** EVUS shows a complex right adnexal mass with mural irregularity *(arrow)* felt to be an ovarian neoplasm. **B,** T1-weighted MR image shows a high–signal intensity mass *(white arrow)* anterior to the uterus *(u).* Small black arrows indicate corresponding mural nodularity. **C,** On T2-weighted MRI the mass decreases in signal intensity. Internal chemical-shift artifact is seen *(black arrows).* *c,* Left ovarian cyst. **D,** Water-suppressed T1-weighted image shows no suppression of signal from the bright area on **B** *(arrow),* confirming the presence of fat within the mass.

masses. Togashi et al[202] have reported that MRI was more sensitive than US, diagnosing 20 of 23 dermoids in their series, 4 more than were seen on US. The relative accuracy of MRI in detecting dermoids in comparison to CT is not known. However, since most dermoids occur in women of reproductive age, CT is not the screening modality of choice because it exposes the patient to ionizing radiation. An occasional dermoid, usually a dermoid comprised primarily of neuroectodermal tissue, will not contain fat. Such dermoids will have signal behavior and morphological characteristics indistinguishable from simple cysts on MR (and CT) examination and therefore may not be prospectively diagnosed.[117,202]

Ovarian Neoplasms

Ovarian carcinoma is the most lethal gynecological malignancy. The American Cancer Society estimates that 25,400 women will be diagnosed with and 14,500 will die from ovarian carcinoma in 1998.[151]

Risk factors for the development of ovarian carcinoma include a positive family history, older age, and high socioeconomic class, as well as factors that increase the number of ovulatory cycles, such as late-onset menopause, early menarche, and nulliparity. Oral contraceptive use and pregnancy may have a protective effect. Ovarian carcinoma is rare in the African-American population. The peak incidence is in the seventh decade.[134,192]

Approximately 70% of ovarian neoplasms and 80% to 90% of ovarian cancers arise from the surface coelomic epithelium of the ovary.[134,192] The most frequently encountered epithelial tumors are serous, mucinous, endometrioid, clear cell, Brenner, and undifferentiated tumors. Epithelial neoplasms may be benign (cystadenomas) or malignant (cystadenocarcinomas) or be of borderline malignant potential. Serous neoplasms are more common than mucinous tumors and more apt to be malignant (30% to 50%) and bilateral (10% to 15%). Serous neoplasms are predominantly cystic; less than 8% are solid. Papillary excrescences, which may be visualized on MRI or endovaginal ultrasound (EVUS), are often present in serous tumors. Although such mural nodules raise suspicion for malignancy, they may be present in benign lesions as well. Serum CA-125 levels may be elevated in both benign or malignant serous tumors.[64] Mucinous epithelial neoplasms tend to be larger than their serous counterparts, and although predominantly cystic, they contain numerous thick septations (Figure 28-68). Mural nodularity is less common, and 77% to 87% of mucinous tumors are benign. Patients with malignant mucinous tumors are more likely to have stage I disease than patients with serous tumors, and therefore the overall 5-year survival rate is slightly higher.[64,134] Serum CA-125 levels may not be elevated in patients with mucinous tumors. Germ cell tumors, including dysgerminomas, immature teratomas, embryonal cell carcinomas, endodermal sinus tumors, and mixed germ cell tumors, account for 5% to 10% of ovarian neoplasms. Malignant germ cell tumors are less aggressive than epithelial-derived malignancies.[134] Stromal cell tumors, namely fibromas, fibrothecomas,

granulosa cell tumors, and Sertoli-Leydig cell tumors, are the least common type of ovarian neoplasm (Figure 28-69). Metastases to the ovary occur most often from breast or gastrointestinal primary tumors (Figure 28-70). Germ cell tumors, stromal cell tumors, and metastases are likely to be solid, although areas of necrosis may be present.

Ovarian carcinoma usually spreads by direct shedding into the peritoneal cavity, local extension, or lymphatic dissemination. Hematogenous spread is rare. Ovarian carcinoma is staged surgically according to the FIGO staging system[49] (Table 28-4), and aggressive debulking

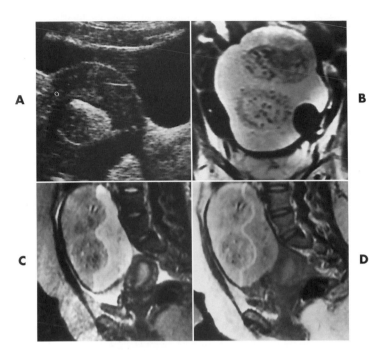

FIGURE 28-67   Cystic teratoma of the ovary. **A,** Transverse transabdominal US shows a complex adnexal mass containing a central echogenic focus with good through transmission. **B,** T1-weighted coronal MR image shows a large adnexal mass isointense to fat. The low–signal intensity mural nodule attached to the inner cyst wall is the Rokitansky's protuberance. **C,** Two hair balls are seen floating at the fat–fluid interface on this T2-weighted image. **D,** The bright line outlining the hair balls represents an internal chemical-shift artifact.

Table 28-4   FIGO Staging of Ovarian Carcinoma

STAGE		PATHOLOGY
I		Limited to ovaries
	A	One ovary/no tumor on external surface
	B	Both ovaries/no tumor on external surface
	C	Malignant ascites/positive peritoneal washings/tumor on surface of ovaries
II		Pelvic extension
	A	Uterus or fallopian tube involved
	B	Extension to other pelvic tissues
	C	Malignant ascites/positive peritoneal washings
III		Intraperitoneal metastases outside of pelvis, including small bowel and omentum, positive retroperitoneal or inguinal lymph nodes
	A	Microscopic seeding
	B	Implants <2 cm
	C	Implants >2 cm and/or positive lymph nodes
IV		Distant metastases, including positive pleural fluid, parenchymal liver metastases

From reference 49.

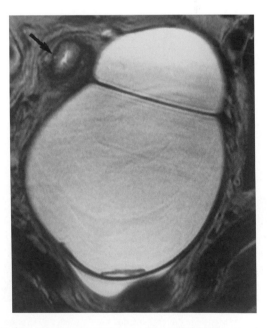

FIGURE 28-68   Mucinous cystadenoma. T2-weighted MR image shows a septated, homogeneous high–signal intensity (cystic) mass without mural nodularity. The mass is located posterior to the uterus *(arrow)*.

surgery followed by combination chemotherapy is the gold standard of treatment. The prognosis is dependent on the stage of the tumor at presentation, the volume of tumor remaining after debulking surgery, histological grade, and the age of the patient.[64,134]

The 5-year survival rate for stage I invasive epithelial carcinoma is nearly 80% to 91%.[220] However, the overall 5-year survival rate for ovarian carcinoma is under 38%, reflecting the fact that there are no early presenting clinical signs or symptoms for ovarian carcinoma; hence the majority of patients who present have advanced disease. The 5-year survival rate for FIGO stages III and IV ovarian carcinoma is estimated at less than 15%.[64,134] The clinical challenge, then, is to diagnose ovarian carcinoma early (stages I and II) when cure is possible, but tumors are clinically silent. Currently, ovarian cancer screening programs for high-risk populations focus on EVUS and serological tumor markers, usually CA-125. However, CA-125 levels may not be elevated in stage I tumors (because the capsule is intact) or in mucinous tu-

mors[47,134]; also elevated CA-125 levels are not specific. CA-125 levels are frequently elevated in premenopausal women with endometriosis, leiomyomas, and pelvic inflammatory disease. Patients with cirrhosis may also have elevated CA-125 levels. However, an elevated CA-125 level is more suspicious in a postmenopausal woman or in a woman who has had therapy for ovarian carcinoma. Markedly elevated or rising titers are also of more concern than minimally elevated titers.[47,134,192]

Because of low cost and ready availability, EVUS is the primary imaging modality used for screening for ovarian cancer and evaluation of adnexal masses. Nonetheless, the ultrasound features of adnexal masses, including Doppler analysis, are nonspecific, and differentiation of benign and malignant lesions is not always possible.* This differentiation is clinically of extreme importance. Although complex or solid ovarian masses (except endometriomas or pelvic inflammatory disease) are generally surgically removed, less invasive (laparoscopic) or elective surgery without a gynecological oncological surgeon in attendance can be planned if a lesion is prospectively considered highly likely to be benign.

The major contribution of MRI in evaluating adnexal masses lies in its ability to determine whether a mass is truly ovarian in origin, accurately identify certain benign entities (e.g., dermoid cysts, endometriomas/hemorrhagic cysts, fibromas), and more precisely define the internal architecture of ovarian masses.† Several studies have demonstrated that subserosal leiomyomas can be accurately differentiated from ovarian masses on MRI by their typical signal intensity (low signal intensity on T1-weighted and T2-weighted images), direct visualization of either pedicle or myometrial attachment, and identification of the ovaries separate from the mass.[86,172,213] On postcontrast T1-weighted sequences, subserosal leiomyomas will be isointense to myometrium.[195,196] Scoutt et al[172] reported that MRI had a 99% accuracy in differentiating subserosal leiomyoma from ovarian lesions. Prospective identification of a leiomyoma in a woman with a clinically suspected ovarian mass can eliminate unnecessary surgeries, thereby reducing health care costs.[168] Non–contrast-enhanced MRI has been shown to be highly accurate in diagnosing dermoid cysts (99%), endometriomas (91%), and hemorrhagic cysts (94%) in patients with clinically suspected adnexal masses[172] (see previous section for criteria). Authors have suggested that a benign fibroma may be diagnosed on MRI when a solid, well-marginated ovarian mass is predominantly low signal intensity on both T1- and T2-weighted images[172,189,204,214] (Figure 28-71). Ovarian fibromas have a similar MR appearance to leiomyomas. Lack

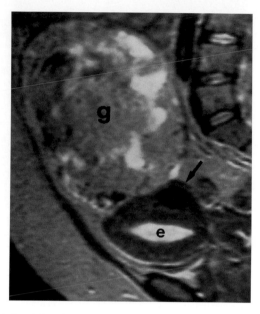

FIGURE 28-69 Granulosa cell tumor. T2-weighted MR image shows a large heterogeneous solid mass *(g)* above the uterus. The endometrium *(e)* is thickened. A small subserosal leiomyoma is noted *(arrow)*. Stromal cell tumors are typically solid.

---

*References 16, 86, 97, 106, 166, 197, 214.
†References 86, 172, 195, 196, 213, 214.

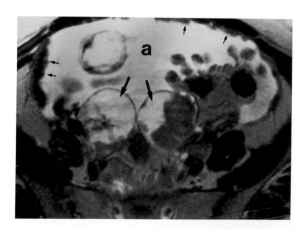

FIGURE 28-70 Metastases to both ovaries from a small cell carcinoma of the vagina. T2-weighted MR image shows complex cystic and solid masses involving both ovaries *(large arrows)*. There are diffuse peritoneal metastases *(small arrows)*. *a,* Ascites.

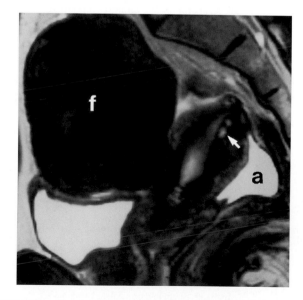

FIGURE 28-71 Ovarian fibroma. T2-weighted MR image shows a low–signal intensity mass *(f)* anterior to the uterus. *a,* Free fluid in the cul-de-sac. Small subendometrial cysts *(arrow)* within uterine fundus are an incidental finding.

of visualization of the ovary and absence of attachment to the uterus are differential features.[204] In a study comparing contrast-enhanced with non–contrast-enhanced MR images, simple cysts, complex cysts, and cystadenomas were more accurately diagnosed with contrast-enhanced imaging, whereas there was no difference in the accuracy of precontrast and postcontrast MRI in diagnosing endometriomas.[214] In this study, precontrast MRI was slightly better for diagnosing dermoids.[214]

Differentiation of benign from malignant cystic epithelial ovarian neoplasms is more difficult. Most authors agree that the presence of solid components or vegetations; thick, irregular walls or septations; and other associated findings, such as ascites, enlarged lymph nodes, peritoneal implants, and infiltration of adjacent organs, increases suspicion for malignancy* (Figures 28-69 through 28-73). Mucinous lesions tend to be more complex than serous lesions. However, architectural findings are nonspecific. Papillary vegetations and thick walls are occasionally seen with benign cystadenomas,[57,189,195,196] and implants or peritumoral infiltration may be seen with endometriosis or pelvic inflammatory disease.[195] Accuracy rates on non–contrast-enhanced MRI for identifying malignancy have been reported to range from 83% to 86%.[57,86,189]

Most authors agree that the addition of contrast-enhanced T1-weighted sequences improves the accuracy of MRI in diagnosing ovarian malignancy[189,196,214] because of both improved visualization of architectural detail, allowing differentiation of debris/clot/necrosis from solid tumor nodules, as well as increased sensitivity in detecting small nodules, septations, or wall irregularity† (Figure 28-73). How-

---

*References 57, 86, 97, 147, 172, 189, 195, 196, 214.
†References 97, 176, 189, 195, 196, 214.

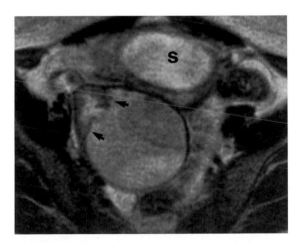

FIGURE 28-72   Stage I serous cystadenocarcinoma presenting in the first trimester of pregnancy as an ovarian mass. T2-weighted MR image shows thick septations and mural irregularity *(arrows),* suggesting malignancy. There is an intrauterine gestational sac *(s)* anterior to the right ovarian mass.

ever, contrast-enhanced imaging is less useful when lesions are hyperintense on T1-weighted images, since enhancement may then make architectural features less conspicuous.[214] Nonetheless, such architectural features remain nonspecific, and accuracy rates for distinguishing benign from malignant lesions with contrast-enhanced MRI have been reported to range from 78% to 95% in recent series.[189,214] Using the presence of solid tissue (i.e., any enhancing internal structure, excluding septations) as the sole criterion for diagnosing malignancy, MRI has been reported to be 89% accurate in identifying ovarian malignancy.[97] Most authors agree that contrast-enhanced MRI is more specific than EVUS in evaluating internal architecture and diagnosing malignancy in ovarian masses.[97,123,214] In a single paper, though, EVUS has been reported to be more sensitive and more accurate than non–contrast-enhanced MRI in diagnosing ovarian cysts and endometriomas, as well as identifying malignancy and evaluating the internal architecture of adnexal masses.[86] However, none of these US studies included Doppler analysis.[86,97,123,214]

The role of preoperative CT or MRI in patients with primary ovarian carcinoma before surgical staging and cytoreduction remains controversial and continues to be actively investigated. Surgical staging frequently results in a higher disease stage than would otherwise be suspected because of the detection of microscopic disease. Aggressive surgical debulking or primary cytoreduction clearly has been shown to improve the prognosis, provided that the residual tumor measures less than 2 cm.[127,137,140,221] Thus surgical staging has an extremely important therapeutic as well as prognostic role, and some clinicians therefore feel that preoperative imaging is unnecessary.

However, surgical understaging has been reported to occur in up to 30% to 40% of patients[52,221] and is particularly problematic in the upper abdomen. Furthermore, when adjacent structures such as the bowel or bladder are invaded by ovarian carcinoma, debulking surgery becomes complex. In addition, recent studies have suggested that patients with nonresectable disease may have a better outcome when chemotherapy precedes surgical debulking.[138,140,206] Therefore a role for preoperative imaging may exist to alert the surgeon to the presence of disease in regions either that are difficult to surgically assess or that require assistance from a gynecological or gastrointestinal oncological surgeon and to identify patients with extensive nonresectable disease who might benefit from preoperative chemotherapy.

In recent studies the overall accuracy of MRI for staging ovarian carcinoma has been reported to range from 75% to 89%[51,123,189] and to be equivalent if not superior to CT.[18,51,111,176] Reported criteria for extraovarian spread include plaquelike or nodular enhancing lesions on peritoneal or serosal surfaces; low–signal intensity regions on T1- and T2-weighted images within the mesentery, which enhance after adminstration of intravenous Gd; lymph nodes larger than 1 cm on short axis; tumor approaching within 3 mm of the pelvic side wall or distorting the iliac vessels; loss of fat plane between the tumor and the bowel and bladder or frank disruption of the bladder or bowel wall; and distortion or encasement of adjacent structures more than 90 degrees[51,111,176] (Figures 28-74 and 28-75). Contrast enhancement,[51,176,189] fast imaging,[110] and fat suppression[51,111,176] have all been reported to improve the sensitivity and accuracy of MR imaging. In addition, Low et al[111] have recently reported that the use of an oral contrast agent, per-

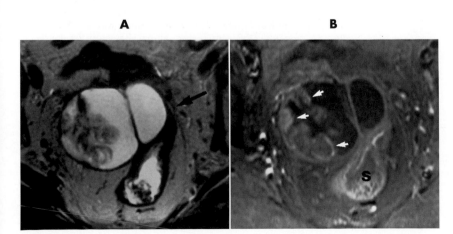

FIGURE 28-73   Ovarian carcinoma. **A,** T2-weighted MR image shows a septated cystic mass deviating the sigmoid colon *(arrow).* The low–signal intensity area within mass may represent debris, hemorrhage, or tumor nodules. **B,** Gd enhancement (fat-suppressed MRI) of internal structures and mural nodularity *(arrows)* confirms the diagnosis of tumor nodules. *s,* Sigmoid colon.

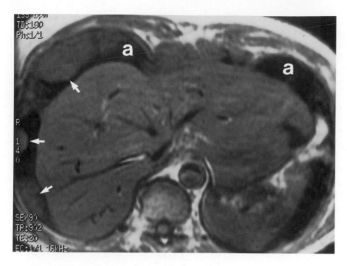

FIGURE 28-74 Peritoneal implants *(arrows)* from ovarian carcinoma. *a,* Ascites.

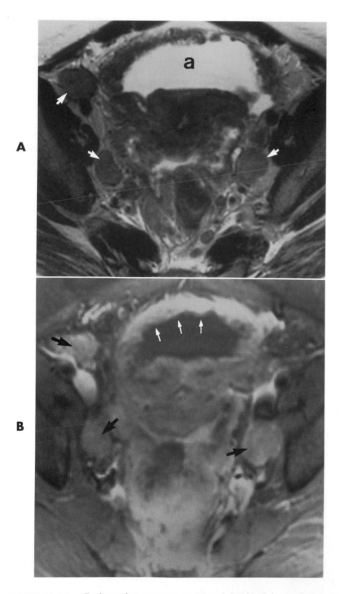

FIGURE 28-75 Peritoneal metastases. **A,** T2-weighted MR image in a patient with advanced disease shows ascites *(a)* and enlarged lymph nodes *(arrows).* **B,** Peritoneal metastases and lymphadenopathy are more easily identified *(white arrows)* on T1-weighted, fat-suppressed Gd-enhanced image.

fluorocarbon, also improves detection of bowel implants on MRI. Forstner et al[51] have reported that both CT and MRI are highly accurate in predicting surgical nonresectability with a PPV of 100% for CT and 91% for MRI and an NPV of 92% for CT and 97% for MRI. However, all authors agree that neither CT nor MRI is accurate in detecting microscopic disease or implants smaller than 1 to 2 cm,[18,51,111,123,176] particularly within the mesentery or on the serosal surface of the small bowel, where lesions as large as 3 cm may be missed.[51] Detection of disease is also reportedly more accurate in the pelvis than in the upper abdomen.[18,51] Two small studies have suggested that MRI is slightly better than CT at assessing colonic and uterine invasion.[51,176] MRI may be better at depicting diaphragmatic and liver implants.[52] Given the ready availability and lower cost, CT therefore remains the primary imaging modality of choice for staging ovarian carcinoma and predicting successful surgical cytoreduction.[125,137] MRI is emerging as a problem-solving modality and may be particularly useful in assessing colonic or uterine invasion.[51,176]

The workup of patients for recurrence of ovarian carcinoma is also controversial. Although routine second-look surgery with secondary cytoreduction has been the standard follow-up procedure, recent studies have demonstrated that tumor eventually recurs in many patients who initially had stage III or IV disease, despite negative findings at routine second-look laparotomy.[56,69,126,156] Furthermore, recent studies have suggested that secondary surgical cytoreduction of tumor recurrence larger than 2 cm may not improve prognosis when compared with chemotherapy alone.[127,155] Also, the serum CA-125 assay is not adequately sensitive to identify recurrence; up to 60% of patients with normal serum CA-125 levels will have persistent or recurrent tumor noted at second-look laparotomy.[142,164] However, as the clinical use and efficacy of second-look surgery are questioned, the role of noninvasive imaging potentially becomes more significant. For patients in clinical remission, distinguishing between women with low-volume recurrent or residual tumor and those in true remission is important to determine both the prognosis and the end point for chemotherapy.[111] Identification of recurrent tumor ($\geq$2 cm) may obviate an extensive second-look surgery, thereby reducing patient morbidity as well as health care costs. Forstner et al[50] have reported that whereas MRI had an overall accuracy of 59% in identifying recurrent tumor, the accuracy of MRI was 82% for detecting macroscopic (i.e., nonresectable) tumor larger than 2 cm. MRI has been shown to be at least equivalent to CT.[158] However, neither modality is judged to be sensitive in detecting small implants or microscopic disease.[50,158]

FALLOPIAN TUBE

Paratubal cysts (Figure 28-76) are located adjacent to the ovary and have the same signal characteristics as ovarian cysts but an oval or elongated configuration.[91] After pelvic inflammatory disease, scarring within the fallopian tube and subsequent accumulation of fluid may result in a cystically dilated fallopian tube, termed *hydrosalpinx*. Although readily identified on US examination, the serpiginous dilated fallopian tube, low signal intensity on T1-weighted images and high signal intensity on T2-weighted images, also is easily identified on MRI. Multiplanar imaging is key, since the distorted tube can appear as an aggregate of cysts in a single imaging plane (Figure 28-77).

On MRI a mature tuboovarian abscess (Figure 28-78) has a nonspecific appearance. Typically an irregular, thick-walled adnexal collection encompassing the ovary is seen. Signal characteristics consistent with hemorrhage are identified in up to 40% of cases.[130] A dilated fallopian tube, diffuse edema in the surrounding pelvic fat, and adhesions may be noted. These findings may mimic the MR appearance of endometriosis or other hemorrhagic lesions, including malignancy. However, the clinical presentation of pain and fever in a nonpregnant, sexually active woman usually establishes the diagnosis.

Primary adenocarcinoma of the fallopian tube is the rarest of gynecological malignancies, accounting for approximately 0.3% of all cancers of the female genital tract. This cancer presents insidiously in older women. Nonspecific symptoms of abdominal pain and abnormal vaginal bleeding develop late in the course of the disease. The 5-year survival rate is low. Primary carcinoma of the fallopian tube is almost never accurately diagnosed before surgery because of its rarity and nonspecific presentation.[39] On MRI, primary fallopian tube carcinoma typically appears as a small, solid adnexal mass, usually high signal intensity on T2-weighted images (Figure 28-79) with homogeneous

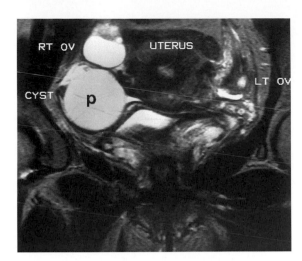

FIGURE 28-76   Paratubal cyst *(p)* is located adjacent to the right ovary.

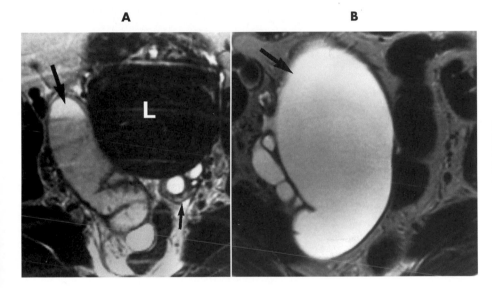

FIGURE 28-77   Hydrosalpinx presenting with pelvic pain and a palpable mass. **A,** T2-weighted MR image shows a dilated right fallopian tube *(long arrow). L,* Leiomyoma; *short arrow,* left ovary. **B,** T2-weighted FSE MR image in another patient shows a markedly distended right hydrosalpinx *(arrow).*

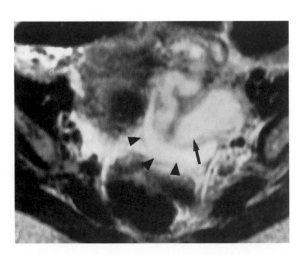

FIGURE 28-78   Tuboovarian abscess. Dilated left fallopian tube *(arrow)* has a thick wall and surrounding free fluid *(arrowheads).*

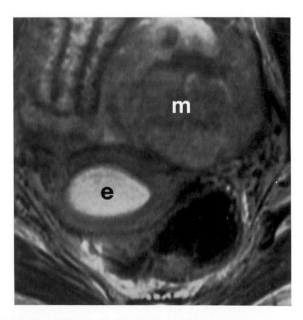

FIGURE 28-79   Primary carcinoma of the fallopian tube. T2-weighted MR image shows a large, heterogeneous solid mass *(m),* superior to the uterus. *e,* Thickened endometrium.

enhancement after Gd administration. Hydrosalpinx, peritumoral ascites, and intrauterine fluid collections are frequently associated.[89] When cystic or associated with hydrosalpinx, fallopian tube carcinoma may be impossible to distinguish from ovarian carcinoma.

REFERENCES

1. American Fertility Society: Revised American Fertility Society classification of endometriosis, Fertil Steril 43:351, 1985.
2. Arrive L, Hricak H, and Martin MC: Pelvic endometriosis: MR imaging, Radiology 171:687, 1989.
3. Ascher SM, Arnold LL, Patt RH, et al: Adenomyosis: prospective comparison of MR imaging and transvaginal sonography, Radiology 190:803, 1994.
4. Ascher SM, Agrawal R, Bis KG, et al: Endometriosis: appearance and detection with conventional and contrast-enhanced fat-suppressed spin-echo techniques, J Magn Reson Imaging 5:251, 1995.
5. Ascher SM, Johnson JC, Barnes WA, et al: MR imaging appearance of the uterus in postmenopausal women receiving tamoxifen therapy for breast cancer: histopathologic correlation, Radiology 200:105, 1996.
6. Ascher SM, Scoutt LM, McCarthy SM, et al: Uterine changes after dilation and curettage: MR imaging findings, Radiology 180:433, 1991.
7. Bacelar AC, Wilcock D, Powell M, et al: The value of MRI in the assessment of traumatic intra-uterine adhesions (Asherman's syndrome), Clin Radiol 50:80, 1995.
8. Bagshawe KD: Trophoblastic tumors: diagnostic methods, epidemiology, clinical features, and management. In Coppleson M, ed: Gynecologic oncology, ed 2, London, 1992, Churchill Livingstone.
9. Balfe DM, et al: Computed tomography in malignant endometrial neoplasms, J Comput Assist Tomgr 7:677, 1983.
10. Barbieri R, and Kistner RW: Endometriosis. In Kistner RW, ed: Gynecology: principles and practice, St Louis, 1986, Mosby.
11. Barton JW, McCarthy SM, Kohorn EI, et al: Pelvic MR imaging findings in gestational trophoblastic disease, incomplete abortion, and ectopic pregnancy: are they specific? Radiology 186:163, 1993.
12. Belloni C, Vigano R, delMaschio A, et al: Magnetic resonance imaging in endometrial carcinoma staging, Gynecol Oncol 37:172, 1990.
13. Berkowitz RS, and Goldstein DP: Management of molar pregnancy and gestational trophoblastic tumors. In Knapp RC, and Berkowitz RS, eds: Gynecologic oncology, New York, 1986, Macmillan.
14. Berman ML, et al: Prognosis and treatment of endometrial cancer, Am J Obstet Gynecol 136:679, 1980.
15. Boronow RC, et al: Surgical staging in endometrial cancer: clinical pathology findings of a prospective study, Obstet Gynecol 63:825, 1984.
16. Brown DL, Frates MC, Laing FC, et al: Ovarian masses: can benign and malignant lesions be differentiated with color and pulsed Doppler US? Radiology 190:333, 1994.
17. Brown HK, Stoll BS, Nicosia SV, et al: Uterine junctional zone: correlation between histologic findings and MR imaging, Radiology 179:409, 1991.
18. Buist MR, Golding RP, Burger, CW, et al: Comparative evaluation of diagnostic methods in ovarian carcinoma with emphasis on CT and MRI, Gynecol Oncol 52:191, 1994.
19. Burghardt E, and Pikel H: Local spread and lymph node involvement in cervical cancer, Obstet Gynecol 52:138, 1978.
20. Buttram VC, and Gibbons WE: Müllerian anomalies: a proposed classification (an analysis of 144 cases), Fertil Steril 32:40, 1979.
21. Buttram VC: Müllerian anomalies and their management, Fertil Steril 40:159, 1983.
22. Buy JN, et al: Cystic teratoma of the ovary: CT detection, Radiology 171:697, 1989.
23. Callen PW: Ultrasound evaluation of gestational trophoblastic disease. In Callen PW, ed: Ultrasonography in obstetrics and gynecology, Philadelphia, 1988, WB Saunders.
24. Carrington BM, Hricak H, Nuruddin RN, et al: Müllerian duct anomalies: MR imaging evaluation, Radiology 176:715, 1990.
25. Chang YC, et al: Vagina: evaluation with MR imaging. II. Neoplasms, Radiology 169:175, 1988.
26. Chen SS, Rumancik WM, and Spiegel G: Magnetic resonance imaging in Stage I endometrial carcinoma, Obstet Gynecol 75:274, 1990.
27. Clarke-Pearson DL, and Dawood MY: Disorders of the anovulatory cycles. In Clarke-Pearson DL, and Dawood MY, eds: Green's gynecology, Boston, 1990, Little, Brown.
28. Clarke-Pearson DL, and Dawood MY: Endometriosis. In Clarke-Pearson DL, and Dawood MY, eds: Green's gynecology, Boston, 1990, Little, Brown.
29. Clement PB, and Scully RE: Pathology of uterine sarcomas. In Coppleson M, ed: Gynecologic oncology, ed 2, London, 1992, Churchill Livingstone.
30. Coleman BG, Arger PH, and Mulhern CB: Endometriosis: clinical and ultrasonic correlation, Am J Roentgenol 132:747, 1979.
31. Coppleson M, Atkinson KH, and Dalrymple JC: Cervical squamous and glandular intraepithelial neoplasia: clinical features and review of management. In Coppleson M, ed: Gynecologic oncology, Edinburgh, 1992, Churchill Livingstone.
32. Creasman WT, and Weed JC: Carcinoma of the endometrium (FIGO Stages I and II): clinical features and management. In Coppleson M, ed: Gynecologic oncology, ed 2, Edinburgh, 1992, Churchill Livingstone.
33. Creasman WT, Morrow CP, and Bundy L: The surgical pathologic spread pattern of endometrial cancer: a Gynecologic Oncology Group study, Cancer 60:2035, 1987.
34. Creasman WT: Disorders of the uterine corpus. In Scott JR, DiSaia PJ, Hammond CB, et al, eds: Danforth's obstetrics and gynecology, 1994, Lippincott.
35. Creasman WT: New gynecologic cancer staging, Obstet Gynecol 75:287, 1990.
36. Davis WK, et al: Computed tomography of gestational trophoblastic disease, J Comput Assist Tomgr 8:1136, 1984.
37. DelMaschio A, Vanzulli A, Sironi S, et al: Estimating the depth of myometrial involvement by endometrial carcinoma: efficacy of transvaginal sonography vs. MR imaging, Am J Roentgenol 160:533, 1993.
38. Demas BE, Hricak H, and Jaffe RB: Uterine MR imaging: effects of hormonal stimulation, Radiology 159:123, 1986.
39. DiSaia PJ: Tumors of the fallopian tube. In Scott JR, DiSaia PJ, Hammond CB, et al, eds: Danforth's obstetrics and gynecology, ed 6, Philadelphia, 1990, Lippincott.
40. Dooms GC, et al: Characterization of lymphadenopathy by magnetic resonance relaxation times: preliminary results, Radiology 155:691, 1985.
41. Dooms GC, Hricak H, and Tscholakoff D: Adnexal structures: MR imaging, Radiology 158:639, 1986.
42. Dudiak CM, et al: Uterine leiomyomas in the infertile patient: preoperative localization with MR imaging versus US and hysterosalpingography, Radiology 167:627, 1988.
43. Ebner F, et al: Tumor recurrence versus fibrosis in the female pelvis: differentiation with MR imaging at 1.5T, Radiology 166:333, 1988.
44. Edelman DA: DES/diethylstilbestrol: new perspectives, Boston, 1986, MTP Press.
45. Fedele L, et al: Magnetic resonance evaluation of double uteri, Obstet Gynecol 74:844, 1989.
46. Fedele L, Dorta M, Brioschi D, et al: Re-examination of the anatomic considerations for hysteroscopic metroplasty, Eur J Obstet Gynecol Reprod Biol 39:127, 1991.
47. Finkler NJ, et al: Comparison of serum CA 125, clinical impression, and ultrasound in the preoperative evaluation of ovarian masses, Obstet Gynecol 72(4):659, 1988.
48. Fishman EK, et al: Computed tomography of endometriosis, J Comput Assist Tomgr 7:257, 1983.
49. Folke Pettersson, ed: Annual report on the results of treatment in gynecological cancer, vol 20, Stockholm, 1988, Panorama Press.
50. Forstner R, Hricak H, Powell CB, et al: Ovarian cancer recurrence: value of MR imaging, Radiology 196:715, 1995.
51. Forstner R, Hricak H, Occhipinti KA, et al: Ovarian cancer: staging with CT and MR imaging, Radiology 197:619, 1995.
52. Forstner R, Hricak H, and White S: CT and MRI of ovarian cancer: review, Abdom Imaging 20:2, 1995.
53. Fried AM, Rhodes RA, and Morehouse R: Endometrioma: analysis and sonographic classification of 51 documented cases, South Med J 86:297, 1993.
54. Friedman AJ, et al: Treatment of leiomyomata with intranasal or subcutaneous leuprolide, a gonadotropin-releasing hormone agonist, Fertil Steril 48:560, 1987.
55. Friedman H, et al: Endometriosis detection by US with laparoscopic correlation, Radiology 157:217, 1985.
56. Friedman JB, and Weiss NS: Second thoughts about second-look laparotomy in advanced ovarian cancer, N Engl J Med 322:1079, 1990.
57. Ghossain MA, Buy JN, Ligneres C, et al: Epithelial tumors of the ovary: comparison with MR and CT findings, Radiology 181:863, 1991.
58. Golan A, et al: Congenital anomalies of the müllerian system, Fertil Steril 51:747, 1989.
59. Gordon AN, Fleischer AC, and Reed GW: Depth of myometrial invasion in endometrial cancer: preoperative assessment by transvaginal ultrasonography, Gynecol Oncol 39:321, 1990.
60. Griffiths CT, and Berkowitz RS: The ovary. In Kistner RW, ed: Gynecology: principles and practice, St Louis, 1986, Mosby.
61. Gross BH, Silver TM, and Jaffe MH: Sonographic features of uterine leiomyomas: analysis of 41 proven cases, J Ultrasound Med 2:401, 1983.
62. Ha HK, Lim YT, Kim HS, et al: Diagnosis of pelvic endometriosis: fat-suppressed T1-weighted vs conventional MR images, Am J Roentgenol 163:127, 1994.
63. Hamlin DJ, et al: MR imaging of uterine leiomyomas and their complications, J Comput Assist Tomgr 9(5):902, 1985.
64. Hart WR: Pathology of malignant and borderline (low malignant potential) epithelial tumors of the ovary. In Coppleson M, ed: Gynecologic oncology, Edinburgh, 1992, Churchill Livingstone.
65. Hawnaur JM, Johnson RJ, Buckley CH, et al: Staging: volume estimation and assessment of nodal status in carcinoma of the cervix: comparison of magnetic resonance imaging with surgical findings, Clin Radiol 49:443, 1994.
66. Hayes CE, Dietz MJ, King BF, et al: Pelvic imaging with phased-array coils: quantitative assessment of signal-to-noise ratio improvement, J Magn Reson Imaging 2:321, 1992.
67. Haynor DR, et al: Changing appearance of the normal uterus during the menstrual cycle: MR studies, Radiology 161:459, 1986.
68. Hirano Y, Kubo K, Hirai Y, et al: Preliminary experience with gadolinium-enhanced dynamic MR imaging for uterine neoplasms, Radiographics 12:243, 1992.
69. Ho AG, et al: A reassessment of the role of second-look laparotomy in advanced ovarian cancer, J Clin Oncol 5:1316, 1987.
70. Ho C-M, Chien T-Y, Jeng C-M, et al: Staging of cervical cancer: comparison between magnetic resonance imaging, computed tomography and pelvic examination under anesthesia, J Formosan Med Assoc 91(10):982, 1992.
71. Hricak H, and Kim B: Contrast-enhanced MR imaging of the female pelvis, J Magn Reson Imaging 3:297, 1993.
72. Hricak H, Chang YCF, and Thurnher S: Vagina: evaluation with MR imaging. I. Normal anatomy and congenital anomalies, Radiology 169:169, 1988.
73. Hricak H, Quivey JM, Campos Z, et al: Carcinoma of the cervix: predictive value of clinical and magnetic resonance (MR) imaging assessment of prognostic factors, Int J Rad Oncol Biol Phys 27:791, 1993.
74. Hricak H, Hamm B, Semelka RC, et al: Carcinoma of the uterus: use of gadopentetate dimeglumine in MR imaging, Radiology 181:95, 1991.
75. Hricak H, et al: Endometrial carcinoma staging by MR imaging, Radiology 162:297, 1987.
76. Hricak H, et al: Gestational trophoblastic neoplasm of the uterus: MR assessment, Radiology 161:11, 1986.
77. Hricak H, et al: Invasive cervical carcinoma: comparison of MR imaging and surgical findings, Radiology 166:623, 1988.
78. Hricak H, Powell CB, Yu KK, et al: Invasive cervical carcinoma: role of MR imaging in pretreatment work-up. cost minimization and diagnostic efficacy analysis, Radiology 198:403, 1996.

79. Hricak H, Swift PJ, Campos Z, et al: Irradiation of the cervix uteri: value of unenhanced and contrast-enhanced MR imaging, Radiology 189:381, 1993.

80. Hricak H, et al: Magnetic resonance imaging of the female pelvis: initial experience, Am J Roentgenol 141:1119, 1983.

81. Hricak H, Rubenstein LV, Gherman GM, et al: MR imaging evaluation of endometrial carcinoma: results of an NCI cooperative study, Radiology 179:829, 1991.

82. Hricak H, Finck S, Honda G, et al: MR imaging in the evaluation of benign uterine masses, Am J Roentgenol 158:1043, 1992.

83. Hricak H, et al: Uterine leiomyomas: correlation of MR, histopathic findings, and symptoms, Radiology 158:385, 1986.

84. Innocenti P, Fiumicelli D, Agostini S, et al: Magnetic resonance imaging in the measurement of clinical stage IB cervical carcinoma, Eur J Radiol 23:222, 1996.

85. Itoh K, et al: Assessing myometrial invasion by endometrial carcinoma with dynamic MRI, J Comput Assist Tomogr 18:77, 1994.

86. Jain KA, Friedman DL, Pettinger TW, et al: Adnexal masses: comparison of specificity of endovaginal US and pelvic MR imaging, Radiology 186:697, 1993.

87. Janus CL, Wiczyk HP, and Laufer N: Magnetic resonance imaging of the menstrual cycle, Magn Reson Imaging 6:669, 1988.

88. Kawakami S, Togashi K, Kojima N, et al: MR appearance of malignant lymphoma of the uterus, J Comput Assist Tomogr 19(2):238, 1995.

89. Kawakami S, Togashi K, Kimura I, et al: Primary malignant tumor of the fallopian tube: appearance at CT and MR imaging, Radiology 186:503, 1993.

90. Kier R, Smith RC, and McCarthy SM: Value of lipid- and water-suppression MR images in distinguishing between blood and lipid within ovarian masses, Am J Roentgenol 158:321, 1992.

91. Kier R: Nonovarian gynecologic cysts: MR imaging findings, Am J Roentgenol 158:1265, 1992.

92. Kim SH, Kim HD, Song IS, et al: Detection of deep myometrial invasion in endometrial carcinoma: comparison of transvaginal ultrasound, CT, and MRI, J Comput Assist Tomogr 19:766, 1995.

93. Kim SH, Choi BI, Han JK, et al: Preoperative staging of uterine cervical carcinoma: comparison of CT and MRI in 99 patients, J Comput Assist Tomogr 17(4):633, 1993.

94. Kim SH, Choi BI, Lee HP, et al: Uterine cervical carcinoma: comparison of CT and MR findings, Radiology 175:45, 1990.

95. Kim SH, Kim SC, Choi BI, et al: Uterine cervical carcinoma: evaluation of pelvic lymph node metastasis with MR imaging, Radiology 190:807, 1994.

96. Kimura I, Togashi K, Babcock CJ, et al: Ovarian torsion: CT and MR appearances, Radiology 190:337, 1994.

97. Komatsu T, Konishi I, Mandai M, et al: Adnexal masses: transvaginal US and gadolinium-enhanced MR imaging assessment of intratumoral structure, Radiology 198:109, 1996.

98. Krinsky GA, et al: Fast MR imaging of the uterus: comparison of four T2-weighted sequences for diagnosis of adenomyosis and leiomyoma, Radiology 197:322, 1995.

99. Lagasse LD, et al: Results and complications of operative staging in cervical cancer: experience of the Gynecologic Oncology Group, Gynecol Oncol 9:90, 1980.

100. Laing FC, et al: Dermoid cysts of the ovary: their ultrasonographic appearances, Obstet Gynecol 57:99, 1981.

101. Lancet M, and Kessler I: A review of Asherman's syndrome and results of modern treatment, Int J Fertil 33:14, 1988.

102. Langman J: Medical embryology, Baltimore, 1975, Williams & Wilkins.

103. Lee JK, et al: Magnetic resonance imaging of abdominal and pelvic lymphadenopathy, Radiology 153:181, 1984.

104. Lee JK, et al: The uterus: in vitro MR anatomic correlation of normal and abnormal specimens, Radiology 157:175, 1985.

105. Letterie GS, Haggerty M, and Lindee G: A comparison of pelvic ultrasound and magnetic resonance imaging as diagnostic studies for müllerian tract abnormalities, Int J Fertil 40:34-38, 1995.

106. Levine D, Feldstein VA, Babcock CJ, et al: Sonography of ovarian masses: poor sensitivity of resistive index for identifying malignant lesions, Am J Roentgenol 162:1355, 1994.

107. Lien HH, Blomlie V, Trope C, et al: Cancer of the endometrium: value of MR imaging in determining depth of invasion into the myometrium, Am J Roentgenol 157:1221, 1991.

108. Lien HH, Blomlie V, Iversen T, et al: Clinical stage I of the cervix: value of MR imaging in determining invasion into the parametrium, Acta Radiol 34:130, 1993.

109. Lin MC, Gosink BB, Wolf SI, et al: Endometrial thickness after menopause: effect of hormone replacement, Radiology 180:427, 1991.

110. Low RN, and Sigeti JS: MR imaging of peritoneal disease: comparison of contrast-enhanced fast multiplanar spoiled gradient-recalled and spin-echo imaging, Am J Roentgenol 163:1131, 1994.

111. Low RN, Carter WD, Saleh F, et al: Ovarian cancer: comparison of findings with perfluorocarbon-enhanced MR imaging, In-111-CYT-103 immunoscintigraphy, and CT, Radiology 195:391, 1995.

112. Lurai JR, and Piver MS: Uterine sarcomas: clinical features and management. In Coppleson M, ed: Gynecologic oncology, ed 2, London, 1992, Churchill Livingstone.

113. Lutz MH, et al: Endometrial carcinoma: a new method of classification of therapeutic and prognostic significance, Gynecol Oncol 6:83, 1978.

114. Maldjian C, and Schnall MD: Magnetic resonance imaging of the uterine body, cervix, and adnexa, Semin Roentgenol 31:257, 1996.

115. Malini S, Valdes C, and Malinak R: Sonographic diagnosis and classification of anomalies of the female genital tract, J Ultrasound Med 3:397, 1984.

116. Mark AS, et al: Adenomyosis and leiomyoma: differential diagnosis with MR imaging, Radiology 163:527, 1987.

117. Mawhinney RR, et al: Magnetic resonance imaging of benign ovarian masses, Br J Radiol 61:179, 1988.

118. Mayr NA, Magnotta VA, Ehrhardt JC, et al: Usefulness of tumor volumetry by magnetic resonance imaging in assessing response to radiation therapy in carcinoma of the uterine cervix, Int J Radiat Oncol Biol Phys 35:915, 1996.

119. McCarthy S, et al: Uterine junctional zone: MR study of water content and relaxation properties, Radiology 171:241, 1989.

120. McCarthy S, Tauber C, and Gore J: Female pelvic anatomy: MR assessment of variations during the menstrual cycle and with use of oral contraceptives, Radiology 160:119, 1986.

121. McCauley TR, McCarthy SM, and Lange R: Pelvic phased array coil: image quality assessment for spin-echo MR imaging, J Magn Reson Imaging 10:513, 1992.

122. McCausland AM, and McCausland VM: Depth of endometrial penetration in adenomyosis helps determine outcome of rollerball ablation, Am J Obstet Gynecol 174:1786, 1996.

123. Medl M, Kulenkampff KJ, Stiskal M, et al: Magnetic resonance imaging in the preoperative evaluation of suspected ovarian masses, Anticancer Res 15:1123, 1995.

124. Mendelson EB, et al: Transvaginal sonography in gynecologic imaging (review), Semin Ultrasound CT MR 9:102, 1988.

125. Meyer JI, Kennedy AW, Fiedman R, et al: Ovarian carcinoma: value of CT in predicting success of debulking surgery, Am J Roentgenol 165:875, 1995.

126. Miller DS, et al: A critical reassessment of second-look laparotomy in epithelial ovarian carcinoma, Cancer 57:530, 1986.

127. Miller DS, Spirtos NM, Ballon SC, et al: Critical reassessment of second look laparotomy for epithelial ovarian cancer, Cancer 69:502, 1992.

128. Mintz MC, and Grumbach K: Imaging of congenital uterine anomalies, Semin Ultrasound CT MR 9:167, 1988.

129. Mintz MC, et al: MR evaluation of uterine anomalies, Am J Roentgenol 148:287, 1987.

130. Mitchell DG, et al: Adnexal masses: MR imaging observations at 1.5T, with US and CT correlation, Radiology 162:319, 1987.

131. Mitchell DG, et al: Polycystic ovaries: MR imaging, Radiology 160:425, 1986.

132. Mittl RL, Yeh I-T, and Kressel HY: High-signal intensity rim surrounding uterine leiomyomas on MR images: pathologic correlation, Radiology 180:81, 1991.

133. Monaghan JM: Invasive tumors of the vagina: clinical features and management. In Coppleson M, ed: Gynecologic oncology, New York, 1992, Churchill Livingstone.

134. Morrow CP: Malignant and borderline epithelial tumors of ovary: clinical features, staging, diagnosis, intraoperative assessment, and review of management. In Coppleson M, ed: Gynecologic oncology, Edinburgh, 1992, Churchill Livingstone.

135. Mutch DG, et al: Role of computed axial tomography of the chest in staging patients with nonmetastatic gestational trophoblastic disease, Obstet Gynecol 68:348, 1986.

136. Muto MG, and Friedman AJ: The uterine corpus. In Ryan KJ, Berowitz RS, and Barbieri RL, eds: Kistner's gynecology, St Louis, 1995, Mosby.

137. Nelson BE, Rosenfield AT, and Schwartz PE: Preoperative abdominopelvic computed tomographic prediction of optimal cytoreduction in epithelial ovarian carcinoma, J Clin Oncol 11:166, 1993.

138. Ng L, et al: Aggressive chemosurgical debulking in patients with advanced ovarian cancer, Gynecol Oncol 38:358, 1990.

139. Nghiem HV, Herfkens RJ, Francis IR, et al: The pelvis: T2-weighted fast spin-echo MR imaging, Radiology 185:213, 1992.

140. NIH Consensus Conference: Ovarian cancer: screening, treatment, and follow-up, JAMA 273:491, 1995.

141. Niloff JM, et al: Malignancy of the uterine corpus. In Knapp RC, and Berkowitz RS, eds: Gynecologic oncology, New York, 1986, Macmillan.

142. Niloff JM, et al: Predictive value of CA 125 antigen levels in second-look procedures for ovarian cancer, Am J Obstet Gynecol 151:981, 1985.

143. Nishimura K, et al: Endometrial cysts of the ovary: MR imaging, Radiology 162:315, 1987.

144. Nyberg DA, et al: MR imaging of hemorrhagic adnexal masses, J Comput Assist Tomogr 11:664, 1987.

145. Oguchi O, Mori A, Kobayashi Y, et al: Prediction of histopathologic features and proliferative activity of uterine leiomyoma by magnetic resonance imaging prior to GnRH analogue therapy: correlation between T2-weighted images and effect of GnRH analogue, J Obstet Gynecol 21:107, 1995.

146. Outwater E, Schiebler ML, Owen RS, et al: Characterization of hemorrhagic adnexal lesions with MR imaging: blinded reader study, Radiology 186:489, 1993.

147. Outwater EK, and Dunton CJ: Imaging of the ovary and adnexa: clinical issues and applications of MR imaging, Radiology 194:1, 1995.

148. Outwater EK, and Mitchell DG: Normal ovaries and functional cysts: MR appearance, Radiology 198:397, 1996.

149. Panageas E, Kier R, McCauley TR, et al: Submucosal uterine leiomyomas: diagnosis of prolapse into the cervix and vagina based on MR imaging, Am J Roentgenol 159:555, 1992.

150. Paraduras FJ: Pathology and classification of trophoblastic tumors. In Coppleson M, ed: Gynecologic oncology, ed 2, London, 1992, Churchill Livingstone.

151. Landis SH, Murray T, Bolden S, et al: Cancer statistics, CA Cancer J Clin 48:6, 1998.

152. Pattani SJ, et al: MRI of uterine leiomyosarcoma, Magn Reson Imaging 13(2):331, 1995.

153. Pellerito JS, et al: Diagnosis of uterine anomalies: relative accuracy of MR imaging, endovaginal sonography, and hysterosalpingography, Radiology 183:795, 1992.

154. Piver MS, and Chung WS: Prognostic significance of cervical lesion size and pelvic node metastases in cervical carcinoma, Obstet Gynecol 46:507, 1975.

155. Podratz KC, and Kinney WK: Second-look operation in ovarian cancer, Cancer 71(4):1551, 1993.

156. Podratz KC, et al: Recurrent disease after negative second-look laparotomy in stages III and IV ovarian carcinoma, Gynecol Oncol 29:274, 1988.

157. Powell MC, et al: Magnetic resonance imaging and hydatidiform mole, Br J Radiol 59:561, 1986.

158. Prayer L, Kainz C, Kramer J, et al: CT and MR accuracy in the detection of tumor recurrence in patients treated for ovarian cancer, J Comput Assist Tomgr 17:626, 1993.

159. Preidler KW, Luschin G, Tamussino K, et al: Magnetic resonance imaging in patients with gestational trophoblastic disease, Invest Radiol 31:492, 1996.

160. Reinhold C, McCarthy S, Bret PM, et al: Diffuse adenomyosis: comparison of endovaginal US and MR imaging with histopathologic correlation, Radiology 199:151, 1996.

161. Reinhold C, Hricak H, Forstner R, et al: Primary amenorrhea: evaluation with MR imaging, Radiology 203:383, 1997.

162. Reuter K, Daly D, and Cohen S: Septate versus bicornuate uteri: errors in imaging diagnosis, Radiology 172:749, 1989.

163. Rubens D, et al: Stage 1B cervical carcinoma: comparison of clinical, MR and pathologic staging, Am J Roentgenol 150:135, 1988.

164. Rubin SC, et al: Serum CA 125 levels and surgical findings in patients undergoing secondary operations for epithelial ovarian cancer, Am J Obstet Gynecol 160:667, 1989.

165. Russell AH, Shingleton HM, Jones WB, et al: Diagnostic assessments in patients with invasive cancer of the cervix: a national patterns of care study of the American College of Surgeons, Gynecol Oncol 63:159, 1996.

166. Salem S, White LM, and Lai J: Doppler sonography of adnexal masses: the predictive value of the pulsatility index in benign and malignant disease, Am J Roentgenol 163:1147, 1994.

167. Sandler MA, Silver TM, and Karo JJ: Gray-scale ultrasonic features of ovarian teratomas, Radiology 131:705, 1979.

168. Schwartz LB, Panageas E, Lange R, et al: Female pelvis: impact on MR imaging on treatment decisions and net cost analysis, Radiology 192:55, 1994.

169. Schwartz P: Gynecologic cancer in clinical medicine. In Spittell JA, ed: Clinical medicine, Philadelphia, 1985, Harper Collins.

170. Scoutt LM, McCarthy SM, Flynn SD, et al: Clinical Stage I endometrial carcinoma: pitfalls in preoperative assessment with MR imaging, Radiology 194:567, 1995.

171. Scoutt LM, Flynn SD, Ruthinger DJ, et al: Junctional zone of the uterus: correlation of MR imaging and histologic examination of hysterectomy specimens, Radiology 179:403, 1991.

172. Scoutt LM, McCarthy SM, Lange R, et al: MR evaluation of clinically suspected adnexal masses, J Comput Assist Tomogr 18(4):609, 1994.

173. Scoutt LM, McCauley TR, Flynn SD, et al: Zonal anatomy of the cervix: correlation of MR imaging and histologic examination of hysterectomy specimens, Radiology 186:159, 1993.

174. Scully RE: Tumors of the ovary and mal-developed gonads. In Hartmann WH, ed: Atlas of tumor pathology, ed 3, Washington, DC, 1979, Armed Forces Institute of Pathology.

175. Secaf E, Hricak H, Gooding CA, et al: Role of MRI in the evaluation of ambiguous genitalia, Pediatr Radiol 24:231, 1994.

176. Semelka RC, Lawrence PH, Shoenut JF, et al: Primary ovarian cancer: prospective comparison of contrast-enhanced CT and pre- and postcontrast, fat-suppressed MR imaging with histologic correlation, J Magn Reson Imaging 3:99, 1993.

177. Shapeero LG, and Hricak H: Mixed müllerian sarcoma of the uterus: MR imaging findings, Am J Roentgenol 153:317, 1989.

178. Shingleton HM, and Orr JW: Cancer of the cervix: diagnosis and treatment, London, 1983, Churchill Livingstone.

179. Siegelman ES, Outwater E, Wang T, et al: Solid pelvic masses caused by endometriosis, MR imaging features, Am J Roentgenol 163:357, 1994.

180. Sironi S, Belloni C, Taccagni GL, et al: Carcinoma of the cervix: value of MR imaging in detecting parametrial involvement, Am J Roentgenol 156:753, 1991.

181. Sironi S, DeCobelli F, Scarfone G, et al: Carcinoma of the cervix: value of plain and gadolinium-enhanced MR imaging in assessing degree of invasiveness, Radiology 188:797, 1993.

182. Sironi S, Taccagni GL, Gorancini P, et al: Myometrial invasion by endometrial carcinoma: assessment by MR imaging, Am J Roentgenol 158:565, 1992.

183. Sironi S, Colombo E, Villa G, et al: Myometrial invasion by endometrial carcinoma: assessment with plain and gadolinium-enhanced MR imaging, Radiology 185:207, 1992.

184. Smith RC, Reinhold C, Lange RC, et al: Fast spin-echo MR imaging of the female pelvis. I. Use of a whole-volume coil, Radiology 184:665, 1992.

185. Smith RC, Reinhold C, McCauley TR, et al: Multicoil high-resolution fast spin-echo MR imaging of the female pelvis, Radiology 184:671, 1992.

186. Smith RC, Lange RC, and McCarthy SM: Chemical-shift artifact: dependence on shape and orientation of the lipid-water interface, Radiology 181:225, 1991.

187. Smith RC: Magnetic resonance imaging of the female pelvis: technical considerations, Top Magn Reson Imaging 7:3, 1995.

188. Stevens SK, Hricak H, and Campos Z: Teratomas versus cystic hemorrhagic adnexal lesions: differentiation with proton-selective fat-saturation MR imaging, Radiology 186:481, 1993.

189. Stevens SK, Hricak H, and Stern JL: Ovarian lesions: detection and characterization with gadolinium-enhanced MR imaging at 1.5 T, Radiology 181:481, 1991.

190. Subak LL, Hricak H, Powell CB, et al: Cervical carcinoma: computed tomography and magnetic resonance imaging for preoperative staging, Obstet Gynecol 86(1):43, 1995.

191. Sugimura K, Okizuka H, Imaoka I, et al: Pelvic endometriosis: detection and diagnosis with chemical shift MR imaging, Radiology 188:435, 1993.

192. Taylor KJW, and Schwartz PE: Screening for early ovarian cancer, Radiology 192:1, 1994.

193. Taylor KJW, Schwartz PE, and Kohorn EI: Gestational trophoblastic neoplasia: diagnosis with Doppler US, Radiology 165:445, 1987.

194. Thomas L, Chacon B, Kind M, et al: Magnetic resonance imaging in the treatment planning of radiation therapy in carcinoma of the cervix treated with the four-field pelvic technique, Int J Radiat Oncol Biol Phys 37:827, 1997.

195. Thurnher S, Hodler J, Baer S, et al: Gadolinium-DOTA enhanced MR imaging of adnexal tumors, J Comput Assist Tomogr 14(6):939, 1990.

196. Thurnher SA: MR imaging of pelvic masses in women: contrast-enhanced vs unenhanced images, Am J Roentgenol 159:1243, 1992.

197. Timor-Tritsch IE, et al: Transvaginal ultrasonographic characterization of ovarian masses by means of color flow-directed Doppler measurements and a morphologic scoring system, Am J Obstet Gynecol 168:909, 1993.

198. Togashi K, et al: Adenomyosis: diagnosis with MR imaging, Radiology 166:111, 1988.

199. Togashi K, et al: Carcinoma of the cervix: staging with MR imaging, Radiology 171:245, 1989.

200. Togashi K, Nishimura K, Kimura I, et al: Endometrial cysts: diagnosis with MR imaging, Radiology 180:73, 1991.

201. Togashi K, et al: Enlarged uterus: differentiation between adenomyosis and leiomyoma with MR imaging, Radiology 171:531, 1989.

202. Togashi K, et al: Ovarian cystic teratomas: MR imaging, Radiology 162:669, 1987.

203. Togashi K, et al: Vaginal agenesis: classification by MR imaging, Radiology 162:675, 1987.

204. Troiano RN, Lazzarini KM, Scoutt LM, et al: Fibroma and fibrothecoma of the ovary: MR imaging findings, Radiology 204:795, 1997.

205. Valie RF, and Sciara JJ: Hysteroscopic treatment of the septate uterus, Obstet Gynecol 67:253-257, 1986.

206. van der Burg ME, van Lent M, Buyse M, et al: The effect of debulking surgery after induction chemotherapy on the prognosis in advanced epithelial ovarian cancer, N Engl J Med 332:629, 1995.

207. van Gils AP, et al: Abnormalities of the uterus and cervix after diethylstilbestrol exposure: correlation of findings on MR and hysterosalpingography, Am J Roentgenol 153:1235, 1989.

208. Van Nagell JR, Roddick JW Jr, and Lowin DM: The staging of cervical cancer: inevitable discrepancies between clinical staging and pathologic findings, Am J Obstet Gynecol 110:973, 1971.

209. Walsh JW, and Goplerund DR: Computed tomography of primary, persistent, and recurrent endometrial malignancy, Am J Roentgenol 139:1149, 1982.

210. Walsh JW, et al: Gray-scale ultrasound in 204 proven gynecologic masses: accuracy and specific diagnostic criteria, Radiology 130:391, 1979.

211. Weber G, Merz E, Bahlmann F, et al: Assessment of myometrial infiltration and preoperative staging by transvaginal ultrasound in patients with endometrial carcinoma, Ultrasound Obstet Gynecol 6:362, 1995.

212. Weber TM, Sostman HD, Spritzer CE, et al: Cervical carcinoma: determination of recurrent tumor extent versus radiation changes with MR imaging, Radiology 194:135, 1995.

213. Weinreb JC, Barkoff ND, Megibow A, et al: The value of MR imaging in distinguishing leiomyomas from other solid pelvic masses when sonography is indeterminate, Am J Roentgenol 154:295, 1990.

214. Yamashita Y, Torashima M, Hatanaka Y, et al: Adnexal masses: accuracy of characterization with transvaginal US and precontrast and postcontrast MR imaging, Radiology 194:557, 1995.

215. Yamashita Y, Mizutani H, Torshima M, et al: Assessment of myometrial invasion by endometrial carcinoma: transvaginal sonography vs. contrast-enhanced MR imaging, Am J Roentgenol 161:595, 1993.

216. Yamashita Y, Takahashi M, Sawada T, et al: Carcinoma of the cervix: dynamic MR imaging, Radiology 182:643, 1992.

217. Yamashita Y, Torashima M, Takahashi M, et al: Hyperintense uterine leiomyoma at T2-weighted MR imaging: differentiation with dynamic enhanced MR imaging and clinical implications, Radiology 189:721, 1993.

218. Yamashita Y, Harada M, Sawada T, et al: Normal uterus and FIGO Stage I endometrial carcinoma: dynamic gadolinium-enhanced MR imaging, Radiology 186:495, 1993.

219. Yazigi R, et al: Magnetic resonance imaging determination of myometrial invasion in endometrial carcinoma, Gynecol Oncol 34:94, 1989.

220. Young RC, Walton LA, Ellenberg SS, et al: Adjuvant therapy in stage I and stage II epithelial ovarian cancer: results of two prospective randomized trials, N Engl J Med 322:1021, 1990.

221. Young RC, Perez CA, and Hoskins W: Cancer of the ovary. In De Vita VT, Hellman S, and Rosenberg SA, eds: Cancer: principles and practice of oncology, ed 4, vol 1, Philadelphia, 1993, Lippincott.

222. Zawin M, McCarthy S, Scoutt L, et al: Monitoring therapy with a gonadotropin-releasing hormone analog: utility of MR imaging, Radiology 175:503, 1990.

223. Zawin M, et al: Endometriosis: appearance and detection at MR imaging, Radiology 171:693, 1989.

224. Zawin M, McCarthy S, Scoutt LM, et al: High-field MRI and US evaluation of the pelvis in women with leiomyomas, Magn Reson Imaging 8:371, 1990.

29 Obstetrics

**Brian S. Worthington, William T.C. Yuh, David D. Stark,
Jeffrey C. Weinreb, and Penny A. Gowland**

 KEY POINTS

- Guidelines permit the use of MRI in pregnancy when medically indicated.
- Maternal indications include conditions where ultrasound has known limitations, as in characterization of pelvic masses, and where ionizing radiation can be avoided, as in MR pelvimetry.
- In assessment of fetal anomalies, MRI can both clarify equivocal ultrasound results and often provide additional useful information.
- There is an emerging role for MRI in the assessment of the compromised pregnancy, including the identification of fetal growth restriction.

Early studies investigating the role of magnetic resonance imaging (MRI) in obstetrics[76-80] were carried out using relatively slow imaging protocols, and the major applications that emerged related to the assessment of maternal anatomy. Attempts to image the fetus were frustrated by motion even in the third trimester. Achieving an optimal imaging plane was entirely fortuitous. The use of sedation and muscle relaxants to reduce or eliminate fetal movement has now been rendered totally unnecessary by the development of fast imaging strategies, including echo-planar imaging (EPI).[35]

SAFETY CONSIDERATIONS

A large number of studies have now been carried out in an attempt to identify any significant biological effects associated with the exposure of living systems to static magnetic fields and varying radiofrequency fields both alone and in combination (see Chapter 14). No definite genotoxic or oncogenic effect has been identified, and either the results of the studies have been largely negative or the studies identified possible nonspecific effects or short-term responses that are not thought to be harmful.[35,37,57] Even with the now large number of studies reported, it has to be recognized that they do not cover every possible exposure condition that could be met in clinical MRI, so the possibility of adverse effect at some particular "imaging window" cannot be ruled out. In the United Kingdom the current advice of the National Radiological Protection Board[58] states that "although there is no good evidence that mammalian embryos are sensitive to the magnetic fields encountered in magnetic resonance systems, it is prudent until further information becomes available, to exclude women during the first three months of pregnancy. However, MR diagnostic procedures should be considered where the only reasonable alternative requires the use of x-ray procedures. There is no need to exclude women for whom a termination of pregnancy has been indicated. It is advised that pregnant women should not be exposed above the advised lower levels of restriction." In the United States the Food and Drug Administration[83] requires labeling of magnetic resonance (MR) systems to indicate that "the safety of MRI when used to image fetuses and the infant has not been established; however, MRI during pregnancy is not specifically contraindicated." The National Institutes of Health Consensus Development Conference on MRI[46] stated that "MRI, as with all interventions during pregnancy should be used during the first trimester only when there are clear medical indications and when it offers a definite advantage over other tests." Currently the generally accepted medical practice in the United States requires that MRI of the pregnant patient and fetus be restricted to the following conditions:
1. Research protocols approved by local institutional research boards
2. Instances in which evaluation of the patient or fetus is critical before delivery, when ultrasound does not provide the necessary information, and when MRI has a reasonable possibility of providing the diagnostic information required to direct appropriate management

The present knowledge base suggests that all the foreseeable applications of MRI in obstetrics will be during the second half of pregnancy. In each case, before proceeding with a study, the clinician must weight the potential benefits of the examination against the possible but as yet unknown and therefore unquantifiable risk of the procedure.

MATERNAL ANATOMY AND PATHOLOGY
Uterus

During pregnancy, the uterus changes in size and shape, becoming progressively more rounded or oval and extending to longer than 20 cm by full term.[32] These changes are well shown with MRI. The wall of the corpus uterus (i.e., myometrium) is composed of smooth muscle with a relatively long T1, and it is seen as a relatively low–signal intensity stripe that increases in intensity with T2 weighting.[51] Although there is an increase in the collagen content and hypertrophy of smooth muscle fibers within the body of the uterus during pregnancy, no consistent change in the signal characteristics of the myometrium has been noted.

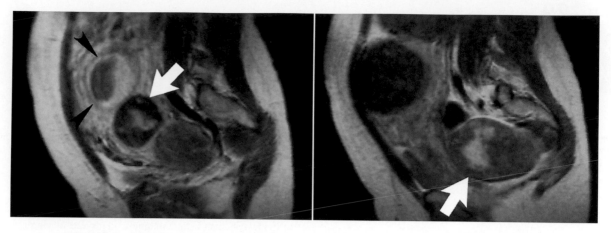

FIGURE 29-1   Multiple uterine leiomyomas in the fourteenth week of pregnancy. There are multiple low-intensity round masses. Some *(arrows)* contain high-intensity regions representing areas of degeneration. SE 2000/30. *Arrowheads,* Conceptus.

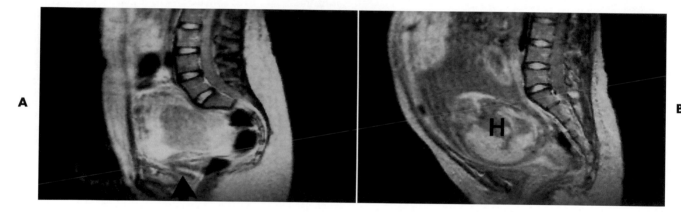

FIGURE 29-2   **A,** Fourteenth week of pregnancy. The laminar appearance of the cervix *(arrow)* is visible. SE 2000/60. **B,** Thirty-sixth week of pregnancy (different patient from **A**). SE 2000/30. The high-intensity cervical zone is wider, and the low-intensity stromal zone is less distinct. *H,* Fetal head.

Because they are stimulated by estrogens, uterine leiomyomas may enlarge during pregnancy.[23] With rapid growth they may outstrip the vascular supply and undergo infarction and necrosis, which may be silent but can also be painful. Leiomyomas can also compromise the ability of the uterus to contract, and if they are in the lower uterine segment, they may preclude vaginal delivery and be associated with an increased incidence of retained placenta.[23,44] Leiomyomas located within the body of the uterus can be associated with early abortion, and multiple leiomyomas are accompanied by a high frequency of malpresentation and premature contractions.[44] Therefore knowledge of the presence, number, and location of uterine leiomyomas in pregnancy can be important. With ultrasound, the evaluation of leiomyomas in the gravid uterus may be difficult because the posterior uterine wall may be obscured by the conceptus. This restriction does not apply with MRI, when they are always clearly identified, and a distinction can be made between degenerate and nondegenerate leiomyomas[90] (Figure 29-1). As in the nonpregnant uterus, MRI is more accurate than ultrasound in assessing the size and localization of leiomyomas.

Serial MR examinations have been used to document the normal process of involution of the postpartum uterus after vaginal delivery.[93] The mean length of the uterine body is 13.8 cm within 30 hours of delivery, which decreases to 5 cm at 6 months, with the greatest change occurring during the first week. The junctional zone is not visible before 2 weeks after birth and even at 6 months appears consistently broad and ill defined, which indicates that caution should be exercised in diagnosing adenomyosis during this period. With ultrasound the cervix is readily visible during pregnancy, but it may be difficult to determine its precise relationship to other structures. Overdistension of the bladder may compress the uterine walls, resulting in an apparent elongation of the cervix[99] or even a false diagnosis of placenta previa.[48] On ultrasound the isthmus of the uterus and cervix cannot be distinguished because of their similar echo textures[41]; furthermore, the external os is not routinely visualized. With MRI the degree of bladder filling has no effect on the ability to visualize the cervix.[51] On sagittal images the position of the internal-external os and the relationship of the cervix to the placenta, lower uterine segment, and presenting fetal parts superiorly and the vagina inferiorly are well seen. The central zone, which has the highest signal intensity, represents cervical mucus and glandular tissue. It is surrounded by a low-intensity zone representing collagen-containing cervical stroma, and around this is an outer muscular layer that returns an intermediate signal.

Cervix

The cervix undergoes important changes during pregnancy (Figure 29-2). Although the cervix does not elongate appreciably, the central high-intensity zone thickens, primarily as a result of proliferation of the endocervical mucosa. The formation of a viscous mucous plug that fills the cervical canal also contributes to the central high intensity zone in the later stages of pregnancy. As cervical connective tissue stroma becomes edematous and undergoes hypertrophy and hyperplasia, the low-intensity stromal zone becomes more prominent. When parturition

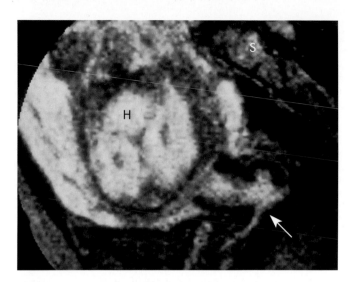

FIGURE 29-3   Cervical incompetence in the thirty-second week of pregnancy. The cervix is seen to be widely dilated (*arrow,* external os). *H,* Fetal head in vertex presentation; *S,* Maternal saccrum. SE 2000/80.

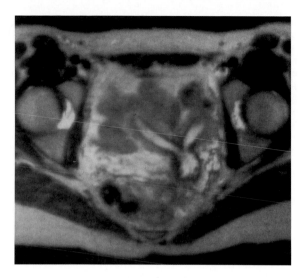

FIGURE 29-4   Bicornuate uterus anteverted. SE 2000/80.

approaches, the cervix begins to efface and dilate. This ripening process is reflected in a widening and shortening of the cervical lumen and a loss of distinction of the fibrous stoma on MR images. In idiopathic cervical dystocia, there is a failure of the ground substance of the cervix to soften in later pregnancy; this is primarily a condition occurring in primigravidas and may necessitate delivery by cesarean section. The ability to use MRI to observe physiological changes in the cervix during pregnancy may provide an opportunity to study abnormalities of cervical function and to evaluate the efficacy of cervical-ripening agents. The postpartum changes in the cervix after uncomplicated vaginal delivery have now been documented by serial MR imaging.[93] The whole cervix shows a high intensity on T2-weighted images obtained less than 30 hours after delivery and an intermediate signal intensity thereafter; the rapid decrease in size and signal intensity probably represents resolving edema.

Cervical incompetence occurs in between 0.05% and 1% of all pregnancies, and the condition is usually considered as a cause of recurrent abortions occurring during the second trimester when no other cause can be identified. Previous trauma to the cervix and in utero exposure to diethylstilbestrol are known causal factors, as are certain congenital abnormalities such as cervical hypoplasia. Detection of an open cervix during pregnancy can be treated by means of cerclage, in which a nonabsorbable suture is placed around the cervix 1.5 cm above the external os at 11 to 18 weeks. The suture is removed at 38 weeks, before the onset of labor. An MR study has been carried out to examine the cervix in a group of patients with a history of cervical incompetence, and the findings have been compared with those from a normal control group.[34] The authors conclude that a cervical length greater than 3.1 cm and an internal os with a width greater than 4.2 mm or an abnormal signal intensity in the cervical stroma are all highly suggestive of an incompetent cervix (Figure 29-3).

Congenital Anomalies of the Female Genital Tract

Congenital anomalies of the female genital tract are relatively rare, but they are found more commonly in women with infertility or a history of repeated miscarriage. Embryologically the fallopian tubes, uterus, and cervix are derived from the fusion and descent of the paired müllerian ducts. Failure of the ducts to fuse may be partial or complete, resulting in a spectrum of anomalies that involve the vagina, cervix, and uterus. From the standpoint of clinical practice the essential distinction that has to be made is between the anomalies in which pregnancy remains possible, with or without surgical intervention, and those in which it is precluded. In the past, the investigation would have been carried out by hysterosalpingography supplemented by laparoscopy to study the external contour of the uterus. Because of MRI, these procedures are now redundant; MRI is the optimal technique for evaluating these condi-

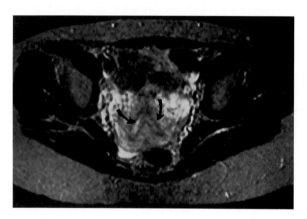

FIGURE 29-5   Bicornuate uterus, retroverted. T2-weighted image shows a Y-shaped endometrial canal and two cornua *(curved arrow).* (From reference 98.)

tions. A series of T2-weighted images is taken parallel to and at right angles to the long axis of the uterus, whereby the internal anatomy and external contour can be displayed. The more common anomalies of septate or subseptate uterus, caused by failure of the sagittal uterine septum to resorb, can be readily distinguished from a bicornuate uterus using MRI. This distinction is of practical importance because the presence of a septum can prevent proper placental implantation and leads to recurrent miscarriages in as many as 67% of pregnancies, whereas implantation may proceed satisfactorily in a bicornuate uterus (Figures 29-4 and 29-5). The diagnosis of an unsuspected subseptate uterus may be made in late pregnancy when a persistent transverse lie of the fetus is found (Figure 29-6).

Placenta

The placenta has been seen as a focal thickening along the periphery of the gestational sac as early as 12 weeks' gestation (Figure 29-7). As pregnancy progresses, the placenta grows and thickens so that by the end of the fourth month, it has attained its final thickness, but circumferential enlargement continues into the third trimester.[96] The placenta may be enlarged in cases of transfusion incompatibility, maternal diabetes, and maternal anemia, whereas the placenta may be smaller than normal in preeclampsia.[94] On T2-weighted spin-echo images, placental tissue returns a high signal intensity, and on T1-weighted spin-echo images, it returns a relatively low signal intensity, slightly greater than that of the myometrium (Figure 29-8). Usually the placenta has a fairly homogeneous appearance, and the internal architecture cannot be appreciated.

Endometrial veins are present along the base of the placenta and in the septa, draining blood from the placenta. These vascular channels occasionally are visible on MR scans.

The normal physiological placental calcifications that occur throughout pregnancy are not visible with MRI. Placenta previa is a most important pathological condition involving the lower uterine segment. It usually presents with painless vaginal bleeding during the third trimester. In the past decade, ultrasound has become the procedure of choice for reevaluating patients with suspected placenta previa. Ultrasound, however, is operator dependent and occasionally is inaccurate, with a reported false-positive rate in the second trimester of 0.4% and a false-negative rate of less than 2%.[11,29] Because sagittal T2-weighted images precisely depict the relationship of the lower edge of the placenta to the internal cervical os, MRI can be used as a test complementary to ultrasound in those patients in whom the lower limit of the placenta is not clearly seen (Figure 29-9). In one study, 25 women with a diagnosis of placenta previa on ultrasound examination underwent MRI.[67] There was complete agreement of placental localization, but significant differences were found in the degree of placenta previa (i.e., total placenta previa, marginal placenta previa, low-lying placenta). In seven of these patients the results of the MRI were more accurate and directly altered patient management.

Anomalies of the placenta, though rare, can be identified by MRI. An example of an abnormal cord insertion in a placenta with a second succenturiate lobe has been reported. The blood vessels running between the two were clearly demonstrated lying between the fetal head and the os.[59]

Placental Migration. By the fourth month of pregnancy the placenta covers half of the uterine surface, but this decreases to less than a third in the final trimester. So that the higher incidence of placenta previa found on ultrasound studies in the second trimester of pregnancy compared with the final trimester could be explained, the concept of placental migration was introduced. One proposal is that this occurs by the placenta becoming detached and then reattached to the uterine wall in a mechanism called *dynamic placentation,* but most authors attribute the apparent migration of the placenta to the formation of the lower uterine segment.[2] The findings of an MRI study support the more recent work with ultrasound and have shown that placental migration exists only in the sense that a placenta situated on the lower uterine segment will appear to move because of the growth of the latter. Placentas adjacent to or on the cervix will not migrate unless effacement occurs.[65]

Gestational Trophoblastic Neoplasia

This spectrum of disease includes hydatidiform mole, invasive mole, and choriocarcinoma.[55] The condition has an incidence of approximately 1 in 2000 pregnancies in the United Kingdom, and 1% to 4% of patients have a recurrence of a molar pregnancy. Clinically a molar pregnancy is considered in a patient with severe preeclampsia before 24 weeks' gestation, a large-for-date uterus, or bleeding in the first trimester. Laboratory findings are usually diagnostic, with an elevated level of the ß-subunit of human chorionic gonadotropin (ß-hCG) in the serum.[97] Often, ultrasound can accurately identify the neoplasm within the uterus and can be useful in combination with serial ß-hCG assays in the evaluation of tumor volume.[70] The sonographic features of hydatidiform mole and its variants are usually diagnostic.[68] Ultrasound can also be valuable in the evaluation of the liver for metastatic disease in patients with choriocarcinoma, and MRI may have similar capabilities. Several cases of hydatidiform mole have been reported with MRI[50,66,90] (Figure 29-10). In some cases the vesicular nature of the mass was appreciated, and areas of hemorrhage were readily identified. Because of its excellent soft tissue contrast resolution, MRI may be particularly useful for demonstrating macroscopic invasion of the myometrium and documenting the return of normal uterine appearances after successful chemotherapy. It may also prove useful in the primary search for metastases in patients with gestational trophoblastic neoplasia.

Nontrophoblastic Neoplasia

Chorioangioma is the most common primary nontrophoblastic tumor of the placenta. It is a vascular malformation that macroscopically appears as a proliferation of capillaries in a loose fibrous stroma.[26] Small tumors are usually incidental findings and have no clinical significance. Large chorioangiomas appear as intraplacental masses that may protrude from the fetal side of the placenta and may be associated with fetal hydrops, congestive heart failure, intrauterine growth restriction

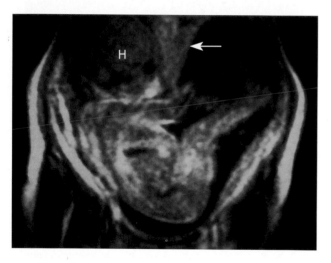

FIGURE 29-6 Coronal scan of a breech presentation with extended legs. A septum is seen arising from the fundus of the uterus *(arrow). H,* Head.

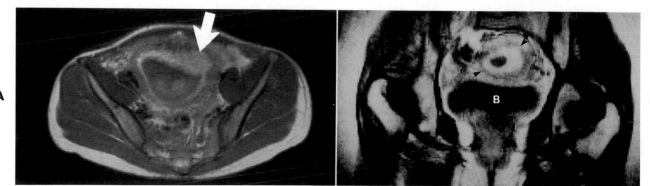

FIGURE 29-7 **A,** Gestational sac with focal thickening *(arrow),* which represents the developing placenta. Twelfth week of gestation, SE 2000/30 transverse image. **B,** In the sixth week of gestation, the gestational sac appears as a dark region surrounded by a bright decidual reaction. Beneath the decidua is a dark zone of myometrium *(arrowheads).* The fetal pole is not visible. *B,* Urinary bladder. SE 500/30 coronal image.

(IUGR) (also called *intrauterine growth retardation*) or fetal death. One case of chorioangioma has been described with MRI[90] (Figure 29-11). It appeared as a slightly inhomogeneous rounded mass on the fetal side of the placenta, with a signal intensity slightly greater than the surrounding placenta on both T1-weighted and T2-weighted images. It was separated from the placenta by a low-intensity capsule that on histological examination represented a thick fibrous capsule. Other macroscopic lesions within the placenta, such as subchorionic fibrin deposition, intervillous thrombosis, perivillous fibrin deposition, and infarcts, have not yet been reported on MR scans.

Pelvic Masses

Ovarian neoplasms occur in 0.1% to 0.4% of pregnancies and are usually incidental findings. During pregnancy, however, they can cause pain as a result of torsion, internal hemorrhage, extrinsic compression of the pelvic organs, or even rupture. During the first trimester, the most common pelvic mass is a corpus luteum cyst (Figure 29-12), which usually undergoes regression by the fifteenth week. They are usually less than 6 cm in size, but occasionally these cysts persist and even grow (Figure 29-13). Although not entirely diagnostic, the ultrasound findings of an anechoic mass with smooth, thin walls and a prominent acoustic enhancement suggest a diagnosis of a corpus luteal cyst and may allow for conservative management.[24] An ovarian cystic mass larger than 10 cm in diameter or one that appears to enlarge during pregnancy should be excised during the second trimester to avoid the complications. Excision is also performed because it may be very difficult to completely exclude neoplastic changes in the wall of the cyst.

Dermoid cysts appear on ultrasound as a complex mass with echogenic components.[62] Occasionally the sebum within a dermoid cyst may appear so echogenic that it can simulate a gas-filled loop of bowel and evade thorough sonographic assessment.[31] MRI will accurately depict dermoid cysts, and usually a precise diagnosis is possible by using sequences with spectral fat saturation (Figure 29-14). In a study of 17 patients with a suspected pelvic mass at ultrasound, the correct origin of the masses was determined by MRI in all but only in 12 on ultrasound. In three cases the MR results led to a change in management. This study emphasizes that MRI is of value when ultrasound results are not definitive.[38]

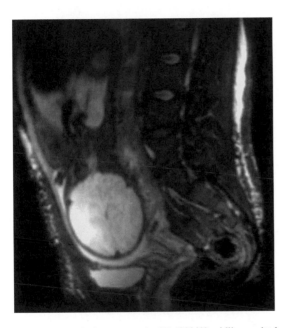

FIGURE 29-8   Marginal placenta previa. SE 4000/60 midline sagittal scan.

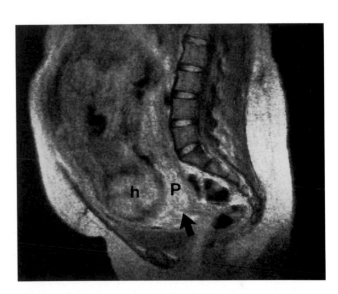

FIGURE 29-9   Complete placenta previa in the thirtieth week of gestation. The placenta *(P)* completely covers the internal cervical os *(arrow)*. h, Fetal head. SE 2000/28.

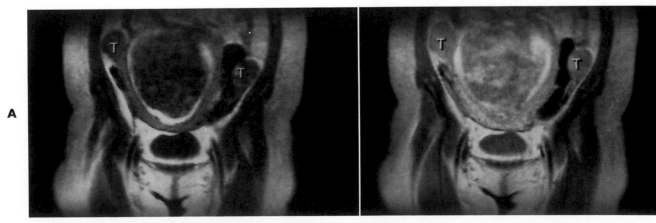

FIGURE 29-10   SE 1000/28 **(A)** and SE 2000/28 **(B)** coronal images. Hydatidiform mole demonstrate the vesicular nature of the intrauterine mass. Areas within and around the mass that demonstrate high signal intensity on T1-weighted and proton density–weighted images are hemorrhage. There are also bilateral theca lutein cysts *(T)*.

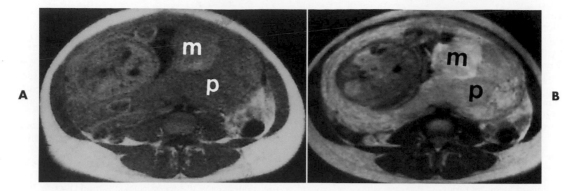

FIGURE 29-11 SE 500/28 **(A)** and SE 1500/56 **(B)** images. Chorioangioma in the thirtieth week of pregnancy. The chorioangioma appears as a slightly inhomogeneous mass *(m)* that arises from the fetal side of the placenta *(p)*. It demonstrates a signal intensity greater than the placenta.

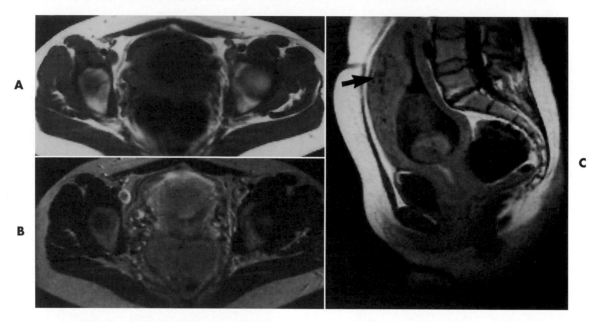

FIGURE 29-12 Corpus luteum cyst in the sixteenth week of pregnancy. **A,** 500/30. **B,** 2000/80. **C,** 500/40. Multilocular cystic mass with long T1 and T2 values is seen posterior to the uterus. In **C,** numerous vascular channels are seen at the placenta–uterine interface *(arrow)*.

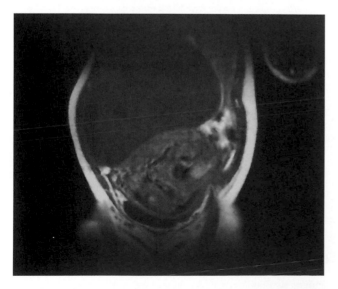

FIGURE 29-13 Giant corpus luteum cyst, superior to the uterus, in the twenty-seventh week of pregnancy. SE 500/28.

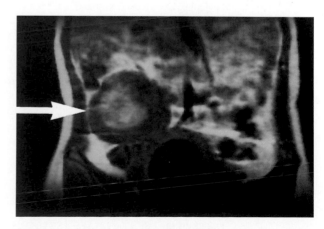

FIGURE 29-14 Dermoid tumor of the right ovary in the fourteenth week of pregnancy. There is a large fat-containing mass *(arrow)* superior to the gravid uterus. SE 500/30

Ectopic Pregnancy

A major role for MRI in the diagnosis of ectopic pregnancy has not been defined. Pelvic or transvaginal ultrasound in conjunction with hCG determinations will probably remain the most useful diagnostic approach.[47] In one reported case, MRI was helpful in identifying the relative position of the fetus, placenta, and uterus in a patient with a viable abdominal pregnancy[13] (Figure 29-15). There is a further report in which MRI correctly diagnosed an incarcerated pregnancy in a bicornuate uterus, which had been misdiagnosed on ultrasound and computed tomography as an abdominal pregnancy.[98] Usually, however, the ectopic gestation is very small and located within the isthmus or ampullary portion of the fallopian tube. As with ultrasound, this would probably be difficult to reliably identify with MRI. Fluid in the cul-de-sac, a secondary finding in some ectopic pregnancies, can be identified with both MRI and ultrasound, but MRI has the additional capability of specifically identifying the fluid as hemorrhagic in nature (Figure 29-16). Nonetheless, this will probably have very limited use, because

hemorrhagic fluid could just as easily have arisen from rupture of a hemorrhagic ovarian cyst or another process.

Maternal Spine and Vessels

Back pain is a common complaint during pregnancy, and it has been claimed that there is an increased incidence of herniation at the L5/S1 interspace in pregnant patients.[9] On the other hand, a more recent study in which a group of 41 asymptomatic parous and nulliparous nonpregnant women were compared with a group of 45 pregnant patients, the prevalence of disk bulge or herniation at one or more levels on MRI was almost identical (54% versus 53%).[89] A study comparing the appearances of the lumbar spine in a series of patients with lumbar backache during pregnancy with the appearance of the spine 1 year later revealed that there had been no significant change in the appearances.[64,66] It is reasonable to conclude that pregnancy does not appear to induce, accelerate, or produce reversible changes in the lumbar disks. MR evidence of disk abnormalities is therefore useful only in the context of the patient's symptomatic complaints, and MR findings must be carefully correlated with clinical findings before therapeutic intervention is considered.

When the pregnant patient is placed in the supine position for imaging, the inferior vena cava may be so compressed by the gravid uterus that it appears virtually occluded.[51] As a result of the impeded venous return by the inferior vena cava and normal physiological changes of pregnancy, dilated venous channels are frequently visualized in the pelvis of pregnant patients (Figure 29-17).

Pelvimetry

For some time there has been evidence to suggest that irradiation of the fetus, even at the low levels used in x-ray pelvimetry, may cause an increased risk of childhood cancer.[33] Nevertheless, as late as 1980, pelvimetry was used in almost 7% of live births in the United States.[86] Despite the widespread belief among clinicians that knowledge of pelvic measurement is of little value in cephalic presentations (since soft tissue dystocia is a more significant factor), overall pelvimetry rates remain between 5% and 7%. Pelvimetry does have a definite place, however, in the management of breech presentations to determine the adequacy of the maternal pelvis to accommodate the unmolded fetal head.[14,84] In some institutions, x-ray pelvimetry has been replaced by computed tomographic pelvimetry to decrease the radiation dose.[21] Because MRI can clearly depict pelvic soft tissue and bony landmarks, it can be used to accurately measure maternal pelvic dimensions, obtaining traditional pelvimetric measurements without the exposure to ionizing radiation[80,88] (Figure 29-18). In one study, a midline sagittal section allowed for measurements of the anteroposterior diameter of the

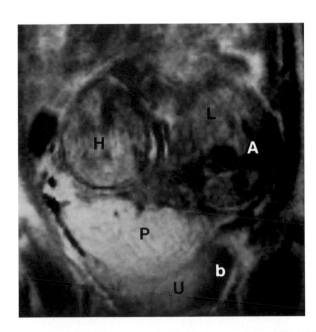

FIGURE 29-15   Viable full-term abdominal pregnancy. Coronal SE 1500/28 image. Transverse fetal lie with the fetal head *(H)* and abdomen *(A)* visible. There is scant amniotic fluid, and the maternal bladder *(b)* is compressed by the maternal uterus *(U)* and placenta *(P). L,* Fetal liver.

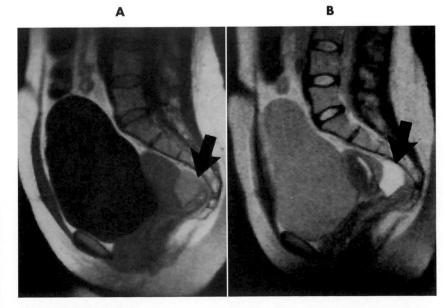

FIGURE 29-16   Ectopic pregnancy with blood in the cul-de-sac. An ectopic gestational sac was not identified. Spin-echo (500/28) **(A)** and spin-echo (2000/50) **(B)** sagittal images show fluid in the cul-de-sac *(arrows),* which demonstrates intermediate high signal on the T1-weighted image and very high signal with more T2 weighting, consistent with hemorrhage.

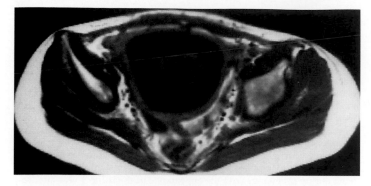

FIGURE 29-17   Twentieth week of pregnancy. Numerous venous channels are visible in the maternal pelvis. This is a normal finding in pregnancy. SE 500/30.

pelvic inlet and outlet, and the multisection set of four transverse axial sections 1 cm in thickness obtained 3 cm above the symphysis pubis allowed assessment of the interspinous diameter. By using spin-echo pulse sequences with short repetition times, the examination can be carried out in less than 10 minutes. Although there is a good correlation between the x-ray and the MRI measurements, account must be taken of the fact that standard x-ray pelvimetry is usually performed in the erect position, whereas MRI is carried out supine.[64]

FETAL ANATOMY AND PATHOLOGY
Technique

Initial attempts to image the fetus using conventional spin-echo sequences[48] were frustrated by fetal motion even during the third trimester[36,61,73,92] and the inability to always achieve an optimal imaging plane (Figure 29-19). Many groups have found that pregnant patients

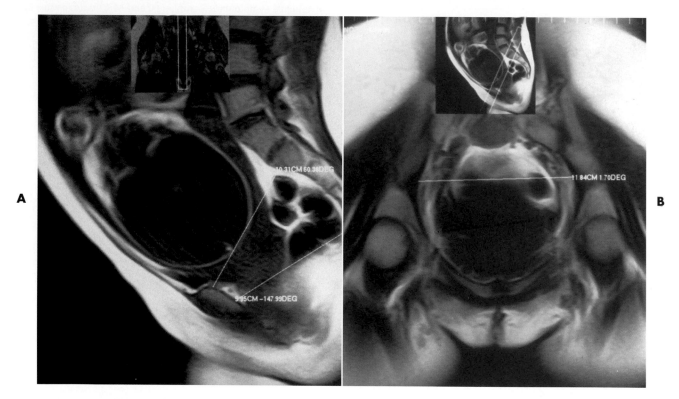

FIGURE 29-18   MR pelvimetry showing midline sagittal section (**A**) and a coronal oblique section through the pelvic inlet (**B**).

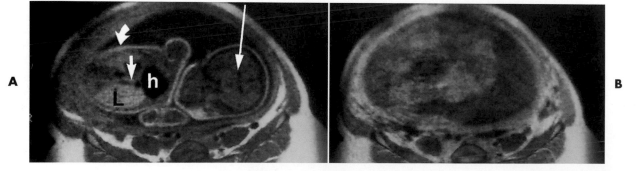

FIGURE 29-19   Polyhydramnios and the normal fetus in the thirty-fourth week of gestation. **A,** Spin-echo (500/28) T1-weighted image with a relatively short repetition time shows cerebral ventricles *(long arrow),* the heart *(h),* the inferior vena cava *(short arrow),* the liver *(L),* and subcutaneous fat *(curved arrow).* **B,** Spin-echo (1500/28) image with a longer repetition time (and longer T1); the fetal anatomical detail is degraded by fetal motion. Note that the maternal anatomical detail is not noticeably changed.

are best imaged while lying in the left lateral decubitus position because they feel more comfortable, the fetus is less likely to move, and the resultant image quality is improved.[75] Others routinely image patients in the supine position, often with the knees flexed and supported by pillows.[87]

The development of fast imaging strategies, particularly EPI, has rendered obsolete the use of sedation* or muscle relaxant[74] to reduce fetal movement (Figures 29-20 and 29-21). Similarly, attempting to capitalize on the effect of maternal posture, meals, and time of day on fetal movements is also unecessary.[27,52,53] On heavily T2-weighted images, details of the placenta, umbilical cord, and surface features of the fetus are highlighted against the high signal of the amniotic fluid. In the thorax the lungs, which have a relatively high fluid content, are contrasted against the heart (Figure 29-21). All the major abdominal organs are well seen, and in the limbs the diaphyses and apophyses of long bones, as well as soft tissue detail, are noted.[35] T1-weighted images provide for an assessment of the subcutaneous fat stores.[79] As expected, the fetal anatomy is better delineated as pregnancy progresses and organ size and tissue contrast increase.[78] Because MRI can demonstrate many fetal structures and morphological abnormalities, it has been used to perform noninvasive autopsies of stillborn fetuses to provide information about anomalies for genetic counseling[82] (Figures 29-22 and 29-23). Ultrasound remains as the primary technique for identifying and evaluating fetal abnormalities in utero, however, but in some cases, additional useful information may be provided by MR examination.

Central Nervous System

Fetal brain architecture can be visualized in utero in the third trimester of gestation.[35,87] The cerebral hemispheres, ventricles, and eyes are almost always identifiable, whereas the posterior fossa, cerebellum, midbrain, brainstem, and craniocervical junction and systems have been depicted less frequently (Figures 29-24 and 29-25). As in adults, the cerebrospinal fluid in the ventricles has a low signal on T1-weighted images, showing an increase in intensity with more T2 weighting.[48] The brain substance itself demonstrates intermediate to low signal intensity on T1-weighted images and a higher signal intensity on more T2-weighted images.[64] The relatively long T1 and T2 relaxation times of the brain probably reflect its high water content.[48] Myelination has been reported within the basal ganglia as early as 34 weeks' gestation; most

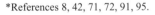

*References 8, 42, 71, 72, 91, 95.

myelination, however, occurs during the first year of postnatal life,[16] and there is generally an absence of demonstrable distinction between gray and white matter in utero.

Excellent anatomical detail has been shown[54] in the brain of aborted fetuses of varying gestational ages imaged at 1.5 Tesla. Three distinct intensity zones seen on MRI were not visualized on gross specimens. These correlated with the germinal matrix internally, the future white matter centrally, and the outer future cortex (Figure 29-26). The unmyelinated white matter demonstrated a low signal intensity on T1-weighted images and a high signal intensity on T2-weighted images. This work suggests that with improvements in imaging capabilities, MRI may allow far better visualization of normal structures of the fetal central nervous system and normal neural development than other imaging techniques. A number of cerebral anomalies have been imaged with MRI (Figures 29-27 to 29-38). These include anencephaly[88] (Figure 29-27), ventriculomegaly,[50,81] cystic hygroma,[50] Dandy-Walker cyst,[81] autolysis,[81] and hydranencephaly.[85] Furthermore, fetal brain metabolism has been evaluated in utero with MR spectroscopy.[56] MR spectroscopy could develop into a powerful research method and eventually a useful clinical tool for the evaluation of in utero brain metabolism. Although occasionally a large portion of the spinal cord can be visualized on a single sagittal image of the fetus,[35,48] more commonly only a segment of the vertebral column and spinal cord is visualized (Figure 29-39), but this can be circumvented by using oblique imaging planes or interrogating a three-dimensional acquisition of the whole fetus.

Thorax

The fetal heart is always visible after 25 weeks' gestation, appearing dark in contrast with surrounding tissues as a result of the flow-void phenomenon[35,49] (Figures 29-21 and 29-40). The atria, ventricles, and intraventricular septum have been resolved on EPI studies, and pulmonary vessels can also be demonstrated. On T2-weighted images the fetal lungs return a high signal, contrasting with the dark vascular structures centrally and the liver inferiorly[35] (Figures 29-8 and 29-21). An accurate and reliable method of estimating fetal lung volume would be valuable in cases in which there was suspected compromised lung growth, such as when a diaphragmatic hernia (Figures 29-41 and 29-42) results in lung hypoplasia and also when premature delivery is contemplated. When computer planimetry of contiguous EPI sections was used, the fetal lung volume was estimated in 20 singleton pregnancies. This study showed that lung volumes increased exponentially with gestational age from 21 ml at 23 weeks' gestation to a maximum of 94 ml

Text continued on p. 608

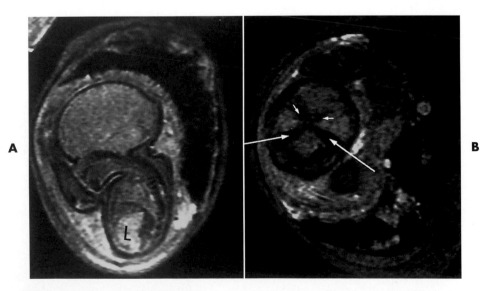

FIGURE 29-20   Fast scanning of normal fetus. **A,** Gradient-recalled acquisition in the steady state (GRASS) parasagittal image with breath-holding technique shows an excellent fetal outline as a result of susceptibility of artifacts from the bony structures. The fetal liver *(L)* is shown as a high–signal intensity structure. However, in these particular pulse sequences, there is poor tissue contrast and anatomical detail, especially within intracranial structures. **B,** Fetal transverse GRASS image through the head shows low signal intensity of temporal bone *(long arrows)* and sphenoid wing *(short arrows)*. (From reference 91.)

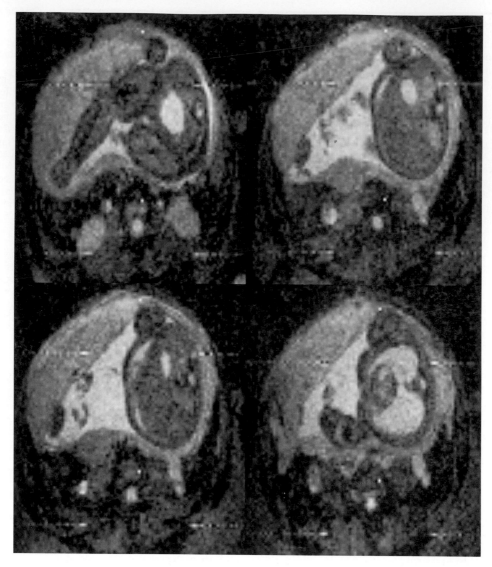

FIGURE 29-21   EPI (transverse T2-weighted) images through the thorax and abdomen of the fetus in a 38-week pregnancy. The placenta, umbilical cord, and surface features of the fetus are highlighted against the high signal of the amniotic fluid.

FIGURE 29-22   Aborted fetus. Coronal MRI shows detailed bronchial and vascular anatomy in the lungs. (Courtesy E. Trefelner and S. McCarthy.)

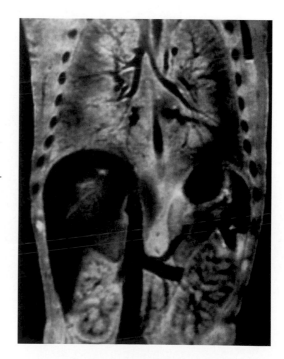

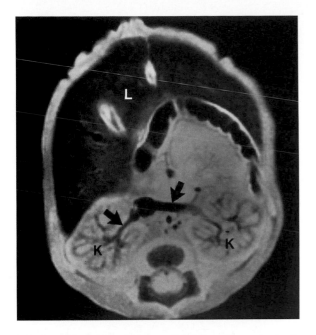

FIGURE 29-23   Aborted fetus. Transverse MRI shows the renal veins *(arrows)* and anatomical details in the kidneys *(K)* and liver *(L)*.

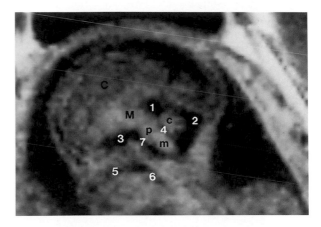

FIGURE 29-24   Fetal head in the twenty-eighth week of gestation. SE 500/28 parasagittal image. *C,* Cerebrum; *c,* cerebellum; *M,* midbrain; *p,* pons; *m,* medulla; *1,* superior cerebellar cistern; *2,* cisterna magna; *3,* suprasellar cistern; *4,* fourth ventricle; *5,* nasopharynx; *6,* oropharynx; *7,* prepontine cistern.

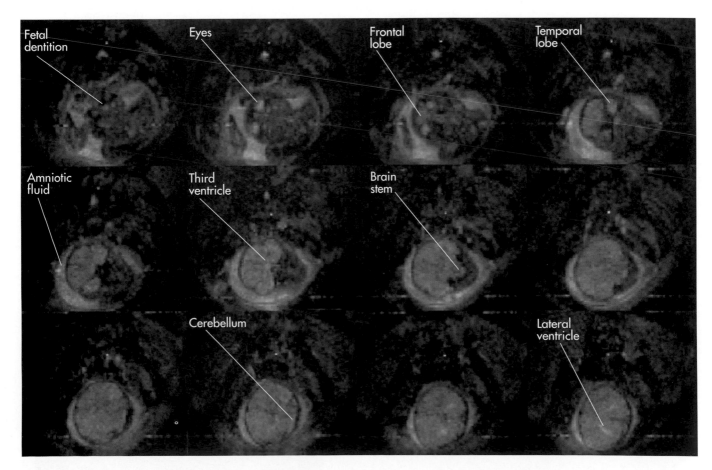

FIGURE 29-25   EPI (T2-weighted) coronal sections through the brain of a 37-week fetus.

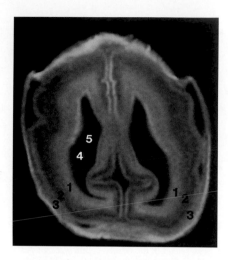

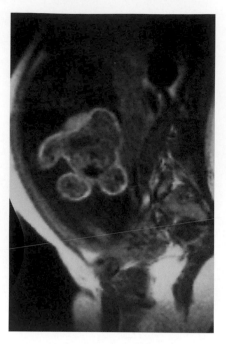

FIGURE 29-26 Aborted fetus at the level of the lateral ventricles in the seventeenth week of gestation. *1,* Germinal (matrix) zone; *2,* intermediate zone (future white matter); *3,* cortical zone (future cortex); *4,* choroid plexus; *5,* lateral ventricle. (Courtesy M. Mintz.)

FIGURE 29-27 Anencephaly and polyhydramnios in the twenty-ninth week of gestation. No head is present above the neck. SE 500/28.

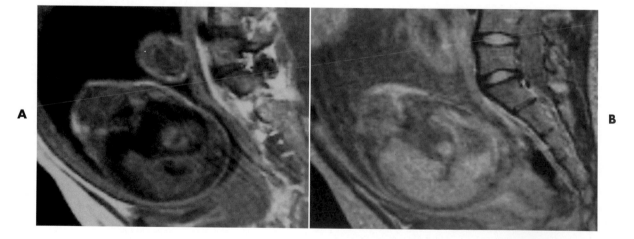

FIGURE 29-28 Hydrocephalus in the thirty-sixth week of gestation. Large cerebrospinal fluid–filled ventricles are dark in **A** (SE 500/30) and show a relative increase in the signal intensity on the SE 2000/40 image **(B).** Note similar signal of amniotic fluid.

FIGURE 29-29 Dandy-Walker cyst in the thirty-fifth week of gestation. There is a symmetrical fluid collection in the posterior fossa of the fetal brain. SE 500/28.

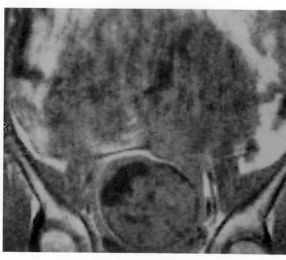

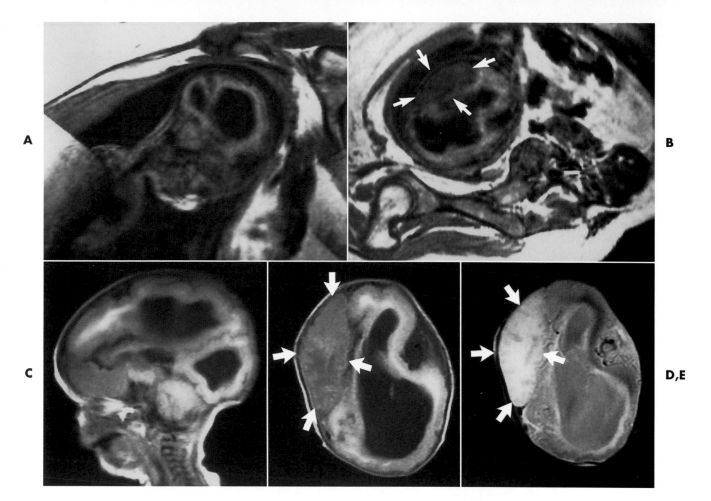

FIGURE 29-30 Hemimeganencephaly. Fetal parasagittal **(A)** and axial **(B)** T1-weighted images show the dilated ventricular system of the left hemisphere. The white matter of the left hemisphere appears to have a much higher signal intensity than that of normal parenchyma (*arrows* in **B**) in the right cerebral hemisphere. This may represent hypermyelination or accelerated myelination of the white matter in the involved hemisphere. Pachygyria of the involved hemisphere is also noted. Neonatal parasagittal T1-weighted image **(C)** corresponding to **A,** axial T1-weighted image **(D)** corresponding to **B,** and axial T2-weighted image **(E)** show enlarged left cerebral hemisphere with a dilated ventricular system. Normal neonatal brain parenchyma (*arrows* in **D** and **E**) shows hypointensity on the T1-weighted image and hyperintensity on the T2-weighed image **(E),** which is a typical finding in an infant during the first year of life. The parenchymal signal intensity of the abnormal left hemisphere is similar to that of a typical adult brain **(D).** Note the pachygyria of the left cerebral hemisphere. (From reference 91.)

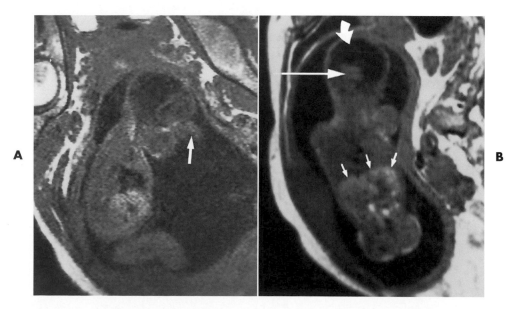

FIGURE 29-31 Alobar holoprosencephaly. T1-weighted fetal parasagittal image **(A)** shows a large proboscis *(large arrow)*. Coronal image **(B)** shows a dilated single ventricle *(curved arrow)*, a fused thalamus *(long arrow)*, and high–signal intensity meconium in the transverse colon *(small arrows)*. (From reference 91.)

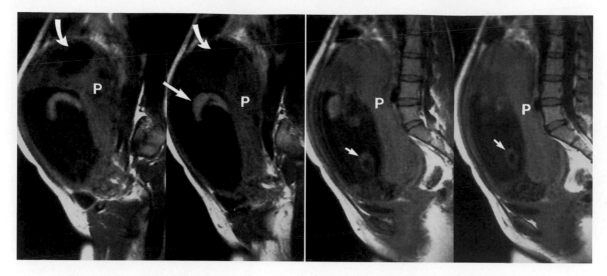

FIGURE 29-32 Hydranencephaly *(curved arrow)* without identifiable intracranial structure. Breech presentation, anhydramnios, and fetal ascites. The fetal liver, shown as a high–signal intensity structure *(large arrow),* and an edematous intestine *(small arrow)* are suspended in fetal ascites. *P,* Placenta.

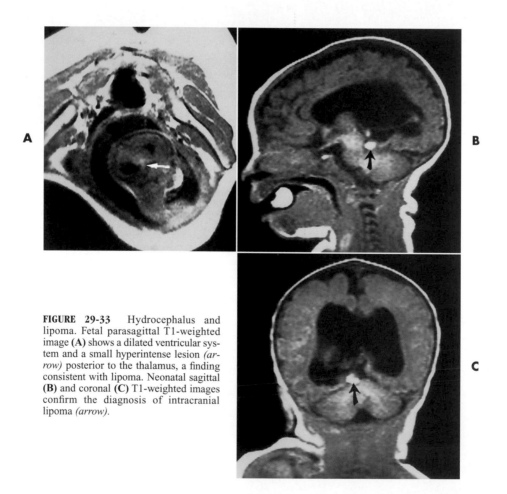

FIGURE 29-33 Hydrocephalus and lipoma. Fetal parasagittal T1-weighted image **(A)** shows a dilated ventricular system and a small hyperintense lesion *(arrow)* posterior to the thalamus, a finding consistent with lipoma. Neonatal sagittal **(B)** and coronal **(C)** T1-weighted images confirm the diagnosis of intracranial lipoma *(arrow).*

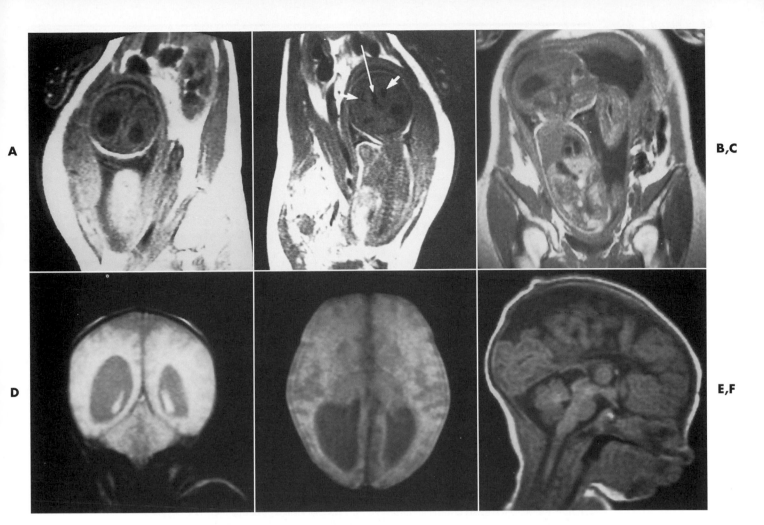

FIGURE 29-34 Colpocephaly, partial agenesis of the corpus callosum, and enlarged massa intermedia. Fetal coronal T1-weighted images from posterior **(A)** to anterior **(B)** show dilated ventricular system **(A)** near the trigone of the lateral ventricle posteriorly. Ventricular dilatation is not noted in the more anterior images **(B)**, in which the body of the lateral ventricles *(small arrows)* appears to be tilted upward. The third ventricle *(long arrow)* is interposed between the lateral ventricles that are tilted upward. This is consistent with partial or complete agenesis of the corpus callosum. Fetal parasagittal **(C)** demonstrates an enlarged ventricle posteriorly (colpocephaly). Note the breech presentation of the fetus. Neonatal coronal T2-weighted image **(D)** corresponding to **A** and axial T2-weighted image **(E)** demonstrate colpocephaly. Parasagittal T1-weighted image **(F)** confirms the partial agenesis of the corpus callosum. The massa intermedia is enlarged. (From reference 91.)

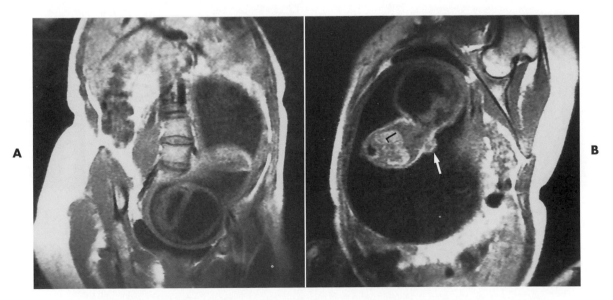

FIGURE 29-35 Hydrocephalus and hypoplastic extremities. **A,** Fetal coronal T1-weighted image of the brain shows a dilated ventricular system. **B,** Fetal T1-weighted image approximating the coronal section of the fetal body shows a small remnant of the upper extremity *(arrow)* and hydrocephalus. The fetal liver *(L)* is normal.

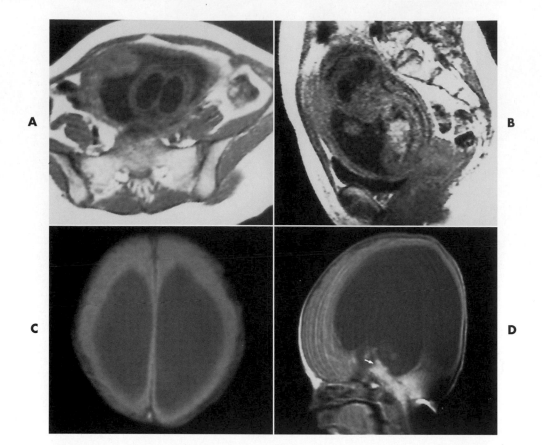

FIGURE 29-36 Aqueductal stenosis and hydrocephalus. **A,** Transverse T1-weighted image shows dilated lateral ventricles. **B,** Sagittal image demonstrates a dilated ventricular system with a relatively intact fourth ventricle. Aqueductal stenosis is therefore suspected. The fetus is in the breech position. **C,** Neonatal transverse image corresponding to **A** demonstrates a dilated ventricular system. **D,** Neonatal sagittal image corresponding to **B** shows the dilated lateral and third ventricles and the proximal dilatation of the aqueduct *(arrow)* consistent with aqueductal stenosis.

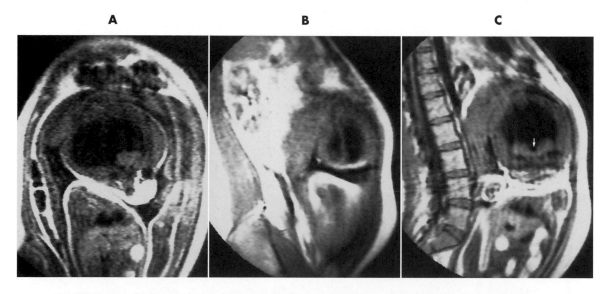

FIGURE 29-37 Hydrocephalus. **A,** Fetal parasagittal T1-weighted image shows a dilated ventricular system. **B,** Axial T1-weighted image near the convexity shows a midline structure (falx), excluding the diagnosis of alobar holoprosencephaly. However, semilobar holoprosencephaly cannot be completely excluded. **C,** Coronal T1-weighted image clearly demonstrates the existence of a third ventricle *(arrow)* and a separate thalamus, confirming the diagnosis of simple hydrocephalus.

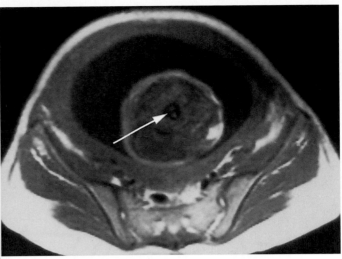

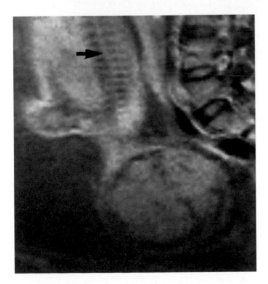

FIGURE 29-38 Iniencephaly and diastematomyelia. **A,** Fetal parasagittal T1-weighted image shows a dilated ventricular system and a hyperextended neck (stargazer). The cerebellum *(small black arrow)* and brainstem *(small white arrow)* appear to be intact. **B,** Fetal axial T1-weighted image shows a division of the cervical spinal cord *(long arrow)*. **C,** More cranially, a linear structure *(small white arrow)* may represent a bony spicule or a fibrous band dividing the cord, supporting the diagnosis of diastematomyelia. (From reference 92.)

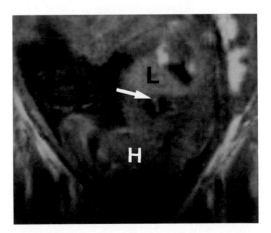

FIGURE 29-39 Dorsal spine is normal and well seen *(arrow)*. Polyhydramnios is present at the thirty-first week of pregnancy. SE 2000/30.

FIGURE 29-40 Cardiac intervention septum *(arrow)* is well seen in this SE 500/28 image of a fetus in the vertex presentation in the thirty-first week of gestation. *H,* Head; *L,* liver.

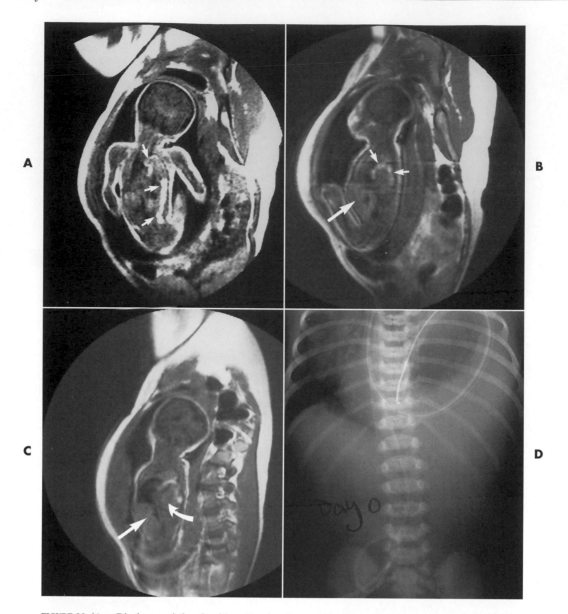

FIGURE 29-41   Diaphragmatic hernia without liver involvement. Fetal coronal **(A)**, parasagittal **(B)**, and oblique **(C)** T1-weighted images show the bowel herniating into the chest cavity (*small arrows* in **A** and **B**). Meconium is shown as a high-signal intensity area within the gastrointestinal tract. The liver (*large arrow* in **B** and **C**) is located anteriorly without evidence of herniation. Herniation is located posteriorly (Bochdalek's hernia). The stomach is shown as an isointense structure (*curved arrow* in **C**) and is also displaced into the chest cavity. Neonatal plain film **(D)** of the chest and abdomen shows the stomach herniating into the chest wall; the soft tissue density next to the stomach may represent the herniated bowel contents.

at term.[4] Recent studies of lung volume using three-dimensional ultrasound have reported similar results.[15,43]

The events that take place in the late canalicular and early terminal sac phase of maturation (between 20 and 30 weeks' gestation) are determinants of gestational age–related survival. These include dilatation of the terminal air sacs, vascularization of the terminal tubules, and formation of type 1 and type 2 pneumocytes, which secrete a lipoprotein complex called *surfactant*[63] that reduces airway surface tension. The most common cause of neonatal death is severe prematurity, and 90% of fetuses delivered before 28 weeks suffer from respiratory distress syndrome resulting from global immaturity of the lungs. With improvements in intensive care and the development of artificial surfactants, an increasing number of infants delivered between 23 and 28 weeks' gestation can be resuscitated. In the third trimester, amniocentesis allows the surfactant content of the amniotic fluid to be measured, which assists in the assessment of lung maturity, but the procedure is in-

vasive and is not without risk. Therefore a noninvasive alternative is greatly needed. Serial measurements of T1 and T2 relaxation times of the fetal lung show pronounced changes around 30 weeks, and refinement of such measurements may allow an estimate of lung maturity to be made.[30]

Abdomen

The liver, which occupies most of the upper abdomen in the fetus, is routinely visible in the second and third trimesters[35,66] (Figure 29-43). Signal changes within the liver have been shown to occur between 20 and 26 weeks in a series of 16 pregnant women studied by contiguous transverse axial EPI sections of the fetus. The T2*-weighted pulse sequence used would be sensitive to the presence of iron-containing moieties, which alter local tissue susceptibility, leading to signal attenuation. The signal changes that are observed can best be explained on the

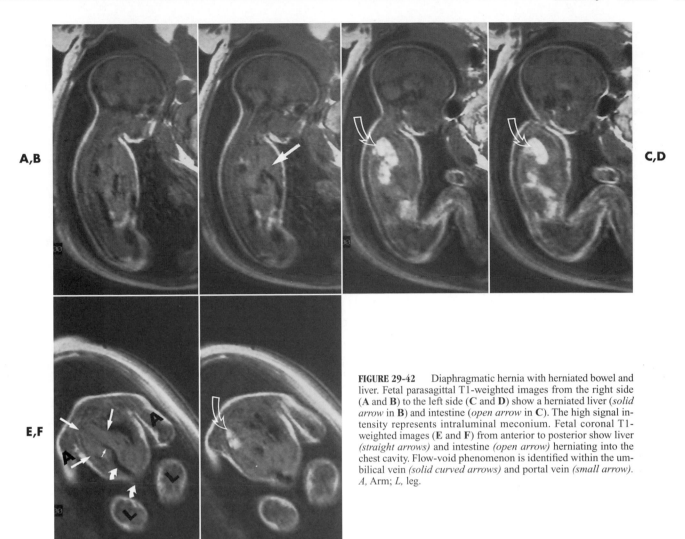

A,B

C,D

E,F

FIGURE 29-42   Diaphragmatic hernia with herniated bowel and liver. Fetal parasagittal T1-weighted images from the right side (**A** and **B**) to the left side (**C** and **D**) show a herniated liver (*solid arrow* in **B**) and intestine (*open arrow* in **C**). The high signal intensity represents intraluminal meconium. Fetal coronal T1-weighted images (**E** and **F**) from anterior to posterior show liver *(straight arrows)* and intestine *(open arrow)* herniating into the chest cavity. Flow-void phenomenon is identified within the umbilical vein *(solid curved arrows)* and portal vein *(small arrow).* *A,* Arm; *L,* leg.

basis of a progressive decrease in red cell production by the liver and a consequent reduction in the liver iron levels as the spleen and bone marrow take over hemopoiesis.[19]

The fetal spleen and pancreas have not yet been assessed with MRI. The fluid-filled stomach is sometimes seen as a high signal intensity in the fetal left upper quadrant on T2-weighted images. Discrete loops of bowel are occasionally discernible. Segments of the umbilical cord are frequently visible. In the final trimester, multiple 3- to 10-mm high–signal intensity areas can be seen in the fetal abdomen and pelvis on both T1- and T2-weighted spin-echo images. The precise origin of these areas has not been established, but it is thought that they represent a normal accumulation of adipose tissue and meconium in the fetal abdomen. Omphalocele (Figure 29-44) and gastroschisis (Figure 29-45) have both been demonstrated on MR examinations.

Genitourinary Tract

The fetal kidneys may be difficult to identify because of the paucity of the surrounding fat and the small size of the organs themselves. The appearances of hydronephrosis (Figure 29-46) and renal cysts (Figure 29-47) have been reported[88] (Figures 29-48 and 29-49). A fetal bladder containing urine can be demonstrated (Figure 29-50) as a central high signal area on T2-weighted images.[35] Delineation of the fetal male genitalia has also been reported.[48]

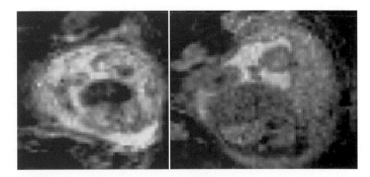

FIGURE 29-43   Liver maturation. EPI (transverse axial T2*-weighted) images through the upper abdomen of a fetus at 20 weeks and 26 weeks, showing the change in signal intensity of the liver.

Musculoskeletal System

Parts of the extremities can be seen in most fetuses during the third trimester. Cortical bone marrow containing bone and apophyseal cartilage, as well as surrounding muscle and subcutaneous fat, can be identified.[35] A fetus with sirenomelia (fused limbs) has been visualized with MRI.[22]

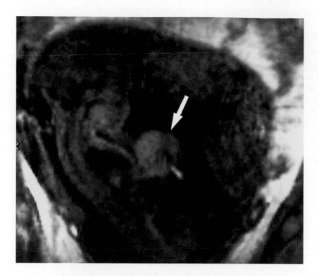

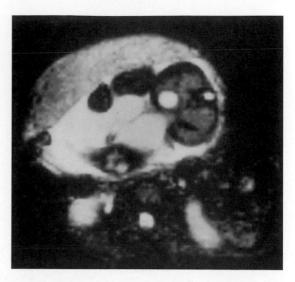

FIGURE 29-44   Omphalocele in the twenty-ninth week of gestation. Sagittal SE 500/30 image through the fetus shows a mass *(arrow)* protruding through the anterior abdominal wall.

FIGURE 29-45   Gastroschisis. The abdominal defect is well shown with loops of bowel within the amniotic fluid.

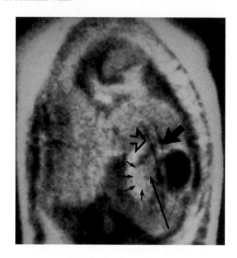

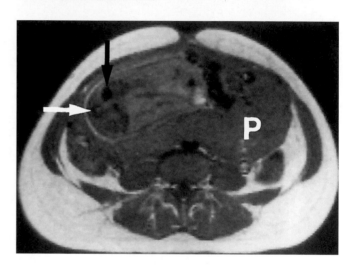

FIGURE 29-46   Hydronephrosis in the thirtieth week of gestation. Inferior vena cava *(closed arrow)*, aorta *(open arrow)*, left renal artery *(long arrow)*, and left kidney *(small arrows)*. The ovoid low-intensity structure is the dilated renal pelvis.

FIGURE 29-47   Renal cyst *(black arrow)* shown at the thirtieth week of gestation. *White arrow,* Fetal spine ; *P,* placenta.

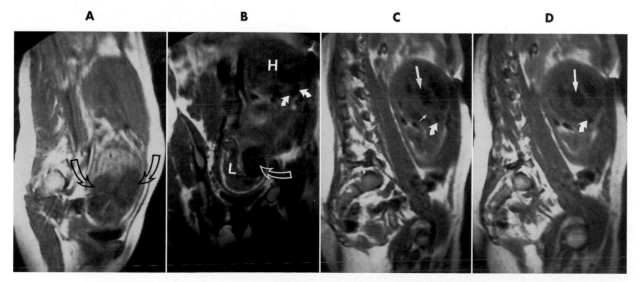

FIGURE 29-48   Meckel-Gruber syndrome. Bilateral polycystic kidneys appear as low–signal intensity structures *(open arrows* in **A** and **B**). Quadrigeminal plate cistern cyst *(long arrow* in **C** and **D**) is identified as a low–signal intensity structure between the lateral ventricles and just above the cerebellum *(small arrow)*. Note the small occipital encephalocele *(solid curved arrows* in **B** to **D**). *H,* Head; *L,* leg.

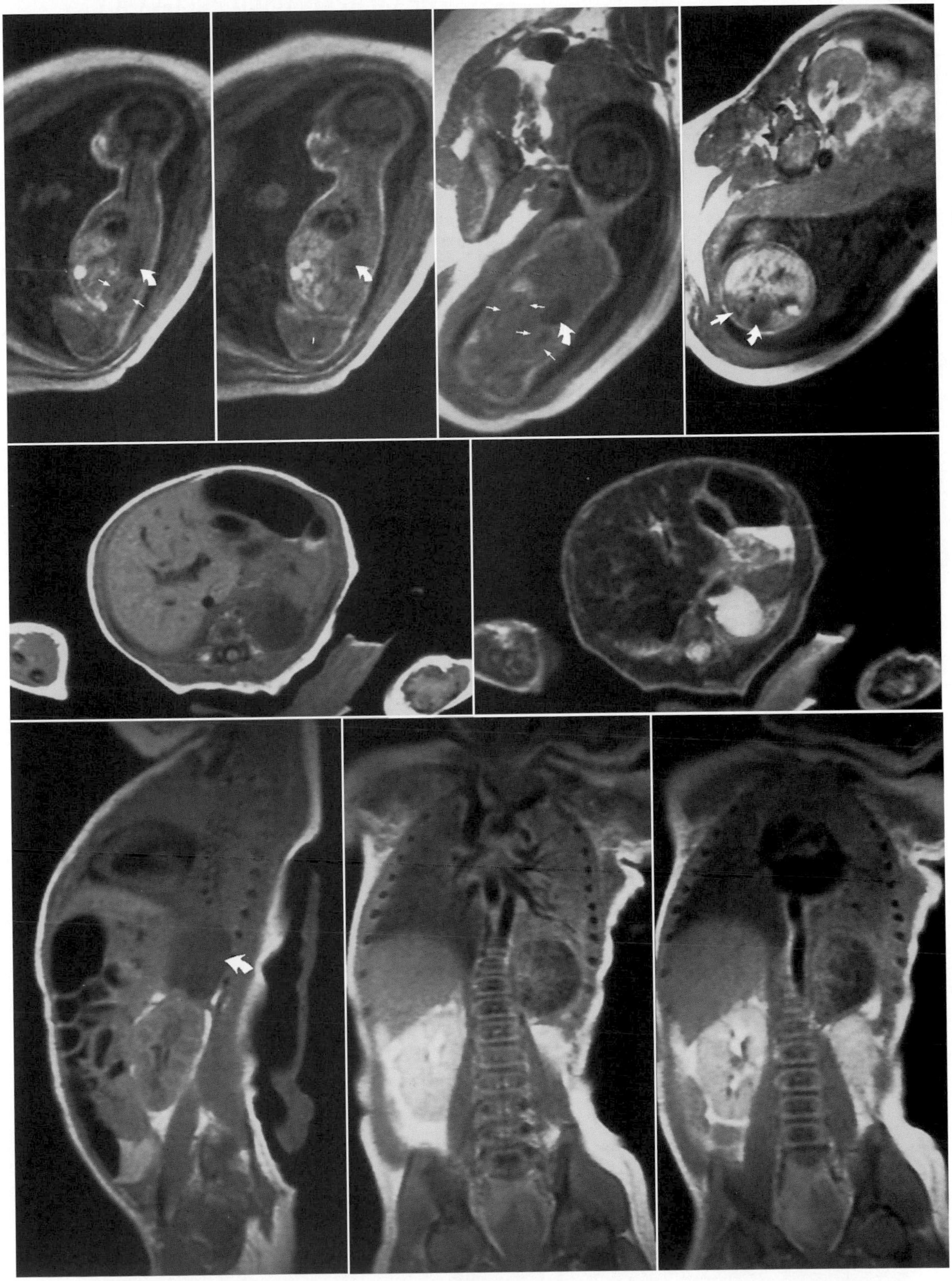

FIGURE 29-49   Extrapulmonary sequestration (infradiaphragmatic). Fetal parasagittal (**A** and **B**), coronal (**C**), and axial (**D**) T1-weighted images show an infradiaphragmatic mass *(curved arrow)* with effacement of the kidney *(small arrows)*. *Straight arrow* in **D,** Fetal spine. Neonatal axial T1-weighted (**E**) and T2-weighted (**F**) images corresponding to **D** demonstrate an infradiaphragmatic mass with low signal intensity on T1-weighted imaging and high signal intensity on T2-weighted imaging. Parasagittal T1-weighed image (**G**) corresponding to **A** demonstrates this mass *(curved arrow)* with effacement of the kidney. Coronal T1-weighted postcontrast-enhanced image (**H**) corresponding to **C** shows arborizing patterns of enhancement similar to those of the pulmonary bronchovascular tree. Lung is compressed posteriorly.

Amniotic Fluid

Amniotic fluid has a relatively low signal on T1-weighted images, reflecting a long T1 relaxation time.[25] On heavily T2-weighted images, however, it returns a high signal.[35] Because it is so well displayed by MRI, it can be quantitatively assessed in a manner like that assessed by ultrasound, and oligohydramnios and polyhydramnios are readily detected (Figure 29-51). Because amniotic fluid reflects fetal renal function in the second half of gestation,[45] in vivo MR spectroscopy of amniotic fluid may provide a technique for evaluating fetal status. Some physiologically relevant compounds related to fetal acidosis and disorders of the central nervous system have been studied with MR spectroscopy using amniotic fluid obtained by amniocentesis.[28] Estimates of the amniotic fluid–meconium concentration, an indicator of fetal distress, have also been obtained from T2 values measured ex vivo.[7,10]

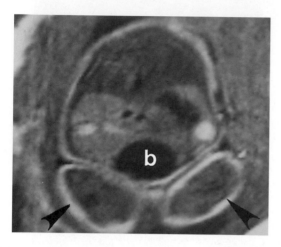

FIGURE 29-50   Urinary bladder *(b)* at thirty-six weeks of gestation. *Arrowheads,* Lower extremities.

THE COMPROMISED PREGNANCY
Estimation of Fetal Weight and Volume

A recent survey of more than 2 million births has demonstrated that fetal mortality rates are more closely related to birth weight than to gestational age, and this puts a premium on the accurate assessment of predelivery fetal weight. Fetal macrosomia is associated with an increased incidence of brachial plexus injuries, meconium aspiration, and shoulder dystocia. IUGR is associated with an increased perinatal mortality rate (4 to 10 times higher than normal). There is an increased incidence of intrapartum fetal distress, meconium aspiration, neonatal hyperglycemia, pneumonia, and hyperviscosity syndrome. Epidemiological studies have shown that there is a strong association between IUGR and a later increased susceptibility to coronary heart disease,[6,60] stroke, and type 2 insulin-dependent diabetes. These long-term effects may result from a "programming" whereby a nutritional deficiency in utero results in a permanent effect on a number of physiological processes.

A large number of clinical and ultrasonographic methods of estimating fetal weight have been described. Overall, reported error rates are in the range of 7% to 10%, with a tendency to overestimate low birth weights and underestimate high birth weights. It should be noted that not all small babies have significant growth restriction. The use of the so-called individualized birth weight ratio provides a better discriminant. This ratio is obtained by comparing the actual birth weight with a predicted birth weight, which is calculated using independent coefficients for gestation at delivery, parity, fetal gender, maternal height, ethnic origin, and booking weight. In a recent study using EPI, fetal volume was estimated close to term by a stereological technique applied to multiple contiguous images of the fetus. A linear relationship was found between fetal volume and birth weight, and the results indicated that this method could provide a more accurate estimate of fetal weight than ultrasound methods. The mean and median differences between actual and estimated birth weights were 3.7% and 3%, respectively, which were significantly less than those obtained using ultrasound.[3]

Subcutaneous fat storage commences in the third trimester,[20] and it is clearly visible on T1-weighted spin-echo or inversion-recovery images because of its high signal intensity in contrast to the adjacent low-

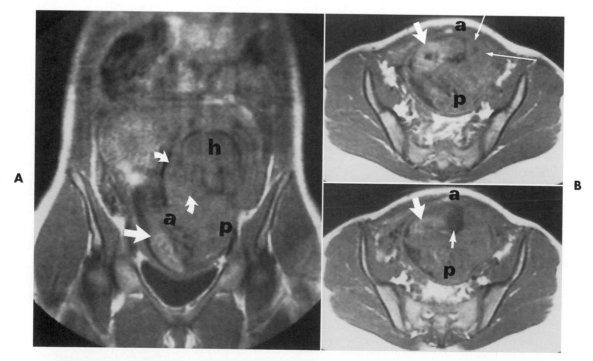

FIGURE 29-51   Pentalogy of Cantrell. Fetal parasagittal **(A)** and axial **(B)** T1-weighted images show the absence of amniotic fluid and the breech presentation of the fetus. Anteriorly, the herniated fetal heart *(curved arrows),* liver *(straight, thick arrow),* kidney *(long, thin arrows),* and stomach *(straight, short arrow)* are demonstrated. *a,* Anterior aspect of the fetus; *h,* head; *p,* posterior aspect of the fetus.

intensity amniotic fluid. It has been suggested that quantitation of subcutaneous fat may be a means of diagnosing IUGR.[17,79] In a study of a series of 11 fetuses in the third trimester, estimates of fetal fat stores using MRI correlated better with neonatal outcomes than sonographic measurements of fetal growth parameters or actual birth weight. Similarly, macrosomic fetuses of diabetic mothers were readily identified by the abundance of subcutaneous fat[75] (Figure 29-52). A case report showed a marked difference in subcutaneous fat on MRI in a pair of twins with a 20% birth discordancy.[12]

The volume of the fetal brain, liver, and placenta has been measured in utero using a stereological technique applied to multiple contiguous echo-planar fetal images. These images showed that the liver volume in growth-restricted fetuses fell on or outside the 95% confidence limits of a normal growth group, whereas no such discrimination was provided by the brain and placental measurements. These preliminary results suggests that a single measurement of fetal liver volume could allow an early diagnosis of IUGR.[5]

Intrauterine Growth Restriction and Preeclampsia

IUGR may occur as a result of toxins such as drugs, infection, or malnutrition, although in the majority of cases, it is thought to be a consequence of abnormal placentation. Preeclampsia, a multisystem disorder characterized by hypertension and proteinuria, carries a number of risks to both mother and fetus. It is unpredictable in onset and progression, and there is no specific diagnostic test. It is thought to reflect a cascade of events that can be traced back to defective placentation.

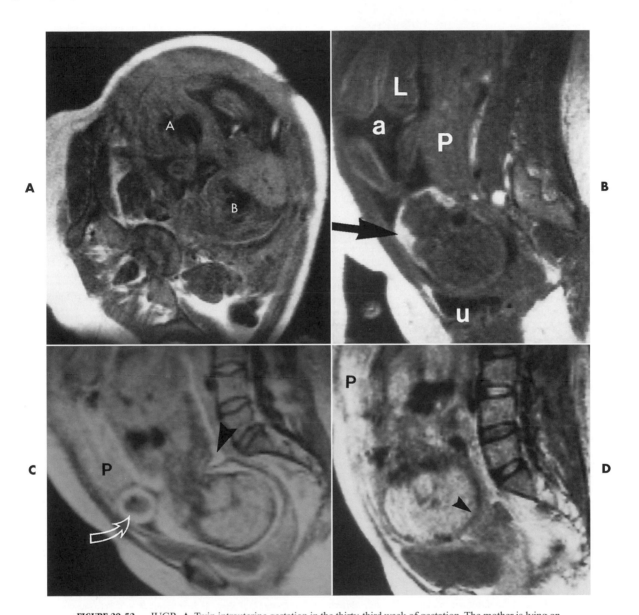

FIGURE 29-52   IUGR. **A,** Twin intrauterine gestation in the thirty-third week of gestation. The mother is lying on her left side. In contrast to fetus *B,* fetus *A* has no appreciable subcutaneous fat. At birth, baby *A* had IUGR, and baby *B* was normal. **B,** Normal, single fetus, third trimester. T1-weighted acquisition time was 5 min. The fetal head is seen in coronal section. Subcutaneous facial fat *(arrow)* has signal intensity similar to that of maternal fat and muscle. Subcutaneous fat is clearly delineated from the amniotic fluid *(a),* muscle (lower extremity *[L]*), posterior placenta *(P),* and maternal urinary bladder *(u).* **C,** Macrosomic fetus of a diabetic mother showing a large amount of subcutaneous fat. Oligohydramnios is present; a small amount of amniotic fluid (dark) is seen surrounding the upper extremity. *Curved, open arrow,* Upper extremity; *arrowhead,* shoulder; *P,* anterior placenta. **D,** IUGR diagnosed by the absence of subcutaneous fat. Bony calvarium *(arrowhead)* is seen immediately adjacent to the internal cervical os without intervening subcutaneous fat. MR diagnosis was confirmed by sonographic, birth weight, and clinical criteria. *P,* Anterior placenta. (From reference 79.)

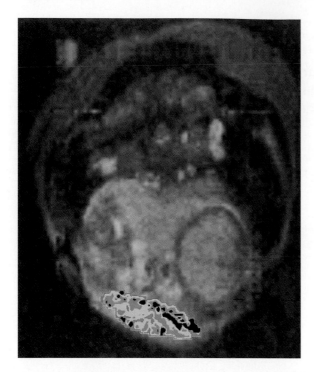

FIGURE 29-53 Perfusion map of the placenta in a normal 38-week pregnancy. *Red,* More than 1000 ml/kg/min; *orange,* 400 to 1000 ml/kg/min; *yellow,* 100 to 400 ml/kg/min; and *blue,* less than 100 ml/kg/min.

IUGR and preeclampsia frequently coexist, and despite the fact that several diagnostic methods have been investigated, none has been found to be accurate or reliable in predicting the development of these conditions. In both IUGR and preeclampsia, there is defective endovascular trophoblastic invasion of the spiral arteries, which are shallow and do not proceed in the myometrial segments; furthermore, fewer vessels show evidence of trophoblastic invasion, which should be complete by 22 weeks of gestation. As a consequence, there are relatively high resistance within the placental vascular bed and secondary reduction of blood flow.

In established disease, Doppler ultrasound can detect changes in the velocity waveform from the uterine artery, reflecting the high resistance in the vascular bed. However, it cannot reliably predict the development of preeclampsia or IUGR earlier in pregnancy.

During normal pregnancy, the placenta increases in both diameter and weight, and the size of the villous surface increases 25 times between 14 weeks and term. In addition, the thickness of the placental barrier becomes progressively smaller closer to term. With defective placentation, however, multiple areas of infarction, reduced areas of exchange, and lower volumes of parenchymal tissue are found. At term the maternal blood supply to the placenta is estimated to be 600 ml/min, and assuming the mass of the placenta to be 550 g, this would give an approximate expected placental perfusion rate of 110 ml/kg/min of tissue.

Perfusion studies using contrast agents have been carried out in animals[1,40] but are precluded during pregnancy. However, perfusion measurements in vivo have been measured using EPI (Figure 29-53) by comparing the T1 measured during an inversion-recovery sequence with a selective and nonselective inversion pulse.[39] The former gives a measure of the true T1 value and the latter the apparent T1 value, which then allows one to calculate the perfusion.[18] The mean placental perfusion rate estimated by this method was 158 ml/kg/min, which is higher than the expected uteroplacental perfusion rate given earlier. The difference between the two estimates reflects both the inclusion of the smaller umbilical placental perfusion and the fact that a large fraction of blood in the placenta is moving in random directions within the placental sinusoids and has a relatively high residence time. Thus MR-measured rates of placental perfusion, which include this component, will exceed the expected classic perfusion rate, which simply reflects the fresh blood delivered to the tissue. With further studies it is anticipated that absolute quantification of the flow through the placenta and definition of the pattern of flow in different parts of the placenta will be achievable. These may allow for early recognition of both IUGR and preeclampsia.

SUMMARY

There are now a growing number of specific indications for the use of MRI during the second half of pregnancy, in particular when equivocal results on ultrasound must be clarified or when ultrasound has known limitations. It has become apparent that MRI offers a powerful research tool in obstetrics, and further work can be anticipated to facilitate the assessment of compromised fetal development.

REFERENCES

1. Angtuaco T, Mattison DR, Thomford PJ, et al: Effect of manganese (Mn+2) on human placental spin lattice (T1) and spin-echo (T2) relaxation times, Annual Meeting of the Radiologic Society of North America, Chicago, Nov 1985.
2. Artis AA, Bowie JD, Rosenberg ER, et al: The fallacy of placental migration: effect of sonographic techniques, Am J Roentgenol 144:79, 1985.
3. Baker PN, Johnson IR, Gowland P, et al: Fetal weight estimation of echo-planar magnetic resonance imaging, Lancet 343(L):644, 1994.
4. Baker PN, Johnson IR, Gowland PA, et al: Estimation of fetal lung volume using echo-planar magnetic resonance imaging, Obstet Gynecol 83:951, 1994.
5. Baker PN, Johnson IR, Gowland PA, et al: Measurement of fetal liver, brain and placental volumes with echo-planar magnetic resonance imaging, Br J Obstet Gynaecol 102:35, 1995.
6. Barker DJ, Winter PD, Osmond C, et al: Weight in infancy and death from ischaemic heart disease, Lancet ii:577, 1989.
7. Bene GJL: The NMR proton relaxation in biological fluids: a good way to identify precisely healthy or pathological states, Ann 1st Super Sanita 19(1):121, 1983.
8. Birger M, Homburg R, and Insler V: Clinical evaluation of fetal movements, Int J Gynecol Obstet 18:337, 1980.
9. Bishop E, and Cefalo R: Signs and symptoms of pregnancy, Philadelphia, 1983, Lippincott.
10. Borcard B, Hiltbrand E, Magnin P, et al: Estimating meconium (fetal feces) concentration in human amniotic fluid by nuclear magnetic resonance, Physiol Chem Phys 14:181, 1982.
11. Bowie JD, Rochester D, Cadkin AV, et al: Accuracy of placental localization by ultrasound, Radiology 128:177, 1985.
12. Brown CE, and Weinreb JC: Magnetic resonance imaging appearance of growth retardation in a twin pregnancy, Obstet Gynecol 71:987, 1988.
13. Cohen JM, Weinreb JC, Lowe TW: MR imaging of a viable full-term abdominal pregnancy, Am J Roentgenol 145: 407, 1985.
14. Collea JV, Chein C, and Quilligan EJ: The radiological management of frank breech presentations: a study of 208 cases, Am J Obstet Gynecol 137:235, 1980.
15. D'Arcy TJ, Hughes SW, Chiu SW, et al: Estimation of fetal lung volume using enhanced three dimensional ultrasound, Br J Obstet Gynaecol 103:1015, 1996.
16. Davidson AM, and Peters A: Myelination, Springfield, 1970, Charles C Thomas.
17. Deter RL, Hadlock FP, and Harrist RB: Evaluation of normal fetal growth and the detection of intrauterine growth retardation. In Callen PW, ed: Ultrasonography in obstetrical gynecology, Philadelphia, 1982, Saunders.
18. Detre JA, Leigh JS, Williams DS, et al: Perfusion imaging, Magn Reson Med 23:37, 1992.
19. Duncan K, Moore R, Issa B, et al: The use of EPI to demonstrate changes in fetal liver physiology, vol 1, New York, 1996, Proceedings of the International Society of Magnetic Resonance in Medicine.
20. England MA: Color atlas of life before birth: normal fetal development, St Louis, 1983, Mosby.
21. Federle MP, Cohen HA, Rosenwein FM, et al: Pelvimetry by digital radiography: a low dose examination, Radiology 143:733, 1982.
22. Fitzmorris-Glass R, Mattrey RF, Cantrell CJ, et al: MRI as an adjunct to ultrasound in oligohydramnios: detection of sirenomelia, J Ultrasound Med 8:159, 1989.
23. Fleischer AC, Boehm FH, and James AE: Sonographic evaluation of pelvic masses and maternal disorders occurring during pregnancy. In Sanders R, ed: The principles and practice of ultrasonography in obstetrics and gynecology, ed 3, New York, 1985, Appleton-Century-Crofts.
24. Fleischer A, James AE, Millis JB, et al: Differential diagnosis of pelvic masses by gray scale sonography, Am J Roentgenol 131:469, 1978.
25. Foster MA, Knight CH, Rimmington JE, et al: Fetal imaging by nuclear magnetic resonance: a study in goats, Radiology 149:193, 1983.
26. Fox H: Pathology of the placenta. In Bennington JL, ed: Major problems in pathology, Philadelphia, 1978, WB Saunders.
27. Gelman SR, Spellacy WN, Wood S, et al: Fetal movements and ultrasound effects of intravenous glucose administration, Am J Obstet Gynecol 137:459, 1980.
28. Gillies RJ, Powell DA, Nelson TR, et al: High resolution proton NMR spectroscopy of human amniotic fluid. Abstracts of Society of Magnetic Resonance in Medicine, fourth annual meeting, London, Aug 1985.
29. Gillieson MS, Winer-Muram HT, and Muran D: Low lying placenta, Radiology 144: 577, 1982.
30. Gowland P, Moor R, Freeman A, et al: Monitoring fetal lung maturation using echo-planar imaging, Proceedings of the International Society of Magnetic Resonance in Medicine, New York, 1:157, 1996.

31. Guttman P: In search of the elusive benign cystic teratoma: "tip of the iceberg sign," J Clin Ultrasound 5:403, 1977.

32. Harrison RG: The urogenital system. In Romanes GF, ed: Cunningham's textbook of anatomy, ed 10, London, 1984, Oxford University Press.

33. Harvey EB, Boice JB, Honeyman M, et al: Prenatal x-ray exposure and childhood cancer in twins, N Engl J Med 312(9):541, 1985.

34. Hricak H, Chang YC, Cann CE, al: Cervical incompetence: preliminary evaluation with MR imaging, Radiology 174:821, 1990.

35. Johnson IR, Stehling MK, Blamire AM, et al: Study of internal structure of the human fetus in-utero by echo-planar magnetic resonance imaging, Am J Obstet Gynecol 163:601, 1990.

36. Jouppila P: Fetal movements diagnosed by ultrasound in early pregnancy, Acta Obstet Gynecol Scand 55:131, 1976.

37. Kay HN, Herfkins RJ, and Kay BK: Effect of MRI on xenopus laevis embryogenesis, Magn Reson Imaging 6:501, 1988.

38. Kier R, McCarthy SM, Scoutt LM, et al: Pelvic masses in pregnancy: MR imaging, Radiology 176:709, 1996.

39. Kim SG: Quantifying relative cerebral blood flow change by flow sensitive alternating inversion recovery technique (FAIR): application to functional mapping, Magn Reson Med 34:293, 1995.

40. Knopp RH, et al: MR placental and fetal imaging: placental contrast enhancement following MN+2 infusion in primates and rats, Washington, DC, Nov 1984, Annual Meeting of the Radiological Society of North America.

41. Laing FC: Ultrasound evaluation in obstetric problems relating to the lower uterine segment and cervix. In Saunders R, ed: The principles and practice of ultrasonography in obstetrics and gynecology, ed 3, New York, 1985, Appleton-Century-Crofts.

42. Lean TH, Rafnam SS, and Sivamboo R: Use of benzodiazepines in the management of eclampsia, J Obstet Gynaecol Br Cwlth 75:856, 1968.

43. Lee A: Fetal lung volume determination by three dimensional ultrasonography, Am J Obstet Gynecol 175:588, 1996.

44. Lev-Toaff AS, et al: Leiomyomas in pregnancy: sonographic study, Radiology 164:375, 1987.

45. Lind T: Biochemistry of amniotic fluid. In Sandler M, ed: Amniotic fluid and its clinical significance, New York, 1981, Marcel Dekker.

46. Magnetic Resonance Imaging Consensus Conference, JAMA 259(14):2132, 1988.

47. Mahoney BJ, Coleman BG, Arger PH, et al: Sonographic evaluation of ectopic pregnancy, J Ultrasound Med 4:222, 1985.

48. McCarthy SM: Obstetrical magnetic resonance imaging: fetal anatomy, Radiology 154:427, 1985.

49. McCarthy SM, Stark DD, Higgins CB, et al: Case report: demonstration of the fetal cardiovascular system by MR imaging, J Comput Assist Tomogr 8(6):1168, 1984.

50. McCarthy SM, Filly RA, Stark DD, et al: Magnetic resonance imaging of fetal anomalies in utero: early experience, Am J Roentgenol 145:677, 1985.

51. McCarthy SM, Stark DD, Filly RA, et al: Obstetrical magnetic resonance imaging: maternal anatomy, Radiology 154:421, 1985.

52. Miller FC, Skiba H, and Klapholz H: The effect of maternal blood sugar levels on fetal activity, Obstet Gynecol 52:662, 1978.

53. Minors DS, and Waterhouse JM: The effect of maternal posture, meals, and time of day on fetal movements, Br J Obstet Gynaecol 86:717, 1979.

54. Mintz M, Grossman RI, Isaacson G, et al: MR imaging of the fetal brain, J Comput Assist Tomogr 11(1):120, 1987.

55. Munyer TP, Callen PW, Filly RA, et al: Further observation on the sonographic spectrum of gestational trophoblastic disease, J Clin Ultrasound 9:349, 1981.

56. Heerachap A, and Van den Berg P: Proton MRS of human fetal brain, Am J Obstet Gynecol 170:1150, 1994.

57. National (British) Radiological Protection Board: Revised guidelines on acceptable limits of exposure during NMR clinical imaging, Br J Radiol 56:974, 1983.

58. National (British) Radiological Protection Board: Statement on clinical magnetic resonance diagnostic procedures, vol 2, no 1, 1991.

59. Nimmo MJ, Kinsella D, and Andrews HS: The diagnosis of vasa previa by MRI, Bristol Med Chirurgi J 103:12, 1988.

60. Osmond C, Barker DJ, Winter PD, et al: Early growth and death from cardiovascular disease in women, Br Med 307:1519, 1993.

61. Patrick J, et al: Human fetal breathing movements and gross fetal body movements at 34 to 35 weeks of gestation, Am J Obstet Gynecol 130:693, 1978.

62. Pennes DR, Bowerman RA, and Silver TM: Echogenic adnexal masses associated with first trimester pregnancy: sonographic appearance and clinical significance, J Clin Ultrasound 13:391, 1985.

63. Possmayer F: The prenatal lung. In Jones C, ed: The biochemical development of the fetus and neonate, Amsterdam, 1982, Elsevier Biomedical Press.

64. Powell MC, and Worthington BS: MRI: a new milestone in modern OB care, Diagn Imaging 86, April 1986.

65. Powell MC, Symonds EM, and Worthington BS: Magnetic resonance imaging of the placenta. In Chamberlain G, ed: Contemporary obstetrics and gynaecology, Oxford, England, 1988, Butterworth-Heinemann.

66. Powell M, Worthington BS, and Symonds EM: MRI in obstetrics and gynaecology, Oxford, England, 1993, Butterworth-Heineman.

67. Powell MC, Buckley J, Price H, et al: Magnetic resonance imaging and placenta previa, Am J Obstet Gynecol 154(3):565, 1986.

68. Powell MC, Buckley J, Worthington JS, et al: Magnetic resonance imaging and hydatidiform mole, Br J Radiol 54:561, 1986.

69. Reid MH, McGahan JP, and Oi R: Sonographic evaluation of hydatidiform mole and its look-alikes, Am J Roentgenol 140:307, 1983.

70. Requard CK, and Mettler FA: The use of ultrasound in the evaluation of trophoblastic disease and its response to therapy, Radiology 135:419, 1980.

71. Rocker I, and Lawerence RM, eds: Fetoscopy, New York, 1981, Elsevier Press.

72. Sadovsky E, et al: Correlation between electromagnetic recording and maternal assessment of fetal movement, Lancet 1:1141, 1979.

73. Sadovsky E, and Polishuk WZ: Fetal movements in utero: nature, assessment, prognostic value, timing of delivery, Obstet Gynecol 50:49, 1977.

74. Seeds JW, Corke BC, and Speilman FJ: Prevention of fetal movement during invasive procedures in pancuronium bromide, Am J Obstet Gynecol 155:818, 1986.

75. Smith FW: Magnetic resonance imaging of human pregnancy, Abstracts of Fourth Annual Meeting of Society of Magnetic Resonance in Medicine, London, England, Aug 1985.

76. Smith FW: The potential use of nuclear magnetic resonance imaging in pregnancy, J Perinat Med 13:265, 1985.

77. Smith FW, Kent C, Abramovich DR, et al: Nuclear magnetic resonance imaging: a new look at the fetus, Br J Obstet Gynaecol 92:1024, 1985.

78. Smith FW, and Sutherland HW: Short T1 inversion recovery (STIR) imaging in human pregnancy, Magn Reson Imaging 4:137, 1986.

79. Stark DD, McCarthy SM, Filly RA, et al: Intrauterine growth retardation: evaluation by magnetic resonance: work in progress, Radiology 155:425, 1985.

80. Stark DD, McCarthy SM, Filly RA, et al: Pelvimetry by magnetic resonance imaging, Am J Roentgenol 144:947, 1985.

81. Thickman D, Mintz M, Mennuti M, et al: MR imaging of cerebral abnormalities in utero, J Comput Assist Tomogr 8(6):1058, 1984.

82. Trefelner E, McCarthy S, and Kier R: Developmental fetal anatomy with MRI, Magn Reson Imaging 7:710, 1989 (abstract).

83. US Food and Drug Administration: Magnetic resonance diagnostic device: panel recommendation and report of petitions for MR reclassification, Fed Reg 53:7575, 1988.

84. Varner MW, Cruikshand DP, and Laube DW: X-ray pelvimetry in clinical obstetrics, Obstet Gynecol 56:296, 1980.

85. Villa-Coro AA, and Dominguez R: Intrauterine diagnosis of hydranencephaly by magnetic resonance, Magn Reson Imaging 7:105, 1989.

86. Villforth JC: Medical radiation protection: a long view, Am J Roentgenol 145:1114, 1985.

87. Weinreb JC, Lowe TW, Cohen JM, et al: Human fetal anatomy: MR imaging, Radiology 157:715, 1985.

88. Weinreb JC, Lowe TW, Santosamos R, et al: Magnetic resonance imaging in obstetric diagnosis, Radiology 154: 157, 1985.

89. Weinreb JC, Wolbarsht LB, Cohen JM, et al: Prevalence of lumbosacral intervertebral disk abnormalities on MR images in pregnant and asymptomatic nonpregnant women, Radiology 170:125, 1989.

90. Weinreb JC, Brown CE, Lowe TW, et al: Pelvic masses in pregnant patients: MR and US imaging, Radiology 159:717, 1986.

91. Wenstrom KD, Williamson RA, Weiner CP, et al: Magnetic resonance imaging of fetuses with intracranial defects, Obstet Gynecol 77:529, 1991.

92. Williamson RA, Weiner CP, Yuh WTC, et al: Magnetic resonance imaging of anomalous fetuses, Obstet Gynecol 73:952, 1989.

93. Willms AB, Brown ED, Kettritz UI, et al: Anatomic changes in the pelvis after uncomplicated vaginal delivery, Radiology, 195:91, 1995.

94. Winsurg F: Echogenic changes with placental aging, J Clin Ultrasound 1:52, 1973.

95. Yeh S, et al: A study of diazepam during labor, Obstet Gynecol 43:363, 1974.

96. Yiu-Chui Y, and Chiu L: Sonographic features of placental complications of pregnancy, Am J Roentgenol 138:879, 1982.

97. Yuen BH, Cannon W, Benedet JL, et al: Plasma beta-subunit human chorionic gonadotropin assay in molar pregnancy and choriocarcinoma, Am J Obstet Gynecol 127:711, 1977.

98. Yuh WTC, Demarino GB, Ludwig WD, et al: MR imaging of pregnancy in bicornate uterus, J Comput Assist Tomogr 12(1):162, 1988.

99. Zemlyn S: The length of the uterine cervix and its significance, J Clin Ultrasound 9:267, 1981.

30 Prostate and Seminal Vesicles

Caroline Pangie Schwartz, Thomas R. McCauley, and Matthew D. Rifkin

 KEY POINTS

- Combined endorectal—phased-array RF-coil, high-resolution, T1- and (CSE or FSE) T2-weighted—images are required.
- Transrectal ultrasound (TRUS) equals MRI for cancer detection, both having sensitivity and positive predictive values somewhat better than 60%.
- The staging accuracy of MRI at 80% is somewhat better than that of TRUS and CT.

The prostate is a small organ situated deep in the male pelvis and is the organ most prone to pathological change. Indeed, all men who live past the age of 50 will develop histological changes within the prostate gland. The most common process is benign prostatic hyperplasia, commonly known as *BPH*.[18] As men age, all will have some histological change consistent with BPH. Many older men also develop prostate cancer, the most common malignancy worldwide and, after skin cancer, the most frequently diagnosed cancer in America.[1-4,33,60] Inflammation of the prostate, or prostatitis, can also affect many men and may occasionally be subclinical. In these cases the diagnosis may be made by imaging studies performed for a variety of other reasons.

A clear understanding of the anatomy of the prostate, seminal vesicles, and their surrounding structures, as well as the pathophysiological changes that affect these organs, is required to appropriately use and interpret imaging studies, such as magnetic resonance imaging (MRI).

NORMAL ANATOMY

The normal prostate gland is a conical organ typically measuring $3 \times 3.5 \times 4$ cm and weighing approximately 20 g (Figure 30-1). The apex of the organ lies inferiorly, adjacent to the urogenital diaphragm. The anterior portion of the prostate is separated from the symphysis pubis and the pubic bones by the anterior prostatic fat, fascia, and a venous plexus known as *Santorini's plexus*. The posterior margin of the gland is separated from the rectum by Denonvillier's fascia. The prostate's lateral margins, along with the levator ani muscles inferiorly and the obturator internus muscles superiorly, are bordered by fat. The superior portion of the prostate, known as the *base of the gland*, borders the inferior margin of the bladder, known as the *base of the bladder*. The prostate is surrounded by a fibrous membrane or capsule that is thin posteriorly and laterally and somewhat thicker anteriorly. The capsule is perforated at its posterior-lateral margins bilaterally by the paired neurovascular bundles, which include the lateral venous plexuses. The vessels of Santorini's plexus, located anteriorly, also perforate the capsule but not as extensively as the lateral venous plexuses (Figure 30-2).

The seminal vesicles are located at the superoposterior aspect of the prostate. The vas deferens are paired structures that arise from the epididymis within the scrotum and course through the inguinal canal with the spermatic cord. The vas deferens insert into the medial portion of the seminal vesicles, forming the ejaculatory ducts (Figure 30-3). The ejaculatory ducts then traverse the prostate just lateral to the midline and course parallel to the proximal prostatic urethra. Both ejaculatory ducts insert into the urethra at the verumontanum.*

For nearly the past century, the prostate has been divided anatomically into lobes. This anatomical description, termed *Lowsley's lobar anatomy*, divided the gland into five major lobes. The lobes included (1) the anterior lobe, the portion of the prostate from its anterior margin to the prostatic urethra; (2) the middle or median lobe, the portion of the prostate between the proximal prostatic urethra and the ejaculatory ducts; (3) the posterior lobe, bordered by the ejaculatory ducts and the inferior portion of the prostatic urethra anteriorly and the posterior margin of the prostate posteriorly; and (4 and 5) the two bulky lateral lobes, which had ill-defined medial margins but included the bulk of the prostate laterally (Figure 30-1). Also described were two usually insignificant minor lobes, known as the *subtrigonal* and the *subcervical lobes*, which were variably present. Lowsley's concept of lobar anatomy of the prostate was based on extensive data obtained from fetal prostates. It has since become apparent that the adult prostate gland differs significantly in anatomical structure from the fetal prostate. Lowsley's description of the prostate also is of limited use in determining the origin and spread of disease.

During the past 30 years, the concept of zonal anatomy has gradually replaced the previously described lobar anatomy of the prostate (Table 30-1). This anatomical description was initially reported in the mid-1960s by McNeal and has been refined over the past decades as more knowledge has been gathered.[25] The zonal anatomy of the prostate divides the gland into four basic anatomical regions, with the urethra as a central point of reference (Figure 30-4). It is therefore most useful to begin the description of zonal anatomy with the urethra.

The prostatic urethra forms at the bladder neck and transects the central portion of the prostate gland. It is important to note that the prostatic urethra does not take a straight course through the prostate

The authors thank Doris Eve Jensen for her assistance in preparing this manuscript.

*References 15, 22, 25, 35, 53, 59.

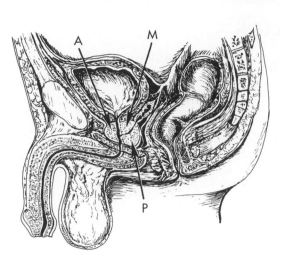

FIGURE 30-1   Lobar anatomy of the prostate. Historically the prostate has been divided into five major lobes. The anterior lobe *(A)* is situated anterior to the prosthetic urethra. The middle or median lobe *(M)* is situated toward the base of the prostate between the prostatic urethra and ejaculatory ducts. The posterior lobe *(P)* is situated in the posterior portion of the prostate. The lateral lobes compose the bulk of the lateral portions of the gland.

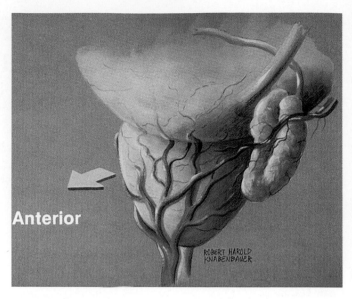

FIGURE 30-2   Normal male pelvis. Anterolateral view of the prostate showing the periprostatic venous plexus anteriorly and laterally. The seminal vesicles and vas deferens are shown in relationship to the bladder and urethra.

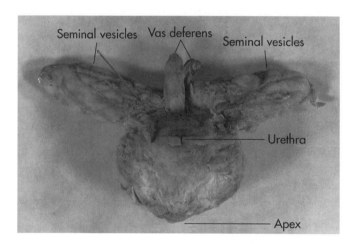

FIGURE 30-3   Normal male pelvis. Formalin-fixed specimen. The prostate, bilaterally paired seminal vesicles, and vas deferens are seen. The apex of the prostate is conically shaped, and the broad-based superior portion adjacent to the urinary bladder (not shown) is the entrance of the (prostatic) urethra.

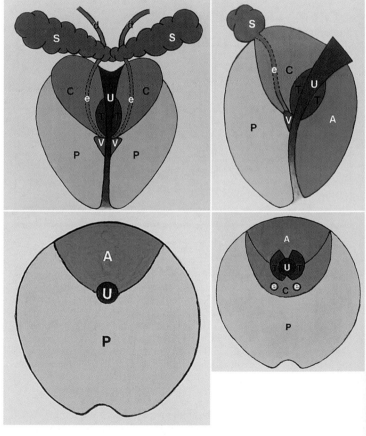

FIGURE 30-4   Zonal anatomy of the prostate. Coronal **(A)** and sagittal **(B)** diagrams. *P,* Peripheral zone; *e,* ejaculatory ducts *C,* central zone; *V,* verumontanum; *T,* transition zone; *U,* urethra; *S,* seminal vesicles; *d,* vas deferens; *A,* anterior fibromuscular stroma. Axial sections through the midportion **(C)** and apex **(D)** of the gland. Axial diagrams of zonal anatomy demonstrate the peripheral zone *(P)* to be situated in the posterior, right, left, and anterolateral aspects of the prostate. The anterior portion of the prostate is composed of anterior fibromuscular stroma *(A).*

Table 30-1 Zonal Anatomy of the Prostate	
ZONE	**CHARACTERISTICS**
Anterior fibromuscular tissue	No prostatic acinar tissue
Inner (central) gland	All prostatic acinar tissue
	Transition zone
	Periurethral glandular tissue
Outer (peripheral) gland	All prostatic acinar tissue
	Central zone
	Peripheral zone

but rather is kinked or curved at the level of the verumontanum (Figure 30-4, *B*). As a result, the prostatic urethra proximal to the verumontanum is angulated approximately 35 degrees anteriorly compared with the more distal prostatic urethra and courses in an oblique coronal plane. The smooth muscle of the internal urethral sphincter is a continuation of the smooth muscle of the urinary bladder base, which extends to surround the proximal portion of the prostatic urethra. The external urethral sphincter is located immediately distal to the prostatic apex at the level of the urogenital diaphragm.

Adjacent to the proximal prostatic urethra and anatomically following in a similar oblique coronal plane as the urethra are small periurethral ducts. The development of these periurethral ducts is felt to be limited by a cylindrical smooth muscle sphincter that extends from the bladder neck to the base of the verumontanum. At the most inferior aspect of this smooth muscle sphincter, the periurethral ducts are able to extend beyond the smooth muscle rings and continue their development. This focal area of periurethral duct development is known as the *transition zone* and is found at the junction of the proximal and distal urethral segments. The transition zone in the normal young male patient constitutes less than 5% of the glandular prostate (Figure 30-4, *C*). In the original description of zonal anatomy, the transition zone, the periurethral ducts, and the periurethral smooth muscle sphincter composed the preprostatic region. This area is also known as the *central* or *inner gland.*

A second area described in the zonal anatomy of the prostate is the central zone (not to be confused with the central gland, which is distinctly different). The central zone is a funnel-shaped segment of gland located at the posterior lateral aspect of the proximal urethra and transition zone. Its apex is at the upper level of the verumontanum, and it extends superiorly to form the base of the gland (Figure 30-4, *A* and *B*). The ejaculatory ducts are contained within the central zone. In the normal young male patient the central zone constitutes approximately 25% of the glandular prostate.

Posterior, lateral, and inferior to the central zone is the peripheral zone, which is a third area described in the zonal anatomy of the prostate. Superior to the verumontanum, the peripheral zone borders the posterior lateral aspect of the central zone. Inferior to the verumontanum, the peripheral zone borders the posterior aspect of the distal prostatic urethra. In the normal young male patient the peripheral zone constitutes approximately 70% of the glandular prostate. The central and peripheral zones together make up what is known as the *peripheral* or *outer gland.*

The fourth and final area described in the zonal anatomy of the prostate is the anterior fibromuscular stroma (Figure 30-4, *B*). This area, which is devoid of glandular tissue, is composed of fibrous and muscular elements. Anteriorly this area is quite thick. As it extends laterally and posteriorly, the fibromuscular stroma thins to form the fibrous capsule.

Two sets of vascular structures surround the prostate and seminal vesicles. As mentioned earlier, Santorini's plexus is a collection of veins situated in the fat between the pubic bones and the anterior portion of the prostate. These vessels perforate through the anterolateral portion of the capsule bilaterally but to a minimal degree. Posterolateral to the prostate is a far more important collection of vessels, the lateral venous plexuses. These veins and arteries are also accompanied by nerves with important physiological functions, including continence and potency. Thus these structures have been termed the *neurovascular bundles.* These bundles perforate through the prostate capsule to a significant degree, and these areas of perforation are a major site for the spread of disease.*

ORIGINS OF DISEASE

Defining the origins of disease within the prostate gland is difficult and inconsistent when Lowsley's concept of lobar anatomy is used. The development of the concept of zonal anatomy has clarified the origins of disease within the prostate. It is now recognized that 80% of prostate cancer (99% of which is adenocarcinoma) originates in the outer gland; approximately 70% arises within the peripheral zone, with 10% in the central zone. The remaining 20% of prostate cancer originates in the

*References 15, 22, 25, 35, 53, 59.

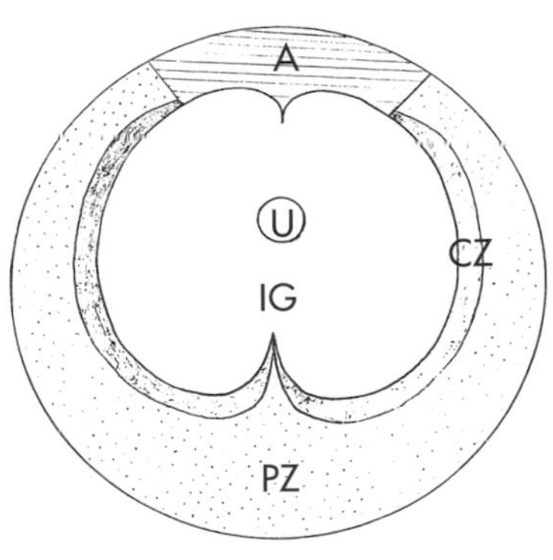

FIGURE 30-5   BPH. Transverse section diagram demonstrates massive enlargement of the inner gland *(IG)*. BPH of the inner gland compresses the central zone *(PZ)*. *U,* Urethra; *A,* anterior zone (fibromuscular stroma).

transition zone.[25] The propensity for prostate cancer to develop in certain zones is not directly related to the volume of each zone. For example, the peripheral zone is three times larger in volume than the central zone. However, prostate cancer is seven times more common within the peripheral zone compared with the central zone.

The origination and spread of prostate cancer often follow a general scheme. It usually originates as a small, histologically well-differentiated lesion. As the cancer enlarges, it frequently dedifferentiates and becomes more anaplastic. Tumors that originate in the peripheral zone can (1) spread within the zone, (2) infiltrate into the ejaculatory ducts and seminal vesicles, (3) spread into the inner gland, or (4) erode through the capsule to involve the neurovascular bundles or periprostatic structures.

BPH, a process that occurs independent of any other pathological process involving the prostate, arises exclusively from the inner gland. Approximately 95% of cases arise within the transition zone, and the remaining 5% arise in the thin lining of the prostatic urethra, the periurethral glandular tissue.[18] This enlargement is similar to the previously termed *median lobe hypertrophy* when Lowsley's concept of anatomy was used. Whereas transition zone enlargement compresses the outer gland, periurethral enlargement affects the bladder base as the prostatic tissue enlarges in a cephalad direction. BPH may cause massive enlargement of the inner gland, compressing and distorting the central and peripheral zones (Figure 30-5). It is important to remember that BPH does not originate in the central or peripheral zones; these areas are only secondarily involved.

Benign inflammatory processes also occur within the prostate. As with prostate cancer, inflammation involves the prostatic acinar tissue and can involve either the inner or the outer gland. The inner gland is most prone to develop inflammatory change after manipulation, such as after cystoscopy, transurethral resection, or another similar types of surgical manipulation. Blood-borne infection can involve either the inner or the outer gland with equal risk. Histologically, prostatitis can be diffuse or focal. The former is the more common presentation. Although most cases of inflammation will be self-limited, some cases will continue to abscess, which can involve either the inner or the outer gland.

MAGNETIC RESONANCE TECHNIQUE

MRI of the prostate has evolved along with developments in magnetic resonance (MR) coils and in MR pulse sequences. Earlier studies used the body-coil and conventional spin-echo pulse sequences. The endorectal surface coil was first developed in 1988[45] (Figure 30-6). The use of the endorectal surface coil increases signal-to-noise ratios; however, this is at the expense of a small field of view and inhomogeneous sensitivity. Inhomogeneous sensitivity results in the signal decreasing with distance from the coil. This can make interpretation of images more difficult for inexperienced readers, as demonstrated in a recent multicenter trial in which use of the endorectal surface coil decreased accuracy compared with use of the body coil for inexperienced readers but increased accuracy for experienced readers.[57] The endorectal surface coil has recently been combined with external coils in an integrated endorectal external phased-array coil, which allows more homogeneous signal over a larger field of view and likely will result in

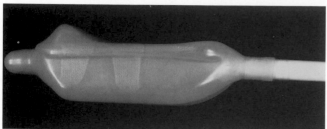

FIGURE 30-6   Endorectal surface coil. An endorectal surface coil that is placed in the rectum has a shape similar to that of a Foley catheter. Flattened on one side, the inflated balloon cups the prostate anteriorly. Flexible wires are embedded in the balloon itself.

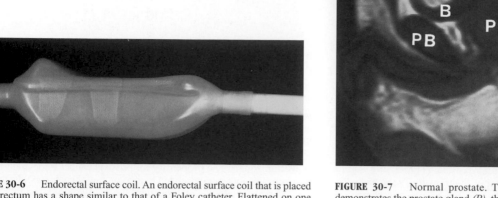

FIGURE 30-7   Normal prostate. T1-weighted spin-echo (600/20) image demonstrates the prostate gland *(P)*, the fluid-filled urinary bladder *(B)*, and the seminal vesicles *(S)*. The prostate is situated between the pubic cones *(PB)* and the rectum *(R)*.

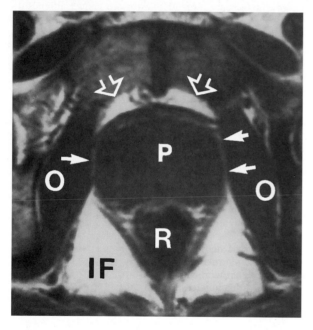

FIGURE 30-8   Normal anatomy. Body-coil technique. The internal structures of the prostate *(P)* are not identified on T1-weighted spin-echo (600/20) images. The anterior *(open arrows)*, lateral *(arrows)*, and ischiorectal fossa *(IF)* fat is identified. The rectum *(R)* and obturator internus muscles *(O)* are also seen.

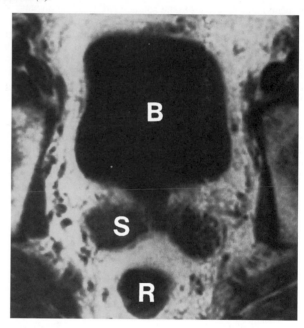

FIGURE 30-9   Normal seminal vesicles. T1-weighted spin-echo (600/20) image demonstrates the low-signal intensity seminal vesicles *(S)* between the rectum *(R)* and fluid-filled urinary bladder *(B)*.

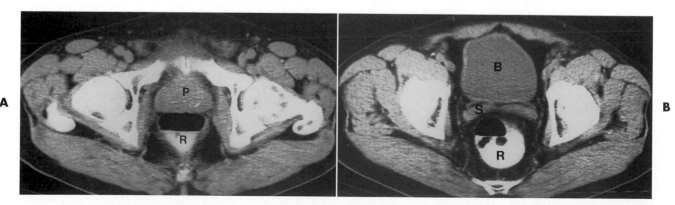

FIGURE 30-10   Normal CT. Fatty tissue planes are well seen; however, there is poor definition of internal structure within the prostate *(P)* (seen in **A**) and seminal vesicles *(S)* (seen in **B**). *B,* Bladder; *R,* rectum.

improved accuracy for both inexperienced and experienced readers.[50] An external phased-array coil has been shown to provide higher image quality than the body coil,[21] and in a separate study the integrated endorectal external phased-array coil has been shown to provide higher accuracy for staging than an external phased-array coil without an endorectal surface coil.[16] Thus an endorectal external phased-array coil currently provides the highest image quality for evaluation of the prostate.

Imaging of the prostate is generally performed with pulse sequences that provide T1-weighted and T2-weighted images. Spin-echo pulse sequences were initially used for both T1- and T2-weighted images; however, fast spin-echo imaging has replaced spin-echo imaging for T2-weighted images at most centers. Fast spin-echo imaging provides a higher available signal-to-noise ratio per unit of imaging time, which can be used to increase resolution, decrease imaging time, or improve signal-to-noise ratio, resulting in higher image quality than conventional spin-echo imaging.[21] Fat suppression and use of gadolinium have both been studied; however, neither has been shown to significantly improve accuracy for staging prostate carcinoma, and thus they are not routinely used.[17,27,28]

In a typical imaging protocol for the evaluation of prostate carcinoma, patients are scheduled at least 3 weeks after transrectal biopsy because of the lower accuracy seen in the first few weeks after biopsy, presumably related to postbiopsy artifacts.[58] If possible, imaging is done with an integrated endorectal external phased-array coil. The balloon of the endorectal surface coil is inflated with 60 to 90 ml of air (as tolerated by the patient) because increased air in the balloon appears to decrease motion artifact. Glucagon is injected intramuscularly immediately before imaging to decrease rectal contractions, which has been shown to improve image quality.[21] A sagittal T1-weighted spin-echo sequence is obtained using the body coil with a large field of view (Figure 30-7). An axial spin-echo T1-weighted sequence is then obtained through the prostate and seminal vesicles (Figures 30-8 and 30-9). This is followed by a fast spin-echo T2-weighted sequence at the same locations. The axial images are similar in orientation to those from conventional computed tomography (CT) of the prostate (Figure 30-10). A coronal oblique fast spin-echo T2-weighted sequence is obtained parallel to the long axis of the prostate. A 12-cm field of view and 4-mm sections with a 1-mm skip are used for all of these sequences, with matrixes of 256 × 192 to 256 × 256 with two excitations. An axial fast spin-echo double-echo sequence with a large field of view (20 to 26 cm) is then obtained, with thicker sections (7 mm with 3-mm skip) from the aortic bifurcation through the pelvis to assess for lymph node enlargement. The entire study can be completed in less than 1 hour.

NORMAL PROSTATE

One of the great advantages of MRI is its ability to image structures in the sagittal, transverse (axial), and coronal planes. This multiplanar imaging capability is useful when evaluating the prostate and periprostatic structures.

Sagittal images can be used to "localize" the prostate and to plan subsequent diagnostic imaging (Figure 30-7). In addition, sagittal images obtained off the midline demonstrate the inner and outer glands as well as the anterior fibromuscular stroma. Midsagittal images are useful in evaluating the relationship between the prostate and the rectum, which are normally separated by Denonvillier's fascia. The prostatic venous plexuses, particularly the venous plexus of Santorini, which is located anterior to the prostate, can also be identified on sagittal imaging. The cephalocaudal dimension of the prostate can be measured in this plane, and intravesical extension of BPH (periurethral glandular enlargement) can be determined.

Transverse (axial) images are useful in delineating the structures surrounding the prostate and the internal zonal anatomy of the gland itself (Figure 30-11). Differentiation can be made between the urethra and the inner and outer glands (Figures 30-12 and 30-13). The lateral margins of the prostate, the lateral and anterior venous plexuses, and the seminal vesicles (Figure 30-14) are well demonstrated on transverse images. The neurovascular bundles, which contain sympathetic nerves, arteries, and veins, course along the posterior lateral aspect of the prostate and can be seen at approximately the 5 and 7o'clock positions on transverse images (Figure 30-13). The prostatic capsule can be seen best with the endorectal surface-coil images as a thin, low–signal intensity region surrounding the gland (Figure 30-15).

Coronal imaging demonstrates the lateral margins of the prostate and surrounding structures. The apex and base of the gland are well defined on the coronal views (Figure 30-16). In addition, the interface between the base of the prostate and the seminal vesicles, as well as the external sphincter, is best delineated on the coronal sequences. Some periprostatic and pelvic conditions, such as adenopathy (Figure 30-17), may be further defined in this plane.

On T1-weighted spin-echo images the prostate appears relatively homogeneous, without differentiation or delineation between the different zones of the gland (Figure 30-11, *C*). These images are insensitive for the detection of many pathological processes within the

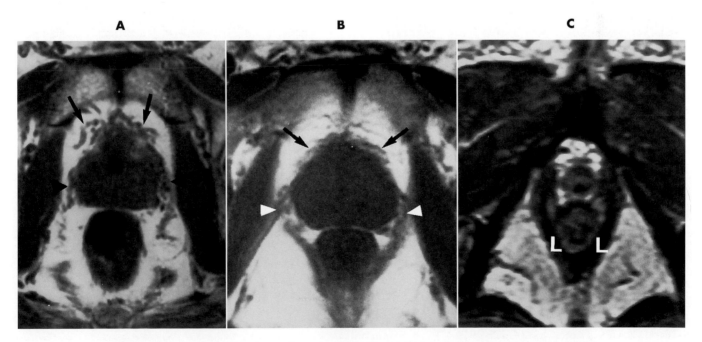

A   **B**   **C**

FIGURE 30-11   **A** and **B**, Normal prostatic venous plexus. Santorini's plexus *(arrows)* anteriorly and the lateral venous plexus (also termed the *neurovascular bundle*) posterolaterally *(arrowheads)*. **C**, Prostatic apex. The rectum and levator ani *(L)* muscles are seen dorsal to the caudal tip of the prostate gland.

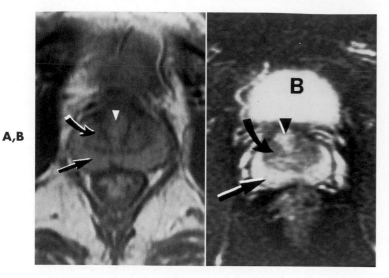

A,B

FIGURE 30-12   Normal zonal anatomy. **A,** Proton density image. The peripheral zone *(straight arrow)* shows high signal intensity relative to the central zone *(curved arrow)*. The signal intensity of the inner gland *(arrowhead)* is intermediate. **B,** T2-weighted spin-echo (2000/80) image with fat suppression. *B,* Urinary bladder.

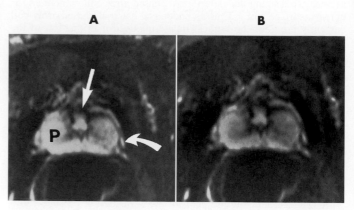

FIGURE 30-13   Normal zonal anatomy. T2-weighted axial spin-echo images (**A,** 2500/120; **B,** 2500/80) demonstrate a high–signal intensity, horseshoe-shaped peripheral zone *(P).* The low–signal intensity fibromuscular stroma *(straight arrow* in **A**) is identified anterior to a high–signal intensity focus from the urethra dilated secondary to a transurethral resection of the prostate. The high–signal intensity periprostatic vasculature *(curved arrow* in **A**) is seen surrounding lateral portions of the prostate, separated from the gland by the low–signal intensity prostatic capsule.

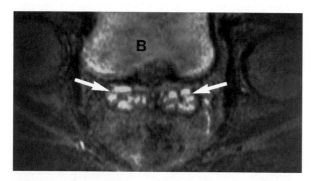

FIGURE 30-14   Normal seminal vesicles. T2-weighted spin-echo (3000/120) image demonstrates a fluid-filled high–signal intensity urinary bladder *(B)* anterior to the paired fluid-filled seminal vesicles *(arrows).*

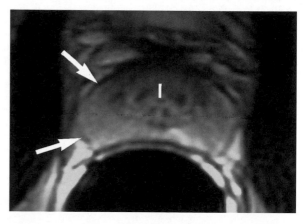

FIGURE 30-15   Normal prostate. Endorectal surface-coil technique. Spin-echo (2500/80) image shows the inner gland *(I)* to be lower in signal intensity than the peripheral zone. The low-signal intensity fibrous capsule *(arrows)* is seen surrounding the entire prostate.

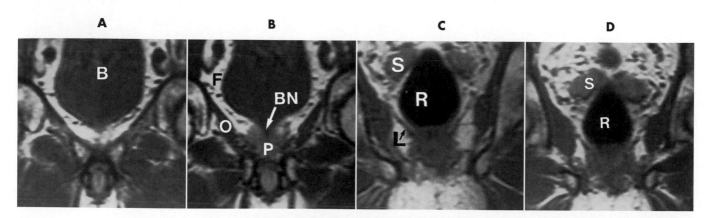

FIGURE 30-16   Normal coronal images spin-echo (600/20) from anterior **(A)** to posterior **(D).** The urinary bladder *(B),* prostate *(P),* perivesical and periprostatic fat *(F),* bladder neck *(BN),* obturator internus muscles *(O),* and levator ani muscles *(L)* are identified, as are the rectum *(R)* and seminal vesicles *(S).*

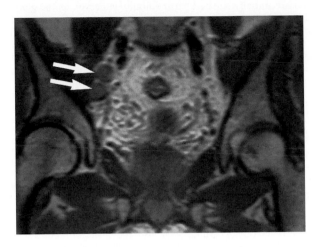

FIGURE 30-17   Pelvic lymphadenopathy.

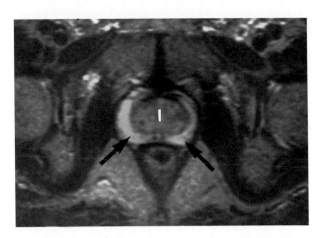

FIGURE 30-18   Mild BPH. *I,* Inner gland; *arrows,* peripheral zone.

prostate. However, T1-weighted MR images are useful for evaluating periprostatic structures. The periprostatic fat is seen as areas of relatively high signal intensity surrounding the gland. Serpentine structures that are decreased in signal intensity may be identified with the periprostatic fat. These areas represent portions of the prostatic venous plexuses. On axial imaging the neurovascular bundles can be identified at approximately the 5 and 7 o'clock positions as small, round areas of decreased signal intensity surrounded by high-intensity fat. The seminal vesicles, seen superior to the prostate on both the axial and the sagittal images, are of low signal intensity and appear similar to the prostate gland. The surrounding musculature of the pelvis, including the levator ani and obturator internus muscles, also demonstrate relatively low signal intensity.[36,40,56]

T2-weighted fast spin-echo images are useful in displaying the internal anatomy of the prostate and surrounding structures. The prostatic urethral lumen, when filled with fluid (urine), has increased signal intensity on T2-weighted images. Surrounding this area of increased signal intensity is a small area of lower signal intensity representing the muscular wall of the urethra (Figure 30-13). In normal men, the central zone is slightly hypointense on T2-weighted images. The adjacent transition zone is isointense relative to the central zone, and therefore these two areas are often indistinguishable. On occasion, the proton density images may demonstrate subtle differences between the transition and central zones (Figure 30-12). The peripheral zone is hyperintense compared with the adjacent inner gland. The anterior fibromuscular stroma is seen as a large area of decreased signal intensity on T2-weighted images. Surrounding the prostate is a thin rim of decreased signal intensity, which represents the prostate capsule. The prostatic venous plexuses are seen as thin tubular areas of increased signal intensity adjacent to the periphery of the prostate. This is best seen on sagittal images, in which the anterior venous plexus of Santorini can be reliably identified. The pelvic musculature is of lower signal intensity than the adjacent prostate gland.[15,22,35,53,59]

BENIGN PROSTATIC HYPERPLASIA

BPH is one of the most common abnormalities affecting the prostate gland. It is estimated that by age 60, approximately 50% of men will have changes of BPH and that this increases to 80% by age 80.[18] Although most older men have changes of BPH within the prostate, the majority do not develop clinically significant symptomatology. When symptoms do occur, they are commonly related to bladder outlet obstruction. The treatment of BPH is directed at relieving this obstruction and may involve either surgical or medical therapy.[18]

BPH develops predominantly within the transition zone. As the transition zone enlarges, it causes compression of the surrounding central zone, as well as the urethra, resulting in varying degrees of bladder outlet obstruction (Figure 30-5). As the disease progresses, the outer gland and the anterior fibromuscular stroma become compressed and appear thinned on MRI (Figures 30-18 to 30-20). Histologically, BPH involves

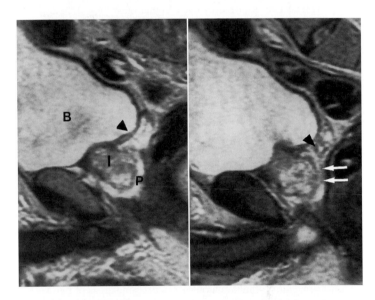

FIGURE 30-19   Abnormal seminal vesicles. Invasion of the left seminal vesicle *(arrowhead)* by prostate carcinoma *(arrows). I,* Inner gland; *arrows,* peripheral gland; *B,* bladder.

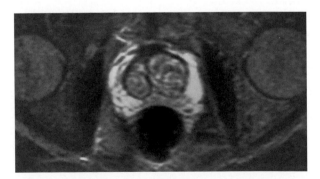

FIGURE 30-20   BPH. Spin-echo (2500/80) image demonstrates nodules separated by a low–signal intensity fibrous halo.

varying degrees of hyperplasia of both the stromal and glandular elements. The two most common forms of BPH that can be identified on MRI are stromal and nonstromal, or glandular, BPH, depending on the predominant tissue element that has become hyperplastic. The appearance of BPH on MRI varies depending on whether stromal or glandular hyperplasia has occurred.[18]

On MRI the overall size of the prostate can be evaluated to determine whether the gland is enlarged. T1-weighted images fail to distinguish BPH from normal prostatic tissue and therefore are of limited use, except to measure the prostate gland. T2-weighted images will demonstrate nodular enlargement of the inner gland.[18] Glandular BPH is characterized as nodular areas of heterogeneously increased signal intensity on T2-weighted images. In contrast, stromal BPH is of more intermediate signal intensity. A very thin rim of low signal intensity can occasionally be identified surrounding these nodules. After the administration of gadolinium, heterogeneous peripheral enhancement may be noted.[18] If the degree of inner gland enlargement is marked, compression and thinning of the central and peripheral zones will be seen, and differentiation of one form of BPH from the other may not be possible. Often, however, a thin, low-signal region separating the hyperplastic, enlarged inner gland from the compressed outer gland may be identified. This region, clinically referred to as the surgical capsule, distinguishes the tissue removed by the surgeon during prostatectomy for BPH (the inner gland) from that which remains (the outer gland) (Figure 30-21).

Currently, transurethral resection of the prostate is the treatment of choice for symptomatic BPH, although suprapubic or retropubic surgery may be required for larger glands. Recently, however, advances have been made in the medical management of BPH using pharmacological agents. The response of BPH to pharmacological therapy appears to depend, at least in part, on the type of tissue elements that have become hyperplastic. Stromal hyperplasia is more effectively treated with α-blockers, whereas glandular hyperplasia responds to androgen deprivation using luteinizing hormone–follicle-stimulating hormone (LH-FSH) antagonist.[18] The signal characteristics of BPH on MRI may therefore play an important role in planning the appropriate medical treatment for patients with symptomatic disease.

PROSTATITIS

Acute prostatitis is usually clinically diagnosed and managed without the aid of imaging studies. Acute infection of the prostate may be secondary to hematogenous spread and involve the inner or outer glands. When prostatitis is secondary to surgical intervention, the periurethral tissues and transition zone are often involved. On T1-weighted images the prostate gland is usually normal in appearance in the setting of acute prostatitis.[5] T2-weighted images may demonstrate areas of increased signal intensity that may be indistinguishable from the normal increased signal of the peripheral zone. If a prostatic abscess develops, the abscess is seen as an area of intermediate signal intensity on T1-weighted images and increased signal intensity on T2-weighted images.[40] Chronic prostatitis, granulomatous prostatitis, and areas of fibrosis after prior infections may all be seen as areas of decreased signal intensity on T2-weighted images.

CALCULI

Prostatic calcifications occur commonly in men of all ages and are often seen in conjunction with BPH. Most calculi are seen within the in-

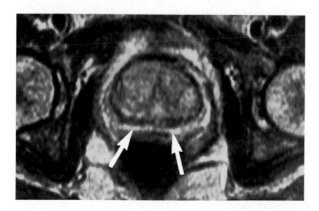

FIGURE 30-21 BPH. Spin-echo (2500/60) image shows compression of the high-signal intensity peripheral zone *(arrows)*. Note the prominent low–signal intensity halo separating the inner gland

ner gland. Calculi are often formed as concretions of corpora amylacea, a proteinaceous material secreted by the periurethral glandular tissues. Calculi are initially situated periurethrally. However, as the gland enlarges secondary to BPH, these calculi may be forced peripherally as the enlarging transition zone pushes the calculi outward. The calculi may then be identified in the area between the enlarged inner gland and the compressed outer gland, the surgical capsule. Occasionally, calcification may be seen in the outer gland. These are considered dystrophic calculi, often the result of previous inflammation or infarction. Dense calcifications are seen as areas of very low signal intensity on both T1- and T2-weighted images.

CYSTIC LESIONS

Cystic lesions of the prostate and periprostatic tissue may be either congenital or acquired in nature. The most common congenital cyst is the utricle cyst, which extends from the posterior urethra at the level of the verumontanum and represents abnormal dilatation of the prostatic utricle. These cysts are midline structures and communicate with the urethra. Müllerian duct cysts are also congenital midline lesions. These cysts, however, do not communicate with the posterior urethra and may occasionally extend superior to the prostate gland. Müllerian duct cysts may rarely be seen in association with renal agenesis. Congenital seminal vesicle cysts may develop as a result of ejaculatory duct atresia. These lesions are typically located superior and posterior to the prostate gland at a variable distance off the midline. Seminal vesicle cysts are commonly associated with ipsilateral renal agenesis. Seminal vesicles cysts can also be associated with adult polycystic disease.[20] In these cases, multiple cysts of varying size will be identified.

Cystic lesions of the prostate typically appear as areas of decreased signal intensity on T1-weighted images and increased signal intensity on T2-weighted images. In the setting of recent hemorrhage or infection, these cysts may develop a more heterogeneous appearance.

Acquired lesions of the prostate include retention cysts, which develop secondary to dilatation of the glandular acini, and ejaculatory duct cysts, which are caused by ejaculatory duct obstruction. These lesions are usually of decreased signal intensity on T1-weighted images and increased signal intensity on T2-weighted images. Occasionally, ejaculatory duct cysts may contain areas of decreased signal intensity on T2-weighted images, representing calculi within the cysts.[24,30,40,47]

CANCER

Prostate cancer is the most common form of cancer to affect American men, and its prevalence is independent of ethnic and racial background.* It is estimated that in 1997, approximately 334,500 new cases of prostate cancer will be diagnosed.[34] The frequency is increasing annually (Figure 30-22). Prostate cancer will account for approximately 41,800 deaths in 1997, making it the second most common cause of death by cancer in American men.[34] It is even more lethal in other groups worldwide (Figure 30-23). Early detection and treatment, although still confined to the prostate gland, can markedly reduce mortality rates.[13] This has led to the increased use of screening techniques, such as prostatic-specific antigen (PSA), digital rectal examination (DRE), transrectal ultrasonography, and MRI, in an attempt to screen for and detect early stages of the disease.[43]

The majority (almost 99%) of prostate cancers are adenocarcinomas. Approximately 70% arise in the peripheral zone, 20% in the transition zone, and the remaining 10% in the central zone.[26] Although cancer may be initially limited to its zone of origin, as the tumor enlarges, it may infiltrate into adjacent zones. As these tumors continue to enlarge, they eventually extend beyond the prostatic capsule and may involve the periprostatic fat, neurovascular bundles, seminal vesicles, or adjacent pelvic structures.

Detection of Prostate Cancer

MRI can be used in the evaluation of prostate cancer for either diagnostic or staging purposes. MRI is in general no better at diagnosing prostate cancer than the less expensive transrectal ultrasound and there-

*References 1-4, 11, 33, 34, 51, 60.

fore is infrequently used for diagnostic purposes. MRI has its major benefit in determining the stage or extent of disease once cancer has been diagnosed. Evaluation of the degree of cancer extension is important when planning appropriate therapy.[13]

Understanding the imaging characteristics of prostate cancer on MRI is essential for evaluating the prostate and periprostatic bed. T1-weighted spin-echo images rarely define prostate cancer well. In general a homogeneous, medium– to low–signal intensity appearance of the entire inner and outer gland is identified. An exception is in the patient after a biopsy, when moderate to high signal intensity, representing postbiopsy hemorrhage, may be identified[58] (Figures 30-24 and 30-25). T2-weighted MR images are useful in differentiating the zones of the prostate. They are also of use in detecting prostate carcinoma. It has been demonstrated that on T2-weighted imaging sequences, prostatic carcinoma is typically seen as an area of decreased signal intensity within the normally high–signal intensity peripheral zone[41] (Figures 30-26 to 30-29). Mucinous adenocarcinomas (which are rare) are an exception and may have increased signal intensity on T2-weighted images, making them difficult to differentiate from the adjacent peripheral

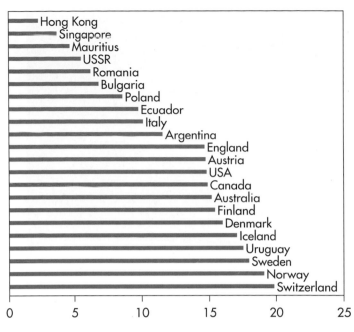

FIGURE 30-23   Mortality rates (age adjusted, per 100,000) of prostate cancer.

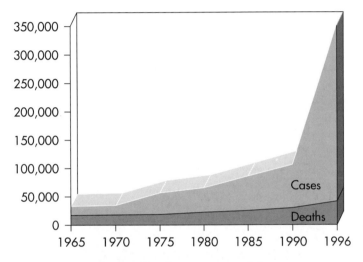

FIGURE 30-22   Prostate cancer statistics.

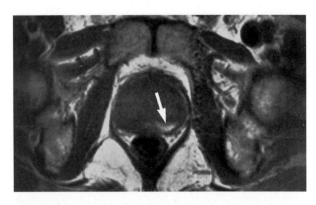

FIGURE 30-24   Hemorrhage secondary to biopsy. T1-weighted image demonstrates high signal intensity *(arrow)*.

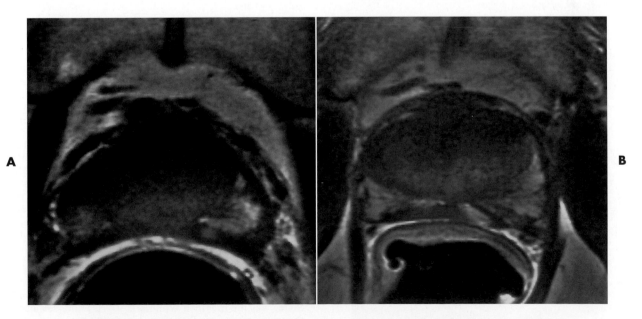

FIGURE 30-25   Postbiopsy hemorrhage. Endorectal surface-coil spin-echo (400/14) MR images in two patients demonstrate focal blood **(A)** in the left posterior peripheral gland in one patient and diffuse blood **(B)** throughout the peripheral gland in another. Blood is identified as high signal intensity in these studies.

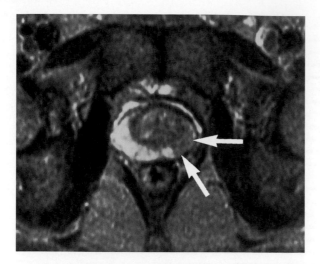

FIGURE 30-26   Prostate cancer *(arrows)* infiltrating and displacing the normal high–signal intensity peripheral zone. The fibrous prostate capsule is seen intact, separating the cancer from the high–signal intensity lateral periprostatic venous plexus.

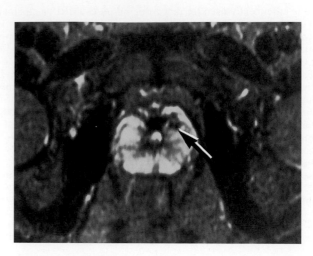

FIGURE 30-27   Prostate cancer. An 8-mm *(arrow)* low–signal intensity cancer in the anterolateral aspect of the peripheral zone.

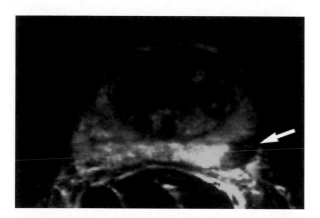

FIGURE 30-28   Prostate cancer *(arrow)*. Fast spin-echo (7000/147, 16 echo train length) endorectal surface-coil image.

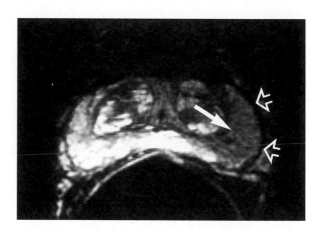

FIGURE 30-29   Prostate cancer *(arrow)*. The capsule *(open arrows)* is not involved by tumor.

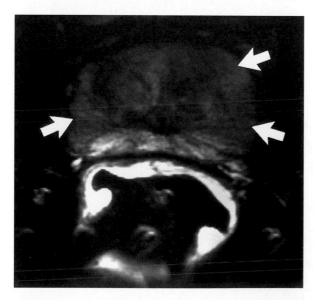

FIGURE 30-30   Prostate cancer *(arrows)* involving the entire gland.

zone.[44] Likewise, prostatic carcinoma originating within the normally lower–signal intensity transition zone may also be difficult to discern from surrounding tissues. When adenocarcinoma involves the entire peripheral zone, a single area of abnormal signal intensity may not be seen (Figure 30-30). Instead the peripheral zone will be diffusely heterogeneous in appearance.

Approximately 60% of lesions larger than 5 mm will be detected on MRI. Larger lesions and lesions located in the posterior half of the gland are more easily detected.[11] Overall the sensitivity of MRI for detecting prostate cancer is approximately 60%.[11] MRI lacks some specificity in the diagnosis of prostate cancer; however, it has a positive predictive value of 68%. This is due to the fact that areas of decreased signal intensity on T2-weighted images may also be seen with benign conditions, such as chronic prostatitis, stromal BPH, infarcts, and areas of fibrosis.

Staging of Prostate Cancer

Until recently, the most commonly used staging system in the United States was the modified Whitmore or Whitmore-Jewett system. Although there are a number of variations of this staging system, prostate cancer usually has been staged into four categories, known as *stages A, B, C,* and *D.* These stages are defined in Table 30-2.

Table 30-2   Prostate Cancer: Whitmore-Jewett Staging System

STAGE		FINDINGS
A*		Cancers are clinically unsuspected and nonpalpable. They are usually diagnosed after a transurethral resection of the prostate for BPH when cancer is incidentally found within chips of prostatic tissue.
	A1	Histologically well-differentiated lesions that are present in less than three "chips" or pieces of the specimen. They are usually localized to the inner gland.
	A2	Lesions that are histologically anaplastic or, if histologically well differentiated, present in more than three pieces of the specimen. They may be localized to the inner gland or involve both the inner and outer glands.
B		Clinically palpable tumors involving the outer gland but also possibly infiltrating into the inner gland.
	B1	Tumors confined to one side of the gland and measuring less than 1.5 cm.
	B2	Tumors that are larger than 1.5 cm or involve both sides of the gland.
C†		Palpable tumors that have extended beyond the confines of the prostate.
	C1	Tumors that have extended into the periprostatic fat alone.
	C2	Tumors that have extended into the seminal vesicles.
D		Tumors having distant metastasis.
	D1	Disease involving the pelvic lymph nodes.
	D2	Metastatic disease involving other organs.

*Both stage A and stage B cancers are believed to be confined to the prostate without extension into the periprostatic fat, adjacent pelvic structures, or pelvic lymph nodes.
†Usually, tumors that involve the seminal vesicles initially extend into the periprostatic fat and subsequently spread to the seminal vesicles. However, tumors can invade the seminal vesicles directly via the ejaculatory ducts without involving the prostatic capsule or periprostatic fat.

The tumor-node-metastasis (TNM) staging system, initially described by the International Union Against Cancer and revised numerous times, is frequently used outside the United States. Although this system has not been used often in North America in the past, it has recently become universally accepted, and its use is now more common. This system divides the stage into tumor extent within the gland (T), lymph node involvement (N), and/or metastatic disease (M). Each patient will have three categories, one from the T, another from the N, and the third from the M. This staging system has a more complex breakdown but is otherwise similar to the Whitmore-Jewett system, and a comparison of the two systems shows similarities. The exact TNM staging system is outlined in Box 30-1.

When prostate cancer is being staged, it is crucial to differentiate disease confined to the prostate gland from disease that has extended beyond the prostate. Treatment may vary depending on the extent of disease.[54] For example, patients with cancer confined to the prostate gland alone may be candidates for radical prostatectomy, a potentially curative procedure. Patients with disease extension beyond the confines of the prostate are generally not surgical candidates and may be offered an alternative therapy. Prognosis also varies with the stage of disease. Patients with prostate carcinoma confined to the gland have a 5-year survival rate of 94%, whereas patients with evidence of extracapsular extension have 5-year survival rates of less than 70%.[60] It therefore becomes crucial in the staging of prostate cancer to determine the exact extent of disease in relation to the prostate capsule.

A variety of imaging tools have been used to stage prostate cancer. Until recently, CT has been considered the most accurate. Unfortunately, there are significant limitations to CT, so accurate staging is limited. Prostate cancer cannot be directly seen by noncontrast or contrast-enhanced CT. The prostate capsule and the neurovascular bundles are not clearly identified on routine CT of the male pelvis. Subtle tumor extension into the periprostatic tissues is not consistently identified. The

BOX 30-1
Prostate Cancer: TNM Staging System

Primary tumor (T)

TX		Primary tumor cannot be assessed
T0		No evidence of primary tumor
T1		Clinically inapparent tumor not palpable or visible by imaging
	T1a	Tumor incidental histological finding in 5% or less of tissue resected (Figure 30-31, *A*)
	T1b	Tumor incidental histological finding in more than 5% of tissue resected (Figure 30-31, *B* and *C*)
	T1c	Tumor identified by needle biopsy (e.g., because of elevated PSA)
T2		Tumor confined within the prostate*
	T2a	Tumor involves half of a lobe or less (Figure 30-31, *D*)
	T2b	Tumor involves more than half of a lobe but not both lobes
	T2c	Tumor involves both lobes (Figure 30-31, *E*)
T3		Tumor extends through the prostatic capsule†
	T3a	Unilateral extracapsular extension (Figure 30-31, *F*)
	T3b	Bilateral extracapsular extension
T4	T3c	Tumor invades the seminal vesicle or vesicles
		Tumor is fixed or invades adjacent structures other than the seminal vesicles
	T4a	Tumor invades bladder neck, external sphincter, or rectum
	T4b	Tumor invades levator muscles and/or is fixed to the pelvic wall

Regional lymph nodes

NX	Regional lymph nodes cannot be assessed
N0	No regional lymph node metastasis
N1	Metastasis in a single lymph node, 2 cm or less in greatest dimension
N2	Metastasis in a single lymph node, more than 2 cm but not more than 5 cm in greatest dimension; or multiple lymph node metastases, none more than 5 cm in greatest dimension
N3	Metastasis in a lymph node more than 5 cm in greatest dimension

Distant metastasis‡

MX		Presence of distant metastasis cannot be assessed
M0		No distant metastasis
M1		Distant metastasis
	M1a	Nonregional lymph node(s)
	M1b	Bone(s)
	M1c	Other site(s)

*Tumor found in one or both lobes by needle biopsy but not palpable or visible by imaging is classified as T1c.
†Invasion into the prostatic apex or into (but not beyond) the prostatic capsule is classified not as T3 but as T2.
‡When more than one site of metastasis is present, the most advanced category (M1c) is used.

major benefit of CT of the prostate is the identification of enlarged regional and extraregional lymph nodes. However, the differentiation between tumor-infiltrated and non–tumor-infiltrated enlarged nodes or the delineation of normal-sized but tumor-infiltrated lymph nodes is not adequate.

Transrectal ultrasound, despite the suggested high accuracy for staging prostate cancer published in the middle of the 1980s, is not able to acceptably stage local prostate cancer. Unlike CT, ultrasound can identify tumor within the prostate, but like CT, it is unable to consistently identify the prostate capsule and subtle infiltration of tumor beyond the prostate.

MRI is unique in its ability to stage prostate cancer. With the use of the endorectal surface coil alone or in conjunction with anteriorly placed surface coils (i.e., in a phased array), MRI is able to routinely identify the tumor, the prostate capsule, the neurovascular bundles, and the surrounding periprostatic structures. Because of this, MRI has the greatest potential to accurately assess tumor extension. Optimal merging of MRI findings with other factors, such as age, PSA level, and Gleason grade, further improves accuracy.[14]

Several criteria can be used to evaluate for extension of tumor beyond the capsule. A systematic approach, such as the following, should be used:

- Identify the tumor (Figures 30-28 to 30-30).
- Identify the capsule and possible invasion (Figures 30-31 to 30-33).
- Evaluate for periprostatic fat infiltration (Figures 30-34 and 30-35).
- Evaluate the neurovascular bundles and other periprostatic vascular structures (Figures 30-36 to 30-38).
- Evaluate abnormalities within the seminal vesicles (Figures 30-19 and 30-39).
- Determine whether the base of the prostate is involved and whether extraprostatic extension at the base is present (Figure 30-40).
- Identify the apex of the prostate and evaluate for possible tumor involvement and apical extension (Figure 30-41).
- Identify any regional or extraregional lymph nodes (Figures 30-17, 30-42, and 30-43, *A*).
- Identify any bone involvement (Figure 30-43, *B*).

Capsule

Examining the prostatic capsule is crucial in evaluating for tumor extension. The capsule, when normal, is routinely identified with the use of an endorectal surface coil. It may not be routinely seen with the use of the body coil. The capsule should be smooth and continuous around the prostate. Disruption of the capsule, as well as areas of focal capsular bulge, may indicate capsular invasion.

Multiple criteria are applied to detect capsular penetration.[31,61] Focal bulge, focal retraction, capsular thickening, loss of the rectoprostatic angle, and periprostatic low signal intensity are all predictive of extracapsular spread. Apparent extension of tumor beyond the capsule on MRI has the highest specificity for tumor extension of all MR findings, (90%) but has a low sensitivity (15%).[31]

Periprostatic Structures

Invasion of the periprostatic venous plexuses causes abnormally decreased signal intensity within these tubular structures. The neurovascular bundles should be carefully evaluated for tumor invasion when staging for prostate cancer. The neurovascular bundles are located at the 5 and 7 o'clock positions on axial images. With tumor invasion,*

---

*References 36, 45, 46, 48, 56, 61.

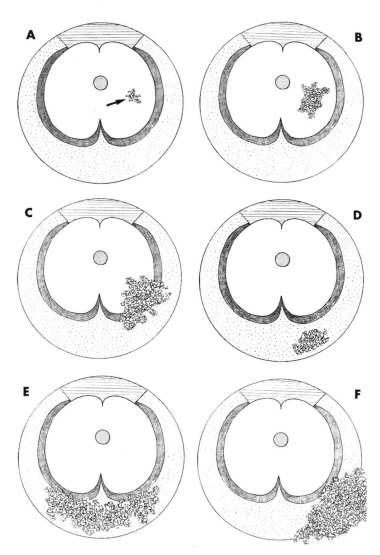

FIGURE 30-31   Diagrams of small (**A**) and large (**B**) cancer confined to the transition zone (inner gland). Cancer invading both the inner and outer gland is illustrated in **C.** Unilateral outer gland confined cancer is illustrated in **D;** bilateral confined outer gland cancer illustrated in **E. F** demonstrates extracapsular extension of cancer.

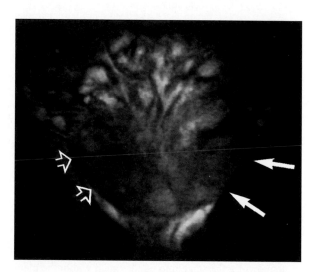

FIGURE 30-32   Prostate cancer with capsule involvement. On the left side, the capsule *(arrows)* is normal, but on the right side *(open arrows),* the capsule is infiltrated by tumor.

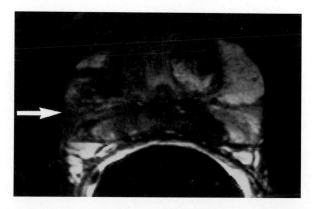

FIGURE 30-33   Prostate cancer with capsule involvement. Tumor involving the right side and posterior aspect of the gland infiltrates *(arrow)* the right capsule.

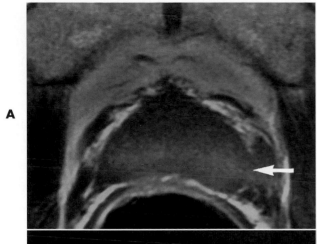

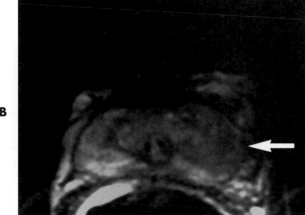

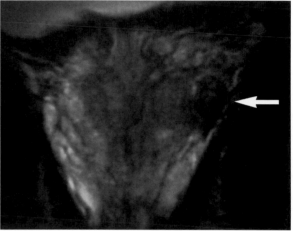

FIGURE 30-34   Prostate cancer with extracapsular involvement. Transverse spin-echo (400/14) image **(A),** fast spin-echo (7000/147, 16 echo train length) image **(B),** and coronal **(C)** image show disruption of the periprostatic fat *(arrow)* and tumor infiltration on the left side.

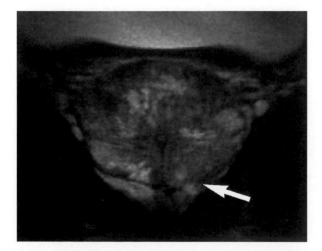

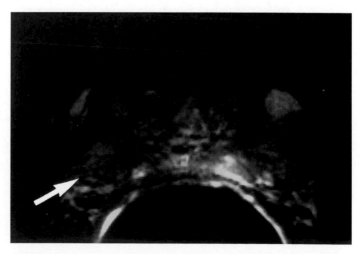

FIGURE 30-35   Prostate cancer with extracapsular tumor extension near the left apex *(arrow)*.

FIGURE 30-36   Diffuse prostate cancer with subtle extension near the right neurovascular bundle. The capsule is disrupted, and a bulge is seen *(arrow)*.

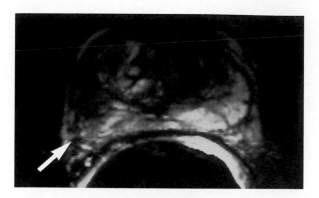

FIGURE 30-37 Prostate cancer with disruption of the right capsule and tumor extension into the right neurovascular bundle *(arrow)*.

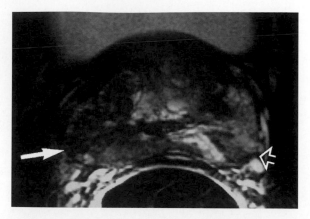

FIGURE 30-38 Bilateral prostate cancer with disruption of the right capsule and neurovascular bundle *(arrow)*. There is subtle tumor extension into the left capsule and neurovascular bundle *(open arrow)*.

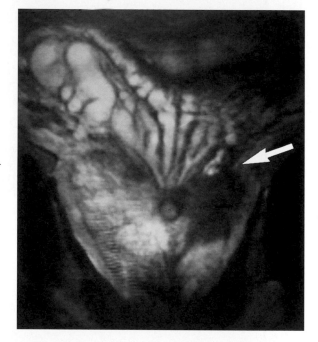

FIGURE 30-39 Prostate cancer with direct extension into the left seminal vesicle *(arrow)*.

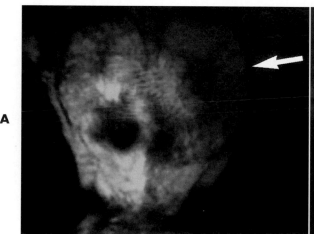

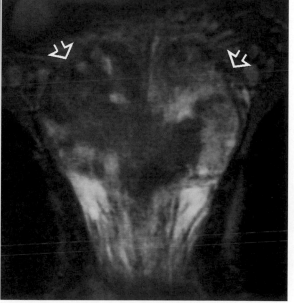

FIGURE 30-40 Prostate cancer with sharp delineation of the capsule *(arrow)* in one patient **(A)** and in another patient **(B)** shows destruction of the capsule bilaterally at the bases *(open arrows)* caused by direct tumor extension.

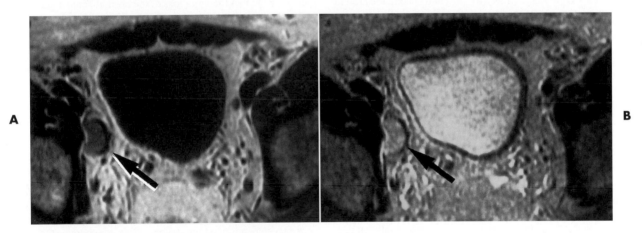

FIGURE 30-41   Prostate cancer with apical involvement. Endorectal surface-coil coronal spin-echo (7000/147, 16 echo train length) images demonstrate the apex to be free of involvement in one patient **(A)** but involved *(arrow)* in the second **(B).**

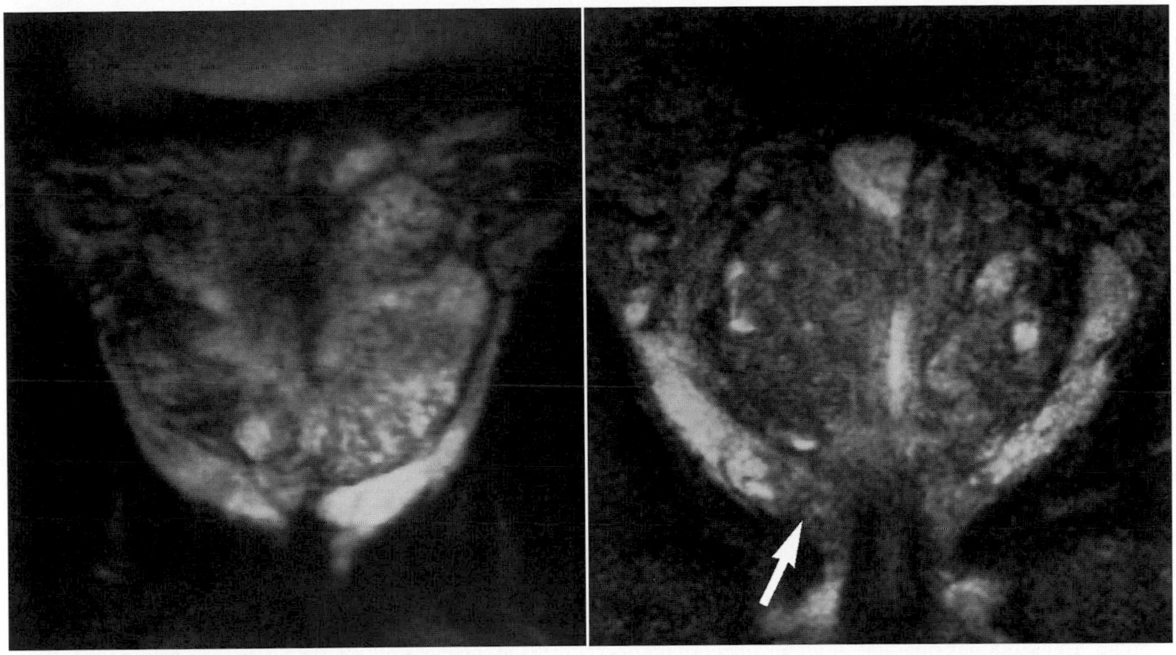

FIGURE 30-42   Stage D1, pelvic lymphadenopathy. Spin-echo (600/20) image **(A)** and spin-echo (2500/60) image **(B)** demonstrate an enlarged lymph node *(arrow)* infiltrated by prostate cancer.

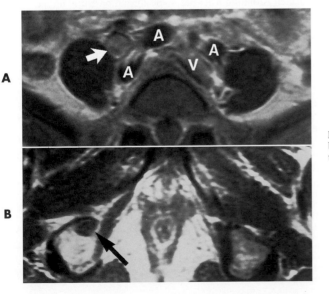

FIGURE 30-43   **A,** Stage D1 retroperitoneal lymphadenopathy *(arrow)* at the bifurcation of the iliac veins *(V)* and arteries *(A).* **B,** Stage D2 bone metastases to the right ilium.

the neurovascular bundles become asymmetrical, and there is a loss of normal signal intensity. Obliteration of the normal rectoprostatic angle is also highly predictive of extracapsular invasion.[61]

Seminal Vesicles

The seminal vesicles are normally of low to intermediate signal intensity on T1-weighted images and increased signal intensity on T2-weighted images. In the setting of prostate cancer, enlargement of one seminal vesicle compared with the other, along with a decrease in the T2 signal intensity of the larger seminal vesicle, is an indication of tumor infiltration.[7,45,48] Asymmetry in size alone is not diagnostic of local tumor extension.

Early infiltration of cancer into the peritubular stroma of the seminal vesicles can occasionally be seen as focal areas of tubular wall thickening.[7] These subtle changes may be seen best on the coronal or sagittal images. The axial orientation alone may not delineate subtle extension into the peritubular stroma of the seminal vesicles.

Apex

Evaluation of the apex, the most difficult area of the prostate to evaluate by clinical or imaging means, requires multiorientation imaging. Detection of tumor within and tumor extension beyond the confines of the prostate at the apex is important because this is a common site of extracapsular spread. Longitudinal imaging in either the coronal or sagittal orientation will demonstrate subtle and on occasion more obvious tumor extension than might otherwise be identified by the axial approach alone.

There has been a wide range of sensitivities and specificities found for identification of extracapsular spread with MR imaging, with accuracies ranging from 51% to 92%.* The largest multicenter trial that examined results with the body coil and with the endorectal surface coil resulted in overall disappointing mean accuracies for all of the readers, ranging from 54% to 61% for different imaging techniques.[57] There were limitations to this study,[23] with the most important being variable experience among the readers, ranging from 1 year to more than 5 years, and the accuracies achieved by the readers, ranging from 50% to 79%. This study along with multiple other studies indicates that staging accuracy appears to be at best in the range of 75% to 85% using current techniques and evaluation by experienced readers. In the future, systems combining radiologists and computers may lead to higher staging accuracy, particularly among less experienced readers.[52]

Although MR staging accuracy is only moderate, it is higher than that found for other imaging techniques and higher than staging accuracy with DRE.[42] Although the information on local spread provided by MRI is imperfect, it is extremely important because the standard for staging accuracy is prostatectomy. Even though it is commonly felt that patients with greater than stage B disease should not be treated with prostatectomy,[45] approximately 40% of patients undergoing prostatectomy are found to have greater than stage B disease at surgery.[29] Predicting stage before prostatectomy is essential because this major surgical procedure can have significant complications, including incontinence in approximately 4% of patients and impotence in approximately 50% of patients.[29] Accurate prediction of the likely benefit from prostatectomy allows patients and physicians to weigh the possible benefits from surgery versus the risks. Recent studies have shown that the addition of MRI improves the prediction of outcome in patients with intermediate risk, as indicated by PSA levels of 10 to 20 ng/ml and Gleason scores of 5 to 7.[9,10] Prostatectomy is an expensive procedure, and identification of patients unlikely to benefit from surgery could decrease the cost of care as well as eliminate the risk of morbidity and mortality rates from surgery. Because prostatectomy is more expensive than MRI, cost savings could be realized, even with a low sensitivity identifying extracapsular spread, as long as this identification could be made with a high degree of confidence (i.e., high specificity) so that patients would not be denied potentially curative surgery.

MRI not only provides information about the presence of extracapsular spread but can also be used to screen for enlarged pelvic lymph nodes and bone metastases. Identification of enlarged lymph nodes with subsequent biopsy using CT guidance was shown to identify lymph node metastases and thus prevent unnecessary surgery in more than 10% of patients in a recent study.[32]

MRI is currently an imperfect method of staging, but it provides additional information for patients and physicians making difficult clinical decisions. MRI is still a rapidly evolving technology, and the use of newer techniques such as three-dimensional fast spin-echo imaging and improved gradient coils and surface coils will result in higher signal-to-noise ratio and resolution, possibly resulting in higher accuracies for staging in the future. Future studies will also need to further define the role of MRI compared with other information, such as Gleason grade, PSA, and tumor deoxyribonucleic acid analysis, for predicting outcome and determining therapeutic choices.

Postbiopsy and Therapy Changes

Patients undergoing MRI for the purpose of staging prostate carcinoma usually have undergone previous prostate biopsy, with hemorrhage frequently occurring at the site of the biopsy. It has been reported that postbiopsy hemorrhage can persist for as long as 4 months.[58] Postbiopsy hemorrhage is seen as areas of increased signal intensity on T1-weighted images and corresponding areas of either high or low signal intensity on T2-weighted images.[58] It can be difficult, if not impossible, to distinguish decreased signal on T2-weighted images caused by postbiopsy hemorrhage from prostatic carcinoma, and postbiopsy hemorrhage can therefore interfere with the accuracy of MR staging. Higher staging accuracy has been found if imaging of the prostate is performed at least 3 weeks after prostate biopsy.[58]

Early reports on the appearance of the prostate after radiation therapy indicate that there is a loss of the normal zonal anatomy within the prostate, with diffuse decreased signal intensity throughout the gland. This loss in signal intensity within the prostate may result in the gland being isointense or even hypointense relative to adjacent fat. Preliminary reports suggest that this loss of signal intensity may be related to prostatic gland atrophy.[6] Hormonal therapy has also been reported to cause diffuse decreased signal intensity within the gland on T2-weighted images.[8,45]

SUMMARY

MRI has allowed great advances to be made in imaging of the prostate gland. The internal zonal anatomy of the prostate is well demonstrated using T2-weighted images. Axial, coronal, and sagittal images are also useful in demonstrating prostatic anatomy, as well as surrounding pelvic structures. MRI can identify prostate cancer. MRI's greatest role, however, is not in the detection of prostate cancer but in its ability to stage the disease. Because the treatment and prognosis for prostate cancer vary depending on the stage of disease, accurate staging is critical. Clinical staging is limited because of its inability to distinguish between localized cancer and disease that has extended beyond the confines of the prostate. Although MRI has some limitations, it is unique among imaging tools in its ability to identify the tumor (which can be done by ultrasound but not CT), identify the capsule (which cannot be done by any other imaging modality), identify the neurovascular bundles (which can be done by ultrasound but not CT), and in most instances demonstrate subtle localized extraprostatic extension of tumor (which cannot be done by any other imaging modality). Although MRI is not perfect, used with clinical parameters it is an important tool in planning appropriate treatment for the most common cancer in the world, the most frequently diagnosed malignancy, and the second most lethal cancer in American men.

REFERENCES

1. Boring C, Squires T, and Tong T: Cancer statistics, 1991, CA Cancer J Clin 41(1):19, 1991.
2. Boring C, Squires T, and Tong T: Cancer statistics, 1992, CA Cancer J Clin 42(1):7, 1992.
3. Boring C, Squires T, and Tong T: Cancer statistics, 1993, CA Cancer J Clin 43(1):7, 1993.
4. Boring C, Squires T, Tong T, et al: Cancer statistics, 1994, CA Cancer J Clin 44(1):7, 1994.
5. Bryan P, Butler H, and Nelson A: Magnetic resonance imaging of the prostate, Am J Roentgenol 146:543, 1986.

---

*References 7, 12, 13, 16, 19, 38, 39, 47, 57.

6. Chan TW, and Kressel HY: Prostate and seminal vesicles after irradiation: MR appearance, J Magn Reson Imaging 1(5):503, 1991.
7. Chelsky MJ, Schnall MD, Seidmon EJ, et al: Use of endorectal surface coil magnetic resonance imaging for local staging of prostate cancer, J Urol 150:391, 1993.
8. Chen M, Hricak H, Kalbhen CL, et al: Hormonal ablation of prostatic cancer: effects on prostate morphology, tumor detection, and staging by endorectal coil MR imaging, Am J Roentgenol 166:1157, 1996.
9. D'Amico A, Whittington R, Malkowicz S, et al: A multivariate analysis of clinical and pathological factors that predict for prostate specific antigen failure after radical prostatectomy for prostate cancer, J Urol 154:131, 1995.
10. D'Amico A, Whittington R, Schnall M, et al: The impact of the inclusion of endorectal coil magnetic resonance imaging in a multivariate analysis to predict clinically unsuspected extraprostatic cancer, Cancer 75:2368, 1995.
11. Ellis JH, Tempany C, Sarin MS, et al: MR imaging and sonography of early prostatic cancer: pathologic and imaging features that influence identification and diagnosis, Am J Roentgenol 162:865, 1994.
12. Epstein J, Carmichael M, and Walsh P: Adenocarcinoma of the prostate invading the seminal vesicles: definition and relation to tumor volume, grade and margin of resection to prognosis, J Urol 149:1040, 1993.
13. Epstein J, Carmichael M, Pizov G, et al: Influence of capsular penetration on progression following radical prostatectomy: a study of 196 cases with long term follow-up, J Urol 150:135, 1993.
14. Getty DJ, Seltzer SE, Tempany CMC, et al: Prostate cancer: relative effects of demographic, clinical, histologic, and MR imaging variables on the accuracy of staging, Radiology 204:471, 1997.
15. Hricak H, Dooms G, McNeal J, et al: MR imaging of the prostate gland: normal anatomy, Am J Roentgenol 148:51, 1987.
16. Hricak H, White S, Vigneron D, et al: Carcinoma of the prostate gland: MR imaging with pelvic phased-array coils versus integrated endorectal-pelvic phased-array coils, Radiology 193:703, 1994.
17. Huch B, Boner J, Lutolf U, et al: Contrast-enhanced endorectal coil MRI in local staging of prostate carcinoma, J Comput Assist Tomogr 19(2):232, 1995.
18. Ishida J, Sugimura K, Okizuka H, et al: Benign prostatic hyperplasia: value of MR imaging for determining histologic type, Radiology 190(2):329, 1994.
19. Jager GJ, Ruijter ETG, van de Kaa CA, et al: Local staging of prostate cancer with endorectal MR imaging: correlation with histopathology, Am J Roentgenol 166:845, 1996.
20. Keenan J, and Rifkin M: Ultrasound diagnosis of seminal vesicle cysts in a patient with ADPKD, J Ultrasound Med 15:343, 1996.
21. Kier R, Wain S, and Troiano R: Fast spin-echo MR images of the pelvis obtained with a phased-array coil: value in localizing and staging prostate carcinoma, Am J Roentgenol 161:601, 1993.
22. Koslin D, Kenney P, Koehler R, et al: Magnetic resonance imaging of the internal anatomy of the prostate gland, Invest Radiol 22:947, 1987.
23. Langlotz C, Schnall M, and Pollack H: Staging of prostatic cancer: accuracy of MR imaging, Radiology 194:645, 1995.
24. McDermott VG, Meakem TJI, Stolpen AH, et al: Prostatic and periprostatic cysts: findings on MR imaging, Am J Roentgenol 164:123, 1995.
25. McNeal J: The zonal anatomy of the prostate. In Liss AR, ed: The Prostate, 2:35, 1981.
26. McNeal J, Redwine E, and Freiha F: Zonal distribution of prostatic adenocarcinoma: correlation with histologic pattern and direction of spread, Am J Surg Pathol 12:897, 1988.
27. Mirowitz S, Brown J, and Heiken J: Evaluation of the prostate and prostatic carcinoma with gadolinium-enhanced endorectal coil MR imaging, Radiology 186(1):153, 1993.
28. Mirowitz S, Heiken J, and Brown J: Evaluation of fat saturation technique for T2-weighted endorectal coil MRI of the prostate, Magn Reson Imaging 12(5):743, 1994.
29. Murphy G, Mettlin C, Menck H, et al: National patterns of prostate cancer treatment by radical prostatectomy: results of a survey by the American College of Surgeons commission on cancer, J Urol 152:1817, 1994.
30. Nghiem H, Kellman G, and Sandberg S: Cystic lesions of the prostate, Radiographics 10:635, 1990.
31. Outwater E, Petersen R, Siegelman E, et al: Prostate carcinoma: assessment of diagnostic criteria for capsular penetration on endorectal coil MR images, Radiology 193:333, 1994.
32. Oyen R, Van Poppel H, Ameye F, et al: Lymph node staging of localized prostatic carcinoma with CT and CT-guided find-needle aspiration biopsy: prospective study of 285 patients, Radiology 190:315, 1994.
33. Parker S, Tong T, Bolden S, et al: Cancer statistics, 1996, CA Cancer J Clin 65:5, 1996.
34. Parker S, Tong T, Bolden S, et al: Cancer statistics, 1997, CA Cancer J Clin 47:5, 1997.
35. Phillips M, Kressel H, Spritzer C, et al: Normal prostate and adjacent structures: MR imaging at 1.5 T1, Radiology 164:381, 1997.
36. Poon PY, Bronskill MJ, Poon CS, et al: Identification of the periprostatic venous plexus by MR imaging, J Comput Assist Tomogr 15(2):265, 1991.
37. Porter A, Blasko J, Grimm P, et al: Brachytherapy for prostate cancer, CA Cancer J Clin 45:165, 1995.
38. Presti J, Hricak H, Narayan P, et al: Local staging of prostatic carcinoma: comparison of transrectal sonography and endorectal MR imaging, Am J Roentgenol 166:103, 1996.
39. Quinn S, Franzini D, Demlow T, et al: MR imaging of prostate cancer with an endorectal surface coil technique: correlation with whole-mount specimens, Radiology 190:323, 1994.
40. Ramchandani P, and Schnall MD: Magnetic resonance imaging of the prostate, Semin Roentgenol XXVIII(1):74, 1993.
41. American Joint Committee for Cancer Staging and End Results Reporting: Manual for staging of cancer, 1978, Chicago, The Committee.
42. Rifkin M, Zerhoiuni E, and Gatsonis C: Comparison of MRI and ultrasonography in staging early prostate cancer: results of a multi-institutional cooperative trial, N Engl J Med 323:621, 1990.
43. Rubens DJ, Gottlieb RH, Maldonado CE Jr, et al: Clinical evaluation of prostate biopsy parameters: gland volume and elevated prostate-specific antigen level, Radiology 199:159, 1996.
44. Schiebler M, Schnall M, and Outwater E: MR imaging of mucinous adenocarcinoma of the prostate, J Comput Assist Tomogr 16(3):493, 1992.
45. Schiebler M, Schnall M, Pollack H, et al: Current role of MR imaging in the staging of adenocarcinoma of the prostate, Radiology 189(2):339, 1993.
46. Schiebler M, Yankaskas B, Tempany C, et al: Efficacy of prostate-specific antigen and magnetic resonance imaging in staging stage C adenocarcinoma of the prostate, Invest Radiol 27(8):575, 1992.
47. Schnall M, Connick T, Hayes C, et al: MR imaging of the pelvis with an endorectal-external multicoil array, J Magn Reson Imaging 2:229, 1992.
48. Schnall M, Imai Y, Tomaszewski J, et al: Prostate cancer: local staging with endorectal surface coil MR imaging, Radiology 178:797, 1991.
49. Schnall M, Lenkinski R, Pollack H, et al: Prostate: MR imaging with an endorectal surface coil, Radiology 172:570, 1989.
50. Schnall M, Tomaszewski J, Pollack H, et al: The bulging prostate gland: a sign of capsular involvement, J Magn Reson Imaging 1:279, 1991.
51. Scott R Jr, Mutchnik D, Laskowski T, et al: Carcinoma of the prostate in elderly men: incidence, growth, characteristics and clinical significance, J Urol 101:602, 1969.
52. Seltzer SE, Getty DJ, Tempany CMC, et al: Staging prostate cancer with MR imaging: a combined radiologist-computer system, Radiology 202:219, 1997.
53. Sommer F, McNeal J, and Carrol C: MR depiction of zonal anatomy of the prostate at 1.5T, J Comput Assist Tomogr 10(6):983, 1986.
54. Steinfeld A: Questions regarding the treatment of localized prostate cancer, Radiology 184:593, 1992.
55. Steyn J, and Smith F: Nuclear magnetic resonance (NMR) imaging of the prostate, Br J Urol 56:679, 1984.
56. Tempany C, Rahmouni A, Epstein J, et al: Invasion of the neurovascular bundle by prostate cancer: evaluation with MR imaging, Radiology 181:107, 1991.
57. Tempany CM, Zhou X, Zerhouni EA, et al: Staging of prostate cancer: results of radiology diagnostic oncology group project comparison of three MR imaging techniques, Radiology 192(1):47, 1994.
58. White S, Hricak H, Forstner R, et al: Prostate cancer: effect of postbiopsy hemorrhage on interpretation of MR images, Radiology 195:385, 1995.
59. White Nunes L, Schiebler MS, Rauschning W, et al: The normal prostate and periprostatic structures: correlation between MR images made with an endorectal coil and cadaveric microtome sections, Am J Roentgenol 164:923, 1995.
60. Wingo P, Tong T, and Bolden S: Cancer statistics, 1995, CA Cancer J Clin 45:8, 1995.
61. Yu KK, Hricak H, Alagappan R, et al: Detection of extracapsular extension of prostate carcinoma with endorectal and phased-array coil MR imaging: multivariate feature analysis, Radiology 202:697, 1997.

SUGGESTED READINGS

Ackerman DA, Barry JM, Wicklund RA, et al: Analysis of risk factors associated with prostate cancer extension to the surgical margin and pelvic node metastasis at radical prostatectomy, J Urol 150:1845, 1993.
Allen K, Kressel HY, Arger PH, et al: Age related changes of the prostate: evaluation by MR imaging, Am J Roentgenol 152:77, 1989.
Allepuz CA, Sanz Velez JI, Gil Sanz MJ, et al: Seminal vesicle biopsy in prostate cancer staging, J Urol 154:1407, 1995.
Bezzi M, Kressel H, Allen K, et al: Prostatic carcinoma: staging with MR imaging at 1.5 T1, Radiology 169:339, 1988.
Biondetti PR, Lee JKT, Ling D, et al: Clinical stage B prostate carcinoma: staging with MR imaging, Radiology 162(2):325, 1987.
Blair A, and Fraumeni J Jr: Geographic patterns of prostate cancer in the United States, J Natl Cancer Inst 61(6):1379, 1978.
Blute ML: Refining the early detection and staging of prostate cancer, J Urol 154:1401, 1995 (editorial).
Brawer M: How to use prostate-specific antigen in the early detection or screening for prostatic carcinoma, CA Cancer J Clin 45:148, 1995.
Breslow N, Chan C, and Dhom G, et al: Latent carcinoma of prostate at autopsy in seven areas, Int J Cancer 20:680, 1977.
Carrol C, Sommer F, and McNeal J, et al: The abnormal prostate: MR imaging at 1.5 T with histopathologic correlation, Radiology 163:521, 1987.
Carter HB, Brem RF, Tempany CM, et al: Nonpalpable prostate cancer: detection with MR imaging, Radiology 178(2):523, 1991.
Chang P: Evaluating the role of transrectal ultrasonography and magnetic resonance imaging in prostate carcinoma, Radiology 3:687, 1991.
Choyke P: Magnetic resonance imaging of the genitourinary tract, Radiology 4(11):24, 1992.
deSouza NM, Flynn RJ, Coutte GA, et al: Endoscopic laser ablation of the prostate: MR appearances during and after treatment and their relation to clinical outcome, Am J Roentgenol 164:1429, 1995.
Drago J: The role of new modalities in the early detection and diagnosis of prostate cancer, CA Cancer J Clin 39(6):326, 1989.
Emory T, Reinke D, Hill A, et al: Use of CT to reduce understaging in prostatic cancer: comparison with conventional staging techniques, Am J Roentgenol 141:351, 1983.
Friedman A, Seidmon E, Radecki P, et al: Relative merits of MRI, transrectal endosonography and CT in diagnosis and staging of carcinoma of prostate, Urology 31(6):530, 1988.

Fritzche R, and Wilvur, M: The male pelvis, Semin Ultrasound CT MR 10:11, 1989.

Gervasi L, Scardino P, and Mata S: The prognostic significance of the extent of nodal metastases in prostate cancer, J Urol 133(S):203A, 1985.

Gleason D, and Mellinger G: Prediction of prognosis for prostatic adenocarcinoma by combined histological grading and clinical staging, J Urol 111:58, 1974.

Golambu M, Morales P, Al-Askari S, et al: CAT scanning in staging of prostatic cancer, Urology 18:305, 1981.

Harris RD, Schned AR, and Heaney AJ: Staging of prostate cancer with endorectal MR imaging: lessons from a learning curve, Radiographics 15:813, 1995.

Herman S, Friedman A, Radecki P, et al: Incidental prostatic carcinoma detected by MRI and diagnosed by MRI/CT-guided biopsy, Am J Roentgenol 146:351, 1986.

Hinkle GH: Current literature: prostate cancer detection and treatment, New Persp Cancer Diag Manag 2(1):37, 1994.

Hricak H, Dooms G, Jeffrey R, et al: Prostatic carcinoma: staging by clinical assessment, CT, and MR imaging, Radiology 162:331, 1987.

Hricak H, Williams R, Spring D, et al: Anatomy and pathology of the male pelvis by magnetic resonance imaging, Am J Roentgenol 141:1101, 1983.

Hutchison G: Incidence and etiology of prostate cancer, Urology 17(Suppl 3): 4, 1981.

Iversen P, Kjaer L, Thomsen C, et al: Magnetic resonance imaging of the prostate, Scand J Urol Nephrol 104:41, 1987.

Lee J, Heiken J, and Ling D: Magnetic resonance imaging of abdominal and pelvic lymphadenopathy, Radiology 153:181, 1984.

Lee J, and Rholl K: MRI of the bladder and prostate, Am J Roentgenol 147:732, 1986.

Ling D, Tee J, Heiken J, et al: Prostatic carcinoma and benign prostatic hyperplasia: inability of MR imaging to distinguish between the two diseases, Radiology 158:103, 1986.

Lovett K, Rifkin M, and Choi H: MR imaging of noncancerous lesions of the prostate gland, Radiology 177(P):266, 1990.

Lowsley O: Embryology, anatomy, and surgery of the prostate gland, Am J Surg 8:526, 1930.

Marshall V: The relation of the preoperative estimate to the pathological demonstration of the extent of vesical neoplasms, J Urol 68:714, 1952.

Martin J, Hajek P, and Baker L, et al: Inflatable surface coil for MR imaging of the prostate, Radiology 167:268, 1988.

Matthay K: Neuroblastoma: a clinical challenge and biologic puzzle, CA Cancer J Clin 45:179, 1995.

McNeal J: Normal anatomy of the prostate and changes in benign prostatic hypertrophy and carcinoma, Semin Ultrasound CT MR 9(5):329, 1988.

McNeal J: The prostate gland, Monogr Urol 4:3, 1983.

McNeal J: Regional morphology and pathology of the prostate, Am J Clin Pathol 49(3):347, 1968.

McNeal J, Kindrachuk R, Freiha F, et al: Patterns of progression in prostate cancer, Lancet 1:60, 1986.

Mukamel E, Hannah J, Barbaric Z, et al: The value of computerized tomography scan and magnetic resonance imaging in staging prostatic carcinoma: comparison with the clinical and histological staging, J Urol 136:1231, 1986.

Papanicolaou N, Pfister R, Stafford S, et al: Prostatic abscess: imaging with transrectal sonography and MR, Am J Roentgenol 149:981, 1987.

Partin A, Yoo J, Carter H, et al: The use of prostate specific antigen, clinical stage and Gleason score to predict pathological stage in men with localized prostate cancer, J Urol 150:110, 1993.

Petersen R: Urologic pathology. In Peterson R, ed: Urologic pathology, Philadelphia, 1986, Lippincott.

Platt J, Bree R, and Schwab R: The accuracy of CT in the staging of carcinoma of the prostate, Am J Roentgenol 149:315, 1987.

Pontes J, Eisenkraft S, and Wantabe H: Preoperative evaluation of localized prostatic carcinoma by transrectal sonography, J Urol 134:289, 1985.

Poon P, McCallum R, Henkelman M, et al: Magnetic resonance imaging of the prostate, Radiology 154:143, 1985.

Rifkin M: Magnetic resonance imaging of the prostate, Radiol Rep 1(2):126, 1989.

Rifkin M: Ultrasound of the prostate, New York, 1988, Raven Press.

Rifkin M, Dähnert W, and Kurtz A: State of the art: endorectal sonography of the prostate gland [review], Am J Roentgenol 154(4):691, 1990.

Rifkin M, Vinitski S, and Mitchell D: Improving prostate MRI with fat suppression, narrow bandwidth and surface coils, Magn Reson Imaging 7(S):86, 1989.

Salo J, Kivisaari L, Rannikko S, et al: Computerized tomography and transrectal ultrasound in the assessment of local extension of prostatic cancer before radical retropubic prostatectomy, J Urol 137:435, 1987.

Schiebler M, McSherry S, Keefe B, et al: Comparison of the digital rectal examination, endorectal ultrasound, and body coil magnetic resonance imaging in the staging of adenocarcinoma of the prostate, Urol Radiol 13:110, 1991.

Schiebler M, Pollack H, and Tomoszewsky J: High resolution MR imaging of prostatic carcinoma and benign prostatic hypertrophy with histologic correlation, Radiology 172:131, 1989.

Schiebler M, Yankaskas B, Tempany C, et al: MR imaging in adenocarcinoma of the prostate: interobserver variation and efficacy for determining stage C disease, Am J Roentgenol 158:559, 1992.

Schnall M, Bezzi M, Pollack H, et al: Magnetic resonance imaging of the prostate, Magn Reson Quart 6(1):1, 1990.

Silverberg E, and Lubera J: Cancer statistics, 1990, CA Cancer J Clin 40:9, 1990.

Slawin K, Ohori M, Dillioglugil O, et al: Screening for prostate cancer: an analysis of the early experience, CA Cancer J Clin 45(3):134, 1995.

Sommer G, Brosnan T, Cao Q, et al: Noise-reduced prostatic MR imaging, Radiology 169:347, 1988.

Sommer F, Nghiem H, Herfkens R, et al: Gadolinium-enhanced MRI of the abnormal prostate, Magn Reson Imaging 11(7):941, 1993.

Thomas M, Narayan P, and Kurhanewicz J: NMR spectroscopy of normal and malignant prostates in vivo, J Urol 63:469, 1989.

Wachsberg RH, Sebastiano LLS, Sullivan BC, et al: Posterior urethral diverticulum presenting as a midline prostatic cyst: sonographic and MRI appearance, Abdom Imaging 20:70, 1995.

Yatani R, Chigusa I, Akazaki K, et al: Geographic pathology of latent prostatic carcinoma, Int J Cancer 29:611, 1982.

31 Scrotum and Testes

Robert F. Mattrey

 KEY POINTS

- Doppler ultrasound is preferred for the initial evaluation of acute scrotal pain.
- MRI is the most specific imaging method for the differential diagnosis of ischemia, inflammation, and tumor.
- MRI is the best technique for localizing and assessing undescended testes and complications of cryptorchidism.
- High-resolution surface-coil T1- and T2-weighted images are essential.

Sonography is the imaging modality of choice in the assessment of scrotal disease.[11,20,31,42,43] Its success is based on its accuracy in distinguishing intratesticular from extratesticular lesions, low cost, easy accessibility, speed, and lack of ionizing radiation. Color Doppler has added both anatomical and functional details to the evaluation of the testis and its surrounding structures, essentially eliminating the need for nuclear scanning in the setting of acute scrotal pain.* However, high-resolution sonography is limited by its small field of view and lack of specificity in many conditions.

Magnetic resonance imaging (MRI) with high field strengths and surface coils provides high contrast as well as a wide field of view.[3,4,59,63,69] Since the first reports,[3,4] the ability of MRI to characterize scrotal disease has been substantiated with added experience.[14,59,63,69] Many disease processes have characteristic appearances that allow their recognition with sufficient specificity. Although the true sensitivity of MRI has not been substantiated, it is likely equal to or may exceed that of sonography.[69] The ability to recognize each intrascrotal structure because of its signal intensity, appearance, and lo-

cation separate from any other structure; the ability to view the right and left hemiscrotum with the inguinal region; and the high contrast afforded by MRI make this modality less subjective than ultrasound. MRI has changed the sonographic diagnosis of testicular disease from benign to cancerous in 4 of 23 (17%) patients[69] and from cancer to benign disease in nearly 6% of our cases.[64] The efficacy of sonography proved over several years, its unlimited access, and its low cost have hindered the ability to assess MRI's impact on patient care.

IMAGING TECHNIQUE
Patient Positioning and Preparation

The patient is positioned supine and feet first on the scan table, and the scrotum is elevated by a support between the thighs to ensure that both testes are in the same horizontal plane for proper coronal imaging. The penis is angled to the side, and the whole region is draped. A 12.5-cm circular surface coil or substitute, such as a shoulder coil, is centered over the scrotum and placed on a 1-cm stand-off. The coil is positioned so that the bottom of the coil is over the caudal tip of the scrotal sac. The entire area is then wrapped with the 14-inch table strap to minimize patient motion. The isocenter is positioned at midscrotum. In infants, the standard 9-cm circular coil is used in lieu of the 12.5-cm coil.

The air surrounding the scrotum could produce susceptibility artifacts at the edge of the testis. The use of an air-displacing support structure that is of equal magnetic susceptibility to water, such as the Sat Pad (Alliance Pharmaceutical Corp., San Diego) could reduce this artifact.[16]

Pulsing Sequence

Multislice imaging begins with a sagittal localizer using a 20-cm field of view. The center of the field of view is shifted anteriorly by 5 cm to ensure that the scrotum is properly centered.

With the advent of the fast spin-echo technique, we now obtain four sequences in addition to the sagittal localizer: a heavily T1-weighted series (repetition time = 400, echo time = 12, 256 × 128, two excita-

*References 10, 29, 30, 37, 44, 52, 53.

tions) and a fast spin-echo T2-weighted series (repetition time = 3500, echo time = 120, 256 × 192, two excitations, 16 echo train) in the coronal and axial planes. Both sequences are obtained with a field of view of 16 cm and slice thickness of 3 mm with a 1.5-mm interslice gap to ensure proper T2 weighting. The coronal series covers from the posterior aspect of the scrotum to the anterior aspect of the external inguinal ring. The testes should be at the center of the imaging volume for proper prescan optimization; otherwise, the scan will be optimized to tissues other than the testes. The axial series covers the area from the inferior aspect of the scrotal sac to the top of the symphysis pubis, again ensuring that the testes are at the center of the volume. Fat suppression is unnecessary because the scrotum contains little fat. Furthermore, because of magnetic field inhomogeneities, water rather than fat could become suppressed, increasing confusion.

The use of intravenous (IV) MR contrast is occasionally needed, as is discussed later. In general, contrast is reserved for patients with subtle, atypical, or complex findings.

Imaging Planes

The coronal plane is ideal for imaging the scrotum.[3,4] It allows the visualization of all important anatomical structures and optimally demonstrates the epididymis and spermatic cord. It also allows comparison of the right and left hemiscrotal and inguinal regions. Because the coronal plane is parallel to the plane of the surface coil, coronal images are the most helpful, since the signal across the field is homogeneous. The sagittal plane can help clarify anatomical structures; however, it is the author's opinion that it can be deleted to save time. Although the coronal series is sufficient in more than 70% of cases, the axial series clarifies complex findings, allows optimal visualization of the anterior and posterior aspect of the testis and the interface between the body of the epididymis and the testis, and allows for the comparison of right and left structures.

ANATOMY

The normal testis (Figures 31-1 to 31-3) on MR images is a sharply demarcated oval structure of homogeneous signal intensity brighter than water and darker than fat on T1-weighted and hydrogen density–weighted images. The testes become darker than water and brighter than fat on T2-weighted images. The intensity of the testis on T2-weighted images is contrasted with the fluid frequently present between the layers of the tunica vaginalis, allowing the assessment of testicular signal behavior. The testis is completely surrounded by the tunica albuginea, a layer of dense fibrous tissue that is of very low signal on T2-weighted

images. The tunica vaginalis, an extension of the peritoneum, is fused to the tunica albuginea except along the "bare area" of the testis, which becomes highlighted by a hydrocele (Figure 31-3). Along the bare area, the tunica albuginea invaginates the testis to produce the mediastinum testis, through which the testis receives part of its blood supply, and delivers the tubules to the epididymis. The mediastinum is a longitudinal structure 1 to 3 cm in length that is isointense with testis on T1-weighted and darker than testis on T2-weighted images (Figure 31-3). Intrinsic testicular signal, although homogeneous, displays the internal texture outlining the lobules and rete testis (Figures 31-3 and 31-4). Transmediastinal vessels are seen in nearly 50% of normal testes and appear as a major bundle emanating from the superior mediastinum toward the lateral aspect of the upper pole to reach the tunica[51] (Figure 31-21).

The epididymis is inhomogeneous with an intermediate intensity less than that of normal testicular tissue on T2-weighted images. The degree of darkening of the epididymis is variable, but when it is much darker than testis, the possibility of fibrosis from prior infection is raised. The head of the epididymis, lying lateral to the upper pole of the testis, drapes the tunica albuginea (Figures 31-1 and 31-4). The normal epididymal tail, best seen when highlighted by fluid, is smaller than the epididymal head (Figures 31-1, 31-2, and 31-4). The body of the epididymis lies in the bare area alongside the mediastinum testis and is therefore extravaginal in location. It can be easily recognized from testis because it has a darker signal on T2-weighted images and is separated from testicular tissue by the dark band of the tunica albuginea (Figure 31-4).

The outer parietal and inner visceral layers of the tunica vaginalis are frequently separated by a small amount of fluid (Figures 31-1, 31-2, and 31-4). On T2-weighted images and in the presence of hydrocele, the fluid completely surrounds the testes except posteromedially along the bare area, where the testis is attached to the scrotal wall (Figure 31-3). The scrotal sac structures, such as fat and dartos muscle, can at times be seen (Figures 31-1 and 31-2).

The spermatic cord is easily imaged in all cases (Figure 31-1). Tortuous tubular structures of low signal intensity located at the posterosuperior aspect of the scrotal sac represent the pampiniform plexus (Figure 31-17), which can be followed into the inguinal canal. At times, the cremasteric reflex causes foreshortening of the cord, which may give the cord a nodular appearance on coronal sections (Figure 31-1). Smooth, undulating tubular structures similar to testis in signal intensity (Figure 31-4) can at times be seen in the cord or epididymis. These may represent a prominent vas deferens, a serpiginous spermatocele, or a varicocele with slow blood flow. The use of IV contrast would allow the distinction of varicocele from the other two structures.

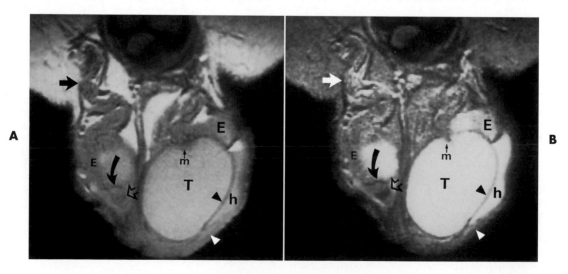

FIGURE 31-1   Normal testes *(T)* and the left mediastinum (*m* in **B**) shown on hydrogen density–weighted **(A)** and T2-weighted **(B)** images in the coronal plane. The accordion-shaped spermatic cord *(thick short arrow)* is seen entering the base of the right hemiscrotum. Note that the small amount of fluid within the tunica vaginalis on the left *(h)* is between the tunica albuginea *(black arrowhead)* and the scrotal wall and outlines the epididymal body (*E* in **A**) and head (*E* in **B**). The epididymal tail is seen on the right *(open arrow)*. The dartos muscle appears as a dark band in the scrotal wall *(white arrowhead)*. (From reference 4.)

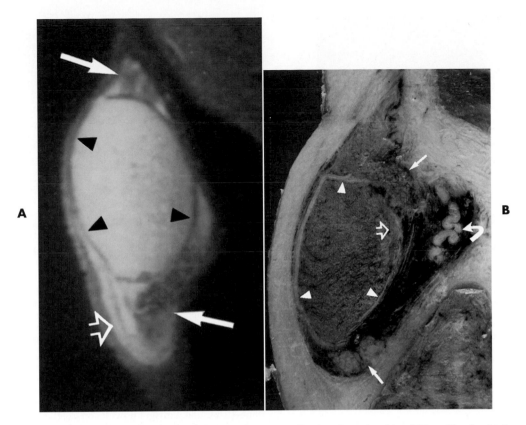

FIGURE 31-2   Normal anatomy. **A,** Clearly delineated tunica albuginea *(arrowheads),* epididymal head and tail *(solid arrows),* and the various layers of the scrotal wall, including the dartos muscle *(open arrow),* on sagittal T2-weighted image. **B,** Cadaveric specimen from a different patient shows similar anatomy. The mediastinum testis *(open arrow)* and the vas deferens *(curved arrow)* can be seen on this particular section of the specimen. (From reference 4.)

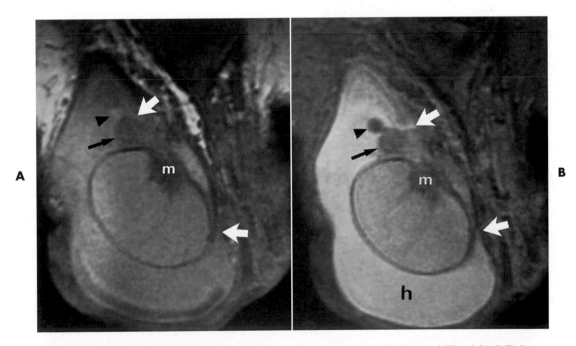

FIGURE 31-3   Acute simple hydrocele is shown on hydrogen density–weighted **(A)** and T2-weighted **(B)** images. The signal of the hydrocele is consistent with water signal (intermediate in **A** and bright in **B**). This sympathetic hydrocele is thought to be caused by torsion of the epididymal appendix *(arrowhead),* shown to be hemorrhagic on MRI (slightly bright in **A** and dark in **B**), and attached to the normal epididymal head *(thin black arrow).* In **B,** the lobular septa can be seen emanating from the mediastinum testis *(m).* Note that the presence of a sizable hydrocele *(h)* demonstrates the "bare area" of the testis, the edges of which are marked by white arrows. (From reference 3.)

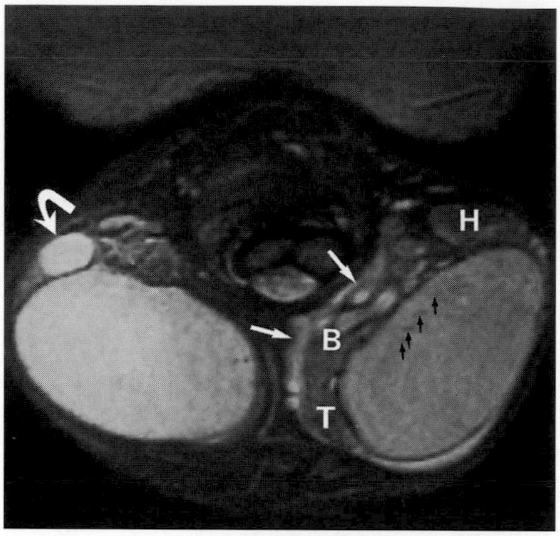

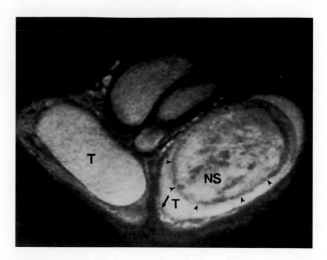

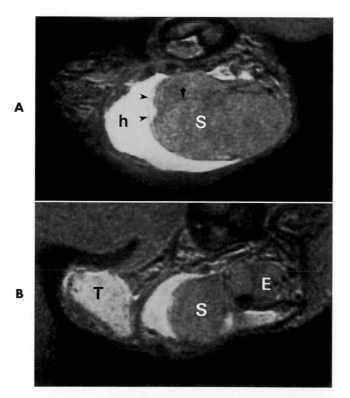

FIGURE 31-4 Dilated ducts (spermatocele) or dilated veins (varicocele) with stagnant blood shown as a prominent serpentine structure *(white arrows)* in the body of the epididymis *(B)* on a coronal T2-weighted image. Its signal was similar to testis on all sequences (not shown). Intravenous contrast could allow this distinction. The entire epididymis, including the head *(H)*, body *(B)*, and tail *(T)*, can be seen. Note the clear delineation of testis from epididymis by the dark tunica albuginea. Small, linear dark signals *(small arrows)* within the testis are interlobular septa converging toward the mediastinum seen on the following slice (not shown). Also note the presence of an epididymal cyst *(curved arrow)* on the right. Because it was dark on the hydrogen density–weighted image (not shown), it behaved similar to water. The difference in right and left testicular signal is caused by coil position. (From reference 49.)

FIGURE 31-5 Left testicular seminoma *(S)* is mildly inhomogeneous on T2-weighted images **(A)** and of markedly lower signal than the remaining normal testicular tissue seen between the tunica albuginea *(arrowheads)* and the tumor margin. A dark band *(arrow)* is a region of cellular condensation and fibrous tissue **(B).** At a more posterior level, at the upper pole of the tesis filled with seminoma *(S)*, epididymal involvement *(E)* is seen. The extratesticular nodules had a similar signal as the intratesticular lesion on all sequences. Note the ipsilateral hydrocele *(h in A)* and the contralateral atrophic testis *(T in B).* (From reference 3.)

FIGURE 31-6 Mixed nonseminomatous tumor *(NS)*, coronal view shows a heterogeneous appearance that reflects the mixed histology, which includes varied mesenchymal elements and blood. Note the normal testicular tissue *(T)* between the tunica albuginea *(arrow)* and a dark band surrounding the tumor *(arrowheads)*, shown pathologically to be a thick, fibrous tumor capsule. The dark regions within the tumor represent islands of hemorrhage and mixed connective tissues.

PATHOLOGY

The homogeneous, relatively high signal intensity of the normal testes on T2-weighted images provides an excellent background for visualizing intratesticular pathology. Except for old blood or epidermoid cysts, all intratesticular pathological conditions have been heterogeneous in signal and generally less intense than normal testicular tissue on T2-weighted images.

The majority of pathological conditions of the scrotum are best visualized on T2-weighted images. T1-weighted images allow for tissue characterization and added specificity. Complete assessment of the scrotum is possible in most cases with coronal sections only. Axial T2-weighted images add confidence, demonstrate to a better advantage small lesions abutting the anterior or posterior surfaces, and help define complex anatomy. The use of IV contrast aids in the assessment of tissue vascularity for greater specificity, but it is infrequently needed.

Neoplasms

General Comments. Testicular neoplasms can be primary or metastatic. Primary cancers can originate from any cell type in normal testes and account for 5000 new cases and 1000 deaths per year in the Unites States.[54] Testicular neoplasms are most frequently detected in people younger than 10 years, between 20 and 40 years, and then older than 60 years of age. They have a peak incidence between the ages of 20 and 34 and are the most common solid tumors in this age group. Primary testicular neoplasms, from the imaging as well as the treatment perspective, are grouped into germ cell and stromal tumors. Germ cell tumors account for 90% to 95% of all primary testicular malignancies, whereas non–germ cell or stromal tumors account for 5% to 10%. Germ cell lesions are in turn grouped into seminomatous and nonseminomatous lesions. Pure seminomas account for nearly 40% of all primary tumors. Spermatocytic seminoma, a subtype accounting for 10% of all detected seminomas, occurs most frequently in people over the age of 50. Nonseminomatous tumors include, in order of occurrence, teratocarcinoma, embryonal cell carcinoma, teratoma, and choriocarcinoma and account for nearly 50% to 55% of all primary testicular neoplasms. Nearly 40% of nonseminomatous tumors are a mixture of two or three cell types. However, since all cell types have a similar prognosis and are treated similarly, the preoperative distinction of the cell type (and whether it is pure or mixed) is not necessary. Seminoma can be mixed with nonseminomatous elements in 10% to 15% of patients, at which time the lesion is regarded and treated as a nonseminomatous tumor. Nonseminomatous lesions have a peak incidence in people in their twenties and early thirties and therefore afflict slightly younger men than seminomatous lesions. Germ cell tumors of yolk sac origin are the predominant lesions of infancy. Testicular lymphoma is the most common neoplasm affecting men older than 50 years of age.[54]

Testicular tumors are bilateral, either at the time of diagnosis or on follow-up, in 1% to 3% of cases.[67] Therefore careful examination of the contralateral testis at the time of diagnosis and close follow-up are mandatory.

Seminomatous and nonseminomatous lesions have different surgical and chemotherapeutic interventions, requiring accurate differentiation of one type from the other. The mode of therapy remains controversial,[54] but a noninvasive approach is favored. Because seminomatous lesions may harbor small islands of nonseminomatous histology in 10% to 15% of cases,[54] treatment is planned after a detailed histological analysis of the resected testis. This is particularly true when there are elevated levels of ß-human chorionic gonadatropin or α-fetoprotein, findings suggesting the presence of nonseminomatous elements.

In this section, the characteristics of each lesion type are presented. Although the preoperative histological diagnosis is less critical for patient management, there are some characteristic findings for seminomatous and nonseminomatous cancers that may allow their specific diagnosis.[34,59,63,69]

Seminomas. Seminomatous lesions are sheets of cells intermixed with fibrous strands or condensations of cells presenting a relatively homogeneous histological pattern. They rarely bleed or necrose centrally. Similarly, the MR appearance of this tumor type is relatively homogeneous. These lesions are rarely visible on T1-weighted images and are consistently of lower signal intensity than normal testicular tissue or hydrocele fluid on T2-weighted images (Figure 31-5). They may contain well-defined regions of low signal intensity, representing the condensation of cells and fibrosis.[34] If there is hemorrhage or necrosis, the affected regions assume a brighter and heterogeneous signal intensity relative to the unaffected portions of the tumor. Therefore the majority of the lesion will have signal behavior typical for seminoma. When metastasis to the epididymis and cord occurs, these structures assume a signal intensity similar to that of the intratesticular mass[3] (Figure 31-5).

A small rim of normal testicular tissue consistently highlights a well-demarcated tumor margin (Figure 31-5). The appearance of the mass in some patients suggests coalescence of multiple nodules. Indeed, when smaller lesions are imaged, "daughter" nodules can be detected (not shown). Although seminomatous lesions have a darker signal than testis, similar to infection or infarction, they have characteristic features that allow the clinician to identify them.

Nonseminomatous Tumors. Nonseminomatous lesions have a heterogeneous histology because of their mixed cellularity; their attempt at tubular formation; the mixed mesenchymal elements, such as bone, cartilage, and muscle, that may be contained in teratomatous lesions; and their high propensity for invading vessels, causing internal hemorrhage and necrosis. The MR appearance is markedly heterogeneous in signal, which represents the most distinctive feature when compared with seminomatous lesions. Over the background that is typically isointense or slightly brighter than normal testis on T2-weighted images, multiple areas of high and low signal intensity on T1- and T2-weighted images are seen representing hemorrhage of various ages or islands of muscle or cartilage within the mass (Figure 31-6). A band of low signal intensity circumscribing the mass in most cases represents the fibrous tumor capsule, a finding also typical for these lesions[34] (Figure 31-6). The remaining normal testicular tissue is easily differentiated from tumor by its homogeneous and characteristic intensity, even when the lesion is very large. Although some lesions may have a dominant signal intensity lower than that of testis, their heterogeneity and visibility on the T1-weighted images distinguish them from seminomatous lesions.

In a study assessing the ability of MRI to distinguish seminomatous from nonseminomatous lesions prospectively,[34] we found that of the 12 patients with sizable lesions that could be characterized, MRI allowed the correct classification of 11 lesions. The thirteenth lesion, shown in Figure 31-7, was too small to characterize. The degree of heterogeneity of signals was the most discriminating factor. A review of the MR literature[3,59,63,69] reveals that tumor signals in figures illustrating tumors match this description, suggesting that MRI may indeed be able to differentiate these two tumor types. Although sonography demonstrates

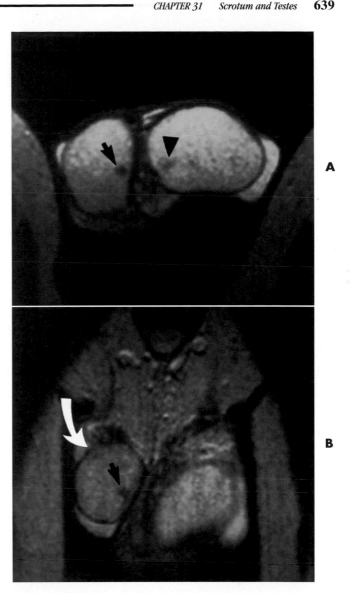

FIGURE 31-7   Embryonal cell tumor with hemorrhage at pathology. Transaxial **(A)** and coronal **(B)** T2-weighted images show a 3-mm focus (*black arrow* in **A** and **B**) in the right testis. The left (*arrowhead* in **A**) and right mediastinum testis (*curved arrow* in **B**) can also be seen. This lesion was too small to allow proper characterization. (From reference 48.)

characteristic echographic findings for seminomatous and nonseminomatous lesions, there is significant overlap in their sonographic appearance.[61]

Stromal Tumors. Stromal tumors occur in persons between 20 and 60 years of age and account for nearly 5% of all primary testicular tumors. They are well circumscribed and rarely exhibit hemorrhage or necrosis. Because these lesions generally produce hormones, prepubertal boys can experience precocious puberty and adults can have gynecomastia. The cell types include Leydig's and Sertoli's cells. These lesions are malignant in 10% of cases. Malignancy is suspected when lesions are large, necrotic, or infiltrative or when they invade blood vessels, but it is clearly established when there are metastases. Given the homogeneous histology and lack of hemorrhage and necrosis, one could hypothesize that their appearance on MRI would mimic seminomatous lesions.[3,69] However, when these tumors are malignant, the appearance of hemorrhage and necrosis mimics that of nonseminomatous lesions. The experience with these lesions is too limited to test this hypothesis.

Two published, proven cases of Leydig's cell tumor show the mass to be of moderately darker signal intensity than normal testis on T2-weighted images.[3,69] One lesion was small, well circumscribed, and ho-

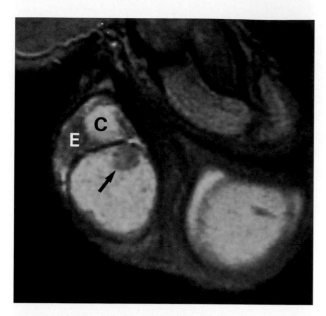

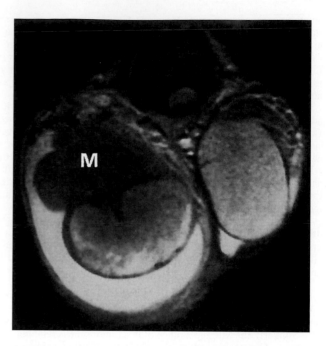

FIGURE 31-8   Leydig's cell tumor *(arrow)* is better seen on the T2-weighted image than the hydrogen density–weighted image (not shown). Mildly inhomogeneous, well-marginated tumor was histologically proved to be Leydig's cell tumor. An epididymal cyst *(C)* within the normal epididymal head *(E)* has MR characteristics similar to water. (From reference 3.)

FIGURE 31-9   Scrotal lymphoma involving the right epididymis and testis is shown on a T2-weighted image. The center of the mass *(M)* is in the epididymis and infiltrates the testis from the hilum. The mass, located along the bare area of the testis, rotated the testis into a horizontal position. The mass within the testis is patchy, and its margins with normal testicular tissue generally are poorly defined. There are mild hypervascularity and a moderate ipsilateral hydrocele. (From reference 49.)

mogeneous[3] (Figure 31-8), and the other totally infiltrated the testis on MRI in a prepubertal boy, causing sonography to miss the lesion.[69]

Other Tumors.   Lymphomatous or leukemic infiltration of the testis is common. Lymphoma accounts for nearly 5% of all testicular neoplasms.[54] It may be primary in the testis, the manifestation of occult disease located elsewhere, or a late manifestation of disseminated disease. The majority of these lesions are infiltrative and may extend into or originate in the epididymis (Figure 31-9). The major cell type is histiocytic lymphoma.

The testis is the prime site of relapse of leukemia in children. A blood-testis barrier similar to the blood-brain barrier exists and limits the chemotherapeutic agent's access to and therefore ability to eradicate disease in the testes. Testicular evaluation and biopsy are commonly performed at the end of chemotherapy to exclude testicular involvement. Although ultrasound can detect leukemic infiltration,[47] it has poor sensitivity.[69] The sensitivity of MRI in this setting has not been determined; however, MRI was more sensitive than sonography in a limited series in which leukemic infiltrates affected the entire testis.[69]

Metastic disease to the testes is rare. The malignancies that can affect the testes are prostate, kidney, and lung cancer and melanoma.

Benign Testicular Lesions

Teratomas.   Although benign testicular tumors are relatively uncommon, intratesticular teratoma is the most common of the benign lesions.[38,57] The sonographic and MR appearance of teratoma would be similar to that of teratocarcinoma, so differentiation may be difficult.

Epidermoid Cysts.   Epidermoid inclusion cysts are benign solitary tumors of germ cell origin accounting for approximately 1% of all testicular tumors.[7,65] They are limited by a fibrous capsule with an epithelial lining. The center contains keratin without teratomatous elements. Epidermoid cysts are typically intratesticular but may be extratesticular. One reported case imaged by MR showed a bull's eye appearance in the testis.[8] We have imaged four cases using MRI, all of which displayed similar findings. The cysts were nearly isointense with testis on all pulsing sequences, with a tendency to be slightly darker on T1-weighted and slightly brighter on T2-weighted images. A low–signal

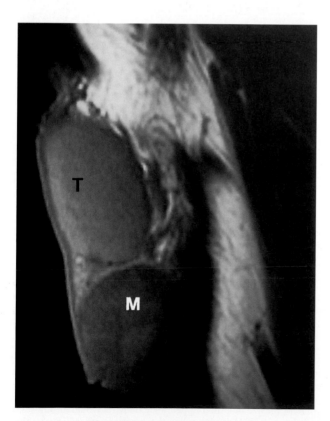

FIGURE 31-10   Extratesticular epidermoid cyst diagnosed at surgery. Sagittal hydrogen density–weighted image through the hemiscrotum shows a spherical extratesticular mass *(M)* inferior to the normal testis *(T)*. This mass, which is slightly darker than testis on hydrogen density–weighted images, was isointense with testis on T2-weighted images (not shown). When IV contrast was given, the mass did not enhance, increasing image contrast relative to the intensely enhanced normal testis (not shown). (From reference 49.)

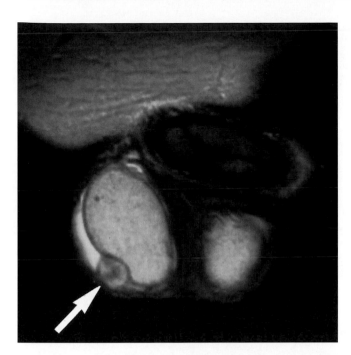

FIGURE 31-11   Adenomatoid tumor *(arrow),* definitively diagnosed at surgery, has signal similar to testis on a T2-weighted image. Its signal was also similar to testis on hydrogen density–weighted images (not shown). Note its extratesticular location as it deviates the tunica albuginea medially. Indentation of the testis suggested that the lesion was between the layers of the tunica albuginea and the tunica vaginalis, which is where it was found at surgery. (From reference 49.)

intensity fibrotic wall was observed on the T2-weighted images in all cases. As expected, the cysts failed to enhance after IV contrast (Figure 31-10). Because normal testicular tissue enhances significantly, the postcontrast images increase not only the conspicuity but also the specificity of these lesions.

Adenomatoid Tumors. Adenomatoid tumors, benign lesions characteristic of the genital tract, consist of fibrous stroma and epithelial cells. These lesions are benign and usually occur in the epididymis but may rarely occur in the testis. We have imaged two such tumors; one was definitively diagnosed at surgery (Figure 31-11). Dependent on the degree of fibrosis, their signal may vary from being similar to testis to darker than testis.

Cysts. Since the advent of high-resolution sonography, simple intratesticular cysts can be detected on 8% to 10% of sonograms.[22, 27,45] Most are 2 to 18 mm and are solitary. They can be intratesticular or tunical. Intratesticular cysts are nonpalpable and are incidental.[38,57] They can occur anywhere within the testis and likely originate from the rete testis, since their histology is similar to that of the rete testis.[70] Another hypothesis includes degeneration after trauma or inflammation.[27] Tunical cysts are palpable and small and are usually detected in middle-aged men. The etiology of these lesions was considered to be posttraumatic or inflammatory degeneration[1]; however, evidence suggests that they may be from an embryological remnant of mesothelial rest or from efferent ductules.[50] MRI displays characteristic findings for cysts. Although they are well depicted when they assume water signal (darker than testis on T1-weighted and brighter than testis on T2-weighted images), they can be isointense with testis, requiring gadolinium diethylene-triamine-pentaacetic acid (Gd-DTPA) to increase their conspicuity.[68]

Dilated Seminiferous Tubules. Dilated seminiferous tubules have been recognized and described on both sonography and MRI.[9,68,73] The findings are somewhat characteristic on sonography, potentially allowing a specific diagnosis to be made to obviate the need for surgery. Among three publications, 48 patients were reported, all of whom had similar sonographic appearances.[9,68,73] The intratesticular process was frequently bilateral, was associated with large ipsilateral spermatoceles, was centered at the mediastinum testis, and was contiguous with the

body of the epididymis. The area of involvement appeared hypoechoic, with a coarse echotexture as a result of multitudes of small reflectors caused by the dilated tubules. Dilated seminiferous tubules may also be associated with mediastinal cysts (Figure 31-12). When this constellation of findings is encountered sonographically, there is no need for further workup; however, short of that, we recommend the use of MRI to confirm the diagnosis. On MRI the findings are specific for this entity and distinguishable from those of neoplastic lesions. The mass of ectatic tubules at the mediastinum is homogeneous and of lower signal intensity than testis on T1-weighted images, is isointense with testis on T2-weighted images, and is identical to the mass of the ipsilateral spermatoceles on all sequences (Figure 31-12). The MR appearance of dilated tubules is different from that of seminomatous tumors in that the latter are typically isointense with testis on T1-weighted and darker than testis on T2-weighted images.[3,34] Nonseminomatous lesions are also different because they are heterogeneous in signal intensity on all pulse sequences, especially on T2-weighted images.[3,34] Because the tubules do not enhance with Gd, their conspicuity and tubular pattern become apparent after contrast administration (Figure 31-12).

Intratesticular Varicoceles. An intratesticular varicocele, which also occurs in the mediastinum testis, may be indistinguishable on gray scale from the dilated seminiferous tubules. If color is visible on Doppler sonography,[74] the distinction is easy. MRI should also allow this distinction, although there have been no reports of such distinction, because of the characteristic MR appearance of flowing blood and because of the fact that slowly flowing or static blood, unlike seminiferous tubules, enhances markedly with IV contrast agents.

Microlithiasis. Testicular microlithiasis is bilateral and is caused by tiny (<2-mm) concentric calcifications within the seminiferous tubules throughout both testes. It is typically incidental to the primary cause that brought the patient to medical attention. It is believed that these concretions form from degenerated tubular epithelial cells. Collagenous lamellae form and offer a nidus for dystrophic calcification. Although an exact cause is not known, diffuse microlithiasis is more frequent in cryptorchidism (delayed testicular descent), a variety of genetic conditions, and pulmonary alveolar microlithiasis. Cancer and infertility have been associated with this condition, but these may be the sequelae of the underlying disorder.[24,33,66]

In our experience, the MR appearance of the testis with microlithiasis has been diffuse and shows poorly demarcated regions of signal loss on T2-weighted images. The tiny calcific regions depicted on sonography were not seen on MRI, either because of the lesser spatial resolution of MRI or more likely because of the presence of mobile protons within these concretions.

Inflammation

Epididymitis. Epididymitis is the most common intrascrotal infection. It may be diffuse or focal and is frequently secondary to prostatitis. Most cases of epididymitis are treated conservatively. Surgery is reserved for complications, such as abscess formation. Therefore diagnostic follow-up in patients with poor response to therapy is warranted.

Patients with clinical evidence of acute epididymitis consistently show epididymal enlargement (Figure 31-13). The epididymis, which is normally of lower signal intensity than the testis on T2-weighted images, maintains a higher signal intensity that can be equal to that of testis. In chronic epididymitis, the epididymis is enlarged in a focal or diffuse manner (Figure 31-14) and assumes a darker signal intensity than normal testis on T2-weighted images. In the setting of chronic epididymitis, acute exacerbation may not affect signal intensity (Figure 31-14).

Acute epididymitis is associated with hypervascularity and thickening and swelling of the spermatic cord, increasing its signal on T2-weighted images (Figures 31-13 and 31-15). Hypervascularity is seen as multiple serpiginous vessels with signal void caused by high flow. This is in contradistinction to normal vessels, which are usually thinner, are less abundant, and lack flow void (Figures 31-1 and 31-4). Hypervascularity of the testis associated with epididymitis has also been observed in some patients (Figure 31-13). Scrotal skin thickening and swelling can be easily seen and were detected in most but not all pa-

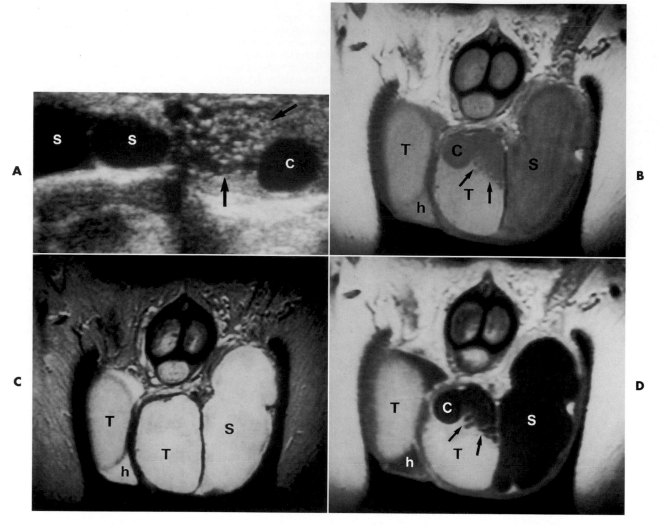

FIGURE 31-12   Spermatocele in a 57-year-old man with an enlarging, symptomatic, left-sided mass. A longitudinal sonogram through the left hemiscrotum **(A)** performed before elective spermatocelectomy shows several locules of a large multilocular spermatocele *(S)*. A mediastinal lesion *(arrows)* has a coarse echotexture, with multiple contiguous tiny cysts and a 1.5-cm intratesticular cyst *(C)*. The mediastinal lesion had no flow on color Doppler (not shown). Hydrogen density–weighted **(B)** and T2-weighted **(C)** coronal MR images show the large spermatocele *(S)*, intratesticular cyst *(C)*, and mediastinal lesion *(arrows)* to be homogeneous and hypointense to testicular parenchyma *(T)* in **B,** becoming isointense with and difficult to distinguish from testis in **C.** Note the small hydrocele *(h)* in the right hemiscrotum. After the infusion of 0.1 mM of Gd-DTPA **(D)** the testes *(T)* enhance markedly, increasing contrast among them and the spermatocele *(S)*, the intratesticular cyst *(C)*, the mediastinal seminiferous tubule ectasia *(arrows)*, and the hydrocele *(h)*. Because of the increased contrast, the recognition of tubular structures at the margin between the abnormal mediastinum and the testis becomes more apparent *(arrows)*. (From reference 68.)

FIGURE 31-13   Acute epididymitis shown on a T2-weighted image in the coronal plane. The testis *(T)* has a slightly lower signal intensity than on the contralateral side and is hypervascular *(arrowheads)*. The epididymis *(E)* is enlarged and assumes a higher signal intensity on T2-weighted images than is normally observed. Note the hypervascularity in the pampiniform plexus *(arrow)*, which is typical of this condition. (From reference 71.)

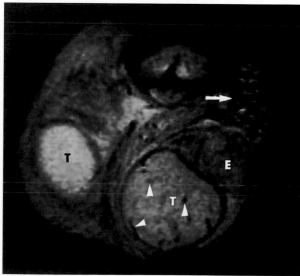

tients (Figure 31-15); however, these findings are not specific to infection. Sympathetic hydrocele was present in most patients and assumed a signal intensity identical to that of water (Figure 31-14). Extensive inguinal adenopathy frequently occurs in these patients (Figure 31-15) but is a nonspecific finding, since it is frequently present in patients with a variety of conditions.

Orchitis.   Orchitis is often the sequela of epididymitis. Pure orchitis without epididymitis suggests a viral or systemic origin. When orchitis accompanies epididymitis, the treatment is extended over a longer time. Orchitis, even when appropriately treated, can develop into an abscess requiring surgical intervention (Figure 31-15). Therefore, when a focus of orchitis is found, follow-up is necessary to ensure its resolution.

Tuberculous orchitis is usually associated with tuberculous epididymitis and typically occurs in patients with known disease. Epididymal changes on MRI are less severe than those seen with bacterial epididymitis, and the degree of hypervascularity is less prominent. Orchitis causes patchy, poorly marginated areas of slightly lower signal than testis (Figure 31-16). In one patient with surgically proven chronic tuberculous orchitis, the testis was diffusely inhomogeneous with low signal intensity on T2-weighted images without mass effect (Figure 31-17).

Trauma

Surgical intervention in scrotal trauma is generally reserved for patients with disruption of the tunica albuginea or patients in whom the intratesticular hematoma is extensive. MRI is well suited to assess both the integrity of the tunica and the degree of intratesticular hematoma.

Intratesticular hematoma is inhomogeneous with high– and low–signal intensity regions compared with normal testicular tissue on both T1-weighted and T2-weighted images (Figure 31-18). Hematocele frequently accompanies trauma and assumes a signal intensity commensurate with the duration since the hemorrhage occurred. Intratesticular trauma, particularly when old, causes more linear than spherical changes, decreasing the chance that it will be confused with mass lesions.

Although clinical and scrotal changes with trauma differ from those of tumors, an underlying tumor, particularly a nonseminomatous lesion, could be masked by the intratesticular hemorrhage. Therefore if the intratesticular change is greater than expected for the degree of trauma that occurred, a follow-up may be warranted to exclude cancer.

Torsion

Intravaginal Spermatic Cord Torsion.   The testis, like other abdominal organs, is retroperitoneal. When descended into the scrotum, the testis is accompanied by a peritoneal reflection, the vaginal process, that forms the tunica vaginalis. This membrane invests the entire contour of the testis except for a strip that extends from the upper to the lower pole, leaving the region of the mediastinum testis, called the *bare area,* uncovered (Figure 31-3). The transverse dimension of the bare area is variable but typically extends for at least one third of the perimeter of the testis (Figure 31-14). This bare area not only serves as a passage for support structures but more important, anchors the testis to the posteromedial scrotal wall. The surface area of this attachment can be variable, depending on the degree the tunica vaginalis invests the testis. The tunica can, however, undermine the support structures and epididymis to a degree that only a thin stalk remains. This anomalous condition, called the *bell-clapper deformity,* predisposes the affected testis to twisting and strangulation. The deformity affects both testes in a large number of patients with torsion, since subsequent contralateral torsion occurs in as many as 40% of patients if the condition is not corrected.[24]

Spermatic cord torsion typically occurs in people in their teens and twenties and affects 1 in 4000 patients younger than 25 years of age.[24] The classic presentation is waking up with testicular pain that radiates to the abdomen, groin, or both structures and that gradually worsens. Torsion may, however, present with an acute onset of pain that can be so severe that it causes nausea and vomiting.[17] The affected hemiscrotum appears indurated, enlarged, and tender, mimicking epididymitis and leading to clinical misdiagnosis in a large number of cases. If torsion is suspected, immediate surgery is required, since salvage of testicular function decreases with time. Nearly all testes can be salvaged if isch-

emic for 5 hours or less, but the salvage rate decreases to 20% if surgery is done at or beyond 12 hours.[32] When the torsion comes to medical attention in the subacute phase (24 hours or later), surgery is still required to remove the torsed testis, control pain, and fix the contralateral testis to the scrotum.

When the testis rotates on its stalk, the veins become occluded and the testis swells. When intratesticular pressure exceeds arterial pressure, blood flow ceases and the testis necroses. Acute torsion can be adequately diagnosed with color Doppler. MR experience has been limited to subacute torsion (>24 hours) in which several characteristic findings have been observed, three of which are specific, allowing for 100% accuracy.[71]

The first finding is the appearance of the point of twist, which is usually located near the posterosuperior aspect of the scrotum. It appears very dark on both T1- and T2-weighted images, presumably because the water is being squeezed out of the tissues (Figures 31-19 and 31-20). From this dark point (point of twist) emanates several curvilinear dark lines, presumably representing the spiraling facial planes resembling a whirlpool, which is best demonstrated when imaged perpendicular to its axis (Figures 31-19 to 31-21). The whirlpool sign was seen in three of six cases with torsion.[71] In an experiment conducted in rats with surgically induced unilateral torsion, the whirlpool sign was the single most accurate finding, allowing the recognition of torsion in all torsed testes from sham controls.[39] In the rat study, the whirlpool sign disappeared 2 weeks after torsion as a result of necrosis and resorption of tissues.[39]

The second finding is the appearance of the testis and epididymis. In all cases, the epididymis was markedly thickened with areas of swelling and subacute hemorrhage (intermediate signal intensity on hydrogen density–weighted images and darker signal intensity on T2-weighted images [Figures 31-19 and 31-20]). The epididymis was in an abnormal position in most patients (superoanterior and transverse orientation rather than posteromedial and longitudinal orientation [Figure 31-19]). The testis in the subacute phase (>5 days) was smaller than the contralateral testis. Its signal was diminished and inhomogeneous, with linear bands of slightly diminished signals separated by thin lines of increased signal emanating from the mediastinum testis (Figures 31-19 and 31-20). A finding seen in some cases was thickening of the tunica albuginea, possibly related to loss of testicular volume in the subacute setting. When imaged beyond 3 weeks after the episode, the loss of testicular volume and tunical thickening become striking (Figure 31-21). The entire testis becomes dark on T2-weighted images without any residual normal tissue (Figure 31-21). The combination of tunical thickening, loss of testicular volume, and loss of signal of the entire testis is characteristic of old torsion.

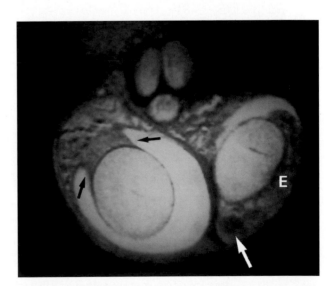

FIGURE 31-14   Diffuse chronic epididymitis involving the entire epididymis on the left and shown in the coronal plane on a T2-weighted image. Note the diffuse enlargement of the entire epididymis *(E)* with possible hemorrhage in the tail *(white arrow).* Mild ipsilateral and moderate contralateral hydroceles are present. The right hydrocele outlines the bare area *(black arrows)* in its transverse direction. (From reference 49.)

The third finding is the appearance of the proximal cord, which was thickened in all cases. All cords had absent or diminished vascularity (Figures 31-19 and 31-20). This is in contradistinction to the hypervascular cord associated with epididymitis (Figures 31-13 and 31-15). It is the discrepancy between the severe epididymal changes and the lack of hypervascularity that is so striking in torsion.

Another helpful finding is a hematocele, which may be seen in torsion (Figures 31-19 and 31-20), in lieu of a hydrocele, which accompanies epididymitis. Furthermore, large hydroceles could demonstrate the bell-clapper deformity or the testicular bare area, allowing the diagnosis of testicular torsion.

With the high competition for MR time and limited access, MRI is not advocated in the acute setting, in which delay in surgery is not appropriate. In this setting, color Doppler has replaced the classic combination of sonography and scintigraphy for the diagnosis of torsion.[53,55] MRI may be helpful in the subacute setting or in missed torsion, when sonography could be equivocal.

Extravaginal Torsion. Extravaginal torsion is a spontaneous event that occurs perinatally during testicular descent and involves the testis, its support structures, and the vaginal process.[24] The torsed vaginal process in the inguinal or spermatic canal can mimic strangulated intestinal hernia. Although the clinical presentation is clear in many cases, at times imaging is required to confirm the diagnosis. This condition generally is not treated surgically, since it is discovered too late to preserve testicular function and is not associated with a developmental anomaly, such as the bell-clapper deformity, which mandates contralateral orchiopexy.[24] Patients are usually monitored for 4 to 6 months until the testis is no longer palpable. If the testis does not regress, imaging is performed to exclude tumor.

Old extravaginal torsion is diagnosed when the testes are small, are dark, and are associated with a thickened tunica albuginea (Figure 31-22), similar to changes seen in chronic torsion in adults (Figure 31-21). As in the adult, the entire testis is dark, without any spared areas.

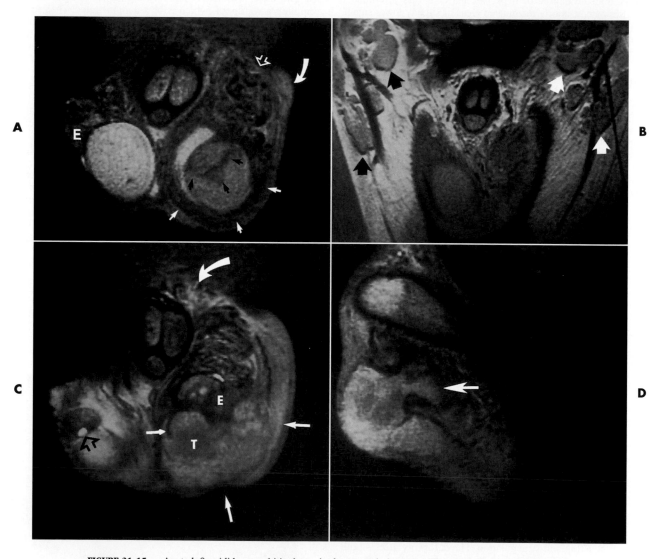

FIGURE 31-15   Acute left epididymoorchitis shown in the coronal plane on a T2-weighted image **(A).** Note the diffuse loss of signal of the affected testis, hypervascular cord, and pampiniform plexus *(open arrow)* at the base of the scrotum; associated skin thickening, including that at the scrotal septum *(white arrows)*; and edema *(curved arrow).* The focus of orchitis *(black arrows)* could be confused with tumor at first, but the associated diffuse loss of testicular signal and the changes in the scrotal wall and cord, in conjunction with the clinical history, should eliminate such confusion. Note the associated bilateral inguinal adenopathy *(arrows)* on a hydrogen density–weighted image **(B)** obtained a few levels posterior to **A.** T2-weighted image **(C)** obtained 10 days after **A** at nearly the same level shows complete destruction of the testis *(T)* and loss of intrascrotal anatomical detail despite antibiotic therapy. Note the cephalic extension of scrotal wall involvement and the spread of edema to the base of the penis *(curved arrow)* compared with **A.** At this time, the changes were due to an epididymal abscess *(arrow),* shown on a T2-weighted sagittal scan **(D)** that involved the testis and pointed along the anterior scrotal wall. There is also a small hemorrhagic cyst *(open arrow)* in the right epididymis **(C).** This cyst was bright on a hydrogen density–weighted image (not shown). *E,* Epididymis. (From reference 3.)

Torsion of Testicular and Epididymal Appendixes. Testicular appendixes are common and represent vestigial remnants of the degenerating embryological müllerian and wolffian ducts. Appendix testis and appendix epididymis were present in 92% and 34% of men at autopsy, respectively.[60] There are four types of appendages[60]: appendix testis, appendix epididymis, paradidymis, and superior and inferior vas aberrans. The appendix testis is located near the upper pole of the testis, outside the tunica albuginea of the normal testis, and has its own tunical covering. The appendix epididymis is attached along the cranial aspect of the epididymis.

Appendix torsion is a common cause of acute painful scrotal swelling in pubescent and adolescent boys and often presents with clinical features similar to those of acute spermatic cord torsion and epididymitis (Figure 31-23). The early diagnosis of a torsed appendage is crucial, since its management is conservative. In a review of 171 patients with acute scrotal pain in whom exploratory surgery was performed, spermatic cord torsion and torsion of an appendage accounted for 89% of cases.[6] Appendix torsion was more frequent than spermatic cord torsion in boys younger than 12 years of age, causing unnecessary exploratory surgery of the scrotum twice as often as in adolescents or adults. Because unnecessary surgery was done in 66% of boys, the authors felt that the delay associated with obtaining an imaging study is warranted.[6]

Although ultrasonography can exclude testicular torsion, the diagnosis of torsed testicular appendage is more difficult, causing nonspecific findings that may be difficult to differentiate from those of epididymoorchitis.[2]

MRI shows the attached mass, containing blood of variable degrees of degradation, which may be accompanied by a hydrocele and inflammation of the epididymis (Figure 31-3). In this setting, MRI can exclude with confidence testicular torsion, infection, or hemorrhage within a tumor, the three clinical conditions that can present with similar signs and symptoms.

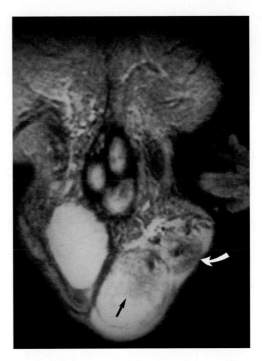

FIGURE 31-16   Acute tuberculous epididymoorchitis involving the upper pole of the left testis *(arrow)* and epididymal head *(curved arrow)* shown in the coronal plane on a T2-weighted image. Note the patchy involvement of the testis, which was seen only on T2-weighted images, and the enlarged epididymis that failed to darken on this T2-weighted image. Note the mild degree of hypervascularity, suggesting subacute inflammation. (From reference 49.)

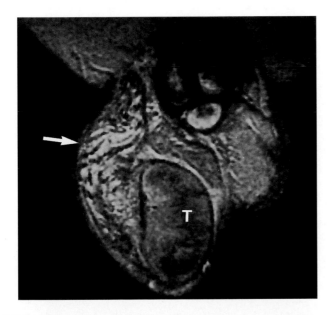

FIGURE 31-17   Chronic tuberculous orchitis shown in the coronal plane on a T2-weighted image. Note the diffuse poorly defined process involving the entire testis *(T)*, which was poorly seen on hydrogen density–weighted images (not shown). Note the prominent pampiniform plexus at the base of the scrotum *(arrow)* compatible with varicocele. The left testis had been removed because of a tuberculous infection. (From reference 3.)

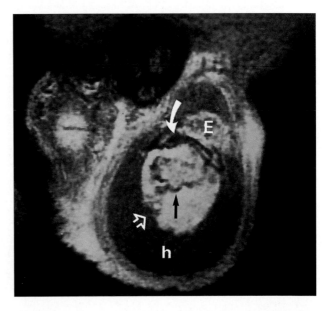

FIGURE 31-18   Trauma, 3 days old, is shown in the coronal plane on a T2-weighted image. The hematoma outlining the tunica albuginea along the upper pole of the testis is very dark *(curved arrow)* and the intratesticular hematoma, although darker than testis, is brighter than the upper pole collection *(arrow)*. The reason for the discrepancy of signals is unclear. The central hemorrhage is incompletely surrounded by a dark band. The tunica is interrupted along the medial lower pole *(open arrow)*. The tunical fluid, a hematocele *(h)*, has signals indicating subacute hemorrhage (intermediate on hydrogen density–weighted images (not shown) and dark on T2-weighted images. The epididymis *(E)* is also enlarged, swollen, and inhomogeneous. (From reference 3.)

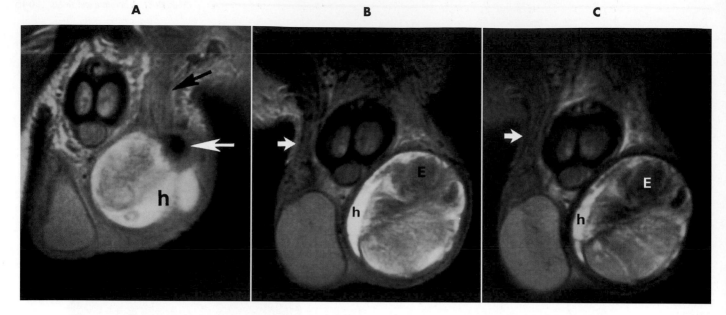

FIGURE 31-19   Torsion, 5 days old, shown on hydrogen density–weighted coronal images (**A** and **B**) and T2-weighted coronal image (**C**) that is the second echo of **B**. This case demonstrates the constellation of findings seen in torsion: the torsion knot (*white arrow* in **A**), a dark region that represents the point of twist and that is hypothesized to be caused by the wringing of water from the cord at the point of twist; a whirlpool pattern (not shown); the swollen hypovascular cord (*black arrow* in **A**) compared with the normal contralateral cord seen in **B** and **C** (*white arrow*); the bell clapper outlined by a hematocele (not shown); the hematocele *(h)* seen as bright fluid in **A**, **B**, and **C**; the enlarged hemorrhagic epididymis *(E)* seen in **B** and **C**; the superior and transverse position of the epididymis seen in **B** and **C**; and the testis with overall signal loss seen in **B**. Note that the intratesticular changes are oriented in the direction of the interlobular septa, emanating from the region of the mediastinum (*arrow* in **B**). (From reference 71.)

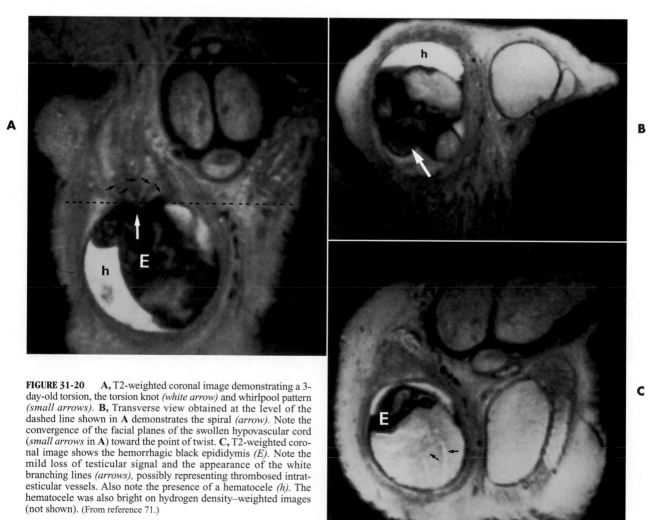

FIGURE 31-20   **A,** T2-weighted coronal image demonstrating a 3-day-old torsion, the torsion knot (*white arrow*) and whirlpool pattern (*small arrows*). **B,** Transverse view obtained at the level of the dashed line shown in **A** demonstrates the spiral *(arrow)*. Note the convergence of the facial planes of the swollen hypovascular cord (*small arrows* in **A**) toward the point of twist. **C,** T2-weighted coronal image shows the hemorrhagic black epididymis *(E)*. Note the mild loss of testicular signal and the appearance of the white branching lines *(arrows),* possibly representing thrombosed intratesticular vessels. Also note the presence of a hematocele *(h)*. The hematocele was also bright on hydrogen density–weighted images (not shown). (From reference 71.)

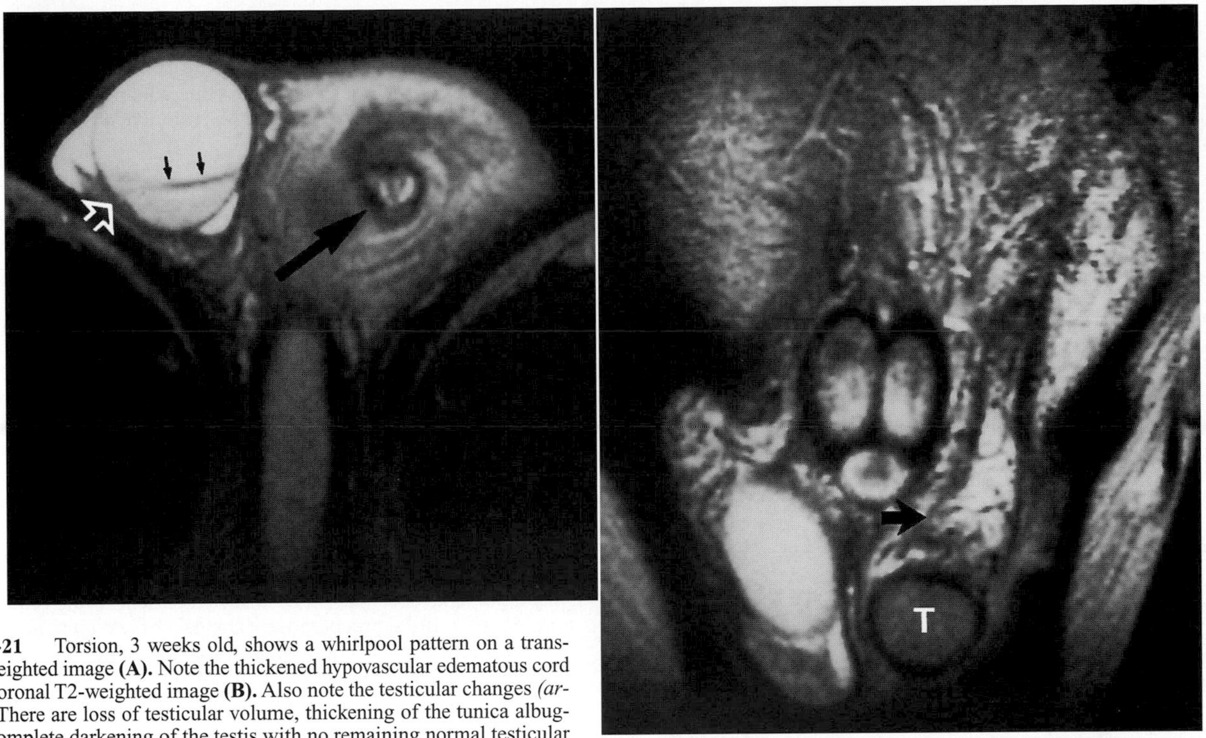

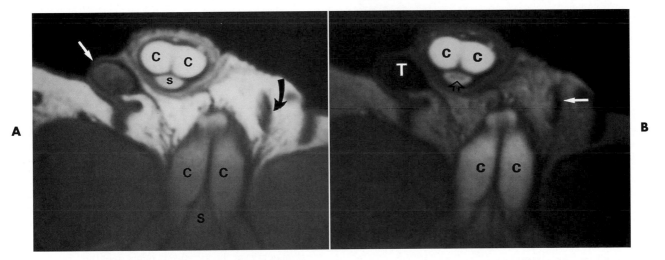

FIGURE 31-21   Torsion, 3 weeks old, shows a whirlpool pattern on a transverse T2-weighted image **(A)**. Note the thickened hypovascular edematous cord seen on a coronal T2-weighted image **(B)**. Also note the testicular changes *(arrow)* in **B**. There are loss of testicular volume, thickening of the tunica albuginea, and complete darkening of the testis with no remaining normal testicular tissue. A dark line *(small arrows)* emanating from the mediastinum *(open arrow)* of the normal contralateral testis in **A** and reaching the tunica albuginea is a vascular structure seen in some normal testes. (From reference 71.)

FIGURE 31-22   Neonatal extravaginal torsion in a 6-month-old infant. Axial hydrogen density–weighted **(A)** and T2-weighted **(B)** images at the level of the affected testis *(arrow)*. Note the loss of testicular volume, the thickened tunica albuginea, and the complete darkening of the testis with no remaining normal testicular tissue similar to the testis seen in Figure 29-21, *B*. Also note that the testis is located in the spermatic canal at the level of the normal contralateral cord *(curved arrow)*. Also well seen is the penile anatomy. The corpora cavernosa *(C)* and spongiosa *(S)* are bright on both images and are surrounded by the tunica albuginea of the penis. The urethra is better seen in **B** *(open arrow)*. The weaker signal of the corpora at the base of the penis is due to increased distance from the surface coil. (From reference 49.)

Ischemia and Infarction

Ischemia and partial infarction can result from intermittent torsion, trauma, infection, embolization, or vasculitis. Acute infarction will likely present as hemorrhage or focal signal loss on T2-weighted images, whereas old infarction will appear as a scar that typically reaches the tunica and deforms the shape of the testicle, assuming a dark, sharply demarcated band on T2-weighted sequences. The specific appearance and distribution depend on the cause of the infarction. Whereas vasculitis typically produces microinfarcts that are diffusely distributed,[28] trauma and infection are more focal.

Ischemic change is more difficult to diagnose, since no definitive study has addressed this process. Changes presumed to represent ischemic injury have been observed in several patients with testicular pain. Sonography has shown hypoechoic bands alternating with normal testicular echogenicity, traversing the testis from the mediastinum to the tunica. On MRI the testis has appeared patchy on T2-weighted images, at times with alternating bands of low and normal signal intensity that follow the rete testis. When IV contrast was given, the dark bands enhanced more prominently than the normal bands. This is presumed to result from the disruption of the blood-testis barrier, which

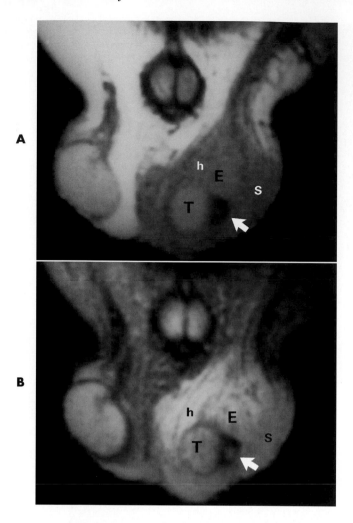

FIGURE 31-23 Torsion of the testicular appendix in a prepubertal boy shown on coronal hydrogen density–weighted **(A)** and T2-weighted **(B)** images. Note the darkened testicular appendix *(arrow)* located between the slightly darkened testis *(T)* and the swollen epididymis *(E)*. Also note the associated hemiscrotal swelling *(S)* and hydrocele *(h)*. Because of MR findings, the condition was treated conservatively. A follow-up MRI 6 weeks later was normal (not shown). (From reference 49.)

provides Gd greater access, analogous to the disruption of the blood-brain barrier.[12,56] In one patient, biopsy showed atrophy and fibrosis. That these changes also occur in other patients with similar MRI findings is not yet certain.

Extratesticular Lesions

Spermatoceles. On MRI, spermatoceles are easily identified within the epididymis. The most frequent site of involvement is globus major (head). Spermatoceles are round, well-circumscribed structures displaying signal intensity similar to hydrocele fluid (Figures 31-4, 31-8, and 31-12). In a minority of cases, the spermatocele can mimic the testicular signal, appearing brighter than water on T1-weighted images (Figure 31-12) and darker than water on T2-weighted images.

Hydroceles. A simple hydrocele has typical fluid characteristics on MRI that are isointense or darker than testis on T1-weighted and high on T2-weighted images (Figure 31-3). Complicated hydroceles will demonstrate signals characteristic of their content (Figures 31-18 and 31-19).

Varicoceles. MRI clearly shows the entire spermatic cord from the inguinal ring to the mediastinum testis. Patients with varicoceles have widening of the spermatic canal and prominence of the pampiniform plexus (Figure 31-17). The plexus is more heterogeneous and has a

greater number of serpiginous structures with increased or decreased signal. The degree of hypervascularity is not prominent, as is seen in epididymitis. Although clinically palpable varicoceles are easily depicted on MRI, it is not clear at this time whether MRI will be able to diagnose subclinical varicoceles with sufficient accuracy.

CRYPTORCHIDISM

Cryptorchidism occurs in 2.7% to 6% of full-term neonates, with a 0.8% prevalence at 1 year of age. Spontaneous descent is unlikely after the first year.[13,26,62] Because the undescended testis is at increased risk of malignancy,[5,58] many techniques have been developed to aid in the diagnosis and treatment so that the clinician can monitor for neoplasia and diminish the incidence of infertility. An undescended testis may be intraabdominal, intracanalicular, ectopic, atrophic, or congenitally absent. Undescended testes may be located anywhere from the renal hilum to the superior scrotum. They may also be found in an ectopic location, such as the perineum or superficial abdominal wall. Testes located proximal to the external inguinal ring are usually not palpable, as may be small or atrophic testes located distal to the external inguinal ring.

Neonatal extravaginal torsion results in complete replacement of testicular tissue with scarring. If neonatal extravaginal torsion is missed at birth, the patient may have a nonpalpable undescended testis but possibly a palpable cord later in life. Such a patient would require surgery for diagnosis. If the preoperative diagnosis of testicular atrophy can be reliably made, surgery could be avoided or limited to patients wanting prosthetic replacement. Therefore the adequate preoperative assessment and localization of the undescended testis are useful in guiding clinical management and surgical exploration, making a more limited operative procedure possible.

Various diagnostic modalities, including sonography,[75,76] computed tomography,[23,41,76] spermatic venography and arteriography,[15,21,23] and MRI,[19,25,36,40,72] have been used to localize the cryptorchid testis. Laparoscopy was introduced to evaluate the nonpalpable testis before exploration.[46] If testicular vessels and the vas deferens end blindly in the abdomen, no exploration is done. If tissue is present at the end of the vas deferens, exploration follows. However, if the vas deferens enters the internal inguinal ring, exploration of the inguinal canal is required to ensure the absence of testicular tissue. Laparoscopy is 100% accurate in localizing the potential location of the testis and may obviate surgery in some patients, but it is not useful if the cord enters the internal inguinal ring. Laparoscopy also does not allow for preoperative planning. Furthermore, it increases anesthesia and operating room time. Although MRI seems to be the most sensitive and specific noninvasive tool, it requires sedation. At present, few imaging studies are done in children.

Magnetic Resonance Techniques

Although high-field systems are ideal, lower fields could be used if thin slices (3 to 5 mm) and heavily T2-weighted sequences can be acquired at an adequate signal-to-noise ratio. Boys between 6 months and 6 years of age require sedation. Patients are placed directly in the head coil if they are small. A standard 5-inch circular surface coil is centered approximately over the symphysis pubis to ensure that the base of the scrotum and lower pelvis are included in the field of view. A 16-cm field of view, a 256 × 256 acquisition matrix, and a 3-mm slice thickness are used (voxel size = 0.63 × 0.63 × 3 mm). In small infants, a 3-inch circular surface coil is used, the field of view is reduced to 12 cm, and other parameters are constant.

T1- and T2-weighted axial and coronal series are sufficient in most cases. Keeping imaging time short is important, since most patients require sedation. The first two series (400/12), T1 weighted and fast spin-echo T2 weighted (3500/120), are obtained in the axial plane with a 3-, 5-, or 10-mm slice thickness (depending on patient size) and an interslice gap of 50% slice thickness. These series are acquired with a 16-cm field of view, 192 matrix, and two acquisitions. Sixteen echo trains are used with the fast spin-echo technique. These series should cover from the base of the scrotum to the middle of the bladder to assess the entire course of the spermatic cord.

The coronal T1- and T2-weighted series are acquired with the same parameters and should cover the area from the posterior aspect of the scrotum to the anterior abdominal wall. The slice thickness for this series is 3 mm in all patients and is obtained with a 50% interslice gap.

This series, which could be obtained with fat suppression if magnetic homogeneity is acceptable, allows further assessment of the cord within the spermatic canal and provides testicular tissue characterization.

If neither the cryptorchid testis nor its cord structures can be seen on the coronal and axial series, T1-weighted and fast spin-echo T2-weighted images are obtained in the transverse plane from the symphysis pubis to the upper pole of both kidneys. Either the head or body coil is used, depending on patient size, with similar imaging parameters except for a different slice thickness and field of view.

Locating the Testis

High-resolution MRI with surface coils clearly delineates the spermatic cord, inguinal canal, inguinal ring, pubic tubercle, testes, and regional lymph nodes.* Both the coronal and axial planes are useful for imaging of the spermatic cords. Undescended testes are best seen and recognized on coronal images.[25,40] The axial plane provides an essential adjunct for more precisely locating the testis relative to the internal or external inguinal rings and femoral vessels. In more than 65% of patients, the two series pairs (axial and coronal T1- and T2-weighted images) were sufficient for complete evaluation, requiring less than 30 min of magnet time.[25] The remainder of cases required imaging of the pelvis and abdomen because the testes were not visualized.

The undescended testes in our series with surgical or clinical proof were found to be intraabdominal in 19%, intracanalicular in 37%, or atrophic within the spermatic canal in 44%. These relationships were nearly similar to those found by others[19,36,72]; however, others referred to the group with atrophic testes as *absent*. All of the four intraabdominal testes were correctly located. Errors made by others were also related to testes in intraabdominal locations.[19,36,72] The overall accuracy of MRI in our prospective series was 93.8% (30 of 32 testes),[25] which is comparable to previously published reports of 94% (15 of 16),[19] 93% (retrospective data) (13 of 14),[36] and 82% (retrospective data done with body coil).[72] Accuracy was lowest for intraabdominal testes. Given the intense enhancement of testes with Gd, data evaluating undescended testes with fat-suppression techniques after the administration of IV contrast are still not available. After Gd administration, accuracy should improve significantly.

Intraabdominal testes located near or at the internal inguinal ring should be easily evaluated by MRI (Figure 31-24). However, because of lack of experience, we missed two of six testes located near the internal inguinal ring that were easily seen in retrospect.

The task of locating intraabdominal testes is the most difficult on MRI.[19,36] There will always be a certain degree of uncertainty when testes are not clearly depicted. Although it is important to visualize these high intraabdominal testes,[18] it is the author's belief that laparoscopy should precede exploration. Therefore the inability to visualize the high intraabdominal testis is less critical for patient management because a patient with absent cord and testis will have to undergo surgical exploration, which would be preceded by laparoscopy. When the testis and cord are well evaluated, laparoscopy is unnecessary. In our series, MRI could have decreased the need for laparoscopy, performed in 100% of patients, to only 13% of cases.

Assessment of the spermatic cord and testis together was essential for proper diagnosis. An empty spermatic canal is visible on MRI. It appears as a thin line extending from the inguinal canal to the base of the scrotum (Figures 31-24 and 31-25), representing the gubernaculum, which is a thin, fibrous strand. This should not be mistaken for an atrophic cord. The latter has significant width but is thinner than the normal contralateral cord (Figure 31-26). Although an empty canal and an absent cord suggested the possibility of an intraabdominal testis, the presence of cord structures in the canal does not exclude this possibility (Figure 31-25). Cord structures may precede the testis, or if attached to a long mesentery, the testis may flip-flop between an intracanalicular and an intraabdominal location.

The majority of intraabdominal testes will be found near the internal inguinal ring, where MRI should be reasonably accurate. Therefore the goal of the imaging schemes should be to maximize the assessment of the internal inguinal ring. The previously described technique would allow such an assessment. The 5-inch surface coil should be centered

*References 3, 4, 19, 25, 36, 40, 59, 63, 69.

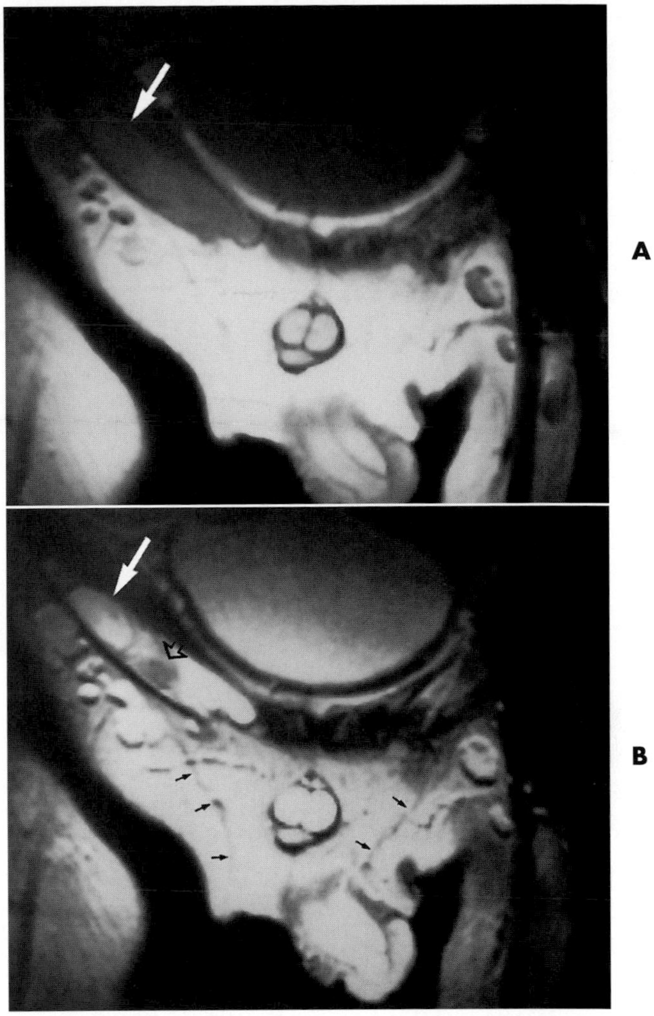

FIGURE 31-24   Undescended nonpalpable right testis in a typical intracanalicular location. The testis has normal signal behavior when seen on hydrogen density–weighted (**A**) and T2-weighted (**B**) images *(arrow)* and has an associated normal epididymis *(open arrow)* and ascites. In this location, fluid is technically ascitic, since the vaginal process is patent. The other testis was intraabdominal (not shown). The gubernaculum is best seen in **B**, and it extends bilaterally from the external inguinal ring to the base of the scrotum *(small arrows)*. Note the presence of inguinal adenopathy lateral to the right and left canals. (From reference 49.)

just below the symphysis pubis to place the testis at an optimal position in the field.

MRI was extremely accurate when testes were located in the inguinal canal. MR image interpretation was simple, since these testes were contrasted with fat, were seen in association with intravaginal fluid in many cases, and were seen with their epididymis (Figure 31-24). The testis had a normal ovoid shape with clear demonstration of the tunica albuginea.

Intracanalicular testes were easily differentiated from lymph nodes. Because their tunica albuginea could be discerned, they were associated with cord structures or epididymis, were surrounded by fluid, and were located in the path of the spermatic cord on axial scans. Lymph nodes, although of similar signal behavior, have a different morphology and are lateral to the cord (Figures 31-24 to 31-26).

Testicular scar most likely related to missed extravaginal torsion is a diagnosis that can be made noninvasively only with MRI. MRI findings are highly specific for this condition, which requires the presence of an atrophic cord that reaches the base of the empty scrotum (Figure 31-26). Surgical resection to eliminate the potential for malignant degeneration is not required in these cases, since viable testicular tissue is no longer present. If further clinical experience shows that MRI can indeed aid in the diagnosis of this entity with no false-positive results, surgical exploration in these patients could be eliminated. This

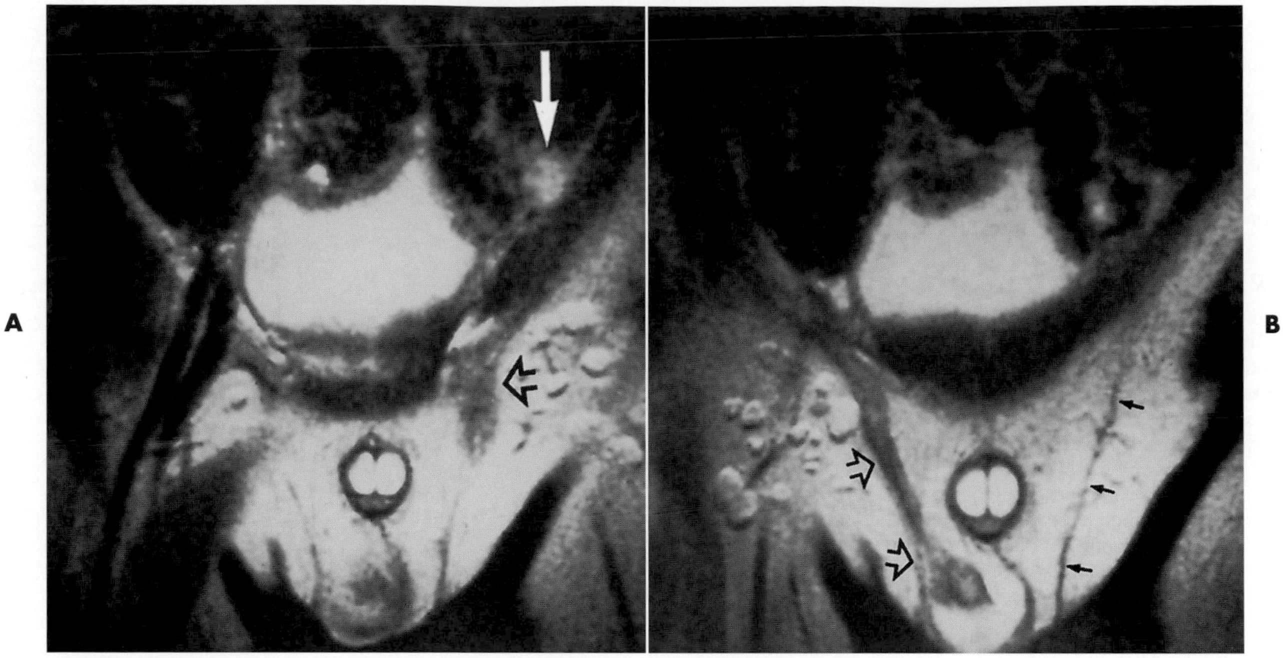

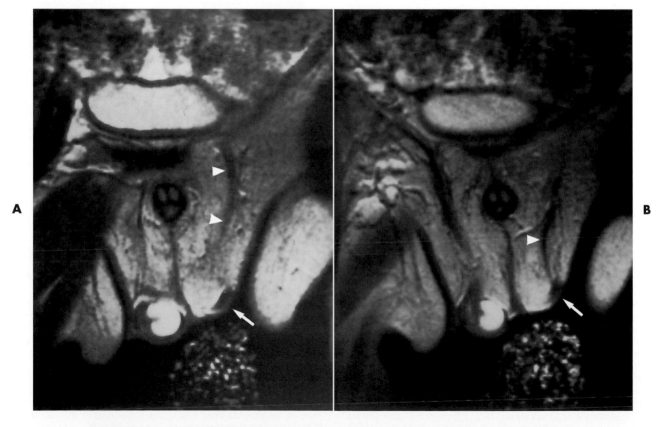

FIGURE 31-25 Left undescended and nonpalpable testis. A dark band thought to be a flattened end of the cord of an atrophic streak testis at the proximal spermatic canal *(open arrow)* is shown in a coronal plane on a T2-weighted image **(A).** The normal right cord and testis *(open arrows)* and the gubernaculum of the left testis *(small arrows)* are also shown on a T2-weighted image **(B).** At surgery the normal left undescended testis was intraabdominal, shown in **A** in a typical intraabdominal location just superior and lateral to the internal inguinal ring *(arrow),* clearly seen in retrospect. The dark region seen on MRI *(open arrow* in **A)** was cord structures preceding the testis. Note the presence of inguinal adenopathy lateral to the cord *(open arrows* in **B).** (From reference 49.)

FIGURE 31-26 Atrophic left testis *(arrow)* seen on T2-weighted images on two consecutive coronal slices **(A** and **B).** Note the presence of an atrophic cord that is thinner than the normal contralateral cord *(arrowheads)* and thicker than the gubernaculum seen in Figures 31-24 and 31-25. The atrophic cord reaches the base of the scrotum and does not end more proximally, as is seen in Figure 31-25. Note the presence of inguinal adenopathy lateral to the right cord. Heterogeneous signal seen below the scrotum is urine in a diaper. (From reference 49.)

ability would have eliminated exploration in 40% of patients in our experience.

INTRAVENOUS CONTRAST

It has been shown that Gd-DTPA significantly enhances the normal testis and epididymis[56] and that the enhancement lasts for a significant time (Figure 31-12). Because the water-soluble agent is eliminated more rapidly from tumors than normal testicular tissue, tumors that are typically invisible on T1-weighted images become more apparent after the administration of contrast.[12,35] However, there is loss of specificity in that seminomatous and nonseminomatous lesions assume a similar appearance. A dose of 0.1 mM/kg of body weight is used. Precontrast and postcontrast images should be obtained with otherwise identical imaging planes and techniques to allow for appropriate comparison. The use of IV contrast does aid in distinguishing cystic from solid lesions (Figure 31-12) and allows the assessment of testicular vascularity and possibly the assessment of epidymitis.[64] Although the enhancement is homogeneous and frequently highlights the rete testis in normal testes, inhomogeneous enhancement patterns have been observed in otherwise asymptomatic male patients, the reason for which remains unclear. It is possible that old ischemic, inflammatory, or traumatic injury might have caused these changes.

SUMMARY

Even with limited experience, certain conditions present with such a consistent constellation of findings that the author believes MRI can be used to differentiate them. MRI can distinguish torsion from epididymitis with very high accuracy and can probably differentiate most tumors from infection. Indeed, in the patient with acute scrotal pain, which can be caused by torsion, epididymitis, or tumor, MRI may prove to be the most specific imaging modality. As experience increases, refinement would be possible, and the efficacy of MRI in scrotal imaging will become better defined. In a retrospective study, we evaluated the specificity of MRI to that of ultrasound in patients who had both studies.[19] MRI was approximately 30% more specific than sonography. Although the study was retrospective and susceptible to selection bias, it does reflect the greater specificity of MRI.

MRI adds a new dimension to the assessment of scrotal disease. It demonstrates exquisite anatomical detail of the entire scrotum and inguinal region. It allows the recognition of each intrascrotal structure on the basis of its characteristic appearance and signal rather than its strict anatomical location. The interpretation of MR images is less subjective than ultrasound, particularly when the normal relationship of the scrotal contents is disturbed. Because it is less subjective, MRI is sufficiently specific to allow differentiation of the various pathological processes, although this hypothesis requires proof. It also appears that MRI may be the most accurate noninvasive tool for localizing undescended testes and guiding the management of patients with nonpalpable testes. In this setting, it can significantly decrease the number of laparoscopies performed, and because of its ability to diagnose old neonatal torsion, it could eliminate the need for surgery in as many as 40% of cases.

REFERENCES

1. Arcadia JA: Cysts of the tunica albuginea testis, J Urol 68:631, 1952.
2. Atkinson GO Jr, Patrick LE, Ball TI Jr, et al: The normal and abnormal scrotum in children: evaluation with color Doppler sonography, Am J Roentgenol 158:613, 1992.
3. Baker LL, Hajek PC, Burkhard TK, et al: Magnetic resonance imaging of the scrotum: pathological conditions, Radiology 163:93, 1987.
4. Baker LL, Hajek PC, Burkhard TK, et al: Magnetic resonance imaging of the scrotum: normal anatomy, Radiology 163:89, 1987.
5. Batata MA, Whitmore WF Jr, Hilaris BS, et al: Cryptorchidism and testicular cancer, J Urol 124:382, 1980.
6. Ben Chaim J, Leibovitch I, Ramon J, et al: Etiology of acute scrotum at surgical exploration in children, adolescents and adults, Eur Urol 21:45, 1992.
7. Berger Y, Srinivas V, Hajdu SI, et al: Epidermoid cysts of the testis: role of conservative surgery, J Urol 134:962, 1985.
8. Brenner JS, Cumming WA, and Ros PR: Testicular epidermoid cyst: sonographic and MR findings, Am J Roentgenol 152:1344, 1989.
9. Brown DL, Benson CB, Doherty FJ, et al: Cystic testicular mass caused by dilated rete testis: sonographic findings in 31 cases, Am J Roentgenol 158:1257, 1992.
10. Burks DD, Markey BJ, Burkhard TK, et al: Suspected testicular torsion and ischemia: evaluation with color Doppler sonography, Radiology 175:815, 1990.
11. Carroll BA, and Gross DM: High frequency scrotal sonography, Am J Roentgenol 140:511, 1983.
12. Cho KS, Auh YH, Lee MG, et al: Testicular tumor: conventional MR imaging and Gd-DTPA enhancement. In Book of abstracts, 77th Scientific Assembly and Annual Meeting, Radiology 181:(S)115, 1991.
13. Cour-Palar IJ: Spontaneous descent of the testicle, Lancet 1:403, 1966.
14. Cramer BM, Schlegel EA, and Thueroff JW: MR imaging in the differential diagnosis of scrotal and testicular disease, Radiographics 11:9, 1991.
15. Diamond AB, Meng CH, Kodroff M, et al: Testicular venography in the non-palpable testis, Am J Roentgenol 129:71, 1977.
16. Eilenberg SS, Tartar VM, and Mattrey RF: Reducing magnetic susceptibility differences using liquid fluorocarbon pads (Sat Pad): results with spectral presaturation of fat, Biomat Art Cells Immob Biotech 22(4):1447, 1994.
17. Finkelstein MS, Rosenberg HK, Snyder HM III, et al: Ultrasound evaluation of scrotum in pediatrics, Urology 27:1, 1986.
18. Friedland GW, and Chang P: The role of imaging in the management of impalpable undescended testis, Am J Roentgenol 151:1107, 1988.
19. Fritzsche PJ, Hricak H, Kogan BA, et al: Undescended testis: value of MRI, Radiology 164:169, 1987.
20. Glazer HS, Lee JKT, Melson GL, et al: Sonographic detection of occult testicular neoplasms, Am J Roentgenol 138:673, 1982.
21. Glickman MF, Weiss RM, and Itzchak Y: Testicular venography for undescended testes, Am J Roentgenol 129:67, 1977.
22. Gooding GAW, Leonhardt W, and Stein R: Testicular cysts: US findings, Radiology 163:537, 1987.
23. Green JR: Computerized axial tomography vs. spermatic venography in localization of the cryptorchid testis, J Urol 26:513, 1985.
24. Gillenwater JY, Grayhack JT, Howards SS, et al: Adult and pediatric urology, St Louis, 1987, Mosby.
25. Gylys-Morin VM, Landa HM, Fitzmorris-Glass R, et al: MR imaging of the cryptorchid testis, Radiology 165(P):59, 1987 (abstract).
26. Hadziselimovic F: Cryptorchidism, New York, 1983, Springer-Verlag.
27. Hamm B, Frobbe F, and Loy V: Testicular cysts: differentiation with US and clinical findings, Radiology 168:19, 1988.
28. Hayward I, Trambert MA, Mattrey RF, et al: Case Report: MR imaging of vasculitis of the testis, J Comput Assist Tomogr 15(3):502, 1990.
29. Horstman WG, Middleton WD, Melson GL, et al: Scrotal inflammatory disease: color Doppler US findings, Radiology 179:55, 1991.
30. Horstman WG, Middleton WD, Melson GL, et al: Color Doppler US of the scrotum, Radiographics 11:941, 1991.
31. Hricak H, and Filly RA: Sonography of the scrotum, Invest Radiol 18:112, 1983.
32. Hricak H, and Jeffrey RB: Sonography of acute scrotal abnormalities, Radiol Clin North Am 21:595, 1983.
33. Janzen DL, Mathieson JR, Marsh JI, et al: Testicular microlithiasis: sonographic and clinical features, Am J Roentgenol 158:1057, 1992.
34. Johnson JO, Mattrey RF, and Phillipson J: Differentiation of seminomatous from nonseminomateous testicular tumors with MR imaging, Am J Roentgenol 154:539, 1990.
35. Just M, Melchior S, Grebe P, et al: MR tomography in testicular processes. The significance of Gd-DTPA enhanced sequence in comparison with plain T2-weighted sequences, ROFO 166:527, 1992.
36. Kier R, McCarthy S, Rosenfield AT, et al: Nonpalpable testes in young boys: evaluation with MR imaging, Radiology 169:429, 1988.
37. Krieger JN, Wang K, and Mack L: Preliminary evaluation of color Doppler imaging for investigation of intrascrotal pathology, J Urol 144:904, 1990.
38. Krone KD, and Carroll BA: Scrotal ultrasound, Radiol Clin North Am 23:121, 1985.
39. Landa HM, Gylys-Morin V, Mattrey RF, et al: Detection of testicular torsion by magnetic resonance imaging in a rat model, J Urol 140:1178, 1988.
40. Landa HM, Gylys-Morin V, Mattrey RF, et al: MRI of the cryptorchid testis, Eur J Pediatr 146(S):S16, 1987.
41. Lee JKT, McClennan BL, Stanley RJ, et al: Utility of CT in the localization of the undescended testis, Radiology 135:121, 1980.
42. Leopold GR, Woo VL, Scheible FW, et al: High resolution ultrasonography of scrotal pathology, Radiology 131:719, 1979.
43. Leopold GR: Superficial organs. In Goldberg B, ed: Ultrasound in cancer, New York, 1981, Churchill-Livingstone.
44. Lerner RM, Mevorach RA, Hulbert WC, et al: Color Doppler US in the evaluation of acute scrotal disease, Radiology 176:355, 1990.
45. Leung ML, Gooding GAW, and Williams RD: High-resolution sonography of scrotal contents in asymptomatic subjects, Am J Roentgenol 143:161, 1984.
46. Lowe DH, Brock WA, and Kaplan GW: Laparoscopy for localization of the nonpalpable testis, J Urol 131:728, 1984.
47. Lupetin AR, King W III, Rich P, et al: Ultrasound diagnosis of testicular leukemia, Radiology 146:171, 1983.
48. Mattrey R: MRI of the male genitalia: testes, seminal vesicles, and urethra. In Goldman SM, and Gatewood OMB, eds: CT and MRI of the genitourinary tract. Contemporary issues in computed tomography, vol 13, New York, 1990, Churchill Livingstone.
49. Mattrey RF: Scrotum and testes. In Edelman RR, Hesselink JR, and Zlatkin MB, eds: Clinical magnetic resonance imaging, Philadelphia, 1996, WB Saunders.
50. Mennemeyer RP, and Mason JT: Non-neoplastic cystic lesions of the tunica albuginea: an electron microscopic and clinical study of 2 cases, J Urol 121:373, 1979.
51. Middleton WD, and Bell MW: Analysis of intratesticular arterial anatomy with emphasis on transmediastinal arteries, Radiology 189(1):157, 1993.
52. Middleton WD, and Melson GL: Testicular ischemia: color Doppler sonographic findings in five patients, Am J Roentgenol 152:1237, 1989.
53. Middleton WD, Siegel BA, Melson GL, et al: Acute scrotal disorders: prospective comparison of color Doppler US and testicular scintigraphy, Radiology 177:177, 1990.

54. Morse MJ, and Whitmore WF: Neoplasms of the testes. In Walsh PC, Gittes RF, Permutter AD, et al, eds: Cambell's urology, ed 5, Philadelphia, 1986, WB Saunders.

55. Mueller DL, Amundson GM, Rubin SZ, et al: Acute scrotal abnormalities in children: diagnosis by combined sonography and scintigraphy, Am J Roentgenol 150:643, 1988.

56. Muller Leisse C, Bohndorf K, Stargardt A, et al: Gadolinium-enhanced T1-weighted versus T2-weighted imaging of scrotal disorders: is there an indication for MR imaging? J Magn Reson Imaging 4(3):389, 1994.

57. O'Mara EM, and Rifkin MD: Scrotum and contents. In Resnick MI, and Rifkin MD, eds: Ultrasonography of the urinary tract, ed 3, Baltimore, 1991, William & Wilkins.

58. Pinch L, Aceto T Jr, and Meyer-Bahlburg HFL: Cryptorchidism. A pediatric review, Urol Clin North Am 1:573, 1974.

59. Rholl KS, Lee JKT, Ling D, et al: MR imaging of the scrotum with a high resolution surface coil, Radiology 163:99, 1987.

60. Rolnick D, Kowanous S, Szanto P, et al: Anatomical incidence of testicular appendages, J Urol 100:775, 1968.

61. Schwerk WB, Schwerk WN, and Rodeck G: Testicular tumors: prospective analysis of real-time ultrasound patterns and abdominal staging, Radiology 164:369, 1987.

62. Scorer CG, and Farrington GH: Congenital deformities of the testis and epididymis, New York, 1972, Appleton-Century-Crofts.

63. Seidenwurm D, Smathers RL, Lo RK, et al: Testes and scrotum: MR imaging at 1.5T, Radiology 164:393, 1987.

64. Semba CP, Trambert MA, and Mattrey RF: Specificity of MRI in scrotal disease versus sonography, RSNA, Chicago, 1990, Radiology 177(P)(S):129, 1990 (abstract).

65. Shah KH, Maxted WC, and Chun B: Epidermoid cysts of the testis: a report of three cases and an analysis of 141 cases from the world literature, Cancer 47:577, 1981.

66. Smith WS, Brammer HM, Henry M, et al: Testicular microlithiasis: sonographic features with pathological correlation, Am J Roentgenol 157:1003, 1991.

67. Sokal M, Peckham MJ, and Hendry WF: Bilateral germ cell tumours of the testis, Br J Urol 53:158, 1980.

68. Tartar VM, Trambert MA, Balsara ZN, et al: Tubular ectasia of the testicle: sonographic and MR imaging appearance, Am J Roentgenol 160:539, 1993.

69. Thurnher S, Hricak H, Carroll PR, et al: Imaging the testis: comparison between MR imaging and US, Radiology 167:631, 1988.

70. Trainer TD: Histology of the normal testis, Am J Surg Pathol 11:797, 1987.

71. Trambert MA, Mattrey RF, Levine D, et al: Subacute scrotal pain: evaluation of torsion versus epididymitis with MR imaging, Radiology 175:53, 1990.

72. Tripathi RP, Jena AN, Gulati P, et al: Undescended testis: evaluation by magnetic resonance imaging, Indian Pediatr 29:433, 1992.

73. Weingarten BJ, Kellman GM, Middleton WD, et al: Tubular ectasia within the mediastinum testis, J Ultrasound Med 11:349, 1992.

74. Weiss AJ, Kellman GM, Middleton WD, et al: Intratesticular varicocele: sonographic findings in two patients, Am J Roentgenol 158:1061, 1992.

75. Weiss RM, Carter AR, and Rosenfield AT: High resolution real-time ultrasonography in the localization of the undescended testis, J Urol 135:936, 1986.

76. Wolverson MK, Houttin E, Heiberh E, et al: Comparison of CT with high resolution ultrasound in the localization of the undescended testis, Radiology 146:133, 1983.

32 Pediatric Body

Rosalind B. Dietrich and Gerald M. Roth

KEY POINTS

- Children under the age of 7 years frequently require sedation and careful monitoring.
- Simple congenital anomalies inaccessible to ultrasound, as well as anatomically complex anomalies, are well imaged by MRI.
- MRI is competitive with CT for staging tumors of the thorax, abdomen, and pelvis.
- Tumor and infection involving musculoskeletal or neural structures are best imaged with MRI.

Although initially slow to become established, magnetic resonance imaging (MRI) now plays a vital role in the diagnostic imaging evaluation of many pediatric diseases and disorders. The ability to produce multiplanar images in a noninvasive manner without the use of ionizing radiation and with only minimal patient preparation has made MRI a useful complement to other cross-sectional modalities such as ultrasound and computed tomography (CT).

The spectrum of pathological conditions in pediatrics is different from that observed in adults, with a higher incidence of congenital anomalies, a different group of neoplasms, and a lower incidence of metastatic and degenerative disorders. When MRI is performed on pediatric patients, the pulse sequences and techniques that are routinely used to evaluate adult disease are often inappropriate for optimal demonstration and characterization of pediatric disease, and therefore optimized pediatric protocols are needed.

PATIENT PREPARATION AND IMAGING TECHNIQUES

A short time spent explaining the procedure to the child before scanning is often helpful. Because children may be apprehensive about the MR study, parents should be encouraged to stay during scanning to give reassurance if necessary (Figure 32-1). Children under age 7 years frequently require sedation. Before sedation, it is important to obtain a history of current or previous illnesses. If a child is suffering from an acute respiratory illness, an elective MRI study should be temporarily postponed. Special care should be taken when sedating children with airway compromise, congenital heart disease, or mental retardation because they have a higher incidence of complication. Children requiring sedation should have nothing by mouth for several hours before the administration of sedation to minimize the risks of aspiration. Many different sedation regimens are being successfully used.[6,15,52,60,75,143] We prefer oral chloral hydrate for children under 18 months of age and rectal thiopental or intravenous pentobarbital (Nembutal) for older children (Table 32-1). General anesthesia may be used if routine sedation fails or in high-risk children.

It is essential to fully monitor all sedated patients. MRI-compatible devices are now available for respiratory, blood pressure, cardiac, and temperature monitoring that are safe and cause minimal or no image degradation when used in conjunction with the MR imager.[3,6,60] The patient should be monitored from the time the sedation is initiated until the child is awake. Sedation flow sheets should be used to document the type and dose of sedation given and to record vital signs periodically. When the child is discharged from the MRI area, postsedation care should be discussed with the parent or caregiver and written instructions given to them.[116]

Surface coils should be used whenever possible when imaging children so that signal-to-noise ratios can be optimized. Several manufacturers now supply specialized pediatric surface coils. When these coils are not available, excellent results can be obtained by placing the bodies of infants snugly into the center of adult head or extremity coils (Figure 32-2). The coil that most approximates the body of the child should be used.

It is imperative that the initial MRI sequences obtained yield maximal information because the study may have to be terminated prematurely if the child awakens or is unable to remain still. Especially small structures are often being evaluated, so it may also be necessary to use contiguous slices or slices thinner than those routinely obtained. Images obtained in nonorthogonal planes may also be useful for better definition of the relationships of adjacent structures and for demonstration of structures and lesions in an oblique orientation.[67]

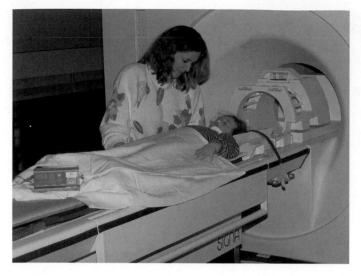

FIGURE 32-1   Parents are encouraged to remain with the child during scanning.

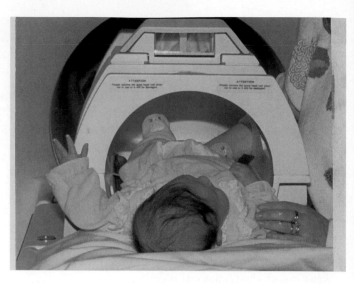

FIGURE 32-2   Infants fit snugly into an adult head or an extremity surface coil.

Table 32-1   Sedation Protocols

SEDATION	AGE*	ROUTE	INITIAL DOSE	ADDITIONAL DOSE	MAXIMUM DOSE
Chloral hydrate	0-18	Oral	75 mg/kg	37.5 mg/kg after 30 min	2000 mg
Pentobarbital (Thiopental)	>18	Rectal	25 mg/kg	12.5 mg/kg after 15 min	—
Pentobarbital sodium (Nembutal)	>18	Intravenous	2.5 mg/kg over 1-2 min	0-3.5 mg/kg titrated as needed	200 mg, or 6 mg/kg

*In months.

Faster imaging techniques such as gradient-echo, fast spin-echo (FSE), and echo-planar imaging, all of which significantly shorten imaging times, can be particularly advantageous when imaging children.[1,21,70,137,142] The role of techniques that demonstrate vascular anatomy, such as MR angiography, remains to be defined in the evaluation of the pediatric patient, but potentially these techniques offer significant advantages over routine sequences in the evaluation of vascular patency[82,92,93,98,159] and in the identification of abnormal vessels.

Gadolinium chelate contrast agents may be useful in the evaluation of vascular lesions. These agents may also prove helpful in defining the borders and internal architecture of any mass lesion[32,126] or in identifying its organ of origin. Oral MR contrast agents have been developed and have been shown to be both safe and effective in children.[9,10]

CONGENITAL DISORDERS

MRI plays an important role in evaluating both complex congenital anomalies, in which ultrasound is inadequate, and simple congenital anomalies, in which sonography is not possible, is incomplete, or is suboptimal. Congenital anomalies are well visualized with MRI because it provides excellent anatomical detail and has multiplanar capabilities. The majority of lesions are adequately assessed using multiplanar T1- and T2-weighted spin-echo (SE) imaging. Occasionally, additional sequences are required, especially if the presence of fat or flowing blood is to be determined.

Thorax

Although the role of MRI in the evaluation of congenital lesions arising in the thorax is at present more limited than in other parts of the body, valid indications for MRI do exist.*

In the evaluation of the mediastinum, the ability of MRI to easily distinguish vessels containing rapidly flowing blood from adjacent mass

*References 12, 40, 73, 131, 132, 135.

lesions without the need for bolus injection of contrast material is useful for distinguishing congenital cysts (bronchogenic, neurenteric, thymic, duplication, and pericardial)[90,91,105,118] (Figure 32-3) from vascular structures. Simple cystic lesions have smooth thin walls of the same signal characteristics as cystic lesions seen elsewhere in the body. They demonstrate low signal intensity on T1-weighted images and high signal intensity on T2-weighted images that increase with prolongation of the relaxation time (TR). Lesions with high protein content or hemorrhage may demonstrate higher signal intensity on T1-weighted sequences, making differentiation between them and well-defined solid lesions more difficult (Figure 32-3). Posterior extension of the thymus may present as a mediastinal mass. On MRI, the "mass" is continuous with the rest of the thymic tissue, does not displace vessels, and has the same signal intensity on all sequences.[101,122]

MR evaluation of intrathoracic extension of lesions primarily arising from the soft tissues of the neck or thorax can also be useful,[17,29,78,134] especially when images are obtained in the coronal and sagittal planes. These masses may arise from any soft tissue component and include lesions such as hemangiomas, lymphangiomas, cystic hygromas, lipomas, and fibromatosis.

The MR appearance of hemangiomas may be varied, depending on the composition of the lesion.[129] Most often they appear as inhomogeneous medium–signal intensity masses containing serpiginous vessels on T1-weighted images, which demonstrate high signal intensity on heavily T2-weighted images. Areas of fat, hemorrhage, or calcification may also be seen within the lesions, and their presence gives the lesions a more inhomogeneous appearance. Occasionally, however, lesions may be entirely homogeneous. In such cases, the absence of surrounding edema and the presence of associated muscle atrophy make a diagnosis of hemangioma more likely than that of an infectious process or a malignant neoplasm.

Cystic hygromas appear as septated cystic masses with high signal intensity on T2-weighted images and signal intensities ranging from low to high on T1-weighted images, depending on the protein and fat content of the loculated fluid within the septations[134,158] (Figure 32-4). Lymphangiomas of the capillary type have similar signal intensities to

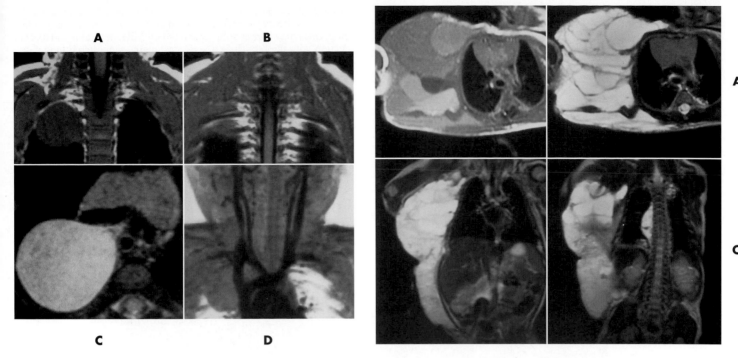

FIGURE 32-3   Bronchogenic cyst. **A** and **B,** Coronal (SE 500/15) image. The medium–signal intensity mass in the apex of the right lung does not extend into the spinal canal. **C,** Axial (SE 3000/160) image. The mass demonstrates very high signal intensity consistent with a cystic lesion. **D,** Coronal two-dimensional time-of-flight (gradient-recalled echo 40/8/15) angiogram. The great vessels are displaced but not involved by the mass.

FIGURE 32-4   Cystic hygroma. **A** and **B,** SE (450/11) and FSE (3000/102Ef) images show a thoracic wall mass that contains cystic spaces of varying signal intensity. **C** and **D,** On FSE (3000/102 eff) images, the mass also has a posterior mediastinal component.

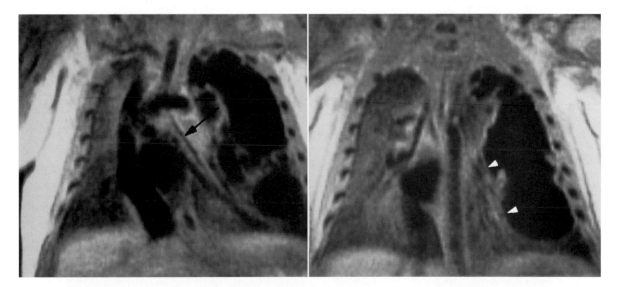

FIGURE 32-5   Cystic adenomatoid malformation on coronal (SE 800/30) images. A large cystic mass fills the left hemithorax, displacing the mediastinum to the right. The bronchus of the left lower lobe is identified *(arrow)* extending into a collapsed left lower lobe *(arrowheads).*

those demonstrated in cystic hygromas but do not contain the large cystic spaces.

Lipomas are fatty tumors that occur in the subcutaneous tissues of the body or in the fascial planes of muscle. They are frequently encapsulated, contain fibrous septations, and have the same signal intensities as fat on all pulse sequences.[47,80] Lipoblastomas, which are also benign, may have imaging characteristics similar to those of lipomas or may have a lower signal intensity on T1-weighted images.[80,128] Differentiation of lipomas from liposarcomas is less of a problem in children than in adults because liposarcomas are rarely seen in the pediatric population.

Juvenile fibromatosis is a rare disorder characterized by infiltrative fibrous lesions that arise from the fascial sheaths of striated muscle.

Histologically, they consist of fibroblasts, a benign cell type that may become locally invasive.[53,79] Initial reports of the MR appearance of juvenile fibromatosis described poorly defined lesions with medium signal intensity on both T1- and T2-weighted images. These lesions may also have high signal intensity on T2-weighted images.[53,79,103]

The most common pediatric abnormalities involving the lung include lobar emphysema, cystic adenomatoid malformation (Figure 32-5), and pulmonary sequestration.[105,109] The first two abnormalities can be evaluated using MRI, although plain-film radiology, CT examination, or both modalities are usually sufficient. Only rarely will MR examination be necessary to supply specific additional information. However, MRI, MR angiography, or both modalities can be very useful

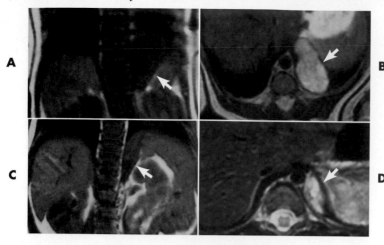

FIGURE 32-6 Intraabdominal extralobar sequestration. **A** and **B,** SE (600/15) and FSE (3000/102 eff) images show a well-defined paraspinal mass *(arrow)* displacing the left adrenal gland laterally. **C** and **D,** Follow-up SE (600/15) and FSE (3000/102 eff) images show the mass becoming smaller.

in cases of sequestration because it may be possible to demonstrate the anomalous feeding vessels and draining veins.[109] The corresponding lung tissue may appear solid or aerated on MRI, depending on its connection with the bronchial tree. Occasionally, sequestered lung tissue may be present below the diaphragm,[22] most frequently located in the paraspinal region medial to the left adrenal gland (Figure 32-6).

Abnormalities of the diaphragm, such as diaphragmatic hernias and eventrations, can also be evaluated using MRI. Coronal and sagittal T1-weighted images are useful in determining the presence or absence of a portion of the diaphragm as well as identifying which, if any, of the normal abdominal contents are in the chest.[156] In patients with defects of the anterior abdominal wall, such as gastroschisis and omphalocele, MRI can be used to determine which abdominal organs have protruded through the defect and to define their position (Figure 32-7).

Great Vessels

The ability of MRI to differentiate vessels containing flowing blood from other mediastinal structures without the use of bolus injection of contrast material makes it an ideal choice for evaluating anomalies of the great vessels.[8,43] Preoperative mapping may alleviate the need for angiography in select patients.[8,43,76] In addition, in lesions such as the

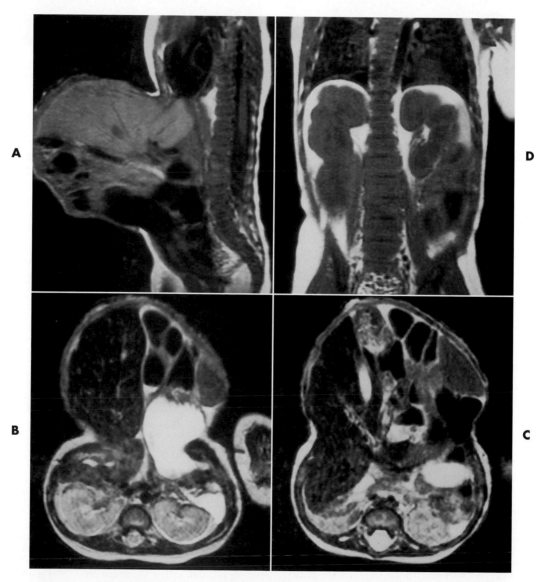

FIGURE 32-7 Omphalocele. **A,** Sagittal (SE 350/11) image shows multiple loops of bowel and a large volume of the liver herniated into the omphalocele sac. **B** and **C,** Axial (FSE 4000/102 eff) images show the liver, gallbladder, bowel, spleen, and stomach in the omphalocele sac. **D,** Coronal (SE 350/12) image shows the kidneys in an abnormally superior position: lying just below the diaphragm.

double aortic arch (Figure 32-8) and the right aortic arch with an aberrant left subclavian artery and a left ligamentum arteriosum, MRI can evaluate for the presence of esophageal and tracheal compression, which may be associated with these lesions. In the entity known as the *pulmonary sling,* in which the left pulmonary artery arises from the right pulmonary artery and passes between the trachea and the esophagus, the presence of tracheal compression may be similarly assessed (Figure 32-9). Other, even less common symptomatic abnormalities, as well as the asymptomatic great vessel anomalies, can also be evaluated. In a patient with a right aortic arch, MRI can determine the presence or absence of mirror-image branching and can demonstrate any associated cardiac anomalies. Cardiac-gated T1-weighted images in the axial and coronal planes can often provide sufficient information for these diagnoses to be made, although sometimes images parallel to the course of the aorta are very useful.

Systemic venous anomalies such as azygous continuation of the inferior vena cava and persistent left superior vena cava are also well evaluated with MRI, again predominantly using combinations of axial and coronal T1-weighted images.[37]

Hepatobiliary System

Congenital anomalies of the hepatobiliary system, such as choledochal cysts, biliary atresia, and polycystic liver disease, can all be evaluated using MRI[2] but are more commonly diagnosed using ultrasound. MRI plays a more important role in the visualization of abnormal vascular anatomy in anomalies such as the Budd-Chiari malformation[98,139] and discontinuity of the inferior vena cava. In the Budd-Chiari malformation, MRI may identify obliteration of the hepatic veins and may help determine whether a congenital web or a thrombus[89] is responsible for the condition.

Kidney

Renal Agenesis and Fusion Anomalies. Abnormal location of the kidneys, whether high (intrathoracic kidney) (Figure 32-7) or low (pelvic kidney), and fusion anomalies such as horseshoe kidney and crossed-fused ectopia are readily seen using MRI.[23,25,26] Although most of these anomalies can be accurately evaluated using ultrasonography, at times it is difficult to differentiate between renal agenesis and an abnormal location of the kidney, especially if air-containing bowel loops are present in the region being scanned. Because visualization of abdominal and pelvic organs using MRI is not limited by the presence of bowel gas or bone, it provides an overall view of the entire area, allowing easy differentiation between renal agenesis (Figure 32-10) and ectopia. In cases of ectopia, possible complications can also be evaluated because ectopic kidneys are more prone to injury or to the development of obstruction.[25]

Most congenital renal anomalies are best evaluated using T1-weighted images obtained in the coronal plane, which provide good

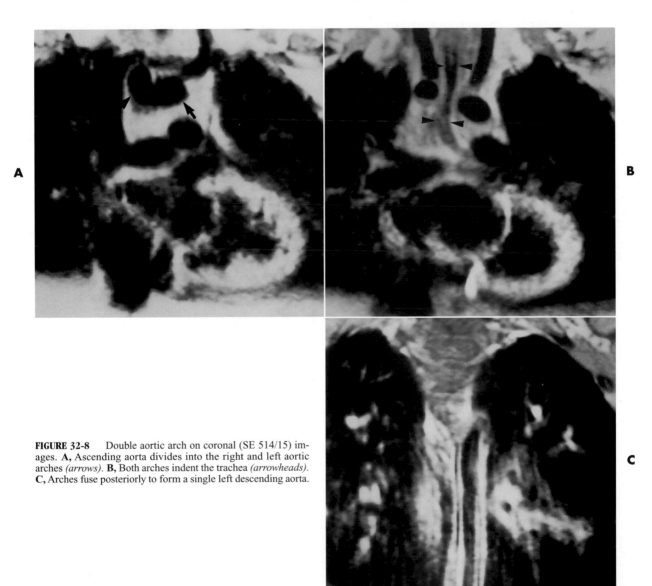

FIGURE 32-8   Double aortic arch on coronal (SE 514/15) images. **A,** Ascending aorta divides into the right and left aortic arches *(arrows).* **B,** Both arches indent the trachea *(arrowheads).* **C,** Arches fuse posteriorly to form a single left descending aorta.

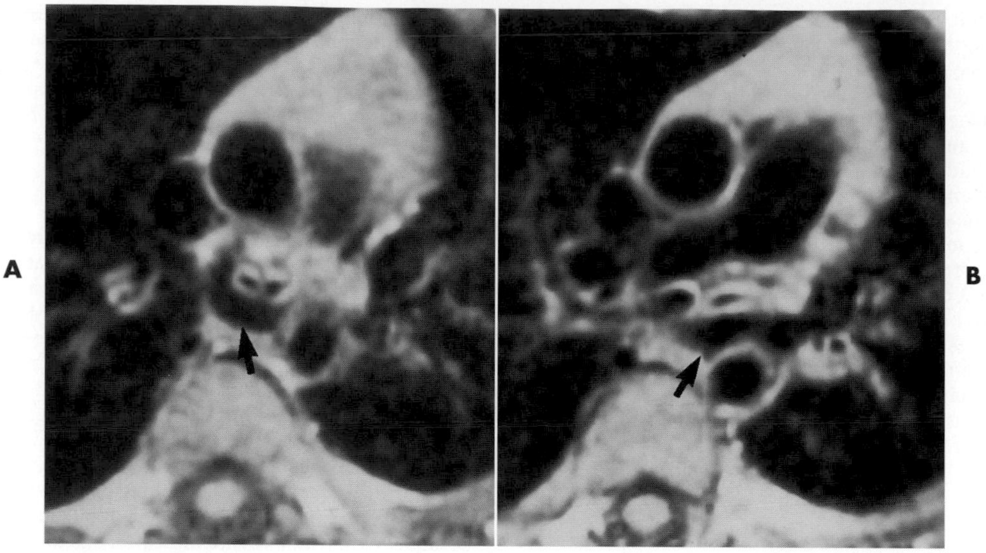

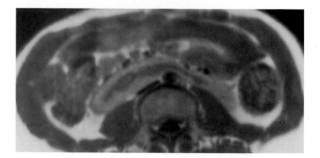

FIGURE 32-9   Pulmonary sling. **A** and **B,** SE (900/12) images show an aberrant left pulmonary artery arising from the right pulmonary artery *(arrow)* and passing between the carina (anteriorly) and the esophagus and aorta (posteriorly).

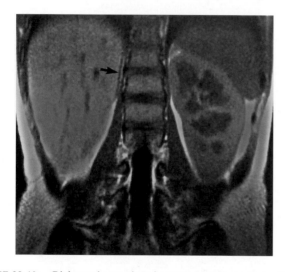

FIGURE 32-10   Right renal agenesis and compensatory hyperplasia of the left kidney. The diskoid adrenal gland is lateral to the crus of the diaphragm *(arrow).*

FIGURE 32-11   Horseshoe kidney. Axial (SE 500/28) image shows fusion of the lower poles of the kidneys across the midline, anterior to the aorta.

anatomical detail. In children with crossed-fused ectopia, such images will demonstrate the abnormally positioned fused kidney on one side and the absence of renal tissue on the contralateral side. Horseshoe kidneys are an exception to this protocol and are easier to diagnose on transverse T1-weighted images (Figure 32-11). On posterior coronal cuts the axes of the kidneys appear normal, and only on more anteriorly positioned cuts can the lower pole fusion be visualized. Because the axes of the kidneys may be angled quite steeply, frequently only a small portion of renal tissue is identified on each slice, and the fusion of the lower poles across the midline can thus easily be missed on coronal images (Figure 32-11).

In children with renal agenesis, the ipsilateral adrenal gland does not develop its characteristic inverted V shape but instead has a diskoid configuration. Discoid adrenal glands can be seen as elongated linear structures on coronal MR images (Figure 32-10).

Cystic Renal Diseases. The classifications of cystic renal disease are often confusing, and many are not directly applicable or helpful to the radiologist. Although early classifications were based on pathological findings, ones more directly related to imaging findings have been established.[54,55] Cystic renal diseases include the polycystic diseases (infantile, juvenile, and adult), multicystic disease, and solitary cysts. Cysts may be confined to the medulla (medullary sponge

kidney and juvenile nephrophthisis) or may be predominantly cortical in distribution (as seen in tuberous sclerosis and in several of the multiple malformation syndromes and the trisomies). Only the more frequently encountered pediatric cystic renal diseases are included in this chapter.

Although all of the renal cystic diseases can be demonstrated using MRI, ultrasound remains the primary imaging modality for this class of diseases. MRI is most useful in clarifying confusing cases and in demonstrating complications such as hemorrhage.

Simple cysts appear as homogeneous, well-defined masses with clearly defined thin walls on the MR image. If the fluid within the cyst is relatively pure, it will demonstrate low signal intensity on SE and inversion-recovery (IR) T1-weighted sequences.[26,65,84,102] On SE T2-weighted sequences, the signal intensity of cyst fluid ranges from medium to high with progressive T2 weighting.[48] The cyst wall and the fluid within the cyst may be indistinguishable. Small amounts of calcification in the wall of the cyst are not readily identified using MRI, but larger amounts may be seen as a rim of signal void.

When the fluid within a cyst has a high protein content or contains subacute hemorrhage, the cyst may demonstrate inhomogeneous high signal intensity on both T1- and T2-weighted sequences.[57,83,84,94] Despite these guidelines, there is a wide range of variability in the appearance of hemorrhagic cysts, even within the same kidney. In some cases, it is not possible to distinguish a hemorrhagic cyst from an infected cyst or even from a neoplasm when current imaging sequences[48,94] or even T1 and T2 values are used.[94] Some authors have suggested that the presence of a fluid-iron level within a cyst correlates with a diagnosis of benign hemorrhage.[57]

Frequently referred to as *infantile polycystic disease,* autosomal recessive polycystic disease is a congenital abnormality affecting both kidneys. Patients with this condition are of varying ages and demonstrate a spectrum of pathological conditions.[87] Associated liver disease ranges from proliferation and dilatation of the biliary radicles (biliary atresia) to severe periportal fibrosis, and the severity of the renal cystic disease and the hepatic fibrosis varies inversely.[55]

In infants with polycystic disease, the kidneys are greatly enlarged bilaterally. Transection of the kidney shows multiple fusiform cysts formed from dilated tubules. In this group, liver disease is rarely a problem. Polycystic disease seen in later childhood tends to have more severe liver involvement and less severe renal involvement. Patients frequently develop portal hypertension and gastrointestinal bleeding from varices. The renal cysts in these children may have a fusiform appearance similar to that of renal cysts in infants or may have a more rounded contour.[87]

MR images show the massively enlarged kidneys and the fusiform cysts contained within them.[26] On SE T1-weighted images, areas of high signal intensity resulting from subacute hemorrhage within the cysts may be identified.[26]

Adult, or autosomal dominant, polycystic disease may be seen in childhood. In the neonate, it may be difficult to distinguish this condition from infantile polycystic disease because the kidneys appear large and contain multiple small cysts in both entities. As the children become older, the cysts become larger and the more characteristic adult-type appearance develops, with multiple asymmetrically positioned cysts involving both kidneys. MRI demonstrates both the simple cysts and the cysts containing hemorrhage.[57,84]

Multicystic dysplasia is the most common form of renal cystic disease occurring in infants. Both the classic and the hydronephrotic forms are caused by obstruction to the ureter in early intrauterine life. In comparison, obstruction occurring after the formation of the functional kidneys results in the development of hydronephrosis.

MR images demonstrate multiple cysts that may vary greatly in size and are separated by a small amount of dysplastic renal tissue.[25] The classic and hydronephrotic types of multicystic kidney can be distinguished using this modality.[25] In the hydronephrotic type, smaller peripheral cysts can be seen surrounding a larger central cyst. Although usually unilateral, multicystic dysplasia may involve both kidneys, and when it does, the patient dies. Neonates with bilateral involvement will demonstrate the classic features of Potter's syndrome.

Cortical cysts may be seen in tuberous sclerosis and von Hippel-Lindau disease.[125] In addition to renal cysts, the kidneys of children with tuberous sclerosis may contain angiomyolipomas. On T1-weighted images, angiomyolipomas may demonstrate homogeneous medium signal intensity but most also contain areas of high signal intensity because of the presence of lipomatous tissue. On routine T1-weighted images, it may not be possible to distinguish this fatty tissue from hemorrhagic cysts, but on images obtained with fat-suppression techniques the lipomatous tissue will demonstrate lower signal intensity than the adjacent cysts. Phase-contrast imaging may also aid in the differentiation of the two types of lesions.

Lower Urinary Tract

Multiplanar T1-weighted imaging is the most useful sequence in the evaluation of congenital abnormalities of the lower urinary tract in children because it provides superior anatomical resolution and clear depiction of fatty planes.[25] Additional sequences may be useful in selected cases. Since both large- and small-capacity bladders can be seen and the wall thickness of the bladder wall can be demonstrated,[36,95] MRI can identify abnormal findings in children with neurogenic bladders. The main role of MRI in these children, however, is to evaluate the lumbosacral spine for possible dysraphic abnormalities or spinal cord tumors that may be the cause of the neurogenic bladder.

MRI shows abnormal location of the bladder with eversion of its posterior wall, separation of the pubic bones, absence of the rectus abdominis muscles, and anterior displacement of the anus in children with bladder exstrophy (Figure 32-18). Other associated anomalies, such as a bifid clitoris and anterior tilting of the vagina in girls and bilateral inguinal hernias in boys, may also be seen. Although these children have normal upper urinary tracts at birth, after surgical closure of the bladder, vesicoureteral reflux usually occurs. Abnormalities of the upper tract may therefore be seen in older children with previously repaired exstrophy. Epispadias may also be seen with exstrophy of the bladder or

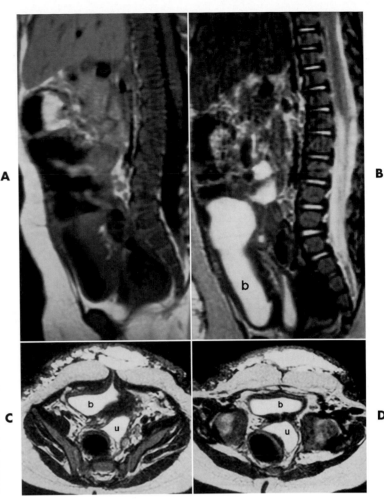

FIGURE 32-12   Cloacal anomaly. **A,** Sagittal (SE 600/12) image. **B** to **D,** Sagittal and axial FSE (3500/102 eff) images show the bladder *(b),* uterus *(u),* and rectum draining into a simple cloaca. The spinal cord is normal.

as an isolated abnormality. In this entity, coronal images obtained at the level of the symphysis pubis demonstrate separation of the corpora cavernosa and displacement of the corpus spongiosum cephalad.[66]

In cloacal malformations, a combination of urinary, genital, and intestinal abnormalities occurs. All three systems drain into a common cloaca.[71] Although these anomalies are usually evaluated using a combination of fluoroscopy with contrast injection and ultrasonography, MRI may be useful to accurately demonstrate the relationship of the pelvic organs to one another before surgery (Figure 32-12).

In prune-belly syndrome, the absence of the abdominal musculature occurs with urinary tract anomalies. Affected children are almost always boys, and two separate groups are identified. In one group an obstructing lesion of the urethra leads to the development of a hypertrophied bladder. In contrast, in the second group a functional abnormality of bladder emptying is present, and the bladder is large and floppy. Severe hydronephrosis and bilateral hydroureter may occur in both groups, and the dilatation of the ureters is frequently disproportionally severe compared to that of the renal pelvises and calyxes. A urachal remnant may also be identified. T1-weighted imaging candemonstrate the entire spectrum of anomalies in children with this disorder.

Genital Tract

MRI is an excellent modality for the evaluation of congenital anomalies of the genital tract. Before the introduction of MRI, diagnostic laparoscopy was often necessary to fully define the abnormal anatomy in patients with such anomalies when other imaging studies proved inconclusive.[64,100]

Congenital anomalies of the genital tract in children are divided into three major groups: (1) disorders of sexual differentiation, (2) müllerian duct anomalies, and (3) aplasia and atresia of the uterus and vagina.

Disorders of Sexual Differentiation. MR images can clearly show the absence or abnormal location of pelvic organs in children with ambiguous genitalia or genetic abnormalities.[46,62] Imaging in both the axial and sagittal planes and with both T1- and T2-weighted sequences is often necessary.

Turner's syndrome is a genetic disorder resulting from complete or partial monosomy of the short arm of the X chromosome. The uterus, cervix, and vagina are always present but are usually hypoplastic, thus demonstrating an infantile configuration. Ovarian anatomy may range from single or (rarely) bilateral normal-appearing ovaries (seen in a small number of patients who menstruate) to bilateral streak ovaries. Both ultrasonography and MRI can clearly define these abnormalities[28] (Figure 32-13). On MRI, streak ovaries are seen as low–signal intensity streaks on both T1- and T2-weighted images. Approximately 4% of patients with Turner's syndrome have 45,XO/46,XY mosaicism. These children are at special risk because they have a 50% chance of developing gonadal neoplasia, particularly gonadoblastoma or dysgerminoma. Because of this possibility, thorough screening of these patients using ultrasound, MRI, or both modalities is essential. When MRI is used, gonadoblastoma appears as an adnexal mass with medium signal intensity on T1-weighted images and high signal intensity on T2-weighted images; thus it has a markedly different appearance from that of streak ovaries.[28,31] The T2-weighted images are particularly important to help define the abnormal tissue and its extent. Associated renal anomalies in children with Turner's syndrome include agenesis, ureteropelvic junction obstruction, ectopia, rotational abnormalities, duplication of the collecting system, and horseshoe kidney.[88]

In 46,XY gonadal dysgenesis, there is failure of testicular differentiation with aberrant gonads and female external genitalia. Female genital ducts are usually present (Figure 32-14).

In children with true hermaphroditism, both ovarian and testicular tissue is present. A uterus is present but may be hypoplastic or unicornuate, and the appearance of the external genitalia ranges from feminine with slight clitoral prominence to fully masculine. MR images obtained in multiple planes can help demonstrate the varied and complex anatomy present in these children.

Pseudohermaphroditism occurs when there is a disturbance in the endocrinological environment of the fetus. Exposure to excessive amounts of androgen in utero leads to varying degrees of masculinization of the external genitalia in children who are genetically female and have normal female internal genitalia. Male pseudohermaphrodites, in contrast, have testes, but the external genitalia are not fully masculin-

ized because of a deficiency of testicular secretions or a failure of target tissues to respond to the secretions elaborated.

Children with testicular feminization have end-organ insensitivity to testosterone. Although they have a male chromosomal pattern of 46,XY, they are phenotypically female. Sagittal MR images show absence of the uterus and cervix, and axial images show primitive gonads either in the adnexal region or in the ectopic position within the inguinal canal. In these patients the vagina ends in a blind pouch.

Müllerian Duct Anomalies. Fusion anomalies of the müllerian ducts are well known.[64] Complete failure of müllerian duct fusion results in the formation of two uteri, two cervixes, and two vaginas (uterus didelphys). Incomplete fusion leads to the development of bicornuate uterus (single vagina and cervix with two uteri) and uterus septus (single vagina, cervix, and uterus with a uterine septum). In children with duplicated systems, one side is occasionally imperforate or obstructed (Figure 32-15).

These uterine abnormalities can frequently be diagnosed and differentiated using MRI, thus avoiding the need for more invasive diagnostic procedures.[16,64,100] MRI is able to differentiate bicornuate and septate uteri in postpubertal girls. This distinction is crucial if surgical intervention is planned. On T2-weighted images in a plane axial to the body of the uterus, a bicornuate uterus will demonstrate a medium–signal intensity strip of myometrium separating the two low–signal intensity junctional zones that the septate uterus will not. MRI can also evaluate the urinary anomalies, such as renal agenesis or renal malposition, that are often associated with müllerian duct anomalies.

Aplasia and Atresia of the Vagina. Absence of both the uterus and the upper vagina is seen in patients with the Mayer-Rokitansky-

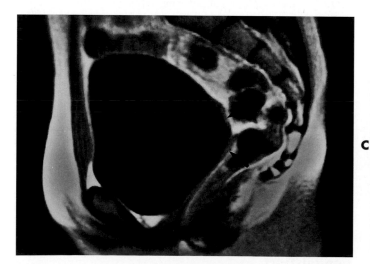

FIGURE 32-13   Turner's syndrome. A hypoplastic uterus and cervix *(arrows)* are present.

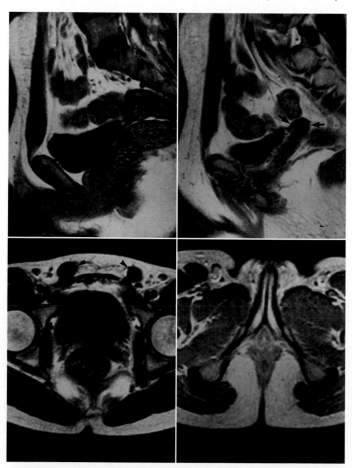

FIGURE 32-14   Mixed gonadal dysgenesis. **A** and **B,** Sagittal (SE 600/20) T1-weighted images demonstrate a phallus and a unicornuate uterus *(arrows* in **B**). **C,** Axial (SE 800/20) image shows bilateral ectopic gonads *(arrowheads).* **D,** Axial (SE 2000/90) image reveals the phallus containing two separate corpora cavernosa.

Küster-Hauser syndrome. Approximately one third of these patients have associated renal anomalies such as unilateral agenesis, malrotation, unilateral or bilateral ectopia, horseshoe kidney, and collecting system abnormalities. Vertebral anomalies have also been reported.[44] Because MRI can be used to evaluate the vagina noninvasively, it is the modality of choice for patients with this disorder as well as for patients with isolated vaginal atresia.[63,68,130,147,151]

In hematometrocolpos, T1- and T2-weighted images can demonstrate a high–signal intensity blood collection within a markedly dilated upper vagina and uterine cavity.[31,147] These dilated structures may compress the adjacent bladder and rectum. The sagittal plane best identifies the location of the fluid collection within the upper vagina and uterine cavity.[25] The fluid collection may extend into the adjoining fallopian tube and a tortuous and dilated, fluid-filled fallopian tube can be seen

extending into the abdomen. In the sagittal plane the undistended lower portion of the vagina may also be identified. In the presence of a müllerian duct anomaly, hematometrocolpos may involve only a portion of the uterine cavity[86] (Figure 32-16).

Undescended Testes. Ultrasonography remains the study of choice in locating the undescended testes, but if it is unsuccessful, then MRI may be performed.[45,77,148] The undescended gonad is usually found in the inguinal canal. If it is positioned within the abdomen or pelvis, it may be located adjacent to the lateral bladder wall, the psoas muscle, or the iliac vessels or in the retroperitoneum or the superficial inguinal pouch. In rare instances the gonad may be prepenile or perineal in position. On T1-weighted images, the ectopic gonad is of medium signal intensity and can frequently be identified if it is surrounded by fat,

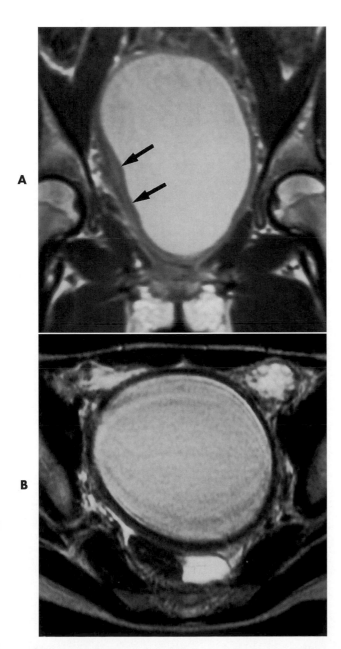

FIGURE 32-15   Hematometros involving one side of a uterus didelphys. **A,** Coronal (SE 600/18) image. High–signal intensity blood products are identified in a markedly distended uterine cavity; a second uterine cavity *(arrows)* with an endometrial stripe is compressed on the right. **B,** Axial (FSE 4000/102 eff) image. The distended left uterine cavity occupies most of the volume of the pelvis, displacing the left ovary anteriorly.

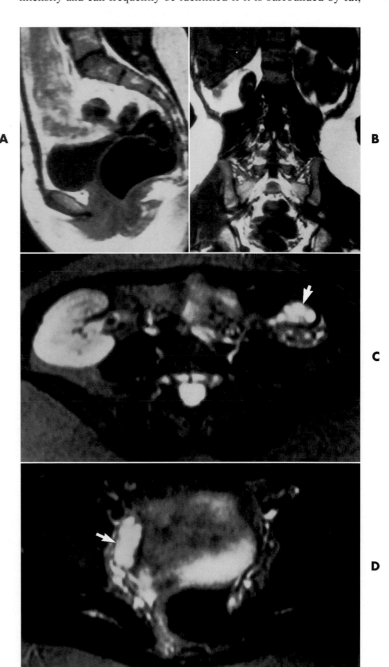

FIGURE 32-16   Mayer-Rokitansky-Kuster-Hauser syndrome. **A,** Sagittal (SE 600/18) image demonstrates a lack of uterus or upper vagina between the bladder and rectum. **B,** Coronal (SE 600/18) image shows absent left and dysplastic right kidneys. **C** and **D,** Axial (SE 2000/9) images show normal right and left ovaries *(arrow)* and a renal transplant.

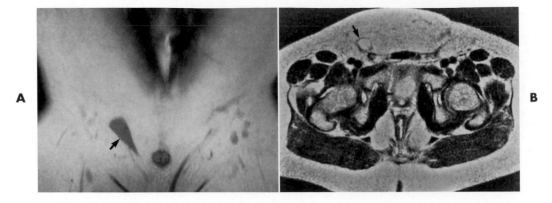

FIGURE 32-17 Undescended testis. **A,** Coronal (SE 300/18) image shows a medium–signal intensity gonad in the inguinal canal *(arrow).* **B,** Axial (SE 1500/60) T2-weighted image demonstrates high signal intensity in the gonad with a medium–signal intensity rim surrounding it *(arrow).*

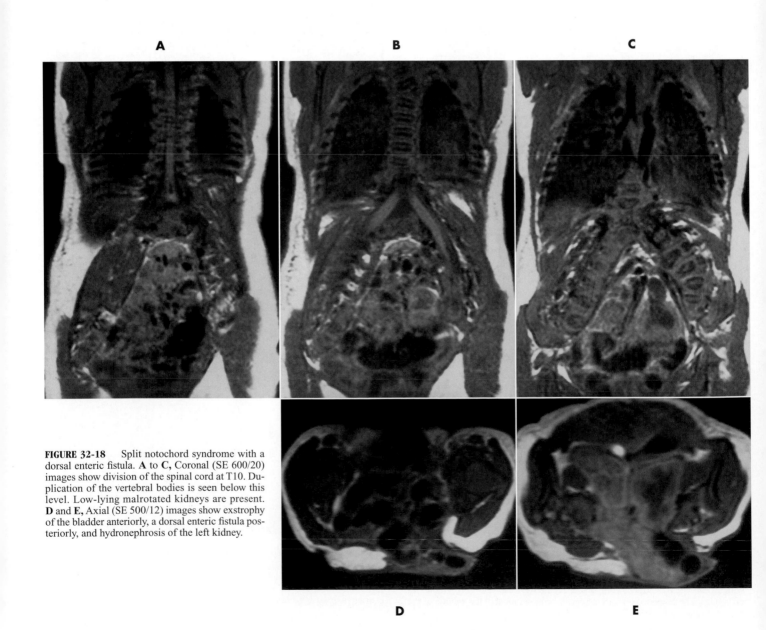

FIGURE 32-18 Split notochord syndrome with a dorsal enteric fistula. **A** to **C,** Coronal (SE 600/20) images show division of the spinal cord at T10. Duplication of the vertebral bodies is seen below this level. Low-lying malrotated kidneys are present. **D** and **E,** Axial (SE 500/12) images show exstrophy of the bladder anteriorly, a dorsal enteric fistula posteriorly, and hydronephrosis of the left kidney.

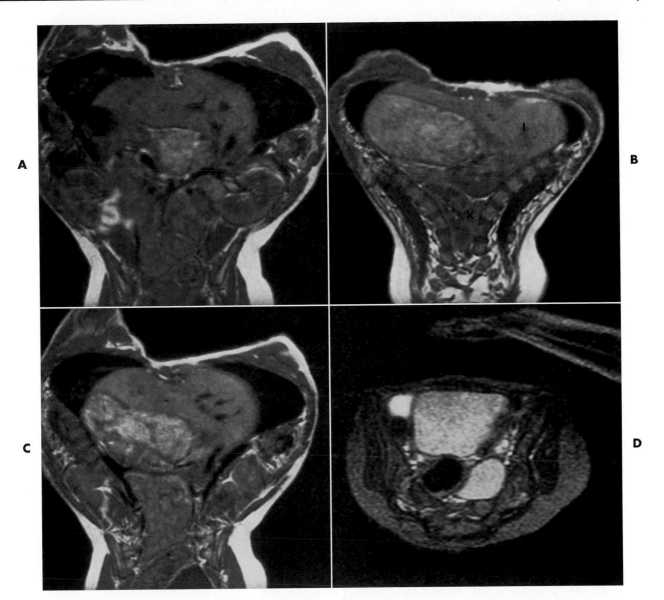

FIGURE 32-19   Conjoined twins. **A** to **C,** Coronal (SE 650/20) images show a single liver *(l)* and single right and left kidneys with a fused third kidney *(k)*. Separate aortas and a joined iliac artery are identified. Separate vertebral columns and spinal cords are seen. **D,** Axial (SE 2000/80) image demonstrates two bladders *(b),* a single uterus *(u),* and a single rectum.

which is of high signal intensity (Figure 32-17). In the search for ectopic gonads, a T2-weighted sequence may add useful information because on such images gonads appear as high–signal intensity structures with a surrounding rim of medium signal intensity and therefore can be easily distinguished from muscles and lymphadenopathy (Figure 32-17). This low–signal intensity rim may be more difficult to see on images obtained at high field strength, on which chemical-shift misregistration is more apparent and may mask the rim.

Anorectal Anomalies

The spectrum of anorectal anomalies includes both imperforate anus and ectopic anus. Both abnormalities result from a failure of descent of the hindgut. In imperforate anus, the rectum terminates in a blind-ending pouch, whereas in ectopic anus, the more common of the two anomalies, there is a fistulous connection between the pouch and another structure such as the perineum, vestibule, vagina, urethra, bladder, or cloaca. Plain-film radiography, contrast fluoroscopy, and ultrasonography have all been helpful in the preoperative evaluation of this group of patients. MRI can noninvasively give a multiplanar view of the hindgut, the puborectalis sling, and the adjacent structures and has been shown to be extremely useful in the evaluation of continuing or re-

current problems in patients after a repair.[96,99,113,124,150] It is less useful in identifying small fistulous tracts[62]; contrast studies performed after decompression colostomy are still necessary to define this anatomy. T1-weighted images in the axial and coronal planes demonstrate the anatomy of the puborectalis sling and can discern whether it is hypoplastic. They can also demonstrate the relationship of the hindgut to the sling. MRI is less useful in children with rectal stenosis and atresia, in which narrowing or complete closure of the rectum is present with a normally formed anus.

Complex Congenital Anomalies

MRI can be extremely useful in the evaluation of complex congenital malformation syndromes. In this group of patients, ultrasonography may be difficult because the routinely used acoustic windows (liver and bladder) may not be present in their usual locations. MRI gives an overview as to the presence or absence of organs and identifies their relationship to one another. The multiple anomalies present can be mapped using SE T1-weighted and FSE T2-weighted images obtained with thin cuts in multiple planes[59,120] (Figures 32-18 and 32-19). Additional modalities may then be used to address specific, more focused questions not answered by the MR examination.

INFECTION AND INFLAMMATION

Children with proven urinary tract infections or with symptoms suggestive of such infections are worked up using a combination of ultrasonography, excretory urography, and nuclear scintigraphy. In this group of patients, MRI should be reserved for the more problematical cases or the cases in which complication develop.

In the evaluation of acute pyelonephritis, the imaging findings are frequently minimal and nonspecific regardless of the modality used. On routine MRI the affected kidney may appear enlarged, and on T1-weighted images the increased water content may cause lower signal intensity and loss of corticomedullary differentiation. Visualization of thickening of the perirenal fascia using MRI has also been described.[4] If the infection affects only part or parts of the kidney, as in acute lobar nephronia and acute focal segmental pyelonephritis, the affected areas may demonstrate lower signal intensity on T1-weighted images than the adjacent normal areas. On T2-weighted images, both normal and abnormal areas may demonstrate similar signal intensity, although infected areas should demonstrate higher signal intensity than the adjacent normal parenchyma if the repetition time is sufficiently long. Recent work using contrast-enhanced fast inversion-recovery and contrast enhanced FSE T2-weighted techniques have shown interesting results in children with acute pyelonephritis.[108] On both of these sequences, normal regions of the kidney show low signal intensity compared to infected, edematous areas, which demonstrate high signal intensity. When these sequences are used, interrenicular septa also appear bright (Figure 32-20).

In children with duplication of the renal collecting system, infection may develop in an obstructed upper-pole moiety. When this occurs, the MR signal intensity of the urine in the obstructed system may vary on T1-weighted images, depending on the protein content of the fluid. A fluid-fluid level may also be seen within the fluid collection on images obtained perpendicular to the dependent plane.

The MR appearance of abscess is variable; the signal intensity of an abscess depends on its content. Abscesses often appear as well-defined mass lesions with fluid centers and thickened irregular walls. At times, fluid-fluid levels or air-fluid levels may be seen within them. Edema may also be identified adjacent to the abscess.[152] After the administration of gadolinium chelates, more information about the internal architecture of the abscess may be gained.[126] Less well-defined areas of infection (phlegma) may be seen as areas of medium signal intensity on T1-weighted images. However, it is usually not possible to distinguish abscess collections from other noninfected fluid collections or from necrotic tumors either from their MR appearance alone or from a measurement of their T1 and T2 values.[14,145,152] Renal abscesses are rare and less commonly seen in children than in adults; pelvic abscesses usually occur in association with an inflammatory process such as appendicitis or inflammatory bowel disease.

TUMORS AND OTHER MASS LESIONS

Because of its multiplanar capability, its ability to distinguish vessels with flowing blood from other structures without the need for bolus injection of contrast material, and its superior contrast resolution compared to CT, MRI is an extremely useful tool in the evaluation of mass lesions, after plain-film radiography in the case of thoracic lesions and ultrasonography in the case of abdominal or pelvic lesions. Multiplanar MRI can be used before surgery to map the tumor. MRI also plays a role in identifying a lesion's organ of origin, characterizing a lesion, defining its extent, evaluating the relationship of the lesion to adjacent vascular structures, and screening for distant metastases. Only when all of these have been addressed is the MR examination complete.

MRI can classify a lesion as cystic, solid, or mixed. Although some solid lesions such as teratomas, lipomas, and hemorrhagic lesions may demonstrate characteristic MR appearances, the majority of solid lesions are impossible to differentiate using only signal intensity. Most solid lesions are of medium signal intensity on T1-weighted images and of high signal intensity on T2-weighted images. However, when the signal characteristics of a lesion are combined with information about its organ of origin, its relationship to adjacent vessels, and its sites of metastasis, a definitive diagnosis can often be made. MRI can be used before treatment to plan a surgical approach or a radiation port and after treatment to assess for residual or recurrent tumor after surgery, chemotherapy, or radiation therapy. Gadolinium-chelate contrast agents may be useful in characterizing masses.[32] In these instances, T1-weighted images obtained dynamically during and immediately after intravenous contrast administration may more clearly define the borders of the lesion, characterize its internal architecture, accentuate surrounding adenopathy, and uniquely define the histology of the lesion.

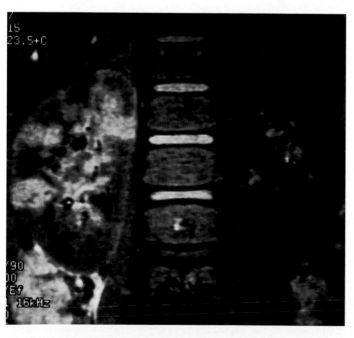

FIGURE 32-20   Pyelonephritis. Coronal (IR 2000/90/17 eff) image after gadolinium contrast. Normally perfused kidney tissue appears dark. Areas of high signal intensity represent underperfused, edematous foci of pyelonephritis. (Courtesy G. Lonergan and D. Pennington, San Antonio.)

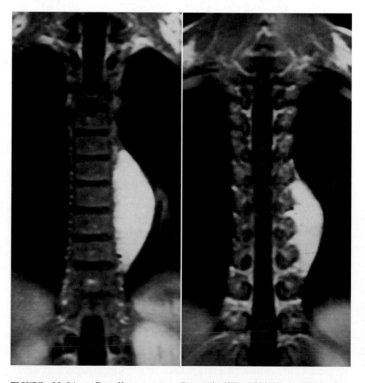

FIGURE 32-21   Ganglioneuroma. Coronal (SE 580/11) images after gadolinium-chelate infusion show a left paraspinal mass with homogeneous enhancement extending into the multiple neural foramens that do not compress the dural sac.

Thorax

MRI is particularly useful in the evaluation of lesions arising in the posterior mediastinum because it may noninvasively demonstrate the presence or absence of intraspinal extension.[27,133] These posterior mediastinal masses are most frequently of neurogenic origin and include entities such as neuroblastomas, ganglioneuroma, and neurofibroma (Figure 32-21). Because they are all of medium signal intensity on T1-weighted images and of high signal intensity on T2-weighted images, they cannot be distinguished from one another using MR signal characteristics alone. Coronal and axial images are useful in demonstrating any intraspinal extension and in clarifying the relationship of the lesion to adjacent vasculature. MR angiography may be used to further assess vascular patency when routine MR images are equivocal.

MRI can also demonstrate lesions in the anterior and middle compartments of the mediastinum and may even have a slight edge over CT in selected cases.[73,101,131,132,135] For example, coronal and sagittal images may help define the extent of neck masses that secondarily involve the mediastinum or lung apices.[29] Multiplanar MRI may also better define the subcarinal area.[111] Fat-selective sequences may also be helpful in distinguishing mediastinal teratomas from other mass lesions (Figure 32-22). In addition, as with posterior compartment masses, MRI may help clarify the relationship of the lesion to adjacent vessels and other structures because of its multiplanar capability, its ability to distinguish vessels with flowing blood from other structures without the need for bolus injection of contrast material, and its superior contrast resolution.

MRI may be useful in the evaluation and staging of all types of lymphoma.[58,106] Lymphomas are classified as either Hodgkin's disease or non-Hodgkin's lymphoma. The latter is more common in young children and includes small noncleaved cell, lymphoblastic, and large cell lymphoma.[97] In the mediastinum, enlarged lymph nodes are easily seen because they are adjacent to low–signal intensity blood vessels and lung parenchyma. Nodes involved with lymphoma demonstrate homogeneous medium signal intensity on T1-weighted images and high signal intensity on T2-weighted images. Unfortunately, neoplastic nodes cannot be distinguished based on MR signal characteristics from inflammatory nodes seen in infectious disorders.[19,106,107] MRI may be helpful in distinguishing residual lymphoma, which demonstrates high signal intensity, from fibrosis, which demonstrates low signal intensity on T2-weighted images.[49]

Abdomen

In the abdomen, MRI is an excellent modality with which to differentiate masses arising from the liver, kidney, adrenal gland, and paraspinal region.

Liver. The most important role of MRI in examination of the liver is in the diagnosis of hepatic neoplasms, the definition of their exact extent, and the assessment of their possible resectability.[11,34,112,114,155]

Children with hemangioendotheliomas, the most common benign hepatic tumor of childhood, present with an abdominal mass or congestive heart failure because of high-output overcirculation. MRI can often demonstrate a well-defined solitary mass in the liver and may identify the feeding and draining vessels. An abrupt caliber decrease in the abdominal aorta distal to the origin of the celiac axis may also be observed. Dynamic imaging after gadolinium-chelate administration can often uniquely identify this hepatic lesion as a hemangioendothelioma because of its distinctive temporal pattern of peripheral to central enhancement. In larger lesions the center of the lesion will frequently contain hemorrhage or fibrosis, preventing uniform contrast enhancement of this area. If the study includes the lower thorax, cardiomegaly or pulmonary edema resulting from the left-to-right shunting associated with this tumor may be identified. Hemangioendotheliomas may occasionally be multifocal. Whether single or multiple, they usually regress with time. In children who have respiratory compromise, chemotherapy or radiation may be given to shrink the size of the tumor or tumors.

Hepatoblastoma and hepatocellular carcinoma are the most common malignant hepatic neoplasms seen in the pediatric population (Figure 32-23). Hepatoblastoma typically is seen in children younger than 3 years of age, whereas hepatocellular carcinoma is most often seen in children older than 3 years. Hepatocellular carcinoma is seen in association with chronic liver diseases such as hepatitis, tyrosinemia, and

α_1-antitrypsin deficiency. Most frequently, affected children have an abdominal mass, weight loss, and fever. Serum α-fetoprotein levels are often elevated. Both lesions generally appear as a single mass lesion; less frequently, these tumors can be multifocal or can diffusely replace hepatic parenchyma. They demonstrate variable signal intensity on T1- and T2-weighted MR images. MRI can be used to assess for vascular invasion by the tumor and can also define the extent of the tumor with respect to the segmental anatomy of the liver, thus aiding in determining resectability of the lesion.[39] Metastatic lesions may be seen in the lymph nodes, lungs, skeleton, and brain.

Less commonly seen primary hepatic lesions include cystic mesenchymal hamartomas,[123,138] lipomas,[11] and lymphoma. Mesenchymal hamartomas are well-circumscribed masses containing multiple cystic spaces separated by fibrous septa.[123] They usually are seen as abdominal masses in children younger than 2 years of age. On T2-weighted images the cystic areas are of high signal intensity and the intervening septa are of low signal intensity. Lipomas may be identified by their characteristic signal intensities, which parallel those of the subcutaneous fat on all sequences. Evaluation of lymphomatous involvement of the liver using MRI has been disappointing. Although localized involvement may be identified in some cases, diffuse involvement is more difficult to appreciate.[19,154] Administration of iron oxide particle contrast agents may aid in the detection of lymphoma involving both the liver and spleen in adults but has not been widely used in children.[110]

In children as in adults, liver metastases can be well visualized using MRI. These can be optimally visualized using either T1-weighted images with short repetition times and echo times or T2-weighted images with long repetition times and echo times, depending on the field strength of the magnet used.[81,117,140] Because the livers of young children have higher T1- and T2-weighted values compared to those of adults, the use of more heavily weighted T2 sequences may be required in this population. In this group, liver metastases are most often caused by neuroblastoma, Wilms' tumor, and rhabdomyosarcoma.

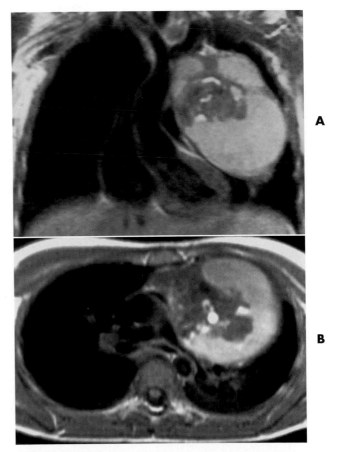

FIGURE 32-22   Mediastinal teratoma. **A,** Coronal and axial (SE 625/11) images. A mediastinal mass is identified with locules of differing signal intensity; a few small foci of bright signal intensity resulting from fat are noted within the mass. **B,** Axial (SE 2000/90) image. The foci of fat have low signal intensity.

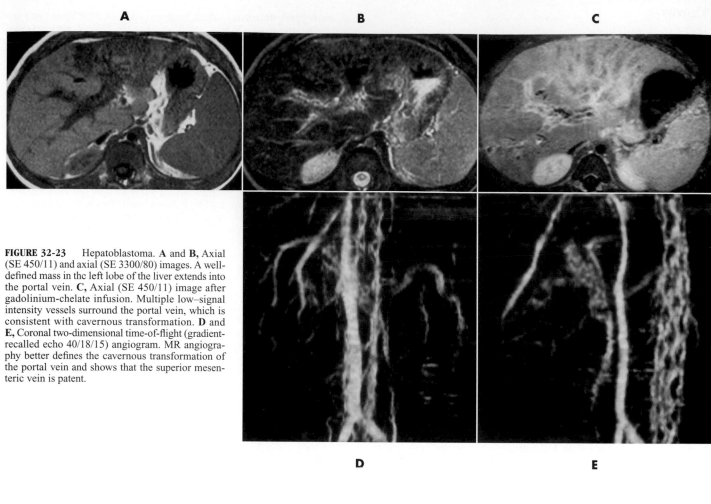

FIGURE 32-23 Hepatoblastoma. **A** and **B,** Axial (SE 450/11) and axial (SE 3300/80) images. A well-defined mass in the left lobe of the liver extends into the portal vein. **C,** Axial (SE 450/11) image after gadolinium-chelate infusion. Multiple low–signal intensity vessels surround the portal vein, which is consistent with cavernous transformation. **D** and **E,** Coronal two-dimensional time-of-flight (gradient-recalled echo 40/18/15) angiogram. MR angiography better defines the cavernous transformation of the portal vein and shows that the superior mesenteric vein is patent.

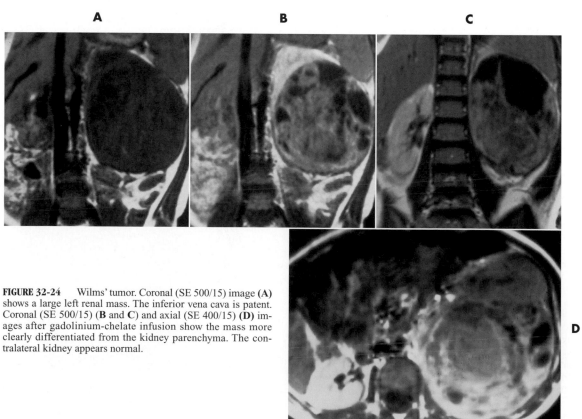

FIGURE 32-24 Wilms' tumor. Coronal (SE 500/15) image **(A)** shows a large left renal mass. The inferior vena cava is patent. Coronal (SE 500/15) **(B** and **C)** and axial (SE 400/15) **(D)** images after gadolinium-chelate infusion show the mass more clearly differentiated from the kidney parenchyma. The contralateral kidney appears normal.

Kidney. The renal neoplasms that occur commonly in children include Wilms' tumor and the various forms of leukemia and lymphoma. Less frequently, renal cell carcinoma, teratoma, clear cell sarcoma, and rhabdoid tumor may be seen. In infants, congenital mesoblastic nephroma can also occur. Most frequently, renal neoplasms demonstrate high signal intensity on T2-weighted images but may be hypointense, isointense, or hyperintense to normal kidney on T1-weighted images.

Wilms' tumor. Wilms' tumor is the most common primary renal neoplasm in children, comprising 95% of cancers affecting the kidney, ureter, and bladder in children under 16.[157] Of these, 90% occur in children younger than 7 years of age, and there is a peak incidence between the ages of 1 and 3. There is also an increased incidence in children with aniridia, hemihypertrophy, genitourinary anomalies, and the Beckwith-Wiedemann syndrome.

Although bilateral tumor involvement is said to occur in approximately 5% to10% of cases of Wilms' tumor, affected children most frequently have a unilateral abdominal mass. Less frequently, children have vague abdominal pain or hematuria. The initial diagnosis is usually made using ultrasonography, which demonstrates a solid mass arising from the kidney. MRI has been shown to be superior to ultrasound and superior or equal to x-ray CT in diagnosing and defining the extent of Wilms' tumor.[5,69,74,153] In this area of the body, coronal T1-weighted images define a lesion's organ of origin and can often separate renal lesions from those arising in the adjacent liver or adrenal gland (Figure 32-24). A combination of T1- and T2-weighted sequences can help define the full extent of the lesion, assess for possible invasion of adjacent organs, and document the presence or absence of associated lymphadenopathy.

The demonstration of the exact margins of a lesion and the identification of any associated adenopathy may be aided through the use of gadolinium chelates. Immediately after the administration of gadolinium chelates, T1-weighted images of the kidney will display corticomedullary differentiation during the early nephrogram phase, but the tumor will be of lower signal intensity. This effect will be especially dramatic on sequential T1-weighted images obtained immediately after administration of gadolinium chelates when a fast dynamic imaging technique is used. On later images, both the kidney and the tumor will have high signal intensity, but the kidney will appear homogeneous, and Wilms' tumor will have an inhomogeneous appearance. Because MRI so clearly defines patent vascular structures, it is extremely useful in demonstrating the presence of tumor thrombus within the renal veins or inferior vena cava, which may be seen in association with Wilms' tumor.[5,20,74] Wilms' tumors may also displace the abdominal aorta, inferior vena cava, or both structures. The direction of displacement and the position of the displaced vessels can be well identified before surgery using MRI, aiding in the planning of the surgical resection of the tumor.[20,121]

Although CT is the modality of choice for the evaluation of lung metastases, Wilms' tumor metastatic to the lung can be appreciated using MRI. These metastases appear as focal regions of high signal intensity against the background of normal low–signal intensity lung tissue. MRI is also a tool for the evaluation of residual or recurrent disease after treatment with chemotherapy or surgical resection.

Nephroblastomatosis. In newborns, small rests of primitive renal parenchyma known as *nephrogenic blastema* are often present within the kidney. These rests usually regress by 4 months of age. In a small number of cases, however, regression does not occur, and the remaining rests have a propensity to develop into Wilms' tumor. Both kidneys are usually affected, and these children frequently have bilateral renal masses. In patients with nodular nephroblastomatosis showing as a unilateral mass, the contralateral kidney should always be very carefully examined. On gross inspection the kidneys are enlarged and lobulated. Enlargement of the kidneys, together with marked distortion and elongation of the pelvocalyceal system, can be seen using MRI. After the administration of gadolinium chelates, rests in nephroblastomatosis do not enhance or enhance only minimally and homogeneously[50] (Figure 32-25). This degree of enhancement is different from that of Wilms' tumor, which demonstrates a more intense heterogeneous enhancement.

Leukemia and lymphoma. Both leukemia and lymphoma may involve the kidney through infiltration of its interstitium with tumor cells. In acute leukemia, involvement is usually diffuse, causing generalized enlargement of the kidneys. In lymphoma, which is most commonly of the non-Hodgkin's type, although diffuse involvement may be seen, involvement is often more focal, appearing as multiple nodules or even as a solitary mass within the kidney. MRI can demonstrate the enlarged kidneys and can identify diffuse or focal disease in both of these entities. Focal disease will appear as one or more masses that are isointense or slightly hypointense compared to the renal parenchyma on SE T1-weighted sequences. Loss of corticomedullary differentiation can also be seen in the involved areas. On T2-weighted sequences the masses are usually of lower signal intensity than the adjacent high-signal intensity normal renal tissue. Involvement of the adjacent vertebral or pelvic bone marrow can also frequently be identified, thus helping differentiate lymphoma from Wilms' tumor because Wilms' tumor rarely metastasizes to the bone marrow.

Adrenal Gland
Neuroblastoma. Neuroblastoma is the most common extracranial solid neoplasm in childhood. Neuroblastoma and its more differentiated forms, ganglioneuroblastoma and ganglioneuroma, arise from primitive sympathetic neuroblasts and may arise from the adrenal gland (most commonly) or from anywhere along the sympathetic chain from the nasopharynx to the presacral region (Figure 32-26). Children with neuroblastoma are seen between 1 and 5 years of age. They may have a palpable abdominal mass or may have symptoms caused by either metastases (such as bone pain) or a paraneoplastic syndrome. The staging of neuroblastoma is based on both the local extent of the tumor and the presence or absence of metastases. Clinically, however, it is more important to determine whether the lesion is operable or inoperable because surgery is the treatment of choice. On MRI, neuroblastoma is usually of medium signal intensity on T1-weighted images and of high signal intensity on T2-weighted images and is less well defined than Wilms' tumor.[18,30,42,127] After gadolinium-chelate administration, neurofibroma most frequently demonstrates moderate inhomogeneous enhancement.[32] If it arises from the adrenal gland, it can displace the kidney inferiorly and laterally. The role of MRI in the evaluation of children with neuroblastoma includes identifying the lesion's organ of origin, defining its extent and its relationship to adjacent vessels, and evaluating the child for the presence of metastasis to the liver, bone marrow, or cortex of bone. The lesion is inoperable if it extends into the spinal canal or around the retroperitoneal vessels (Figure 32-26).

Adrenal hemorrhage. The spectrum of adrenal hemorrhage occurring in the perinatal period is wide, ranging in severity from focal involvement of a portion of one adrenal gland to diffuse involvement of both adrenal glands. When hemorrhage is unilateral, the right adrenal gland is the one more frequently affected, reportedly accounting for 70% of lesions.[72] The specific cause of adrenal hemorrhage is unclear, however, and this entity has been associated with traumatic delivery, sepsis, bradycardia, asphyxia, and liver transplantation. There is also an increased incidence of adrenal hemorrhage in children born to diabetic mothers. Affected children have flank masses, jaundice, and anemia. Rarely, when bleeding is severe, hypotension and shock may occur.

Differentiation of neonatal adrenal hemorrhage from neuroblastoma is crucial. In the majority of cases, differentiation of the two entities using ultrasound or MRI is simple. On ultrasonography neonatal adrenal hemorrhage is usually anechoic and avascular in contradistinc-

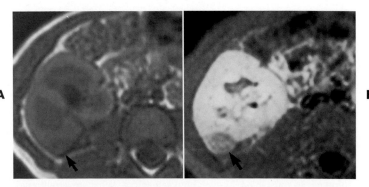

FIGURE 32-25   Nephroblastomatosis. **A,** Axial (SE 500/35) image shows small rests peripherally in the right kidney. **B,** Axial (SE 500/30) image after gadolinium-chelate infusion shows a mild homogeneous enhancement of the rests.

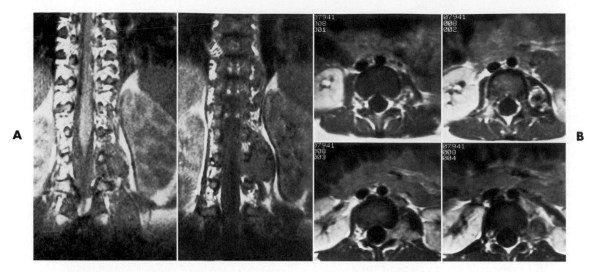

FIGURE 32-26   Neuroblastoma. Coronal (SE 500/20) **(A)** and axial (SE 800/20) **(B)** images after the administration of gadolinium diethylene-triamine-pentaacetic acid. A left paraspinal mass involves the psoas muscle and is extending into the intravertebral foramen and abutting the thecal sac. (Courtesy P. Perry, Morristown, Tennessee.)

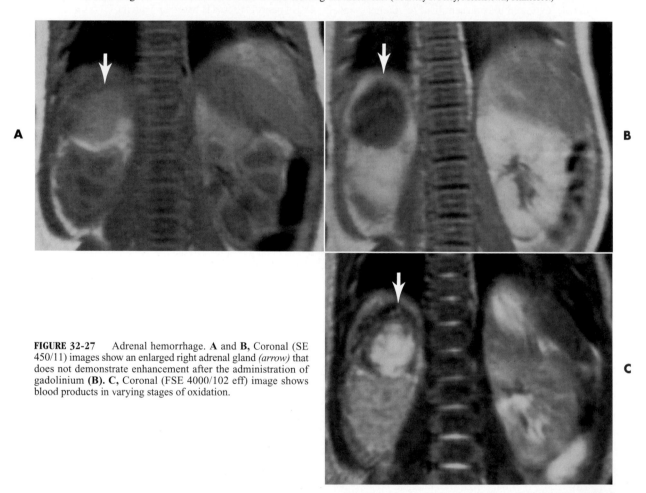

FIGURE 32-27   Adrenal hemorrhage. **A** and **B,** Coronal (SE 450/11) images show an enlarged right adrenal gland *(arrow)* that does not demonstrate enhancement after the administration of gadolinium **(B). C,** Coronal (FSE 4000/102 eff) image shows blood products in varying stages of oxidation.

tion to neuroblastoma, which is usually echogenic and vascular. In some instances, however, adrenal hemorrhage does not appear cystic on ultrasonography, and MRI may be extremely useful in helping make this distinction. The MR appearance of adrenal hemorrhage[25] is similar to that of hematomas seen elsewhere in the body; evolution with time results in a changing MR appearance.[51,149] Whereas acute hematomas are isointense to muscle on T1-weighted sequences, subacute hematomas demonstrate high signal intensity on these sequences. Adrenal hemorrhage does not enhance after the administration of gadolinium chelates (Figure 32-27). Neuroblastoma, in contrast, usually demonstrates

medium homogeneous signal intensity on T1-weighted images, high signal intensity on T2-weighted images, and heterogenous enhancement. Problems of characterization occur in the rare cases of cystic neuroblastoma that contain significant hemorrhage and therefore can demonstrate an appearance identical to that of adrenal hemorrhage in its subacute phase. Careful examination of the liver may be helpful in differentiating these two entities. Children with neuroblastoma at birth frequently also have multiple metastases to the liver. Metastases within the liver appear as low–signal intensity lesions on T1-weighted images obtained with very short repetition and echo times and as high–signal

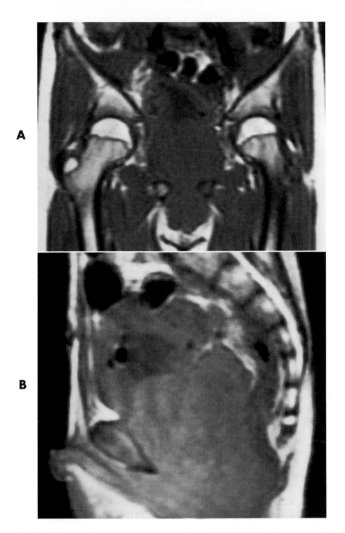

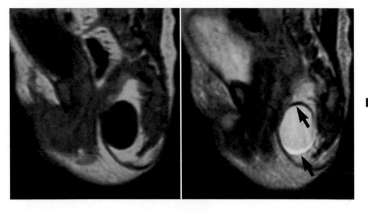

FIGURE 32-29   Presacral teratoma. **A,** Sagittal (SE 800/23) image shows presacral mass with components that are hypointense, isointense, and hyperintense to muscle. **B,** Sagittal (FSE 3000/102 eff) view shows chemical-shift spatial misregistration, which verifies the presence of fat *(arrows);* thus lipid-selective presaturation pulses are not necessary to characterize the lesion.

tion of inferior, lateral, or posterior extension of tumors arising in this region. As with the MR appearance of most neoplasms the MR appearance of this lesion is nonspecific, consisting of a solid mass with medium signal intensity on T1-weighted images, high signal intensity on T2-weighted images,[25] and inhomogeneous enhancement after contrast administration.[32]

Sacrococcygeal Teratoma. Teratomas contain derivatives of all three germinal layers. In young children, teratomas are most commonly found in the presacral region. These are most frequently present at birth when a buttock or perineal mass lesion is identified. However, those that are predominantly internal may not be found until later in childhood, when pressure effects on adjacent structures lead to the development of symptoms. Although the majority of these lesions are benign, some, particularly those in older children, can undergo malignant change. The MR appearance of a teratoma is characteristic: T1- and T2-weighted images demonstrate a large mass containing rounded, well-defined areas of varying signal intensity representing its cystic, solid, and sometimes calcified components. Teratomas frequently displace or distort the overlying sacrum without invading it (Figure 32-29). Sacrococcygeal teratomas can be easily distinguished from lesions arising in the pelvic cavity because like all presacral lesions, they displace the adjacent rectum anteriorly. The differential diagnosis of a mass in this region in a child includes anterior meningocele, rectal duplication, neuroblastoma, and lymphoma.

Ovarian Tumors. Ovarian tumors are uncommon in the pediatric population, especially in children younger than 5 years of age. In older children the most frequent sign is pain, whereas in younger children the more frequent sign is an abdominal mass. In children as in adults, the tumors may be of surface epithelial origin (adenomas and adenocarcinomas), germ cell origin (teratomas, dysgerminomas, and gonadoblastomas), or metastatic origin (lymphomas, leukemia, and neuroblastomas).

Like other imaging modalities, MRI is not always able to give a definitive diagnosis of the type of ovarian tumor present, but it can identify the lesion as cystic, solid, or mixed in nature, narrowing the differential diagnosis.[33,56,61] In cases of ovarian teratoma, however, the MR appearance is characteristic; well-defined smooth areas of differing signal intensities within the lesion are caused by areas of fat, solid tumor, and cysts containing proteinaceous fluid.[144,146] Areas of signal void within the lesions usually represent areas of calcification. In malignant teratomas, metastatic deposits involving the mesentery may be seen in association with liver metastases. The differential diagnosis of a cystic lesion involving the ovary includes ovarian cyst, abscess, cystadenoma, and cystadenocarcinoma. When a large, septated, cystic lesion is seen, cystadenoma or cystadenocarcinoma is the most likely diagnosis (Figure 32-30).

Dysgerminomas, granulosa cell tumors, and embryonal carcinomas are the most frequently seen solid ovarian neoplasms of childhood. On MRI, they are of homogeneous medium signal intensity on T1-weighted images and of high signal intensity on T2-weighted images.

FIGURE 32-28   Rhabdomyosarcoma. Coronal (SE 500/20) **(A)** and sagittal (SE 800/20) **(B)** gadolinium-chelate images show a mass arising from the prostate, filling the pelvis, and invading the bladder. The mass shows moderate enhancement.

intensity lesions on T2-weighted images, and they should not be present in children with adrenal hemorrhage. If focal areas of hemorrhage are seen within the liver in patients with adrenal hemorrhage, these areas should demonstrate the same signal intensity as the adrenal hemorrhage on every pulse sequence, differentiating them from metastases.

Pelvis

Rhabdomyosarcoma. Rhabdomyosarcoma is the most common tumor of the lower urinary tract in children. It may arise from the bladder, urethra, or prostate.[157] It occurs more commonly in boys than in girls and has peak incidences in patients younger than 4 years of age and between 15 and 19 years of age. Children with rhabdomyosarcoma have urinary retention or less commonly, hematuria. Bladder lesions most commonly arise from the submucosa of the trigone or the bladder base and then infiltrate the bladder wall, spreading to adjacent tissues. In girls, invasion of the vagina and uterus may occur. Because of this tumor's propensity for local invasion, it can be difficult to determine whether the primary site was the bladder or the vagina in female patients or the bladder or the prostate in male patients. Prostatic rhabdomyosarcoma tends to infiltrate the bladder neck, posterior urethra, and perirectal tissues early in its course, and tumor arising in this organ is more likely to metastasize distally.

The multiplanar capabilities of MRI are extremely useful in the evaluation of children with rhabdomyosarcoma[25,41] (Figure 32-28). MRI can clearly demonstrate thickening of the bladder wall in patients with bladder neoplasms,[38,119] and use of the sagittal and coronal planes is particularly helpful for evaluation of the bladder base and demonstra-

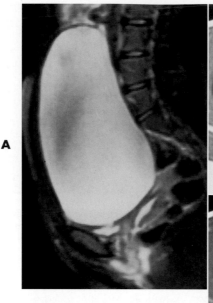

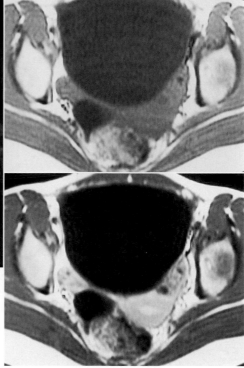

FIGURE 32-30 Cystadenoma. **A,** Sagittal (SE 2100/70) image shows a large cystic mass compressing the bladder and uterus inferiorly. **B** and **C,** Axial (SE 300/12) images before and after gadolinium-chelate infusion show normal enhancement of the endometrium and ovaries but no enhancement of the mass.

MISCELLANEOUS
Chronic Liver Disease

In children with generalized parenchymal liver disease, MRI may demonstrate a small shrunken liver, but in most cases, it cannot determine the cause.[141] Diseases in which deposition of substances within the liver leads to a change in signal intensity of the organ are the exception. These diseases include hemochromatosis and hemosiderosis,[13,104,115,136] in which deposition of iron leads to a reduction in the T2 relaxation time and in which the signal intensity of the liver is diffusely reduced on both T1- and T2-weighted SE sequences. In patients with hemochromatosis, iron is deposited primarily in the hepatocytes and the pancreatic parenchyma, leading to decreased signal intensity in the liver and the pancreas but not the spleen. In patients with hemosiderosis, on the other hand, iron deposition occurs primarily in the reticuloendothelial cells, causing decreased signal intensity in the liver and spleen.[136]

Fatty infiltration of the liver may be focal or diffuse. It represents a nonspecific response and may be seen in patients with cystic fibrosis, Cushing's disease, or malnutrition or in patients undergoing chemotherapy or hyperalimentation. It is best seen using fat-suppression techniques.[85] Occasionally, focal areas of fat may be seen within the liver on T1-weighted images. A high signal intensity of the liver on T1-weighted images resulting from lipid deposition, in conjunction with large adrenal glands, may be seen in Wolman's disease.

In children who are candidates for liver transplantation or shunt procedures, MRI can obviate the need for angiography by documenting the patency of the portal vein and other venous structures, identifying vascular anatomical variants and demonstrating the presence and location of collateral vessels.[7,24,35] MRI may also be useful after liver transplantation for assessment of complications.

SUMMARY

Clearly, significant advances have been made since the first reports of pediatric MRI appeared in the literature in the early 1980s. MRI has now proved itself a vital tool in the evaluation of a wide range of abnormalities seen in infants and children. As MRI technology improves and new contrast agents are developed, the indication for MRI in pediatrics should continue to evolve.

REFERENCES

1. Ahn SS, et al: Rapid MR imaging of the pediatric brain using the fast spin-echo technique, Am J Neuroradiol 13:1169, 1992.
2. Alexander MC, and Haaga JR: MR imaging of a choledochal cyst, J Comput Assist Tomogr 92:357, 1985.
3. American Academy of Pediatrics, Committee on Drugs: Guidelines for monitoring and management of pediatric patients during and after diagnostic and therapeutic procedures, Pediatrics 89:1110, 1992
4. Baumgartner B, et al: Kidneys. In Stark DD, and Bradley WG Jr, eds: Magnetic resonance imaging, ed 2, St Louis, 1992, Mosby.
5. Belt TG, et al: MRI of Wilms', tumor: promise as the primary imaging method, Am J Roentgenol 146:955, 1986.
6. Bissett GS, and Ball WS: Preparation, sedation and monitoring of the pediatric patient in the magnetic resonance suite, Semin US CT MR 12:376, 1991.
7. Bisset GS, Strife JL, and Balistreri WF: Evaluation of children for liver transplantation: value of MR imaging and sonography, Am J Roentgenol 155:351, 1990.
8. Bisset GS, et al: Vascular rings: MR imaging, Am J Roentgenol 149:251, 1987.
9. Bisset GS, et al: Evaluation of potential practical oral contrast agents for pediatric magnetic resonance imaging: preliminary observations, Pediatr Radiol 20:61, 1989.
10. Bisset GS, et al: Perflubron as a gastrointestinal MR imaging contrast agent in the pediatric population, Pediatr Radiol 26:409, 1996.
11. Boechat MI, et al: Primary liver tumors in children: comparison of CT and MR imaging, Radiology 169:727, 1988.
12. Brasch, et al: Magnetic resonance imaging of the chest in childhood, Radiology 150:463, 1984.
13. Brasch RC, et al: Magnetic resonance imaging of transfusional hemosiderosis complicating thalassemia, Radiology 150:767, 1984.
14. Brown JJ, et al: Magnetic resonance relaxation times of percutaneously obtained normal and abnormal body fluids, Radiology 154:727, 1985.
15. Burckart G, et al: Rectal thiopental versus an intramuscular cocktail for sedating children before computerized tomography, Am J Hosp Pharm 37:222, 1980.
16. Carrington MB, et al: Müllerian duct anomalies: MR imaging evaluation, Radiology 176:715, 1990.
17. Cohen EK, et al: MR imaging of soft tissue hemangiomas: correlation with pathologic findings, Am J Roentgenol 150:1079, 1988.
18. Cohen MD, et al: Magnetic resonance imaging of neuroblastoma with a 0.15-T magnet, Am J Roentgenol 143:1241, 1984.
19. Cohen MD, et al: Magnetic resonance imaging of lymphomas in children, Pediatr Radiol 15:179, 1985.
20. Cohen MD, et al: Visualization of major blood vessels by magnetic resonance imaging in children with malignant tumors, Radiographics 5:441, 1985.
21. Crooks LE, et al: Echo-planar pediatric imager, Radiology 166:157, 1988.
22. Daneman A: Disappearing suprarenal masses in the fetus and neonate, Proceedings of 40th annual meeting of the Society for Pediatric Radiology, 1997.
23. Daneman A, and Alton DJ: Radiographic manifestations of renal anomalies, Radiol Clin North Am 29:351, 1991.

24. Day LD, et al: MR evaluation of the portal vein in pediatric liver transplant candidates, Am J Roentgenol 147:1027, 1986.

25. Dietrich RB: Genitourinary system. In Cohen MD, and Edwards MK, eds: Magnetic resonance imaging of children, Philadelphia, 1989, BC Decker.

26. Dietrich RB, and Kangarloo H: Kidneys in infants and children: evaluation with MR, Radiology 159:215, 1986.

27. Dietrich RB, and Kangarloo H: Retroperitoneal mass with intradural extension: value of magnetic resonance imaging in neuroblastoma, Am J Roentgenol 146:251, 1986.

28. Dietrich RB, et al: Role of ultrasonography and magnetic resonance imaging of the Turner syndrome, Radiology 157(P):40, 1985.

29. Dietrich RB, et al: Head and neck MR imaging in the pediatric patient, Radiology 159:769, 1986.

30. Dietrich RB, et al: Neuroblastoma: the role of MR imaging, Am J Roentgenol 148:937, 1987.

31. Dietrich RB, et al: Pelvic abnormalities in children: assessment with MR imaging, Radiology 163:367, 1987.

32. Dietrich RB, et al: MRI of extracranial masses in children: the usefulness of gadolinium-chelate enhancement, Pediatr Radiol 28:322, 1998..

33. Dooms GC, Hricak H, and Tscholakoff D: Adnexal structures: MR imaging, Radiology 158:639, 1986.

34. Finn JP, et al: Primary malignant liver tumors in childhood: assessment of resectability with high-field MR and comparison with CT, Pediatr Radiol 21:34, 1990.

35. Finn JP, et al: Liver transplantation: MR angiography with surgical validation, Radiology 179:265, 1991.

36. Fisher MR, Hricak H, and Crooks LE: Urinary bladder MR imaging. I. Normal and benign conditions, Radiology 157:467, 1985.

37. Fisher MR, Hricak H, and Higgins CB: Magnetic resonance imaging of developmental venous anomalies, Am J Roentgenol 145:705, 1985.

38. Fisher MR, Hricak H, and Tanagho EA: Urinary bladder MR imaging. II. Radiology 157:471, 1985.

39. Fisher MR, et al: Hepatic vascular anatomy on magnetic resonance imaging, Am J Roentgenol 144:739, 1985.

40. Fletcher BD, Dorr GB, and Mulopulos GP: MR imaging in infants with airway obstruction: preliminary observations, Radiology 160:245, 1986.

41. Fletcher BD, and Kaste SC: Rhabdomyosarcoma, Urol Radiol 14:263, 1992.

42. Fletcher BD, et al: Abdominal neuroblastoma: magnetic resonance imaging and tissue characterization, Radiology 155:699, 1985.

43. Fletcher BD, et al: MRI of congenital anomalies of the great arteries, Am J Roentgenol 146:941, 1986.

44. Fore SR, et al: Urologic and genital anomalies in patients with congenital absence of the vagina, Am J Obstet Gynecol 46:410, 1975.

45. Fritzsche PJ, et al: Undescended testis: value of MR imaging, Radiology 164:169, 1987.

46. Gambino J: Congenital disorders of sexual differentiation: MR findings, Am J Roentgenol 158:383, 1992.

47. Gelinek J, et al: Evaluation of lipomatous soft-tissue tumors by MR imaging, Acta Radiol 35:367, 1994.

48. Glazer GM: MR imaging of the liver, kidneys, and adrenal glands, Radiology 166:303, 1988.

49. Glazer HS, et al: Radiation fibrosis: differentiation from recurrent tumor by MR imaging, Radiology 156:721, 1985.

50. Gylys-Morin V, et al: Wilms' tumor and nephroblastomatosis: imaging characteristics at gadolinium-enhanced MR imaging, Radiology 188:517, 1993.

51. Hahn PF, et al: Intraabdominal hematoma: the concentric-ring sign in MR imaging, Am J Roentgenol 148:115, 1987.

52. Harckle HT, Grissom LE, and Meisler MA: Sedation in pediatric imaging using intranasal midazolam, Pediatr Radiol 25:341, 1995.

53. Hartman TE, Berquist TH, and Fetsch JF: MR imaging of extraabdominal desmoids: differentiation from other neoplasms, Am J Roentgenol 158:581, 1992.

54. Hayden CK, and Swischuk LE: The urinary tract. In Hayden CK, and Swischuk LE, eds: Pediatric ultrasonography, Baltimore, 1987, Williams & Wilkins.

55. Hayden CK, et al: Renal cystic disease in childhood, Radiographics 6:97, 1986.

56. Heiken JP, and Lee JKT: MR imaging of the pelvis, Radiology 166:11, 1988.

57. Hilpert PL, et al: MRI of hemorrhagic renal cysts in polycystic kidney disease, Am J Roentgenol 146:1167, 1986.

58. Hoane BR, Shields AF, Porter BA, et al: Comparison of initial lymphoma staging using computed tomography (CT) and magnetic resonance (MR) imaging, Am J Hematol 47:100, 1994.

59. Hoffman CH: Split notochord syndrome with dorsal enteric fistula, Am J Neuroradiol 14:622, 1993.

60. Holshauser BA, Hinshaw DB, and Shellock FG: Sedation, anesthesia and physiologic monitoring during MR imaging: evaluation of procedures and equipment, J Magn Reson Imaging 3:553, 1993.

61. Hricak H: MRI of the female pelvis: a review, Am J Roentgenol 146:1115, 1986.

62. Hricak H: Pelvic fistulas: appearances on MR images, Abdom Imaging 22(1):91, 1997.

63. Hricak H, Chang YCF, and Thurnher S: Vagina: evaluation with MR imaging. I. Normal anatomy and congenital anomalies, Radiology 169:169, 1988.

64. Hricak H, and Chang YCF: The female pelvis. In Higgins CB, and Hricak H, eds: Magnetic resonance imaging of the body, New York, 1987, Raven.

65. Hricak H, et al: Nuclear magnetic resonance imaging of the kidney, Radiology 146:425, 1983.

66. Hricak H, et al: Normal penile anatomy and abnormal penile conditions: evaluation with MR imaging, Radiology 169:683, 1988.

67. Huber DJ, Mueller E, and Heubes P: Oblique magnetic resonance imaging of normal structures, Am J Roentgenol 145:843, 1985.

68. Hugosson C, Jorulf H, and Bakri Y: MRI in distal vaginal atresia, Pediatr Radiol 21:281, 1991.

69. Hugosson C, et al: Imaging of solid kidney tumours in children, Acta Radiol 36:254, 1995.

70. Jaramillo D, Laor T, and Mulken RV: Comparison between fast spin-echo and conventional spin-echo imaging of normal and abnormal musculoskeletal structures in children and young adults, Invest Radiol 29:803, 1994.

71. Jaramillo D, Lebowitz RL, and Hendren WH: The cloacal malformation: radiologic findings and imaging recommendations, Radiology 177:441, 1990.

72. Johnston JH: Vascular lesions of the adrenal and kidney. In Rickham PP, Lister J, and Irving IM, eds: Neonatal surgery, St Paul, Minn, 1978, Butterworth.

73. Kangarloo H: Chest MRI in children, Radiol Clin North Am 26:263, 1988.

74. Kangarloo H, et al: Magnetic resonance imaging of Wilms tumor, Urology 28:203, 1986.

75. Keeter S, et al: Sedation in pediatric CT: national survey of current practice, Radiology 175:745, 1990.

76. Kersting-Sommerhoff BA, et al: MR imaging of congenital anomalies of the aortic arch, Am J Roentgenol 149:9, 1987.

77. Kier R, et al: Nonpalpable testes in young boys: evaluation with MR imaging, Radiology 169:429, 1988.

78. Kransdorf MJ, Jelinek JS, and Moser RP Jr: Imaging of soft tissue tumors, Radiol Clin North Am 31:359, 1993.

79. Kransdorf MJ, et al: Magnetic resonance appearance of fibromatosis, Skeletal Radiol 19:495, 1990.

80. Kransdorf MJ, et al: Fat-containing soft-tissue masses of the extremities, Radiographics 11:81, 1991.

81. Kressel HY: Strategies for magnetic resonance imaging of focal liver disease, Radiol Clin North Am 26:607, 1988.

82. Lee BC, Park TS, and Kaufman BA: MR angiography in pediatric neurologic disorders, Pediatr Radiol 25:409, 1995.

83. Leichter HE, et al: Acquired cystic kidney disease in children undergoing long-term dialysis, Pediatr Nephrol 2:8, 1988.

84. Leung AW-L, et al: Magnetic resonance imaging of the kidneys, Am J Roentgenol 143:1215, 1984.

85. Levenson H, Greensite F, Hoefs J, et al: Fatty infiltration of the liver: quantification with phase-contrast MR imaging at 1.5T vs. biopsy, Am J Roentgenol 156:307, 1991.

86. Li YW, Sheih CP, and Chen WJ: Unilateral occlusion of duplicated uterus with ipsilateral renal anomaly in young girls: a study with MRI, Pediatr Radiol 25:S54, 1995.

87. Lieberman E, et al: Infantile polycystic disease of the kidneys and liver: clinical, pathological and radiological correlations and comparison with congenital hepatic fibrosis, Medicine 50:277, 1971.

88. Lippe B, et al: Renal malformations in patients with Turner syndrome: imaging in 141 patients, Pediatrics 82:852, 1988.

89. Lois JF, et al: Budd-Chiari syndrome: treatment with percutaneous transhepatic recanalization and dilation, Radiology 170:791, 1989.

90. Lupetin AR, and Dash N: MRI appearance of esophageal duplication cyst, Gastrointest Radiol 12:7, 1987.

91. Lyon RD, and McAdams HP: Mediastinal bronchogenic cyst: demonstration of a fluid-fluid level at MR imaging, Radiology 186:427, 1993.

92. Maas KP, et al: Selected indications for and applications of magnetic resonance angiography in children, Pediatr Neurosurg 20:113, 1994.

93. Mann CL, et al: Post traumatic carotid artery dissection in children: evaluation with MR angiography, Am J Roentgenol 160:134, 1993.

94. Marotti M, et al: Complex and simple renal cysts: comparative evaluation with MR imaging, Radiology 162:679, 1987.

95. McCarthy S, and Fritzsche PJ: Male pelvis. In Stark DD, and Bradley WG Jr, eds: Magnetic resonance imaging, ed 1, St Louis, 1988, Mosby.

96. McHugh K, Dudley NE, and Tarr P: Pre-operative MRI of anorectal anomalies in the newborn period, Pediatr Radiol 25:33, 1995.

97. Merten DF, and Gold SH: Radiologic staging of thoracoabdominal tumors in childhood, Radiol Clin North Am 32:133, 1994.

98. Meyer JS, and Fellows KE: Vascular imaging in children, Semin Pediatr Surg 3:79, 1994.

99. Mezzacappo PM, Price AP, Haller JD, et al: MR and CT demonstration of levator sling in congenital anorectal anomalies, J Comput Assist Tomogr 11:273, 1987.

100. Mintz MC, et al: MR evaluation of uterine anomalies, Am J Roentgenol 148:287, 1987.

101. Molina PL, Siegel MJ, and Glazer HS: Thymic masses on MR imaging, Am J Roentgenol 155:495, 1993.

102. Moon KL Jr, and Hricak H: NMR imaging of the urinary tract, Appl Radiol 21:34, 1984.

103. Moore SG: The musculoskeletal system. In Cohen MD, and Edwards MK, eds: Magnetic resonance imaging of children, Philadelphia, 1989, BC Decker.

104. Murphy FB, and Bernadino ME: MR imaging of focal hemochromatosis, J Comput Assist Tomogr 10:1044, 1986.

105. Naidich DP, et al: Congenital anomalies of the lungs in adults: MR diagnosis, Am J Roentgenol 151:13, 1988.

106. Negendank WG, et al: Lymphomas: MR imaging contrast characteristics with clinical-pathologic correlations, Radiology 177:209, 1990.

107. Nyman R, et al: Magnetic resonance imaging, chest radiography, computed tomography and ultrasonography in malignant lymphoma, Acta Radiol 28:253, 1987.

108. Pennington DJ, et al: Enhanced T2-weighted fast SE MR imaging in the diagnosis of pyelonephritis in children, Proceedings of the 40th annual meeting of the Society for Pediatric Radiology 53, 1997.

109. Pessar ML, et al: MRI demonstration of pulmonary sequestration, Pediatr Radiol 18:229, 1988.

110. Petersein J, Saini S, and Weissleder R: Liver. II. Iron oxide–based reticuloendothelial contrast agents for MR imaging: a clinical review, MRI Clin North Am 4:53, 1996.

111. Platt JF, et al: Radiologic evaluation of the subcarinal lymph nodes: a comparative study, Am J Roentgenol 151:279, 1988.

112. Pobiel RS, and Bisset GS III: Pictorial essay: imaging of liver tumors in the infant and child, Pediatr Radiol 25:495, 1995.

113. Pomeranz SJ, et al: Magnetic resonance of congenital anorectal malformations, Magn Reson Imaging 4:69, 1986.
114. Powers C, et al: Primary liver neoplasms: MR imaging with pathologic correlation, Radiographics 14:459, 1994.
115. Querfeld U, et al: Magnetic resonance imaging of iron overload in children treated with peritoneal dialysis, Nephron 50:220, 1988.
116. Rawson JV, and Seifel MJ: Techniques and strategies in pediatric body MR imaging, MRI Clin North Am 4:589, 1996.
117. Reinig JW, et al: Liver metastases: detection with MR imaging at 0.5 and 1.5T, Radiology 170:149, 1989.
118. Rhee RS, et al: Cervical esophageal duplication cyst: MR imaging, Comput Assist Tomogr 12:693, 1988.
119. Rholl KS, et al: Primary bladder carcinoma: evaluation with MR imaging, Radiology 163:117, 1987.
120. Richardson RJ, Applebaum H, Taber P, et al: Use of magnetic resonance imaging in planning the separation of omphalopagus conjoined twins, J Pediatr Surg 24:683, 1989.
121. Robinson JD, et al: Preoperative mapping of pediatric pathology with MR imaging, Radiology 109(P):265, 1988.
122. Rollins NK, and Currarino G: Case report: MR imaging of posterior mediastinal thymus, J Comput Assist Tomogr 12:518, 1988.
123. Ros PR, et al: Mesenchymal hamartoma of the liver: radiographic-pathologic correlation, Radiology 158:619, 1986.
124. Sato Y, et al: Congenital anorectal anomalies: MR imaging, Radiology 168:157, 1988.
125. Sato Y, et al: Hippel-Lindau disease: MR imaging. Radiology 166:241, 1988.
126. Schmiedl U, et al: MR imaging of liver abscesses; application of Gd-DTPA, Magn Reson Imaging 6:9, 1988.
127. Schultz CL, et al: Magnetic resonance imaging of the adrenal glands: a comparison with computed tomography, Am J Roentgenol 143:1235, 1984.
128. Schultz E, et al: Detection of a deep lipoblastoma by MR imaging and ultrasound, Pediatr Radiol 23:409, 1993.
129. Sebag GH, Moore SC, and Parker BR: Magnetic resonance imaging of pediatric musculoskeletal hemangioma, Am J Roentgenol 153:202, 1989.
130. Secaf E: Role of MRI in the evaluation of ambiguous genitalia, Pediatr Radiol 24:231, 1994.
131. Siegel MJ, and Luker GD: Pediatric chest MR imaging, MRI Clin North Am 4:599, 1996.
132. Siegel MJ: Mediastinal lesions in children: comparison of CT and MR, Radiology 160:241, 1986.
133. Siegel MJ, et al: MR imaging of intraspinal extension of neuroblastoma, J Comput Assist Tomogr 10:593, 1986.
134. Siegel MJ, et al: Lymphangiomas in children: MR imaging, Radiology 170:467, 1989.
135. Siegel MJ, et al: Normal and abnormal thymus in childhood: MR imaging, Radiology 172:367, 1989.
136. Siegelman ES, et al: Parenchymal vs. reticuloendothelial iron overload in the liver: distinction with MR imaging, Radiology 179:361, 1991.
137. Sigmund G, et al: RARE-MR-urography in the diagnosis of upper urinary tract abnormalities in children, Pediatr Radiol 2:416, 1991.
138. Stanley P, et al: Mesenchymal hamartomas of childhood: sonographic and CT findings, Am J Roentgenol 147:1035, 1986.
139. Stark DD, et al: MRI of the Budd-Chiari syndrome, Am J Roentgenol 146:1141, 1986.
140. Stark DD: MR imaging of focal liver masses, Radiology 168:323, 1988.
141. Stark DD, et al: Chronic liver disease: evaluation by magnetic resonance, Radiology 150:149, 1984.
142. Stehling MK, et al: Whole-body echoplanar MR imaging at 0.5T, Radiology 170:257, 1989.
143. Strain JD, et al: IV Nembutal: safe sedation for children undergoing CT, Am J Radiol 151:975, 1988.
144. Surratt JT, and Siegel MJ: Imaging of pediatric ovarian masses, Radiographics 11:433, 1991.
145. Terrier F, et al: MR imaging of body fluid collections, J Comput Assist Tomogr 10:953, 1986.
146. Togashi K, et al: Ovarian cystic teratomas: MR imaging, Radiology 162:669, 1987.
147. Togashi K, et al: Vaginal agenesis: classification by MR imaging, Radiology 162:675, 1987.
148. Troughton AH, et al: The role of magnetic resonance imaging in the investigation of undescended testes, Clin Radiol 41:178, 1990.
149. Unger EC, et al: MRI of extracranial hematomas: preliminary observations, Am J Roentgenol 146:403, 1986.
150. Vade A, et al: The anorectal sphincter after rectal pull-through surgery for anorectal anomalies: MR evaluation, Pediatr Radiol 19:179, 1989.
151. Vainright JR, Fulp CJ, and Schiebler ML: MR imaging of vaginal agenesis with hematocolpos, J Comput Assist Tomogr 12:891, 1988.
152. Wall SD, et al: Magnetic resonance imaging in the evaluation of abscesses, Am J Roentgenol 144:1217, 1985.
153. Weese DL, Applebaum H, and Taber P: Mapping intravascular extension of Wilms' tumor with magnetic resonance imaging, J Pediatr Surg 26:64, 1991.
154. Weinreb JC, Brateman L, and Masavilla KR: Magnetic resonance imaging of hepatic lymphoma, Am J Roentgenol 143:1211, 1984.
155. Weinreb JC, et al: Imaging the pediatric liver: MRI and CT, Am J Roentgenol 147:785, 1986.
156. Yeagar BA, et al: Magnetic resonance imaging of Morgagni hernia, Gastrointest Radiol 12:296, 1987.
157. Young JL, and Miller RW: Incidence of malignant tumors in U.S. children, J Pediatr 86:254, 1975.
158. Yuh WTC, et al: MR imaging of pediatric head and neck cystic hygromas, Ann Otol Rhinol Laryngol 100:54, 1991.
159. Zimmerman RA, Bogdan AR, and Gusnard DA: Pediatric magnetic resonance angiography: assessment of stroke, Cardiovasc Intervent Radiol 15:60, 1992.

Index